COMPARATIVE PULMONARY PHYSIOLOGY

LUNG BIOLOGY IN HEALTH AND DISEASE

Executive Editor: **Claude Lenfant**

Director, National Heart, Lung, and Blood Institute
National Institutes of Health
Bethesda, Maryland

Volume 1 IMMUNOLOGIC AND INFECTIOUS REACTIONS IN THE LUNG, *edited by Charles H. Kirkpatrick and Herbert Y. Reynolds*

Volume 2 THE BIOCHEMICAL BASIS OF PULMONARY FUNCTION, *edited by Ronald G. Crystal*

Volume 3 BIOENGINEERING ASPECTS OF THE LUNG, *edited by John B. West*

Volume 4 METABOLIC FUNCTIONS OF THE LUNG, *edited by Y. S. Bakhle and John R. Vane*

Volume 5 RESPIRATORY DEFENSE MECHANISMS (in two parts), *edited by Joseph D. Brain, Donald F. Proctor, and Lynne M. Reid*

Volume 6 DEVELOPMENT OF THE LUNG, *edited by W. Alan Hodson*

Volume 7 LUNG WATER AND SOLUTE EXCHANGE, *edited by Norman C. Staub*

Volume 8 EXTRAPULMONARY MANIFESTATIONS OF RESPIRATORY DISEASE, *edited by Eugene Debs Robin*

Volume 9 CHRONIC OBSTRUCTIVE PULMONARY DISEASE, *edited by Thomas L. Petty*

Volume 10 PATHOGENESIS AND THERAPY OF LUNG CANCER, *edited by Curtis C. Harris*

Volume 11 GENETIC DETERMINANTS OF PULMONARY DISEASE, *edited by Stephen D. Litwin*

Volume 12 THE LUNG IN THE TRANSITION BETWEEN HEALTH AND DISEASE, *edited by Peter T. Macklem and Solbert Permutt*

Volume 13 EVOLUTION OF RESPIRATORY PROCESSES: A COMPARATIVE APPROACH, *edited by Stephen C. Wood and Claude Lenfant*

Volume 14 PULMONARY VASCULAR DISEASES,
edited by Kenneth M. Moser

Volume 15 PHYSIOLOGY AND PHARMACOLOGY OF THE AIRWAYS,
edited by Jay A. Nadel

Volume 16 DIAGNOSTIC TECHNIQUES IN PULMONARY DISEASE (in two parts),
edited by Marvin A. Sackner

Volume 17 REGULATION OF BREATHING (in two parts),
edited by Thomas F. Hornbein

Volume 18 OCCUPATIONAL LUNG DISEASES:
RESEARCH APPROACHES AND METHODS,
edited by Hans Weill and Margaret Turner-Warwick

Volume 19 IMMUNOPHARMACOLOGY OF THE LUNG,
edited by Harold H. Newball

Volume 20 SARCOIDOSIS AND OTHER GRANULOMATOUS
DISEASES OF THE LUNG,
edited by Barry L. Fanburg

Volume 21 SLEEP AND BREATHING,
edited by Nicholas A. Saunders and Colin E. Sullivan

Volume 22 *PNEUMOCYSTIS CARINII* PNEUMONIA:
PATHOGENESIS, DIAGNOSIS, AND TREATMENT,
edited by Lowell S. Young

Volume 23 PULMONARY NUCLEAR MEDICINE:
TECHNIQUES IN DIAGNOSIS OF LUNG DISEASE,
edited by Harold L. Atkins

Volume 24 ACUTE RESPIRATORY FAILURE,
edited by Warren M. Zapol and Konrad J. Falke

Volume 25 GAS MIXING AND DISTRIBUTION IN THE LUNG,
edited by Ludwig A. Engel and Manuel Paiva

Volume 26 HIGH-FREQUENCY VENTILATION IN INTENSIVE CARE
AND DURING SURGERY,
edited by Graziano Carlon and William S. Howland

Volume 27 PULMONARY DEVELOPMENT: TRANSITION
FROM INTRAUTERINE TO EXTRAUTERINE LIFE,
edited by George H. Nelson

Volume 28 CHRONIC OBSTRUCTIVE PULMONARY DISEASE, second edition, revised and expanded,
edited by Thomas L. Petty

Volume 29 THE THORAX (in two parts),
edited by Charis Roussos and Peter T. Macklem

Volume 30 THE PLEURA IN HEALTH AND DISEASE,
edited by Jaques Chrétien, Jean Bignon, and Albert Hirsch

Volume 31 DRUG THERAPY FOR ASTHMA: RESEARCH AND CLINICAL PRACTICE,
edited by John W. Jenne and Shirley Murphy

Volume 32 PULMONARY ENDOTHELIUM IN HEALTH AND DISEASE,
edited by Una S. Ryan

Volume 33 THE AIRWAYS: NEURAL CONTROL IN HEALTH AND DISEASE,
edited by Michael A. Kaliner and Peter J. Barnes

Volume 34 PATHOPHYSIOLOGY AND TREATMENT OF INHALATION INJURIES,
edited by Jacob Loke

Volume 35 RESPIRATORY FUNCTION OF THE UPPER AIRWAY,
edited by Oommen P. Mathew and Giuseppe Sant'Ambrogio

Volume 36 CHRONIC OBSTRUCTIVE PULMONARY DISEASE: A BEHAVIORAL PERSPECTIVE,
edited by A. John McSweeny and Igor Grant

Volume 37 BIOLOGY OF LUNG CANCER: DIAGNOSIS AND TREATMENT,
edited by Steven T. Rosen, James L. Mulshine, Frank Cuttitta, and Paul G. Abrams

Volume 38 PULMONARY VASCULAR PHYSIOLOGY AND PATHOPHYSIOLOGY,
edited by E. Kenneth Weir and John T. Reeves

Volume 39 COMPARATIVE PULMONARY PHYSIOLOGY: CURRENT CONCEPTS,
edited by Stephen C. Wood

Volume 40 RESPIRATORY PHYSIOLOGY: AN ANALYTICAL APPROACH,
edited by H. K. Chang and Manuel Paiva

Volume 41 LUNG CELL BIOLOGY,
edited by Donald Massaro

Additional Volumes in Preparation

HEART–LUNG INTERACTIONS IN HEALTH AND DISEASE,
edited by Steven M. Scharf and Sharon Cassidy

COMPARATIVE PULMONARY PHYSIOLOGY

CURRENT CONCEPTS

Edited by

Stephen C. Wood

Lovelace Medical Foundation
Albuquerque, New Mexico

MARCEL DEKKER, INC. New York • Basel

Library of Congress Cataloging-in-Publication Data

Comparative pulmonary physiology.
(Lung biology in health and disease ; v. 39)
Includes bibliographies and indexes.
1. Lungs--Physiology. 2. Respiratory organs--Physiology. 3. Respiration. 4. Physiology, Comparative. I. Wood, Stephen C. II. Series.
[DNLM: 1. Physiology, Comparative. 2. Respiration. 3. Respiratory System--physiology.
W1 LU62 v.39 / WF 102 C737]
QP121.C685 1989 599'.0121 88-25771
ISBN 0-8247-7961-4

Marcel Dekker, Inc.
270 Madison Avenue, New York, New York 10016

Current printing (last digit):
10 9 8 7 6 5 4 3 2 1

Printed in the United States of America

To Kjell Johansen
Viking and Physiologist
Mentor, Colleague, and Friend

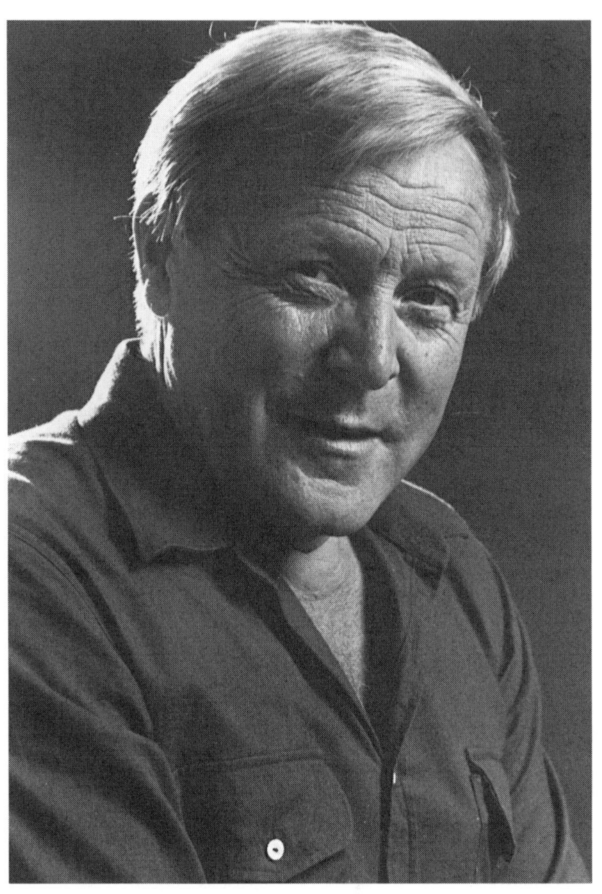

Kjell Johansen
1932–1987

MEMORIAL

Eye of Newt, and toe of hog,
Wood of bat, and tongue of dog,
Adder's fork, and blind-worm's sting
Lizard's leg and howlet's wing . . .

Macbeth

All these topics and many others were of interest to Kjell Johansen. There was no limit to his intellectual curiosity, and his laboratory was the world.

This volume comprises 28 chapters, but it should have had 29. The missing one, "Heart Structure and Function," was to have been written by Kjell. When he died suddenly in France on March 5, 1987, he was working on it.

Kjell Johansen was born in Norway on September 30, 1932. His research career began in 1956, when he became a research fellow at the University of Oslo, and continued when he became a research associate at the University of Washington in 1960. In 1971, when he had advanced to Professor of Zoology at the University of Washington, he returned to Europe to become Professor and Chairman of Zoophysiology at Aarhus, Denmark. Typically, there were intervals when he was visiting professor: in 1964 at the University of Saõ Paulo in Brazil, and in 1973 at the University of Nairobi in Kenya. But he remained at Aarhus until his untimely death.

My first contact with Kjell was in 1959, when I wrote to him to ask about a recent publication of his in *Acta Physiologica Scandinavica*. He had written an article on polarographic determination of intramuscular oxygen tensions in vivo, an interest of mine at that time. His response was marvelous, a warm and detailed letter that ended with an invitation to write again if I needed more help, and that expressed the hope we would meet soon. Clearly, this letter was written by a generous person. Although in 1959 Kjell was in Norway and I was in France, by chance we both moved to Seattle in 1960. But it took three more years before we met. It was in Miami, on the occasion of the fall meeting of the American Physiological Society. One afternoon I decided to forgo listening to papers to take a short cruise and to enjoy the sunshine and the beautiful sea. Well, there was another passenger on the boat who also wanted to relax in the warm Florida weather–Kjell Johansen. (Perhaps this was because we both were from Seattle!) And so we met, not knowing that we had been working a few hundred feet apart, but both remembering vividly our previous correspondence.

Kjell's research interests were comparative cardiovascular physiology; mine were human respiratory function in health and disease. We quickly realized that our interests were more than complementary and that we would both gain from working together. And so an exchange of research ideas that began on the deck of a yacht off Miami led to a friendship and collaboration that lasted more than 25 years. While we were both in Seattle, we worked, wrote papers, and traveled together, but our collaboration was only a small part of Kjell's many undertakings and pursuits. Frankly, I don't recall having ever met another person with such energy and curiosity. Kjell's physical strength was obvious; his scientific inquisitiveness was a marvel. Because he knew so well the animal kingdom and the habits and habitats of so many species, he could pose many questions that he would address relentlessly. I do remember our long days in the equatorial regions on land and on sea, and in the two polar regions. Birds and snakes, aquatic and terrestial mammals, air- and water-breathing fishes, and amphibians were all to be studied. Of course, mollusks and worms would also be part of the program. At the end of the day, when rest was to be anticipated, Kjell's vitality would rejuvenate and spill over, revealing another of his characteristics, his *joie de vivre*. Indeed, Kjell knew no limits.

This book is dedicated to Kjell Johansen. His *curriculum vitae* and his rich bibliography attest to the breadth of his interests. Kjell left behind a legacy of landmark observations. His scientific contributions are evident not only from his writings but also from the work of his many colleagues. He enjoyed working with others, and never hesitated to share his knowledge and his ideas.

In addition to being a great researcher, Kjell Johansen was a generous and compassionate human being. He loved his family and his friends. He had concerns for the world, and he was deeply affected by social injustice. Over the years he traveled extensively, on his own or with organized scientific expeditions. Although the purpose was to explore and study new biological phenomena, wherever he was, he spent time to learn about the local people and to try to understand the society of which they were part.

Kjell's premature death is a great loss to science as well as to those who knew him and were his friends. But in many ways, the "*Current Concepts*" described in this volume are a testimony to his legacy.

Claude Lenfant, M.D.
Bethesda, Maryland

INTRODUCTION

Since the very beginning of biology research, comparative physiology has played an important role in the many advances that have been achieved. The animal kingdom constitutes a laboratory with endless perspectives and, if well used, can provide biologists with unlimited ideas for human studies and tools. Indeed, biological mechanisms and processes that are normal under the ecological and environmental conditions of some species often mirror human pathological situations. Without question, a comparative approach can shed light on many obscure aspects of human biology in health and disease.

It has been nine years since Wood and Lenfant published *Evolution of Respiratory Processes: A Comparative Approach*, the thirteenth volume in the Lung Biology in Health and Disease series. Much has happened since then: New observations have been made; more species have been studied; and the impact of different environments has been noted. In short, many concepts have evolved and newer ideas have emerged.

Hence, I am grateful that Stephen C. Wood agreed to edit this volume, *Comparative Pulmonary Physiology: Current Concepts*. The table of contents of this monograph is impressive. Virtually the entire animal world is represented.

Structure is coupled with function, and responses to varied environments or stresses are evaluated. The breadth of the content is equaled only by the expertise of the authors. Recognizing that the animal kingdom has no frontiers, Steve Wood selected contributors representing a similar diversity: They come from three continents and seven countries. They include physiologists, biologists, biochemists, and zoologists, as well as honest-to-goodness clinical doctors! The common thread is their excellence and long reputation as creative researchers.

Steve Wood has put together a superb volume that will be a true asset to this series of monographs. I am grateful to him and to his authors for such an important contribution.

Claude Lenfant

PREFACE

Scientists have abnormally high levels of curiosity. For physiologists, the curiosity is about how animals work. This intense curiosity has been a vital force in the field of comparative physiology. This book provides some new ideas about how animals work. I hope that it also provides some new *questions* about how animals work.

Concepts in science are continuously evolving. The emphasis on "current" concepts in this book is not intended to imply that old concepts are not enduring or that the concepts presented herein are replacements. Rather, the aim of the book is to present a current synthesis of older and newer ideas that represent the state of knowledge in comparative pulmonary physiology and to provide new insights from comparative studies that are relevant to all branches of lung biology.

Chapter 1, by Pierre Dejours, provides an overview and summarizes the main fields explored in the book. The remaining 25 chapters of this book are divided into six parts. In the first part, "Energy Demand," Chapter 1 covers the upper and lower limits of energy demand. Chapter 2 describes scaling of energy demand and the important new concept of symmorphosis, i.e., that structure is developed to match functional requirements.

Part Two, "Structure and Function of the Gas Exchange Organ," provides a superb collection of chapters that describe the structure-function relationships of nonmammalian vertebrate gas exchange organs, namely fish gills (Chapter 4), amphibian larval gills (Chapter 5), amphibian lungs (Chapter 6), reptile lungs (Chapter 7), and bird lungs (Chapter 8). As the concept of symmorphosis would predict, all these organs are developed to the extent necessary for the level of aerobic function that has evolved in each group.

Part Three comprises seven chapters related to the dynamic field of gas exchange and transport. Chapter 9 presents current insights into the development of respiratory function, particularly oxygen transport, in mammals. Chapter 10 describes structure-function relationships for hemoglobin, the courier of oxygen, and how these relations are manifested in whole-blood oxygen transport. Chapter 11 offers some current ideas on homeostasis of oxygen transport in lower vertebrates, emphasizing animals with normally occurring intracardiac shunts. Some recent and exciting concepts about blood flow, oxygen homeostasis, and temperature regulation in the brain of birds are provided in Chapter 12. Chapter 13 presents recent theory, models, and experimental data about gas exchange that are quantitative and universally applicable. The concept of symmorphosis surfaces again in Chapter 14, where the role of diffusing capacity in gas exchange is considered. Chapter 15 also deals with respiratory homeostasis; in this case, homeostasis of carbon dioxide.

Part Four covers an area that historically has been ignored in most comparative physiology texts: fluid balance. This is unfortunate, and I am grateful to the authors of Chapters 16-18 for contributing to this volume because, as readers will discover, many principles of fluid balance and acid-base regulation in mammals do not apply or are modified in fascinating ways in other animals.

Part Five covers the respiratory pumps of vertebrate breathing. Chapter 19 discusses comparative aspects of pulmonary mechanics in which the common requirement of pumping air is solved in interesting ways. Chapter 20 deals with the control of respiratory pumps. Here again, readers accustomed to medical physiology principles will discover new, and teleologically sensible, departures from the mammalian "standard."

The last section, "Diving Physiology," is one I was especially pleased to compile for this volume. This is an area that most teachers of applied physiology find very useful in their classes because so many important physical, chemical, and physiological concepts can be illustrated and exemplified. This section presents, for the first time in one volume, the diving physiology of each vertebrate group: fish that "dive" into air (Chapter 21); amphibians, the obligatory divers (Chapter 22); reptiles, the longest divers of all (Chapter 23); marine mammals, the deepest divers (Chapter 24); and birds, the triathletes of diving (Chapter 25). Chapter 26 focuses on man, which, as a species, has no need to ever enter the water but can do remarkably well when he tries.

This book started as a collection of topics that I thought were the most interesting, revealing, informative, and exciting. I was most fortunate in having the leading authorities for each topic agree to contribute to this volume. As I had hoped, the collected topics are more than the sum of the parts. The book should be interesting and informative for anyone interested in lung biology. This volume, like its predecessor in this series, *Evolution of Respiratory Processes: A Comparative Approach* by Wood and Lenfant, applies lung biology widely across taxonomic lines and lifestyles and, by so doing, provides many unifying concepts. The book will be useful not only for pulmonologists but for graduate students in biology, zoology, and physiology, as well as for their teachers. By fortunate coincidence, many of the chapters have been written at a time when new insights of textbook-level caliber have just developed, making this volume one of not only current but important concepts in comparative pulmonary physiology.

Stephen C. Wood

CONTENTS

Part One ENERGY DEMAND

Part Two STRUCTURE AND FUNCTION OF THE GAS EXCHANGE ORGAN

CONTRIBUTORS

Marvin H. Bernstein, Ph.D. Professor, Department of Biology, New Mexico State University, Las Cruces, New Mexico

Robert G. Boutilier, B.Sc., M.Sc., Ph.D. Assistant Professor, Department of Biology, Dalhousie University, Halifax, Nova Scotia, Canada

Warren W. Burggren, Ph.D. Professor, Department of Zoology, University of Massachusetts, Amherst, Massachusetts

Pierre Dejours, M.D. Research Director, Laboratoire d'Etude des Régulations Physiologiques, Centre National de la Recherche Scientifique, Strasbourg, France

Alfred P. Fishman, M.D. William Maul Measey Professor of Medicine and Director, Cardiovascular-Pulmonary Division, Department of Medicine, University of Pennsylvania, and Hospital of the University of Pennsylvania, Philadelphia, Pennsylvania

R. J. Galante, B.S. Research Specialist, Cardiovascular-Pulmonary Division, Department of Medicine, University of Pennsylvania, and Hospital of the University of Pennsylvania, Philadelphia, Pennsylvania

Mogens L. Glass, Ph.D.* Department of Zoophysiology, University of Aarhus, Aarhus, Denmark

Alan R. Hargens, Ph.D.† Professor, Department of Surgery–Orthopaedics and Rehabilitation, University of California, and Veterans Administration Medical Center, San Diego, California

Norbert Heisler, M.D. Professor, Department of Physiology, Max Planck Institute for Experimental Medicine, Göttingen, Federal Republic of Germany

James W. Hicks, Ph.D.‡ NIH Postdoctoral Fellow, Physiological Research Laboratory, Scripps Institution of Oceanography, University of California at San Diego, La Jolla, California

Peter W. Hochachka, Ph.D., F.R.S.C. Professor, Department of Zoology and Division of Sports Medicine, Faculties of Science and of Medicine, University of British Columbia, Vancouver, British Columbia, Canada

Suk Ki Hong, M.D., Ph.D. Professor, Department of Physiology, State University of New York, Buffalo, New York

Hans Hoppeler, M.D. Department of Anatomy, University of Berne, Berne, Switzerland

Donald C. Jackson, Ph.D. Professor, Division of Biology and Medicine, Brown University, Providence, Rhode Island

David R. Jones, B.Sc., Ph.D. Professor, Department of Zoology, University of British Columbia, Vancouver, British Columbia, Canada

---

Present affiliations:

*Department of Physiology, Max Planck Institute for Experimental Medicine, Göttingen, Federal Republic of Germany

†Chief, Space Physiology Branch, NASA–Ames Research Center, Moffett Field, California

‡Assistant Professor, Department of Physiology, Creighton University School of Medicine, Omaha, Nebraska

Richard H. Karas, M.D., Ph.D.* Research Associate, Department of Organismic and Evolutionary Biology, Museum of Comparative Biology, Harvard University, Cambridge, Massachusetts

Gerald L. Kooyman, Ph.D. Research Physiologist, Physiological Research Laboratory, Scripps Institution of Oceanography, University of California at San Diego, La Jolla, California

Pierre Laurent, D.Sc. Research Director, Laboratoire de Morphologie Fonctionelle et Ultrastructurale des Adaptations, Centre National de la Recherche Scientifique, Strasbourg, France

Gary M. Malvin, Ph.D. Research Associate, Department of Physiology and Biophysics, University of Washington School of Medicine, Seattle, Washington

James Metcalfe, M.D. Professor, Department of Medicine, Oregon Health Sciences University, and Assistant Chief of Staff, Vancouver Campus, Portland Veterans Administration Medical Center, Portland, Oregon

William K. Milsom, Ph.D. Associate Professor, Department of Zoology, University of British Columbia, Vancouver, British Columbia, Canada

A. I. Pack, M.B., Ch.B., Ph.D. Associate Professor and Director, Pulmonary Diagnostic Services, Cardiovascular-Pulmonary Division, Department of Medicine, University of Pennsylvania, and Hospital of the University of Pennsylvania, Philadelphia, Pennsylvania

Steven F. Perry, Ph.D. Associate Professor, Fachbereich 7 (Biologie), Universität Oldenburg, Oldenburg, Federal Republic of Germany

Johannes Piiper, M.D. Professor, Department of Physiology, Max Planck Institute for Experimental Medicine, Göttingen, Federal Republic of Germany

Frank L. Powell, Ph.D. Associate Professor, Department of Medicine, University of California at San Diego, La Jolla, California

Peter Scheid, M.D., Ph.D. Professor, Department of Physiology, Ruhr-Universität, Bochum, Federal Republic of Germany

---

Present affiliation:
*Junior Medical Resident, Department of Medicine, Brigham and Women's Hospital, Boston, Massachusetts

Roger S. Seymour, Ph.D. Senior Lecturer, Department of Zoology, University of Adelaide, Adelaide, South Australia, Australia

Allan W. Smits, M.A., Ph.D.* Parker B. Francis Fellow in Pulmonary Research, Department of Zoology, University of Massachusetts, Amherst, Massachusetts

Richard Stephenson, B.Sc., Ph.D. Research Fellow, Department of Zoology, University of British Columbia, Vancouver, British Columbia, Canada

Michael K. Stock, Ph.D.† Research Instructor, Heart Research Laboratory, Oregon Health Sciences University, and Portland Veterans Administration Medical Center, Portland, Oregon

C. Richard Taylor, Ph.D. Alexander Agassiz Professor of Zoology, Museum of Comparative Zoology, Harvard University, Cambridge, Massachusetts

Roy E. Weber, Ph.D.‡ Professor, Biology Institute, Odense University, Odense, Denmark

Ewald R. Weibel, M.D. Professor and Chairman, Department of Anatomy, University of Berne, Berne, Switzerland

Rufus M. G. Wells, Ph.D., D.Sc., F.R.S.N.Z. Associate Professor, Department of Zoology, University of Auckland, Auckland, New Zealand

Fred N. White, Ph.D. Director, Physiological Research Laboratory, Scripps Institution of Oceanography, University of California at San Diego, La Jolla, California

Stephen C. Wood, Ph.D. Senior Scientist, Lovelace Medical Foundation, Albuquerque, New Mexico

---

Present affiliations:

*Assistant Professor, Division of Natural Sciences, University of Texas, Arlington, Texas

†Research Assistant Professor

‡Professor, Zoophysiology Department, Institute for Zoology and Zoophysiology, University of Aarhus, Aarhus, Denmark

COMPARATIVE PULMONARY PHYSIOLOGY

1

Current Concepts in Comparative Physiology of Respiration
An Overview

PIERRE DEJOURS

Laboratoire d'Etude des Régulations Physiologiques
Centre National de la Recherche Scientifique
Strasbourg, France

I. Introduction

This overview aims to define certain ideas–and to give a summary of the recent main fields of exploration. What are the concepts? What gave rise to them? Must they be amended? Will new concepts evolve with further research? A "state-of-the-art" exposition, as this book intends to be, may point the way to the future.

This book is part of a series devoted to lung biology. The lung is a component of the respiratory system, the definition of which must be given first, because the concepts that will be alluded to here concern not only the lung but other respiratory structures as well. Nevertheless, the content of this volume and of another volume of the same series (Wood and Lenfant, 1979) covers much more than pulmonary physiology.

II. The Respiratory System

Lavoisier (1743-1794), in making his famous analogy between the processes of respiration in the animal body and the combustion of coal, immediately raised the fundamental question of where respiration takes place. Over the years, four sites were successively proposed: "combustion" occurred (1) in the lungs, (2) in the circulating blood, (3) in capillary blood, and (4) in the cells of the tissues. Pflüger (1829-1910) is credited with the statement that the elementary process of respiration takes place in the cell (1872). The role of the intracellular pigments, the histohematins which MacMunn (1852-1911) discovered in 1886, was not understood at this time and would not be until the work of Keilin (1887-1963), who named the pigments cytochromes (see references in Keilin, 1966).

The discovery of the true nature of respiration was probably impeded because Lavoisier, and many of his successors, studied complex mammalian organisms. Had they turned their attention to lungless, bloodless animals, the site of the respiratory process would probably have been recognized much sooner. Indeed, Spallanzani (1729-1799), the founder of comparative physiology of respiration, observed that preparations he examined—leeches, earthworms, insects in their three life stages, vertebrates, and various tissues studied in vitro—all use oxygen and produce carbon dioxide. Unfortunately, his experiments, buried in a rare three-volume work published by Senebier (1807), were overlooked for many years.

Paul Bert (1833-1886) seems to have been the first to have clearly enunciated the concept of a gas-exchange system within the body (1870):

> There are two distinct chapters in the story of respiration. In the first, the environment, air or aerated water, meets and conflicts with the blood, gives up oxygen and receives carbon dioxide. This is what is commonly called respiration, and it is carried out in special body structures. But there follow more essential phenomena, for the first is but a means to an end: oxygen is in the blood, and it is taken up by the tissues. This fundamentally is respiration.

To this may be added that O_2 and CO_2 transfer can occur by diffusion through an air-to-blood or water-to-blood barrier, and also by diffusion from the systemic capillaries to the cells; by convection through aquatic or aerial ventilation; and by blood circulation. Thus, the respiratory system may be viewed as a sequence of apparatuses, ventilatory and circulatory, and of barriers; this compartmental system is normally the seat of a net influx of O_2 and of a net efflux of CO_2. By an unhappy convention, these two vectorial quantities were given a positive sign; hence, the respiratory quotient is positive. Unfortunately, the term *the respiratory system* has recently been used in an incorrect sense because the authors dealt only with pulmonary respiration.

III. The Principles of Transfer of O_2 and CO_2 Molecules

Diffusion and convection are defined by the two *Fick equations*. They apply to and among all milieus: waters, gas, blood, or any body fluids. These equations cannot be used blindly because they are valid for only simple models. In particular, for the Fick equation of diffusion between two milieus, one cannot use the concentration gradient as it appears in the equation; but the equation must be transformed by introducing a partial pressure gradient and a Krogh's constant.

Under certain conditions, and if the gas exchange model is simple enough, the Fick equations then may be applied. This is particularly true at the macroscopic level, but on a microscopic scale, it may be difficult to know if the gas exchanges are diffusive or convective. In the terminal bronchioles and in the air sacs of the alveolar lung, convection is slight, and diffusion may not be sufficient to obtain a homogenized gas: some *stratification*, generally minor, may exist. At high altitude, it may be negligible, but it may be important in hyperbary.

Often it is not easy to know what the actual partial pressure gradient across a membrane or a sheet of tissue is. Indeed, some *unstirred layers* (USL), also called boundary layers, may lengthen the actual diffusion path. The USL effects may be very complex (see Barry and Diamond, 1984); they may exist between the blood and the alveolar gas, between the blood and the interstitial fluid, and between the interlamellar water and the blood in the gills.

A. Facilitated Diffusion

Facilitated diffusion of O_2 and CO_2 was discovered in the early 1960s. Facilitated diffusion takes place in many organs or tissues, but its actual role remains to be evaluated. It should be most important when O_2 and CO_2 fluxes are intense, i.e., during exercise and in poikilotherms at relatively high temperatures.

B. Kinetics of Loading and Unloading of O_2 and CO_2 by Blood

Sixty years ago, it was tacitly assumed that the loading and unloading of O_2 and CO_2 by blood were instantaneous or, at least, very fast in comparison with the time spent by blood in the systemic, branchial, or pulmonary capillaries; but the reactions are not intantaneous. The hydration of CO_2 is accelerated by carbonic anhydrase in many tissues, but CO_2 loading and unloading are not particularly rapid. The loading and unloading of O_2 and CO_2 in blood are concomitant, and the kinetics for both gases must be approached simultaneously because they are tied by the Bohr–Haldane effect.

If the O_2 and CO_2 reactions with the blood are incomplete by the time the blood has reached the termination of the capillaries, certain reactions will continue in the outflowing blood. The question is raised: What kind of arterial blood does the brain of the smallest homoiotherms, some shrews and hummingbirds (body mass of the adult 2.5 g) receive, considering that the lung-to-brain circulation time is less than 1 second? It may happen that the arterial blood that is collected, and analyzed later, is different from the actual arterial blood perfusing the brain.

The kinetics of CO_2 loading by water, which requires equilibrations between the various forms of CO_2, especially in buffered water such as seawater and most freshwater, is a similar problem. It seems that the equilibration is rapid, perhaps because carbonic anhydrase is present at the gill-water interface.

The *allosteric modulations* of oxygen-hemoglobin affinities have been, for the last 20 years, a major subject of research, and a large quantity of data have been accumulated. But what one really needs to know is what the oxygen affinity of blood is in vivo, at a given temperature, at the actual values of P_{O_2}, P_{CO_2}, and pH. It is probably safe to say that the air breathers, who live in an environment rich in oxygen, have a lower O_2 affinity than do those who breathe in water. Are these differences a result of different conformations of the O_2-carrying pigment, of allosteric factors, or of both? The same kind of problem is raised for the commonly observed drop in the blood O_2 affinity when embryos or larvae become adults that have a more direct access to the environmental oxygen.

IV. Design and Function

Comparative physiology, anatomy, and chemistry are closely related. Certainly, function is no longer inferred from the anatomy, generally by analogy. A physiological phenomenon requires a direct demonstration. In the last 25 years a new science, morphometry, has appeared in respiratory studies. Gross anatomy, histology, and cytology are basic, but details of form and dimension are now particularly important. This approach has been applied to gills, lungs, systemic circulation, blood, tissues, and cellular organelles. From morphometric studies of the lung, calculation of the pulmonary diffusing conductance to oxygen has been attempted. The estimated values differ from those obtained by so-called physiological methods. The search for the reason for the discrepancy is rewarding because it points out the assumptions, and maybe the limitations, of both approaches.

Anatomical features and functions vary with body size, zoological group, and environment. One can try to relate variables; many relationships can be expressed by equations, one term of which is a power function. For example, the oxygen consumption, $\dot{M}_{O_2}$, in a given animal group, at a given temperature, in other well-defined conditions, is proportional to the body mass, B, to the power 0.75 ($\dot{M}O_2 = a\,B^{0.75}$). The exponent, 0.75 in the equation, is "other" than 1 which characterizes an isometric, proportional relationship; hence, the terms allometric and allometric equations. That there are many allometric relationships does not mean that all of them make sense and by no means, implies a direct cause-and-effect relationship. Nevertheless, when the relationships are not spurious, but mean something, they may suggest further research.

Comparative anatomy and physiology, including the allometric approach, show that human respiration is nothing unique. It is no different from that of quadrupeds and other bipeds, except for one organ: the brain, whose size and respiration intensity are above the usual range. Comparative studies put human physiology in its normal perspective.

V. Models and Mathematical Approaches

The respiratory system of any animal species has its own characteristics, and there are more than a million species. The physiological diversity parallels the phenotypic diversity. From the body plan and from the main characteristics of the respiratory system, some simplifying models may be constructed that lead to clarification of the main general dispositions and to their possible working mechanisms. To be useful, models must be general enough to avoid a sterile cumbersome variety. Everyone who tries to understand respiration, and other functions, more or less consciously uses the modelistic approach. With models, it is possible to understand how the O_2 and CO_2 exchanges take place. The first step is qualitative. The second is formal and takes a mathematical expression. However, to be rewarding, this advanced modelistic approach requires (1) a good model, one neither too simple nor too complex; (2) an expression of all assumptions or simplifications made; (3) the correct use of the physicochemical concepts; (4) an accurate use of symbols and the relevant proper units, in other words, the right language. Any modelistic description permanently raises the everlasting problem "models versus biological reality" and is threatened on both sides by oversimplification and by an excess of complexity. Actually, one finds in nature a great variety of complex respiratory dispositions, in particular of breathing mechanisms (Tenney, 1979).

VI. Regulations

The study of respiratory regulations has been concentrated on the control of external breathing, at rest, at high altitude, in exercise; mainly in mammals, especially humans. The examination of these problems in vertebrates other than mammals is a recent move of the last 20 years. The history of respiratory regulations suffered, and still suffers, from the anthropocentric approach of the respiration physiologists at the beginning of the twentieth century. Certainly, the study of pulmonary physiology in humans is satisfactory as long as it applies in a general way to all mammals, but it is not valid, for instance, for birds and their parabronchial lungs. The study of human blood as a typical O_2- and CO_2-carrying milieu has a more general value because blood may be regarded as a physicochemical system, and the general principles that apply to human blood are valid for most bloods and hemolymphs. Important differences exist, however, particularly in the conditions of the CO_2 tension and the acid-base balance. An intriguing problem is that in invertebrates, the respiratory pigment is generally dissolved, whereas in vertebrates it is located in erythrocytes, nucleated in all vertebrate classes but mammals. The reasons for these differences are not obvious.

The respiratory function that is primarily controlled is the oxygenation of the tissues. The acid-base balance is subordinate, because it may be changed, more or less permanently, by the change of oxygenation of the body (see Dejours et al., 1987). This is contrary to the belief, at the beginning of the twentieth century, that was based on the study of humans living at sea level in a milieu rich in oxygen. It is probably safe to say that external respiration aims at maintaining two intensive variables, namely the O_2 tension and the pH (an expression of the proton activity, which is an intensive variable). The P_{CO_2} adjusts to maintain the pH value, but P_{CO_2} is not the regulated signal. In fish, birds, and mammals, the arterial blood that is delivered to the tissues has a unique composition. Thus, because the needs of the different organs and tissues vary, two mechanisms may satisfy these needs: (1) variations of the local blood flow, which may change the average composition of the local interstitial fluid; (2) particular activities of the cells to satisfy their specific requirements.

The control of breathing during exercise has been studied almost exclusively in humans. One principle has emerged: no single factor can explain this control. Because many factors are known to influence breathing and because all of these factors may change in the course of exercise, it is unavoidable to look for a multifactorial theory, such as the neurohumoral theory. Certainly the complexity of the situation has led to a profusion of theories, some based on elaborated applications of control theory, as used by engineers, and very remote from the biological facts. It is not certain that the time is ripe for this formalization. Nevertheless, what must be understood is how O_2 is delivered to the cells and how CO_2 is cleared from the body. All steps of the O_2 and CO_2 transfer system are involved, and each one has its own control. It is rarely easy to recognize what the regulated signals of the various subsystems are.

VII. Respiration and Environment

Quite naturally, the study of animals in their relationships with the environment is the most rewarding of comparative physiological questions. Environments are infinite; moreover, except rarely, they change. By necessity animals are adapted to their milieus and must cope with daily and seasonal variations. These comments are limited to two milieus, water and air. It is an oversimplified division, because there are many kinds of water: seawater, more or less diluted, and an immense variety of freshwaters, whereas air is a relatively simple milieu. Soil is another kind of multifarious environment, intermediary between water and air. However, the differences between air and any kind of water are so marked that all air breathers have respiratory characteristics quite different from those of water breathers.

In water the solubility of O_2 is much lower than that of CO_2, it therefore follows that the uptake of a given amount of O_2 from the water and the output of the same amount of CO_2 into the water ($RQ = 1$) entail completely different changes of the partial pressures of O_2 and CO_2 between inspired and expired waters. For example, PO_2 fails from 150 torr in inspired water to 110 torr in expired water, a decrease of 40 torr, whereas PCO_2 increases by only 2 torr, or even much less if the respired water contains buffers, which are mainly carbonates. The situation is completely different in air because the O_2 and CO_2 solubilities (capacitances) are the same and close to the CO_2 solubility in water. In air, for a respiratory quotient of 1, a fall of PO_2 by 40 torr will be accompanied by an identical increase of PCO_2. This relative hypercapnia is because for the same partial pressure of O_2, the O_2 concentration is much higher in air than in water, hence, to take in a unit quantity of O_2 the air breathers breathe much less O_2 than water breathers do; in short, the *specific ventilation* is lower in air breathers than in water breathers. As a consequence, in water breathers, PCO_2 in the body fluids is never much different from the inspired PCO_2, whereas it is many tens of torr higher in the body fluids of air breathers (Rahn, 1966). This is a general law, with dual breathers occupying an intermediate position. The same phenomena are observed in amphibians; for example, blood PCO_2 in the dual-breathing adult frog may be 10 torr and in the aquatic tadpole 2 torr. Amphibians are excellent examples of the transition from aquatic breathing to air breathing.

However, water breathers and air breathers have the same blood pH values. The $[HCO_3]$ increases in direct proportion to the PCO_2 increase in the course of the transition from aquatic to aerial breathing, leading to the assertion that air breathers are in a state of *compensated hypercapnic acidosis* compared with their ancestral water breathers. Thus, it is not the PCO_2 that is regulated, but the pH value. However, pH may be upset by a change of environmental oxygenation, so that the pH regulation must be considered as subordinate to the regulation of the body oxygenation.

Another major discovery of comparative physiology is that a pH value cannot be considered alone, but must be accompanied by mention of the *temperature* at which it is measured. Indeed pH values change with temperature and are lower the higher the temperature. For example, in the turtle, blood pH is 8.0 at 5°C and 7.45 at 37°C, a fall of -0.017 pH unit for an increase of 1°C. This *pH temperature-dependency* is particularly common in air breathers as well as in water breathers and, as far as we know, the intracellular pHs follow the same rule. Furthermore, the difference between the blood pH values and the corresponding pHs of neutral water, which are also temperature-dependent, is more or less constant; hence, the concept of *constant relative alkalinity* (Rahn, 1967).

Many factors in the environment may vary simultaneously: oxygenation, carbon dioxide conditions, water availability, ionic composition of water, food quality, temperature; all these factors interact with respiration and may change the pH values. Probably exceptions to physiological rules should not be considered a priori as real because they may correspond to a different set of environmental conditions.

The discovery of the completely different specific ventilations and acid–base balances of air and water breathers have suggested further investigations regarding the physiological traits that can be affected by other and very marked differences that exist between air and water (Dejours, 1979; Little, 1983; Schmidt-Nielsen, 1983). In fact, one observes many common types of adaptation in terrestrial animals: snails, spiders, insects, terrestrial vertebrates, compared with their aquatic kindred (see Dejours et al., 1987).

VIII. Summary

The field covered by the comparative physiology of respiration is broad because it encompasses (1) all the functions that allow an adequate O_2 delivery to the cells, a proper clearance of CO_2, and a correct acid–base balance of the body fluids; (2) all species of the entire animal kingdom; (3) the diverse and usually varying environments; and (4) the ontogeny, growth, and aging of the animal. Moreover, the respiratory functions cannot be considered separately from all of the other functions of the organism: nutrition, excretion, endocrine, and nervous controls. When ambient conditions change, all the functions cannot continue to run at their optimal pace and some may be spared at the expense of the others; in other words, there exists a hierarchy of functions.

Comparative physiology is extremely close to environmental physiology, but environmental physiology may not be comparative. We have considered here the relationships between respiration and environment and studied briefly the very important differences in the respiratory functions of air breathers versus water breathers. In the Cambrian period, some invertebrates existed and in the late Cambrian some agnaths are recorded. However, the first recorded land animals were scorpions, living about 400 million years ago when the ambient PO_2 is believed to have been some 12 torr. Why did terrestrial life not appear earlier, because even if the atmospheric pressure of O_2 was low compared with today, its concentration was much higher than in water? The answer is that one cannot enter the atmosphere without first solving two problems: one concerns the nature of the nitrogenous-end products, the other, the water economy. Most wholly aquatic animals are ammoniotelic. They can afford to be because water is a sink for ammonia owing to its extreme solubility, whereas the capacitance of air for ammonia is 1/700th that of water. Thus, it is impossible for ammoniotelic animals to remain so when they leave water, because ammonia is highly toxic. Certainly in terrestrial animals some ammonia can be excreted from the body through the cutaneous or pulmonary routes and through urine and feces, but most organic nitrogen catabolism yields uric acid or urea, which are not particularly toxic. Uric acid does not require much water to be eliminated because it precipitates. Urea needs more, but its solubility in water is rather high. However, to become a completely terrestrial animal, to be able to invade dry environments where little water may be available, (1) water vaporization must decrease, in particular a dry tegument must be developed; (2) salts and nitrogenous-end products must be concentrated. This is what is achieved by some insects, reptiles, birds, and mammals. These arguments involve three large research fields: chemistry, anatomy, and physiology. They are crucial to the problem of the *evolution* of life. Thus, it turns out that starting from comparative respiratory physiology, one must deal with the comparative physiology of all functions, with the relationship between life and environment, and finally the problems of evolution.

More observations and a different intellectual attitude about the biological problems will lead to new concepts or to alterations of today's concepts. Many examples could be given of concepts that at one time were deeply rooted and seemed untouchable. At the beginning of the century, the concept of alveolar gas seemed to be well established, and although Krogh and Lindhard, on the one hand, and Haldane, on the other, expressed some doubts about the actual composition of alveolar gas, the problem was not attacked until the concept of a ventilation/perfusion ratio was formalized in 1949. Since then, this concept has been extensively developed and has not yet reached its final expression. Sixty years ago, blood as a O_2 and CO_2 carrier was sufficiently understood that the difference between arterial and venous blood was known. Yet the kinetics of O_2 and CO_2 loading and unloading were unknown or, more exactly, were assumed to be instantaneous. The discovery of modulators of the O_2-pigment relation is only 20 years old.

There is no doubt that new concepts will emerge as a result of new observations and of the reevaluation of known facts.

References

Barry, P. H., and Diamond, J. M. (1984). Effects of unstirred layers on membrane phenomena. *Physiol. Rev.* 64:763-872.

Dejours, P. (1979). La vie dans l'eau et dans l'air (Life in water and in air). *Pour Sci.* 20:87-95.

Dejours, P., Bolis, L., Taylor, C. R., and Weibel, E. R. (eds.) (1987). *Life in Water and on Land*. Liviana Press. Distributed by Springer-Verlag, New York, p. 556.

Keilin, D. (1966). *The History of Cell Respiration and Cytochrome*. Cambridge, Cambridge University Press, p. 416.

Little, C. (1983). *The Colonisation of Land, Origins and Adaptations of Terrestrial Animals*. Cambridge, Cambridge University Press, p. 290.

Rahn, H. (1966). Aquatic gas exchange: Theory. *Respir. Physiol.* 1:1-12.

Rahn, H. (1967). Gas transport from the external environment to the cell. In *Development of the Lung*. Edited by A. V. S. De Reuck and R. Porter. A Ciba Foundation Symposium. London, J. & A. Churchill, pp. 3-23.

Schmidt-Nielsen, K. (1983). *Animal Physiology. Adaptation and Environment*, 3rd ed. Cambridge, Cambridge University Press, p. 619.

Tenney, M. (1979). A synopsis of breathing mechanisms. In *Evolution of Respiratory Process. A Comparative Approach*. Edited by S. C. Wood and C. Lenfant. New York, Marcel Dekker, p. 370.

Wood, S. C., and Lenfant, C. (1979). *Evolution of Respiratory Process. A Comparative Approach*. New York, Marcel Dekker, p. 370.

Part One

Energy Demand

2

Upper and Lower Limits to Energy Demand in Homoiotherms

PETER W. HOCHACHKA

University of British Columbia
Vancouver, British Columbia, Canada

I. Introduction

Because gas exchange is considered the raison d'être of the mammalian lung, a good starting point for a book dealing with comparative pulmonary biology is the problem of limits to O_2 flux and to adenosine triphosphate (ATP) turnover rates. What are the highest energy demands that must be supported by the respiratory (and cardiovascular) systems? Are there lower limits below which energy metabolism cannot be reduced? What biochemical factors cause, or at least contribute to, the upper and lower limits of energy metabolism? Because among endotherms, the highest metabolic rates are found in the smallest animals, whereas the lowest rates are found in the largest species, one way to analyze the problem of limits to energy metabolism is to treat animal size as a fundamental experimental variable in its own right. Such allometric approaches, of course, are common in biology, and it is well known that mass-specific basal metabolic rates are inversely related to body size. The equation relating body mass (M_b) and metabolism is often given as

$$\dot{V}O_2/M_b = 0.676\, M_b^{-0.25}$$

where $\dot{V}O_2/M_b$ is the mass-specific rate of basal metabolism in liters·h^{-1}·kg^{-1} of O_2 and M_b is body mass in kilograms. The allometric exponent (-0.25) may vary for different rate processes or different groups of organisms. If replotted as log $\dot{V}O_2$ versus log body mass, the allometric exponent, which is the slope of the line, is about 0.75. In both kinds of plots, the allometric exponents are the same for basal or maximum aerobic metabolism (Schmidt-Nielsen, 1984), which means that the scope for activity (the step-up from basal to maximum metabolic rate) is about the same in large and small animals—about 10-fold.

Interestingly, the difference between resting and maximum rates within a species is modest relative to the magnitude of the scaling impact on O_2 consumption of organisms. Compared with a 10- to 20-fold aerobic scope for activity in mammals, the mass specific resting $\dot{V}O_2$ values in milliliters per gram per hour (ml·g^{-1}·h^{-1}) for shrews, humans, and elephants differ by a full 100-fold (7.4, 0.21, and 0.07, respectively). Extrapolating these numbers to whales of 10^5-kg mass yields VO_2/M_b of only 0.02 ml·g^{-1}·h^{-1} O_2 (Schmidt-Nielsen, 1984; Coulson and Hernandez, 1983). This VO_2 value is only 1/400 the rate in shrews, and only one-fifth the rate in permanently hypometabolic bathypelagic fishes measured at 5°C (Torres et al., 1979)!

Because these scaling effects are of such large magnitude, we reasoned that they may supply useful insights into limits to energy metabolism and to regulation of normal rest → work transitions. Unfortunately, the metabolic biochemistry of scaling has been almost totally ignored, with only two studies being exceptional. First, Somero and Childress (1980) examined the scaling of enzymes in oxidative and anaerobic metabolism in the skeletal muscle and brain of 13 species of teleosts. They found that, in contrast to enzymes in aerobic metabolism, there was a direct relationship between body mass and the catalytic potential of enzymes working in anaerobic muscle metabolism. At the same time, Emmett (1980) independently showed that for a series of 10 species of mammals, varying in size by a factor of between 10^5 and 10^6, the catalytic activities of muscle anaerobic enzymes [in μmol·g^{-1}·min^{-1} or units (U)·g^{-1}] scale directly with body mass, whereas the catalytic activities of muscle oxidative enzymes scale inversely (see Fig. 1-3; and Emmett and Hochachka, 1981). More recent assessment (Hochachka et al., 1988) indicates that enzymes in aerobic metabolism of cardiac muscle also scale with a slope similar to that for skeletal muscle enzymes (Fig. 1). What is the meaning of such size-related partitioning of energy metabolism between aerobic and anaerobic pathways? What are the limits and constraints to these scaling patterns?

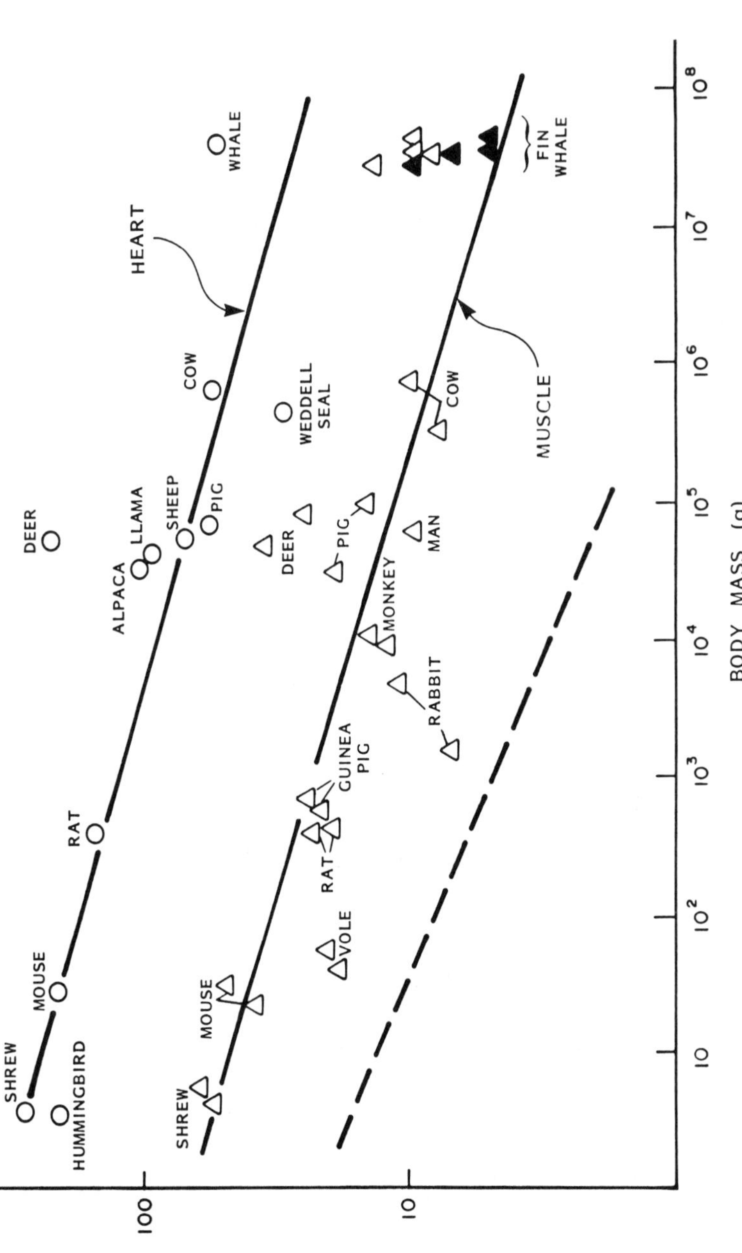

Figure 1 Activity of citrate synthase (U·g^{-1}) in the gastrocnemius muscle (triangles) and heart (circles) of homoiotherms as a function of body size. Data from Emmett and Hochachka (1981) and Hochachka et al. (1982). Data for fin whales (open triangles for longissimus dorsi, closed triangles for hypaxial muscle) from Hochachka et al. (1988). The slope of the dashed line is –0.2, equivalent to the slopes for basal or maximum whole-organizm metabolic rates, and to the slopes for mass-specific cardiac output. Hummingbird data from Suarez et al. (1986).

II. Metabolic Meaning of Scaling of Heart Oxidative Enzymes

It is important to begin by considering the heart data on oxidative enzymes because of a provocative theory (Coulson and Hernandez, 1983; Coulson, 1986) which proposes that the main determinant of metabolism–size relationships in vertebrates is simply blood flow (proportional to cardiac output). This model suggests that shrews, for example, have much higher mass-specific metabolic rates than large animals, simply and solely because they perfuse their tissues at much higher rates; 70-kg alligators are sluggish by comparison with a 70-kg man because they sustain lower average flow rates to their tissues. For the Coulson model, it is necessary to assume that enzyme and substrate concentrations in any given tissue are much the same. For enzymes, such an assumption is now known to be too simplistic, and ample data are available indicating systematic scaling of both enzyme activities (Hochachka et al., 1988) and of mitochondrial volume densities (Taylor, 1987). Coulson and his coworkers may have been unduly influenced by studies of glycolytic enzymes (which are influenced by body mass to a lesser degree) and by studies of reptiles, in which oxidative capacities are limited.

To properly understand the heart enzyme data, it is important to remember that the mass of the heart in mammals scales directly with body mass, but cardiac output (i.e., work of the heart) scales with an allometric exponent of 0.8, the same as resting and maximum metabolic rates. During rest-to-maximum aerobic activity, heart rate and cardiac output increase by factors that are apparently independent of size (see Calder, 1984, and Schmidt-Nielsen, 1984, for literature covering these problems). The scaling of heart citrate synthase activities (see Fig. 1) is thus entirely consistent with data on heart work and heart metabolic rates. Because of the relatively small size of the heart, however, its own energy demands only modestly influence the scaling of whole-organism metabolic rate. For this reason, our main concern is necessarily skeletal muscle.

III. Meaning of Muscle Oxidative Enzyme Activities (in Units per Gram) Scaling Inversely with Mass

At least under one set of conditions—maximum aerobic exercise—about 90% of $\dot{V}O_2$ is due to the metabolism of skeletal muscle which, with few exceptions in mammals, constitutes about 40 to 45% of the body mass. Therefore, enzyme scaling patterns in muscle are of particular interest. Assuming that the allometric exponent for maximum and basal aerobic metabolism is statistically the same, -0.20 to -0.25 (Schmidt-Nielsen, 1984), there are only two ways of scaling oxidative enzyme activities: either in parallel with the metabolism curves or with a slope even closer to zero. The former strategy ensures that carbon flux can be

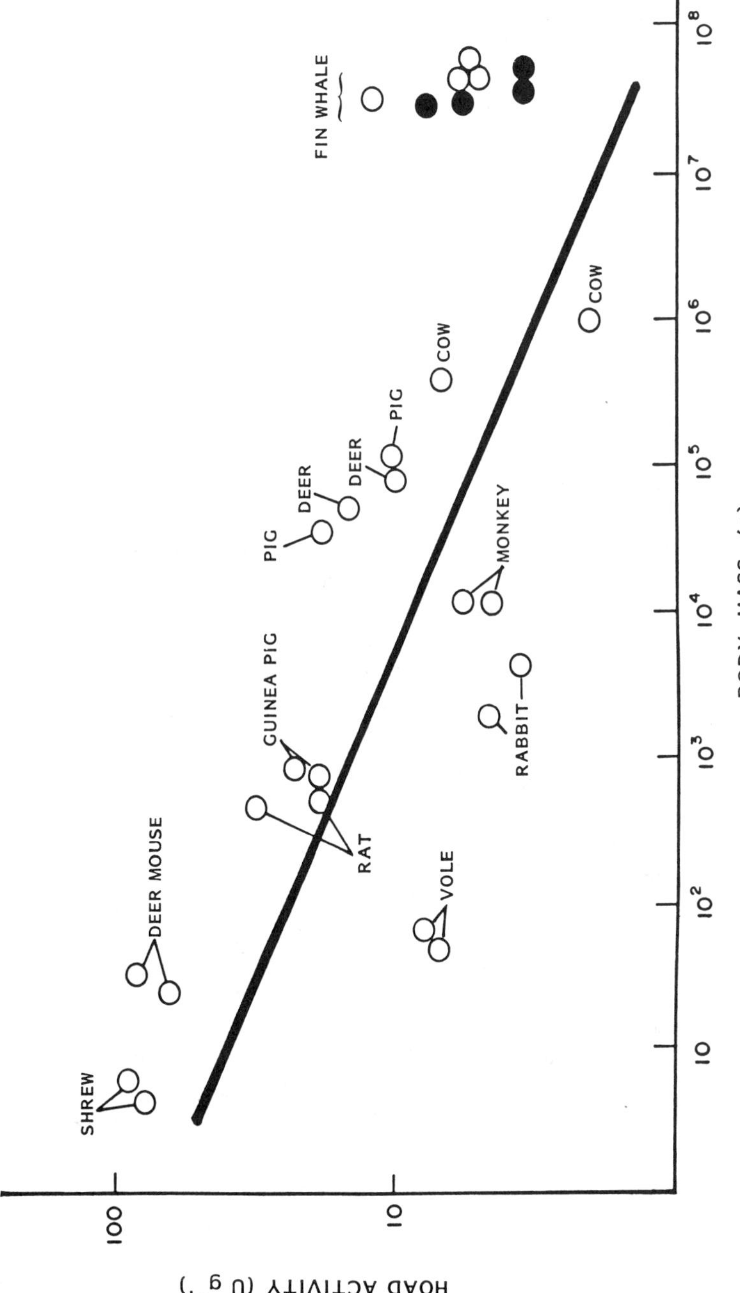

Figure 2 Activity of β-hydroxybutyrylCoA dehydrogenase (HOAD) in the gastrocnemius muscle of several mammals as a function of body size. Data from Emmett and Hochachka (1981). Data for fin whales (open circles for longissimus dorsi, closed circles for hypaxial muscle) from Hochachka et al. (1988). The slope of the HOAD line is −0.21, from Emmett and Hochachka (1981).

increased such that the aerobic scope is amplified to about the same degree in all mammals, without sustaining unacceptably high steady-state substrate levels at any given size range. As substrate concentrations are apparently independent of size (Coulson and Hernandez, 1983), this scaling pattern allows enzyme function where it is most easily regulated: at low substrate concentrations (Atkinson, 1977), irrespective of animal size.

In the second kind of scaling pattern—catalytic potential is scaled by an exponent smaller than -0.20, as observed for citrate synthase in the 10 mammalian species studied by Emmett (1980) and in teleost muscle (Somero and Childress, 1980)—the metabolic consequences are different. Here, as body mass increases, the catalytic potential is in excess of that needed to pace flux without compromising any regulatory constraints. That is, *enzymes scaling with exponents less than those obtained for* $\dot{V}O_{2max}/M_b$ *cannot determine the latter.* By the same token, enzymes that scale with exponents equal to that observed for $\dot{V}O_{2max}/M_b$ could, in principle, cause the scaling pattern observed for maximum oxidative metabolism. Such causal connection may be implied from the data for β-hydroxybutyrylCoA dehydrogenase (HOAD; Fig. 2). The same idea of a causal connection arises from mitochondrial volume density measurements, showing (1) that plots of log mitochondrial volume density versus those of log body mass display slopes of -0.20, and (2) that a given volume, say 1 ml, of muscle mitochondria during maximum aerobic exercise consumes the same amount of O_2 (4-5 ml·min^{-1}), irrespective of source. Systematic downward adjustments of mitochondrial volume densities with increasing body size are, thus, taken to be a fundamental mechanism underlying the scaling of maximum aerobic metabolism in mammals (see Taylor, 1987, for a recent discussion of this area). Whether or not a given enzyme in mitochondrial metabolism displays the same pattern depends upon its role in regulating overall flux of substrates in oxidative phosphorylation; in the species examined by Emmett and Hochachka (1981), citrate synthase clearly does not fit this pattern, whereas HOAD does, which may imply a predominant dependence upon fat catabolism in the 10 species studied.

There is an additional important implication of these data: Because log-log plots for resting and maximum metabolic rates have a similar slope, it is evident that either the same general control mechanisms in mitochondrial metabolism are used, independent of animal size (which we consider most probable) or, if different mechanisms are used, their net effect *in moving fluxes from resting to maximum rates must be the same*. Because of this constraint, and only because of it, can resting and maximum metabolic rates be scaled similarly. This regulatory constraint may also be the explanation for why muscle mitochondria respire at essentially the same rate when animals are at $\dot{V}O_{2(max)}$, again irrespective of size.

IV. The Upper Limit in Aerobic Enzyme Scaling Patterns and the Minimal Size of Homoiotherms

What are the upper limits to plots such as those in Figures 1 and 2? Do oxidative enzyme activities play a role in setting these limits? Or, rephrasing the question, is the lower-size limit set by the amount of oxidative enzyme machinery that can be packed into muscle cells, or any other cells, for that matter? Nature may have come close to such a limit in the design of the fastest muscle currently known, the tymbal muscle of cicadas. This muscle can operate at a contraction frequency of 550 Hz, and it may well be at a limit determined by the approximately 1:1:1 volume density ratios of mitochondria/sarcoplasmic reticulum (SR)/myofilaments (Josephson and Young, 1985). It is probable, although not yet proved, that any further increase in oxidative enzyme capacity (i.e., in mitochondrial volume densities) would be counterproductive because it would simultaneously require reductions either in SR or myofilaments. The near 1:1:1 ratio observed represents a classic example of compromise and coadaptation when contraction frequency is the property under selective pressure.

Interestingly, the ultrastructures of skeletal muscle and heart of the smallest mammal (the shrew) and of the smallest bird (the hummingbird) indicate amplification of mitochondrial volume densities and of SR that approach but do not reach the same optimization point expressed in tymbal muscle. Although the three volume densities (mitochondria, SR, and myofilaments) have not been quantified systematically, most workers in this field estimate mitochondrial volume density at 45 to 50%, about equal to that of the myofilaments, and consistent with recent measurements showing particularly high levels of oxidative enzymes (Suarez et al., 1986). This allows for less than a 10% volume density for SR, a value substantially lower than that for the fast tymbal muscles of cicadas or other very fast vertebrate muscles.

The difference in ultrastructural design of the two (mammalian and insect) muscle types can be rationalized in terms of their different functions. In mammalian skeletal and heart muscles, power output is directly proportional to contraction frequency (for any given system) because the maximum force that can be exerted, maximum percentage of shortening of myofilaments, the number of myofilaments per cross-sectional area of muscle, the maximum overlap between thick and thin filaments, and the number of cross bridges, all are size-independent (see Schmidt-Nielsen, 1984; Taylor et al., 1985). In heart and skeletal muscles of the smallest homoiotherms, maximum oxidative metabolism (and presumably maximum power output) is achieved during hovering flight at contraction frequencies of about 20 Hz for the heart and of about 60 to 80 Hz for the flight muscle of hummingbirds (see Suarez et al., 1986, for literature in this area). The tymbal muscles of cicadas, on the other hand, are adapted for very high-frequency sound production and thus for much higher-frequency contraction; however, power output is *not* inordinately high, presumably because these muscles need not shorten by more than a fraction of that required in hummingbird or shrew muscles (Schmidt-Nielsen, 1984; Josephson and Young, 1985). Because of the role of the SR in modulating Ca^{2+} fluxes during contraction–relaxation cycles, maximizing muscle for frequency in this system would be expected to require SR amplification: The limit appears to be close to the 1:1:1 ratios mentioned earlier.

We propose that, given the constraint that power output is proportional to contraction frequency, as in other vertebrates, the mitochondrial volume densities in hummingbird and shrew muscles also are close to their upper limits; further increases would require decreases in myofilament or SR volume densities. The former would reduce the maximum forces that could be exerted, whereas the latter would reduce the possible contraction frequencies. Thus, there seems to be little room left for adaptation (at least expressed as upward regulation of mitochondrial abundance). If this conclusion is correct, it supplies another reason why hummingbirds and shrews are at the lower-size limit for homoiotherms; further reductions in size would require drastic qualitative adjustments either in skeletal muscle or in cardiac muscle design. Many workers believe that even attaining their current small size requires significant cardiovascular adjustments; in particular, the time required for the systole–diastole cycle must be minimized (this requires about 50 msec and sets the maximum contraction frequency at 20 Hz, substantially less than can be achieved by the flight muscle), the heart/body ratio is elevated, and the blood O_2-carrying capacity is tightly (and perhaps precariously) balanced relative to viscosity (Schmidt-Nielsen, 1984).

V. The Lower Limit in Aerobic Enzyme Scaling Patterns at the Maximum Size of Homoiotherms

Just as allometric plots (Figs. 1 and 2) raise the question of the lower limit to size, they also raise the question of the upper limit to the size of homoiotherms. What roles, if any, do oxidative enzyme activities play in setting these limits? Is there a minimum level of mass-specific oxidative metabolism below which homoiotherms cannot go? These questions are much more difficult to address than one of minimal size; the answers may depend upon the state of the organism or on environmental conditions (see Hochachka and Guppy, 1987). Although direct measurements are unavailable, extrapolations indicate that the mass-specific $\dot{V}O_2$ of a 10^5-kg whale is already down to 0.02 $ml \cdot g^{-1} \cdot h^{-1}$ of O_2. That is equivalent to an ATP turnover rate of 0.013 $\mu mol \cdot g^{-1} \cdot mm^{-1}$. By comparison, the resting metabolic rate of humans turns over ATP about 10 times faster (0.14 $\mu mol \cdot g^{-1} \cdot min^{-1}$). Marathon runners turn over muscle ATP at about 30 μmol $g^{-1} min^{-1}$, whereas the muscles of a hovering hummingbird turn over ATP at over 600 $\mu mol \cdot g^{-1} \cdot min^{-1}$ (Suarez et al., 1986), or nearly 50,000 times faster than in the whale at rest (whatever that means for this animal!). Could a mammal get much bigger? How much more could it slow down? Unfortunately, we do not know, but again, there are reasons for thinking the largest whales are close to a lower metabolic limit. In fact, at this rate of oxidative energy metabolism, the difference between ectotherms and endotherms begins to get blurry. Two examples illustrate the point. In the first place, the mass-specific metabolic rate of 3°C of a torpid turtle (one of the most hypometabolic ectotherms known) is about 0.001 $ml \cdot g^{-1} \cdot h^{-1}$ of O_2 (Herbert and Jackson, 1985), not too different from the projected estimate for whales of a 10^5-kg mass. Second, excluding varanids, which for reptiles display unusually high metabolic rates, and snakes, which display unusually low metabolic rates (Chappell and Ellis, 1987), reptiles are thought to display resting metabolic rates of about one-fourth to one-third those of mammals of the same size (Schmidt-Nielsen, 1979). The allometric exponent, on the other hand, is higher than in mammals (Andrews and Pough, 1985); extrapolating log–log plots of aerobic metabolic rate versus body mass for mammals and reptiles indicates that they intersect at about the mass of the largest dinosaurs or of whales (approximately 10^5 kg). If this analysis is correct, it implies that the argument about whether or not dinosaurs were endotherms may be rather academic; allometric constraints may have led to metabolic rates that, in any event, would be almost indistinguishable from those of the present-day largest whales.

These arguments refer to the resting state. As far as we know, whales retain a typically mammalian (about 10-fold) scope for activity. In fact, under active conditions, whales are apparently confronted with overheating problems, which may represent another brake upon further increases in body mass for mammals as well as dinosaurs (Schmidt-Nielsen, 1984). According to Coulson and Hernandez (1983) and Coulson (1986), the heart/body ratio of reptiles is much lower than in mammals and, unlike mammals, reptiles sustain a further drop in this ratio as size increases. In relative terms, large reptiles have small hearts; that is presumably why they are unable to generate flows and tissue perfusion rates (Coulson, 1986) commensurate with the active metabolic rates typical of mammals. The implication, then, is that the largest dinosaurs, even if homoiothermic in a formal sense, could not have developed mammalian performance capacities.

VI. Lower Limits of the Glycolytic Enzyme Scaling Pattern and the Aerobic Function of Anaerobic Enzymes

Are there limits to how low muscle glycolytic enzyme levels can be reduced in small homoiotherms? Hummingbird and shrew skeletal muscles retain some

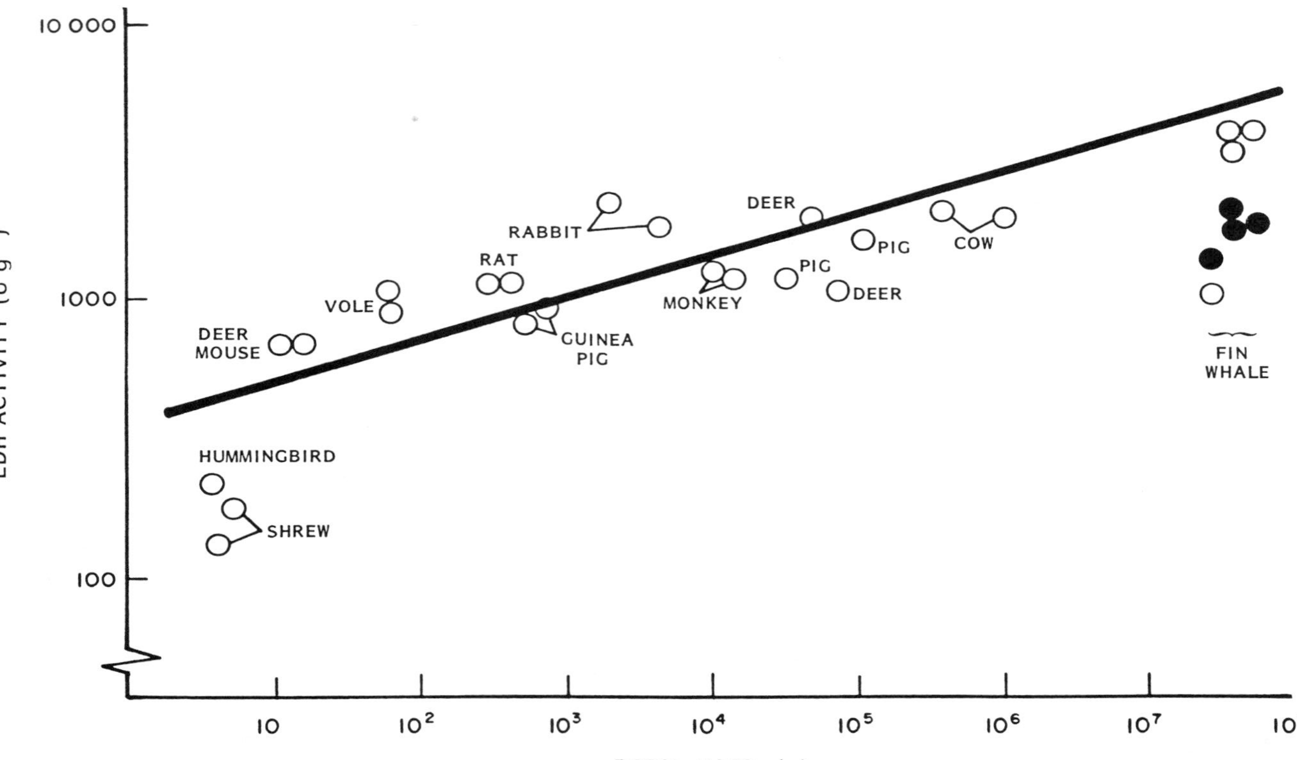

Figure 3 Activity of lactate dehydrogenase in the gastrocnemius muscle of several mammals as a function of body size. Data for fin whales from Hochachka et al. (1988); (open circles for longissimus dorsi; closed circles for hypaxial muscle). Methods and other mammalian data from Emmett and Hochachka (1981). Hummingbird flight muscle data are included for comparison (Suarez et al., 1986).

lactate dehydrogenase (LDH) activity (Fig. 3), for example; hence, one is tempted to look for reasons why these kinds of enzymes are not deleted. Because such deletion of LDH occurs, in fact, in some insect flight muscles (Sacktor, 1976), we may conclude that muscle cells can work perfectly well without any LDH. However, in insect flight muscle, LDH deletion is considered particularly crucial because these muscles depend upon α-glycerophosphate dehydrogenase (α-GPDH) for cycling reducing equivalents from NADH into the mitochondria. Under aerobic conditions it is imperative to avoid α-GPDH–LDH competition for NADH, because with glucose as a carbon source, a 50:50 split of NADH between these two reaction pathways would mean zero net ATP formation in glucose conversion to lactate (see Hochachka and Somero, 1984; Hochachka, 1980).

In contrast, vertebrate skeletal muscles, including hummingbird and shrew muscles, seem to depend mainly upon the malate–aspartate cycle for shuttling hydrogen between cytosol and mitochondria (see Suarez et al., 1986, for relative enzyme activities). Connett et al. (1985) argue that, in these kinds of muscles, the LDH reaction serves as a kind of safety mechanism buffering the cytosolic $NADH/NAD^+$ ratios during activated aerobic muscle metabolism. Such an aerobic function for LDH (which may be exaggerated in the phenomenal rest-to-work transitions typical of hummingbird flight muscle) may well explain why this enzyme is retained even in muscles as aerobic as those of the shrew and hummingbird.

The redox buffering function proposed for LDH during otherwise totally oxidative work is analogous to the function proposed for creatine phosphokinase (CPK) in buffering the cell's ATP reserves during rest-to-work transitions (see Kushmerick, 1985). Again, the need for this function may be exaggerated in muscles of very small homoiotherms, which may explain why hummingbird flight muscle sustains some 2000 U of CPK per gram (Suarez et al., 1986), a level clearly at variance with the scaling patterns for enzymes that are normally thought to be involved mainly in anaerobic metabolism.

VII. The Upper Limits to Glycolytic Enzyme Scaling Pattern

The final question of limits concerns how far large mammals can go in upward scaling of enzymes such as muscle LDH. Is there a limit to how much LDH or other anaerobic enzymes large animals can incorporate into their muscle cells? Because anaerobic glycolysis, particularly in burst working muscles, operates as an effectively closed system, there are several critical constraints necessarily built into the system. Perhaps the most important of these serve to protect against the generation of potentially harmful end products, particularly protons. Overproduction of H^+ ions, in fact, is generally thought to be the most serious hazard of reliance upon anaerobic glycolysis, which may explain why glycogen is stored in muscle at maximally about 100 μmol·g^{-1}, *far below possible levels*. We know it is possible to pack in glycogen to well over 1 M levels (!); this is commonly observed in liver of hypoxia-tolerant animals such as turtles. Here, however, the end product of glycogen mobilization is glucose (for export to the rest of the body) not lactate, and there is no net generation of protons. The need to avoid problems of proton overproduction is also an important reason why several properties—stored glycogen, catalytic capacities of glycolytic enzymes, myosin ATPase capacities (or volume densities of myofilaments), and muscle buffering power—all coadapt; upward adjustment in any one of these factors, as occurs in fast-twitch or white muscles, means upward adjustment in all of them (Hochachka, 1985). This suggests that the upper limit to LDH incorporation into muscle cells of large mammals really represents a kind of maximization process: maximizing the amount of myosin ATPase capacity without sacrificing the amounts of glycogen, buffers, and glycolytic enzymes that can simultaneously be maintained. At the limit, the maximum glycolytic ATP generating capacity, in effect, must at least equal the in vivo maximum myosin ATPase capacity, and there should be little cellular room left for further upward scaling of myofilaments. Whether or not this is approached, or actually reached, in the muscles of the largest whales, unfortunately, is not currently known. We know that this limit is not reached in fin whales of about 3×10^4 kg because the LDH levels in their muscles can be surpassed by adaptation of white muscles for speed in very fast swimming fishes (Hochachka, 1980; 1985).

VIII. Conclusions

It is well documented that basal and maximum O_2-uptake rates of homoiotherms scale approximately to the 0.75 power; log-log plots of mass-specific metabolic rates versus body mass yield slopes of -0.20 to -0.25. Recent studies of 11 mammalian species and the hummingbird indicate that marker enzymes of mitochondrial muscle and heart metabolism (citrate synthase, for example) scale inversely with body mass. Hummingbirds and shrews are near the upper limit in the degree to which the oxidative capacity of heart and skeletal muscles can be elevated; further increase in mitochondrial volume densities would sacrifice myofilament or sarcoplasmic reticulum (SR) volume densities. Whales of about 10^5-kg mass may be near the limit at the opposite extreme because mass-specific resting metabolic rates are predicted to be already about as low as those of extremely hypometabolic ectotherms (torpid turtles). In contrast to oxidative enzyme-scaling patterns, enzyme activities, such as lactate dehydrogenase (LDH), normally functional in muscle anaerobic glycolysis, increase directly with body mass. Hummingbirds and shrews are considered to have reduced muscle LDH levels close to a lower limit, commensurate with buffering of cytosolic redox, an aerobic LDH function. The upper limit for packing anaerobic glycolytic potential into muscle cells appears to be set by a compromise between myofilament volume densities and the combined volume densities of glycogen granules, intracellular-buffering components, and glycolytic enzymes. This limit is not reached in muscles of fin whales, which are about one-third the mass of the largest mammals.

References

Andrews, R. M., and Pough, F. H. (1985). Metabolism of squamate reptiles: Allometric and ecological relationships. *Physiol. Zool.* 58:214-231.

Atkinson, D. E. (1977). *Cellular Energy Metabolism and Its Regulation*. New York, Academic Press.

Calder, W. A. (1984). *Size, Function, and Life History*. Cambridge, Harvard University Press, pp. 1-215.

Chappell, M. A., and Ellis, T. M. (1987). Resting metabolic rates in boid snakes: Allometric relationships and temperature effects. *J. Comp. Physiol.* 157: 227-236.

Connett, R. J., Gayeski, T. E. J., and Honig, C. R. (1985). Energy sources in fully aerobic rest-work transit: A new role for glycolysis. *Am. J. Physiol.* 248:H922-H929.

Coulson, R. A. (1986). Metabolic rate and the flow theory: A study in chemical engineering. *Comp. Biochem. Physiol.* 84A:217-229.

Coulson, R. A., Hernandez, T., and Herbert, J. D. (1977). Metabolic rate, enzyme kinetics in vivo. *Comp. Biochem. Phsyiol.* 56A:251-262.

Coulson, R. A., and Hernandez, T. (1983). Alligator metabolism. Studies of chemical reactions in vivo. *Comp. Biochem. Physiol.* 74:1-182.

Emmett, B. (1980). The metabolic biochemistry of the wandering shrew (*Sorex vagrans*). M.Sc. Thesis, Univ. of British Columbia.

Emmett, B., and Hochachka, P. W. (1981). Scaling of oxidative and glycolytic enzyme in mammals. *Respir. Physiol.* 45:261-272.

Herbert, C. V., and Jackson, D. C. (1985). Temperature effects on the responses to prolonged submergence in the turtle *Chrysemys picta bellii*. II. Metabolic rate, blood acid-base and ionic changes, and cardiovascular function in aerated and anoxic water. *Physiol. Zool.* 58:670-681.

Hochachka, P. W. (1980). *Living without Oxygen*. Cambridge, Harvard University Press, pp. 1-237.

Hochachka, P. W. (1985). Fuels and pathways as designed systems for support of muscle work. *J. Exp. Biol.* 115:149-164.

Hochachka, P. W., and Somero, G. N. (1984). *Biochemical Adaptation*. Princeton, Princeton University Press, pp. 1-537.

Hochachka, P. W., and Guppy, M. (1987). *Metabolic Arrest and the Control of Biological Time*. Cambridge, Harvard University Press, pp. 1-227.

Hochachka, P. W., Stanley, C., Merkt, J., and Sumar-Kalinowski, J. (1982). Metabolic meaning of elevated oxidative enzymes in high altitude adapted animals: An interpretive hypothesis. *Respir. Physiol.* 52:303-313.

Hochachka, P. W., Emmett, B., and Suarez, R. K. (1988). Limits and constraints in the scaling of oxidative glycolytic enzymes in homeotherms. *Can. J. Zool.* (in press).

Josephson, R. K., and Young, D. (1985). A synchronous insect muscle with an operating frequency greater than 500 Hz. *J. Exp. Biol.* 118:185-208.

Kushmerick, M. (1985). Patterns in mammalian muscle energetics. *J. Exp. Biol.* 115:165-177.

Sacktor, B. (1976). Biochemical adaptations for flight in the insect. *Biochem. Soc. Symp.* 41:111-131.

Schmidt-Nielsen, K. (1979). *Animal Physiology, Adaptation and Environment*, 2nd ed. Cambridge, Cambridge University Press, pp. 1-560.

Schmidt-Nielsen, K. (1984). *Scaling. Why Is Size So Important*? Cambridge, Cambridge University Press, pp. 1-241.

Somero, G. N., and Childress, J. J. (1980). A violation of the metabolism-size scaling paradigm: Activities of glycolytic enzymes in muscle increase in larger-size fish. *Physiol. Zool.* 53:322-337.

Suarez, R. K., Brown, G. S., and Hochachka, P. W. (1986). Metabolic sources of energy for hummingbird flight. *Annu. Rev. Physiol.* 251:R537-R542.

Taylor, C. R. (1987). Structural and functional limits to oxidative metabolism: Insights from scaling. *Annu. Rev. Physiol.* 49:135-146.

Taylor, C. R., Weibel, E., and Bolis, L. (eds.). (1985). *Design and Performance of Muscular Systems. J. Exp. Biol.* 115:1-412.

Torres, J. J., Belman, B. W., and Childress, J. J. (1979). Oxygen consumption rates of midwater fishes off California. *Deep-Sea Res.* 26A:185-197.

3

Matching Structures and Functions in the Respiratory System
Allometric and Adaptive Variations in Energy Demand

C. RICHARD TAYLOR
and RICHARD H. KARAS*

Museum of Comparative Zoology
Harvard University
Cambridge, Massachusetts

EWALD R. WEIBEL
and HANS HOPPELER

University of Berne
Berne, Switzerland

I. Symmorphosis: A Principle of Economic Design

A. A "Common Sense" Hypothesis

In this chapter we will consider and evaluate evidence for a general principle of economic animal design as it may apply to the mammalian respiratory system. Common sense dictates that animals should not be wasteful in building and maintaining structures that they do not use. It is also clear that the structural components of the body respond to functional demands placed upon them,

---

**Current affiliation*: Brigham and Women's Hospital, Boston, Massachusetts.

Dedicated to Pierre Dejours on the occasion of his 65th birthday, March 29, 1987.

The preparation of this chapter was supported by grants from the Swiss National Science Foundation (3.036.84) and the U.S. National Science Foundation (DCB-8612294).

both during growth and in adult life. Structures must be continually renewed. and they change to reflect the functional demands they experience. For example, with training, athletes can finely tune the structures of their muscles and their cardiovascular system to the functional demands of a particular athletic event, and these structural modifications are soon lost when the training is stopped (Saltin and Gollnick, 1983; Hoppeler and Lindstedt, 1985; Howald, 1985; Goldspink, 1985; Saltin, 1985). The skeletal system provides another familiar example of the dynamic nature of structures. The amount and type of bone our body builds reflects the force regimens experienced by individual bones. For example, the long bones in the serving arm of a professional tennis player may have twice the cross-sectional area of the nonserving arm, and it has proved extremely difficult to prevent a continued atrophy of bone in astronauts subjected to the absence of gravity forces in space (Lanyon and Rubin, 1985). Structural design and maintenance is clearly a dynamic process that responds to functional demands.

If animals are built reasonably, we would, therefore, expect that they should build and maintain just enough, but no more, structure than they need to meet functional requirements. We have proposed calling this principle of economic design *symmorphosis*, defining it as the state of structural design whereby the formation of structural elements (morphogenesis) that occurs both during growth and during maintenance of structures in adults, should be regulated to satisfy, but not exceed, the functional requirements of the system (Taylor and Weibel, 1981).

B. The Mammalian Respiratory System: A Test Case For Symmorphosis

The flow of O_2 through the respiratory system provides an excellent test case for the principle of symmorphosis. Oxygen flows through a series of linked steps on its way from the environmental air to the mitochondria where it is consumed in the process of oxidative phosphorylation (Fig. 1). The transfer of O_2 at each step is determined by a combination of functional and structural variables that can be assigned, in first approximation, to the pressure gradients as the driving force, or to the conductances, respectively (Dejours, 1981; Weibel, 1984).

There is a clearly defined upper limit to O_2 consumption ($\dot{V}O_{2max}$), at which one, or more, of these steps becomes limiting. The rate of O_2 consumption increases with exercise intensity up to this limit. Further increases in exercise intensity are no longer accompanied by an increase in O_2 consumption; instead additional energy is supplied anaerobically and the duration of exercise becomes limited by metabolic acidosis (Margaria, 1976). From this observation we can conclude that the limitation to endurance exercise is not the result of the

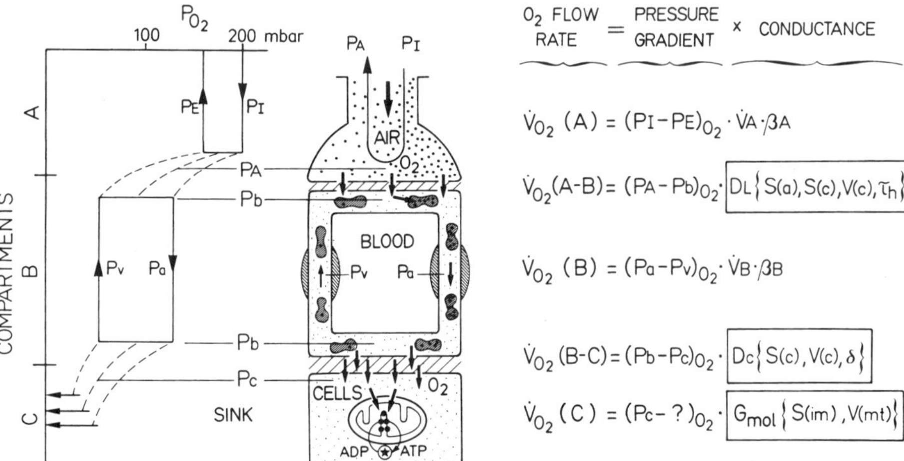

Figure 1 Model of respiratory system indicating O_2 flow rates, partial pressure differences, and conductances. At levels A (air) and B (blood) the conductances are related to mass flow rates $\dot{V}$ multiplied with the capacitance (β) of the medium for O_2. At the transfer levels A–B and B–C the conductances are "diffusing capacities" determined in part by morphometric properties (enclosed in boxes, see text for definitions). In the mitochondria (C) the conductance is related to the molecular make-up (respiratory chains) of the mitochondrial membranes. (From Taylor and Weibel, 1981.)

limited power of the muscles' contractile machinery. It is, rather, related to the capacity of muscles to utilize O_2 in the mitochondria or of the respiratory system to transfer O_2 to the mitochondria.

It is evident that the performance of this multistep respiratory system depends upon a large number of structural and functional variables. Each of these variables potentially can be a limiting factor for O_2 flow. In its simplest formulation, symmorphosis predicts that once the upper limit of O_2 uptake is reached, all of the available structure for O_2 transfer or uptake is utilized. Thus, the limits should be reached simultaneously at all steps, and the design of each part of the respiratory system should be matched to that at all others.

C. A Comparative Approach: Evaluating Nature's Experiments

How do we approach the problem of testing this hypothesis? Each part of the entire interlinked system must be considered in the context of the entire system.

Accordingly, there is no simple, straightforward approach to test the hypothesis: we must utilize a strategy that allows the variations in design and functional properties within the respiratory system to be studied in an integrated fashion. The general approach adopted in this chapter is that of comparative systems physiology.

The fundamental reference parameter is oxidative capacity. We consider how the different parts of the respiratory system differ in response to large differences in oxidative capacity observed in the animal kingdom by exploiting two types of variations.

Allometric Variations in $\dot{V}O_{2max}$

Allometry, or the scaling of structures and functions to body mass, provides a basic tool for this type of comparative systems approach. Size has profound consequences for animal design, and much can be learned about fundamental relationships between biological structures and functions by studying how they scale over a size range of animals. This area of biology has recently received a great deal of attention, and several excellent books on the subject have been published recently (McMahon and Bonner, 1983; Schmidt-Nielsen, 1984; Calder, 1984).

Morphological and physiological variables can be scaled relative to body mass (M_b) using allometric equations of the general form:

$$y = a \cdot M_b{}^b$$

The exponent b is called the scaling factor. The logarithmic transformation of this equation:

$$\log y = \log a + b \log M_b$$

is generally used by the biologist because b then becomes simply the slope of the linear regression line on a double logarithmic plot, allowing the regression and statistical confidence intervals to be calculated (Draper and Smith, 1966).

Our fundamental reference parameter for the study of O_2 transport in the respiratory system, $\dot{V}O_{2max}$, has a scaling factor of about 0.81 in mammals (Taylor et al., 1981). This means that under rate-limiting conditions each gram of a 30-g mouse consumes O_2 at about six times the rate of a 300-kg cow. It is evident that this "experiment of nature" presents us with large enough differences in the maximal flow rates of O_2 through the respiratory system to study the question of whether or not structural and functional components of the system are matched to maximal O_2 flow.

Adaptive Variations in $\dot{V}O_{2max}$

Different species have become adapted for different levels of endurance performance. Husky dogs, for example, sustain for hours metabolic rates more than twice the maximal rate predicted for an animal of their size as they pull sleds across the arctic tundra (Van Citters and Franklin, 1969), whereas goats and sheep of the same size, being much more sedentary in their habits, are not even able to reach the predicted rates (Taylor et al., 1987a). Adaptive variations of this kind have been shown to provide two- to threefold differences in $\dot{V}O_{2max}$ between animals of the same size in size classes of mammals from small rodents to large horses and cows (Seeherman et al., 1981; Weibel et al., 1987b). Adaptive variation, therefore, provides a second approach for testing the predictions of the principle of symmorphosis.

In this chapter we use these two variations in $\dot{V}O_{2max}$ to address the question of how, and to what extent, the serial components of the respiratory system vary when it adapts as a whole to meet the higher energetic demands of the muscles. We dissect the pathway for O_2 from the lung to muscle mitochondria into the various structural and functional components shown in Fig. 1 and ask how each differs to provide the large differences in O_2 transfer capacity at each level.

II. Mitochondria in Skeletal Muscles: An Invariant Building Block?

A. Mitochondria and the Demand for Oxygen

Oxygen is consumed by the mitochondria as they product ATP by oxidative phosphorylation. The phosphorylation is carried out by respiratory chain enzymes that are built into the mitochondria's multiply infolded inner membrane, the cristae (Fig. 2). The area of inner membrane per unit volume of mitochondria in skeletal muscle is relatively constant at about 40 $m^2 \cdot ml^{-1}$ of mitochondria (Hoppeler et al., 1981a); and the concentrations of the respiratory chain enzymes in the inner membrane are also relatively constant (Schwerzmann et al., 1986). Thus, as a first approximation, the volume of mitochondria in skeletal muscles is a valid estimate of the quantity of respiratory chain enzymes present (Hoppeler et al., 1987b).

Under conditions of heavy exercise where the limiting conditions of $\dot{V}O_{2max}$ are reached, more than 90% of the O_2 is consumed by the mitochondria of the skeletal muscles (Mitchell and Blomqvist, 1971). Thus, the rate of O_2 consumption of the animal is approximately equal to the volume of mitochondria in skeletal muscle, $V_{(mt)}$, times the average rate that each unit volume consumes O_2 under these conditions, $\dot{v}O_{2(mt)}$, i.e:

$$\dot{V}O_{2max} = V_{(mt)} \cdot \dot{v}O_{2(mt)} \tag{1}$$

The question to address then is whether the large differences in $\dot{V}O_{2max}/M_b$ resulting from allometric and from adaptive variation are due to differences in

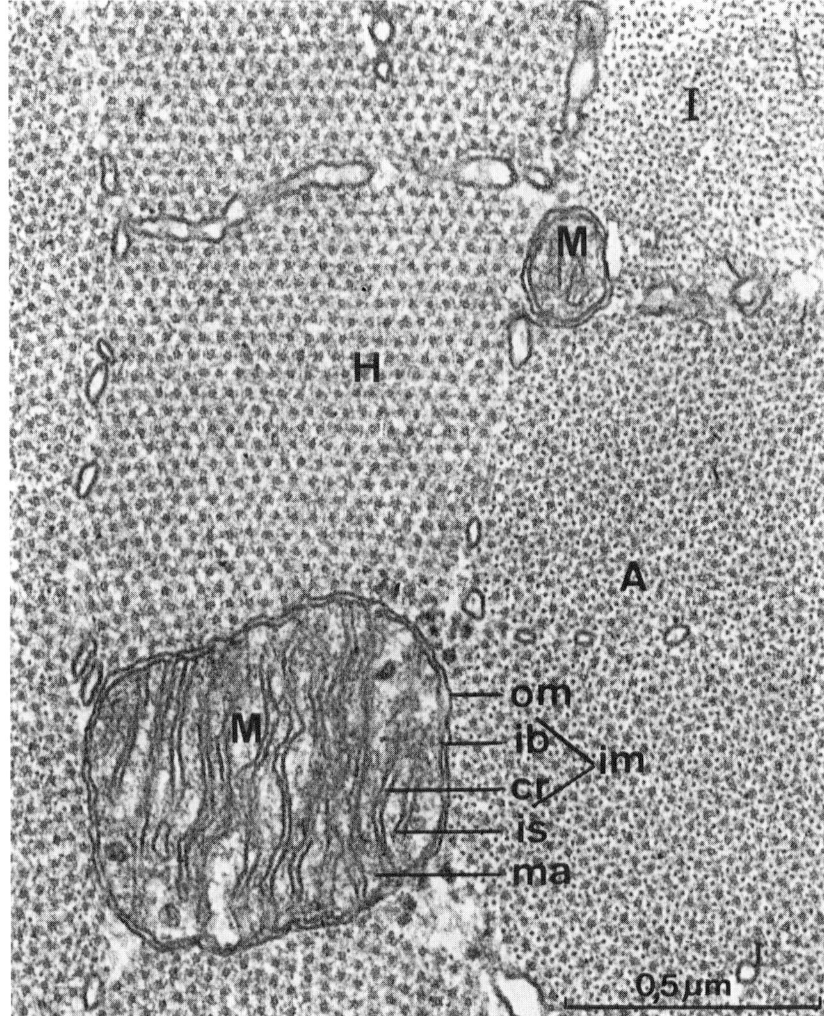

Figure 2 Cross section of a portion of a muscle fiber showing two mitochondria (M). The A-, H-, and I-band part of the sarcomere can be distinguished because of the presence or absence of myosin (thick) and actin (thin) filaments (om, outer membrane; im, inner membrane, consisting of ib, inner boundary membrane and cr, cristae membrane; ma, matrix space, is, intermembrane space; sr, sarcotubular system). (From Hoppeler et al., 1987b.)

$V_{(mt)}$, or whether they are the result, either wholly or in part, of differences in the rate at which the mitochondria carry out phosphorylation as evidenced by $\dot{v}O_{2(mt)}$.

B. Allometric Variations in Mitochondria at $\dot{V}O_{2max}$: $V_{(mt)}$ and $\dot{v}O_{2(mt)}$

Small animals have more mitochondria in each gram of their muscles than large animals (Mathieu et al., 1981). The higher mitochondrial density of small animals is obvious in Figure 3 in which cross-sections of the semitendinosus muscle of a 400-g dwarf mongoose and a 250-kg eland are compared. Both Mathieu et al. (1981) and Else and Hulbert (1985) found that the mitochondrial volume, $V_{(mt)}$, of selected skeletal muscles had about the same scaling factor with body mass as $\dot{V}O_{2max}$. This agrees with the findings of Emmett and Hochachka (1981) that the catalytic capacities of several oxidative enzymes in skeletal muscle also scale with the same factor as $\dot{V}O_{2max}$.

Recently, a morphometric technique for estimating the total volume of mitochondria in skeletal muscles of an animal has been developed (Hoppeler et al., 1984). Data obtained using this technique indicate that measurements of mitochondrial volume densities of semitendinosus and vastus medialis muscles are representative of the skeletal muscles of the whole body. Because these two muscles have been used in allometric studies of mitochondria (Mathieu et al., 1981), this finding enables us to calculate a total volume of mitochondria of skeletal muscles in animals spanning a range of body size.

The top panel of Figure 4 compares how total volume of mitochondria in skeletal muscles and maximal O_2 uptake change with body size on the same allometric plot. To reduce the "biological noise" in this comparison, we have used only data for which the measurements of both parameters have been made on the same animals. Although the absolute values of the scaling factors for these parameters calculated from this limited data base may differ from published values derived from larger data bases, the comparison of the two scaling factors provides better information about the relationship between these two parameters. The scaling factors for $\dot{V}O_{2max}$ and $V_{(mt)}$ with M_b are virtually identical (0.85 vs 0.87). Thus, the higher demand for O_2 in smaller animals appears to be met simply by building more mitochondria.

An average value for the O_2 consumption of each milliliter of mitochondria when animals exercise at $\dot{V}O_{2max}$ can be obtained by dividing $\dot{V}O_{2max}$ by total $V_{(mt)}$ in skeletal muscle. Using this approach, Hoppeler and Lindstedt (1985) calculated that under these exercise conditions, each milliliter of skeletal muscle mitochondria consumes 3-5 ml $\cdot$ min^{-1} of O_2 in all mammals. This finding is supported by mounting evidence from a wide variety of species (Taylor, 1987; Taylor et al., 1987b).

Figure 4b uses the data on $\dot{V}O_{2\,max}$ and $V_{(mt)}$ presented in Figure 4a to calculate an average mitochondrial oxygen consumption for skeletal muscles when animals exercise at $\dot{V}O_{2\,max}$. It graphically confirms the independence of mitochondrial O_2 consumption and body size over a size range of mammals from 21-g wood mice to 500-kg steers and horses. Thus, the 5- to 10-fold allometric differences in maximal O_2 consumption in each gram of muscle appear to be matched by corresponding differences in the amount of mitochondrial structure that animals build, whereas the functional parameter, the rate at which each unit of structure consumes O_2, appears to be invariant.

C. Adaptive Variations in Mitochondria at $\dot{V}O_{2\,max}$: $V_{(mt)}$ and $\dot{v}O_{2\,(mt)}$

In a recent study, Hoppeler et al. (1987b) addressed the question of how mitochondria respond to differences in maximal aerobic capacity resulting from adaptive variation. They compared two of nature's endurance athletes, dogs and ponies, with similarly sized goats and calves. The $\dot{V}O_{2\,max}$ differed by a factor of 2.5-fold within each of these adaptive size-pairs.

The total muscle mass of the dog and the horse was about 1.3 times larger than in the goat and the steer (44% vs 32% of M_b). An increase in muscle mass is therefore an important mechanism for increasing both the mechanical and the aerobic power of athletic animals. This is strikingly demonstrated in the "elite" animal athletes (Snow, 1985), such as the greyhound, in which muscle mass constitutes 57% of M_b (Gunn, 1978).

The volume density of mitochondria was also higher in the athletic animals, contributing in part to their higher aerobic capacity. Thus, both increases in muscle mass and increases in mitochondrial density must be taken into account in evaluating the match between structure and function of the mitochondria in the adaptive pairs. Figure 5 presents a box plot that graphically indicates the relative contribution of volume density of mitochondria, $V_{V(mt,f)}$, and muscle mass to increasing total mitochondrial volume of aerobic compared with less aerobic species of the adaptive pairs. The shaded areas represent the total mitochondrial volume for each of the species (i.e., total volume equals density times muscle mass). The line drawn from the origin through the corner of

---

Figure 3 Cross section of two portions of adjacent muscle fibers showing considerable differences in their content in subsarcolemmal (ms) and in interfibrillar or central (mc) mitochondria in M. semitendinosus of two mammals of different body size: (a) dwarf mongoose (500 g), and (b) eland (220 kg). (From Mathieu et al., 1981.)

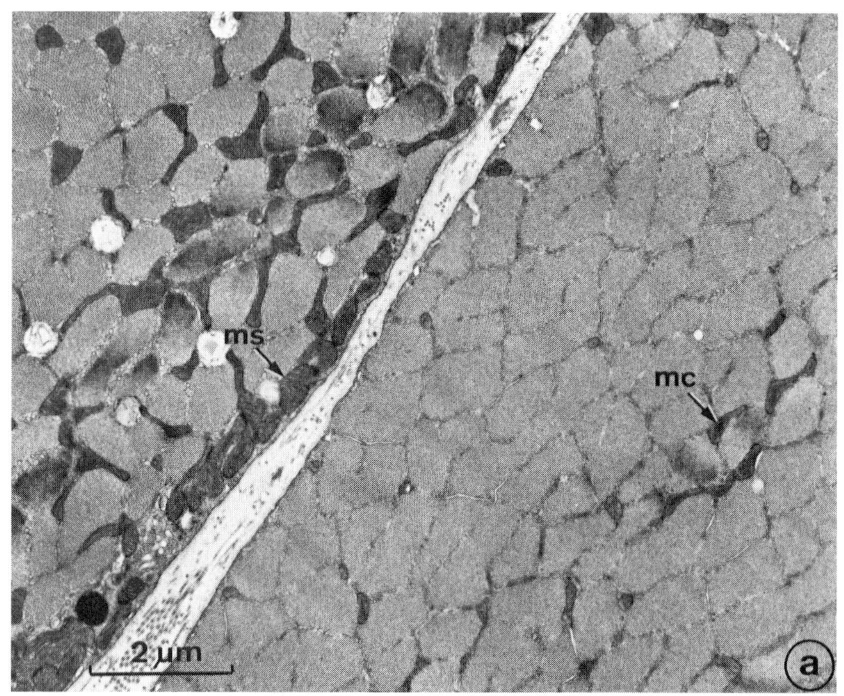
ms
mc
2 µm
a

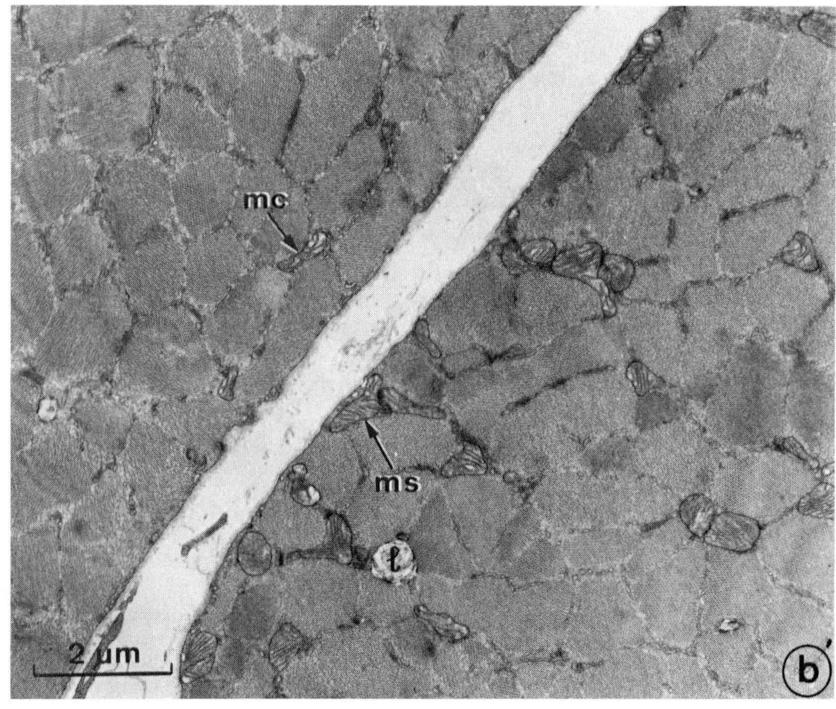
mc
ms
ℓ
2 µm
b

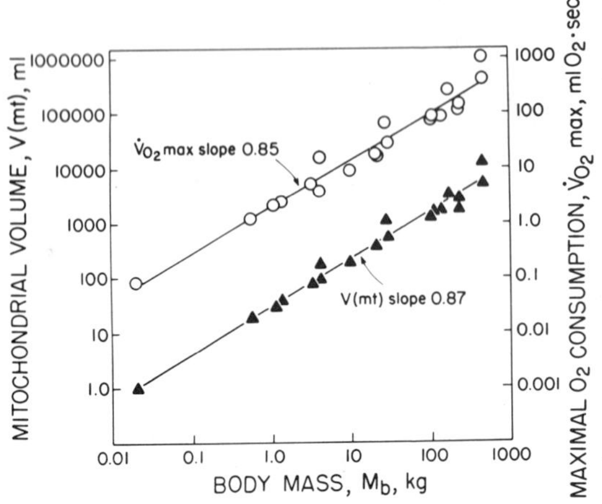

Figure 4a The $\dot{V}O_{2max}$ and whole-body muscle mitochondrial volume $V_{(mt)}$, plotted as a function of body mass, M_b, on logarithmic coordinates have nearly equal slopes. The equations for these functions, calculated by the method of least square, are: $\dot{V}O_{2max} = 1.79\ M_b{}^{0.854}$, where VO_{2max} has the units for $O_2 \cdot sec^{-1}$ and Mb is in kilograms; 95% confidence intervals: intercept 1.30, 2.48; slope 0.772, 0.936; and $V_{(mt)} = 30.12\ M_b{}^{0.865}$, where $V_{(mt)}$ is in milliliters and M_b is in kilograms; 95% confidence intervals: intercept 23.71, 38.77; slope 0.804, 0.926. (From Taylor et al., 1987b.)

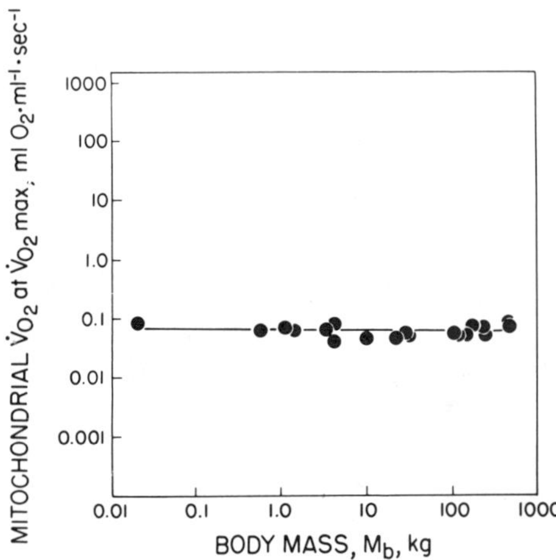

Figure 4b Mitochondrial O_2 consumption at $\dot{V}O_{2max}$ is independent of body mass: $\dot{v}O_{2(mt)}$ (calculated as $\dot{V}O_{2max}/V_{(mt)}$ using data from Fig. 4a) is plotted as a function of M_b on logarithmic coordinates. The slope of the regression is not significantly different from zero. The mean $\dot{v}O_{2(mt)}$ for all other species is 0.050 ml $O_2 \cdot ml^{-1} \cdot sec^{-1} \pm$ S.E. 0.003 (3.54 ml $O_2 \cdot ml^{-1} \cdot min^{-1}$). (From Taylor et al., 1987b.)

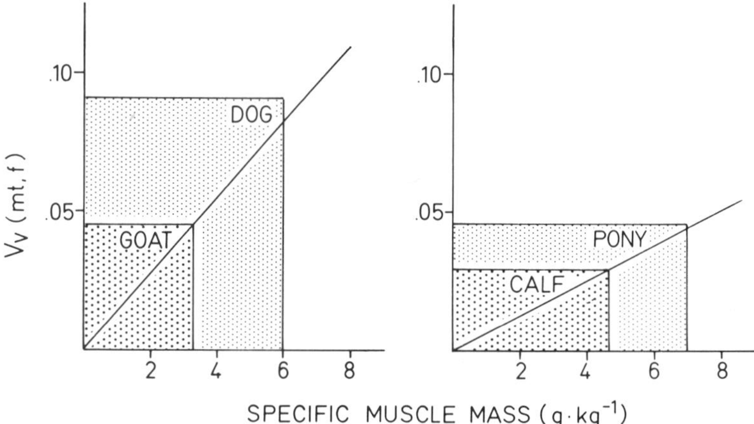

Figure 5 Box plots indicating the relative contribution of volume density of mitochondria, $VV_{(mt,f)}$, and muscle mass to the difference in total mitochondrial volume in locomotor muscles of aerobic vs. less aerobic animals. (From Hoppeler et al., 1987b.)

the box that represents the less aerobic goat and calf extends through the corner of the box that represents the athletic dog and pony. This indicates that both muscle mass and mitochondrial density contribute nearly equally to the higher mitochondrial volume of the more aerobic species.

A relatively good match was found between total mitochondrial volume and $\dot{V}O_{2\,max}$ of the dog-goat and pony-calf pairs. Dividing $\dot{V}O_{2\,max}$ by total mitochondrial mass in skeletal muscle yielded a similar value for all species, namely 3.4–4.6 ml · min^{-1} of O_2 for each milliliter of mitochondria. It is immediately evident that this is the same value as that obtained for the allometric comparison, supporting the concept that the basic mitochondrial building block is invariant relative to the demand for O_2 among mammalian species, regardless of whether the changes in demand result from allometric or from adaptive variations.

D. Mitochondrial Oxygen Consumption and Symmorphosis

What then can we conclude about symmorphosis and the mitochondrial step in the respiratory system? The conclusion seems to be both simple and general: higher maximal rates of O_2 uptake are achieved by building more of the same structural units, and the amount of structure varies 1:1 with maximal rate of oxygen consumption. Figure 6 illustrates this general conclusion both for allometric (top) and adaptive variation (bottom), showing that increases in the

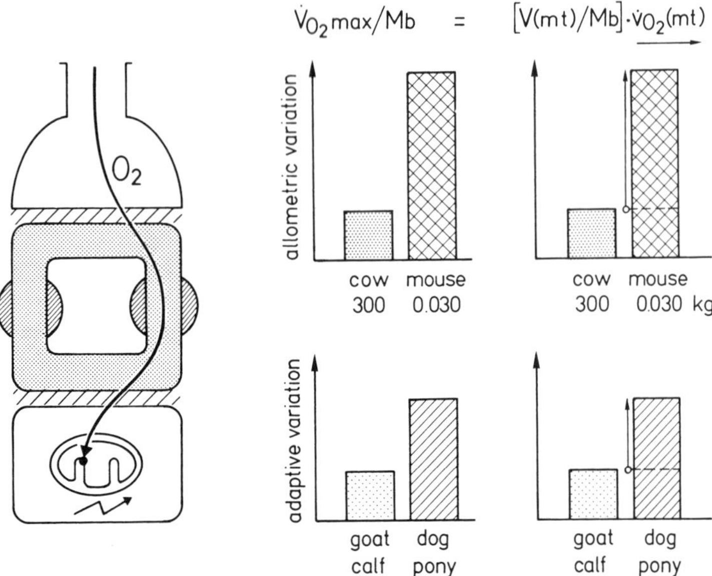

Figure 6 Comparing structural adaptation of muscle mitochondria to allometric (top) and adaptive variation (bottom) in $\dot{V}O_{2\,max}$, respectively. In both cases total mitochondrial volume per unit body mass, $V_{(mt)}/M_b$ is proportional to $\dot{V}O_{2\,max}$, hence, O_2 consumption per unit mitochondrial volume at $\dot{V}O_{2\,max}$, $\dot{v}O_{2\,(mt)}$ is invariant.

amount of structure, $V_{(mt)}$ (depicted as the height of the two histograms in the right-hand panels) account almost entirely for the increases in $\dot{V}O_{max}/M_b$ (the area of the left-hand histograms), whereas the rate at which each unit volume of structure consumes O_2, $\dot{v}O_{2\,(mt)}$ (depicted as the width of the histograms on the right), is invariant of either body size or adaptation. In both instances the findings of a match between structure and function at this level are in accord with the predictions of symmorphosis.

Despite the similarities, however, there is an important difference in the manner in which the match is achieved. The relative volume of skeletal muscle does not change in a systematic manner with body mass, being similar in large and small animals (Schmidt-Nielsen, 1984). However, it does increase with adaptation for higher aerobic capacity among animals of the same size, and this increase in muscle mass accounts for approximately half the increase in mitochondrial volume in the athletic animals of the adaptive pairs.

III. Capillaries in Skeletal Muscle: Variations in Structure and Function

A. The Tissue Gas Exchange: A Diffusive Step

The O_2 must diffuse from the capillaries to the mitochondria where it is consumed (Fig. 7). To consider symmorphosis as it applies to this step in the respiratory system, we must define a relevant descriptor of the O_2 delivery capacity of the capillary network. Because O_2 delivery to the muscles is a diffusive process, it can be described by the following equation (Conley et al., 1987):

$$\dot{V}O_2 = (\bar{P}bO_2 - \bar{P}cO_2) \cdot DTO_2 \tag{2}$$

where $\bar{P}bO_2$ is the mean capillary and $\bar{P}cO_2$ is the mean intracellular PO_2, and DTO_2 is the diffusive conductance of the tissue gas exchanger. The mean capillary PO_2 is determined by the PO_2 in arterial and venous blood and by the off-loading reaction kinetics of the blood, whereas $\bar{P}cO_2$ depends on the rate of oxygen consumption of the mitochondria and the O_2-buffering capacity of the myoglobin.

The conductance DTO_2 extends from the erythrocytes in the capillaries to the mitochondrial O_2 sinks and is determined by a series of resistances: an off-loading resistance of the erythrocytes; a resistance of the plasma barrier; a "membrane" resistance that comprises the endothelium and the interstitial space; and a myocyte resistance that extends from the sarcoplasm to the mitochondria. We do not as yet have a model at hand that allows us to formulate the dependence of DTO_2 on functional and structural variables. The matter is complicated particularly for the myocytic resistance, which depends on the variable myoglobin content of muscle cells, as well as on the uneven distribution of mitochondria.

In general terms, however, the conductance must somehow be related to the density of capillaries, because this factor determines the volume of capillary blood that can deliver O_2 to the mitochondria. Because the capillaries form networks of partially oriented tubes (Mathieu et al., 1983), we use the length density of capillaries related to the unit volume of muscle fibers, Jv(c,f), as a basic morphometric variable from which we calculate the total capillary length, J(c), and the total capillary volume, V(c), of the locomotor muscles. The capillary volume also determines the mean transit time, t_c, of blood through the muscles.

In analogy to the mitochondrial step, we can then, at least in a first approximation express the total maximal flow of O_2 from the capillaries, $\dot{V}O_{2max}$, as the product of a structural component, $V_{(c)}$, and a functional component, $\dot{v}O_{2(c)}$, the rate at which O_2 flows from the unit capillary blood volume at $\dot{V}O_{2max}$:

$$\dot{V}O_{2max} = V_{(c)} \cdot \dot{v}O_{2(c)} \tag{3}$$

We will see that hemoglobin concentration, a structural value of the blood, can dramatically affect $\dot{v}O_{2(c)}$. Still this relationship proves useful in analyzing the structural and functional contributions in accounting for differences in $\dot{V}O_{2max}$ until we have formulated a better characterization of DTO_2.

B. Allometric Variations in Capillaries at $\dot{V}O_{2max}$: $V_{(c)}$, $\dot{v}O_{2(c)}$, and t_c

Small animals have more capillaries in each gram of their muscles than large animals, thus the structural component, $V_{(c)}$, appears important in providing the faster mass-specific rates of O_2 delivery at this step (Eq. 3). In an allometric study of African mammals, capillary length density was found to scale with a factor of 0.9 in selected limb muscles (Hoppeler et al., 1981b). We can estimate the total capillary volume of the skeletal muscles of these animals, $V_{(c)}$, from the capillary volumes of two skeletal muscles used in this allometric study, because Hoppeler et al. (1984) found that the capillary volume of these muscles was representative of that measured for total skeletal muscle mass. Figure 8a plots $V_{(c)}$ and $\dot{V}O_{2max}$ as a function of body mass on logarithmic coordinates using data for which both measurements have been made on the same animal. This figure shows that $V_{(c)}$ has a slope of 0.89, which is not significantly different from the slope of 0.86 for the $\dot{V}O_{2max}$ of these animals.

The rate at which O_2 flows out of each milliliter of capillaries at $\dot{V}O_{2max}$, $\dot{v}O_{2(c)}$, can be calculated according to Equation 3 by dividing $\dot{V}O_{2max}$ by $V_{(c)}$. An allometric plot of $\dot{v}O_{2(c)}$ calculated in this manner for each of the data points in Figure 8a is given in Figure 8b. It shows that $\dot{v}O_{2(c)}$ tends to be higher in smaller animals, contributing to their higher rate of O_2 delivery. For example using the regression equation for the data in Figure 8b we calculate that a 30-g mouse would have a $\dot{v}O_{2(c)}$ about 1.5 times that of a 300-kg cow. More data is necessary to reach a definitive conclusion, but it appears that although a higher $\dot{v}O_{2(c)}$ may contribute to the higher $\dot{V}O_{2max}$ of smaller animals at this step in the respiratory system, the structural component $V_{(c)}$ accounts for most of the difference.

A higher $\dot{v}O_{2(c)}$ in smaller animals could be accomplished by a faster blood flow through the capillaries, a higher concentration of hemoglobin in the blood, or a more complete extraction of O_2. The concentration of hemoglobin

---

Figure 7 Cross section of muscle fibers, shown under low power, from M. semitendinosus of dog: (a) shows distribution of capillaries (fat arrows) and of interfibrillar (mc) and subsarcolemmal (ms) mitochondria. (b) Capillary (cap) with erythrocyte (ec) at higher magnification, showing interstitial space (if) and lipid droplets (i) in relation to mitochondria. (From Hoppeler et al., 1987b.)

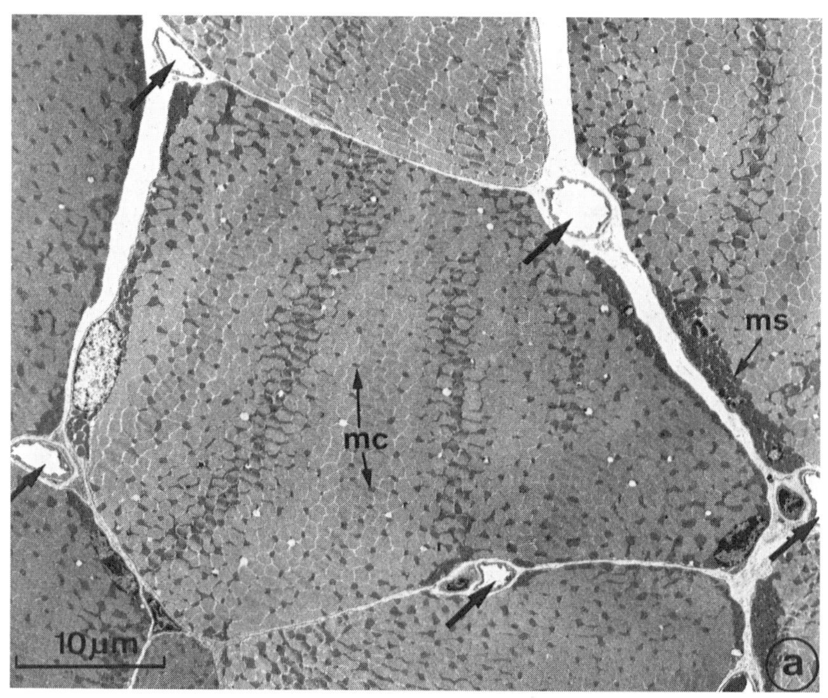
ms
mc
10 µm
a

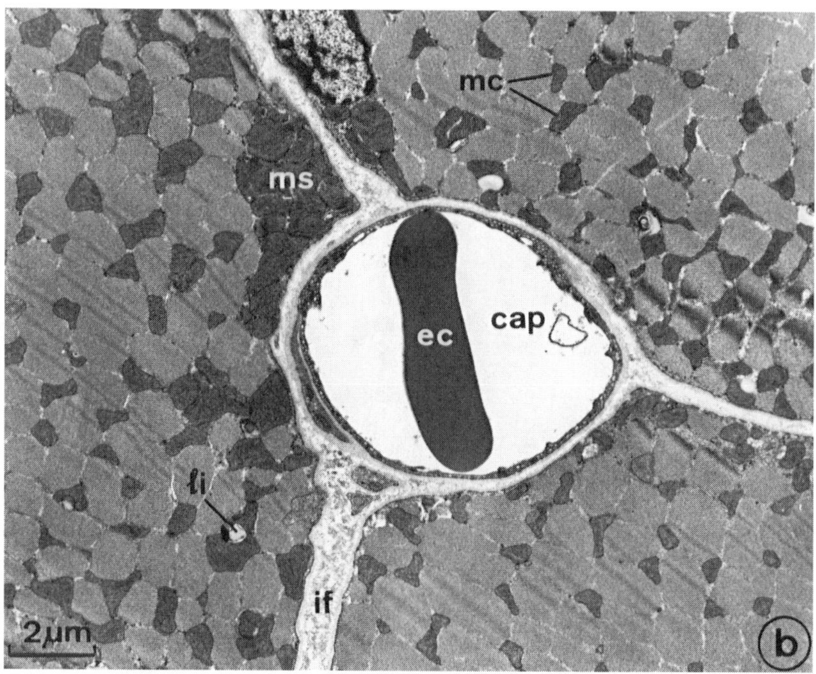
mc
ms
ec
cap
li
if
2 µm
b

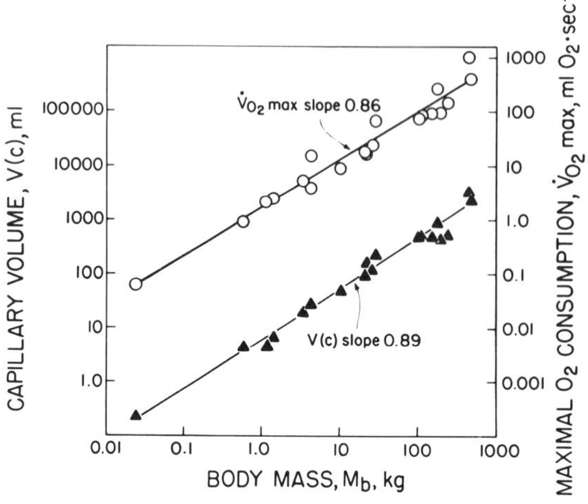

Figure 8a $\dot{V}O_{2max}$ and whole-body muscle capillary volume, $V_{(c)}$, plotted as a function of body mass, M_b, on logarithmic coordinates, have similar slopes. The equations for these functions, calculated by the method of least squares, are: $\dot{V}O_{2max} = 1.77\ M_b^{0.857}$, where $\dot{V}O_{2max}$ has the units of $ml \cdot sec^{-1}\ O_2$ and M_b is in kilograms; 95% confidence intervals: intercept 1.28, 2.45; slope 0.775, 0.939; and $V_{(c)} = 7.15\ Mb^{0.891}$ where $V_{(c)}$ has the unit milliliters and M_b is in kilograms; 95% confidence intervals: intercept 5.46, 9.54; slope 0.820, 0.961. (From Taylor et al., 1987b.)

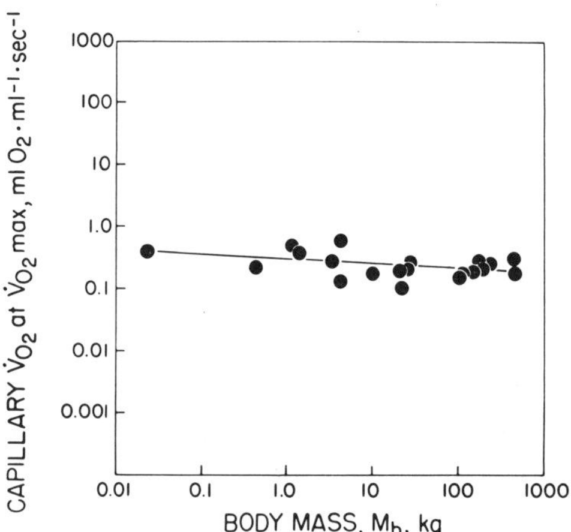

Figure 8b Oxygen delivery per milliliter of muscle capillary, $\dot{v}O_{2(c)}$, tends to increase with a decrease in M_b: $\dot{v}O_2(c)$ is calculated at $\dot{V}O_{2max}/V_{(c)}$, using data from Figure 4a. The equation for the regression is $\dot{v}O_{2(c)} = 0.258\ M_b^{-0.046}$, where $\dot{v}O_{2(c)}$ has the units $ml \cdot ml^{-1} \cdot sec^{-1}$ for O_2 and M_b is in kilograms; 95% confidence intervals: intercept 0.197, 0.337; slope −0.114, 0.022. The regression predicts a value of 0.303 $ml \cdot ml^{-1} \cdot sec^{-1}$ of O_2 for a 30-g mouse compared with 0.198 $ml \cdot ml^{-1} \cdot sec^{-1}$ of O_2 predicted for a 300-kg cow.

in, and the extraction of oxygen from the blood are reported to be independent of body size (Schmidt-Nielsen, 1984). Therefore, the blood flow through the capillaries must be more rapid in the smaller animals. Average transit time, calculated by dividing $V_{(c)}$ by cardiac output, has been found to decrease from about 0.9 s in 500-kg horse and steer (Kayar et al., 1987), to about 0.5 s in the 20- to 30-kg goat and dog (Conley et al., 1987) to about 0.3 s in the 3- to 4-kg fox (Bicudo, personal communication).

The higher $\dot{v}O_{2(c)}$ must also be associated with a faster rate of diffusion of O_2 from the capillaries to the mitochondria. This could be accomplished by a larger DTO_2 or by a larger pressure head for diffusion according to Equation 2. The average diffusion distance between capillaries and mitochondria will decrease with decreasing body size as a result of the volume density of both capillaries and mitochondria increasing. Other things being equal, the shorter diffusion path will result in a larger DTO_2. However, it is possible to find pairs of animals, such as goat versus cow (Conley et al., 1987; Kayar et al., 1987), in which mean muscle mitochondrial and capillary density are approximately the same (indicating a similar diffusion distance), although O_2 flow from and transit time through the capillaries differs. Thus, diffusion distance alone cannot account for all differences in mass-specific O_2 delivery rates, and it is quite possible that a larger pressure gradient of O_2 also contributes to a more rapid diffusion of O_2 from capillaries to mitochondria in smaller animals.

C. Adaptive Variations in Capillaries with $\dot{V}O_{2max}$: $V(c)$, $\dot{v}O_{2(c)}$, and t_c

The 2.5-fold difference in $\dot{V}O_{2max}$ between dog-goat and pony-calf adaptive pairs is associated with only a 1.7-fold difference in capillary volume of their skeletal muscles (Conley et al., 1987). Thus, by using Equation 3, we can calculate that $\dot{v}O_{2(c)}$ must also be higher by a factor of 1.7 in the athletic species. In contrast to the situation observed with allometric variation in which hemoglobin concentration does not change, the 1.7 times higher $\dot{v}O_{2(c)}$ of the two athletic species can be accounted for entirely by 1.7 times higher hemoglobin concentrations (Fig. 9).

Interestingly, the minimal transit time through capillaries, t_c, is about the same for both the athletic and the less athletic species of each pair. This can be calculated starting with the Fick equation:

$$\dot{V}O_{2\,max}(CaO_2 - C\bar{v}O_2) \cdot \dot{Q}_{max} \tag{4}$$

Because almost all of the cardiac output at $\dot{V}O_{2max}$ flows through the skeletal muscle capillaries:

$$V_{(c)}/\dot{Q}_{max} = t_c \tag{5}$$

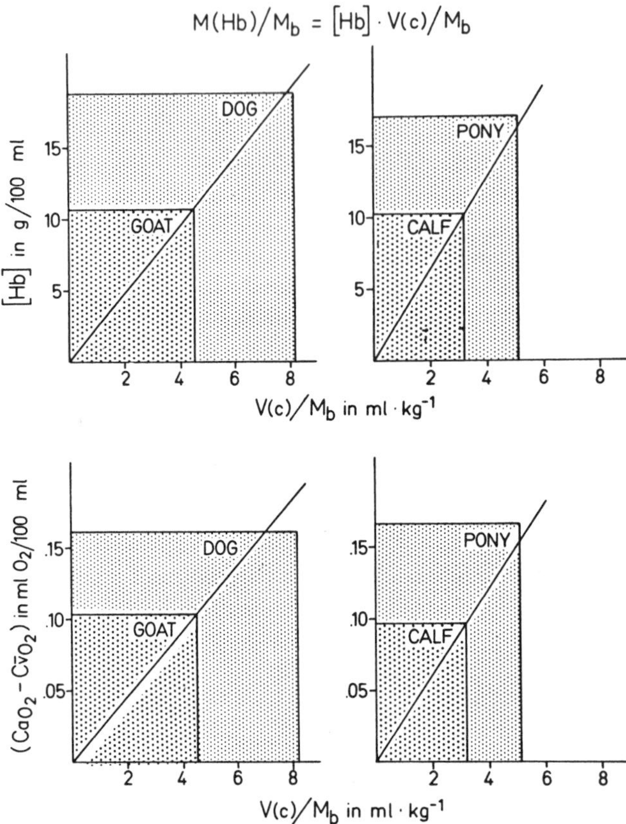

Figure 9 Capillary volume, $V_{(c)}$, and hemoglobin concentration (Hb) contribute about equally to the higher O_2 capacity of muscle capillary blood in the athletic species. The amount of O_2 discharged is larger in the athletic species because of a larger capillary volume combined with a larger arteriovenous O_2 concentration difference. (From Conley et al., 1987.)

and because almost all of the oxygen is consumed by the skeletal muscle we can combine Equations 4 and 5 to give:

$$t_c = V_{(c)} \cdot (CaO_2 - C\bar{v}O_2)/\dot{V}O_{2max} \tag{6}$$

Because both the product of $V_{(c)}$ times $(CaO_2 - C\bar{v}O_2)$ and $\dot{V}O_{2max}$ change by the same factor of 2.5 in our adaptive pairs, t_c does not change.

The mean path for diffusion of O_2 between capillaries and mitochondria is shorter in the athletic species as a consequence of the higher density of both capillaries and mitochondria in their muscles. Other things being equal, this will

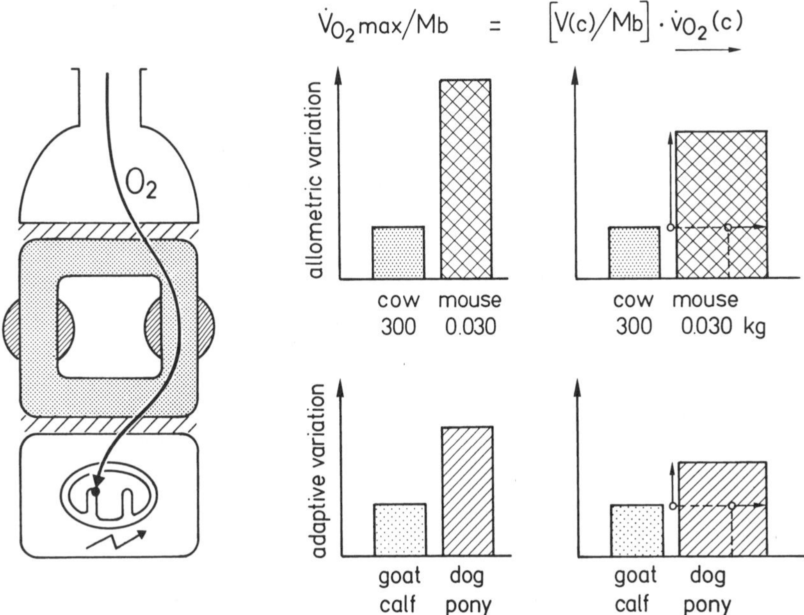

Figure 10 Comparing structural adaptation of muscle capillaries with allometric (top) and adaptive (bottom) variation in $\dot{V}O_{2max}$, respectively. Total capillary volume per unit body mass, $V_{(c)}/M_b$, contributes most of the adaptation to higher values of $\dot{V}O_{2max}$ with allometric variation but only half with adaptive variation. The other half is contributed by an elevated O_2 discharge rate from the capillary blood, resulting from a higher hemoglobin concentration.

result in a larger DTO_2, helping to account for the higher rate of O_2 diffusion (see Equation 2). The role played by the pressure head remains to be evaluated.

D. The Tissue Gas Exchanger and Symmorphosis

What can we conclude about the tissue gas exchanger and symmorphosis? It is clear that we still need to develop a better model linking structures and functions at this level of the respiratory system, similar to the model of pulmonary gas exchanger that has been developed by Weibel (1970/71). We are lacking precise information about the mean diffusion path length from capillaries to the mitochondria and about the relative roles of the two diffusive paths for O_2 transfer (molecular O_2 and oxymyoglobin). Although this information is necessary to formulate a good biophysical model linking structures and functions, we still have enough information using our basic descriptor, the length density of capillaries, to provide some important insights into the match between structures and function.

Differences in capillary volume account for about half of the difference in mass-specific maximal rates of O_2 consumption with adaptive variations (Fig. 10), i.e., there is a 1.7-fold difference in capillary volume for a 2.5-fold difference in $\dot{V}O_{2max}$. The endurance athletes of the adaptive pairs have a higher hemoglobin concentration, hence, the difference in amount of O_2 per volume of capillaries matches the 2.5-fold difference in $\dot{V}O_{2max}$ between the species of the adaptive pairs. This results in the same transit time through the capillaries in athletic and normal animals.

A similar match is achieved at this level with allometric variations in $\dot{V}O_{2max}$, but the means of achieving it are different (see Fig. 10). The hemoglobin concentration does not change with body size and the higher O_2 delivery to the capillaries of smaller animals is, for the most part, achieved simply by building more capillaries, i.e., a larger $V_{(c)}$. A faster transit time of the blood through the capillaries also contributes, but more data are necessary to evaluate this possibility. The higher O_2 consumption of both small and athletic animals is associated with a shorter mean diffusion path between the capillaries and mitochondria, and this should result in a greater DTO_2. Therefore, we can conclude that there is a reasonably good match between structures and maximal O_2 flow at this level of the respiratory system, although much work still remains before we can reach definitive quantitative conclusions.

IV. Convective Transport of Oxygen by the Circulation

A. Cardiac Output and Arteriovenous Oxygen Difference: Two Ways to Adjust Oxygen Delivery to Demand

Oxygen is transported from the capillaries in the lung to the capillaries in the muscle by the circulation. Matching O_2 flow to differences in maximal demand could be accomplished by variations in maximal cardiac output, $\dot{Q}_{max}$, in the difference in arteriovenous O_2 concentration, $(CaO_2 - C\bar{v}O_2)$, or some combination of the two, according to the Fick equation:

$$\dot{V}O_{2\,max} = \dot{Q}_{max} \cdot (CaO_2 - C\bar{v}O_2) \tag{7}$$

This convective step is often considered to be the limiting step in O_2 transport during strenuous exercise, and it is assumed that there is excess capacity at other steps (see Rowell, 1974, Scheuer and Tipton, 1977, Blomqvist,

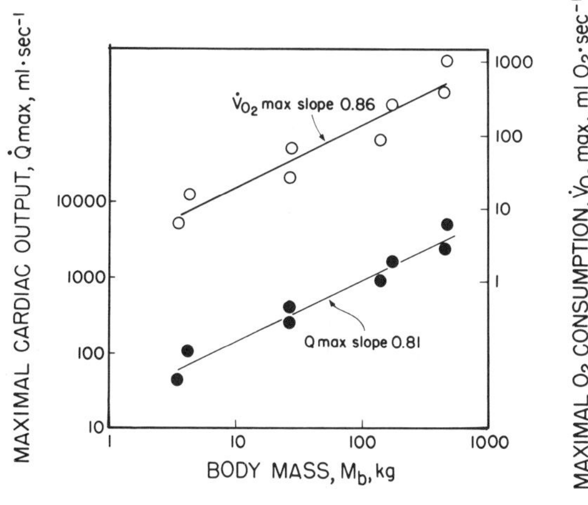

Figure 11a Plots of $\dot{V}O_{2max}$ and maximal cardiac output, $\dot{Q}_{max}$, as a function of M_b on logarithmic coordinates have nearly equal slopes. The equations for these functions calculated by the method of least squares are: $\dot{V}O_{2max} = 2.60\ M_b^{0.857}$, where $\dot{V}O_{2max}$ has the units of ml · sec^{-1} for O_2 and M_b is in kilograms; 95% confidence intervals: intercept 0.86, 8.37; slope 0.589, 1.124; and $\dot{Q}_{max} = 21.90\ M_b^{0.810}$, where $\dot{Q}_{max}$ has the units ml · sec^{-1} and M_b is in kilograms; 95% confidence intervals: intercept 10.80, 44.41; slope 0.648, 0.972.

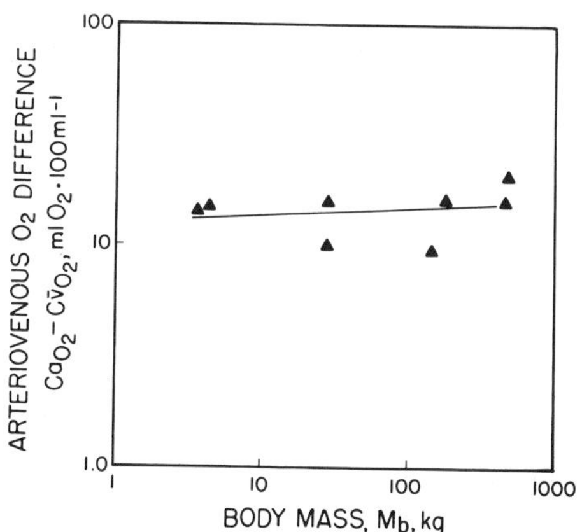

Figure 11b Arteriovenous O_2 concentration difference, $CaO_2 - C\bar{v}O_2$, plotted as a function of M_b on logarithmic coordinates, is nearly independent of body mass. The slope of the regression is not significantly different from zero. The mean $CaO_2 - C\bar{v}O_2$ is 14.9 ml · 100 ml^{-1} ± S.E. 1.3 for O_2. (From Taylor et al., 1987b.)

1983). To test the concept of symmorphosis as it applies to O_2 delivery by the circulation, we will consider whether this step operates at or near its maximal capacity for O_2 delivery as $\dot{V}O_{2max}$ varies with allometry and adaptation for high levels of aerobic performance. We will also consider the role played by structural and functional variables in matching O_2 delivery to demand.

Cardiac output can be varied to meet differences in maximal demand by varying a functional value, the maximal frequency of contraction of the heart pump, f_H, a structural variable, the size of the heart and thereby the amount of blood pumped with each contraction, V_S, or some combination of these variables. This is expressed in the following equation:

$$\dot{Q}_{max} = f_H \cdot V_S \qquad (8)$$

Arteriovenous O_2 concentration difference can also be varied by varying functional or structural values. The O_2 carrying capacity of the blood is

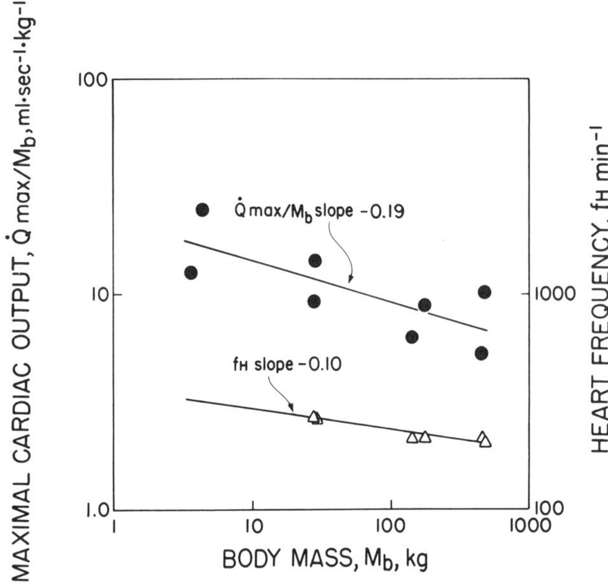

Figure 12 Allometric plots of mass specific cardiac output at $\dot{V}O_{2max}$, $\dot{Q}_{max}/M_b$, and heart frequency at $\dot{V}O_{2max}$, f_H, illustrates that these two functions scale differently with M_b: $\dot{Q}_{max}/M_b = 21.90\ M_b^{-0.190}$; 95% confidence intervals: intercept 10.80, 44.41; slope -0.028, 0.352; and $f_H = 368.3\ M_b^{-0.097}$, where f_H has the unit of min^{-1} and M_b is in kilograms; 95% confidence intervals: intercept 285.9, 474.5; slope -0.046, 0.148. (From Taylor et al., 1987b.)

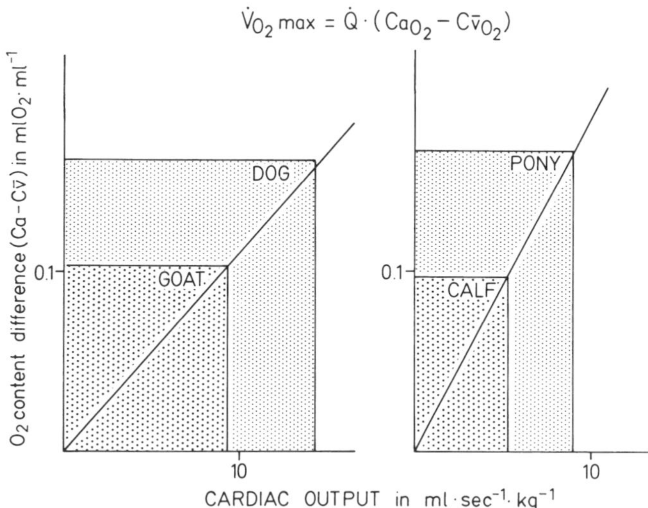

Figure 13 Box plots indicating the relative contribution of the arteriovenous difference in O_2 concentration and cardiac output to the 2.5-fold difference in $\dot{V}O_{2max}$ between dog and goat (left box) and between pony and calf (right box). The smaller boxes represent the $\dot{V}O_{2max}$ values of the less aerobic goat and calf while the larger boxes represent the $\dot{V}O_{2max}$ values of the athletic dog and pony. The diagonal line from the origin and the corner of the box representing $\dot{V}O_{2max}$ of the less aerobic species would intersect the corner of the box representing $\dot{V}O_{2max}$ of the athletic species if a higher O_2 concentration difference and a higher cardiac output contributed equally to the higher rates of O_2 transport in the circulation of the athletic species and this is seen to be the case. (From Karas, et al., 1987a.)

dependent primarily upon the concentration of hemoglobin, and this is determined by the number of erythrocytes, a structural factor that can be varied. Functionally, the completeness of saturation of the blood with O_2 as it passes through the lung, and the completeness of extraction of O_2 as it passes through the muscles, can also be varied. We will consider the relative importance of each of these factors in matching O_2 delivery to differences in maximal O_2 demand.

B. Allometric Variations in $\dot{Q}_{max}$ and $(CaO_2 - C\bar{v}O_2)$

When animals exercise at $\dot{V}O_{2max}$, O_2 must be transported from the capillaries of the lung to each gram of muscle four times faster in a 30-g mouse than in a 300-kg steer (Fig. 11a). The higher rate of convective transport is accomplished almost entirely by a higher $\dot{Q}_{max}$ as seen in the allometric plot in Figure 11a, in which both $\dot{Q}_{max}$ and $\dot{V}O_{2max}$ are seen to have the same scaling factors with M_b. Thus, each gram of the mouse muscle is perfused at four times the rate that of the steer, whereas the arteriovenous O_2 concentration difference at $\dot{V}O_{2max}$ is invariant with size. The structural variable of hemoglobin concentration and the functional variables of completeness of saturation and extraction of O_2 to and from the hemoglobin do not appear to be utilized in matching O_2 delivery by the circulation to allometric differences in demand (Fig. 11b).

The higher $\dot{Q}max/M_b$ of smaller animals appears to be, in part, due to higher frequencies of contraction and, in part, to larger mass-specific stroke volumes. The data base for which f_H and $\dot{Q}_{max}/M_b$ have been measured in different-sized animals is still too meager to draw definitive conclusions; however, when they are plotted on an allometric plot (Fig. 12), we find that a higher frequency can account for only half of the difference in $\dot{Q}_{max}/M_b$ with body size, thus, according to Equation 8 a larger V_S/M_b must account for the other half. The reason that we have some reservations about this conclusion is that allometric relationships for resting heart rates are found to scale in direct proportion to $\dot{Q}_{max}/M_b$, and resting V_S/M_b is found to be in-

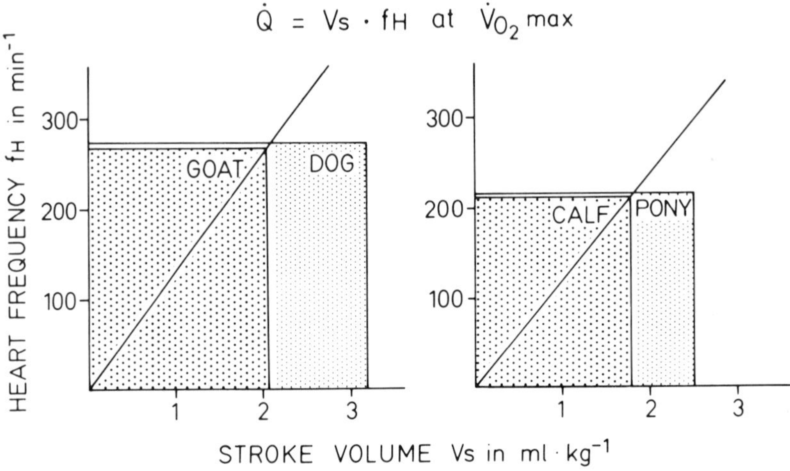

Figure 14 Box plots indicating the relative contribution of heart frequency (f_H) and stroke volume (V_S) to the higher cardiac outputs ($\dot{Q}_{max}$) of the athletic dog and pony compared with the goat and calf. The heart frequencies of the species are seen to be the same within each size pair, so that the higher $\dot{Q}_{max}$ values (the areas denoted by the box) are entirely the result of larger V_S in the dog and pony. (From Karas et al., 1987a.)

variant with body size (Schmidt-Nielsen, 1984). This could indicate different scaling factors for resting values or a distortion of the relationships by the selection of animals included in the allometric relationships. More data are necessary to resolve these uncertainties.

C. Adaptive Variations in $\dot{Q}_{max}$ and $(Ca_{O_2} - C\bar{v}_{O_2})$

The 2.5-fold higher rates of O_2 delivery of the athletic dog and pony in comparison with the goat and calf appear to be met in about equal parts by a higher $\dot{Q}_{max}/M_b$ and a higher $Ca_{O_2} - C\bar{v}_{O_2})$ (Karas et al., 1987b). This is illustrated in the box plots of Figure 13 on which $Ca_{O_2} - C\bar{v}_{O_2}$ is plotted against $\dot{Q}_{max}/M_b$ for each adaptive pair. The areas of the small boxes represent $\dot{V}_{O_2max}/M_b$ of the less aerobic member of each pair and the larger box, that of the more aerobic member. The relative contribution of the two parameters to the difference in $\dot{V}_{O_2max}$ is indicated by the diagonal line. A nearly equal contribution of both parameters to the higher $\dot{V}_{O_2max}$ would be indicated if it extended from the origin through the corners of the two boxes. This is seen to be true for both species pairs.

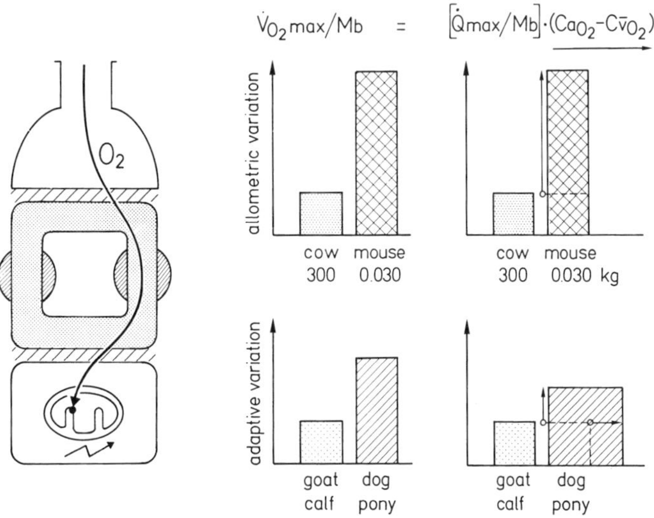

Figure 15 Comparing adaptation of O_2 delivery by the circulation to allometric (top) and adaptive (bottom) variation in $\dot{V}_{O_2max}$, respectively. With allometric variation, higher levels of $\dot{V}_{O_2max}/M_b$ are achieved by increasing $\dot{Q}_{max}/M_b$ proportionately. In adaptive variation the adaptive effort is shared by cardiac output and arteriovenous O_2 concentration difference, the latter resulting from higher hemoglobin concentration in the blood.

The higher $\dot{Q}_{max}/M_b$ of the athletic species is entirely the result of their larger stroke volumes, for the heart frequency of each member of a size pair (i.e., goat-dog, pony-calf) at $\dot{V}O_{2max}$ is identical. This reliance entirely on the structural variable for both adaptive pairs is shown graphically in the box plots of Figure 14, where f_H is plotted against V_S/M_b.

By turning now to (CaO_2 - $C\bar{v}O_2$), we find that both the dog and the pony have much higher (50-70%) arterial O_2 concentrations than the goat and calf (Karas et al., 1987b). This is the result of higher hemoglobin concentrations. The O_2 concentration of the mixed venous blood reached similar levels and the percentage extraction showed no consistent pattern with aerobic capacity of the adaptive pairs.

D. Circulatory Transport of Oxygen and Symmorphosis

The higher maximal rates of O_2 transport by the circulation are met in different ways with allometric and adaptive variations in demand. Allometric variations involve entirely a higher $\dot{Q}_{max}/M_b$ (Fig. 15 top), whereas both a higher $\dot{Q}_{max}/M_b$ and a higher arteriovenous O_2 difference contribute almost equally to the difference with adaptive variations (Fig. 15 bottom).

The higher $\dot{Q}_{max}/M_b$ in smaller animals is the result of differences in both the functional variable, higher frequency, and the structural variable, larger stroke volume. In contrast, two structural variables are involved in meeting the differences in demand with adaptive variation (erythrocyte concentration and stroke volume), whereas maximal heart frequencies appear to be tightly determined by an animal's body size and to be independent of cardiac output and $\dot{V}O_{2max}$ for a given-sized animal.

What can we conclude about whether or not all of the structural capacity for convective transport of O_2 is utilized by a given animal? The studies, to date, indicate that animals are operating at, or close to, the upper limit of their structural capacity for convective transport of O_2 in the circulatory system at $\dot{V}O_{2max}$ (Taylor et al., 1987a). Available structures (stroke volume and hemoglobin concentration) for both $\dot{Q}_{max}$ and (CaO_2 - $C\bar{v}O_2$) appear fully exploited by the time an animal has increased its O_2 consumption from resting to maximal levels. Thus, at this step of O_2 transport in the respiratory system, there appears to be a match between maximal rates of O_2 delivery and the structures involved, a finding in accord with the predictions of symmorphosis.

V. The Pulmonary Gas Exchanger: A Safety Factor at the Environmental Interface?

A. The Pulmonary Gas Exchanger: A Diffusive Step

Oxygen uptake in the lung is governed by diffusive O_2 flow from alveolar air (A) to capillary blood (b) in the pulmonary gas exchanger (Fig. 16). The rate of flow is governed by the PO_2 difference between the air in the lungs and the blood in the capillaries and a diffusion conductance or diffusing capacity, DLO_2, according to the Bohr equation (1909):

$$\dot{V}O_2 = (PAO_2 - \bar{P}bO_2) \cdot DLO_2 \tag{9}$$

The PO_2 difference is a functional variable, whereas the diffusion conductance is mainly determined by structural properties of the lung. A model has been developed describing DLO_2 in terms of lung structure (Weibel, 1970/71). The diffusion path from alveolar air to the O_2 site in the hemoglobin (Fig. 16b) is divided into three serial resistances: the reciprocals of the conductances for tissue (t), plasma (p), and erythrocytes (e):

$$DLO_2^{-1} = DtO_2^{-1} + DpO_2^{-1} + DeO_2^{-1} \tag{10}$$

Each of these partial conductances are dependent on morphometric measurements that can be quantified:

$$DtO_2 = ktO_2 \cdot (SA + Sc)/(2 \cdot \tau_{ht}) \tag{11}$$

$$DpO_2 = kpO_2 \cdot Sc/\tau_{hp} \tag{12}$$

$$DeO_2 = \theta O_2 \cdot V_c \tag{13}$$

where SA and Sc are the total alveolar and capillary surface area, V_c is the total capillary blood volume, τ_{ht} and τ_{pt} are the harmonic mean thicknesses of the tissue and plasma barriers, respectively, ktO_2 and kpO_2 are the Krogh diffusion coefficients for O_2 in tissue and plasma, and θO_2 is the reaction rate of the whole blood with O_2.

The various building blocks of the gas exchanger are relatively invariant: the loading of the gas exchange surface with capillary blood, the thickness of the diffusion barrier, and the size of the alveoli show only small variations between species (Gehr et al., 1981a). Therefore, to adjust DLO_2 to variations in demand would seem to involve making more of these building blocks.

B. Allometric Variations in DLO_2 and PAO_2 - PbO_2)

In an allometric study of DLO_2, measured and calculated according to this morphometric model, Gehr et al. (1981a) compared lungs of mammals, ranging in body size from shrew and mouse to cow and horse, and found that the DLO_2 increased linearly with body mass, i.e., with a scaling factor of 1.0. This is consistent with the scaling factor obtained with physiological estimates of the diffusing capacity of the lung measured using carbon monoxide (Stahl, 1967; Weibel et al., 1983). It, therefore, appears in these allometric studies that DLO_2 is not proportional to maximal rates of O_2 uptake, and that the pressure head for diffusion must increase as mass-specific O_2 consumption

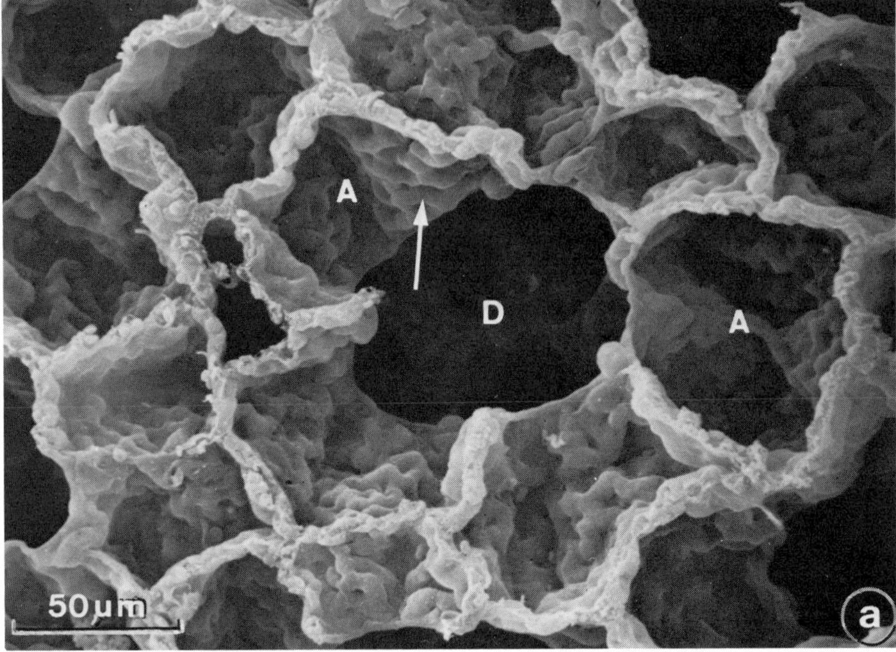

Figure 16a Scanning electronic micrograph of lung parenchyma in gazelles showing a cross section of an alveolar duct (D) surrounded by alveoli (A). Note the dense loading of the alveolar septa with a network of bulging capillaries (arrow).

increases with decreasing body size (Weibel et al., 1981; Weibel, 1987).

By using only data for which $\dot{V}O_{2max}$ and DLO_2 have been measured on the same animals (Fig. 17), we find that $\dot{V}O_{2max}$ scales with the 0.86 power of M_b, whereas DLO_2 scales with the 1.1 power of M_b. Thus, according to the Bohr equation, $PAO_2 - PbO_2$) will scale with the -0.20 power. This scaling of the pressure head could result from a lower mean alveolar PO_2 in larger animals according to a series ventilation and parallel perfusion model of the lung as proposed by Weibel et al. (1981; Fig. 18). According to this model the mean alveolar PO_2 would fall as O_2 is continuously extracted along the acinus of the lung (a region where O_2 moves by diffusion rather than convection). The longer acinus of the larger animals would result in a lower mean alveolar PO_2 or to a greater $\dot{V}A/\dot{Q}$ inhomogeneity. Preliminary measurements of acinar length indi-

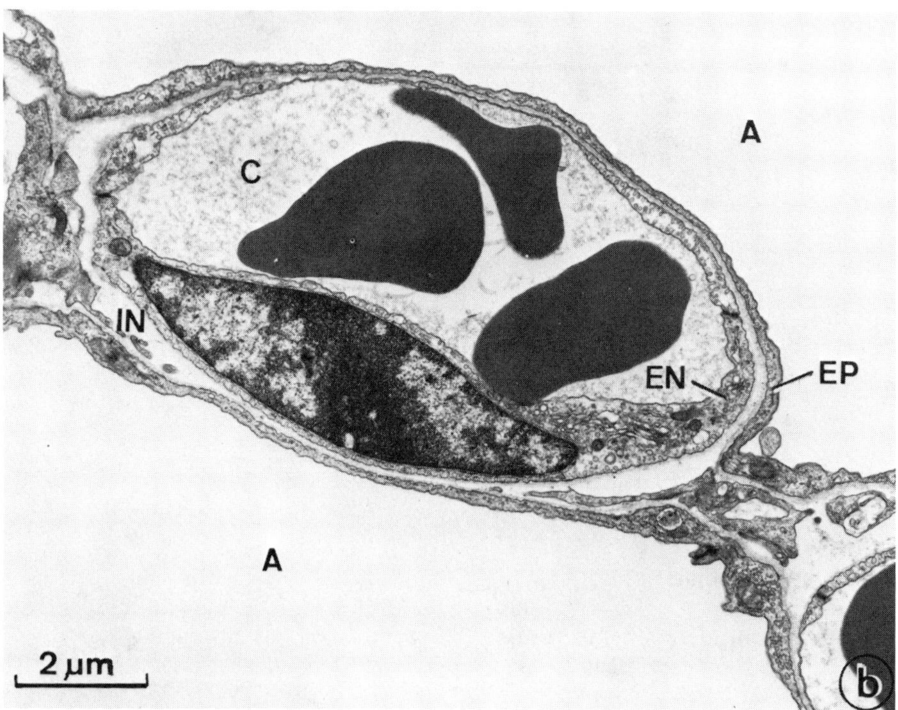

Figure 16b Capillary of dik-dik lung at higher power reveals the barrier made of endothelium (EN), epithelium (EP) and interstitial space (IN) separating the capillary blood (C) from the alveolar space (A). (From Gehr et al., 1981a.)

cate a scaling factor for acinar length of the magnitude necessary for such a model to be feasible (Weibel, 1987).

An alternative explanation for the lower pressure head in larger animals is that the capillary blood in their lungs equilibrates with the PO_2 in the alveolar air, well before the blood exits the lung, and that progressively less of the lung is used for O_2 exchange as animal size increases. This would result in a higher mean capillary PO_2 as the blood spends more of the transit time equilibrated with alveolar PO_2. In essence this explanation involves large animals having a structural capacity of O_2 diffusion far in excess of the demand for O_2 at this step in the respiratory cascade. Then, progressively, more of the diffusing capacity of the lung would be utilized as O_2 demand increases with decreasing body size.

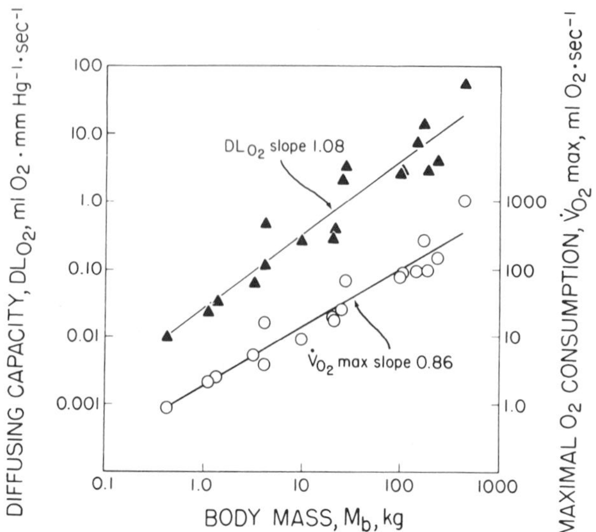

Figure 17 Allometric plots of $\dot{V}O_{2max}/M_b$ and mass-specific diffusing capacity of the lung for O_2 (DLO_2/M_b) illustrate that these two functions scale differently with M_b: $DLO_2 = 0.0258\ M_b^{1.084}$, where DLO_2 has the units for O_2 of ml · $mmHg^{-1}$ · sec^{-1} and M_b is in kilograms; 95% confidence intervals: intercept 0.0129, 0.0517; slope 0.895, 1.272; and $\dot{V}O_{2max} = 1.78\ M_b^{0.864}$, where $\dot{V}O_{2max}$ has the units for O_2 of ml · sec^{-1} and M_b is in kilograms; 95% confidence intervals: intercept 1.15, 2.75; slope 0.752, 0.980. The pressure head for diffusion, ΔPO_2, is equal to the ratio VO_{2max}/DLO_2; therefore it increases with a decrease in M_b. (From Taylor et al., 1987b.)

Recent measurements on 3-kg foxes (Longworth et al., 1986) enable us to calculate the time course of the change in PO_2 and O_2 concentration as blood transits the lung under conditions of $\dot{V}O_{2max}$. Oxygen exchange appears to be complete after the blood has passed through two-thirds of their lungs. If one uses the foxes' DLO_2/M_b and V_c/M_b, and adjusts the transit time to account for the allometric increase in $\dot{Q}_{max}/M_b$, one finds that the DLO_2 of the fox would be just sufficient to meet the higher O_2 demands of a 3-g shrew (calculated using the allometric equation for $\dot{V}O_{2max}$), if all of the structural diffusing capacity of the lung were used for O_2 exchange.

C. Adaptive Variation in DLO_2 and ($PAO_2 - \bar{P}bO_2$)

In a recent study, Weibel et al. (1987a) addressed the question of whether or not the 2.5-fold difference in $\dot{V}O_{2max}$ between athletic dogs and ponies and simi-

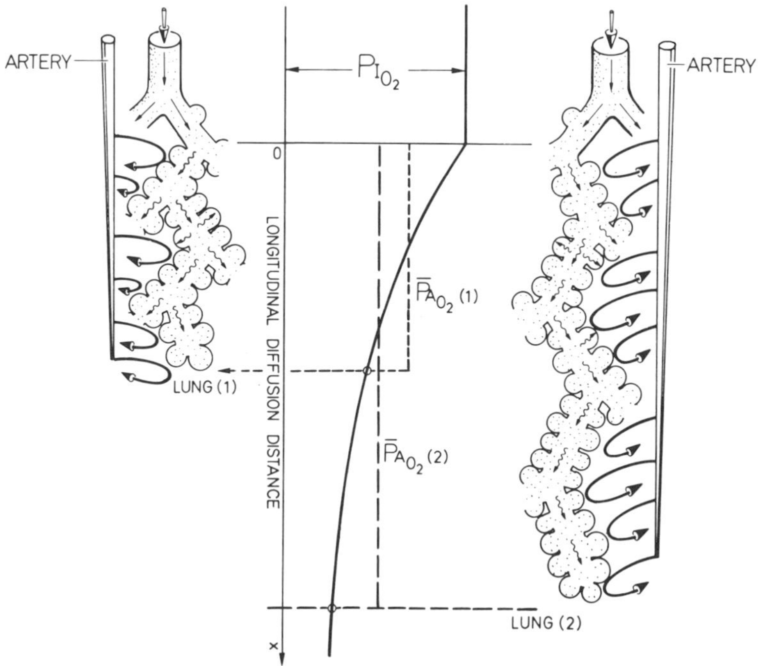

Figure 18 Hypothetical gradients of alveolar PO_2 along axis of acinus in small (1) and large (2) lung. Capillary network units related to vascular "loops" are exposed to different alveolar PO_2. Mean alveolar PO_2 will be lower in larger lung. (From Weibel et al., 1981.)

larly sized goats and calves was matched by a proportional change in DLO_2. They found that half of the difference in O_2 consumption could be accounted for by a 1.6-fold difference in DLO_2 and about half by a 1.6-fold difference in $(PAO_2 - P\bar{b}O_2)$. This is graphically illustrated in the box plots of Figure 19 in which $(PAO_2 - P\bar{b}O_2)$ is plotted against DLO_2/M_b for the goat-dog and calf-pony pairs. The areas of the boxes represent $\dot{V}O_{2max}$ and an equal contribution of the two parameters to the higher aerobic capacities of the more athletic species would be indicated by the diagonal line intersecting the corners of the boxes of both species of a pair; a situation that we find to be approximately in accord with the measurements.

Using physiological data measured on the same animals of these adaptive pairs while they exercised at $\dot{V}O_{2max}$, together with the morphometric DLO_2 discussed in the previous paragraph, Karas et al. (1987a) calculated the change in O_2 concentration and PO_2 as blood transits the lung of these four species (Fig.

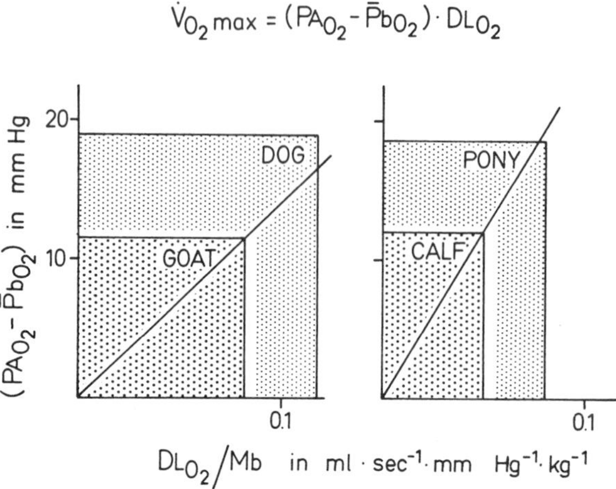

Figure 19 The 2.5-fold increases of $\dot{V}O_{2max}$ of dog and pony over the goat and calf (area of rectangle) is achieved by increasing both the diffusing capacity and the driving force by about equal amounts. (From Weibel et al., 1987b.)

20). According to these calculations, most of the O_2 exchange at $\dot{V}O_{2max}$ is completed by the time the blood has finished about 40% of its transit through the lung in the goat and the calf, whereas about 70% of the transit time is utilized for O_2 exchange in the athletic dog and pony. Thus, all four species appear to have excess pulmonary diffusing capacity, and the excess is much greater in the less aerobic species.

D. The Pulmonary Gas Exchanger and Symmorphosis

One cannot reach an unequivocal conclusion after reviewing the evidence of the proportionality between maximal O_2 consumption and the structures determining the diffusion rate of O_2 in the lung. The different scaling factors for DLO_2 and $\dot{V}O_{2max}$ indicate that the pressure head for diffusion of O_2 increases to account for the higher O_2 consumption of smaller animals, whereas the mass-specific diffusing capacity of the lung is invariant (Fig. 21 top). It is possible to explain at least part of this difference by the change in a structural component, the size of the acinus, which increases with body size (Weibel et al., 1981). However, it seems likely that the fraction of the lung utilized for gas exchange increases with decreasing body size. We calculate that the smallest mammal, the shrew, may have just enough lung structure to meet its maximal O_2 consumption if it utilizes all of its diffusing capacity and that progressively less of the lung is required to meet O_2 diffusion needs as maximal rates of O_2 consumption decrease with increasing body size.

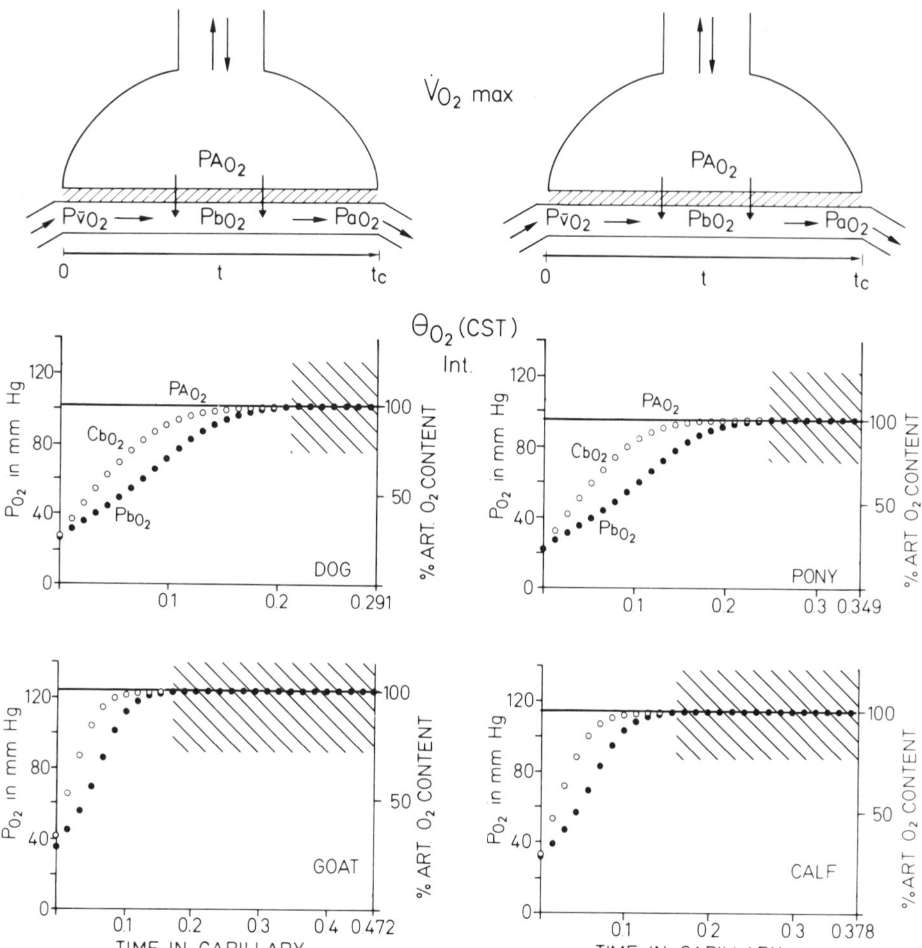

Figure 20 Bohr integrals reflecting the increase in O_2 concentration, CO_2, and PO_2 of the blood during the time it transits the pulmonary capillary bed when animals exercise at $\dot{V}O_{2\,max}$. Note the PO_2 reaches arterial levels after different fractions of transit time in the various species, so that the redundant part of the capillary path (shaded area) is smaller in the dog and pony than in the goat and calf. (From Karas et al., 1987a.)

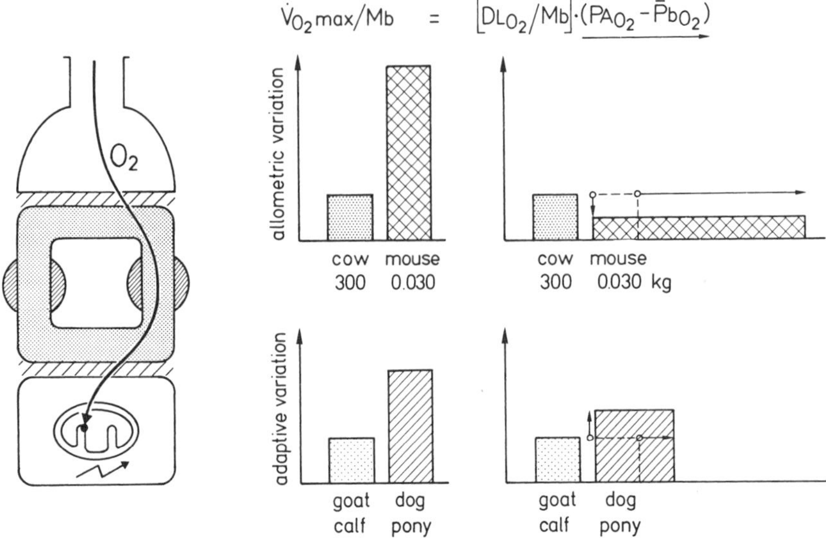

Figure 21 Comparison of the structural adaptation of the pulmonary gas exchanger with allometric and adaptive variation in $\dot{V}O_{2max}$, respectively. With adaptive variation DLO_2 is increased by about half the amount required to match the increase in $\dot{V}O_{2max}$, resulting in a higher PO_2 difference as driving force. In allometric variation DLO_2 is not increased in small animals with higher $\dot{V}O_{2max}$; a higher O_2 flow rate is achieved entirely by increasing the driving force.

The results of the study in which maximal O_2 consumption differs because of adaptive variation also indicate only a partial match between structure and fraction at the level of the lung. The diffusing capacity increases by a factor of only 1.6 in the athletic species, accounting for just half of the increase in $\dot{V}O_{2max}$. The other half is accounted for by using a larger fraction of the available lung structure for O_2 exchange (Fig. 21 bottom). The oxygen content of the blood of the normal species reaches arterial values after passing through only one-half of the capillary distance in the lungs, and the athletic species utilize three-fourths of the capacity of the pulmonary gas exchanger at $\dot{V}O_{2max}$. None of the species utilize the entire capillary length for equilibrating capillary blood with alveolar air, and the redundancy is less in the athletic species.

These findings lead to the conclusion that the principle of symmorphosis does not strictly hold in the lung: the structural variables that determine the O_2 diffusion conductance are not varied in simple proportion to $\dot{V}O_{2max}$. All four species of the adaptive pairs, and for that matter, all but perhaps the smallest mammals, have an excess diffusing capacity. This might be thought of as a "safety factor" which could be important because the pulmonary gas exchanger forms the interface between the body and the environment and is, therefore, not only imperiled by various outside effects but also exposed to different levels of ambient PO_2. However, this still leaves open the question of why such a safety factor should be smaller in athletic species and in smaller animals.

VI. A New Look at Symmorphosis

The concept of symmorphosis, as originally formulated (Taylor and Weibel, 1981), was too simple. Only in one instance in this review of O_2 flow through the respiratory system do we find the simple proportionality between one structural element and maximal rate of O_2 consumption that we initially sought. However, this does not invalidate the principle. There are clearly several instances in which symmorphosis does apply but in a more complex manner. The definition must be expanded to include changes in both structural and functional variables and also take into account the observation that more than one factor can vary to bring about the match between structure and function required for economic design.

VII. Conclusions

The conclusions we draw are the following:

Symmorphosis applies in its simplest form with respect to the mitochondria. The volume of mitochondria varies directly in proportion to $\dot{V}O_{2max}$, regardless of how the energetic demand is varied (see Fig. 6).

Symmorphosis seems to apply at the level of O_2 flow from the capillaries to the mitochondria, but both structural [$V_{(c)}$, erythrocyte concentration, and DTO_2] and functional (t_c) variables are involved in matching O_2 flow to $\dot{V}O_{2max}$ at this level (see Fig. 10).

Symmorphosis also applies at the level of transport of oxygen in the circulatory system; however, there is an added level of complexity. Again, it involves both structural and functional variables but the match is accomplished in a different manner with adaptations for high levels of aerobic performance within animals of the same size (V_S and erythrocytes being involved but not t_c), and with allometric variations in $\dot{V}O_{2max}$ across the size range of mammals (V_S and t_c being involved but not erythrocytes (see Fig. 15).

Finally, we find that symmorphosis is only partially fulfilled at the level of the lung. Two structural elements change with $\dot{V}O_{2max}$: acinar length with allometry; and DLO_2 with adaptive variation. However, the magnitude of the change in both accounts for only about half of the difference in $\dot{V}O_{2max}$ (see Fig. 21). It appears that only the smallest animals utilize all of the diffusing capacity of their lungs for O_2 exchange at $\dot{V}O_{2max}$.

The principle of symmorphosis depends on "regulated morphogenesis." There is a great deal of evidence that the lung's structure is not very malleable, hence, "making more lung" is not easy, nor, perhaps, even possible. This may explain why symmorphosis does not apply to the lung.

References

Blomqvist, C. G. (1983). Cardiovascular adaptations to physical training. *Annu. Rev. Physiol. 45*:169-189.

Bohr, C. (1909). Ueber die spezifische Tätigkeit der Lungen bei der respiratorischen Gasaufnahme. *Scand. Arch. Physiol. 22*:221.

Calder, W. A. III (1984). *Size, Function, and Life History*. Cambridge, Harvard University Press, 431 pp.

Conley, K. E., Kayar, S. R., Rösler, K., Hoppeler, H., Weibel, E. R., and Taylor, C. R. (1987). Adaptive variation in the mammalian respiratory system in relation to energetic demand: IV. Capillaries and their relationship to oxidative capacity. *Respir. Physiol. 69* (in press).

Dejours, P. (1981). *Principles of Comparative Respiratory Physiology*, 2nd ed. Amsterdam, Elsevier/North-Holland, 265 pp.

Draper, N. R., and Smith, H. (1966). *Applied Regression Analysis*. New York, John Wiley & Sons.

Else, P. L., and Hulbert, A. J. (1985). Mammals: An allometric study of metabolism at tissue and mitochondrial level. *Am. J. Physiol. 248*:R415-R421.

Emmett, B., and Hochachka, P. W. (1981). Scaling of oxidative and glycolytic enzymes in mammals. *Respir. Physiol. 45*:261-272.

Gehr, P., Mwangi, D. K., Ammann, A., Sehovic, S., Maloiy, G. M. O., Taylor, C. R., and Weibel, E. R. (1981). Design of the mammalian respiratory system. V. Scaling morphometric pulmonary diffusing capacity to body mass: Wild and domestic mammals. *Respir. Physiol. 44*:61-86.

Goldspink, G. (1985). Malleability of the motor system: A comparative approach. *J. Exp. Biol. 115*:375-391.

Gunn, H. M. (1978). The proportions of muscle, bone and fat in two different types of dog. *Rest. Vet. Sci. 24*:277-282.

Hoppeler, H., Mathieu, O., Krauer, R., Claassen, H., Armstrong, R. B., and Weibel, E. R. (1981a). Design of the mammalian respiratory system. VI. Distribution of mitochondria and capillaries in various muscles. *Respir. Physiol. 44*:87-111.

Hoppeler, H., Mathieu, O., Weibel, E. R., Krauer, R., Lindstedt, S. L., and Taylor, C. R. (1981b). Design of the mammalian respiratory system. VIII. Capillaries in skeletal muscles. *Respir. Physiol. 44*:129-150.

Hoppeler, H., Lindstedt, S. L., Uhlmann, E., Niesel, A., Cruz-Orive, L. M., and Weibel, E. R. (1984). Oxygen consumption and the composition of skeletal muscle tissue after training and inactivation in the European woodmouse (*Apodemus sylvaticus*). *J. Comp. Physiol. B 155*:51-61.

Hoppeler, H., and Lindstedt, S. L. (1985). Malleability of skeletal muscle tissue in overcoming limitation: Structural elements. *J. Exp. Biol. 115*:355-364.

Hoppeler, H., Kayar, S. R., Claassen, H., Uhlmann, E., and Karas, R. H. (1987b). Adaptive variation in the mammalian respiratory system in relation to energetic demand: III. Skeletal muscles: setting the demand for oxygen. *Respir. Physiol. 69*:27-46.

Howald, H. (1985). Malleability of the motor system: Training for maximizing power output. *J. Exp. Biol. 115*:365-373.

Karas, R. H., Taylor, C. R., Jones, J. H., Reeves, R. B., and Weibel, E. R. (1987a). Adaptive variation in the mammalian respiratory system in relation to energetic demand: VII. Flow of oxygen across the pulmonary gas exchanger. *Respir. Physiol. 69*:101-115.

Karas, R. H., Taylor, C. R., Rösler, K., and Hoppeler, H. (1987b). Adaptive variation in the mammalian respiratory system in relation to energetic demand: V. Limits to oxygen transport by the circulation. *Respir. Physiol. 69*:65-79.

Kayar, S. R., Hoppeler, H., Armstrong, R. B., Lindstedt, S. L., and Jones, J. H. (1987). Minimal blood transit time in muscle capillaries. *Fed. Proc. 46*: 210.

Lanyon, L. E., and Rubin, C. T. (1985). Functional adaptation in skeletal structures. In: *Functional Vertebrate Morphology*. Edited by M. H. Hildebrand, D. M. Bramble, K. L. Liem, and D. B. Wake. Cambridge, Belknap Press of Harvard University Press. pp. 1-25.

Longworth, K. E., Jones, J. H., Bicudo, J. E. P. W., Karas, R. H., and Taylor, C. R. (1986). Scaling pulmonary diffusion with body mass in mammals. Physiologist 29*:142*.

Margaria, R. (1976). *Biomechanics and Energetics of Muscular Exercise*. Oxford, Clarendon Press, 146 pp.

Mathieu, O., Krauer, R., Hoppeler, H., Gehr, P., Lindstedt, S. L., Alexander, R. McN., Taylor, C. R., and Weibel, E. R. (1981). Design of the mammalian respiratory system. VII. Scaling mitochondrial volume in skeletal muscles to body mass. *Respir. Physiol. 44*:113-128.

Mathieu, O., Cruz-Orive, L. M., Hoppeler, H., and Weibel, E. R. (1983). Estimating length density and quantifying anisotrophy in skeletal muscle capillaries. *J. Microsc. (London) 131*:131-146.

McMahon, T. A., and Bonner, J. T. (1983). *On Size and Life*. New York, Scientific American Library, W. H. Freeman and Company, 255 pp.

Mitchell, J. H., and Blomqvist, G. (1971). Maximal oxygen uptake. *N. Engl. J. Med. 284*:1018-1022.

Rowell, L. B. (1974). Human cardiovascular adjustments to exercise and thermal stress. *Physiol. Rev. 54*:75-159.

Saltin, B., and Gollnick, P. D. (1983). Skeletal muscle adaptability: Significance for metabolism and performance. In *Handbook of Physiology, Skeletal Muscle*. Edited by L. D. Peacy, R. H. Adrian and S. R. Geiger. Baltimore, Williams & Wilkinson, pp. 555-631.

Saltin, B. (1985). Malleability of the system in overcoming limitations: Function elements. *J. Exp. Biol. 115*:345-354.

Scheuer, J., and Tipton, C. M. (1977). Cardiovascular adaptations to physical training. *Annu. Rev. Physiol. 39*:221-251.

Schmidt-Nielsen, K. (1984). *Scaling: Why is Animal Size So Important*? Cambridge, Cambridge University Press, 241 pp.

Schwerzmann, K., Cruz-Orive, L. M., Eggmann, R., Sanger, A., and Weibel, E. R. (1986). Molecular architecture of the inner membrane of mitochondria from rat liver: A combined biochemical and sterological study. *J. Cell. Biol. 102*:97-103.

Seeherman, H. J., Taylor, C. R., Maloiy, G. M. O., and Armstrong, R. B. (1981). Design of the mammalian respiratory system. II. Measuring maximum aerobic capacity. *Respir. Physiol. 44*:11-23.

Snow, D. H. (1985). The horse and dog, elite athletes–why and how. *Proc. Nutr. Soc. 44*:267-272.

Stahl, W. R. (1967). Scaling of respiratory variables in mammals. *J. Appl. Physiol. 22*:453-460.

Taylor, C. R. (1987). Structural and functional limits to oxidative metabolism: Insights from scaling. *Ann. Rev. Physiol. 49*:135-46.

Taylor, C. R., and Weibel, E. R. (1981). Design of the mammalian respiratory system. I. Problem and strategy. *Respir. Physiol. 44*:1-10.

Taylor, C. R., Mahoiy, G. M. O., Weibel, E. R., Langman, V. A., Kamau, J. M. Z. Seeherman, H. J., and Heglund, N. C. (1981). Design of the mammalian respiratory system. III. Scaling maximum aerobic capacity to body mass: Wild and domestic mammals. *Respir. Physiol. 44*:25-37.

Taylor, C. R., Karas, R. H., Weibel, E. R., and Hoppeler, H. (1987a). Adaptive variation in the mammalian respiratory system in relation to energetic demand. II. Reaching the limits to oxygen flow. *Respir. Physiol. 69*:7-26.

Taylor, C. R., Longworth, K. E., and Hoppeler, H. (1987b). Matching O_2 delivery to O_2 demand in muscle. II. Allometric variation in energy demand. In *Oxygen Transfer From Atmosphere to Tissue*. Edited by N. Gonzalez. New York, Plenum Publishing Co. (in press).

Van Citters, R. L., and Franklin, D. L. (1969). Cardiovascular performance of Alaska sled dogs during exercise. *Circ. Res. 24*:33-42.

Weibel, E. R. (1970/71). Morphometric estimation of pulmonary diffusion capacity. I. Model and method. *Respir. Physiol. 11*:54-75.

Weibel, E. R., Taylor, C. R., Gehr, P., Hoppeler, H., Mathieu, O., and Maloiy, G. M. O. (1981). Design of the mammalian respiratory system. IX. Functional and structural limits for oxygen flow. *Respir. Physiol. 44*:151-164.

Weibel, E. R., Taylor, C. R., O'Neil, J. J., Leith, D. E., Gehr, P., Hoppeler, H., Langman, V., and Baudinette, R. V. (1983). Maximal oxygen consumption and pulmonary diffusing capacity: A direct comparison of physiologic and morphometric measurements in canids. *Respir. Physiol. 54*:173-188.

Weibel, E. R. (1984). *The Pathway for Oxygen: Structure and Function in the Mammalian Respiratory System*. Cambridge, Harvard University Press, 425 pp.

Weibel, E. R. (1987). Scaling of structure and functional variables in the respiratory system. *Annu. Rev. Physiol. 49*:146-59.

Weibel, E. R., Marques, L. B., Constantinopol, M., Doffey, F., Gehr, P., and Taylor, C. R. (1987a). Adaptive variation in the mammalian respiratory system in relation to energetic demand: VI. The pulmonary gas exchanger. *Respir. Physiol. 69*:81-100.

Weibel, E. R., Taylor, C. R., Hoppeler, H., and Karas, R. H. (1987b). Adaptive variation in the mammalian respiratory system in relation to energetic demand: I. Introduction to problem and strategy. *Respir. Physiol. 69*:1-6.

Part Two

Structure and Function of the Gas Exchange Organ

4

Gill Structure and Function
Fish

PIERRE LAURENT

Laboratoire de Morphologie Fonctionnelle
et Ultrastructurale des Adaptations
Centre National de la Recherche Scientifique
Strasbourg, France

I. Introduction

The gill has been the focus of attention for biologists more than ever during the last decade. The reasons for this interest are multiple. Among many others, the unprecedented risk incurred by inhabitants of dramatically polluted aquatic and marine environments makes it necessary to better understand the functioning of the main water-blood interface in fishes.

In addition to, and probably more than, an academic call for basic knowledge, this practical side appeals for support from the economic community. Actually, the gill is now often designated as the target organ in water pollution studies, for instance, when acidification of the milieu becomes a major threat.

Aquaculture, marine or continental, should also receive a direct benefit from studies concerning gill functions because the gill is the site for permanent exchanges between the fish and its milieu and also the beginning of multiple pathological problems.

More fundamentally, the gill is the site where several functions are superimposed. This is not unique in biology, but here a high degree of complexity is reached. The gill serves primarily as a gas exchanger and, as a consequence of variable respiratory gas partial pressures in the aquatic milieu, it undergoes morphological and functional adaptations (see Chap. 13). Second, the gill is deeply involved in the acid-base regulation that operates differently depending upon the composition of the milieu (see Chap. 20). Third, bathed with a medium in which most of the chemicals are soluble (ions and organic compounds) the gill serves as a chemical exchanger and, therefore, plays a preeminent role in osmoregulation and excretion including carbon dioxide and ammonia. The integration of respiration, acid-base regulation, osmoregulation, and excretion makes the gill a fascinating and useful model in which a strict balance between ions and water fluxes shows adaptation to a milieu varying from almost distilled water to one even more concentrated than seawater. Moreover, in terms of respiratory function, the aquatic milieu shows variations that undoubtedly are far beyond those encountered in the atmosphere, e.g., PO_2 varying from a few torr up to 600 torr.

Very recently, one recognizes a new approach that considers the gill as a metabolic organ similar to the lung. Indeed, gill tissues are able to bind several physiologically active molecules, to activate or to deactivate them. This type of research will probably open new fields in comparative physiological regulation.

Therefore, this chapter will successively consider the following topics:

The organization and control of the gill vasculature

The structure and function of the gill epithelia

The adaptation and maladaptation of the gill to the milieu

This paper will not review in detail what is presently known about gill morphology and physiology, for instance, the mechanical aspects of ventilation and its control are not discussed here (see Hugues, 1984). The reader should refer to the publications listed at the end of the chapter for further reading. However, for clarity some basic knowledge will be reviewed before considering the "state of the art."

II. Perfusion

As with other systems, to understand the exchange of matter across epithelia (lung, kidney, intestine, etc.), a precise knowledge of the organization and regulation of perfusion are essential. This can be simply shown by the application of Fick's principles. Vascular casting techniques using silicone rubber or methacrylate resine have revealed the detailed organization of the gill vasculature (see Laurent 1984).

In all groups of fish (taken in its broader sense): Elasmobranchii, Cyclostomii, Chondrostei, Holostei, and Teleostei, the gill vasculature consists of two distinct but interconnected systems: the systemic and the arteriovenous circulations.

A. Systemic Circulation: The Blood Supply of the Lamellae

The systemic branchial circulation (also called arterioarterial vasculature) has an arterial afferent component supplying the respiratory lamellae with nonoxygenated blood and an efferent arterial component that gathers the oxygenated blood from the lamellae where the respiratory exchanges take place and sends it into the dorsal aorta, and from there into the systemic bed. In lower groups, such as elasmobranchs and Chondrostei, a system of labyrinthic vessels, the cavernous tissue, is interposed between the afferent limb of this system and the lamellae. The function of the cavernous tissue is uncertain. It is generally considered as a structure stiffening the filament in spite of the presence in these species of a cartilage gill rod. The structure of the cavernous tissue has been recently reinvestigated in the dogfish (De Vries and De Jager, 1984). Moreover, the so-called cavernous body cells that line this compartment are able to sequester particulate matter from the blood before it enters the lamellae capillaries (Hunt and Rowley, 1986).

The Lamella: Respiratory Unit

The structure of the lamellae in the different groups of fish has been described in detail in a recent monograph (see Laurent, 1984). In addition to the bilayered epithelium that makes up most of the gill water–blood barrier (see Sec. III) pillar cells are a particular feature of the fish gill. They are endothelial in function because they line the lamellar capillaries just beneath the basement membrne of the lamellar epithelium. But because they contain endocellular bundles of actomyosin filaments (Smith and Chamley-Campbell, 1981) they have characteristics of myoendothelial cells, as do the mesangial cells of the kidney or the interalveolar septa cells of the mammalian lung. It has been repeatedly proposed that they might exert a control on lamellar perfusion. It is clear from model computation (Smith and Johnson, 1977) that contraction or relaxation of pillar cells is able to alter the lamellar blood flow and the diffusion of respiratory gas across the epithelium by changing the pattern of blood distribution within the lamellae. However, there is, as yet, no experimental evidence of such a role for pillar cells that are not innervated. Nevertheless, the myogenic tonicity of the pillar cells probably affects the compliance of the lamellae vascular component (Farrel, 1980). The recently observed communicating junctions between pillar cells, as revealed by freeze-fracture in the Atlantic hagfish gill, are interesting (Bartels and Decker, 1985). These junctions consist of small clusters of packed particles on the P face and pits on the E face of the split plasma membrane of the pillar cells. These observations suggest that these cells behave like a functional syncitium such that coordination of contractile, metabolic, or secretory activity could be achieved by the communicating junctions.

The Vascular Sphincters

Morphological studies have shown two types of typical vascular sphincters. These observations constitute the only evidence for the localization of the gill systemic control. The short vascular segments that drive the blood in and out of the lamellae from the filament afferent arteries are equipped with a well-structured ring of smooth muscle around the vessles in elasmobranchs (Wright, 1973) and the subteleostean groups (Dunel and Laurent, 1980) in which they are not innervated. In teleosts, these sphincters are not so obvious because the arterial wall is more uniform in media thickness and does not display a ring shape.

In addition to fluorescent fibers distributed to both afferent and efferent lamellar arteries (Donald, 1984), recent immunocytochemical studies have shown the presence of neural structures close to the efferent lamellar arteries. They consiste of neurons sending fingerlike extensions around the vessel. At least one neuron is present near each lamellar artery. Neurons that contain serotonin, a potent vasoconstrictor of the branchial vasculature (Ostlund and Fänge, 1962; Reite, 1969), apparently have some connections with the serotoninergic nerve fibers running along the filament from its base to the top (Bailly and Dunel-Erb, personal communication).

The second type of sphincter is located around the efferent filament arteries close to their junction with the efferent branchial artery (Laurent and Dunel, 1976; Dunel and Laurent, 1977; Smith, 1977). These sphincters exist in all groups of fish. They consist of a substantially increased number of smooth-muscle layers. They have an abundant innervation, which has recently been studied in detail. This innervation is supplied by the protrematic branches of the vagus in arches I to IV. Nerve endings filled with cholinergic-type vesicles are located in close association with the adventicial smooth-muscle cells. One observes a strong acetylcholinesterase activity in relation to the nerve membranes (Bailly and Dunel-Erb, 1986). These observations suggest that this innervation derives from postganglionic axons of the parasympathetic system. In addition, other specific techniques have revealed an aminergic component showing a formaldehyde-induced fluorescence. Endings filled with dense-cored vesicles come in contact with the cholinergic endings (Dunel-Erb and Bailly, 1986). Such an organization suggests that a sympathetic innervation modulates the effects of the parasympathetic component. Physiological studies have shown that electrical stimulation of the branchial branches of the vagus constricts the systemic gill vasculature by decreasing the blood flow coming out of the efferent branchial arteries (Nilsson, 1973; Petterson and Nilsson, 1979). This constrictive effect is mimicked by acetylcholine (Ach) and blocked by atropine (Dunel and Laurent, 1977). On the other hand, epinephrine produces a dilation of the branchial vasculature (Dunel and Laurent, 1977; Payan and Girard, 1977; Wood, 1974). Sympathetic nerve stimulation increases the systemic gill blood flow (Nilsson and Pettersson, 1981). It is likely that the final hemodynamic result depends upon the balance between the sympathetic and the parasympathetic activities.

Role of the Sphincter

One might speculate on the role played by the two types of sphincters and how the functioning of these sphincters might alter the pattern of lamellar perfusion. It has been repeatedly said, since Randall et al. (1967), that under certain conditions (e.g., hypoxia) the so-called transfer factors for O_2 and CO_2 are increased.

Several explanations might account for an increased diffusion of respiratory gas: a recruitment of nonperfused lamellae (i.e., an increased exchange surface area) or a thinning down of the blood-water barrier. Both result from the lamellar distension after an increase in intrabranchial blood pressure (see Soivio and Tuurala, 1981). It is clear that this is achieved by contraction of the efferent filament sphincters. Moreover, in teleosts an increased perfusion of the lamellae along the filament is achieved possibly through an activation of the lamellar sphincters. If sphincters progressively close down lamella after lamella from the base to the top of the filament, it would result in a total filling of the lamellae supported by the filament. In this context, the morphological relationships between the neurons located around the lamellar efferent arteries and the neuroepithelial cells described by Dunel-Erb et al. (1982) in the filament epithelium suggest a possible activation of the lamellar efferent arteries by messages generated within the neuroepithelial cells in response to environmental conditions.

B. Arteriovenous Circulation: Blood Supply of the Filaments

The Nutrient Vasculature

A second gill vasculature is located within the body of the filament itself and does not concern the lamellae whatsoever. It consists first of a loose network of narrow but long nutrient arteries, which take their origin from the efferent filament or from the branchial arteries, or both (Laurent and Dunel, 1976). They finally give rise to capillaries vascularizing the different parts of the filament body, especially the striated and smooth-muscle bundles (Laurent, 1984; Dunel-Erb and Bailly, 1987) that put into motion the filament synchroneously with the ventilation (Ballintijn, 1985). Gill smooth-muscle bundles are controlled by adrenergic nerves (Dunel-Erb and Bailly, 1987; Bailly, 1983; Nilsson, 1985). The blood is finally collected into the filament or into the branchial veins joining the internal jugular vein. An abundant adrenergic innervation is present around the nutrient arteries (Donald, 1984).

The Filamental Blood Sinuses

Second, a complex system of sinuses, extending from the core of the filament (central sinus) toward the peripheral veinlike compartment, underlies the filament epithelium (see Laurent, 1984). It is noteworthy that these sinuses are also directly connected with the branchial systemic circulation by arteriovenous anastomoses. Anastomoses have a muscular media, which suggests a vasomotive regulation. Anastomoses are, indeed, constricted by catecholamines by α-type receptors, but they apparently are not innervated (Dunel and Laurent, 1977). In the higher groups of teleosts, anastomoses make communication only between the efferent limb of the filament circulation and the sinuses, in contrast with lower groups of fish (elasmobranchs, Chondrostei, Holostei, and lower Teleostei) in which both afferent (nonarterialized blood) and efferent (arterialized blood) limbs have arteriovenous anastomoses (Laurent and Dunel, 1976; Dunel and Laurent, 1980; Donald and Ellis, 1983).

The sinuses have a veinlike structure. They are lined with a thin layer of endothelial cells with long, thin, loosely interdigitating processes linked to each other and ornamented with surface flaps on the luminal and the abluminal sides. Maculae occludentes are often observed linking the processes. As suggested by Fawcett (1963) flaps may have a pinocytotic function in taking up and passing fluid through the endothelial membrane from the plasma to the tissue, and vice versa. True pinocytotic vesicles are also present. In contrast with the pillar cell lining of the lamellar capillaries, "Weibel and Palad bodies" are present as usual in endothelial cells. Beneath the endothelial cells a matrix of extracellular material separates from a relatively dense basement membrane. Formaldehyde-induced fluorescence has demonstrated the existence of a perisinusal neural network (Bailly, 1983; Laurent, 1984; Donald, 1984).

The Role of Filament Circulation

The function of the system of sinuses is uncertain. Teleologically, it probably does not primarily serve to carry oxygen, albeit in higher groups it might serve this purpose. I suggest that its main function is to drain the extracellular fluids that result from the activity of the gill epithelia (Laurent and Dunel, 1978). Interestingly, in saltwater (SW) fish, and in accordance with the osmotic gradient, the sinuses are generally small in volume contrasting with the dilated aspect in freshwater (FW) species. In this respect the function of the anastomoses is likely to supply or to flush the low pressure compartment, or both.

Recent in vivo measurement indicates that in the resting trout only 7% of the cardiac output was directed from the systemic bed into the venous gill circulation (Iwama et al., 1986). This value departs from previous experiments indicating that about 30% is returned through the venous gill circulation directly to the heart (Hughes et al., 1982). Another point of interest is that the blood pH was lower and CCO_2, PCO_2 higher in the gill venous blood than in the systemic blood (Iwama et al., 1986). These data clearly indicate that the arteriovenous circulation does not represent an efficient systemic shunt, albeit definite metabolic exchanges take place across the wall of this compartment. Further information on the transepithelial ions movements that reflect upon the gill venous blood composition will be given in Section III.

C. Gill Vasculature Control

Nerve

In addition to the localization of sphincters (see under Sec. I.A) and arteriovenous anastomoses (see under Sec. II.B), attempts to present an exhaustive view of the gill vascular control have been undertaken (Nilsson, 1983; Laurent, 1985). Unfortunately, many points are still missing concerning the branchial innervation, and especially the interneuronal connections within the filament where abundant populations of neurons have been observed (Bailly, 1983). On the other hand, little is known about the localization, the structure, and the neural connections of the gill sensory receptors. Nevertheless, the schematic representation in Figure 1 summarizes our present knowledge for teleosts. We have also represented hypothetical localization of innervation resulting from pharmacological and physiological clues.

Humoral Factors

In addition to direct nerve action, we should remind the reader that physiologically active blood-borne molecules have long been considered to be an efficient control of the gill vasculature. This is particularly true for circulating catecholamines (CA) (see Nilsson, 1984, for references and a more complete account). Catecholamines are known to cause not only β-adrenoceptor-mediated vasodilation of the isolated branchial vasculature but also a predominant systemic constriction through α-adrenoceptors. In the conscious unrestrained eel, results have shown that epinephrine injection increases the systemic vascular resistance (and to a lesser extent the cardiac output) but has no consistent effect on branchial vascular resistance (Hipkins, 1985). The variable effects on the gill vasculature in vivo probably have two causes. First, they are the result of an α-adenoreceptor-mediated vasoconstriction of arteriovenous anastomoses and a β-adrenoreceptor-mediated vasodilation of the efferent filamental arteries' sphincters. These effects have been localized and visualized on vascular cast preparations (Dunel

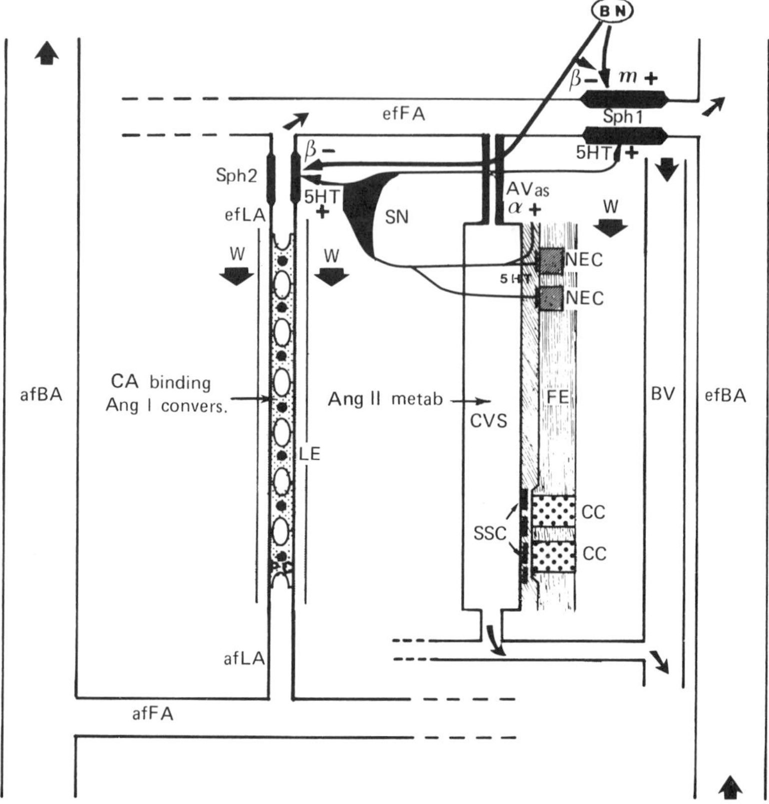

Figure 1 Schematic representation of some aspects of the gill control machinery as suggested by recent findings from ultrastructural, histochemical, and immunocytochemical studies (Bailly, Dunel-Erb, and Laurent, submitted).

These new results mianly relate to the discovery of a rich intramural serotonergic nervous system. This system relates the serotonin-containing neuroepithelial cells (NEC; Dunel-Erb et al., 1982), serotonergic large neurons (Bailly and Dunel-Erb, 1986; Dunel-Erb and Bailly, 1986) and strategically located vascular sphincters (Dunel and Laurent, 1980). Large, short processes of SN, filled up with 5HT, surround the sphincters tunica media, whereas another type of process (dendrites) run close to the NEC. Environmental hypoxia has been shown to "degranulate" the NEC. Thus, this organization suggests that vasoconstriction of sph 1 and sph 2 is mediated by 5HT (a potent vasoconstrictor in fish; Reite, 1969) release from SN, the functioning of which depends, in turn, on transduction of environmental or tissular factors.

Another system consists of small cells containing serotonin (SCC) located within the wall of the central vascular compartment of the filament (CVS) beneath its epithelium and close to chloride cells (CC). This organization raises and Laurent, 1977) and are, in addition, discussed in other reports on more classic methods of study (see Nilsson, 1984, pp. 203-204). Second, in isolated gill preparation a cholinergic vasoconstriction of central origin exerted on the filament sphincter in vivo does not compete with the branchial vasodilation.

Another problem appears when comparing the physiologically active concentrations of CA and their effective plasma level. In *Gadus morhua* there is no good agreement between these two sets of values (Smith et al., 1985) in contrast with previous results (Wahlqvist, 1980; Wahlqvist and Nilsson, 1980). The agreement is no better for *Salmo gairdneri*. Indeed, the concentration response curve for epinephrine extends from 0% of the full response at 10^{-9} mol up to 100% at 10^{-4} mol concentration (Wood, 1974). The plasma epinephrine concentraion ranges from 3×10^{-9} mol in resting, unrestrained, catheterized animals and does not exceed 2×10^{-8} in stressed fish (Ristori et al., 1979; Ristori, 1984; Ristori and Laurent, 1985; Pennec-Le Bras and Pennec, 1986). Generally speaking, the low plasma concentrations of CA, measured with methods that avoided stressful situations by highly sensitive analytical procedures in fish in good physiological conditions make it necessary to reassess the dose-effect relationships in the gill. Many effects on the vasculature and epithelia have been

---

Figure 1 (continued) the hypothesis of a functional link between 5HT and epithelial ion transport by chloride cells by adenylate cyclase activation in a way similar to that recently shown in the mussel (Saintsing and Dietz, 1983) (Scheide and Dietz, 1984).

Finally, the following are also presented: catecholamine binding to lamellae pillar cells (Nekvasil and Olson, in press; Nekvasil and Olson, 1985), angiotension converting activity (Ang I–II) of the lamellar tissues (Galardy et al., 1984; Olson et al., 1986), and angiotensin II metabolism in the arteriovenous bed (Olson et al., 1986).

Abbreviations: af BA, ef BA, af FA, ef FA, af LA, ef LA: respectively, afferent, efferent branchial, filament, lamellar artery. AVas: arteriovenous anastomose. BN: branchial nerve (vagosympathetic branch). BV: branchial vein. CC: chloride cell. CVS: filament central vascular compartment. FE: filament epithelium. LE: lamellar epithelium. NEC: neuroepithelial cell. PC: pillar cell. SCC: small serotonin-containing cell. SN: serotonergic neuron. α^+: α-adrenoceptor (probably noninnervated in the gill) mediating AVas construction. β^-: β-adrenoceptor (presumably innervated) mediating sph 1 and sph 2 dilation. m^+: muscarinic (innervated) receptor: mediating sph 1 cholinergic contraction. $5HT^+$: serotonin receptor (presumably $5HT_2$) mediating sph 1 and sph 2 constriction.

We suppose that serotonin vasoconstriction corresponds with the nonadrenergic, noncholinergic (NANC) effects described by Nilsson (1983); (These abbreviations are in accordance with those recommended and used in W. S. Hoar and D. J. Randall, eds. (1984). Fish Physiology, Vol. XA.

reported for concentrations in the micromolar range, whereas the plasma levels actually fall within the nanomolar range (see Rankin and Bolis, 1984; Ungell et al., 1984).

Metabolism of Active Substances

The metabolism of CA and its extraction from blood is another complication that exists when estimating the role played by circulating CA (or any other hormone). This problem has recently been studied on the trout gill (Nekvasil and Olson, in press). Gill homogenates deaminate catecholamines faster than homogenates of liver, kidney, and skeletal muscle. Branchial *O*-methylation has been found comparable with that of the liver and kidney. During a continuous catecholamine perfusion of the isolated gill, 30% of norepinephrine was removed and only 7% of epinephrine. In the lamprey, high disappearance rates of epinephrine and dopamine have been observed between the ventral and dorsal aorta, suggesting that these molecules are metabolized within the gills (Dashow and Epple, 1985). As shown by autoradiography, the pillar cells of the lamellae and certain endothelial cells in the filament sinuses are the main structures binding catecholamines (Nekvasil and Olson, 1985). In other words, CA determinations from the dorsal aortic blood lead to an underestimate of their potential effects on gill vasculature. Other biological molecules that are active on blood pressure are metabolized during gill perfusion. This is true for angioentsin. The angiotensin-converting enzyme (ACE) is over 30 times more concentrated in the gill and the corpuscles of Stannius than in plasma, whereas the enzyme is almost undetectable in muscle, liver, and kidney (Galardy et al., 1984). It has also been shown that captopril, an inhibitor of ACE, decreases the dorsal aortic pressure by more than 40% and that injection of angiotensin II increases it by 100% (Ristori and Laurent, submitted); it was thus concluded that the gill angiotensin metabolism participates in the regulation of the systemic blood pressure. In addition, the gill systemic pathway is able to convert angiotensin I into angiotensin II, whereas the venous pathway metabolizes either angiotensin I or angiotensin II into inactive metabolites (Olson et al., in press). Autoradiography has demonstrated that on gills perfused with an ^{3}H-labeled ACE inhibitor pillar cells are the major site of ^{3}H accumulation (Olson et al., 1986).

Therefore, it could be concluded that the arteriovenous circulation participates in the clearance of angiotensin from the blood (Olson et al., in press). As pointed out by Olson (personal communication) all of these results point to a new function for gill tissues; the metabolism of circulating hormones in a manner similar to that of the lung (Heinemann and Fishman, 1969; Gaddum et al., 1953; Strum and Junod, 1972).

The branchial clearance of lactate and glucose, two important gill oxydative substrates, has been recently determined in trout (Mommsen, 1984).

III. The Gill Epithelia

Two types of epithelia surround the gill in its entirety. One is thick and envelopes the filament body: the filament epithelium. The other is very thin and covers the lamellae: the lamellar (or respiratory) epithelium.

A simple light microscopic examination of a gill filament cross section offers evidence of organizational relationships between the vasculature and epithelia. The vascularization of the filament epithelium is taken up by the arterio-venous system, whereas the respiratory epithelium is vascularized by the branchial systemic circulation. This functional correspondence is noteworthy because experimental concepts are based on it (Girard and Payan, 1980; Gardaire et al., 1985).

A. The Lamellar Epithelium

The lamellar epithelium is structurally adapted to the transfer of respiratory gas, i.e., it represents a large surface area and is thin enough to allow oxygen, a rather poorly diffusible gas, to cross it. Thorough descriptions have been recently given (e.g., Laurent, 1984). Therefore, we will simply remind the reader of the fundamental points inasmuch as there is a great similarity in organization throughout the different groups of fish.

The lamellar epithelium is separated from the flanged pillar cells by a thick basement membrane. It generally consists of two layers of flat cells separated from each other by extracellular spaces of variable width that often contain lymphocytes. The total thickness of the epithelium ranges from 1 to 5 μm.

The innermost layer comprises nondifferentiated cells, upon which, as yet, little attention has been focused. According to their ultrastructure (Laurent and Dunel, 1980), they probably serve as stem cells for the renewal of the cellular components of the outermost layer. The external layer consists of large pavement cells. They have an apical membrane ornamented with fingerprintlike ridges. Pavement cells are particularly active cells because they have abundant populations of organelles: a rich, rough endoplasmic reticulum, and an exceptionally developed Golgi complex giving rise to numerous coated vesicles rising toward the apical membrane. This apical membrane is externally lined with a thick glycocalix that creates an unstirred layer of charged glycoprotein molecules containing acidic groups (Pisam et al., 1980). The role of the glycocalix, so far, has been somewhat overlooked. It is probably involved in epithelial permeability to ions and to water. The glycocalix undergoes obvious structural modifications according to the milieu in which the fish lives. Pavement cells are linked to each other by long junctions consisting of five to nine anastomosed strands (Sardet et al., 1979). This pattern of arrangement means that the lamellar epithelium is tight according to the classification of Claude and Goodenough (1973), and consequently, it is impermeable to water and electrolytes. Such junctional low permeability is what could be expected from an epithelium bathed with a high-flow, high-pressure blood compartment. This, and several other arguments, contributes to deflection of osmotic exchanges away from the lamellae (Isaia, 1984), albeit paracellular tight pathways allow passages of organic molecules (Masoni and Isaia, 1980) and ions (Zadunaisky, 1984). In addition, it has been shown that the gills are the major site of diffusional water exchanges (Motais et al., 1969) and that the water fluxes occur mainly through the cells of the lamellar epithelium (Isaia, 1982). Freeze-fracture studies have demonstrated the presence of intramembranous particles in different states of organization within the apical plasma membrane of the pavement cells (Sardet et al., 1980; Bartels and Welsch, 1986). Possibly, these structures represent the morphological support for water exchange as suggested by studies on the urinary bladder (Chevalier et al., 1974, 1985).

Interestingly, the basal membrane of these cells are considered to be the limiting barrier for diffusion (Isaia et al., 1978), and water permeability is significantly higher in FW-adapted than in SW-adapted trout (Isaia, 1982) and eel (Motais et al., 1969), a characteristic that probably is due to the higher calcium concentration of the salt water. All of these characteristics separate lamellar from filamental epithelium, which is considered by some authors as the main site of osmotic water fluxes (Isaia, 1984), at least, in saltwater or saltwater-adapted fish.

B. The Filament Epithelium

The multilayered filament epithelium surrounds the filament, including its leading and trailing edges. In addition it intercalates between the lamellae. As noted previously, the core of the filament is occupied by the sinuses of the arteriovenous vasculature. Multiple processes emanating from the central sinuses spread beneath the epithelium; hence, it makes sense to say that the filament epithelium is vascularized by the arteriovenous system. Functionally speaking, this makes an important difference with the lamellar epithelium. Sinuses are low-flow and low-pressure vascular compartments and, in addition, they are differently supplied with blood according to the species. For instance, eel and some other lower groups of fish have their filament sinuses supplied by prebranchial and postbranchial blood. This might be a large consideration with the sphere of ionic or osmotic exchanges across the filament epithelium (Dunel and Laurent, 1980).

The filament epithelium has several types of cellular components. First, it has an external lining of pavement cells which have ultrastructural characteristics not quite similar to those of the lamellae. On the trailing and the leading edges of the filament, there are mucus-secreting cells. The mucous layer is believed to form a protective and unstirred layer, and because of this and the cationic exchange properties (Marshall, 1978), it contributes to the control of epithelial permeability (Kirschner, 1978; Wendelaar-Bonga, 1978). However, in contrast to a broadly accepted opinion, we believe that a mucous curtain does not always cover the whole gill surface in contrast with the pavement cell glycocalix. In fact, mucous secretion occurs in response to drastic conditions: acidification of the milieu, stress, pollutants, mechanical erosion, etc.

Chloride Cell

The chloride cells is the most conspicuous component of the gill epithelium, although it is not always confined to this organ. Chloride cells are also present in different teguments such as the head skin (Lasker and Threadgold, 1968; Zaccone and Licata, 1981), the opercular lining (Karnaky and Kinter, 1977), and the pseudobranch (see Laurent and Dunel-Erb, 1984). All of these localizations are species related. It is important to mention that the chloride cells must be considered as a specific component of the filament epithelium. In seawater fish or seawater-adapted euryhaline species, chloride cells are restricted to the filament and almost exclusively on its afferent half (trailing edge plus interlamellar area of the filament surface) (Laurent, 1982, 1984; Hossler et al., 1985). In freshwater fish we often see trout having chloride cells on their lamellae [on the trailing edge and, very exceptionally, on the leading edge (Laurent and Dunel, 1980; Laurent et al., 1985)]. From scanning electron microscopic observation of several thousands of trout gills, we have concluded that such a lamellar location represents a response to situations linked to environmental or pathological disturbances. However, chloride cell invasion of the lamellar epithelium follows an huge increased density on the filament epithelium.

Chloride cell morphology has been recently reviewed in detail (Laurent, 1984). Since the original work of Keys and Willemer (1932), the chloride cell has been the theme of numerous papers. Briefly, this mitochondria-rich cell possesses an abundant system of tubulelike basolateral membranal invaginations. Its apical surface generally lies in contact with the external milieu; occasionally, however, the cell can be entirely burrowed within the epithelium or separated from the external milieu by a thin sheet of pavement cell cytoplasm. This process of sequestration is rapid and may account for almost instantaneous physiological adaptation (Laurent and Dunel, 1980). The basolateral membrane is close to the sinuses of the arteriovenous filamental circulation. This suggests functional relationships between chloride cells and arteriovenous circulation.

In saltwater stenohaline or saltwater-adapted euryhaline fishes, the discovery of "accessory cell" as an obligatory cell mate of the chloride cell (Dunel and Laurent, 1973; Dunel, 1975; Hootman and Philpott, 1980; Laurent and Dunel, 1980) linked to each other by a short, tight junction (100-200 Å), in comparison with intercellular pavement cells junctions (1000 Å), has prompted specific research. Freeze-fracture studies demonstrate that in SW filament epithelium this junction is leaky and does not exist in FW (Sardet, 1980).

Recent research has confirmed, by autoradiography, that the chloride cell and accessory cell are distinct types (Chretien and Pisam, 1986).

Neuroepithelial Cells

Neuroepithelial cells are another major component of the filament epithelium. They have been described by Dunel-Erb et al. (1982) in all groups of fish thus far examined, including elasmobranchs. In fact, they share many characteristics with the cells forming the neuroepithelial bodies observed within the epithelium of the mammalian airways (Feyrter, 1938; Lauweryns et al., 1972) and in the respiratory mucosa of birds, reptiles, and amphibians (Dunel-Erb et al., 1982). The occurrence of the same type of cell in the respiratory epithelium of aerian and water vertebrates poses an interesting problem of evolution. These cells, which are season-dependent in number (Dunel-Erb et al., submitted) are located on the serosal side of the filament epithelium along the leading edge of the filaments with process facing the inhalant water flow. They are innervated by afferent and efferent innervations. It has been demonstrated by immunocytochemical methods (Bailly et al., submitted) that they contain dense-cored vesicles filled with serotonin, as found in mammals (Lauweryns et al., 1982). Serotonin released by an exocytotic mechanism within the surrounding tissues presumably activates the smooth-muscle cells that control the postlamellar arteries (see Sec. II.A). Exocytosis and degranulation are mediated by environmental hypoxia (Dunel-Erb et al., 1982), an effect that also has been observed in aerian pathway neuroepithelial cells (Lauweryns and Van Lommel, 1982) (see Fig. 1).

Finally, the presence of subepithelial populations of small serotoninergic cells is worth mentioning. These cells contain vesicles of different sizes suggesting possible association of serotonin with other substances (peptides?). Mast cells are also well represented in the leading edge of the filament beneath the epithelium (Bailly, personal communication).

C. Functions and Functioning of Epithelia

Attempts have been made to differentiate the functions of lamellar and filamental epithelia by using the perfused trout head preparation (Payan and Matty, 1975; Girard and Payan, 1980; Gardaire et al., 1985). This useful method has been repeatedly reevaluated and improved (Pärt et al., 1982; Perry et al., 1984a; Bornancin et al., 1985). However, the results are never unequivocal; thus, for the sake of clarity we will review the epithelial functions regardless of their location.

Ionic Movements in Fresh Water

The main problems for freshwater fish are (1) to compensate for the leakage of its vital ions, (2) to oppose the body invasion by osmotic water flux, and (3) to maintain the ionic loss. Gills play a preeminently important role in all of them.

Krogh (1938) and, later, Maetz and Garcia-Romeu (1964), were the first to observe that a net uptake of NaCl occurs through the gills. Then, it was proposed that the lamellar epithelium (the so-called respiratory cell) is the site for coupled sodium-ammonium, sodium-proton, and chloride-bicarbonate exchanges in freshwater fish (Girard and Payan, 1980). Thus, in addition to an active inward transport of Na^+ and Cl^-, the fish benefits from this operation to get rid of wastes: ammonia (or ammonium), protons, and excess bicarbonate. A lamellar respiratory cell localization is still a debated question (Kikuchi, 1977; Evans, 1982a) and has been recently challenged by morphophysiological investigations (Laurent et al., 1985; Gardaire et al., 1985; Avella, 1986). Arguments against a respiratory cell localization are as follows:

First, transporting epithelial cells are distinguished by specific characteristics, namely, huge mitochondrial equipment and multiple basolateral membrane infoldings. Lamellar pavement respiratory cells have none of these characteristics. In contrast, they are distinguished by a cellular ultrastructure involved in glycocalix synthesis (developed rough endoplasmic reticulum), a high transport of vesicles, a extremely active Golgi complex, and membrane fusion (pinocytosis).

Second, recent results suggest that the development of chloride cells correlates with gill ionic uptake. When trout are transferred from water of medium hardness (for instance $Na^+ = 1$, $Cl^- = 0.5$-0.8, $CA^{2+} = 1$-$3\ mEq \cdot L^{-1}$) into poor (soft) water ($Na^+ = 0.05$, $Cl^- = 0.03$, $Ca^{2+} = 0.07\ mEq \cdot L^{-1}$) an intense proliferation of large chloride cells occurs, first on the filament epithelium and later (2-5 days) on the lamellar epithelium. The lack of NaCl and not of Ca^{2+} was proved to be responsible (Laurent et al., 1985). The same conclusion was drawn from experiments with the brown bull-head catfish (Laurent et al., unpublished). In addition, by manipulating the ionic content of the milieu (and consequently the number and the functional state of chloride cells), Na^+ influx was found to be closely related to the chloride cells' development (Avella, 1986). The chloride cells of the filament contribute about 20% to the total sodium uptake in trout kept in low-concentration NaCl fresh water ($< 0.2\ mEq \cdot L^{-1}$) and high Ca^{2+} (Gardaire et al., 1985), the remaining 80% is transported across the lamellar epithelium. It is noteworthy that at NaCl concentrations this low, chloride cells are present on lamellae. Thus, it is likely that the lamellar epithelium participates in the ionic uptake through the proliferating chloride cells, but the question remains unanswered whether or not lamellar pavement cells contribute to this function.

It is interesting that transport of Na^+-H^+ and Na^+-NH_4^+ was primarily present in the gills of seawater ancestors, where it contributed to acid-base regulation and nitrogen excretion (at least Na^+-H^+ in hagfish, Evans, 1984). These branchial mechanisms have made possible an adaptation to fresh water in which they are engated in NaCl regulation, whereas in marine teleosts and elasmobranchs they remain the main routes for the excretion of acid and ammonia (Evans, 1982, 1984; Heisler, 1980). This may be the reason for the presence of numerous chloride cells of the FW type on the gill epithelium of elasmobranchs (Laurent, 1982).

In the hagfish, recent studies have shown evidence for the existence of FW-type chloride cells (i.e., absence of accessory cell; Elger and Hentschel, 1983; Bartels and Welsch, 1986). In this marine hyperosmoregulating fish, characterized by isonatric internal and external media, chloride cell function probably deals with a sodium inward transport as seen in freshwater teleosts.

Evans and Cameron (1986) have reviewed the different pathways for ammonia excretion. In addition to the apical Na^+-NH_4^+ exchange, already mentioned, they have studied four more mechanisms. Among them the nonionic diffusion of NH_3 which obeys the Fick's principle. Ammonia (a gas) follows the partial pressure gradient (and not NH_4 concentration). This is supposed to be the predominant mechanism of transfer across the gill.

Here, the need for a great amoung of blood convection beneath the epithelium is contradictory with the small flow perfusing the filamental chloride cells; thus rendering this type of cell an unlikely candidate in contrast with the thin, large and well-perfused lamellar epithelium, an organization that fits fickian kinetics. This prerequisite for a large exchange surface area might explain recent data from morphometric analysis of the respiration system of trout kept in deionized water (DW). As shown in Table 1, the surface area after 5 days in DW increases by a factor of 2 and the diffusion path decreases by a factor of 1.5. In other words, the conductance should be multiplied by a factor of 3 for NH_3 diffusion in water that is almost free of ions (Laurent, unpublished data). Supposedly, the lack of Na^+ ions hampers the cycle of nitrogen excretion via NH_4^+, then NH_3 becomes the major (if not the sole) end product (see als, Cameron and Heisler, 1983; Wright and Wood, 1985; Cameron, 1986).

The Na^+-NH_4^+ exchange system requires carbonic anhydrase. It is, therefore, necessary to localize the enzyme rather than its end product of the histochemical reaction (Hanson, 1967). Thus, specific antibody has been raised against the gill antigen because antibody raised against fish erythrocyte carbonic anhydrase does not cross-react with gill carbonic anhydrase (Rahim et al., 1988). After immunogold staining, carbonic anhydrase labeling has been found (1) over the apical region of chloride cells; (2) over the apical part of the lamellar pavement cells; and (3) over the apical membrane of the pavement cells, in a way that suggests that the enzyme might operate externally. This latter localization

Table 1 Gill Lamella Morphometry (*Salmo gairdneri*) After 144 h in Deionized Water ($\phi = 8 \times 10^5\ \omega \cdot cm^{-1}$) at 21°C[a]

	Lamella area (mm^2)	Lamella thickness (μm)	Interlamellar space (μm)	Water-blood barrier thickness (μm)	
				Arith. mean	Harmonic mean
DW[b] n = 6 w = 98 ± 6	0.72 ± 0.07	14.02 ± 0.32	32.42 ± 1.72	1.64 ± 0.13	1.28 ± 0.09
FW n = 6 w = 133 ± 2	0.38 ± 0.02	15.12 ± 0.30	25.77 ± 1.09	2.44 ± 0.10	1.94 ± 0.04

[a]Deionized water was renewed twice a day (250 L/kg/12 h).
[b]All values significant, $P < 0.001$.

leads one to think that CO_2 hydration is quite instantaneous in lamellar water (Wright et al., 1986). This fact has some importance for the acid-base balance (see Heisler, 1984).

Ionic Permeability

The balance between salt loss and uptake conditions the survival of hyperosmoregulator fish (FW). Thus, if the salt uptake is relatively limited (for instance 50 $\mu Eq \cdot h^{-1} \cdot 100\ g^{-1}$ in freshwater trout; Payan et al., 1984), the total loss must be kept at the same value by regulating the branchial (and extrabranchial) permeability. This roughly indicates the order of magnitude of the branchial ionic permeability.

Evans (1984) has proposed a series of equations that quantify the interplay between salt uptake and ions loss. He states that the critical minimum salinity (value of the external salinity in which uptake is equal to loss) might be lowered by a decrease in the diffusion coefficient or in the surface area of the exchange surface, or both, to allow the fish to adapt in fresh water. There is no data establishing that the morphometry of lamellae is significantly different in animals adapted to FW or SW, albeit these parameters are very sensitive to deionized water (see under Sec. III.C). In contrast, important variability in the diffusion coefficient D, or more exactly branchial permeability to ions, D/1 (1 = diffusion path length) plays an obvious role in reducing salt efflux when euryhaline fish are transferred from SW into FW [for instance, *Anguilla anguilla*, Na^+ efflux = 1450 (SW), 48 (FW); Cl^- efflux = 1200 (SW), 3-5 (FW); *Tilapia mossambica*, Na^+ efflux = 2937 (SW), 224 (FW); *Salmo gairdneri*, Na^+ efflux = 254 (SW), 23 (FW), values expressed in $\mu mol \cdot 100\ g^{-1} \cdot hr^{-1}$] (Evans, 1984).

Several factors are known to control branchial permeability. The hypophysis is necessary for the survival of killifish in fresh water. Moreover, hypophysectomized animals injected with prolactin survive well. On the other hand, prolactin is released in larger quantity in the blood stream when tilapia are transferred in low-salinity medium (Nicol et al., 1981), a result which has been confirmed in the trout by radioimmunoassays performed with antibody raised against homologous hormone (Prunet et al., 1985). Prolactin receptors have been demonstrated by binding of ^{125}I-labeled ovine prolactin to gill tissue (Edery et al., 1984). Prolactin injection into hypophysectomized fish reduced Na^+ efflux (Potts and Evans, 1966). It has been denied that this effect was due to a stimulated mucous secretion (Marshall, 1978), as was previously believed. The ultrastructure of prolactin cells was studied in animals kept in deionized water. When this milieu is supplemented with $CaCl_2$, the survival does not exceed 40 days, with no change in the apparent stimulation of the prolactin cells, whereas if the milieu is supplemented with NaCl, 50% of the animals are still alive after 45 days. In this latter case, prolactin cells have a structure similar to control-water fish (Dubourg et al., 1983). These results, which do not depend upon external osmolarity, confirm that sodium chloride rather than calcium is the main concern in deionized water (Dubourg et al., 1983; Laurent et al., 1985) and that prolactin controls the blood ion concentrations. It has also been suggested that prolactin is able to block the initiation of gill salt excretion that normally occurs when an euryhaline fish enters seawater (Foskett et al., 1983). Thus, prolactin might have played an important role in the course of evolution during the transitional phases from seawater to fresh water and vice versa.

Epinephrine has also been studied as a factor inhibiting Na^+ and Cl^- efflux by the α-adrenergic receptors (Pic et al., 1975), an inhibition that does not depend upon hemodynamic effects of the drug (Girard, 1976). Epinephrine also inhibits the transepithelial potential across the flounder gills (Shuttleworth, 1978), the short-circuit current, and the net efflux of Cl^- (Degnan and Zadunaisky, 1979). However, all these effects are obtained with supraphysiological concentrations (10^{-6} M) in comparison with the dorsal aortic blood catecholamine levels in resting and even in stressed fish (the plasma concentration in resting and active trout: 10^{-9} M to 10^{-8} M; Ristori and Laurent, 1984). It would thus be of interest to measure the blood-borne concentrations of catecholamines and indolamines in the ventral aortic blood from fish subjected to ionic stress, i.e., before any gill binding or metabolism (see under Sec. II.C). Nevertheless, physiological or even supraphysiological ($8\ \mu g \cdot kg^{-1}$) injections of dopamine, epinephrine, and norepinephrine produce no change in serum osmolarity or in sodium and chloride concentrations, at least in the eel (Epple and Kahn, 1985).

Water Permeability

The branchial epithelium is the major site for diffusional efflux of water. Its measurement is essential because it gives an indication of the fundamental impermeability of animals inhabiting an aquatic milieu. Diffusional permeability coefficients in fishes are among the lowest in vertebrates, including amphibians. It is higher in freshwater or FW-adapted fish than in seawater or seawater-adapted fish.

The osmotic permeability is also lower in fish than in amphibians and higher in freshwater or freshwater-adapted fish (Motais et al., 1969). Consequently, and in spite of a greater osmotic gradient across the gill, osmotic and diffusional water flow are lower in sea water. It is difficult to ascertain the part played, respectively, by the filament and the lamellar epithelia for both types of permeability, although the diffusional exchanges could for obvious reasons (surface area and thinness of the epithelium), be attributed to the lamellae, whereas osmotic water flow might occur across the filament epithelium, at least in sea water, because of its leaky junctions (see under Sec. III.B).

For regulation of the osmotic water movements, a mechanism of rectification has been described (Isaia and Hirano, 1975). During the instantaneous transfer from SW to FW and vice versa, the intensity of the net fluxes measured in one direction (seromucosal) is less than that in the reverse. Arches isolated from eel or trout, adapted to either fresh or sea water, gain water during freshwater incubation faster than they lose water during a saltwater incubation in spite of a much greater gradient in sea water. The raison d'être for this regulation is to limit the branchial osmotic water flux, particularly in euryhaline species entering different milieux. Its intimate mechanism is not known.

Finally, two routes do not appear to have been explored so completely. They might disclose some interesting information about the subcellular mechanisms of permeability control. The first involves the role of the intramembranous particle aggregrates which have been described in the apical membrane of the frog urinary bladder epithelium (Chevalier et al., 1974). These submicroscopic structures are the presumed site for water flow. A preliminary report has demonstrated, by use of the freeze-fracture technique, the existence of a similar type of particle in the apical membrane of the lamellar pavement cells (Sardet, 1977; Bartels and Welsch, 1986). These studies, if continued, might allow the correlation of functional and structural states and, from there, the localization of the site of water movement. The second route involves the role played by the apical cell coat of lamellar cells in water flow control, in rectification of permeability, and in ionic movements resulting from the negative charge of the cell coat. If the mucous coat is often considered as a possible factor intervening in ionic and water exchanges, it seems possible that the glycocalix, a resistant layer of charged molecules firmly anchored in the membrane, is more responsible. As far as we know, no report has been given that concerns a specific role in gill physiology, although an ultrastructural study has been done (Pisam et al., 1980). More generally, the question of gill permeability must now be considered on a microdomain basis at different epithelial levels: apical, basolateral, and basement membrane by using tracer techniques with cationized ferritin and other electron-opaque tracers (reviewed in Herzog and Farquhar, 1983).

The Role of Calcium

The role of Ca^{2+} in gill function has been recently reviewed (Hunn, 1985). This role is many-sided. First, Ca^{2+} decreases gill permeability to water. This has been shown on isolated gill preparations (Ogawa, 1974; Wendelaar-Bonga et al., 1983; Ogasawara and Hirano, 1984) and in intact animals by measuring the urine output (Hunn, 1982; Oduleye, 1975). The high diffusional water permeability in FW fish is considered to be due to the rather low level of Ca^{2+} (approximately 1-mmol) compared with SW (approximately 10-mmol). Second, Ca^{2+} affects ionic regulation through its effect on transepithelial potential and concomitant reduction of Na^+ and Cl^- efflux (Eddy, 1975; Mac Williams and Potts, 1978; Mac Williams, 1980) and an increase of Na^+ influx (Cuthbert and Maetz, 1972, Isaia and Masoni, 1976).

The idea that Ca^{2+} may bond to microdomains of the membrane surface originated from frog skin experiments (Curran et al., 1961). It has been suggested that bound calcium might be lost from the gill epithelium by transferring fish into deionized water (Cuthbert and Maetz, 1972). Conversely, this might explain the high sodium influx rate when the fish is again transferred to water containing sodium (Eddy, 1975). Results also relate passive sodium efflux rates and low Ca^{2+} concentrations at pH < 7, whereas influx was increased only at an acidic pH. In acidified softwater ($Ca^{2+} = 0.15$ mmol) survival is less and loss of ions is much larger than in acidified hard water ($Ca^{2+} = 1$ mmol) (MacDonald et al., 1980; Brown, 1981; MacWilliams, 1982a).

Results from MacWilliams (1983) show that calcium binds to extracellular surfaces and that acidification leaches Ca^{2+} from the gill surface which, in turn, increases the rate of sodium loss from the blood by an increased permeability to Na^{+} (MacWilliams, 1982a). Another interesting set of data concerns the influence of Ca^{2+} and Na^{+} in counteracting the displacement of Ca^{2+} from its binding sites by environmental acidification (MacWilliams, 1983). By measuring $^{45}Ca^{2+}$ efflux from incubated gill arches of *Salmo trutta* in the presence of either Ca^{2+} or Na^{+}, or both, at different concentrations, the efflux curves appear to be made up of two components, suggesting that Ca^{2+} actually binds two different sites and that both Ca–Na and Ca–Ca exchanges are taking place at these sites. These two sites have different relative affinity for Ca^{2+} and Na^{+}. It was concluded from the affinity characteristics that apparently only one type is involved in the control of membrane permeability.

Recently, Flik et al. (1984a) has identified a Ca^{2+}-binding protein very similar to calmodulin in the mucus of trout, catfish, and tilapia. This calmodulin-type activity doubles in response to reduction of ambient Ca^{2+} concentration. These results suggest that gills, when transferred into soft water, are able to create a hard water environment (MacDonald and Rogano, 1984).

It could be of practical interest that an acid-tolerant strain of brown trout (adapted to a low Ca^{2+} environment) has particular calcium-binding characteristics. Surface-bound calcium is lost less rapidly in an acidic environment from the gills of this strain than from the gills of a strain inhabiting an environment high in calcium (Brown, 1981). This acquired resistance indicates that selection might help to solve the ecological problem encountered in populations of trout that have to face adverse conditions, such as very soft water subjected to acidic rainfall and snowmelt. It is noteworthy that acids have a variable ability to displace calcium from its binding sites. At the same pH, the Ca^{2+}-removing activities of the brown trout gill effluxed in deionized water fall in the order $H_2SO_4 > HNO_3 > HCl$ (HNO_3 and HCl being very close) (MacWilliams, 1983). Moreover, the addition of a small quantity of sodium is beneficial in reducing the rate of Ca^{2+} loss and in facilitating sodium uptake. All of these factors increase survival in acidic media (Brown, 1981) because of the inhibiting effect of Na^{+} on Ca^{2+} displacement from its binding sites (MacWilliams, 1983).

Gill Calcium Uptake and Regulation

It is not known if calcium bound to gill cellular membrane is directly taken up from the environment or proceeds from a preliminary internalization and depends upon calcium homeostasis.

In higher vertebrates, calcium homeostasis is achieved by a balance between intestinal absorption and renal excretion (Urist, 1976). Fish, in permanent contact with an external medium wherein calcium concentrations range from 0.01 (soft fresh water) to 20 mEq · 1^{-1} (seawater), obviously face unfavorable gradients for calcium movements either in or out of the body. Several radiotracer studies have demonstrated that the gill is the major site of calcium transport (Milhaud et al., 1977; Milet et al., 1979; Payan et al., 1981; Mugiya and Ishii, 1981). The kinetics of whole-body (Flick et al., 1986) and branchial calcium uptake in freshwater fish have been studied in relation to acclimation to various external levels (Hobe et al., 1984; Perry and Wood, 1985). Acclimation to low external calcium causes a rapid increase of J_{in}^{Ca} ; conversely acclimation to high external calcium causes a reduction of J_{in}^{Ca}. Stanniectomy increases J_{in} of seawater-adapted killifish (Pang et al., 1980). It has been suggested that the lamellar epithelium is the site for Ca^{2+} uptake rather than the filament epithelium because 95% of J_{in}^{Ca} appears in the arterioarterial circulation of the gill (Perry and Wood, 1985).

Transient or permanent proliferation of chloride cells was observed on filament and lamella epithelia as the level of sodium chloride was respectively normal (0.8 mEq · L^{-1}; Perry and Wood, 1985) or low (0.03 mEq · L^{-1}; Laurent et al., 1985). Actually, chloride cell proliferation appears to be related to plasma Na^+ and Cl^- concentrations and indirectly with Ca^{2+} concentration, the lowering of which transitorily enhances the permeability of monovalent ions (Dharmanba and Maetz, 1972). This interpretation is strengthened by the fact that supplementation of ion-poor water with NaCl but not Ca^{2+} cancels proliferation (Laurent et al., 1985). Identical results were obtained from the brown bullhead (*Ictalurus nebulosus*) a stenohaline catfish (Laurent, submitted). In young tilapia placed in low Ca^{2+} water (Ca^{2+} = 0.2 mmol), the number of chloride cells tripled in comparison with high Ca^{2+} water (Ca^{2+} = 2 mmol) (Flik et al., 1986) but in the absence of data for the plasma levels and fluxes of the monovalent ions, the origin of this proliferation remains uncertain.

For several authors (Payan et al., 1981; Mayer-Gostan et al., 1983; Flik et al., 1984) there is little doubt that chloride cells are involved in the branchial calcium uptake, an opinion that has been recently challenged (Perry and Wood, 1985; Laurent et al., 1985). According to Doneen, in *Gillichthys* (1982), and Flik et al., in tilapia (1985) and in American eel (1984b, 1985a), a high-affinity Ca^{2+}-ATPase activity, that is calmodulin sensitive, has been found in the gill plasma membrane. Obviously, this activity increases when external Ca^{2+} concentration decreases and, in addition, is stimulated during prolactin-induced hypercalcemia (Flik et al., 1984c).

Ionic Movements in Sea Water

All marine teleosts have to cope with a loss of water and a net gain of salt. The salt overload results from the saltwater intake to compensate for the osmotic water permeability of all integuments (gill, skin, fins).

H. Smith (1930) first demonstrated that a branchial salt secretion occurs against a chemical gradient in seawater fish. In addition, a net diffusional uptake may also take place but descending an electrochemical gradient. In seawater fish, the transepithelial potential (TEP) lies within the range of 20 to 30 mV (serosal side positive), values that are far below the chloride equilibrium potential and that favor its net influx. Conversely, TEP counters the sodium influx to some extent. Therefore, it might be necessary for the fish to excrete only chloride through active transport.

Owing to high gradients of ion concentration, the branchial epithelium in seawater fish appears to be more permeable to Na^+ and Cl^- than in freshwater fish. On the other hand, as already pointed out (see under Sec. III.C), its water permeability is lower. This might represent an adaptation to this medium. In elasmobranchs the ionic permeability is low, close to that of freshwater teleosts, the reason presumably being that elasmobranchs have no leaky junction such as teleost do in SW (Laurent and Dunel, 1980, and unpublished).

Numerous radioisotope studies in intact animals have demonstrated that sodium and chloride effluxes are coupled and linked with the activity of Na^+-K^+-ATPase, the efflux of Na^+ being sensitive to K^+ (Epstein et al., 1976; Kamiya and Utida, 1968) and probably localized within the chloride cell membrane (Kamya, 1972; Sargent et al., 1975) (see Trigari et al., 1985, for characterization of Na^+-K^+-ATPase). To go further, it has been necessary to use in vitro methods.

The isolated perfused head preparation was introduced by Key and coworkers in the 1930s and later used in conjunction with isotopic tracers (Tosteson et al., 1962; Kirschner, 1969). With progression from eel to trout preparations, further technical refinements were made (Payan and Mathy, 1975). Among others, a crucial improvement in the experimental design was the monitoring of hemodynamic variables (flow, resistance) and use of a perfusate that contained small concentrations of epinephrine. On the other hand, by taking advantage of better anatomical knowledge of the gill vasculature (Laurent and Dunel, 1976), Girard and Payan (1977) were able to partition the arterioarterial (lamellar) and the arteriovenous (filament) blood flow (reviewed in Perry et al., 1984).

The preparation has been used in a variety of experiments on freshwater and seawater-adapted trout. Actually, this technique suffers from several drawbacks: a rapid hemodynamic degradation, and inflow/outflow ratio much often higher than unity (edema), and large discrepancies between in vivo and in vitro effluxes of Na^+ and Cl^- (Ellis and Smith, 1983). More species should be investigated to find those that suffer less from the problems mentioned earlier (Evans et al., 1982).

Soon after the work of H. Smith (Copeland, 1948) it was thought that the chloride cell (see under Sec. III.B) was responsible for Cl^- and Na^+ effluxes in seawater and seawater-adapted fish. Indeed, the shape and density of a cellular population have been shown to correlate with the composition of the external medium (see Laurent, 1984; Hossler et al., 1985). However, localization of chloride cells within the complex structure of the gill rendered direct investigations impractical. Fortunately, morphological studies have demonstrated the presence of chloride cells in several fish integuments: the head skin (Burns and Copeland, 1950) and, later, the opercular epithelium of *Fundulus heteroclitus*, with an ultrastructure identical with that of the chloride cells of the gill epithelium (Karnaky and Kinter, 1977). This flat opercular epithelium allowed the physiologist to investigate the chloride cell function in conditions comparable with those used with other epithelia according to the method developed some years ago by Ussing and coworkers.

In the opercular epithelium of saltwater killifish, 50 to 70% of the lining is composed of chloride cells. Other lining components consist of mucous cells and pavement cells organized in such a way that there is little difference from that of gill filament epithelium. Several layers of "nondifferentiated" cells intermingle with chloride cells and mucous cells. Generally, chloride cells rest on the epithelial basement membrane. Many aspects of this organization have not yet been fully explored. Another feature that is not well documented concerns the vascular system, the function of which is essential to an efficient blood clearance. Similar to the filament epithelium, the opercular epithelium is vascularized by an arteriovenous system, the hemodynamic control of which is unknown.

The opercular epithelium technique has led to clear conclusions concerning the branchial salt secretion (Degnan and Zadunaisky, 1982). The opercular skin is placed in a Ussing-type chamber, bathed on both of its sides with a Ringer solution isotonic with the plasma. In this condition, the epithelium develops a TEP difference negatively oriented in the seromucosal directions (Degnan et al., 1977). This TEP is the result of a net outward transport of Cl^-, with no net transport of Na^+ (Karnaky et al., 1977). It has been shown that chloride cells are the site of this ion transport by demonstrating that cell density correlates with the amplitude of the short-circuit current (SCC) generated by the preparation during Cl^- secretion (Karnaky et al., 1979, 1984). Finally, recent utilization of the vibrating probe method invented by Frömter (1972) has clearly demonstrated that the maximum current generated by a short-circuited opercular preparation clearly corresponds with the apical pit of the chloride cell (Foskett and Scheffey, 1982).

Other studies validate these results for species having similar localization of chloride cells: opercular epithelium of *Sarotherodon mossambicus* (Foskett et al., 1979, 1981), jaw epithelium of *Gillichthys mirabilis* (Marshall and Bern, 1980; Marshall and Nishioka, 1980).

In such preparations, Na^+ fluxes are passive and presumably pass up the leaky junction between the chloride cell and accessory cell (Dunel and Laurent, 1973; Sardet, 1979; Ernst et al., 1980; Hootman and Philpott, 1980; Laurent and Dunel, 1980; Dunel-Erb and Laurent, 1980). Indeed the sodium permeability of the chloride-accessory cell complex is one of the largest that has yet been measured in epithelia (reviewed by Foskett et al., 1983). However, one must remember that the conclusions drawn from the opercular epithelium method, which encompasses only a limited number of species, may be nonvalid for the whole group of marine teleosts, particularly for those species that maintain Na^+ out of an electrochemical gradient (Evans, 1982b).

Nervous and Hormonal Control

If we set aside the neuro- and neurohumoral control of the branchial hemodynamics (see Humoral Factors under Sec. II.C), few papers are strictly concerned with neurocontrol of the epithelia. Transection of the ninth and tenth cranial nerves in the eel brings about a slow demineralization in freshwater-adapted eel that results from an excess loss of Na^+ and Cl^-. On the other hand, the denervated eels are not able to withstand a transfer to seawater because the fish do not drink, and the mechanism for efflux of Na^+ ceases to function. Thus, the integrity of the glossopharyngeal and vagus nerves is necessary for the maintenance of hydromineral balance in seawater. Denervation is followed by an increase in plasma ion concentrations. Sodium fluxes are not modified, and there is no increase of the drinking rate to compensate for osmotic water loss. An interesting hypothesis would be that the sensory pathways afferent to osmoregulatory central machinery are disconnected and that peripheral receptors are unable to send their messages (Mayer-Gostan and Hirano, 1976). In this context, pseudobranchial afferent innervation might represent the afferent limb of such reflexes (Laurent and Rouzeau, 1972).

The hormonal control of the gill is difficult to study in vitro or in vivo because of the interplay of hemodynamic and epithelial effects. When sodium and chloride movements are considered, it again appears to be appropriate to use opercular epithelium or any other type of chloride cell-rich tissue.

The role played by epinephrine and norepinephrine has been discussed earlier (see Humoral Factors under Sec. II.C) (see also Foskett et al., 1982a). Cyclic AMP increases chloride secretion in chloride cells as in other chloride-secreting epithelia. Phosphodiesterase inhibition increases the cAMP level and stimulates a short-circuit current. Other hormones, such as glucagon and vasoactive intestinal peptide (VIP), stimulate chloride secretion through an intracellular increase of cAMP (see Foskett, 1983, for discussion on mechanisms of hormonal action).

Cortisol, the major corticosteroid in fish, restores sodium efflux in the interrenalectomized eel and enhances NA^+-K^+-ATPase (review by Maetz, 1974). It increases the number of chloride cells and stimulates their differentiation, but it is unable to initiate chloride secretion in freshwater fish (Foskett et al., 1981). Cortisol is present in high concentration in smolts (Leloup-Hatey, 1964). In this juvenile form of *Salmo salar*, it is thought to participate in some preadaptation to gill marine environment, but it does not directly stimulate gill N+-K^+-ATPase (Langhorne and Simpson, 1986). In *Salmo gairdneri*, it has been shown that cortisol affects neither branchial Na^+-K^+-ATPase nor the number of chloride cells (Eib and Hossner, 1985), whereas in tilapia, the stimulatory effect of cortisol on gill Na^+-K^+-ATPase was further elevated by thyroxine and was greater in saltwater-adapted than in freshwater-adapted fish (Dange, 1986). Thus, cortisol by itself is unable to induce gill salt secretion in freshwater fish.

In juvenile salmonids there is a correlation between thyroid hormone, gill (Na^+-K^+-ATPase, and salinity tolerance, along with development and smoltification (Boeuf and Prunet, 1984). Actually T_4 seems to depress gill Na^+-K^+-ATPase (Dickhoft et al., 1982), whereas T_3 enhances activity of this enzyme (Omeljanink and Eales, 1986).

It has often been proposed that prolactin, the so-called freshwater-adapting hormone, is the hormone that switches off the gill salt secretion (reviewed in Foskett et al., 1983; Hirano, 1986). For instance, it has been suggested that prolactin "removes" chloride cells from the opercular epithelium in seawater-adapted tilapia because prolactin decreases both short-circuit current and membrane conductance (Foskett et al., 1982b). This "removing" action might be assumed from dedifferentiation, reduction of size and number, or by blocking the differentiation of new chloride cells and lysis of accessory cells (in other words, disappearance of the leaky junction). In seawater-adapted trout retransferred into freshwater, a condition that stimulates prolactin secretion (Prunet et al., 1985), chloride cells lose their apical contact with the external milieu within a few hours, and later on, accessory cells are no longer visible (Laurent and Dunel, 1980; and unpublished). All of these operations are rapid because it has been reported that chloride cells start developing or degenerating a leaky junction within 3 h after transfer from FW to SW, and vice versa (Hwang and Hirano, 1985).

IV. Gill Adaptation and Maladaptation

From what has been presented throughout this review, it is obvious that gills adapt to the total physiological demand of the whole organism to fulfill their proper functions, i.e., gas, ions, and waste products transfer, to keep this organism in equilibrium. But the word "adaptation" should be specified and deserves some comment. Adaptation is involved each time new physiological conditions that depart substantially from those preceding successfully induce morphological and biochemical transformations that allow the organism to reach a new equilibrium. Nevertheless, the boundary between regulation and adaptation remains uncertain. One piece of unquestionable evidence is morphological, when gills show permanent changes in shape and organization without any ultrastructural disorder. For instance, gills might adapt by an increase of exchange surface area, proliferation of cell types, or different distribution of cell organelles.

Maladaptation is concerned in situations that stimulate inadequate regulation or regulation that is adequate from one standpoint but is totally inadequate from another, e.g., the gill secretion of mucus as a protective layer against ion loss but in doing so impedes gas exchanges.

The gill might also respond by adaptation to limited noxious factors, for instance, xenobiotics under their threshold of toxicity. Beyond this limit, which might be variable with species or in the presence of other factors, the gill undergoes reversible or irreversible damages that make it unable to fulfill its functions.

A. Hypoxia

Hypoxia is a common situation encountered in the wild when the oxidation of organic matter consumes more oxygen that that transferred from the atmosphere or delivered by photosynthesis. Such a situation might occur with the release in bulk of sewage and made still worse by elevated temperatures.

Permanent hypoxia in certain areas or during certain geological periods explains the occurrence in a number of species of respiratory adaptation to bimodal breathing. These species developed, besides the gill, aerian respiratory organs or modify the gills to transfer atmospheric oxygen (reviewed in Dutta and Datta Munshi, 1985). Fish that have developed lungs, for instance, present modified gills that are better adapted to efficiently transfer carbon dioxide or ions than oxygen (Laurent et al., 1978).

Functionally speaking, hypoxia consists mainly in an excessive reduction of the ambient oxygen partial pressure. Then the water-blood O_2 gradient decreases in such a way that the gill O_2 uptake becomes diffusion-limited. This situation departs from the normoxic one wherein gill oxygen transfer is, rather, perfusion-limited (Scheid and Piiper, 1976; Malte and Weber, 1985). Long-term hypoxic gill adaptation might consist of changes in the parameter values for the well-known Fick's diffusion law (Piiper et al., 1971; Piiper and Scheid, 1982) wherein morphometric data are considered. The effective gill-diffusing capacity values can be estimated (Scheid et al., 1986), in additon to a rather approximate Krogh' constant of permeability, from the gill surface area (direct proportionality) and the length of the diffusive water-blood pathway (thickness of the barrier: inverse proportionality).

During acute or short-term hypoxia, a significant decrease of the blood-water barrier thickness has been reported, whereas the vascular space/tissue ratio increases (Soivio and Tuurala, 1981). The origin of these changes is still unclear and, rather, might be related to some hemodynamic adjustment of blood pressure than an adaptative morphological change.

A recruitment of lamellae that are nonperfused in resting and well-oxygenated fish can afford a large increase in diffusing capacity when the milieu becomes hypoxic (see Randall and Daxboeck, 1984). A shunting pathway switch-off, which drives the blood closer to the exchange surfaces, during hypoxia has also been considered (Pärt et al., 1984) and questioned (Laurent, 1985b). [Gill anatomical shunts exist in the lungfish *Protopterus* and *Lepidosiren* (Laurent et al., 1978) where they serve to augment the lung circulation. When the fish is surfacing to breath air, the shunts are closed. Conversely, during the periods of submersion the shunts are open. The blood flows through the gill lamellae mainly for CO_2 excretion. Then blood bypasses the lung circulation and goes directly through the open ductus arteriosus into the systemic circulatory system (Laurent, 1981; Fishman et al., 1985)]. An enlargement of the respiratory units (lamellae) has also been suggested, which should be the most direct evidence for a long-term adaptive modification in response to hypoxia. However, no conclusive results are yet available. Such an adaptation seems contradictory with the conclusion drawn from comparative morphometry data in trout, an oxiphilic fish, and in catfish, a species tolerating poorly oxygenated milieux. The measured O_2-diffusing capacity is much higher in the former as is the calculated diffusing capacity. Trout have a much larger gill surface (240 $mm^2 \cdot g^{-1}$) than catfish (150 $mm^2 \cdot g^{-1}$) and a thinner blood-water barrier (6 versus 10 μm; Hughes, 1972). Thus, the morphometric scaling of the gill is probably more related to the scope of activity (O_2 requirement) than to characteristics of the milieu (O_2 availability). This point needs additional investigation.

B. Exercise

Exercise has recently been investigated in an effort to demonstrate its possible effect on gill structure and function. Whereas morphometric data have not yet shown any evidence of adaptative changes, it appears that a long-term (6 weeks) but moderate training of rainbow trout (swimming at a constant speed of one body length per second) increases the growth rate twice as much as that of resting fish and markedly improves the swimming performance (exhaustion time). The protein synthesis rate is much higher in the gill than in any other tissue (heart, red muscle, white muscle excepted), whereas the protein deposition is very low in the gill compared with other tissues. In trained fish, protein synthesis is not affected in the gill, but it increases significantly in other tissues. This means that the turnover rate of protein is exceptionally high in the gill but is not related to an adaptation to exercise. The fate of the synthetized and degraded proteins in gills is still unknown (Houlihan et al., 1986; Houlihan and Laurent, 1987).

C. Salinity

Adaptation of gills to seawater has been extensively described in this paper. The discussion mainly concerns euryhaline species transferred from SW into FW, and vice versa. We just remind the reader that hyperosmotic or hypoosmotic adaptations have manyfold facets. From a morphological viewpoint, they consist in meaningful changes in chloride cell organization, in alteration of Na^+-K^+-ATPase activity, and in biophysical modifications related to diffusional and osmotic permeabilities, transepithelial potentials, and the resulting ion fluxes.

On the other hand, gill adaptation to ion-poor water has raised recent questions, probably because of the close relationships between soft water and acid pollution. Less-buffered, ion-poor waters are dramatically sensitive to acid. Actually, fresh waters are much more variable in ion concentration than is seawater. Some of them are poor in calcium but have a rather elevated NaCl concentration and, conversely, some are rich in calcium but almost devoid of NaCl. Other types are close to deionized water. In terms of adaptive changes, fish may have to face completely different ionic problems.

In rainbow trout transferred to low-Ca^{2+} (25 μmol) low-NaCl (60 μmol) pH 7.5, the whole-body net Na^+ and Cl^- losses (but not Ca^{2+}) occur at a high rate during the first hours of exposure and at a slower rate thereafter. Such losses represent a significant part of the total body content and contribute to a temporary decline of the plasma Na^+ level and a permanent deficit of Cl^-. If the NaCl environmental concentration is higher, the plasma levels remain steady, suggesting a threshold below which there is no possibility of maintaining the ionic balance. As shown by unidirectional flux measurements, the compensatory reduction of whole-body ion losses is mainly of branchial origin and results both from decline in branchial effluxes and from the subsequent increase in Na^+ and Cl^- inward transport (MacDonald and Rogano, 1986).

Proliferation of chloride cells occurs during low ambient NaCl concentrations, irrespective of the Ca^{2+} concentration that probably represents an adaptative increase in the number of transport sites and basically the support of increased Cl^- and Na^+ inward transport (Laurent et al., 1985).

According to MacDonald and Rogano (1986), urine flow, which is directly related to branchial water permeability, increases at the beginning of the transfer period and subsequently returns to a hard water level. This suggests a progressive restoration of the relative gill water impermeability. Interesting, chelation of gill surface-bound Ca^{2+} by EDTA (2 mmol) increases the ionic permeability both in hard and soft water, but this effect is relatively smaller in soft water, suggesting an increased branchial Ca^{2+} binding (MacDonald and Rogano, 1986).

Adaptation to soft water exposure ($Ca^{2+} < 0.4$ mmol) is probably hormonally controlled. Prolactin is known as one of the hormones concerned. The prolactin effects on gills are manyfold and have already been described. Stimulation of hypophyseal prolactin cells as a response to deionized water occurs in some species such as stickelbacks and tilapia (Wendelaar-Bonga and Greven, 1978; Wendelaar-Bonga and Van der Meij, 1981), whereas stimulation of periodic acid-Schiff (PAS)-positive (or so-called "calcium-sensitive") pars intermedia cells occurs in eel and goldfish (Olivereau et al., 1980; Olivereau and Olivereau, 1982). More recent studies have shown that PAS-positive cells do not seem to be involved in ion regulation as a response to acidification in tilapia, but they are in goldfish in which they probably have hypercalcemic activity (Wendelaar-Bonga et al., 1984).

D. Acid Stress

Water acidity develops mainly in an ion-poor environment, particularly when the Ca^{2+} concentration is low (reviewed in Beament et al., 1984). Chester (1984) has classified the Norwegian lakes as fishless and populated ones. It is clear that acidity correlates calcium concentration and that fishless lakes correspond to low pH and low Ca^{2+}.

As pointed out by Wood and MacDonald (reviewed, 1982), fish in acid water have to face three physiological problems: respiratory distress, ionoregulatory failure, and acid-base imbalance. The branchial permeability to protons is very high and passive entry of H^+ occurs along a concentration gradient. A blockade of acid secretion would result from inhibition of Na^+-H^+ and Na^+-$NH_3 + H^+$ exchanges (probably because of competition of H^+ and Na^+ on the transport sites). Elevation of passive permeability of branchial epithelia to Na^+, K^+, Cl^- results from displacement of membrane-bound Ca^{2+} by acids which, in turn, favors an entry of H^+. This effect is interpreted as evidence that calcium controls the access of sodium and chloride to their exchange sites (Cuthbert and Maetz, 1972; MacDonald and Rogano, 1986). All of these mechanisms might account for ionic and acid-base disturbances. In addition, it has been suggested that plasma pH shifts have indirect effects on the hemogloblin dissociation curve via a Bohr and Root shift, with hypoxia as a consequence (Packer and Dunson, 1970). This assumption has been verified in carp at pH 3.5 but not at higher pH values (Ultsch et al., 1981). Nevertheless, severe respiratory problems are observed even in O_2-tolerant species, such as the sucker, when transferred into acidic soft water (Hobe et al., 1984b).

Mucous secretion is increased during acid exposure below pH 5.6 and becomes quite dramatic at pH 4 and lower (reviewed in MacDonald, 1983). The mucous layer creates a diffusion barrier that slows down ion losses (Hobe et al., 1983) but also represents an unstirred layer hampering gas exchanges (Ultsch et al., 1980). The resulting benefit of bulk secretion of mucus at low pH is unclear, and the response might be nonadaptative because it might also impair ionic influxes at the same time.

In soft water it has clearly been seen that fish surviving the "acid toxicity syndrome" show branchial compensation of acidosis with progressive reduction in Na^+ and Cl^- loss and of concomitant uptake of H^+ and progressive increase of NH_4 excretion. The origin of this compensation is still unclear (Wood and MacDonald, 1982) but probably does not result simply from a reduction in branchial permeability, because Na^+ and Cl^- outfluxes were not similarly adjusted (Hobe et al., 1984). It has been shown that gill Na^+-K^+-ATPase and gill carbonic anhydrase are increased after several days at lower pH (MacKeown et al., 1985). This increase is higher in trout than in sucker, a difference that might account for a better ability to limit ion plasma alteration at low pH in the latter, whereas white sucker is more tolerant to water acidity and does not regulate as many plasma electrolytes (Hobe et al., 1983).

The gill structure in acid-stressed fish has been the subject of a limited number of field and laboratory studies. First, light microscopic histopathological study shows that gills (*Salvelinus fontinalis*) are the most sensitive of exposed surfaces to short-term acid exposure (Daye and Garside, 1976). The threshold values are variable with the species: pH 5.2 in *S. fontinalis* (Daye and Garside, 1976), pH 4 in *S. alpinus* (Jagoe and Haines, 1983).

Electron microscopy after long-term acid exposure (pH 5.5 to 5) of the fathead minnows (*Pimephales promelas*) (Leino and Mac Cormick, 1984) shows an increase in the number of chloride cells on the filament epithelium and occurrence of these cells on the lamellar epithelium. Strange, indeed, is the appearance of chloride cells with an apical crypt, usually seen in marine fish but never observed in freshwater teleosts (Laurent, 1984). Nevertheless, the frequency of these changes correlates with acidity level morphometrically. The experimental fish in the study of Leino and MacCormick seemed to be healthy and did not reveal any altered or necrotic structure.

On the contrary, comparative field observations of brook trout caught from acidified (pH 5.5 to 5.2) and nonacidified (pH 6.8 to 7) lakes of the Laurentide Park (Canada) revealed that, in the latter stations (both have around 150 $\mu Eq \cdot L^{-1}$ Ca^{2+}), trout have extensively damaged gills with separation of epithelial layers, lysis of chloride cells, and hyperplasic interlamellar filament epithelium. No accumulation of mucus is detected at this pH (Chevalier et al., 1985).

In the sucker (*Catostomus commersoni*), a freshwater stenohaline species, collected from an acid softwater lake, pH 5.3, and transferred at a lower pH (4) for various periods (up to several weeks), gills do not present any kind of deterioration but, rather, change in the distribution and abundance of mucous and chloride cells. Mucous cell proliferation is particularly important in sucker collected from natural soft water and then exposed for 24 h to the same but acidified water (pH 4.2) (Hobe, 1985; Hobe and Laurent, unpublished). This mucous secretion might be at the origin of severe respiratory problems (Hobe et al., 1984b).

From all of these observations, it might be concluded that the gill morphological response to acid stress is linked to (1) an indirect limitation of Na^+ uptake, which in turn induces a chloride cell proliferation in a way similar to that of fish living in ion-poor water (Laurent et al., 1985); this response should be considered adaptative; (2) an activation of the mucous cell populations, especially in stenohaline species in which they probably act as a protective barrier preventing gill damage. The other symptoms are destructive and do not implicate any form of adaptive process. Damages are reversible, if exposure time and level of acidity are limited. However, and especially in salmonids, destructive effects are so rapidly irreversible that tentative acclimation to low pH has been widely unsuccessful (MacDonald, 1983).

Nevertheless, it is known that certain species are more tolerant than others in acidic water. An Amazonian fish (*Cherodon axelrodi*) is able to withstand pH 3.5 for an indefinite period owing to a particular resistance of its gill ion regulation to acid (Dunson et al., 1977). Another example is the common perch (*Perca fluviatilis*). This species is able to live and to reproduce in humic acid-rich water (peat bog), an ability that might result from a nonacid-sensitive Na^+ transport and low diffusional permeability of gill epithelia (MacWilliams, 1982b).

E. Xenobiotics

The factors hitherto mentioned are, more or less, linked to natural events. We now must briefly consider the most recent results concerning the toxicity of substances that have no relationship with life: xenobiotics (Rankin et al., 1982).

In addition to acid deposition, which has been treated separately, two categories of xenobiotics are of concern within this chapter: metal ions and detergents. Many other noxious substances that are not relevant to these groups accumulate in gills (Gluth et al., 1985). However, we will limit our topic to substances known to interact with gill functions.

The gill uptake of metal ions is often rapid and leads to huge accumulations within the gills (and other tissues as well). Gill cadmium might reach 1000 times the environmental concentration (Sangalang and Freeman, 1979). Metals generally bind particular proteins that regulate their intracellular homeostasis and reduce toxic effects (Thomas et al., 1985). These effects consist in alteration of the main functions of gill: respiration, acid-base regulation, and ion regulation.

Zinc, at elevated doses ($>$ 1.5 ppm), is known to disrupt gill tissues. The result is an irreversible inhibition of gas transfer (hypoxemia) and lactate accumulation (Skidmore and Tovel, 1972; Spry and Wood, 1984). At a lower concentration (0.8 ppm), and particularly in soft water-reared rainbow trout, a small rise of lactate is observed without a decrease of PaO_2. A rise of $PaCO_2$ is also observed, an effect that might be related to carbonic anhydrase inhibition. The net branchial uptake of Na^+ and Cl^- in control animals, becomes net losses after Zn exposure, with concomitant stimulation of both influx and efflux. An increase in chloride cell number is observed (Tuurala and Soivio, 1982). Ammonia excretion and base loss are stimulated. Net Ca^{2+} uptake is abolished, and K^+ loss is considerably augmented. However, neither the resulting acidemia nor ion disturbances might explain the observed mortality. Thus, the nature of the lethal mechanism is still unclear (Spry and Wood, 1985).

The gill is the first target organ affected by copper. At the very low concentration of 12.5 ppb, it causes Na^+, Cl^-, K^+ losses whatever the water pH and hardness. At higher concentration (50 ppb) NaCl losses appear to be due to influx inhibition, and at high concentrations, a stimulation of efflux occurs. Interestingly, influx inhibition is less pronounced in soft water, an effect that might be related to the proliferation of chloride cells (the presumable site for NaCl uptake, Laurent et al., 1985, see under Sec. III.C). Plasma glucose and ammonia correlate with copper concentration. Adaptation to copper might possibly occur in juvenile trout by an increase in copper-binding protein. Adaptation might also be induced by recovery of branchial epithelium, including enhancement of transport enzymes and chloride cell proliferation (Lauren and MacDonald, 1985).

Cadmium severely affects gills from *Fundulus* exposed at lethal concentrations (Gardner and Yevich, 1970) with formation of edema in lamellae, impairing diffusion capacity. Some synergy appears to occur between cadmium and surfactants, some of them increasing the gill transfer of cadmium (anionic surfactant). On a perfused gill preparation, analysis of synergy indicates that nonionic surfactant, when associated with cadmium, increases Na^+ efflux more than cadmium or any surfactant alone (Pärt et al., 1985). The mechanisms of the synergy are still unclear, although some of them include chemical interactions: i.e., binding of Cd by detergents. Anionic detergent alone at relatively high concentration affects the histochemically evaluated activity of gill respiratory enzymes in association with severe deterioration of the gill organization (Zaccone et al., 1985; see also Mommsen, 1984, for biochemical characterization or gill enzymes).

Aluminium is known to be toxic in certain circumstances. For instance, survival of brown trout fry to aluminium exposure decreases when environmental calcium decreases and pH increases. This suggests that the physiological effects of aluminium might be correlated with the functioning of gill ionoregulation (Brown, 1983). However, the formation of nontoxic or nonpenetrating aluminium complexes in environmental water renders any attempt to simply consider its local concentration as a factor of survival very doubtful.

Finally, an interesting problem is raised by the action of nitrite on gills. It is known that nitrite accumulates in fish organs through the gill (Bath and

Eddy, 1980). The toxicity of nitrite is due to formation of methemoglobin: for instance, 1 ppm NO_2N gives rise to 20.7% methemoglobin in *Ictalurus punctatus* (Tomasso et al., 1979). In addition, a hepatotoxicity develops as a consequence of tissular anoxia and also possible interaction with the amino and thio groups of membrane proteins (Arillo et al., 1984; Margiocco et al., 1983). Protective effects are observed when salts are added to the milieu ($CaCO_3$, NaCl, $CaCl_2$), as well as at high pH. Thus, seawater adaptation renders salmon fivefold more resistant (Crawford and Allen, 1977). It has been suggested that NO_2^- competes with Cl^- in the uptake of Cl^- in the gill epithelium of freshwater fish (Bath and Eddy, 1980). A proliferation of chloride cells, similar to what occurs in low NaCl (Laurent and Dunel, 1980; Laurent et al., 1985), is observed in the presence of 0.45 mg · L^{-1} NO_2N. The proliferation is interpreted as an increased activity of chloride cells, the Cl^--HCO_3^- exchange sites being predominantly occupied by NO_2^-. In addition, carbonic anhydrase, which yields the counterion HCO_3^-, is inhibited by nitrite: an additional problem for salt uptake. Curiously, however, no decline in plasma Cl^- is observed (Gaino et al., 1984).

References

Arillo, A., Gaino, E., Margiocco, C., Mensi, P., and Schenone, G. (1984). Biochemical and ultrastructural effects of nitrite on rainbow trout: Liver hypoxia at the root of the acute toxicity mechanism. *Environ. Res. 34*: 135-154.

Avella, M. (1986). Role des cellules à chlorure de la lame secondaire danss l'-entrée branchiale de sodium chez la truite d'eau douce. Importance de l'échange Na^+/H^+. *In thèse 3ème cycle, cytologie.* Univ. de Nice.

Bailly, Y. (1983). Recherches sur quelques innervations dans la branchie des poissons – *Thesis (Cytology)* Univ. P. et M. Curie, Paris.

Bailly, Y., and Dunel-Erb, S. (1986). The sphincter of the efferent filament artery in teleost gills, I: structure and parasympathetic innervation. *J. Morphol. 187*:219-237.

Ballintijn, C. M. (1985). The respiratory function of the gill filament muscles in the carp. *Resp. Physiol. 60*:59-74.

Bartels, H., and Decker, B. (1985). Communicating junctions between pillar cells in the gills of the Atlantic hagfish, *Myxine glutinosa. Experientia 41*:1039-1040.

Bartels, H., and Welsch, V. (1986). Mitochondria-rich cells in the gill epithelium of cyclostomes. A thin section and freeze fracture study. In *Indo-Pacific Fish Biology: Proceedings of the Second International Conference on Indo-Pacific Fishes*, pp. 58-72.

Bath, R. N., and Eddy, F. B. (1980). Transport of nitrite across fish gills. *J. Exp. Zool. 214*:119-121.

Beaument, J., Broadhaw, A. D., Chester, P. F., Holgate, M. W., Sugden, M., and Trush, B. A. (1984). Ecological effects of deposited sulphur and nitrogen compounds. *Phil. Trans. R. Soc. Lond. B. 305*:255-577.

Boeuf, G., and Prunet, P. (1985). Measurement of gill (Na+/K+) ATPase activity and plasma thyroid hormones during smoltification in Atlantic salmon (*Salmo salar* L.). *Aquaculture 45*:11-119.

Bornancin, M., Isaia, J., and Masoni, A. (1985). A re-examination of the technique of isolated perfused trout head preparation. *Comp. Biochem. Physiol. 81A*:35-41.

Brown, D. J. A. (1981). The effects of various cations on the survival of brown trout, *Salmo trutta*, at low pH's. *J. Fish. Biol. 18*:31-40.

Brown, D. J. A. (1983). Effect of calcium and aluminium concentrations on the survival of brown trout, *Salmo trutta*, at low pH. *Bull. Environ. Contamin. Toxicol. 30*:582-587.

Burns, J., and Copeland, D. E. (1950). Chloride excretionin the head region of *Fundulus heteroclitus. Biol. Bull. Mar. Biol. Lab. Woods Hole 99*:381-385.

Cameron, J. N. (1986). Responses to reversed NH_3 and NH_4 gradients in a teleost (*Ictalurus ponctatus*), and elasmobranch (*Raya erinacea*), and a crustacean (*Callinectes sapidus*): Evidence for NH_4^+/H^+ exchange in the teleost and the elasmobranch. *J. Exp. Zool. 239*:183-195.

Cameron, J. N., and Heisler, N. (1983). Studies of ammonia in the rainbow trout: Physico-chemical parameters, acid-base behaviour and respiratory clearance. *J. Exp. Biol. 105*:107-125.

Chester, P. F. (1984). (General discussion). *Phil. Trans. R. Soc. Lond. B. 305*: 565.

Chevalier, J., Bourguet, J., and Huguon, J. S. (1974). Membrane-associated particles: Distribution in frog urinary bladder epithelium at rest and after oxytoxin treatment. *Cell Tissue Res. 152*:129-140.

Chevalier, J., Pinto da Silva, P., Ripoche, P., Gobin, R., Wang, X., Grossette, J., and Bourguet, J. (1985). Structural and cytochemical differentiation of membrane of amphibian urinary bladder epithelial cells. A label fracture study. *Biol Cell 55*:181-190.

Chevalier, G., Gauthier, L., and Moreau, G. (1985). Histopathological and electron microscopic studies of gills of brook trout, *Salvelinus fontinalis*, from acidified lakes. *Can. J. Zool. 63*:2062-2087.

Chretien, M., and Pisam, M. (1986). Cell renewal and differentiation in the gill epithelium of fresh- or salt-water-adapted euryhaline fish as revealed by [^{3}H] thymidine radioautography. *Biol. Cell 56*:137-150.

Claude, P., and Goodenough, D. A. (1973). Fracture faces of zonulae occludentes from "tight" and leaky epithelia. *J. Cell Biol. 58*:390-400.

Copeland, D. E. (1948). The cytology of secretory cells of *Fundulus heteroclitus. J. Morph. 82*:201-218.

Crawford, R. E., and Allen, G. H. (1977). Seawater inhibition of nitrite toxicity to chinook salmon. *Trans. Am. Fish. Soc. 106*:105-109.

Curran, P. F., Zadunaisky, J., and Gill, J. R. (1961). The effect of ethylenediamine tetraacetate on ion permeability of the isolated frog skin. *Biochim. Biophys. Acta 52*:392-395.

Cuthbert, A. W., and Maetz, J. (1972). The effects of calcium and magnesium on sodium fluxes through the gills of *Carassius auratus* (L.). *J. Physiol. 221*: 633-643.

Dange, A. D. (1986). Branchial Na+/K+ ATPase activity in freshwater or saltwater acclimated tilapia, *Oreochromis (Sarotherodon) mossambicus*: Effects of cortisol and thyroxine. *Gen. Comp. Endocrinol. 62*:341-343.

Dashow, L., and Epple, A. (1985). Plasma catecholamines in the lamprey: Intrinsic cardiovascular messengers. *Comp. Biochem. Physiol. 82C*:119-122.

Daye, P. G., and Garside, E. T. (1976). Histopathologic changes in superficial tissues of brook trout *Salvelinus fontinalis* (Mitchill) exposed to acute and chronic levels of pH. *Can. J. Zool. 54*:2140-2155.

De Vries, R., and De Jagger, S. (1984). The gill of the spiny dogfish, *Squalus acanthias*: Respiratory and nonrespiratory function. *Am. J. Anat. 169*: 1-29.

Degnan, K. J., and Zadunaisky, J. A. (1979). Open-circuit sodium and chloride fluxes across isolated opercular epithelia from the teleost *Fundulus heteroclitus. J. Physiol. (Lond.) 294*:483-495.

Degnan, K. J., and Zadunaisky, J. A. (1982). The opercular epithelium: An experimental model for teleost gill osmoregulation and chloride secretion. In *Chloride transport in biological membranes*. Edited by J. A. Zadunaisky, New York, Academic Press, pp. 215-318.

Degnan, K. J., Karnaky, K. J., and Zadunaisky, J. A. (1977). Active chloride transport in the in vitro opercular skin of the teleost *Fundulus heteroclitus*, a gill like epithelium rich in chloride cells. *J. Physiol. (Lond.) 271*: 155-191.

Dharmamba, M., and Martz, J. (1972). Effects of hypophysectomy and prolactin on the sodium balance of *Tilapia mossambica* in fresh water. *Gen. Comp. Endocrinol. 19*:175-183.

Dickhoft, W. W., Folmer, L. C., and Gorbman, A. (1982). Thyroid function during smoltification of salmonid fish. In *Phylogenic Aspects of Thyroid Hormone Actions*, Vol. 19. Gunna Symposium on Endocrinology. Acad. Pub. Tokyo, pp. 45-62.

Donald, J. A. (1984). Adrenergic innervation of the gills of brown and rainbow trout, *Salmo trutta* and *S. gairdneri. J. Morphol. 182*:307-316.

Donald, J. A., and Ellis, A. G. (1983). Arterio-venous anastomoses in the gills of Australian short-finned eel, *Anguilla australis. J. Morphol. 178*:89-93.

Doneen, B. A. (1981). Effects of adaptation to sea water, 170% sea water and to fresh water on activities and subcellular distribution of branchial NA^+/

K^+/ATPase, low and high affinity Ca^{2+}/ATPase, and ouabain insensitive ATPase in *Gillichthys mirabilis. J. Comp. Physiol. 145*:51-61.

Dubourg, P., Chambolle, P., Kah, O., Maïza, S., and Olivereau, M. (1983). Ultrastructure des cellules à prolactine et survie de *Gambusia* sp. (Poisson téléostéen) en eau désionisée enrichie en calcium ou en sodium. *Gen. Comp. Endocrinol. 50*:432-444.

Dunel, S. (1975). Contribution à l'étude structurale et ultrastructurale de la pseudobranchie et de son innervation chez les Téléostéens. DSc thesis, Univ. Louis Pasteur, Strasbourg.

Dunel, S., and Laurent, P. (1973). Ultrastructure comparée de la psuedobranchie chez les Téléostéens marins et d'eau douce. *J. Microsc. (Paris) 16*:53-74.

Dunel, S., and Laurent, P. (1977). La vascularisation branchiale chez l'anguille: Action de l'acétylcholine et de l'adrenaline sur la répartition d'une résine polymérisable dans les différents compartiments vasculaires. *C. R. Hebd. Séances Acad. Sci. 284*:2011-2014.

Dunel, S., and Laurent, P. (1980). Functional organization of the gill vasculature in different classes of fish. In *Epithelial Transport in the Lower Vertebrates*. Edited by B. Lahlou. Cambridge, Cambridge University Press, pp. 37-58.

Dunel-Erb, S., and Bailly, V. (1986). The sphincter of the efferent filament artery in teleost gills.II: Sympathetic innervation. *J. Morphol. 187*:239-246.

Dunel-Erb, S., and Bailly, V. (1987). Smooth muscles in relation to the gill skeleton of *Perca fluviatilis*: Organization and innervation. *Cell Tissue Res. 247*:339-350.

Dunel-Erb, S., Bailly, Y., and Laurent, P. (1982). Neuroepithelial cells in fish gill primary lamellae. *J. Appl. Physiol. 53*:1342-1353.

Dunel-Erb, S., and Laurent, P. (1980). Ultrastructure of marine teleost gill epithelia: SEM and TEM study of chloride cell apical membrane. *J. Morphol. 165*:175-186.

Dunson, W. A., Swarts, F., and Silvestri, M. (1977). Exceptional tolerance to low pH of some tropical blackwater fish. *J. Exp. Zool. 201*:157-162.

Dutta, H. M., and Datta-Munshi, J. S. (1985). Functional morphology of air breathing fishes: A review. *Proc. Acad. Sci. Indian-Anim. Sci. 94*:359-375.

Eddy, F. B. (1975). The effect of calcium on gill potentials and on sodium and chloride fluxes in the goldfish *Carassius auratus. J. Comp. Physiol. 96*: 131-142.

Edery, M., Young, G., Bern, H., and Steiny, S. (1984). Prolactin receptors in tilapia (*Sarotherodon mossambicus*) tissue: Binding sites studies using ^{125}I-labeled ovine prolactin. *Gen. Comp. Endocrinol. 56*:19-23.

Eib, D. W., and Hossner, K. L. (1985). The effects of cortisol and actinomycin D injections in chloride cells and branchial Na+/K+ATPase in rainbow trout (*Salmo gairdneri*). *Gen. Comp. Endocrinol. 49*:449-452.

Elger, M., and Hentschel, H. (1983). Morphological evidence for ionocytes in the gill epithelium of the hagfish, *Myxine glutinosa. Bull. Mt. Desert Isl. Biol. Lab. 23*:4-8.

Ellis, A. G., and Smith, D. G. (1983). Edema formation and impaired O_2 transfer in Ringer-perfused gills of the eel, *Anguilla australis. J. Exp. Zool. 227*: 371-380.

Epple, A., and Kahn, H. A. (1985). Exogenous catecholamines do not affect osmoregulatory parameters in the intact eel. *J. Exp. Zool. 234*:485-488.

Epstein, F. H., Katz, A. I., and Pickford, G. E. (1967). Sodium and potassium-activated adenosine triphosphatase of gills: Role in adaptation of teleost to salt water. *Science 156*:1245-1247.

Ernst, S. A., Dodson, W. C., and Karnaky, K. J. (1980). Structural diversity of occluding junctions in the low-resistance chloride-secreting opercular epithelium of sea-water adapted killifish (*Fundulus heteroclitus*). *J. Cell Biol. 87*:488-497.

Evans, D. H. (1982a). Salt and water exchange across vertebrate gills. In *Gills*. Edited by D. F. Houlihan, J. C. Rankin, and T. J. Shuttleworth. Cambridge, Cambridge University Press, pp. 149-172.

Evans, D. H. (1982b). Mechanisms of acid extrusion by two marine fishes: the teleost *Opsanus beta* and the elasmobranch, *Squalus acanthias. J. Exp. Biol. 97*:289-299.

Evans, D. H. (1984). Gill Na^+/K^+ and Cl^-/HCO_3^- exchange systems evoluted before the vertebrates entered fresh water. *J.*,*Exp. Biol. 113*:465-469.

Evans, D. H., and Cameron, J. N. (1986). Gill ammonia transport. *J. Exp. Zool. 239*:17-24.

Evans, D. H., Claiborne, J. B., Farmer, L., Mallery, C., and Krasny, E. J. (1982). Fish gill ionic transport: Methods and models. *Biol. Bull. 163*:108-130.

Farrell, A. P. (1980). Vascular pathways in the gill of the ling cod, *Ophiodon elongatus. Can. J. Zool. 58*:796-806.

Fawcett, D. W. (1963). Comparative observations on the fine structure of blood capillaries. In *The Peripheral Blood Vessels*. Edited by J. L. Orbison and D. E. Smith. Baltimore, Williams & Wilkins, pp. 17-44.

Feyrter, F. (1938). Uber diffuse endokrine epithelial Organe. *Leipzig E. Ger.* Barth

Fishman, A. P., Delaney, R. G., and Laurent, P. (1985). Circulatory adaptation to bimodal respiration in the dipnoan lungfish. *J. Appl. Physiol. 59*:285-294.

Flik, G., Fenwick, J. C., Kolar, Z., Mayer-Gostan, N., and Wendelaar-Bonga, S. E. (1986). Effects of low ambient calcium levels on whole body Ca^{2+} flux rates and internal calcium pools in the freshwater cichlid teleost, *Oreochromis mossambicus. J. Exp. Biol. 120*:249-264.

Flik, G., Jeanne, H., and Wendelaar-Bonga, S. E. (1985). Evidence for high-affinity Ca^{2+} ATPase activity and ATPase driven Ca^{2+}-transport in membrane preparations of the gill epithelium of the cichlid fish, *Oreochromis mossambicus. J. Exp. Biol. 119*:335-349.

Flik, G., Van Rijs, J. H., and Wendelaar-Bonga, S. E. (1984a). Evidence for the presence of calmodulin in fish mucus. *Eur. J. Biochem. 138*:651-654.

Flik, G., Wendelaar-Bonga, S. E., and Fenwick, J. C. (1984b). Ca^{2+} dependent phosphatase and Ca^{2+} dependent ATPase activities in eel gill plasma membranes. II. Evidence for transport high-affinity Ca^{2+} ATPase. *Comp. Biochem. Physiol. 79B*:9-16.

Flik, G., Wendelaar-Bonga, S. E., and Fenwick, J. C. (1984c). Ca^{2+} dependent phosphatase and Ca^{2+} dependent ATPase activities in eel gill plasma membranes. III. Stimulation of high affinity Ca^{2+} ATPase activity during prolactin-induced hypercalcemia in American eels. *Comp. Biochem. Physiol. 79B*:521-524.

Flik, G., Wendelaar-Bonga, S. E., and Fenwick, J. C. (1985). Active Ca^{2+} transport in plasma membranes of branchial epithelium of the north American eel, *Anguilla rostrata* Leseuer. *J. Cell Biol. 55*:265-272.

Foskett, J. K., Bern, H. A., Machen, T. E., and Conner, M. (1983). Chloride cells and the hormonal control of teleost fish osmoregulation. *J. Exp. Biol. 106*:255-281.

Foskett, J. K., Hubbard, G. M., Machen, T. E., and Bern, H. A. (1982a). Effect of epinephrine, glucagon and vasoactive intestinal polypeptide on chloride secretion by teleost opercular membrane. *J. Comp. Physiol. 146*:72-34.

Foskett, J. K., Logsdon, C. D., Turner, T., Machen, T. E., and Bern, H. A. (1981). Differentiation of the chloride extrusion mechanism during sea water adaptation of a teleost fish, the cichlid *Sarotherodon mossambicus. J. Exp. Biol. 93*:209-224.

Foskett, J. K., Machen, T. E., and Bern, H. A. (1982b). Chloride secretion and conductance of teleost opercular membrane: Effects of prolactin. *Am. J. Physiol. 242*:R380-R389.

Foskett, J. K., and Scheffey, C. (1982). The chloride cell: Definitive identifications as the salt secretory cell in teleosts. *Science 215*:164-164.

Foskett, J. K., Turner, T., Logsdon, C., and Bern, H. (1979). Electrical correlates of chloride cell development in subopercular membrane of tilapia, *Sarotherodon mossambicus* transfrerred to sea water. *Am. J. Zool. 19*: 995.

Fromter, E. (1972). The route of passive ion movement through the epithelium of *Necturus* gallbladder. *J. Membr. Biol. 8*:259-301.

Gaddum, J. H., Hebb, C. O., Silver, A., and Swan, A. A. B. (1953). 5-Hydroxytyrptamine: Pharmacological action and destruction in perfused lungs. *Q. J. Physiol. Cogn. Med. Sci. 38*:225.

Gaino, E., Arillo, A., and Mensi, P. (1984). Involvement of the gill chloride cells of trout under acute nitrite intoxication. *Comp. Biochem. Physiol. 77A*: 611-617.

Galardy, R., Podhasky, P., and Olson, K. R. (1984). Angiotensin converting enzyme activity in tissues of the rainbow trout. *J. Exp. Zool. 230*:155-158.

Gardaire, E., Avella, M., Isaia, J., Bornancin, M., and Mayer-Gostan, N. (1985). Estimation of sodium uptake through the gill of the rainbow trout, *Salmo gairdneri. J. Exp. Biol. 44*:181-189.

Gardner, G. R., and Yevich, P. P. (1970). Histological and haematological responses of an estuarine teleost to cadmium. *J. Fish. Res. Board Can. 27*: 2185-2196.

Girard, J. P. (1976). Salt secretion by the perfused head of trout adapted to sea water and its inhibition by adrenaline. *J. Comp. Physiol. 111*:77-91.

Girard, J. P., and Payan, P. (1977). Kinetic analysis and partitioning of sodium chloride influxes across the gills of sea water adapted trout. *J. Physiol. (Lond.) 267*:519-536.

Girard, J. P., and Payan, P. (1980). Ion exchanges through respiratory and chloride cells in freshwater and seawater adapted teleosteans. *Am. J. Physiol. 238*:R260-R268.

Gluth, G., Freitag, D., Hanke, W., and Korte, F. (1985). Accumulation of pollutants in fish. *Comp. Biochem. Physiol. 81C*:273-277.

Golstein, L. (1982). Gill nitrogen excretion. In *Gills*. Edited by D. F. Houlihan, J. C. Rankin and T. J. Shuttleworth. Cambridge, Cambridge University Press, pp. 193-206.

Hansson, P. J. (1967). Histochemical demonstration of carbonic anhydrase activity. *Histochemie 11*:112-128.

Heinemann, H. O., and Fishman, A. P. (1969). Nonrespiratory functions of mammalian lung. *Physiol. Rev. 49*:1.

Heisler, N. (1980). Regulation of the acid-base status in fishes. In *Environmental Physiology of Fishes*. Edited by M. A. Ali. New York, Plenum Press, pp. 132-162.

Heisler, N. (1984). Acid-base regulation in fishes. In *Fish Physiology*, Vol. XA. Edited by W. S. Hoar and D. J. Randall. New York, Academic Press, pp. 315-400.

Herzog, V., and Farquhar, M. G. (1983). Use of electron opaque tracers for studies on endocytosis and membrane recycling. In *Methods in Enzymology*, Vol. 98. New York, Academic Press, pp. 203-225.

Hipkins, S. F. (1985). Adrenergic responses of the cardiovascular system of the eel, *Anguilla australis*, in vivo. *J. Exp. Zool. 235*:7-20.

Hirano, T. (1986). The spectrum of prolactin action in teleosts. In *Comparative Endocrinology: Developments and Directions*. New York, Alan R. Liss, pp. 53-74.

Hobe, H. (1985). The physiological responses of the stenohaline white sucker, *Catostomus commersoni*, to low environmental pH, particularly in natural soft water. Ph.D. Dissertation. Univ. of Calgary.

Hobe, H., Laurent, P., and MacMahon, B. R. (1984a). Whole body calcium flux rates in freshwater teleosts as a function of ambient calcium and pH levels: A comparison between the euryhaline trout, *Salmo gairdneri* and stenohaline bullhead, *Ictalurus nebulosus. J. Exp. Biol. 113*:237-252.

Hobe, H., Wilkes, P. R. H., Walker, R. L., Wood, C. M., and MacMahon, B. R. (1983). Acid-base balance, ionic status and renal function in resting and acid-exposed white suckers (*Catostomus commersoni*). *Can. J. Zool. 61*: 2660-2668.

Hobe, H., Wood, C. M., and MacMahon, B. R. (1984b). Mechanism of acid-base and ionoregulation in white sucker (*Catostomus commersoni*) in natural soft water. I. Acute exposure to low ambient pH. *J. Comp. Physiol. 154*: 35-46.

Hootman, S. R., and Philpott, C. W. (1980). Accessory cells in teleost bronchial epithelium. *Am. J. Physiol. 238*:R199-R206.

Hossler, F. E., Musil, G., Karnaky, K. J., and Epstein, F. H. (1985). Surface ultrastructure of the gill arch of the killifish, *Fundulus heteroclitus*, from seawater and freshwater, with special reference to the morphology of apical crypts of chloride cell. *J. Morphol. 185*:377-386.

Houlihan, D. F., and Laurent, P. (1987). The effects of exercise training on the performance, growth, and protein turnover of rainbow trout, *Salmo gairdneri. R. Can. J. Fish. Aquat. Sci.* (in press).

Houlihan, D. F., McMillan, D. M., and Laurent, P. (1986). Growth rates, protein synthesis and protein degradation rates in rainbow trout: Effect of body size. *Physiol. Zool. 59*:482-493.

Hughes, G. M. (1972). Morphometrics of fish gill. *Resp. Physiol. 14*:1-25.

Hughes, G. M. (1984). General anatomy of the gills. In *Fish Physiology*, Vol. XA. Edited by W. S. Hoar and D. J. Randall, New York, Academic Press, pp. 1-72.

Hughes, G. M., Peyraud, C., Peyraud Watizenegger, M., and Soulier, P. (1982). Physiological evidence for the occurrence of pathways shunting away from the secondary lamellae of eel gills. *J. Exp. Biol. 98*:277-288.

Hunn, J. B. (1982). Urine flow rates in freshwater salmonids: A review. *Prog. Fish. Cult. 44*:119-125.

Hunn, J. B. (1985). Role of calcium in gill function in fresh water fish. *J. Comp. Biochem. Physiol. 82A*:543-547.

Hunt, T. C., and Rowley, A. F. (1986). Studies on the reticuloendothelial system of the dogfish, *Scyliorhinus canicula*. Endocytotic activity of fixed cells in the gills and peripheral blood leucocytes. *Cell Tissue Res. 244*: 215-226.

Hwang, P. P., and Hirano, R. (1985). Effects of environmental salinity on intercellular organization and junctional structure of chloride cells in early stages of teleost development. *J. Exp. Zool. 236*:115-126.

Isaia, J. (1982). Effects of environmental salinity on branchial permeability of rainbow trout, *Salmo gairdneri. J. Physiol. (Lond.) 326*:297-307.

Isaia, J. (1984). Water and nonelectrolyte permeation. In *Fish Physiologie*, Vol. XB. Edited by W. S. Hoar and D. Randall. New York: Academic Press, pp. 1-38.

Isaia, J., and Hirano, T. (1975). Effect of environmental salinity change on osmotic permeability of the isolated gill of the eel, *Anguilla anguilla* L. *J. Physiol. (Paris) 70*:737-747.

Isaia, J., and Masoni, A. (1976). Effects of Ca^{2+} and Mg^{2+} on water and ionic permeabilities in the SW adapted eel, *Anguilla anguilla. J. Comp. Physiol. 109*:221-233.

Iwana, G. K., Ishimatsu, A., and Heisler, N. (1986). In vivo characterization of the lamellar and CVS comparments in the gill of rainbow trout. *Physiologist 28*:282.

Jagoe, H. J., and Haines, T. A. (1983). Alterations in gill epithelial morphology and yearling Sunapee trout exposed to acute acid stress. *Trans. Am. Fish. Soc. 112*:689-695.

Kamya, M. (1972). Sodium-potassium-activated adenosinetriphosphatase in isolated chloride cells from eel gills. *Comp. Biochem. Physiol. B 43B*:611-617.

Kamya, M., and Utida, S. (1968). Changes in activity of sodium-potassium-activated adenosinetriphosphatase in gills during adaptation of the Japanese eel to sea water. *Comp. Biochem. Physiol. 26*:675-685.

Karnaky, K. J., Jr., Degnan, K. J., and Zadunaisky, J. A. (1977). Chloride transport across isolated opercular epithelium of killifish. A membrane rich in chloride cells. *Science 195*:203-205.

Karnaky, K. J., Jr., Dengan, K. J., and Zadunaisky, J. A. (1979). Correlation of chloride cell number and short-circuit current in chloride-secreting epithelia of *Fundulus heteroclitus. Bull. Mt. Desert. Biol. Lab. 19*:109-111.

Karnaky, K. J., Jr., Degnan, K. J., Garreton, L. T., and Zadunaisky, J. A. (1984). Identification and quantification of mitochondria rich cells in transporting epithelia. *Am. J. Physiol. 246*:R770-R775.

Karnaky, K. J., Jr., and Kinter, W. B. (1977). Killifish opercular skin: A flat epithelium with a high density of chloride cells. *J. Exp. Zool. 199*:355-364.

Keys, A., and Wilmer, E. N. (1932). Chloride secreting cell in the gills of fishes with special reference to the common eel. *J. Physiol. (Lond.) 76*:368-378.

Kikuschi, S. (1977). Mitochondria rich (chloride) cells in the gill epithelia from four species of stenohaline freshwater teleosts. *Cell Tissue Res. 180*:87-98.

Kirschner, L. B. (1969). Ventral aortic pressure and sodium fluxes in perfused eel gills. *Am. J. Physiol. 217*:596-604.

Kirschner, L. B. (1978). External charged layer and Na^+ regulation. In *Osmotic and Volume Regulation*. Edited by E. Parker-Jorgensen, E. Skadhauge, and P. Hess-Taysen. Alfred Benzon Symposium XI, Munksgaard Copenhagen, pp. 310-324.

Krogh, A. (1938). The active absorption of ions in some freshwater animals. *Z. Vgl. Physiol. 25*:335-350.

Langhorne, P., and Simpson, T. (1986). The interrelationship of cortisol, gill (Na^+K^+) ATPase and homeostasis during the parr-smolt transformation of Atlantic salmon *(Salmo salar* L.). *Gen. Comp. Endocrinol. 61*:203-213.

Lasker, R., and Threadgold, L. T. (1968). Chloride cells in the skin of the larval sardine. *Exp. Cell Res. 52*:582-590.

Lauren, D. J., and MacDonald, D. G. (1985). Effects of copper on branchial ionoregulation in the rainbow trout, *Salmo gairdneri* Richardson. *J. Comp. Physiol. 155B*:635-644.

Laurent, P. (1981). Circulatory adaptation to diving in amphibious fish. In *Advances in Animal and Comparative Physiology*, Vol. 20. Edited by G. Pethes and V. L. Frenyo. Pergamon Press Akademiai Kiado, pp. 305-306.

Laurent, P. (1982). Structure of vertebrates gills. In *Gills*. Edited by D. F. Houlihan, J. C. Rankin, and T. J. Shuttleworth. Cambridge, Cambridge University Press, pp. 25-43.

Laurent, P. (1984). Gill internal morphology. In *Fish Physiology*, Vol. XA. Edited by W. S. Hoar and D. J. Randall. New York, Academic Press, 73-183.

Laurent, P. (1985a). A survey of the morphofunctional relationships between epithelia, vasculature and innervation within the fish gill. *Fortschr. Zool. 30*:339-351.

Laurent, P. (1985b). Organization and control of the respiratory vasculature in lower vertebrates: Are there anatomical gill shunts? In *Cardiovascular Shunts*. Edited by K. Johansen and W. W. Burggren. Alfred Benzon Symposium. Munksgaard Copenhagen, pp. 58-70.

Laurent, P., Delaney, R. G., and Fishmann, A. P. (1978). The vasculature of the gills in the aquatic and aestivating lungfish (*Protopterus aethiopicus*). *J. Morphol. 156*:173-208.

Laurent, P., and Dunel, S. (1976). Functional organization of the teleost gill. I. Blood pathways. *Acta Zool. (Stockh.) 57*:189-209.

Laurent, P., and Dunel, S. (1978). Relations anatomiques des ionocytes (cellules à chlorure) avec le compariment veineux branchial: Définition de deux types d'épithélium de la branchie des poissons. *C. R. Hebd. Acad. Sci. Ser. D. 286*:1447-1450.

Laurent, P., and Dunel, S. (1980). Morphology of gill epithelia in fish. *Am. J. Physiol. 238*:R147-R159.

Laurent, P., and Dunel-Erb, S. (1984). The pseudobranch: Morphology and function. In *Fish Physiology*, Vol. XB. Edited by W. S. Hoar and D. J. Randall. New York, Academic Press, pp. 285-323.

Laurent, P., Hobe, H., and Dunel-Erb, S. (1985). The role of environmental sodium chloride relative to calcium in gill morphology of freshwater salmonid fish. *Cell Tissue Res. 240*:675-692.

Laurent, P., and Rouzeau, J. (1972). Afferent neural activity from pseudobranch of teleost. Effects of PO_2, pH, osmotic pressure and Na^+ ions. *Resp. Physiol. 14*:307-331.

Lauweryns, J. M., De Bock, V., Verhofstad, A. A. T., and Steinbusch, H. V. M. (1982). Immunohistochemical localization of serotonin in intrapulmonary neuroepithelial bodies. *Cell. Tissue Res. 226*:215-223.

Lauweryns, J. M., Cokelaere, M., and Theunynck, P. (1972). Neuroepithelial bodies in the respiratory mucosa of various mammals. *Z. Zellforsch. Mikrosk. Anat. 135*:569-592.

Lauweryns, J. M., and Van Lommel, A. (1982). Morphometric analysis of hypoxia-induced synaptic activity in intrapulmonary neuroepithelial bodies. *Cell Tissue Res. 226*:201-214.

Leino, R. L., and McCormick, J. H. (1984). Morphological and morphometrical changes in chloride cells of the gills of *Pimephales promelas* after chronic exposure to acid water. *Cell Tissue Res. 236*:121-128.

Leloup-Hatey, J. (1964). Fonctionnement de l'interrenal anterieur de deux téléostéens, le saumon atlantic et l'anguille européene. *Ann. Inst. Oceanogr. 42*:221-338.

MacDonald, D. G. (1983). The effects of H^+ upon the gills of freshwater fish. *Can. J. Zool. 61*:391-703.

MacDonald, D. G., Hone, H., and Wood, C. M. (1980). The influence of calcium on the physiological responses of the rainbow trout, *Salmo gairdneri*, to low environmental pH. *J. Exp. Biol. 88*:109-131.

MacDonald, D. G., and Rogano, M. S. (1986). Ion regulation by the rainbow trout, *Salmo gairdneri*, in ion-poor water. *J. Physiol. Zool. 59*:318-331.

MacKeown, B. A., Geen, G. H., Watson, T. A., Powell, J. F., and Parker, D. B. (1985). The effect of pH on plasma electrolytes, carbonic anhydrase and ATPase activities in rainbow trout (*Salmo giardneri*) and largescale suckers (*Catostomus macrocheilus*). *Comp. Biochem. Physiol. 80A*:507-514.

MacWilliams, P. G. (1980). Acclimation to an acid medium in the brown trout, *Salmo trutto. J. Exp. Biol. 88*:269-280.

MacWilliams, P. G. (1982a). The effects of calcium on sodium fluxes in the brown trout, *Salmo trutta*, in neutral and acid media. *J. Exp. Biol. 96*: 439-442.

MacWilliams, P. G. (1982b). A comparison of physiological characteristics in normal and acid exposed populations of the brown trout, *Salmo trutta. Comp. Biochem. Physiol. 72*:515-522.

MacWilliams, P. G. (1983). An investigation of the loss of bound calcium from the gills of the brown trout, *Salmo trutta*, in acid media. *Comp. Biochem. Physiol. 74A*:107-116.

MacWilliams, P. G., and Potts, W. T. W. (1978). Effects of pH and calcium concentrations on gill potentials in the brown trout, *Salmo trutta. J. Comp. Physiol. 126*:277-286.

Maetz, J. (1974). Aspects of adaptation to hypoosmotic and hyperosmotic environments. In *Biochemical and Biophysical Perspectives in Marine Biology*, Vol. I. Edited by D. C. Malins and J. R. Sargent. New York, Academic Press, pp. 1-167.

Maetz, J., and Garcia-Romeu, F. (1964). The mechanisms of sodium and chloride uptake by the gills of a fresh water fish, *Carassius auratus*. II. Evidence for NH_4^+/Na^+ and HCO_3^-/Cl^- exchanges. *J. Gen. Physiol. 47*:1209-1227.

Malte, H., and Weber, R. E.(1985). A mathematical model for gas exchange in the fish gill based on non-linear blood gas equilibrium curves. *Resp. Physiol. 62*:359-374.

Margiocco, C., Arillo, A., Mensi, P., and Schenone, G. (1983). Nitrite bioaccumulation in *Salmo gairdneri* Rich and hematological consequences. *Aquat. Toxicol. 3*:261-270.

Marshall, W. S. (1978). On the involvement of mucous secretion in teleost osmoregulation. *Can. J. Zool. 56*:1088-1091.

Marshall, W. S., and Bern, A. H. (1980). Ion transport across the isolated skin of the teleost *Gillichthys mirabilis*. In *Epithelial Transport in the Lower Vertebrates*. Edited by B. Lahlou. Cambridge, Cambridge University Press, pp. 337-350.

Marshall, W. S., and Nishioka, R. S. (1980). Relation of mitochondria rich chloride cells to active chloride transport in the skin of a marine teleost. *J. Exp. Zool. 214*:147-156.

Masoni, A., and Isaia, J. (1980). Mise en évidence du rôle des cellules à chlorure dans le transport des macromolécules organiques. In *Epithelial Transport in the Lower Vertebrates*. Edited by B. Lahlou. Cambridge, Cambridge University Press, pp. 71-80.

Mayer-Gostan, N., Bornancin, M., De Renzis, G., Naon, R., Yee, J. A., Shew, R. L., and Pang, P. K. T. (1983). Extraintestinal calcium uptake in the killifish, *Fundulus heteroclitus. J. Exp. Zool. 227*:329-338.

Mayer-Gostan, N., and Hirano, T. (1976). The effects of transecting the IXth and Xth cranial nerves on hydromineral balance in the eel, *Anguilla anguilla. J. Exp. Biol. 64*:461-475.

Millet, C., Peignoux-Deville, J., and Martelly, E. (1979). Gill calcium fluxes in the eel, *Anguilla anguilla* (L.). Effects of stannius corpuscles and ultimobranchial body. *Comp. Biochem. Physiol. 63A*:63-70.

Milhaud, G., Rankin, J. C., Bolis, L., and Benson, A. A. (1977). Calcitonin: Its hormonal action on the gill. *Proc. Natl. Acad. Sci. USA 74*:4693-4696.

Mommsen, T. P. (1984). Biochemical characterization of the rainbow trout gill. *J. Comp. Physiol. 154*:191-198.

Motais, R., Isaia, J., Rankin, J. C., and Maetz, J. (1969). Adaptative changes of the water permeability of the teleostean gill epithelium in relation to external salinity. *J. Exp. Biol. 51*:529-546.

Mugiya, Y., and Ishii, T. (1981). Effects of estradiol-17β on branchial and intestinal calcium uptake in the rainbow trout, *Salmo gairdneri. Comp. Biochem. Physiol. 70A*:97-101.

Nekvasil, N. P., and Olson, K. R. Extraction and metabolism of circulating catecholamines by the trout gill. (in press).

Nekvasil, N. P., and Olson, K. R. (1985). Localization of [^{3}H] norepinephrine binding sites in the trout gill. *J. Exp. Zool. 235*:309-313.

Nicol, C. S., Farmer, S. W., Nishioka, R. S., and Bern, H. A. (1981). Blood and pituitary prolactin levels in tilapia (*Sarotherodon mossambicus*: Teleostei) from different salinities as measured by homologous radioimmunoassay. *Gen. Comp. Endocr. 44*:365-373.

Nilsson, S. (1983). *Autonomic Nerve Function in the Vertebrates*. Berlin, Springer-Verlag.

Nilsson, S. (1984). Innervation and pharmacology of the gills. In *Fish Physiologie*. Vol. XA. Edited by N. S. Hoar and D. J. Randall. New York, Academic Press, pp. 185-227.

Nilsson, S. (1985). Filament position in fish gills is influenced by a smooth muscle innervated by adrenergic nerves. *J. Exp. Biol. 118*:433-437.

Nilsson, S., and Pettersson, K. (1981). Sympathetic nervous control of blood flow in the gills of the Atlantic cod, *Gadus morhua. J. Comp. Physiol. 144*:157-163.

Oduleye, S. O. (1975). The effects of calcium on water balance of the brown trout, *Salmo trutta. J. Exp. Biol. 63*:343-356.

Ogasawara, T., and Hirano, T. (1984). Effects of prolactin and environmental calcium on osmotic water permeability of the gills in the eel, *Anguilla japonica. Gen. Comp. Endocr. 53*:315-324.

Ogawa, M. (1974). The effects of bovine prolactin, sea water and environmental calcium on water influx in isoated gills of the euryhaline teleosts, *Anguilla japonica* and *Salmo gairdneri. Comp. Biochem. Physiol. 49A*:545-553.

Olivereau, M., Aimar, C., and Olivereau, J. M. (1980). PAS-positive cells of the pars intermedia are calcium sensitive in the goldfish maintained in the hypoosmotic milieu. *Cell Tissue Res. 212*:29-38.

Olivereau, M., and Olivereau, J. (1982). Calcium sensitive cells of the pars intermedia and osmotic balance in the eel. *Cell Tissue Res. 225*:487-496.

Olson, K. R., Evan, A. P., and Ryan, J. W. (1986). Binding of the angiotensin converting enzyme inhibitor RAC-X-65 to trout gills. *Fed. Proc. 45*:641.

Olson, K. R., Kullman, D., Narkates, A. J., and Oparil, S. (1986). Angiotensin extraction by trout tissues in vivo and metabolism by the perfused gill. *Am. J. Physiol. 250*:R532-R538.

Omeljaniuk, R. J., and Eales, J. G. (1986). The effect of 3,5,3′-triiodo-L-thyronine on gill Na^+/K^+/ATPase of rainbow trout, *Salmo gairdneri*, in fresh water. *Comp. Biochem. Physiol. 84A*:427-429.

Ostlund, E., and Fänge, R. (1962). Vasodilation by adrenaline and noradrenaline, and the effects of some other substances on perfused fish gills. *Comp. Biochem. Physiol. 5*:307-309.

Pang, P. T. K., Griffith, R. W., Maetz, J., and Pic, P. (1980). Calcium uptake in fishes. In *Epithelial Transport in the Lower Vertebrates*. Edited by B. Lahlou. Cambridge, Cambridge University Press, pp. 120-132.

Packer, R., and Dunson, W. (1970). Effects of low environmental pH on blood pH and sodium balance of brook trout. *J. Exp. Zool. 174*:65-72.

Pärt, P., Svanberg, O., and Bergstrom, E. (1985). The influence of surfactants on gill physiology and cadmium uptake in perfused rainbow trout gills. *Ecotoxicol. Environ. Safety 9*:135-144.

Pärt, P., Tuurala, H., and Soivio, A. (1982). Oxygen transfer, gill resistance and structural changes in rainbow trout (*Salmo gairdneri* Richardson) gills perfused with vaso-active agents. *Comp. Biochem. Physiol. 71C*:7-13.

Pärt, P., Tuurala, H., Nikinmaa, M., and Kiessling, A. (1984). Evidence for a non-respiratory intralamellar shunt in perfused rainbow trout gills. *Comp. Biochem. Physiol. 79A*:29-34.

Payan, P., Girard, J. P., and Mayer Gostan, N.(1984). Branchial ion movements in teleosts: The roles of respiratory and chloride cells. In *Fish Physiology*, Vol. XB. Edited by W. S. Hoar and D. J. Randall. New York, Academic Press, pp. 39-63.

Payan, P., and Matty, A. J. (1975). The characteristics of ammonia excretion by an isolated perfused head of trout (*Salmo gairdneri*): Effect of temperature and CO_2 free Ringer. *J. Comp. Physiol. 96*:167-184.

Payan, P., Mayer-Gostan, N., and Pang, P. K. T. (1981). Site of calcium uptake in the fresh water trout gill. *J. Exp. Zool. 216*:345-347.

Pennec-Le Bras, Y. M., and Pennec, J. P. (1986). Evaluation et rôle au niveau cardiaque des catécholamines chez la truite lors des transferts d'eau douce en eau de mer. *Ichtyophysiol. Acta 10*:108-117.

Perry, S. F., Davie, P. S., Daxboeck, C., Ellis, A. G., and Smith, D. G. (1984). Perfusion methods for the study of gill physiology. In *Fish Physiology*, Vol. XB. Edited by W. S. Hoar, and D. J. Randall. New York, Academic Press, pp. 325-388.

Perry, S. F., Lauren, D. J., and Booth, C. E. (1984). Absence of branchial edema in perfused heads of rainbow trout (*Salmo gairdneri*). *J. Exp. Zool. 231*: 441-445.

Perry, S. F., and Wood, C. M. (1985). Kinetics of branchial calcium uptake in the rainbow trout: Effects of acclimation to various external calcium level. *J. Exp. Biol. 116*:411-433.

Pettersson, K., and Nilsson, S. (1979). Nervous control of the branchial vascular resistance of the Atlantic cod, *Gadus morhua*. *J. Comp. Physiol. 129*: 179-183.

Pic, P., Mayer-Gostan, N., and Maetz, J. (1975). Branchial effects of epinephrine in the sea water adapted mullet. II. Na and Cl extrusion. *Am. J. Physiol. 228*:441-447.

Piiper, J., Dejours, P., Haab, P., and Rahn, H. (1971). Concepts and basic quantities in gas exchange physiology. *Resp. Physiol. 13*:292-304.

Piiper, J., and Scheid, P. (1982). Physical principles of respiration gas exchange in fish gills. In *Gills*. Edited by D. F. Houlihan, J. C. Rankin, and T. J. Shuttleworth. Cambridge, Cambridge University Press, pp. 45-61.

Pisam, M., Sardet, C., and Maetz, J. (1980). Polysaccharide material in chloride cell of teleostean gill: Modifications according to salinity. *Am. J. Physiol. 238*:R213-R218.

Potts, W. T. W., and Evans, D. H. (1966). The effects of hypophysectomy and bovine prolactin on salt fluxes in fresh water adapted, *Fundulus heteroclitus*. *Biol. Bull. 131*:362-368.

Prunet, P., Boeuf, G., and Houdebine, L. M. (1965). Plasma and pituitary prolactin levels in rainbow trout during adaptation to different salinities. *J. Exp. Zool. 235*:187-196.

Rahim, M. S., Delaunoy, J. P., and Laurent, P. (1988). Identification and immunocytochemical localization of two different carbonic anhydrase isoenzymes in teleostean fish erythrocyte and gill epithelia. *Histochemistry* (in press).

Randall, D., and Daxboeck, C. (1984). Oxygen and carbon dioxide transfer across fish gills. In *Fish Physiology*, Vol. XA. Edited by W. S. Hoar and D. J. Randall. New York, Academic Press, pp. 263-314.

Randall, D. J., Holeton, G. F., and Stevens, E. D. (1967). The exchange of oxygen and carbon dioxide across the gills of rainbow trout. *J. Exp. Biol. 46*: 339-348.

Rankin, J. C., and Bolis, L. (1984). Hormonal control of water movement across the gills. In *Fish Physiology*, Vol. XB. Edited by W. S. Hoar and D. J. Randall. New York, Academic Press, pp. 177-201.

Rankin, J.C., Stagg, R. M., and Bolis, L. (1982). Effects of pollutants on gills. In *Gills*. Edited by D. F. Houlihan, J. C. Rankin, and T. J. Shuttleworth. Cambridge, Cambridge University Press, pp. 207-221.

Reite, O. B. (1969). The evolution of vascular smooth muscle responses to histamine and 5-hydroxytryptamine. *Acta Physiol. Scand. 75*:221-239.

Ristori, M. T. (1984). La concentration plasmatique des catécholamines dans diverses situations physiologiques chez la truite (*Salmo gairdneri*). DSc Thesis, Univ. scientifique et médicale de Grenoble.

Ristori, M. T., and Laurent, P. (1985). Plasma catecholamines and glucose during moderate exercise in the trout: Comparison with burst of violent activity. *Exp. Biol. 44*:247-253.

Ristori, M. T., Rehm, J. C., and Laurent, P. (1979). Dosages des catecholamines plasmatiques chez la truite au cours de l'hypoxie controlée. *J. Physiol. (Paris) 75*:67A (abstr.).

Saintsing, D. G., and Dietz, T. H. (1983). Modification of sodium transport in freshwater mussels by prostaglandins, cyclic AMP and 5-hydroxytryptamine: Effects of inhibitions of prostaglandin synthesis. *Comp. Biochem. Physiol. 76C*:285-290.

Sangalang, G. B., and Freeman, H. C. (1979). Tissue uptake of cadmium in brook trout during chronic sublethal exposure. *Arch. Environ. Contamin. Toxicol. 8*:77-84.

Sardet, C. (1977). Ordered arrays of intramembrane particles on the surface of the fish gills. *Cell Biol. Int. Rep. 1*:409-418.

Sardet, C. (1980). Freeze fracture of the gill epithelium of euryhaline teleost fish. *Am. J. Physiol. 238*:R207-R212.

Sardet, C., Pisam, M., and Maetz, J. (1979). The surface epithelium of teleostean fish gills. Cellular and junctional adaptations of the chloride cell in relation to salt adaptation. *J. Cell Biol. 80*:96-117.

Sardet, C., Pisam, M., and Maetz, J. (1980). Structure and function of gill epithelium of euryhaline teleost fish. In *Epithelial Transport in the Lower Vertebrates*. Edited by B. Lahlou. Cambridge, Cambridge University Press, pp. 59-68.

Sargent, J. R., Thomson, A. J., and Bornancin, M. (1975). Activities and localization of succinic dehydrogenase and Na^+/K^+-activated adenosine triphosphatase in the gill of the eels (*Anguilla anguilla*) adapted to fresh water and sea water. *Comp. Biochem. Physiol. B 51B*:75-79.

Scheid, P., and Piiper, J. (1976). Quantitative functional analysis of branchial gas transfer: Theory and application to *Scyliorhinus stellaris* (Elasmobranchii). In *Respiration of Amphibious Vertebrates*. Edited by G. M. Hughes. New York, Academic Press, pp. 17-38.

Scheid, P., Hook, C., and Piiper, J. (1986). Model for analysis of countercurrent gas transfer in fish gills. *Resp. Physiol. 64*:365-374.

Scheide, J. E., and Dietz, T. H. (1984). The effects of calcium on serotonin stimulated adenylate cyclase in freshwater mussels. *Biol. Bull. 166*:594-607.

Shuttleworth, T. J. (1978). The effect of Adrenalin on potentials in the isolated gills of the flounder (*Platichthys flessus* L.). *J. Comp. Physiol. 124*:129-136.

Silva, P. R., Solomon, R., Spokes, K., and Epstein, F. H. (1977). Ouabain inhibition of gill Na^+/K^+/ATPase. Relationship to acid chloride transport. *J. Exp. Zool. 199*:419-427.

Skidmore, J. F., and Tovell, P. W. A. (1972). Toxic effects of zinc sulphate on the gills of rainbow trout. *Water Res. 6*:217-230.

Smith, H. W. (1930). The absorption and excretion of water and salts by marine teleost. *Am. J. Physiol. 93*:485-505.

Smith, D. G., and Chamley-Campbell, J. (1981). Localization of smooth-muscles myosin in branchial pillar cells of snapper (*Chrysophys auratus*) by immunofluorescence histochemistry. *J. Exp. Zool. 215*:121-124.

Smith, D. G., and Johnson, D. W. (1977). Oxygen exchange in a simulated trout gill secondary lamella. *Am. J. Physiol. 233*:R145-R161.

Smith, D. G., Nilsson, S., Wahlqvist, I., and Eriksson, B. M. (1985). Nervous control of the blood pressure in the atlantic cod, *Gadus morhua. J. Exp. Biol. 117*:335-347.

Soivio, A., and Tuurala, H. (1981). Structural and circulatory responses to hypoxia ins the secondary lamellae of *Salmo gairdneri* gills at two temperatures. *J. Comp. Physiol. 145*:37-43.

Spry, D. J., and Wood, C. M. (1984). Acid-base, plasma ion and blood gas changes in rainbow trout during short term toxic zinc exposure. *J. Comp. Physiol. 154B*:149-158.

Spry, D. J., and Wood, C. M. (1985). Ion fluxes rates, acid-base status and blood gases in rainbow trout, *Salmo gairdneri*, exposed to toxic zinc in natural soft water. *Can. J. Fish. Aquat. Sci. 42*:1332-1341.

Strum, J. M., and Junod, A. F. (1972). Radioautographic demonstration of 5-hydroxytriptamine-^{3}H uptake by pulmonary endothelial cells. *J. Cell Biol. 54*:456-467.

Thomas, D. G., Brown, M. W., Shurben, D., Solbe, J. F., Del, G., Cryer, A., and Kay, J. (1985). A comparison of the sequestration of cadmium and zinc in the tissues of rainbow trout (*Salmo gairdneri*) following exposure to the metals singly or in combination. *Comp. Biochem. Physiol. 82C*:55-62.

Tomasso, J. R., Smico, B. A., and Davis, K. B. (1979). Chloride inhibition of nitrite-induced methemoglobinemia in channel catfish (*Ictalurus punctatus*). *J. Fish. Res. Board Can. 36*:1141-1144.

Tosteson, D. C., Spivacks, S., and Nelson, D. (1962). Sodium and chloride transport by the isolated perfused eel gill. *J. Gen. Physiol. 45*:620.

Trigari, G., Borgatti, A. R., Pagliarani, A., Ventrella, V. (1985). Characterization of gill (Na^+/K^+) ATPase in the sea bass (*Dicentrarchus labrax* L.). *Comp. Biochem. Physiol. 80B*:23-33.

Tuurala, H., and Soivio, A. (1982). Structural and circulatory changes in the secondary lamellae of *Salmo gairdneri* gills after sublethal exposures to dehydroabietic acid and zinc. *Aquat. Toxicol. 2*:21-29.

Ultsch, G. R., Ott, M. E., and Heisler, N. (1980). Standard metabolic rate, critical oxygen tension and aerobic scope for spontaneous activity of trout (*Salmo gairdneri*) and carp (*Cyprinus carpio*) in acidified water. *Comp. Biochem. Physiol. 67*:329-335.

Ultsch, G. R., Ott, M. E., and Heisler, N. (1981). Acid-base and electrolyte status in carp (*Cyrpinus carpio*) exposed to low environmental pH. *J. Exp. Biol. 93*:65--80.

Ungell, A. L., Kiessling, A., and Nilsson, S. (1984). Transfer changes in fish gills during stress. In *Toxins, Drugs and Pollutants in Marine Animals*. Edited by Bolis et al. Berlin, Herdelberg, Springer-Verlag, pp. 115-121.

Urist, M. R. (1976). Biogenesis of bone calcium and phosphorus in the skeleton and blood in vertebrate evolution. In *Handbook of Physiology*, Sect. 7, Vol. VII. Edited by R. D. Greep, E. B. Atwood, and G. D. Aurback. Baltimore, Williams & Wilkins, pp. 183-213.

Wahlqvist, I. (1980). Effects of catecholamines on isolated systemic and branchial vascular beds of the cod, *Gadus morhua. J. Comp. Physiol. 137*:139-143.

Wahlqvist, I., and Nilsson, S. (1980). Adrenergic control of the cardiovascular system of the Atlantic cod, *Gadus morhua* during stress. *J. Comp. Physiol. 137*:145-150.

Wendelaar-Bonga, S. E. (1978). The effects of changes in external sodium, calcium and magnesium concentrations on prolactin cells, skin and plasma electrolytes of *Gasterosteus aculeatus. Gen. Comp. Endocrinol. 34*:265-275.

Wendelaar-Bonga, S. E., and Graven, S. A. A. (1978). The relationship between prolactin cell activity, environmental calcium and plasma cadmium in the teleost, *Gastereosteus aculeatus*: Observations on stanniectomized fish. *Gen. Comp. Endocrinol. 36*:90-101.

Wendelaar-Bonga, S. E., Lowick, C. J. M., and Van der Meij, J. C. A. (1983). Effects of external Mg^{2+} and Ca^{2+} on branchial osmotic water permeability and prolactin secretion on the teleost fish, *Sarotherodon mossambicus. Gen. Comp. Endocrinol. 52*:222-231.

Wendelaar-Bonga, S. E., and Van der Meij, J. C. A. (1981). Effect of ambient osmolarity and calcium on prolactin cell activity and osmotic water permeability of the gills in the teleost fish, *Sarotherodon mossambicus. Gen. Comp. Endocrinol. 43*:432-442.

Wendelaar-Bonga, S. E., Van der Meij, J. C. A., Van der Krabben, W. A., and Flik, G. (1984). The effect of water acidification on prolactin cells and pars intermedia PAS-sero positive cells in the teleost fish *Oreochromis* (formerly *Sarotherodon*) *Mossambicus* and *Carassius auratus. Cell Tissue Res. 238*:601-609.

Wood, C. M. (1974). A critical examination of the physical and adrenergic factors affecting blood flow through the gills of the rainbow trout. *J. Exp. Biol. 60*:241-265.

Wood, C. M., and MacDonald, D. G. (1982). Physiological mechanisms of acid toxicity to fish. In *Acid Rain Fisheries*. Edited by R. E. Johnson. Bethesda, Am. Fish. Soc. (Publ.), pp. 157-226.

Wright, D. E. (1973). The structure of the gills of the elasmobranch, *Scyliorhinus canicula* L. *Z. Zellforsch. 144*:489-509.

Wright, P., Heming, T., and Randall, D. (1986). Downstream pH changes in water flowing over the gills of rainbow trout. *J. Exp. Biol. 126*:499-512.

Wright, P. A., and Wood, C. M. (1985). An analysis of branchial ammonia excretion in the freshwater rainbow trout: Effects of environmental pH change and sodium uptake blockade. *J. Exp. Biol. 114*:329-353.

Zaccone, G., Fasulo, S., Lo Cascio, P., and Licata, A. (1985). Patterns of enzyme activities in the gills of the catfish *Heteropneustes fossilis* (Bloch) exposed to anionactive detergent *N*-alkyl-benzene sulphonate (LAS). *Histochemistry 82*:341-343.

Zaccone, G., and Licata, A. (1981). Histoenzymorphology and fine structure of the ionocytes in the head epidermis of a marine teleost, *Xyrichthys novacula* L. (Labridae, Pisces). *Arch. Biol. 92*:451-465.

Zadunaisky, J. A. (1984). The chloride cell: The active transport of chloride and the paracellular pathways. In *Fish Physiology*, Vol. XB. Edited by W. S. Hoar and D. J. Randall, New York, Academic Press, pp. 130-176.

5

Gill Structure and Function
Amphibian Larvae

GARY M. MALVIN

University of Washington
School of Medicine
Seattle, Washington

I. Introduction

The amphibian gill is an aquatic respiratory organ used by embryonic, larval, and neotenic amphibians. In contrast to the gills of most fish, the amphibian gill is seldom the primary gas exchange organ. Rather, it functions in conjunction with skin, with lungs, and with the buccopharyngeal cavity in exchanging gases. The amphibian gill also participates in nonrespiratory functions such as salt and water balance and feeding. Gills disappear during metamorphosis at a time when most amphibians become more reliant on aerial gas exchange. The shapes and sizes of amphibian gills span a wide range from small epithelium-covered capillary tufts, to large arborescent organs, to sheetlike structures that extend longer than the length of the body. Their respiratory importance is also variable. Branchial gas exchange varies from a few percent to about 60% of total gas exchange among different species. Large changes also occur within an individual under different conditions.

Despite its ubiquitous nature, the amphibian gill is one of the least studied of vertebrate respiratory organs. It is estimated that anatomists and physiologists have examined no more than 0.5% of the approximately 4000 amphibian species. Consequently, information is fragmentary and may not be representative of this diverse vertebrate class. Nevertheless, our understanding of this organ has grown considerably over the past few years. This chapter attempts to convey an appreciation for the unique structures of several types of gills and to present a partial picture of branchial gas exchange and its regulation. Because of the paucity of information, only a few species of anurans and urodeles will be discussed.

II. Structure

A. Urodeles

Morphology

The gills of urodeles begin development early in the embryonic stage (Harrison stage 35; approximately 7 days after fertilization in *Ambystoma punctatum* at 20°C; Harrison, 1969) and probably participate in gas exchange well before hatching. Urodeles that go through an aquatic larval stage after hatching retain the gills, with only minor modifications. Typically, urodele larvae have three pairs of external gills protruding from the body into the aquatic environment. Each gill comprises a cartilagenous and a respiratory section. The cartilagenous section, a rigid arch, runs in a ventrodorsal direction forming a portion of the sides of the posterior buccal cavity. The medial surface of the cartilagenous bars are often serrated to aid in feeding. The branchial respiratory section extends outward from the cartilagenous section and forms a fingerlike primary gill bar. Two rows of respiratory lamellae protrude at right angles from the ventral surface of the gill bar. The lamellae are small leaflike structures with a large surface area. Thus, most branchial gas exchange probably occurs there. The length of the primary gill bar and the number of lamellae increase from the first (most anterior) to the third gill. Generally, the gills of larvae that inhabit fast-flowing streams are smaller than those of pond-dwelling species (Duellman and Trueb, 1986). This difference probably reflects an adaptation to enhance mobility in swift currents. It may also reflect an adjustment to the high PO_2 of streams, which reduces the need for a large respiratory surface area. However, even within a species, gill size may vary. Chronic exposure to hypoxic water increases the size of the primary gill bar and lamellae, whereas hyperoxia has the opposite effect (Babak, 1907; Bond, 1960; Drastich, 1925). Long-term exposure to increased temperature also enlarges the respiratory section of the gill (Babek, 1907). The degree of responsiveness to these environmental factors varies considerably among species.

The core of the primary gill bar contains loose connective tissue, blood vessels, and bands of striated muscle which insert upon the cartilagenous gill arch. Above is a basement membrane supporting an epithelium consisting of several cell layers. The respiratory lamellae, in contrast, lack striated muscle and have a much thinner epithelium (Bond, 1960; Hackford et al., 1977). The lamel-

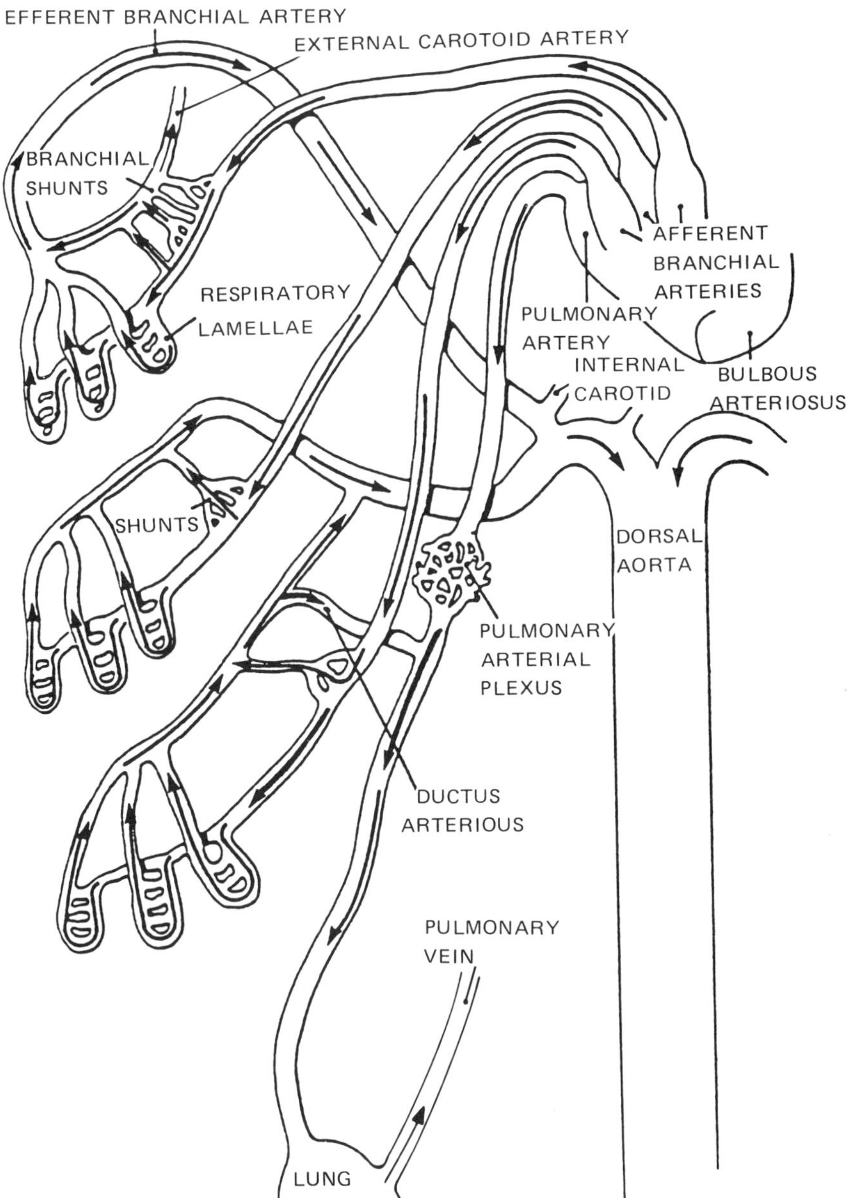

Figure 1 Vascular organization of the aortic arches, gills, and lung in *A. tigrinum*. (From Malvin, 1985a,c.)

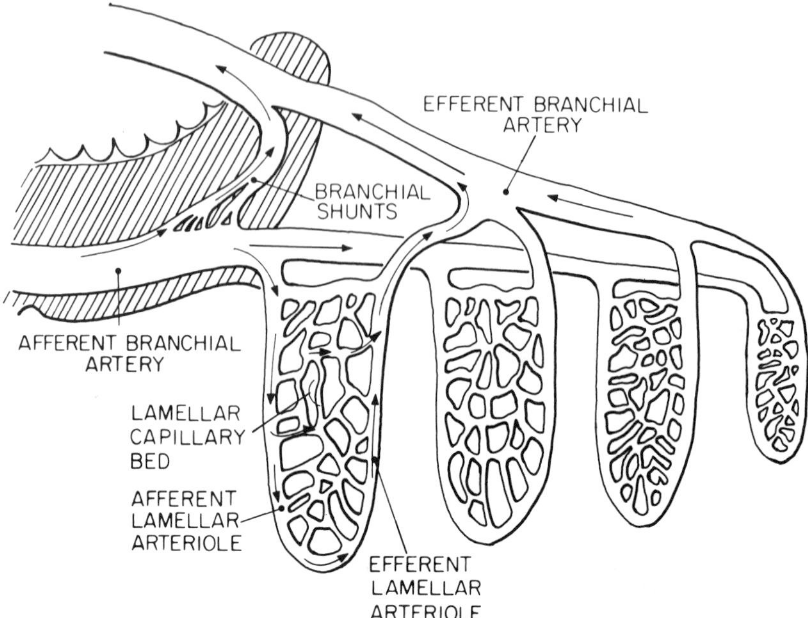

Figure 2 Vascular organization of the gills in *A. tigrinum*. (Adapted from Figge, 1936.)

lar blood-water diffusion barrier is approximately 5 to 15 μm in neotenic *A. mexicanum* (Hackford et al., 1977) and as little as 1 μm in *Salamandra salamandra* larvae (Greven, 1980). There are several cell types in the gill epithelium including ciliated cells and cells with numerous mitochondria (Greven, 1980; Hackford et al., 1977). The mitochondria-rich cells are considerably more numerous in the primary gill bar than in the lamellae. In *S. salamandra*, these cells have been shown to contain carbonic anhydrase, suggesting specialization for CO_2 transport (Lewinson et al., 1984). That enzyme is also present in the gills of *Necturus maculosus*, but is absent from *A. tigrinum* gills (Toews et al., 1978).

Vascular Organization

Each gill receives blood directly from the heart through an afferent branchial artery (Fig. 1: Baker, 1949; Figge, 1934; Gilmore and Figge, 1929; Hackford et al., 1977; Malvin, 1985a; McIndoe and Smith, 1984a). Afferent branchial arteries usually emerge directly from the bulbus arteriosus, but in *N. maculosus* the third afferent branchial artery splits from the second between the heart and the gill (Baker, 1949). These vessels are the ventral portions of aortic arches III,

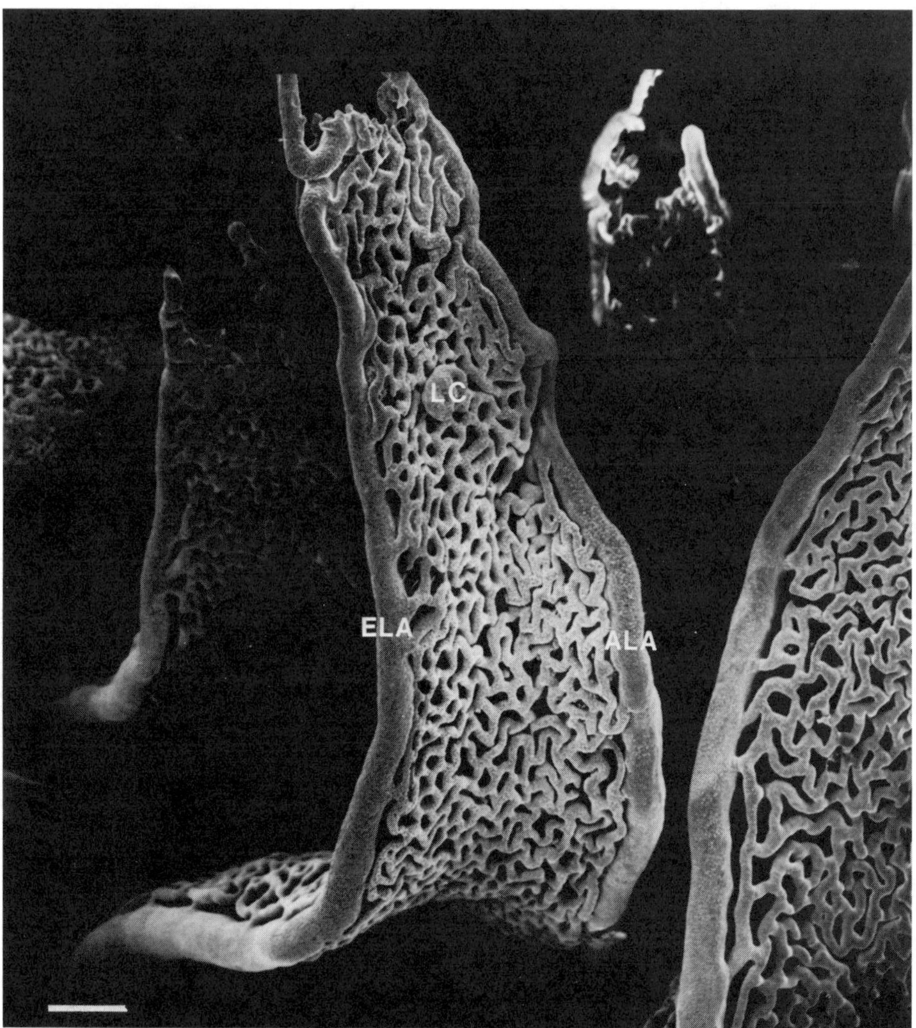

Figure 3 Scanning electron micrograph of a vascular corrosion cast of the respiratory lamellae in *A. tigrinum*. ALA = afferent lamellar arteriole, ELA = efferent lamellar arteriole, LC = lamellar capillaries. Bar = 100 μm.

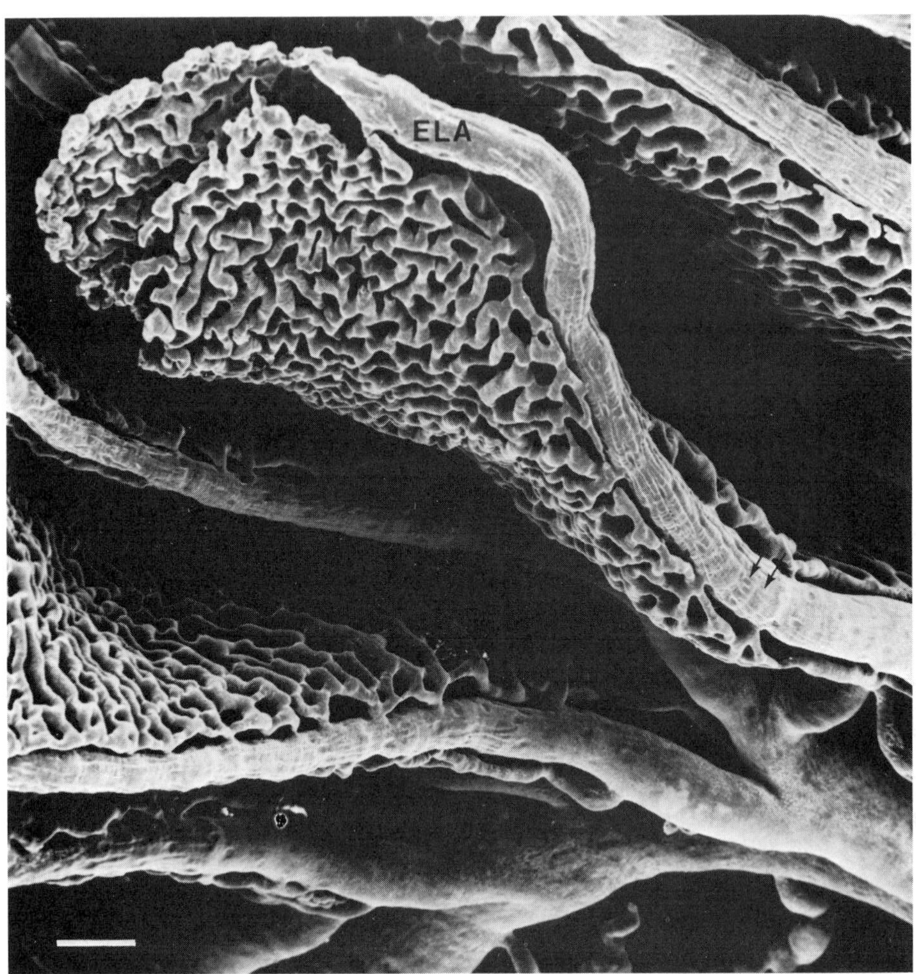

Figure 4 Scanning electron micrograph of a vascular corrosion cast of a respiratory lamella in *A. tigrinum*. The cast has been broken to reveal two sheets of capillaries. Note constrictions (arrows) in the efferent lamellar arteriole (ELA). Bar = 100 μm.

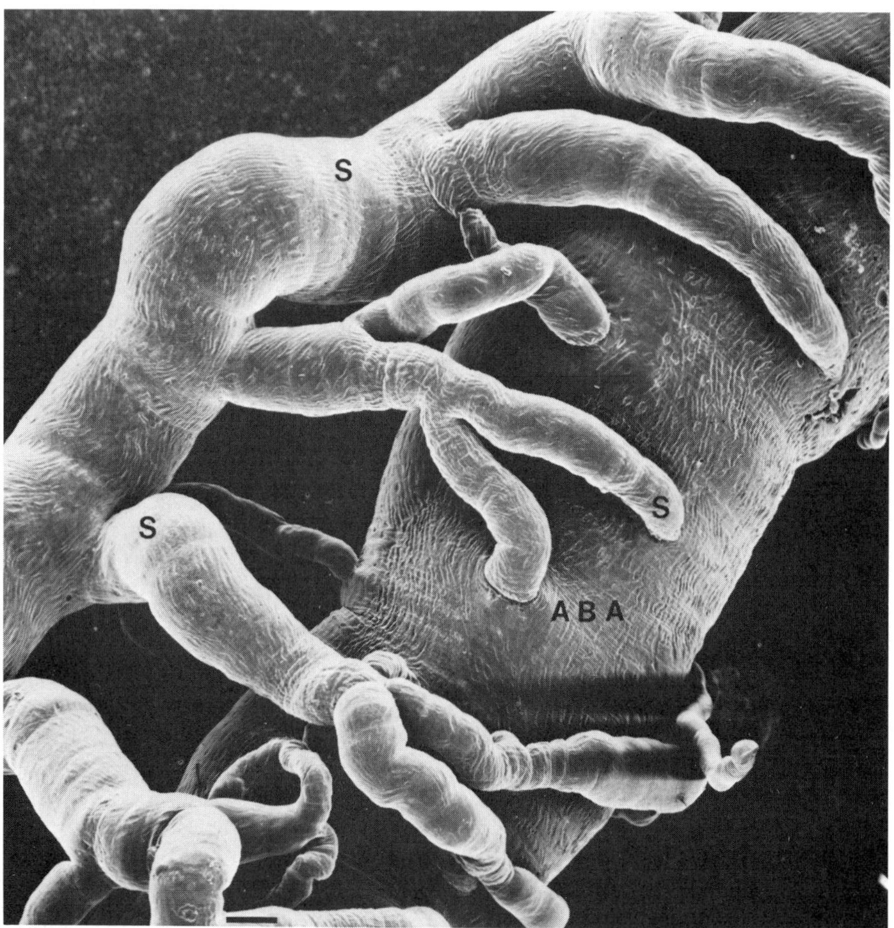

Figure 5 Scanning electron micrograph of a vascular corrosion cast of the shunt vessels (S) and afferent branchial artery (ABA) of the second gill in *A. tigrinum*. Bar = 100 μm.

IV, and V. Within most urodele gills are two major circulatory pathways: a respiratory pathway and a shunt (Fig. 2). In the respiratory pathway, blood flows from the afferent branchial artery into the respiratory section of the gill and then into the respiratory lamellae via afferent lamellar arterioles (Fig. 3). Each afferent lamellar arteriole courses along one edge of a lamella, tapering as it approaches the lamellar tip. The efferent lamellar arteriole is a continuation of the afferent arteriole on the opposite edge of the lamella. A double-sheeted

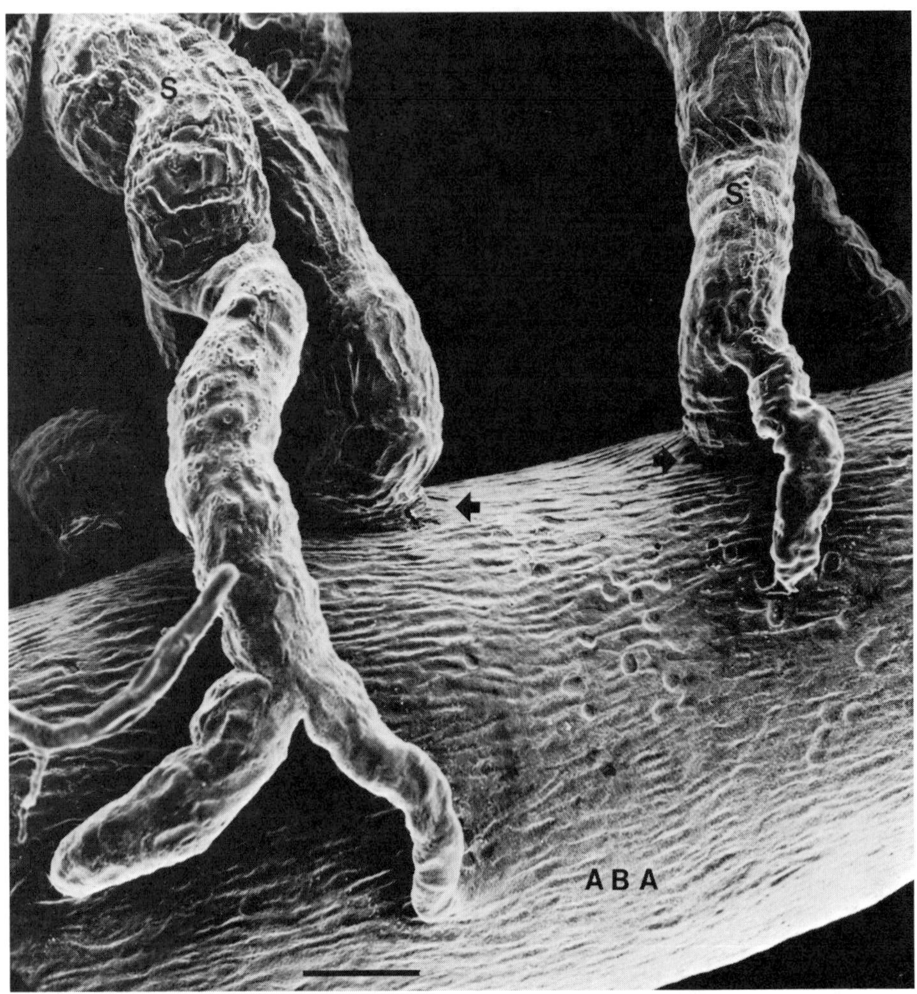

Figure 6 Scanning electron micrograph of a vascular corrosion cast of the shunt vessels (S) of the first gill in *A. tigrinum*. Note constrictions (arrows) in the shunt vessels where they anastomose with the afferent branchial artery (ABA). Bar = 100 μm.

capillary mesh spans each lamella between the arterioles (Fig. 4). This arrangement allows for two intralamellar perfusion pathways. Blood can flow between the arterioles through the capillary mesh, or it can remain in the arterioles completely bypassing the capillary bed. Regardless of the pathway, the efferent arteriole carries blood from the lamella into the primary gill bar. Adjacent efferent arterioles then join to form small efferent branchial arteries, which drain into larger arteries. Blood leaves the branchial respiratory section through a single efferent branchial artery. Each gill bar also contains a venous sinus (Hackford et al., 1977), and in *A. mexicanum*, there is a vascular space between the lamellar capillary sheets (McIndoe and Smith, 1984a).

The other major pathway in the gill allows blood to bypass the branchial respiratory section by flowing directly from the afferent to the efferent branchial artery through a collection of shunt vessels at the cartilagenous base of the gills (Figs. 5 and 6). The shunt vessels are more numerous in the first gill than in the others and in *N. maculosus* the third gill completely lacks shunt vessels (Baker, 1949). Efferent branchial arteries are the dorsal portions of the aortic arches, and they eventually anastomose to form the dorsal aorta.

In air-breathing larval urodeles, the pulmonary circulation is closely associated with the branchial vasculature (see Fig. 1). In *A. tigrinum*, the pulmonary artery (aortic arch VI) emerges directly from the heart just posterior to the third afferent branchial artery. Approximately half-way to the lung, the ductus arteriosus joins the pulmonary artery with the efferent branchial artery of the third gill. Over 75% of pulmonary blood flows first to the third gill and then to the lung through the ductus arteriosus (Malvin, 1985c). Thus, the lungs and gill are largely perfused in series. The pulmonary artery is also characterized by a vascular plexus in the proximal segment of the pulmonary artery (see Fig. 1; Figge, 1934; Malvin, 1985a) which is probably a remnant of a once-present fourth gill (Malvin, 1985c). However, there is little information on its occurrence among the urodele species.

Although this description may be considered as the usual, vascular connections with the lung vary considerably among species. For example, in *N. maculosus* the pulmonary artery emerges from a vessel formed by the union of the second and third efferent branchial arteries and, thus, is missing a direct connection with the heart (Baker, 1949). Other variations are found in *Siren lacertina* (Baker, 1949) and *Salamandra salamandra* (Boas, 1907).

B. Anurans

Anuran larvae utilize two types of gills: external gills that function for only a few days and internal gills that develop after degeneration of the external gills.

External Gills

Morphology

At approximately the time of hatching (Gosner stage 19), small outpouchings appear on the first three branchial arches (visceral arches III, IV, and V). They develop into feathery filaments that quickly degenerate as the operculum grows backward from the hyoid arch to envelope the branchial region. In *Rana pipiens*, degeneration begins after the gills have functioned for only a few days; degeneration taking from 5 to 7 days (Rugh, 1951). During their brief existence, the external gill filaments consist of capillary loops covered by a thin epithelium of variable thickness. The minimum blood-water distance is approximately 1 μm. Two cell types are found in the epithelium: a characteristic epithelial cell containing mucus and a ciliated cell without mucus (Michaels et al., 1971). The branchial arch supporting the filaments functions as a filter for suspended food particles.

As in urodeles, the structure of the external gills may be altered by environment factors. Exposure to environmental hypercapnia (3-5% CO_2) between Gosner stages 14 and 23 causes an increase in both filament length and number in *R. pipiens* and *R. temporaria*. Hyperoxic conditions (40% O_2) decrease filament length in developing *R. pipiens* (Lovtrup and Pigon, 1968).

Vascular Organization

As the external gill filaments develop, capillary loops emerge from the third, fourth, and fifth aortic arches. The capillaries run between the ventral and dorsal segments of the aortic arches, which thus become the afferent and efferent branchial arteries, respectively. As the capillary loops elongate during development of the filament, the section of the aortic arch between the loop becomes thinner but remains patent (Rugh, 1951). Thus, like the urodele gill, two branchial perfusion pathways exist: a route through the respiratory capillaries and a shunt through the original aortic arch. Presumably, shunt flow increases as the filaments degenerate.

Internal Gill

Morphology

Simultaneously with degeneration of the external gill filaments, a new branchial respiratory surface develops at a more ventral position on all four branchial arches. During this time, the operculum grows to enclose completely the gills within the branchial chamber (Rugh, 1951). This second respiratory surface is formed by a bushy row of tufts on the ventral surface of each branchial arch (Fig. 7). The number of tufts per arch is variable (between approximately six and 30), but the fourth gill always has the fewest. Each tuft has a stem giving rise to a branching system of blood-filled epithelial tubes. There are at least three orders of branches, and the terminal branch (Fig. 8) is roughly 20 μm in diam-

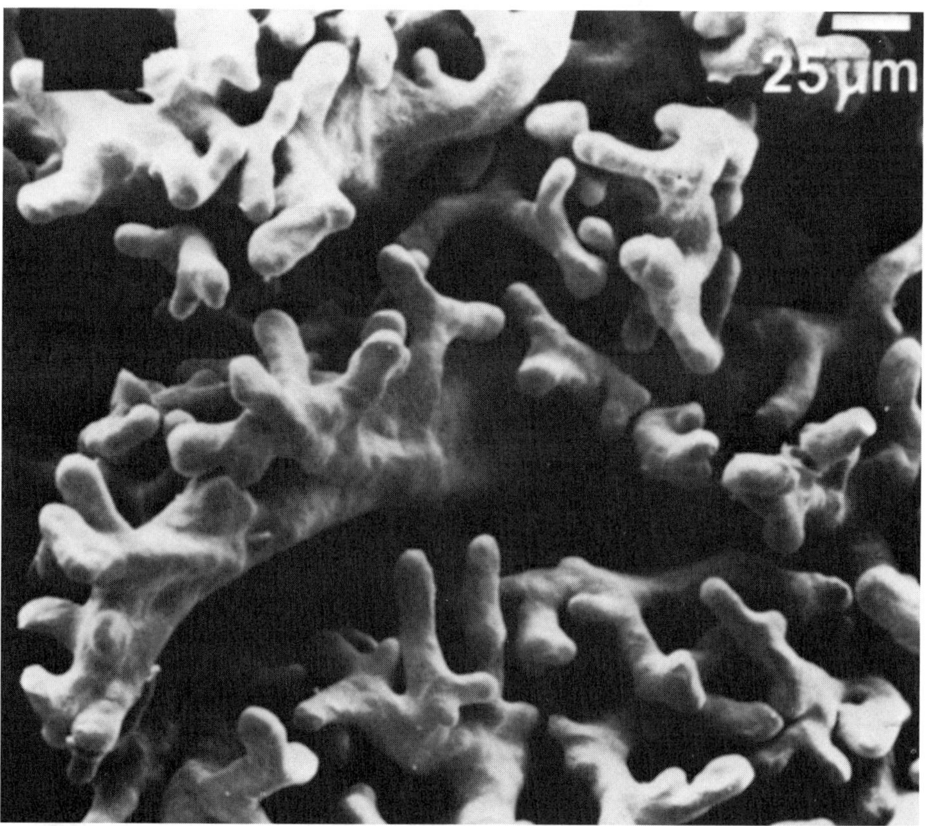

Figure 7 Scanning electron micrograph of the epithelial surface of gill tufts in *Litoria ewingii*. (From McIndoe and Smith, 1984b.)

eter (Burggren and Mwalukoma, 1983; Gradwell, 1971; Hourdry, 1974; McIndoe and Smith, 1984b). In some species (pipids, *Rhinophrynus*, and several microhylids), the branchial arches are devoid of respiratory tufts.

As with the other gill types, environmental factors can affect gill morphology. In *R. catesbiana* tadpoles, chronic hypoxia (water PO_2 between 70 and 80 torr for approximately 4 weeks) elicits increases in the number, height, and width of the gill tufts plus the length of the entire gill arch. Long-term exposure to an environmental PO_2 above 275 torr has the opposite effect (Burggren and Mwalukoma, 1983).

In *Discoglossus pictus*, the epithelium covering the stem and larger branches of the tufts comprises one or two layers of cuboidal cells. Many of

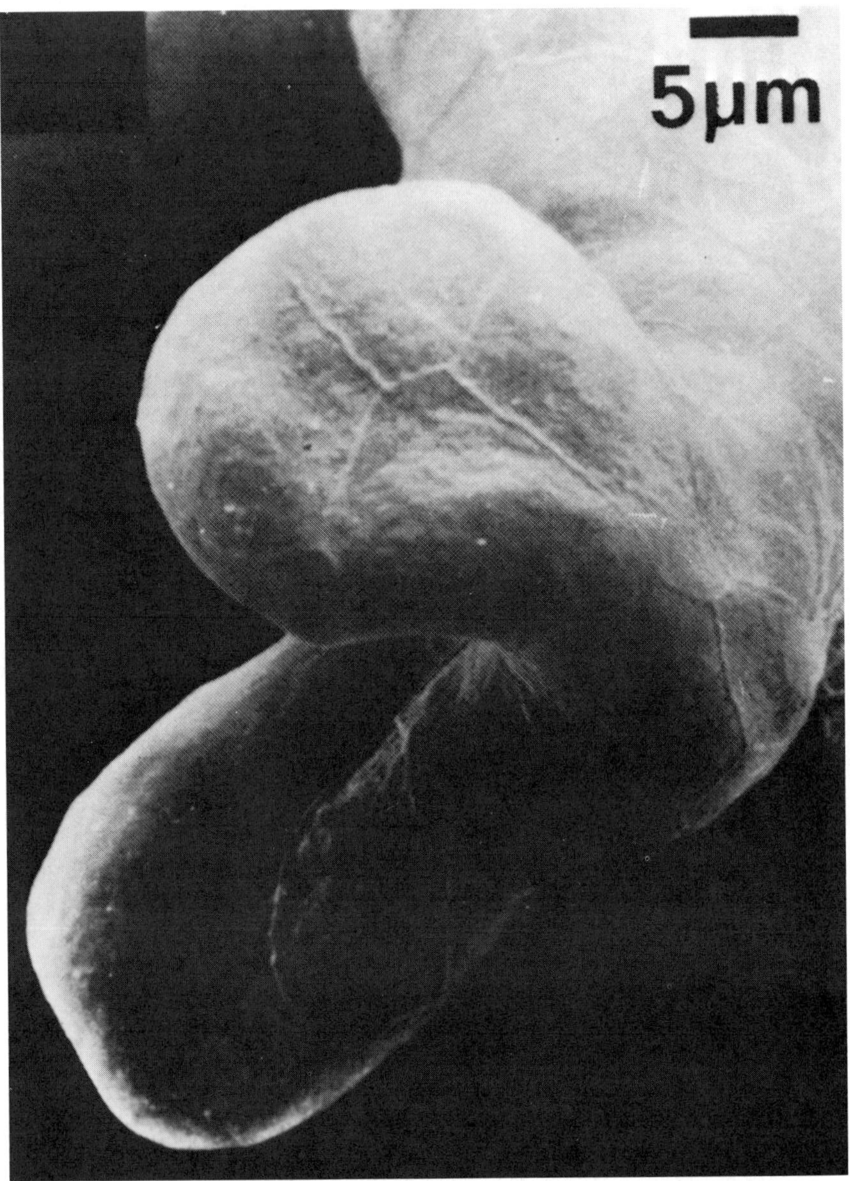

Figure 8 Scanning electron micrograph of the epithelial surface of a terminal branch of a gill tufts in *L. ewingii*. (From McIndoe and Smith, 1984b.)

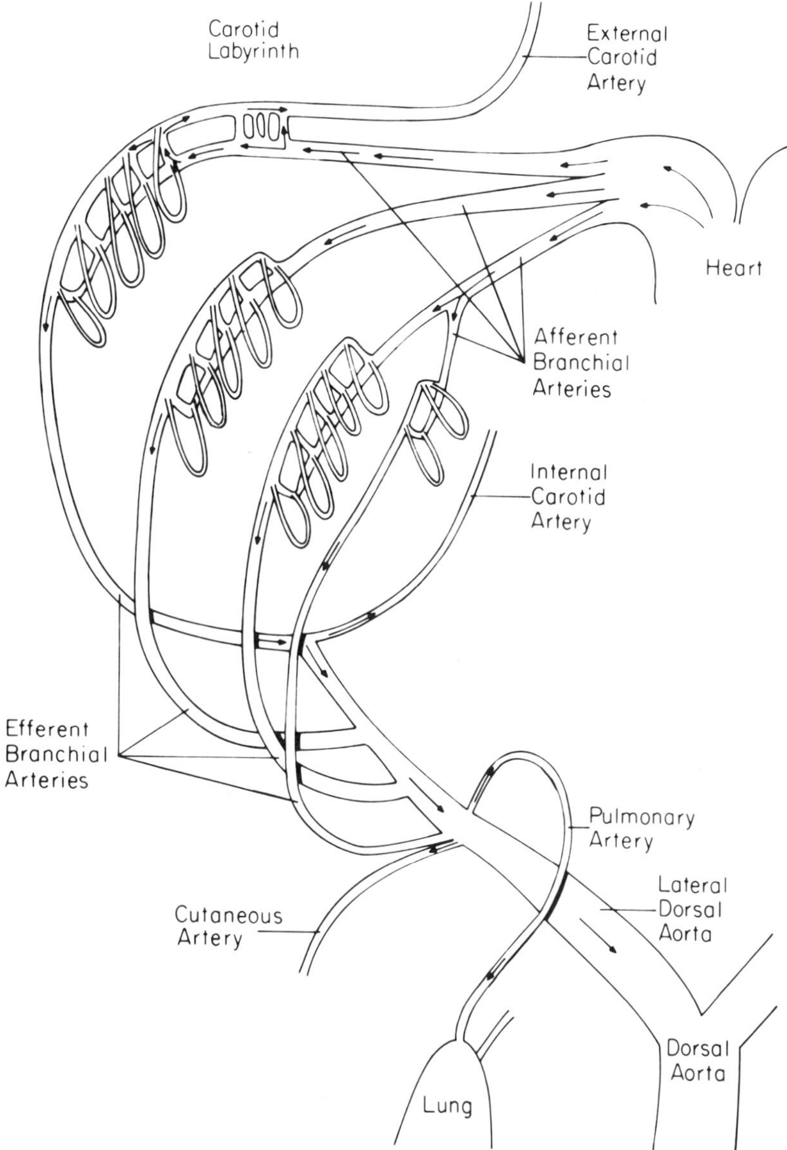

Figure 9 Vascular organization of the aortic arches, gills, and lungs in *L. ewingii*. (Adapted from McIndoe and Smith, 1984b.)

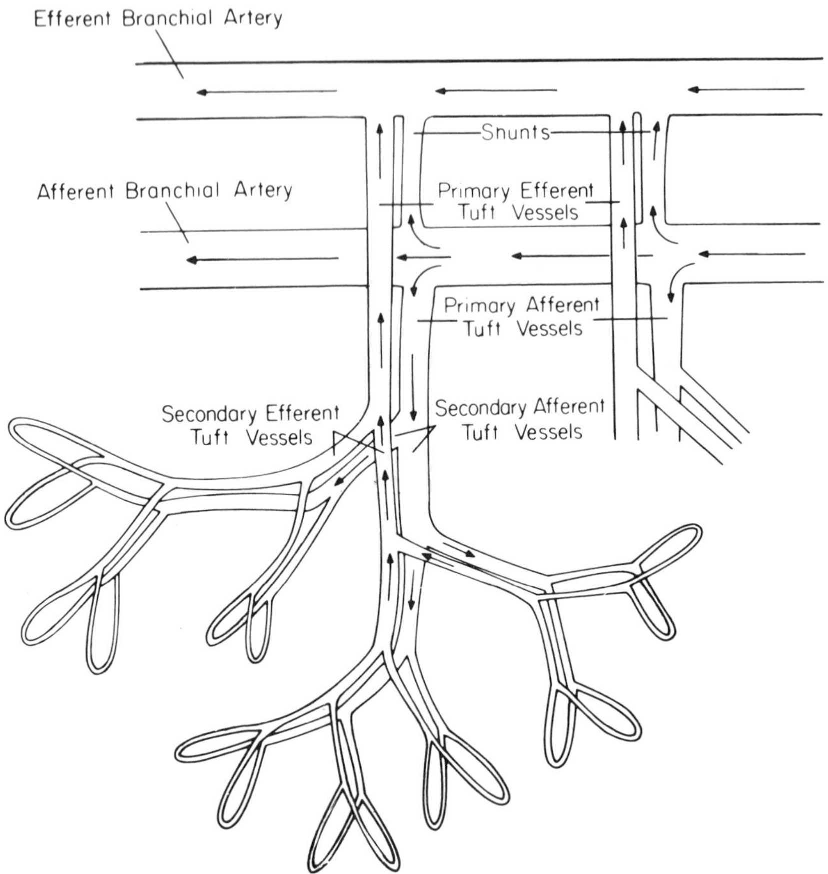

Figure 10 Vascular organization of the gill tufts in *L. ewingii*. (Adapted from McIndoe and Smith, 1984b.)

these cells contain numerous mitochondria suggesting that they function in active transepithelial transport. The epithelium is exclusively one layer in the terminal branches where very thin pavement cells are interspersed with cuboidal cells that are not rich in mitochondria. Here the thickness of the blood-water barrier is quite variable—the thinnest sections being approximately 2 μm across the pavement cells (Hourdry, 1974).

It is noteworthy that the dorsal surface of the gill arch functions primarily as a filter for the entrapment of food particles rather than as a respiratory organ. The filters are parallel epithelial ridges supported by the cartilage within the branchial arch. Each ridge is highly folded into a lattice of smaller ridges and grooves (Gradwell, 1971; McIndoe and Smith, 1984b; Wassersug, 1972).

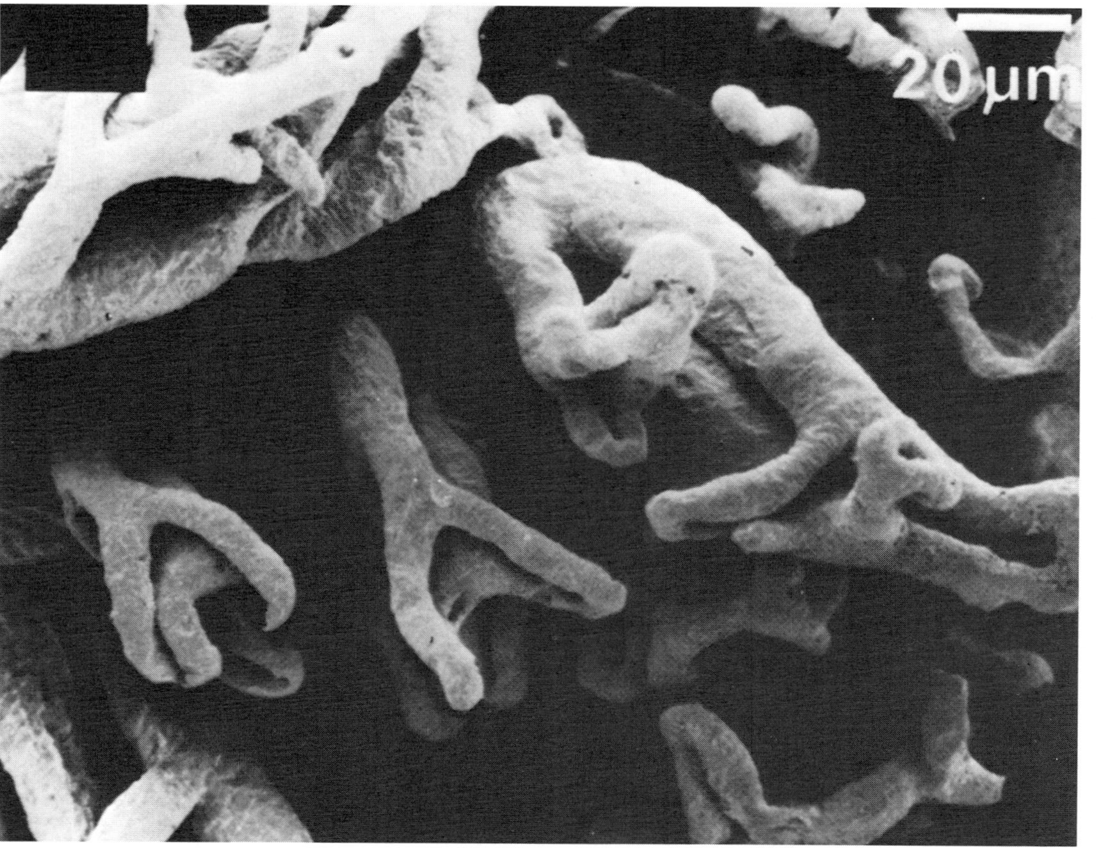

Figure 11 Scanning electron micrograph of a vascular corrosion cast of the terminal capillary loops in the gill tufts of *L. ewingii*. (From McIndoe and Smith, 1984b.)

Vascular Organization

As in other types of amphibian gills, the internal anuran gill has both a respiratory circulation and a shunt pathway (Figs. 9 and 10). Branchial respiratory blood courses from the afferent branchial artery (ventral portion of the aortic arch) into afferent primary tuft vessels that branch into progressively smaller tuft vessels and finally into capillaries. The capillaries form a loop in the smallest branches of the tufts (Figs. 10 and 11), and blood flows out of the tufts through efferent tuft vessels. The afferent and efferent tuft vessels run side by side carrying blood in opposite directions, forming a countercurrent system. In *D. pictus*, less than 7 μm may separate these vessels (Hourdry, 1974); an arrangement that may allow diffusion of gases between the efferent and afferent vessels. Such countercurrent exchange would be expected to depress the respiratory efficiency of the gills, but this possibility has not yet been evaluated. The efferent branchial tuft vessels drain into efferent branchial arteries that converge to form a lateral dorsal aorta on each side of the animal. The two lateral aortae then fuse to become the dorsal aorta (McIndoe and Smith, 1984b). Anastomoses between the afferent and efferent branchial arteries at the base of the tufts allow blood to be shunted past the respiratory vasculature (Figs. 10 and 12: Huxley, 1883; McIndoe and Smith, 1984b; de Saint-Aubain, 1981). In addition, the carotid labyrinth at the base of the first gill provides another respiratory bypass (McIndoe and Smith, 1984b).

Beneath the gill filter epithelium is a dense capillary mesh supplied by vessels branching from afferent branchial arteries. The capillaries drain directly into systemic veins rather than the systemic arterial system, which receives blood from the tufts. It is possible that the filter surface may also function in gas exchange, although the epithelium there is several times thicker than the tuft epithelium (McIndoe and Smith, 1984b).

As in urodeles, the pulmonary circulation in lunged larval anurans is associated with the gills. In *Litoria ewingii*, the pulmonary artery emerges from the lateral dorsal aorta (see Fig. 9). The cutaneous artery, a vessel supplying a substantial fraction of the skin, originates adjacent to the origin of the pulmonary artery (McIndoe and Smith, 1984b). Thus, blood reaching the skin and lungs, the other major gas exchange surfaces, first passes through the gills.

III. Gas Exchange

A. Urodeles

Gas Exchange

Only two studies have measured branchial gas exchange in urodeles. Guimond and Hutchison (1972) reported that the large gills of *Necturus maculosus*, which has only rudimentary lungs, account for approximately 60% of total O_2

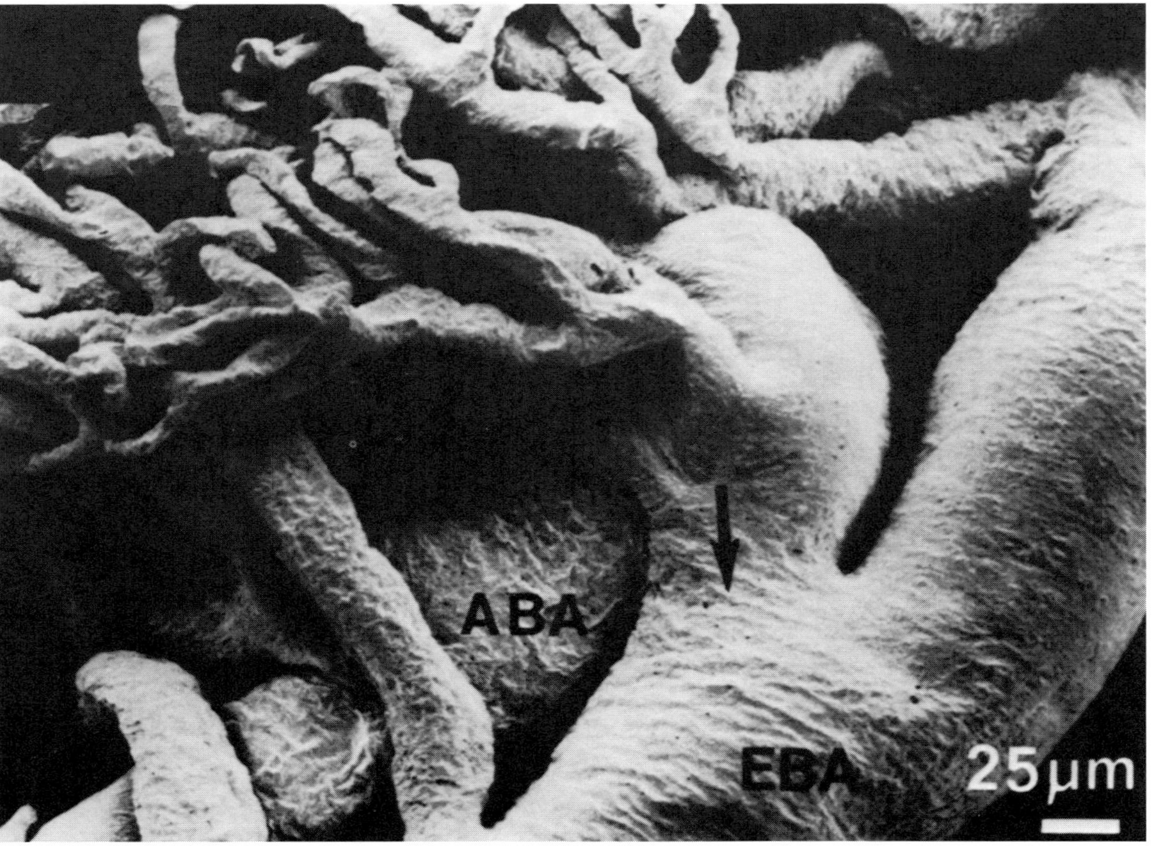

Figure 12 Scanning electron micrograph of a vascular corrosion cast of a branchial shunt vessel in *L. ewingii*. ABA = afferent branchial artery, EBA = efferent branchial artery. (From McIndoe and Smith, 1984b.)

uptake and CO_2 excretion at 25°C. In contrast *Siren lacertina*, heavily reliant on pulmonary respiration, exchanges only 2.5% of total O_2 and 11.3% of total CO_2 across the gills at the same temperature (Guimond and Hutchison, 1973). As temperature falls, the fraction of total gas exchange occurring across the gills rises in *Siren*, but declines slightly in *Necturus*. These measurements were performed on restrained animals with the gills protruding into a water-tight chamber. It is not known how these values relate to undisturbed animals.

Other investigators have sought to assess the respiratory importance of urodele gills by comparing total O_2 uptake between intact animals and animals with the gills either ligated or removed. In larval *A. tigrinum* (Heath, 1975), *A. punctatum* (Boell et al., 1963), and *S. lacertina* (Shield and Bentley, 1973), gill ligation does not alter total O_2 uptake during normoxic conditions, although it causes a 40% decrease in *N. maculosus* (Shield and Bentley, 1973). In environmental hypoxia, elimination of the gills decreases O_2 uptake and survival in *A. tigrinum* (Heath, 1975) and *A. punctatum* (Boell et al., 1963). These results are consistent with a greater importance of the gills during hypoxic than during normoxic conditions. Studies documenting branchial hypertrophy during chronic hypoxia (Babak, 1907; Bond, 1960; Drastich, 1925) support this idea. However, ligation experiments are difficult to interpret because the results reflect not only the loss of branchial gas exchange but also compensatory changes in the other respiratory organs and major trauma to the circulatory system.

Regulation of Gas Exchange

Gill Ventilation

Gill ventilation is probably not an important factor in gas exchange among urodeles because most of these animals do not have specialized mechanisms to produce a large water flow across the lamellar surface. The gills of most urodeles simply "hang" in the water. Environmental water currents will certainly ventilate the gills, but there is no evidence that urodeles seek them out. Gill ventilation will also occur when the animal moves, and this may be a passive mechanism to augment branchial gas exchange during activity. Some ventilation of the lamellar surface may also be accomplished by cilia on the branchial epithelium. In larval *Cryptobranchus allegheinsis*, strong ciliary movements produce observable water currents around the gills (Smith, 1912). However, it is not known to what degree ciliary motion aids in gas exchange or if ciliary activity is regulated to meet different respiratory requirements.

One urodele that does have a specialized branchial ventilatory mechanism is *N. maculosus*, which rhythmically moves its gills back and forth through the water. The frequency of gill movements is regulated to meet changes in metabolic demands and environmental conditions. An increase in temperature from 5 to 25°C causes frequency to increase from 9 to 55 min^{-1}. Activity, physical restraint, and water hypoxia also increase the frequency of gill movements (Guimond and Hutchison, 1972). The physiological pathways and receptors involved in these responses are largely unknown.

Branchial Blood Flow

Because gill ventilation does not appear to be a primary respiratory factor in most urodeles, regulation of branchial gas exchange probably occurs mostly through the changes in blood flow.

The complex organization of the respiratory vasculature allows for many possible patterns of blood flow both within the gills and between the gills and lungs. Information about the distribution of respiratory blood flow comes from studies on *A. tigrinum* involving radiolabeled microspheres (Malvin, 1985c), direct microscopic observation of the gill circulation (Figge, 1936), and vascular resistance measurements on isolated-perfused gills (Figge, 1936; Malvin, 1985a; Malvin, 1985b).

In experiments designed to characterize blood flow patterns in vivo, differently radiolabeled microspheres were simultaneously infused into the systemic and pulmonary venous systems (Malvin, 1985c). Of the microspheres infused into the systemic venous system, 5, 16, and 20% became trapped in the first, second, and third gills, respectively. In contrast, 9, 13, and 6% of the pulmonary venous microspheres lodged in gills 1 through 3, respectively. The difference in microsphere distributions indicates that the heart can selectively distribute the two types of venous blood into the three pairs of branchial arches. Blood entering the first branchial arch is rich in oxygenated pulmonary venous blood, whereas the third branchial arch receives blood enriched in systemic venous blood. Because the lung derives most of its blood from the efferent artery of the third gill through the ductus arteriosus, this pattern of distribution reduces recirculation of pulmonary and systemic venous blood to the lung and systemic vasculatures, respectively. This distribution also indicates that during normoxic conditions, approximately 30 to 40% of total cardiac output flows through capillaries in the respiratory section of the gills.

Microsphere experiments also indicate that respiratory blood flow patterns change during severe aquatic hypoxia (water $PO_2 < 10$ torr) when all O_2 uptake is through the lungs and O_2 may actually be lost across the gills (Malvin, 1985c). Microspheres infused into the venous sytems under these conditions indicate that the fraction of cardiac output perfusing the respiratory section of the first gill is 50% less than during normoxic conditions, and the fraction reaching the head, which receives most of its blood from the first branchial arch, is reduced by 30%. In contrast, there is no change in the fraction of cardiac output perfusing the respiratory sections of the other two gills. This suggests that resistance in the first branchial arch had increased relative to the other arches. Such a change may be adaptive to the hypoxic challenge for two reasons. First, blood will be shunted away from the first arch into the other two branchial arches. Because the third arch is in series with the lung, an increase in its flow will make more blood available for lung perfusion through the ductus arteriosus. Second, a decrease in first gill perfusion will probably reduce O_2 loss from blood to water across that gill during severe aquatic hypoxia. This may be particularly important in the first gill because blood entering the first branchial arch should be high in oxygenated pulmonary venous blood.

The distribution of branchial blood flow also changes in response to alterations in lung O_2 content (Figge, 1936). Lung inflation with 100% O_2 causes flow through the respiratory lamellae to fall and shunt flow to increase. In addition, blood that does flow through the lamellae is redistributed away from the lamellar capillaries and through the entire lamellar arteriolar loop. Lung inflation with 15% CO_2 appears to have the opposite effect. These responses do not seem to be neurally mediated, inasmuch as they are not affected by cutting the ninth and tenth cranial nerve.

Altered perfusion patterns in the gill may also result from long-term exposure to certain environmental conditions. Changes in gill size (Babak, 1907; Bond, 1960; Drastich, 1925) suggest that lamellar blood flow may increase during chronic hypoxia, decrease during long-term hyperoxia, and vary directly with temperature.

Although mechanisms mediating changes in gill perfusion patterns are not known, the vasoactive properties of the gill have been studied. These studies indicate that many physiological systems have the ability to regulate branchial blood flow. Adrenergic control over gill perfusion is possible because epinephrine (EPI) and norepinephrine (NE) are both vasoactive in the gill. In the isolated-perfused gill of *A. tigrinum*, NE is predominantly a vasodilator in the respiratory section of the gill, although at high doses a brief vasoconstriction precedes dilation. Shunt resistance, however, is not responsive to NE. In contrast to NE, EPI is a pressor agent in the shunt vasculature (Figge, 1936; Malvin, 1985a). In a recent study, the primary response to EPI of the respiratory vasculature was vasoconstriction, although at very high doses, a slight vasodilation followed the vasoconstriction (Malvin, 1985a). Earlier work of Figge (1936), also using isolated-perfused gills, found EPI to be solely a vasodilator in that vascular bed. This discrepancy is probably because the EPI available at the time of his study was impure. It was a mixture of both EPI and NE (Goldenberg et al., 1946) so that the dilation observed might have been due to the NE. Pharmacological studies indicate that in the respiratory section of the gill, α- and β-adrenoceptors mediate catecholamine-induced vasoconstriction and vasodilation, respectively (Malvin, 1985b).

Responsiveness to catecholamines in the isolated gill suggests that blood flow distribution between the shunt and respiratory circulations may be regulated by circulating catecholamines and by direct adrenergic innervation of the blood vessels. An increase in circulating NE, for example, should dilate the respiratory section of the gill but have no effect on shunt resistance. This should increase blood flow through the respiratory section. An increase in circulating EPI, on the other hand, should increase vascular resistance in both sections of the gill. However, both the ED_{50} and threshold of the constrictor response to EPI are higher in the shunts than in the respiratory vasculature, and the maximum increase in vascular resistance produced by EPI is nearly four times greater in the respiratory circulation (Malvin, 1985a). Thus, a constrictor response to EPI should be more pronounced in the respiratory section than in the shunts, causing blood to be directed away from the branchial gas exchange surface. The effects of simultaneous increases in EPI and NE are difficult to predict. It is unfortunate that there are no data relating circulating levels of catecholamines to different environmental conditions. Such information would allow a better understanding of the control of gill blood flow.

Histofluorescent-staining for catecholamines has revealed direct adrenergic innervation of the shunt but no such innervation in the respiratory section of the gill (Malvin and Dail, 1986). Because EPI is the major transmitter of amphibian adrenergic nerves (Burnstock, 1969), an increase in adrenergic outflow to the gills should selectively increase shunt resistance and augment branchial respiratory perfusion.

Regulation of branchial blood flow by cholinergic nerves and the renin-angiotensin system is also possible. Acetylcholine is a very effective constrictor agent in both gill circulations, and angiotensin II causes vasoconstriction in the respiratory section of the gill (Malvin, 1985a). Branchial vascular resistance may also be affected directly by environmental or by intravascular PO_2, PCO_2, and pH. However, alterations of these factors in the isolated-perfused gill have, at most, only a slight effect on vascular resistance (Malvin, 1985a). It is possible that responsiveness to these factors is lost when the gill is isolated and artificially perfused, but this is speculative.

The precise vascular segments that participate in the resistance changes are not known. However, vascular corrosion casts of the branchial circulation display prominent constrictions in the shunt vessels where they anastomose with the afferent branchial artery (see Fig. 6). This suggests that regulatory smooth-muscle sphincters may be present at that location. Constrictions in vascular casts are also visible along the efferent lamellar arteriole.

Although it appears that the patterns of gill perfusion are regulated, the impact of these circulatory changes on gas exchange is unknown. There have been neither experimental nor theoretical studies to assess the role of blood flow changes on gas exchange in urodele gills.

B. Anurans

Branchial Gas Exchange

Gas flux across the external gills of anurans has never been measured; thus, little can be said. On the other hand, gas exchange across internal anuran gills has been measured in *Rana catesbiana* (Burggren et al., 1983; Burggren and West, 1982; West and Burggren, 1982) and *R. berlandieri* (Burggren et al., 1983) by cannulating the opercular spout, collecting the expired water, and then analyzing the inspiratory and expiratory water. In lungless *R. catesbiana* tadpoles (Gosner stages 29 to 30; Gosner, 1960) at 20°C during normoxic conditions, the gills account for approximately 40% of total O_2 and CO_2 exchange, the remainder occurring across the skin. As lungs develop, both the branchial respiratory surface area and gill ventilation fall, causing a reduction in branchial O_2 uptake. When tadpoles are obligate air breathers (stages 40 to 41), the gills contribute less than 20% of the total O_2 consumed. The percentage of total CO_2 excreted by the gills in lunged tadpoles remains at approximately 40%, despite the reduction in gill surface area and ventilation, primarily because blood P_{CO_2} rises with air breathing. This difference between O_2 and CO_2 exchange causes the respiratory quotient, R, for the gills to rise during larval development (Burggren and West, 1982).

The P_{O_2} of inspired water and temperature affect O_2 uptake across the gills. Between inspired P_{O_2}s of approximately 96 and 650 torr, branchial O_2 uptake by *R. catespiana* tadpoles (stages 40 to 41) remains constant. However, at an inspired P_{O_2} of 41 torr, branchial O_2 uptake is only 40% of that at normoxic levels, and at an inspired P_{O_2} of 21 torr, O_2 is actually lost across the gill to the water. Animals in hypoxic water compensate for the reduction in branchial gas exchange by increasing aerial respiration (West and Burggren, 1982). Branchial O_2 uptake of air-breathing tadpoles increases with temperature. The rate of increase parallels that of the entire animal; hence, the fraction of total O_2 uptake by the gills is unaffected (Burggren et al., 1983).

The amount of O_2 normally extracted from the inspired water by the gills of *R. catesbiana* is high. In both lungless and air-breathing tadpoles in normoxic water, the P_{O_2} of expired water is between approximately 50 and 60 torr. This represents an O_2 utilization by the gills of approximately 60%, which is comparable with that of fish and almost twice that of mammalian lungs. The O_2 utilization increases in hyperoxic and decreases in hypoxic waters (Burggren and West, 1982).

The degree of perfusion and diffusion limitation for O_2 in the gills of *R. catesbiana* tadpoles has been addressed by Burggren and West (1982). They artificially increased gill ventilation by increasing the hydrostatic pressure gradient across the gill and measured a rise in expired water P_{O_2} but no change in branchial O_2 uptake. The increase in expired P_{O_2} probably reflected an increase in the P_{O_2} of the water surrounding the gill tufts, suggesting that the P_{O_2} gradient across the branchial epithelium between blood and water decreased. Assuming that blood and water flow patterns were not disrupted by the increased ventilation, the steady uptake of O_2 in the face of a smaller O_2 diffusion gradient indicates that the diffusion of O_2 from water to blood does not limit O_2

flux. Instead, the limiting factor is most likely the volume of blood perfusing the gill tufts per time. Thus, O_2 uptake in the amphibian gill, like in the mammalian lung, but unlike the fish gill, appears to be largely perfusion limited under normoxic conditions.

Regulation of Gas Exchange

Gill Ventilation

Mechanics of Ventilation. Internal anuran gills are ventilated by a unidirectional and nearly continuous flow of water propelled by muscles acting on the buccal and pharyngeal cavities (see Fig. 13). In *R. catesbiana* during inspiration, the mouth opens, the buccal floor moves downward, and the pharynx constricts. This causes hydrostatic pressure to fall below ambient pressure within the buccal cavity and to rise in the pharyngeal cavity. Water moves into the buccal cavity through the mouth and nares because of the pressure difference between the buccal cavity and the environment. The increase in pharyngeal pressure propels water downward across the gills and into the branchial chamber, which is bounded on the outside by the operculum. Water leaves the animal by a spiracle on the ventral surface of the body. Flow from the pharynx to the buccal chamber is prevented by a thin flap of tissue, the ventral velum, which forms a seal between the two cavities when pharyngeal pressure exceeds buccal pressure. During the first part of expiration, the mouth closes, the buccal floor is elevated, and the pharynx relaxes. Pressure in the buccal cavity rises as pharyngeal pressure falls, causing a reversal of the bucco-pharyngeal pressure gradient. Consequently, the ventral velum opens, allowing water to flow into the pharynx from the buccal cavity. Flow out through the nares is prevented by a narial valve, which closes when the buccal pressure exceeds the ambient. Early expiratory flow from the buccal cavity expands the pharyngeal cavity and during this time flow across the gills stops. As water continues to move into the pharynx, pressure there rises and flow is resumed across the gills. After the early part of expiration, some water flows directly from the buccal cavity through the first gill slit (Gradwell 1971a; Gradwell, 1971b; Wassersug and Hoff, 1979).

The gill filters are the first part of the gill to come into contact with the ventilated water. Suspended particulate matter becomes entrapped on this feeding apparatus, and then it is transported to the esophagus by a flow of mucus. Water cleared of particulate matter passes across the capillary tufts on the other side of the gill (Wassersug, 1972).

The ventilatory rate is normally quite high in *R. catesbiana.* At 20°C under normoxic conditions in *R. catesbiana* tadpoles (stages 29 to 30), pump frequency is approximately 93 min^{-1} and stroke volume is 3 $\mu l \cdot g^{-1}$ body weight, which produces a net flow of approximately 0.27 $ml \cdot g^{-1} \cdot min^{-1}$ (Burggren and West, 1982). At rest, ventilatory frequency is synchronized with the heart beat in a number of species (Wassersug et al., 1981).

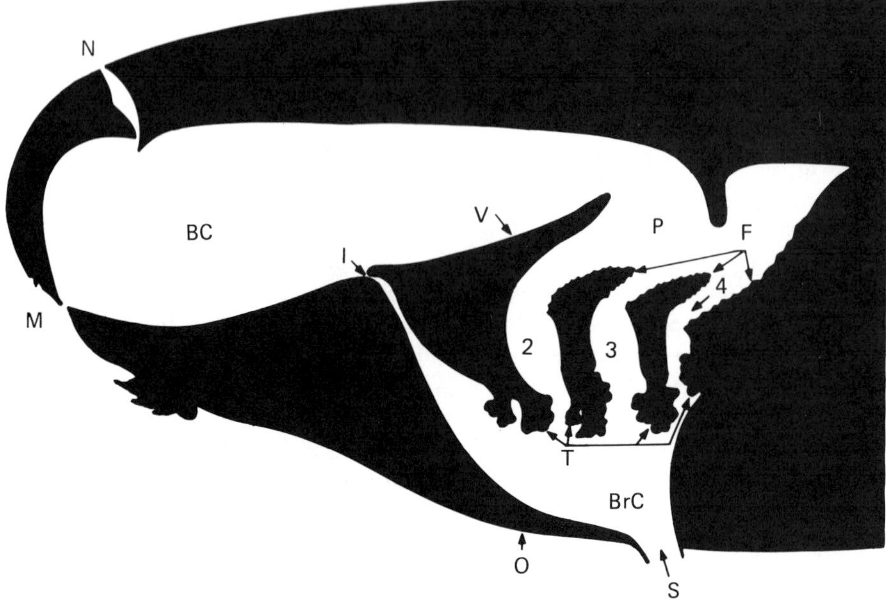

Figure 13 Diagram of the structures associated with gill ventilation in *R. catesbiana*. BC = buccal cavity, BrC = branchial chamber, F = gill filters, M = mouth, N = nares, O = operculum, P = pharynx, S = spiracle, V = ventral velum, 1–4 = gill slits 1–4. (From Gradwell, 1970.)

Control of Gill Ventilation. In contrast to urodeles, gill ventilation is probably an important regulator of branchial gas exchange in anurans. Ventilation in many, but not all, species is influenced by development, the PO_2 of inspired water, lung ventilation, and temperature. In *R. catesbiana*, stroke volume of the bucco-pharyngeal pump decreases during development so that total gill ventilation is approximately 50% less in air-breathing tadpoles (stages 39 to 40) than in younger water breathers (stages 26 to 29; Burggren and West, 1981). The PO_2 of inspired water exerts a strong influence over gill ventilation in *R. catesbiana*. Above a water PO_2 of approximately 80 to 90 torr at 20°C, both buccopharyngeal pump frequency and stroke volume are inversely related to inspired PO_2 (West and Burggren, 1982; West and Burggren, 1983). The threshold for this hypoxic ventilatory drive is between 200 and 300 torr (West and Burggren, 1983). Gill ventilation would probably continue to increase below an inspiratory PO_2 of 80 to 90 torr if lung ventilation did not increase. However, lung ventilation exerts a strong inhibition on gill ventilation and the high frequency of air breathing in hypoxic water acts to override the branchial hypoxic drive, causing a net reduction in gill ventilation (West and Burggren, 1982; West

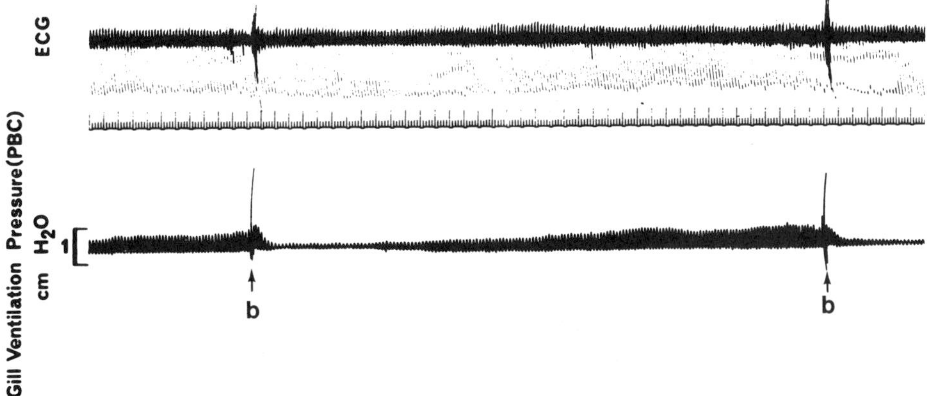

Figure 14 Inhibition of gill ventilation by an air breath in a *R. catesbiana* larva in hypoxic water (PO_2 = 80 torr). Upper trace is an electrocardiogram, middle trace is a 1-s and 5-s time marker, and lower trace is buccal pressure recorded via a narial cannula. (From West and Burggren, 1982.)

and Burggren, 1983). Inhibition by an air breath is characterized by a rapid decrease in both the frequency and pressure generated by the buccopharyngeal pump followed by a gradual return to prebreath levels (Fig. 14). The onset of inhibition is extremely rapid (< 0.1 s). Because it is unaffected by intrapulmonary PO_2, it is likely that pulmonary stretch receptors are involved. The magnitude and duration of inhibition are larger in hypoxic water than in water high in O_2. In addition, the degree of inhibition is directly related to intrapulmonary PO_2. This suggests that an O_2 sensor acts in conjunction with pulmonary stretch receptors to modulate the response (West and Burggren, 1982).

Control of gill ventilation has also been demonstrated in other species. As in *R. catesbiana*, aquatic hypoxia stimulates buccopharyngeal pump frequency in *R. berlandieri* (Feder, 1983; Wassersug et al., 1981) and also in *Xenopus laevis*, but only when these species are denied access to air (Feder and Wassersug, 1984). In *R. pipiens*, aquatic hypoxia depresses gill ventilatory frequency at stage 41, but it has no effect during stages 29-1/2 and 34. Ventilatory frequency in *Scaphiopus bombifrons* does not respond to alterations in aquatic PO_2 (Wassersug and Seibert, 1975). Pulmonary inhibition of gill ventilation may also occur in *R. berlandieri* (Feder, 1983). In some species, feeding regulates ventilation. Buccopharyngeal pump frequency in *X. laevis* varies inversely with the concentration of suspended food particles in water (Feder et al., 1984), and in *S. bombifrons*, frequency increases when the tadpole moves along the bottom where it feeds (Wassersug and Seibert, 1975).

Control of Blood Flow

Perhaps the largest gap in our understanding of anuran gills is in their perfusion. There have been no measurements of blood flow, vascular resistance, vascular innervation, vasoactivity, or blood pressures within either the internal or external gills. However, indirect observations suggest a few characteristics of branchial perfusion. In vascular corrosion casts of *Litoria ewingii*, the diameters of the shunt vessels are several times larger than those of the primary tuft vessels, suggesting that the shunts are able to carry a substantial fraction of the branchial blood flow (see Fig. 12; McIndoe and Smith, 1984b). The actual distribution of flow and its regulation between the respiratory and shunt vessels is not known. However, hypertrophy of the respiratory surfaces during chronic hypercapnia (Lovtrup and Pigon, 1968) or hypoxia (Burggren and Mwalukoma, 1983) indicates that these conditions may augment branchial respiratory perfusion. Rapid matching of blood flow to ventilation or the PO_2 of the respiratory medium is common among vertebrate respiratory organs. If such regulation also exists in amphibian gills, sudden changes in branchial flow or in its distribution would be expected during alterations in inspired PO_2 and lung ventilation. This remains to be evaluated.

IV. Nonrespiratory Functions

In addition to gas exchange, amphibian gills are used extensively in feeding and in ion regulation. They may also be involved in chemoreception.

The gills are probably the primary site for ion regulation in anuran larvae. Considerable active uptake of Na^+ and Cl^- occurs across the gills (Alvarado and Moody, 1970; Boonkoom and Alvarado, 1971; Dietz and Alvarado, 1974) that is intensified by salt depletion (Alvarado and Moody, 1970). In addition, NH_4^+, the primary end product of nitrogen metabolism in larvae, is excreted by the gills, and branchial excretion of lactate following exercise appears to be important in acid-base regulation (Quinn and Burggren, 1983). During larval development, transepithelial ion transport decreases across the gills, whereas it increases across the skin (Alvarado and Moody, 1970; Gonzalez et al., 1979), which is the major organ for salt and water balance in adults. Urodele gills also take up Na^+ and Cl^- (Whittouck, 1972), but their importance in total ion exchange is questionable because gill ligation in urodeles has no effect on total body Na^+ flux (Baldwin and Bentley, 1982; Whittouk, 1974) or on Ca^{2+} flux (Baldwin and Bentley, 1981). It has been suggested that the mitochondria-rich cells of the gill epithelium are involved in ion exchange (Greven, 1980; Hackford et al., 1977; Hourdry, 1974; Lewinson et al., 1984). If this is correct, then ion transport is probably restricted to areas containing these cells (i.e., the primary gill bar in urodeles and the stem and primary divisions of the anuran tufts).

A chemoreceptive role for the gills is suggested by the close association of the first gill with the carotid labyrinth. In anurans, the carotid labyrinth is located at the base of the first gill (McIndoe and Smith, 1984b; Rugh, 1951). Urodele larvae do not have a carotid labyrinth, but the shunt vasculature of the first gill develops into that organ during metamorphosis. Although the function of the larval carotid labyrinth has never been studied, there is evidence that in the adult it is involved in sensing blood PO_2 (Ishii et al., 1966). Cells similar to the putative chemoreceptive cells of the adult carotid labyrinth have been identified in the shunt vasculature of the first gill (Malvin and Dail, 1986), suggesting chemoreception in that circulation.

V. Metamorphosis

During metamorphosis, the gills disappear and aerial gas exchange increases. In *R. catesbiana*, branchial respiration decreases with lung development (Burggren and West, 1982) and probably falls precipitously during metamorphic climax. The gills completely disappear by stage 44. Although never measured, branchial gas exchange in urodeles probably quickly declines early in metamorphosis inasmuchas branchial respiratory perfusion falls approximately 85% 10 days after initiation of thyroxine-induced metamorphosis in *A. tigrinum* (Malvin, 1985c). The first signs of gill regression are a reduction in the size of the respiratory surfaces, thickening and cornification of the epithelium, and a decrease in capillary diameter (Hackford et al., 1977; Hourdry, 1974; Michaels et al., 1971). All of these changes must act to reduce gas flux. Late in metamorphosis, the gill slits close and the branchial arches are incorporated into the sides of the buccal cavity. Tissue destruction is accomplished, in part, by macrophages that invade the gills (Hackford et al., 1977; Hourdry, 1974). In anurans, autolysis by acid phosphotase probably contributes to tissue resorption (Hourdry, 1974), although no evidence for autolysis in urodeles has been found (Hackford et al., 1977). While the branchial respiratory vasculature disappears, gill blood flow is maintained by the shunt vessels, which enlarge and eventually coalesce into the tubular aortic arches of the adult. Aortic arch V disappears or becomes much reduced. Aortic arch VI enlarges to become the pulmocutaneous artery in anurans, whereas it remains as the pulmonary artery in urodeles, but the pulmonary arterial plexus is replaced by a single tube. The ductus arteriosus usually disappears, although in some species (e.g., *A. tigrinum*) it is retained but in a smaller form. In urodeles the shunt vasculature of the first gill is transformed into the carotid labyrinth (Gilmore and Figge, 1929; Malvin, 1985c).

VI. Summary

In summary, the amphibian gill is an extremely complex organ. Not only does it have a complex structure, but the gill performs several functions simultaneously (i.e., gas exchange, ion regulation, and feeding). In addition, most amphibian gills are transitory organs, arising in the embryo and disappearing at metamorphosis.

Gas exchange across the gill is affected by many factors including temperature, environmental gas tensions, and lung ventilation. Many of the changes in gas exchange involve alterations in blood flow and in gill ventilation. The mechanisms regulating gill perfusion and ventilation are still largely unknown, but they appear to involve many different physiological systems.

At present, information on all aspects of the amphibian gill is scarce and much must be acquired for a full understanding of the structure and function of this organ.

References

Alvarado, R. H., and Moody, A. (1970). Sodium and chloride transport in tadpoles of the bullfrog *Rana catesbiana. Am. J. Physiol. 218*:1510-1516.

Baker, C. L. (1949). The comparative anatomy of the aortic arches of the urodeles and their relation to respiration and degree of metamorphosis. *J. Tenn. Acad. Sci. 24*:12-40.

Baldwin, G. F., and Bentley, P. J. (1981). Calcium exchanges in two neotenic urodeles: *Necturus maculosus* and *Ambystoma tigrinum*. Role of the integument. *Comp. Biochem. Physiol. 70A*:65-68.

Baldwin, G. F., and Bentley, P. J. (1982). Roles of the skin and gills in sodium and water exchanges in neotenic urodele amphibians. *Am. J. Physiol. 242*: R94-R96.

Boas, J. E. V. (1882). Uber den Conus Arteriosus und die Arterieren der Amphibien. *Morphol. Jahrb. 7*:488-572.

Boell, E. J., Greenfield, P., and Hille, B. (1963). The respiratory function of gills in the larvae of *Amblystoma punctatum. Dev. Biol. 7*:420-431.

Boonkoom, V., and Alvarado, R. H. (1971). Adenosinetriphosphatase activity in gills of larval *Rana catesbiana. Am. J. Physiol. 220*:1820-1824.

Bond, A. N. (1960). An analysis of the response of salamander gills to changes in the oxygen concentration of the medium. *Dev. Biol. 2*:1-20.

Burggren, W. W., Feder, M. E., and Pinder, A. W. (1983). Temperature and the balance between aerial and aquatic respiration in larvae of *Rana berlandieri* and *Rana catesbiana. Physiol. Zool. 56*:263-273.

Burggren, W., and Mwalukoma, A. (1983). Respiration during chronic hypoxia and hyperoxia in larval and adult bullfrogs (*Rana catesbiana*). I. Morphological responses of the lungs, skin, and gills. *J. Exp. Biol. 105*:191-203.

Burggren, W. W., and West, N. H. (1982). Changing importance of gills, lungs and skin during metamorphosis in the bullfrog *Rana catesbiana. Respir. Physiol. 47*:151-164.

Dietz, T. H., and Alvarado, R. H. (1974). Na and Cl transport across the gill chamber epithelium of *Rana catesbiana* tadpoles. *Am. J. Physiol. 226*: 764-770.

Drastich, L. (1925). Ueber das Leben der Salamandra-Larvan bei hohem und niedrigen Sauerstoffpartialdruck. *Z. Vgl. Physiol. 2*:632-657.

Duellman, W. E., and Trueb, L. (1986). *Biology of Amphibians*. New York, McGraw-Hill Book Co., pp. 156-158.

Feder, M. E. (1983). Responses to acute hypoxia in larvae of the frog, *Rana berlandieri. J. Exp. Biol. 104*:79-95.

Feder, M. E. (1984). Aerial versus aquatic oxygen consumption in larvae of the clawed frog, *Xenopus laevis. J. Exp. Biol. 108*:231-245.

Figge, F. H. J. (1934). The effect of ligation of the pulmonary arch on amphibian metamorphosis. *Physiol. Zool. 7*:149-177.

Figge, F. H. J. (1936). The differential rection of the blood vessels of a branchial arch of *Amblystoma tigrinum* (Colorado axolotl) I. The reaction to Adrenalin, oxygen, and carbon dioxide. *Physiol. Zool. 9*:79-101.

Gilmore, R. J., and Figge, F. J. (1929). Morphology of the blood vascular system of the tiger salamander, (*Ambystoma tigrinum*). Heart and aortic arches. *Col. Coll. Publ. Gen. Ser. 161*:2-14.

Gonzalez, M., Morales, M., and Zambrano, F. (1979). Sulfatide content and $(Na^+ + K^+)$-ATPase activity in skin and gill during development of the Chilean frog, *Calyptocephalella caudiverbera. J. Membr. Biol. 51*:347-359.

Gosner, K. L. (1960). A simplified table for staging anuran embryos and larvae with notes on identification. *Herpetologica 16*:183-190.

Gradwell, N. (1970). The function of the ventral velum during gill irrigation in *Rana catesbiana. Can. J. Zool. 48*:1179-1186.

Gradwell, N. (1972). Gill irrigation in *Rana catesbiana*. Part II. On the musculoskeletal mechanism. *Can. J. Zool. 50*:501-521.

Greven, H. (1980). Ultrastructural investigations of the epidermis and the gill epithelium in the intrauterine larvae of *Salamandra salamandra* (L.) (Amphibia, Urodela). *Z. Mikrosk. Anat. Forsch. Leipz. 94*:196-208.

Guimond, R. W., and Hutchison, V. H. (1972). Pulmonary, branchial and cutaneous gas exchange in the mud puppy, *Necturus maculosus maculosus* (Rafinesque). *Comp. Biochem. Physiol. 42A*:367-392.

Guimond, R. W., and Hutchison, V. H. (1973). Trimodal gas exchange in the large aquatic salamander, *Siren lacertina* (Linnaeus). *Comp. Biochem. Physiol. 46A*:249-268.

Hackford, A. W., Gillies, C. G., Eastwood, C., and Goldblatt, P. J. (1977). Thyroxine-induced gill resorbtion in the axolotl (*Ambystoma mexicanum*). *J. Morphol. 153*:479-504.

Harrison, R. G. (1969). Harrison stages and description of the normal development of the spotted salamander, *Ambystoma punctatum* (Linn.). In *Organization and Development of the Embryo*. Edited by R. G. Harrison. New Haven, Yale University Press, pp. 44-66.

Heath, A. G. (1975). Respiratory responses to hypoxia by *Ambystoma tigrinum* larvae, paedomorphs, and metamorphosed adults. *Comp. Biochem. Physiol. 55A*:45-49.

Hourdry, J. (1974). Etude des branchies "internes" puis de leur regression au moment de la metamorphose, chez la larve de *Discoglossus pictus* (Otth), amphibien anoure. *J. Microsc. 20*:165-182.

Huxley, T. H. (1883). *The Anatomy of the Vertebrated Animals*. New York, D. Appleton and Co., pp. 165.

Lewinson, D., Rosenberg, M., and Warburg, M. R. (1984). "Chloride-cell"-like mitochondria-rich cells of the salamander larva gill epithelium. *Experientia 40*:956-958.

Lovtrup, S., and Pigon, A. (1968). Observations on the gill development in frogs. *Ann. Embryol. Morphol. 2*:3-13.

Malvin, G. M. (1985a). Vascular resistance and vasoactivity of gills and pulmonary artery of the salamander. *Ambystoma tigrinum. J. Comp. Physiol. 155*:241-249.

Malvin, G. M. (1985b). Adrenoceptor types in the respiratory vasculature of the salamander gill. *J. Comp. Physiol. 155*:591-596.

Malvin, G. M. (1985c). Cardiovascular shunting during amphibian metamorphosis. In *Cardiovascular Shunts, Alfred Benzon Symposium* 21. Edited by K. Johansen and W. W. Burggren. Copenhagen, Munskgaard, pp. 163-178.

Malvin, G. M., and Dail, W. G. (1986). Adrenergic innervation of the gills, pulmonary arterial plexus and dorsal aorta in the neotenic salamander, *Ambystoma tigrinum. J. Morphol. 189*:67-70.

McIndoe, R., and Smith, D. G. (1984a). Functional morphology of gills of larval amphibians. In *Respiration, and Metabolism of Embryonic Vertebrates*. Edited by R. S. Seymour. Dordrecht, Dr. W. Junk Publishers, pp. 55-69.

McIndoe, R., and Smith, D. G. (1984b). Functional anatomy of the internal gills of the tadpole of *Litoria ewingii* (Anura, Hylidae). *Zoomorphology 104*: 280-291.

Michaels, J. E., Albright, J. T., and Patt, D. I. (1971). Fine structural observations on cell death in the epidermis of the external gills of the larval frog, *Rana pipiens. Am. J. Anat. 132*:301-318.

Quinn, D., and Burggren, W. W. (1983). Lactate production, tissue distribution, and elimination following exhaustive exercise in larval and adult bullfrogs *Rana catesbiana. Physiol. Zool. 56*:597-613.

Rugh, R. (1951). *The Frog.* New York, McGraw-Hill Book Co.

Saint-Aubain, M. L. de (1981). Shunts in the gill filament in tadpoles of *Rana temporaria* and *Bufo bufo* (Amphibia, Anura). *J. Exp. Zool. 217*:143-145.

Shield, J. W., and Bentley, P. J. (1973). Respiration of some urodele and anuran amphibia–I. In water, role of the skin and gills. *Comp. Biochem. Physiol. 46A*:17-28.

Smith, B. G. (1912). The embryology and larval development of *Cryptobranchus allegheniensis*, including comparisons with some other vertebrates. II. General embryonic and larval development, with special reference to external features. *J. Morphol. 23*:455-579.

Toews, D., Boutilier, R., Todd, L., and Fuller, N. (1978). Carbonic anhydrase in the amphibia. *Comp. Biochem. Physiol. 59A*:211-213.

Wassersug, R. J. (1972). The mechanism of ultraplanktonic entrapment in anuran larvae. *J. Morphol. 137*:279-288.

Wassersug, R. J., and Hoff, K. (1979). A comparative study of the buccal pumping mechanism of tadpoles. *Biol. J. Linn. Soc. 12*:225-259.

Wassersug, R. J., Paul, R. D., and Feder, M. E. (1981). Cardiorespiratory synchrony in anuran larvae (*Xenopus laevis, Pachymedusa dacnicolor*, and *Rana berlandieri*). *Comp. Biochem. Physiol. 70A*:329-334.

Wassersug, R. J., and Siebert, E. A. (1975). Behavioral responses of amphibian larvae to variation in dissolved oxygen. *Copeia* 1975:86-103.

West, N. H., and Burggren, W. W. (1982). Gill and lung ventilation to steady-state aquatic hypoxia and hyperoxia in the bullfrog tadpole. *Respir. Physiol. 47*:165-176.

West, N. H., and Burggren, W. W. (1983). Reflex interactions between aerial and aquatic gas exchange organs in larval bullfrogs. *Am. J. Physiol. 244*:R770-R777.

Wittouck, P. J. (1972). Intensification par la prolactine de l'absorbtion d'ions sodium au niveau des branchies isolees de larves d'*Ambystoma mexicanum. Arch. Int. Physiol. Biochim. 80*:825-827.

6

Lung Structure and Function
Amphibians

WARREN W. BURGGREN

University of Massachusetts
Amherst, Massachusetts

I. Introduction

The structure and function of amphibian lungs have been investigated since the seventeenth century (Malpighi, 1671; Linnaeus, 1758). Several reasons account for this long-standing interest. First, amphibians have the simplest lungs of any tetrapod in terms of both morphology and physiology. Such relative simplicity can greatly facilitate investigation of phenomena basic to the vertebrate lung, although this is not always recognized by mammalian physiologists. Another basis for the interest in amphibian lungs lies in the radical adjustments in respiratory physiology that accompany amphibian metamorphosis. Many amphibians undergo an ontogenetic transition from what is essentially an aquatic larval existence to a semiterrestrial or fully terrestrial adult life-style supported largely by pulmonary gas exchange. The morphological and physiological basis for such transitions is of interest to a wide range of developmental biologists. Finally, to under-

---

Financial support was provided by National Science Foundation grant DCB8608658.

stand structural and functional aspects of living amphibians is to gain important insights into the evolution of the tetrapod lung. The extant amphibian orders consist of the Anura (frogs, toads), Urodela (salamanders), and Apoda (caecilians). These amphibian orders probably bear only limited resemblance to the ancestors of the amniotes (Gans, 1970), but they do remain the closest living representative of the archtypical tetrapods that we have to examine.

The intent of this chapter is to present a general review of current information of pulmonary structure and function in the amphibians and to identify important areas for future research. The reader is also directed to other chapters in this volume that contain detailed information on particular aspects of amphibian lung biology.

II. Pulmonary Gross Structure

A. Embryonic Origin of the Lungs

In most amphibian embryos the lungs first arise as paired pouches in the endoderm immediately behind the last pair of gill slits. Noble (1931), interpreting embryological studies of Marcus (1908, 1922) on the apodan *Hypogeophis* and other amphibians, clearly identifies these pouches as branchial pouches and not intestinal diverticula that have secondarily taken over a respiratory function. The enlarging lung pouches soon join a median ventral depression in the pharynx, which is the rudimentary larynx and trachea. This respiratory complex eventually closes off from the pharynx to leave the glottis as the sole communication with the enlarging lungs. A similar developmental pattern occurs in reptiles, birds, and mammals and leaves little doubt about the homology of tetrapod lungs (see Goodrich, 1930). Further growth and differentiation of the larva produce the adult amphibian condition of specialized glottis, well-defined larynx, and a relatively stiff trachea, distinct from the lung parenchyma.

B. The Trachea and Bronchi

In many amphibian species, particularly the Anura, the trachea cannot easily be resolved at the point on the pharynx where the bronchus from each lung coalesce (Fig. 1). In those species in which a trachea occurs, it frequently is extremely short, sometimes the equivalent of only two or three of its diameters in length. In some Apoda and Urodela, the trachea is often quite clearly formed, and in *Siren, Amphiuma*, and *Ichthyophis* it is strengthened by a series of paired cartilages similar to the semirings of the amniote trachea (Noble, 1931; Pattle et al., 1977). The trachea is usually a nondifferentiated, poorly vascularized airway. The microvillus luminal surface of the trachea of *Salamandra salamandra, Rana temporaria, R. esculenta*, and *Bufo bufo* contains cilia in small groups or individually, and the epithelium is pseudostratified and contains granular cells

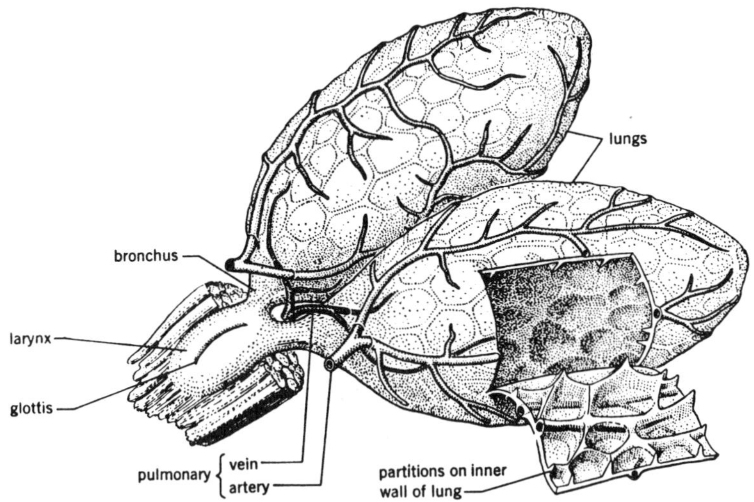

Figure 1 Diagrammatic representation of the pulmonary system of a ranid frog.

(Tesik, 1978). Interesting exceptions to this general tracheal structural pattern are the apodans *Typhlonectes* (Fuhrman, 1914), *Uraeotyphlus* (Baer, 1937), *Hypogeophis* (Gaymer, 1971), and *Ichthyophis* (Pattle et al., 1977), which have a trachea that appears morphologically specialized for respiratory gas exchange.

In amphibians with a clearly developed trachea, the trachea usually bifurcates into bronchi connecting with two anatomically distinct lungs. The length of the bronchus varies considerably among species, being comparatively long in *Xenopus laevis* and virtually nonexistent in *B. marinus* (Smith and Rapson, 1977). Unlike in many reptiles, the bronchi rarely persist to any depth within the lung parenchyma.

C. Lungs

The general form of the amphibian lung has probably departed little from that of ancestral tetrapods. Relative to the lungs of amniote vertebrates (and even the lungfishes), amphibian lungs tend to be simple, saclike structures. Pulmonary division beyond tertiary septation does not occur, and alveoli, if present, are large and distantly spaced. Yet, given the limitation of this basic morphological simplicity, pulmonary gross structure still shows considerable interspecific variation (Fig. 2). Many authors have attempted to relate the extent of lung differentiation to the behavioral, ecological, or physiological specializations of particular groups of amphibians. Although some generalizations no doubt hold, exceptions abound and frequently cut sharply across systematic divisions, obviating a phylo-

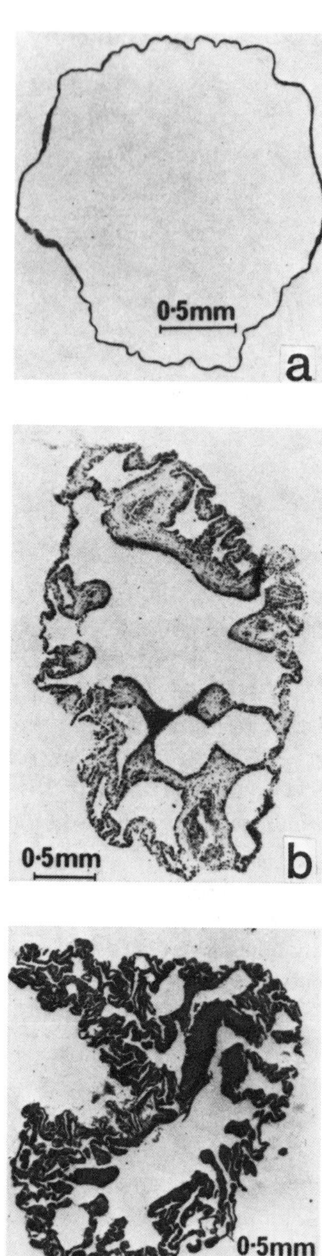

Figure 2 Transverse sections through the lung of the newt, *Triturus vulgaris* (a), the apodan, *Ichthyophis orthoplicatus* (b), and the frog, *Rana temporaria* (c). (From Pattle et al., 1973.)

genetic approach to the problem. Moreover, the pulmonary morphology has been described in detail for only a few dozen of the nearly 3100 species of extant amphibians, and frequently those that have been examined have been chosen because they are unusual, rather than typical, for their group. The reader is thus urged to view the so-called morphological adaptions that follow with some degree of caution.

In many aquatic urodeles (e.g., *Amphiuma, Siren*) and adopans (e.g., *Tylphlonectes*), the lungs are very large, extending for two-thirds of the body length (Goodrich, 1930; Guimond and Hutchison, 1972, 1973, 1974, 1976). In some species, extensive septation greatly increases the internal surface area of the lung and, not surprisingly, such animals rely heavily upon pulmonary gas exchange (see Guimond and Hutchison, 1976). In other aquatic urodeles, however, most gas exchange occurs across buccopharyngeal and cutaneous surfaces (Guimond and Hutchison, 1976; Boutilier et al., 1980; Moalli et al., 1981). In such species, typified by *Proteus, Triturus, Necturus, Cryptobranchus*, and newts such as *Triton*, there is little or no septation of the inner lung surface (Marcus, 1927; Goodrich, 1930; Brodowa, 1956; Czopek, 1959b; Guimond and Hutchison, 1976). Although rigorous experimental evidence frequently is lacking (see Sec. V.C), the large lungs are thought to be of primary importance in regulation of buoyancy (Noble, 1931; Guimond and Hutchison, 1972, 1976).

Relatively simple, nondifferentiated lungs are also found in the ambystomid salamander *Rhyacotriton olympicus*, which inhabits rapidly flowing mountain streams containing cold, oxygen-rich water. In addition, however, the lungs of this species are greatly reduced in size compared with many other aquatic urodeles. Presumably, most gas exchange occurs across the skin, and the reduction in lung size purportedly reduces buoyancy to aid movement in fast-water currents (Porter, 1972). As Goodrich (1930), Noble (1931), and others have emphasized, reduction in pulmonary complexity and in size in extant amphibians most likely represents either a retained larval feature or a secondary evolutionary degeneration of the lung associated with nonrespiratory functions. This view is underscored by consideration of the terrestrial salamander family Plethodontidae (e.g., *Plethodon, Spelerpes, Batrachoseps, Manculus, Aneides, Desmognathus*). Embryos of this family develop only a small "pulmonary" depression on the floor of the esophagus. Consequently, the lungs, trachea, and larynx are completely absent in adults (Camerano, 1896; Luhe, 1900; Mekeel, 1926), and respiration in plethodontids is carried out entirely through the skin (see Feder and Burggren, 1985a). The terrestrial family Salamandridae (e.g., *Salamandra*), represents an intermediate condition of secondary lung degeneration. In some terrestrial salamanders, the lungs are not greatly reduced in size, but the anterior regions of the lung are highly septate, whereas the posterior portion remains more saccular.

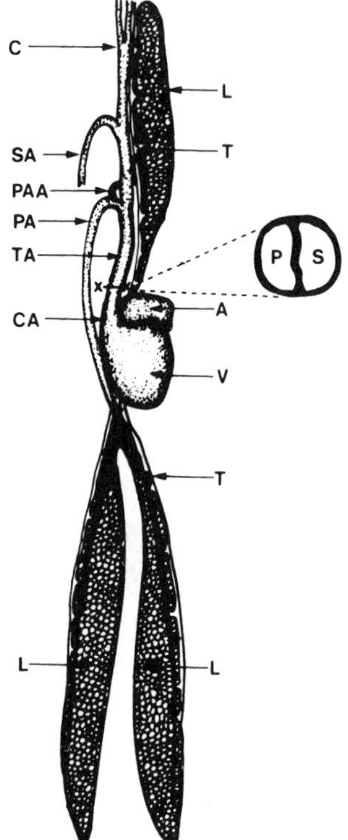

Figure 3 The pulmonary and central cardiovascular system of the apodan amphibian, *Typhlonectes compressicauda*. Note that about three-fourths of the length of the posterior lobes of the lung have not been drawn. A, atrium; C, carotid artery; CA, conus arteriosus; L, lung; P, pulmonary side of truncus; PA, pulmonary artery; PAA, anterior branch of pulmonary artery; S, systemic side of truncus; SA, systemic arch; T, trachea; TA, truncus arteriosus. (From Toews and MacIntyre, 1978.)

Many variations in pulmonary gross anatomy also occur in the Anura, which generally have globular rather than elongate lungs in conformation with their reduced spinal column and stout body (see Fig. 1). Anurans typically inhabiting hypoxic water, or terrestrial species with comparatively thicker, more gas-impermeable skin, tend to have more complex lungs, although again there are many exceptions. In aquatic anurans such as *Xenopus laevis* and *Pipa pipa*, for example, the lungs, although still essentially saclike, show extensive septation of their inner surfaces and small, densely packed alveoli lead to a high respiratory surface area (Marcus, 1937; Czopek, 1955a,b; Bieniak and Watka, 1962; Andrzejewski et al., 1962; Smith and Rapson, 1977). A similarly complex lung is found in many members of the terrestrial anuran family Bufonidae, in which the highly vascularized pulmonary septa branch extensively (Marcus, 1937; Smith and Campbell, 1976; Smith and Rapson, 1977). The Lake Titicaca frog, *Telmatobius culeus*, represents an interesting exception to the pattern of well-developed lungs in Anura. Although exposed to chronic hypoxia by virtue of the high altitude of Lake Titicaca (3812 m), the lungs are very small (Macebo, 1960) and, apparently, are never ventilated (Hutchison et al., 1976; Hutchison, 1982). Large folds of skin greatly increase the surface area of the body, across which all gas exchange occurs.

In many apodans, only the right lung has any degree of alveolarization and the left lung is much reduced in length (Noble, 1931; Pattle et al., 1977), as occurs in most snakes. Nobel (1931) suggests that asymmetric lung reduction in amphibians, as also evident in the urodele *Amphiuma* (Guimond and Hutchison, 1974), may be a response to body elongation. The lungs of *Siren* are of equal length, however. In any event, the very elongate apodan, *Typhlonectes compressicauda* demonstrates yet another pattern of pulmonary organization (Fig. 3). The lung extends virtually the entire length of the body cavity, but it is divided into two caudal lobes only posteriorly to a major pulmonary constriction at the level of the heart.

D. Lung Vascularization

Blood entering the pulmonary arterial circulation of amphibians is derived primarily from the right atrium. In most amphibians, right atrial blood is partially oxygenated because the venous drainage of oxygenated blood leaving the skin mixes with the venous drainage from the deeper tissues before entering the right atrium. Pulmonary arterial blood also contains some left atrial blood because both atrial outflows enter the single ventricle, where some admixture can occur (see Shelton, 1976, Chap. 24 for details). The pulmonary arterial circulation in amphibians arises from the distal end of the bulbus arteriosus, which is the major outflow channel from the ventricle. In anuran amphibians, a pulmocutaneous trunk bifurcates distally to yield paired pulmonary arteries and smaller cutaneous arteries that supply some of the skin.

In accordance with the length and structure of the trachea, bronchi, and lungs, themselves, the pulmonary arteries are variously very short (e.g., *Bufo marinus*), of intermediate length (e.g., *Xenopus laevis*), or elongate in those amphibians with a fusiform shape (e.g., *Typhlonectes compressicauda*; see Fig. 3). In *T. compressicauda*, the pulmonary artery gives rise to a small anterior pulmonary artery that perfuses the anterior lobe of the lung, whereas the pulmonary artery itself continues on to the two posterior lobes.

The gross pattern of distribution of pulmonary arterial blood within the lung has been described for very few amphibians (Kuttner, 1874, 1875; Konigstein, 1903; Smith and Campbell, 1976; Smith and Rapson, 1977) and, unfortunately, has not been described for those species with simple lungs used primarily for flotation. Major differences exist in the perfusion patterns evident in the lungs of the two anurans, *B. marinus* and *X. laevis*. In *Xenopus*, which has a relatively elongate lung for an anuran, the pulmonary artery runs as an axial trunk posteriorly along most of the length of the lung, giving off perpendicular circumferential vessels at regular intervals (Fig. 4). A third generation of radial

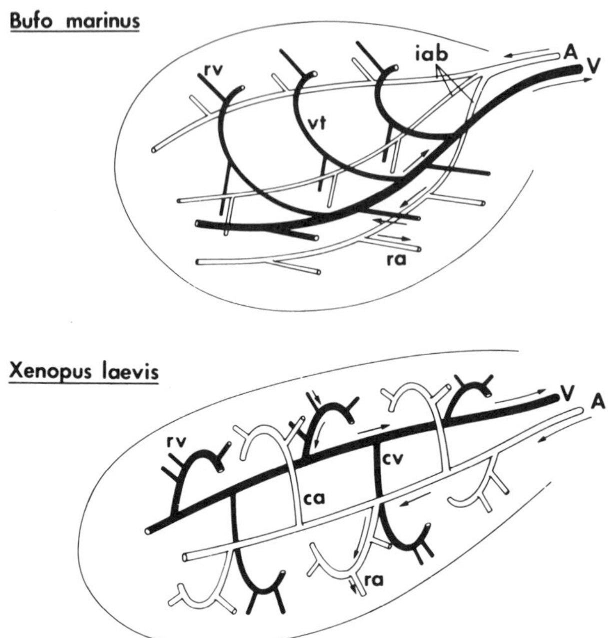

Figure 4 Diagrammatic representation of the major vascular branching patterns in the marine toad *B. marinus* and the African clawed toad *X. laevis*. Directions of blood flow are indicated by arrows. A, pulmonary artery; ca, circumferential artery; cv, circumferential vein; iab, intrinsic arterial branches; ra, radial artery; rv, radial vein; vt, venous tributary; V, pulmonary vein. (From Smith and Rapson, 1977.)

arteries arising from the circumferential vessels gives off short arterioles, which supply the respiratory capillaries of the lung wall and its septa (Smith and Rapson, 1977). A similar arrangement, in which radial arteries branch at right angles from an axial artery running the length of the lung, is found in some apodans (see Fig. 3) and in urodeles with highly elongate lungs (Konigstein, 1903). In *B. marinus*, however, which has a more globular lung, the pulmonary artery divides immediately upon entering the lung parenchyma (see Fig. 4). Three major arteries then course in parallel, more or less, over the lung surface, giving off radial arteries at regular intervals. A similar division of the pulmonary artery into three major branches, serving three longitudinal zones, has been described for the lungs of *Rana esculenta* (Kuttner, 1874) and *R. temporaria* (Konigstein, 1903), although Offman (1875) described a single axial pulmonary arterial distribution in the latter species.

The venous drainage in both *Bufo* and *Xenopus* is essentially a mirror image of the arterial distribution of vessels. In an exhaustive study of more than 25 amphibians (and about 50 reptiles), Willnow and Willnow (1971) frequently observed pulmonary arterial, but never arteriovenous, anastomoses. However, no anastomoses of any description were found in the lungs of bufonids, including *B. marinus*. Interestingly, Smith and Rapson (1977) described relatively large-diameter peribranchial vessels in *Bufo* that connect the extrinsic pulmonary artery and the pulmonary vein across the lung surface. Smith and Rapson (1977) suggest a hemodynamic justification for the existence of these nonrespiratory shunts, based on the utility of having an "intrapulmonary", as well as a central cardiovascular mechanism, for bypassing the pulmonary capillary bed.

The lungs of some amphibians appear to receive collateral vessels from the systemic circulation (Konigstein, 1903). Systemic collateral vessels have been described in the lungs of *R. temporaria*, but these were in purportedly abnormal specimens (Wateson, 1896; Mudge, 1898; Warren, 1898, 1900). Smith and Rapson (1977) identified a systemic arterial supply to the base of the trachea of *B. marinus*, but no systemic vascular supply to the lung parenchyma.

Not surprisingly, considerable simplification of the circulation occurs in the lungless salamanders (Hopkins, 1896; Bruner, 1900, 1914). The bulbus is greatly simplified, and the interatrial septum is poorly developed, if present at all.

No treatment of a vascular system is complete without consideration of lymphatic vessels. Unfortunately, current knowledge of the general amphibian lymphatic system is very rudimentary, with most studies concentrating on the endolymphatic organs and the lymphatic heart. Information on the pulmonary lymphatic system, in particular, is virtually nonexistent for any amphibian species (see Kampmeier, 1969). Rates of plasma filtration in amphibian lungs are high compared with those of mammals or birds (see Chap. 19), and the pulmonary lymphatics must play a critical role in maintaining appropriate fluid balance in the lungs. The morphology and physiology of the pulmonary lymphatic system is a prime area for future investigation, not only in amphibians, but in all lower vertebrates.

E. Lung Innervation

Motor Fibers

The autonomic innervation of the respiratory organs of lower vertebrates has been extensively investigated (see Nilsson, 1985). Considerable information exists on the efferent innervation to the smooth muscle and, to a lesser extent, the vasculature of the amphibian lungs. It should be noted, however, that most studies have been on anurans, particularly *B. marinus*.

Both excitatory and inhibitory fibers reach the lungs by so-called vagosympathetic trunks. Urodeles appear to differ from anurans in that their lungs do not have excitatory fibers (Luckhardt and Carlson, 1920, 1921). In anurans, cholinergic excitatory fibers have been reported to originate both from the sympathetic chains (Shimada and Kobayasi, 1966; Wood and Burnstock, 1967; Campbell, 1971) and the vagus nerve (Wood and Burnstock, 1967; Campbell and Duxson, 1978), but this requires further work to be fully resolved (see Nilsson, 1985 for discussion). Adrenergic fibers cause contraction of the smooth muscle of the lung wall and of the vasculature (Shimada and Kobayasi, 1966; McLean and Burnstock, 1967; Wood and Burnstock, 1967; Campbell, 1971a,b; Campbell et al., 1978; Campbell and Duxson, 1978; Holmgren and Campbell, 1978). Paradoxically, relaxation, in addition to contraction, can be obtained in whole-lung preparations by stimulation of the cervical sympathetic chain. Differences between lung regions in response to sympathetic chain stimulation and catecholamines may complicate interpretation. For example, Holmgren and Campbell (1978) reported that α-adrenergic receptors were involved in mediating contraction of smooth muscle located in the free margins of the septa of the lung of *B. marinus* (see Sec. III for distribution of pulmonary smooth muscle), whereas both α-adrenergic and β-adrenergic receptors were involved in mediating relaxation of the smooth muscle in immediately adjacent regions of the lung wall. These regional differences may have important physiological consequences, and require further investigation.

Notwithstanding these observations of relaxation produced by sympathetic stimulation or adrenergic pharmacological stimulation, the major inhibitory fibers to the smooth muscle of the septa and lung wall appear to be of vagal origin and are nonadrenergic, noncholinergic (NANC) (Campbell, 1971; Campbell et al., 1978; Campbell and Duxson, 1978; Holmgren and Campbell, 1978).

The role of the efferent innervation to the lung is less clear, although its morphological and pharmacological features have been well described (at least for some anurans). As described in detail in Section III, regional smooth-muscle contraction may play a role in adjusting the surface area of the lung alveoli. Tonically active autonomic fibers relax the lung wall, whereas excitatory fibers contract it (Carlson and Luckhardt, 1920; Luckhardt and Carlson, 1920, 1921). Action of these muscles during inspiration and expiration may facilitate lung ventilation (see Chap. 21; and Nilsson, 1985).

Sensory Fibers

Compared with our considerable knowledge of the efferent innervation, the afferent innervation of the amphibian lung largely remains to be described. Neither the exact sites and structure of sensory receptors in the lung, nor the route of these fibers back to the CNS, are clearly established. As with so many aspects of their pulmonary structure and function, most of what is known has been derived from anurans.

Numerous studies indicate that anuran lungs contain mechanoreceptors stimulated by adjustments in lung volume (Neil et al., 1950; Bonhoeffer and Kolatat, 1958; Downing and Torrance, 1961; Taglietta and Casella, 1966, 1968; McKean, 1969; Milsom and Jones, 1977; Fedde and Kuhlmann, 1978; Kuhlman and Fedde, 1979; West and Burggren, 1983). Experimental evidence arises either from an observed modulation of some physiological function after perturbation of lung pressure or volume, or recording from vagal fibers between the lungs and CNS.

Receptors that are primarily sensitive to changes in local O_2 or CO_2 levels have not been identified in the lungs of anurans, but mechanoreceptors sensitive to CO_2 and O_2 are thought to occur in the lungs of adult ranid frogs (Milsom and Jones, 1977; Fedde and Kuhlman, 1978; Kuhlman and Fedde, 1979) as well as their larvae (West and Burggren, 1983). Reptiles are known to have both chemosensitive mechanoreceptors and stretch-insensitive chemoreceptors (see Jones and Milsom, 1982 for references) and, thus, appear to represent an evolutionary stage more aligned with the higher vertebrates than with the amphibians. This is in accordance with the more elaborate pulmonary structures in many reptiles compared with amphibians (see Chap. 7).

III. Pulmonary Fine Structure

The most detailed accounts of pulmonary fine structure are for anuran amphibians (*Rana*—Gaupp, 1904; Sprumont, 1969; *Pipa*—Marcus, 1926, 1937; *Bufo*—Smith and Campbell, 1976; Smith and Rapson, 1977; Okada et al., 1962; *Xenopus*—Smith and Rapson, 1977; Meban, 1973). The following account is based largely on these studies, to which the reader is referred for details. Only limited studies have been made of apodans (*Ichthyophis*—Okada et al., 1962; Pattle et al., 1977).

In all amphibians showing pulmonary septation, primary septa arise from the internal lung wall to form relatively large, open cavities (Fig. 5), variously described as *gas sacs, cava*, and *alveoli*. In some species (e.g., *B. marinus*), secondary and tertiary septa of lesser heights also arise from the internal lung wall, tremendously increasing lung surface area (Smith and Campbell, 1976). Importantly, Smith and Campbell (1976) conclude that levels of septation in amphibian lungs are distinguished on the basis of their different heights from a common base on the internal lung wall. Patterns of septation in which successive branching of septa occur perpendicular to each other yet horizontal to the lung wall have not been reported in amphibians (with one uncomfirmed exception—

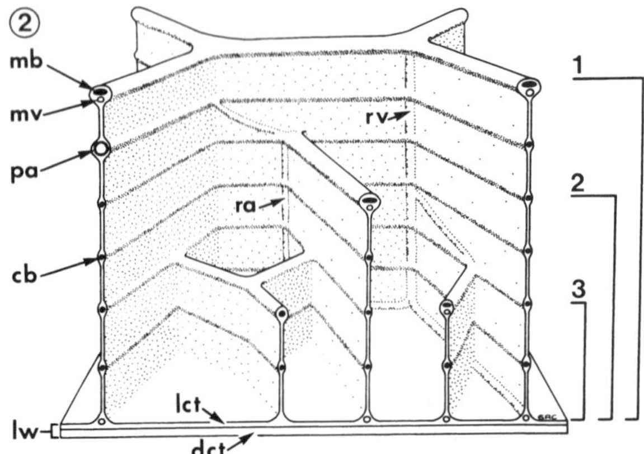

Figure 5 Patterns of pulmonary septation in *B. marinus*. Primary (1), secondary (2) and tertiary (3) septa are indicated, and are differentiated on the basis of height from the common pulmonary wall. A branch of the pulmonary artery (pa) runs within the wall of a primary septum and distributes to the lung wall (lw) and other septa by one of the many radial arteries (ra). A radial vein (rv) drains toward a marginal vein (mv) lying at a primary septal border just below the large marginal smooth-muscle bundle (mb). A layer of loose (lct) and dense connective tissue (dct) can be distinguished within the lung wall. Numerous circumalveolar smooth-muscle bundles (cb) enscribe the alveoli at regular intervals within the septa. (From Smith and Campbell, 1976.)

see Renault's description for *Rana* in Krogh, 1941). Unfortunately, it is this latter pattern of septal branching, typical of reptiles and mammals (see Chap. 7), that erroneously is diagrammed for amphibians in most general morphological treatises (e.g., Goodrich, 1930; Romer, 1970).

The pattern of pulmonary septation in amphibians (see Fig. 5) may limit total lung surface area compared with the pattern of septation evident in the lungs of amniotes. The alveoli in amphibian lungs cannot be stacked in multiple layers because essentially each elongate alveolus must open at some point into the lung lumen. However, as Smith and Campbell (1976) indicate, this anatomical arrangement may promote diffusive mixing of gases during the characteristic periods of apnea, because the tertiary alveoli are not situated at the ends of long narrow tubes, as in the lungs of mammals and some reptiles.

Primary, secondary, and tertiary septa form a dense alveolar lining of the lung wall. The larger arteries, arterioles, veins, and venuoles lie within the connective tissues of the walls and septa. In ranids, these vessels lie relatively close to the surface, but in bufonids they are deeply imbedded within the lung wall and septa (Smith and Campbell, 1976; Smits, unpublished). A single sheet of respiratory capillaries lies on the inner lung wall (Fig. 6A,C), whereas each septum (whether primary, secondary, or tertiary) bears two parallel sheets of capillaries facing out in either direction into the alveoli (see Fig. 6B,D) (Ludike, 1955; Czopek, 1957, 1959a, 1962, 1965; Smith and Campbell, 1976; Smith and Rapson, 1977). The alveolar capillaries form a dense network of anastomosing channels approximately 7-15 μm in diameter (see Fig. 6C,D). Whereas in *B. marinus* respiratory capillaries frequently pass from the septal walls to connect parallel capillary sheets on either side of the septa, in *X. laevis* the parallel capillary sheets form two distinct layers (Smith and Rapson, 1977).

The alveoli delineated by the septa are lined by a, more or less, continuous layer of epithelial cells (Meban, 1973; Atkinson and Just, 1975). In spite of numerous studies, there is still disagreement on alveolar cell structure, perhaps aggravated by real differences between congeners. Several cell types have been described in the anurans *Rana nigromaculata* and *R. temporaria*, the urodeles *Taricha pyrrhogaster* and *T. vulgaris*, and the apodan *Ichthyophis* (Okada et al., 1962; Pattle et al., 1977), but these cells are not so easily classified into the type I and type II cells described for mammalian lungs. In *X. laevis, R. pipiens* and *Necturus* there is purportedly just one epithelial cell type, which is thought to be homologous to the alveolar cells in the mammalian lung, although not so highly differentiated (Meban, 1973). In all species, the squamous epithelial cells have numerous microvilli on the free cell surface (see Fig. 6E). The lateral cell walls have interdigitating cytoplasmic processes and numerous desmosomes. Meban (1973) concluded that for *Xenopus* the alveolar cells appear specialized for secretion of surface-active materials because these cells contain numerous lamellated osmiophilic bodies (LOPBs), which are generally regarded as intracellular deposits of surfactant. Large numbers of large LOPBs were also observed in *Rana* and *Ichthyophis*, but very rarely in *Triturus vulgaris* (Pattle et al., 1977).

Ciliate and mucous cells in the lung are limited to the septal margins in *Bufo, Rana*, and *Ichthyophis* (Marcus, 1937; Atkinson and Just, 1975; Smith and Campbell, 1976). The free margins of the septa are enlarged to make the septa appear "blub like" in cross-section (see Fig. 5). The marginal smooth-muscle bundles tend to be arranged like a drawstring about the medial opening of each alveolus. Additional smooth-muscle bundles are distributed in the loose connective tissues of the lung.

The function of these various muscle bundles in the amphibian lung has yet to be determined experimentally. Adjustment in the degree of tonic contraction might alter the diameter of the alveolar opening into the lung lumen and, thus, alter diffusion dead space, but Smith and Campbell (1976) suggest that for *Bufo* contraction of this smooth muscle might reduce septal height and, thus, reduce the total surface area of exposed capillaries. Holmgren and Campbell (1978) have shown that, on the basis of different populations of adrenergic receptors, the lung wall muscle can relax simultaneously with contraction of the

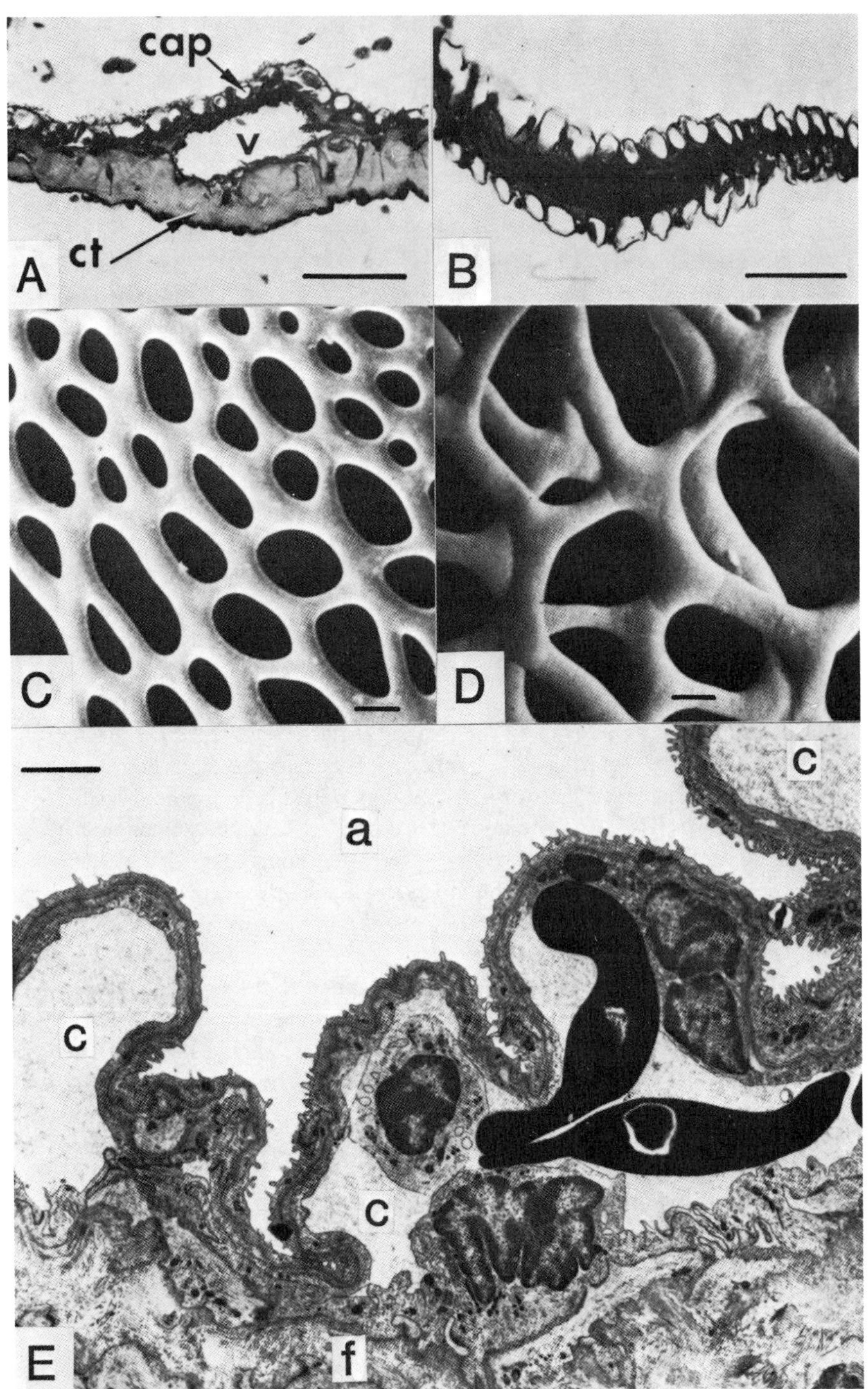

cap
v
ct
A
B
C
D
E
a
c
c
c
f

septal muscle, which might act to raise the free margins of the septa and thus increase alveolar surface area. Coordinated phasic contraction of the visceral smooth muscle in the lungs also might generate some convective flow of gas to eliminate stagnant boundary layers in the large alveoli. Rhythmic lung contractions occurring once every few minutes have been recorded both in vivo and in vitro in the Japanese toad (Tsuchiya, 1959), although the function of these contractions was not determined. Finally, contractions produced by pulmonary smooth muscle may have a role in lymphatic pumping (see Chap. 19). In *Bufo*, smooth-muscle fibers circumscribe each alveolus at regularly spaced intervals and appear to regulate the distribution of blood within the alveolus (Smith and Campbell, 1976).

The distribution of smooth muscle within the lungs of urodeles and apodans has not been described in any detail. The regulation of smooth-muscle contraction and its function in the lungs of amphibians and other lower vertebrates is in great need of additional study.

IV. Pulmonary Morphometrics

Extensive quantitative data on pulmonary morphometrics have been compiled for many amphibian species. Comparisons between studies are problematic, however, because there have not been uniform methods for dissection, preservation, or analysis. Moreover, different aspects of pulmonary structure change at different rates as body mass varies (Tenney and Tenney, 1970), further complicating comparisons between different studies where different-sized animals have been used. In spite of these limitations, differences between the lungs of various amphibians apparent at the gross anatomical level are supported by the available morphometric data.

Figure 6 (A) Transverse section of the lung wall of *Bufo marinus* showing the single layer of capillaries (cap) above the thick envelope of connective tissue (ct) that surrounds the entire lung. A small vein (v) can be seen running outside the capillary net. Scale bar = 100 μm. (B) Transverse section of septum in the lung of *B. marinus*. The double layer of capillaries is separated by a layer of connective tissue containing smooth muscle cells. Scale bar = 100 μm. (C) Face view of single-layered lung wall capillaries from a corrosion vascular cast of a moderately inflated lung of *B. marinus*. Scale bar = 10 μm. (D) Face view of double-layered septal capillaries. Scale bar = 10 μm. (E) Electron micrograph showing a transverse section through a pulmonary septum in a lung of *Xenopus laevis*. A, air space; C, lumen of capillary; F, fibrous, connective tissue septum. Scale bar = 2 μm. (Figs. 6A–6D from Smith and Campbell, 1976. Fig. 7E from Meban, 1973.)

Table 1 Lung Morphometrics in Selected Amphibia

Species	n	Body mass (g)	Alveolar diameter (mm)	Blood–gas diffusion distance (μm)	Total pulmonary surface area ($cm^2 \cdot g$ body $mass^{-1}$)	Septal surface area/ Lung wall surface area	Ref.
Bombina bombina	n.r.	6.6	–	–	1.97	0.25	Czopek, 1955a
Pelobates fuscus	n.r.	16.0	–	–	1.66	0.76	Czopek, 1955a
Bufo marinus	4	108	2.3	–	13.03	–	Tenney and Tenney, 1970
B. bufo	n.r.	48.0	–	–	3.08	5.09	Czopek, 1955a
B. americanus	7	46	1.35	–	–	–	Tenney and Tenney, 1970
Hyla arborea	n.r.		–	–	–	1.62	Andrzejewski and Maciaszek, 1960
N. arborea	n.r.	6.8	–	–	6.87	3.28	Czopek, 1955a
H. Cinerea	3	4.0	–	–	2.33	–	Tenney and Tenney, 1970
Rana temporia		1.9	–	–	–	1.24	Andrzejewski and Maciaszek, 1960

R. temporia	n.r.	28.0	–	–	2.68	3.93	Czopek, 1955a
R. terrestris	n.r.	17.3	–	–	2.52	2.67	Czopek, 1955a
R. esculenta	n.r.	53.0	–	–	2.86	4.50	Czopek, 1955a
R. esculenta	?	250	–	–	–	8.19	Andrzejewski et al., 1962
R. pipiens	14	35	1.45	–	2.15	–	Tenney et al., 1970
R. pipiens	n.r.	127	–	–	–	3.68	Andrzejewski et al., 1962
R. catesbeiana	22	97	0.3–0.5	2.3		–	Burggren and Mwalutioma, 1983
R. catesbeiana	9	214	2.3	–	2.47	–	Tenney and Tenney, 1970
Xenopus laevis	n.r.	32.3	–	–	–	5.3	Czopek, 1955b
X. laevis	n.r.	"adults"	0.15–0.30	0.7–1.5	–	–	Meban, 1973
X. laevis	7	60	0.85	–	7.80	–	Tenney and Tenney, 1970
Amphiuma means	2	398	–	–	1.25	–	Tenney and Tenney, 1970
Ichthyophis orthoplicatus	*n.r.*	14	0.25–1.0	1.0	–	–	Pattle et al., 1977

nr = Not reported.

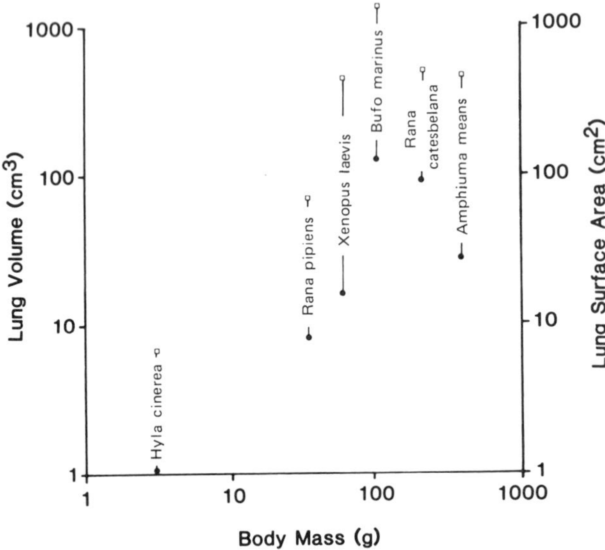

Figure 7 Absolute values of lung volume (●) and lung surface area (□) as a function of body mass in six amphibians species. (Unpublished data courtesy of S. M. Tenney and J. B. Tenney.)

A. Lung Volume

Although interspecific differences in lung volume associated with various respiratory and nonrespiratory adaptations have frequently been proposed (discussed earlier), this parameter has not yet been quantified for a sufficiently broad range of species from which to make conclusions. Certainly, no consistent pattern in either absolute or mass-specific lung volume emerges, even though there is more than an order of magnitude difference in either of these variables when comparing different species (Table 1, Fig. 7). Measured lung "volume" depends upon transmural pressure at time of measurement, as well as whether the lungs are in situ (and thus confined by the body wall) or isolated from the body. The value of measurements of lung volume or compliance in excised, isolated lungs is probably quite limited. Tenney and Tenney (1970) argue that data acquired on dried, isolated lungs of amphibians might be considered equivalent to "real maximal lung volumes," and comparison of their data with that for the same species measured in intact animals with physiological inflation pressure does not refute their contention.

Pooling data for seven amphibian species, Tenney and Tenney (1970) were able to predict that absolute lung volume in amphibians scaled nearly proportionally with body mass (lung vol. = mass$^{1.05}$ over the range of 35 to 398 g).

This is quite distinct from reptiles, in which lung volume scaled to body mass to the exponent 0.75, but is similar to the change in lung volume with body mass in mammals (exponent = 1.02).

With the exception of those relatively few amphibians with secondary lung reduction, mass-specific lung volume in many amphibians is generally larger than in mammals. The pattern of alveolar septation generally prevents multiple stacking of alveoli to enhance surface area. Consequently, a disproportionately large lung is one structural modification that could increase surface area. Many amphibians also use lungs to enhance buoyancy (see Sec. V.C), and this may also have resulted in generally larger lungs in amphibians than in higher vertebrates.

B. Lung Compliance

As with measurement of lung volume, the measurement of lung compliance depends greatly upon whether the lungs are in situ or are isolated. Hughes and Vergara (1978), investigating *Rana pipiens*, found that even removal of the liver and heart from an otherwise intace carcass shifted the pressure–volume curves toward greater compliance, whereas A. Smits (personal communication) has found that pulmonary compliance in *Bufo* varies considerably with whether the animal's dorsal or ventral side is up. Compliance curves on isolated lungs, as opposed to the in situ pulmonary system, may be most useful when investigating relative changes, for example, when considering developmental changes (Dupre et al., 1985) or the role of pulmonary surfactants in pressure–volume curve hysteresis (Hughes and Vergara, 1978).

Lung compliance for both in situ and isolated lungs of some anuran amphibians are presented in Table 1. Generally, lung compliance in amphibians (and lower vertebrates generally) is nearly an order of magnitude lower than in mammals, over a wide range of lung inflation. In mammals, low lung compliances frequently are associated with reduced levels of pulmonary surfactants acting to reduce surface tension during lung inflation. Pulmonary surfactants have been described in amphibians (see Sec. V.B), and calculated surface tensions in anuran lungs are only slightly higher than in many mammals (Miller and Bondurant, 1961; Hughes and Vergara, 1978). However, the radically different structure of mammalian and amphibian lungs, particularly in alveolar diameter, may obviate direct comparisons of the contributing components to pulmonary compliance.

C. Surface Area

Pulmonary surface area is one of the most important, yet one of the most difficult to measure, of the various lung variables. Few data are available for amphibians compared with other vertebrates, and some studies have provided only relative, rather than absolute, measures of pulmonary surface area. As for lung volume, comparison between studies is frustrated by lack of standardization of lung inflation and preservation techniques.

Table 2 Pulmonary Volume and Compliance in Selected Amphibia

Species	n	Body mass (g)	Preparation	Inflation pressure (cm H_2O)	Total respiratory volume ($ml \cdot g^{-1}$ body mass)	Respiratory compliance ($ml \cdot cmH_2^{-1} \cdot g^{-1}$ body mass)	Comments	Ref.
Rana pipiens	7	35	Isol.	8.2	0.05	.023	Compliance at midcapacity volume during air inflation	Price and Pierce, 1963
R. pipiens						–		Guimond and Hutchison, 1968
R. pipiens	14	26	Isol.	20	0.24	–		Tenney and Tenney, 1970
R. pipiens	n.r.	26	Isol.	8.4	0.22	0.049	Compliance during air inflation	Hughes and Vergara, 1978
R. pipiens	34	80	In situ	6.0	0.08	0.022	Living animal, compliance during air inflation	West and Jones, 1975
R. catesbiana (adult)	n.r.	300	In situ	–	0.1–0.2	–	Technique not described	Gans et al., 1969
R. catesbiana (adult)	7	260	In situ	–	0.09	–	Respiratory mass spectrometry, living animals	Glass et al., 1981
R. catesbiana (adult)	7	97	In situ	6.0	0.27	–	Freshly killed young adult	Burggren and Mwalukoma, 1983

R. catesbiana (larvae)	16	28	In situ	6.0	0.03	–	Freshly killed stage 15–20 larvae	Burggren and Mwalukoma, 1983
R. catesbiana (adult)	9	214	Isol.	20	0.44	–		Tenney and Tenney, 1970
R. catesbiana (adult)	6	n.r.	Isol.	4.0	–	0.55–0.60	Volume-specific compliance ($ml \cdot cmH_2O^{-1}$)	Dupre et al., 1985
R. catesbiana (larvae)	6	n.r.	Isol.	4.0	–	0.35–0.40	Volume-specific compliance ($ml \cdot cmH_2O^{-1} \cdot ml^{-1}$) stage 2 larvae	Dupre et al., 1985
Xenopus laevis	7	60	Isol.	20	0.27	–		Tenney and Tenney, 1970
Hyla cinerea	3	3	Isol.	20	0.39	–		Tenney and Tenney, 1970
Bufo marinus	4	108	Isol.	20	1.22	–		Tenney and Tenney, 1970
Amphiuma	2	398	Isol.	20	0.068	–	Living animal, based on respiratory gas analysis	Toews et al., 1971
A. tridactylum	25	250–1000	In situ	–	0.06–0.07	–		Toews et al., 1971
Ichthyophis orthoplicatus	n.r.	14	n.r.	n.r.	0.047	–		Pattle et al., 1977

n.r. = Not reported.

One of the most critical morphological factors contributing to total pulmonary surface area is the magnitude of septation of the lung. Obviously, the more extensive the septation, the greater the surface area. More extensive septation results in smaller alveolar diameter, and the latter gives an indirect measure of the degree of specialization of the lung. As has been noted previously for other pulmonary variables, there is considerable difference in alveolar diameter between amphibian species and also in values reported for a particular species in different studies (Table 2). No clear pattern emerges from the limited data available on the influence of systematics, habitat, or body mass on alveolar diameter when comparing various studies.

Tenney and Tenney (1970) made an extensive study of alveolar diameter and lung surface area in seven amphibian and 15 reptilian species. Although it should be emphasized that they studied isolated, dried lungs probably expanded well beyond physiological volumes, their data do provide for interesting allometric comparisons. Alveolar diameter in amphibians increased to a small extent as body mass increased. The exponent *b* from the allometric equation relating the two variables was only 0.2, which is a value similar to that in mammals. Importantly, alveolar diameter in amphibians was larger (indicating a lesser degree of pulmonary subdivision) than in reptiles over a wide range of body mass.

In considering lung volume, the considerable interspecific differences defy categorization on the basis of habitat or systematics (see Table 2). Lung surface area for several species, all from a single study (Tenney and Tenney, 1970), are presented in Figure 7. Comparing lung surface areas with lung volume over a range of body mass, it becomes apparent that there is only a very loose correlation between lung volume and the surface area it presents, with discrepancies almost certainly because of the extent of internal septation.

Finally, it should be emphasized that it is possible that lung surface area may be actively adjusted through the action of the pulmonary smooth muscle raising and lowering the height of the septa (see Secs. II.E and III). This variable has not yet been taken into account in morphometric studies. Moreover, we know nothing of the patterns or magnitude of pulmonary capillary recruitment, and thus have no information on how "physiological" surface area (i.e., that area of the lung laying over perfused capillaries) relates to anatomical surface area. This begs further investigation not only in amphibian lungs but in the gas exchange organs of all lower vertebrates.

D. Lung Microvasculature

Although the total surface area of a lung is a useful morphometric index of pulmonary structure, the pattern and density of capillarization of the lung wall and septa is perhaps more directly related to the actual capability for exchange of respiratory gases. Numerous investigators have carried out extensive quantitative studies of the capillary networks in both larval and adult amphibian lungs (and other respiratory surfaces). The reader is referred to early morphological work reported by Czopek (1965). Subsequent studies have tended to be more functionally inclined (Hillman and Withers, 1979; Burggren and Mwalukoma, 1983).

Given the vast quantity of available data, an exhaustive reporting of the quantitative aspects of the pulmonary microvasculature is well beyond the scope of the present review. In reviewing data from more than 20 anurans, Czopek (1965) reported a capillary density (expressed as number of "capillary meshes", i.e., the number of separate tissue areas each enclosed within an anastomosing capillary network) on lung septa that ranged from a low of 280 meshes per square millimeter in *Bombina bombina*, to a high of 1723 meshes per square millimeter in *Rana esculenta*. Expressing pulmonary capillarization in terms of total meters of capillaries per gram of body mass, values ranged from 3.4 meshes per gram in *Leipelma hochstetteri* to 34.4 meshes per gram in *Hyla arborea*. As Czopek (1965) emphasizes, the sometimes large differences in pulmonary vascularization cannot be explained by systematic position of a species; nor can differences in habitat be evoked to explain differences in pulmonary capillary density. Feder and Burggren (1985a), examining the literature on vascularization of the skin of amphibians, similarly concluded that differences cannot readily be explained by habitat or systematics.

Recent studies of respiratory capillaries in amphibian skin have underscored the importance of distinguishing between the total number of capillaries and those that are actually being perfused at a given point in time (Burggren and Moalli, 1984; Feder and Burggren, 1985a,b, 1986; Burggren and Feder, 1986). Functional surface area, i.e., that surface area underlain by perfused capillaries, is significantly less than total surface area when not all capillaries are recruited. Applying this concept to vascularization of lung surfaces, it is possible that the actual recruitment of pulmonary capillaries under a given set of physiological conditions varies among species. In terms of pulmonary gas exchange, interspecific differences in recruitment patterns could either nullify or exacerbate apparent differences based simply on morphometric studies. Unfortunately, pulmonary capillary recruitment, obviously much more difficult to quantify than total numbers and lengths of capillaries, has yet to be measured in amphibian lungs.

V. Lung Function in Amphibians

A. Gas Exchange and Acid-Base Balance

It might be considered paradoxical that this review, having spent considerable time discussing pulmonary structure, will now spend little time specifically discussing what purportedly is the major raison d'etre for the lungs of amphibians –respiratory gas exchange. In fact, this aspect of amphibian lung biology has been reviewed on numerous occasions (see Shelton and Boutilier, 1982 and the papers they cite) and is covered in great detail in several other chapters in this volume, which place the respiratory function of amphibian lungs in a comparative context with the lungs of other vertebrates. Thus, Chapter 21 describes the mechanisms for lung ventilation in amphibians, while Chapters 14-16 describe gas exchange theory and actual performance. Chapter 2 discusses the control of breathing in amphibians. The respiratory physiology of diving in amphibians, a common situation in many species, is dealt with in Chapter 24.

If anything, what might not emerge from the multifaceted treatment of amphibian gas exchange in this volume is an answer to the simple question: How efficient are amphibian lungs in exchanging respiratory gases—relative to the lungs of other vertebrates? Unfortunately, several factors prevent easy comparisons with other air-breathing animals.

First, metabolic rates in amphibians generally are substantially lower than those of many reptiles (which tend to have higher preferred body temperatures) and are at least an order of magnitude lower than birds and mammals. Consequently, the total gas exchange requirements of amphibians are comparatively nondemanding.

Second, although many species do take up a considerable proportion if not most, of their oxygen through the lungs, it must be emphasized that almost all amphibians normally supplement pulmonary oxygen uptake with uptake across additional respiratory surfaces. Importantly, CO_2 elimination by nonpulmonary routes almost always greatly exceeds that through the lungs, reflected in pulmonary respiratory quotients that rarely rise above 0.2 (Fig. 8). What are the alternatives to pulmonary gas exchange? Amphibian larvae and neotenic adults, almost all of which are aquatic, generally possess either internal or external gills (see Chap. 5). These gills are functionally as effective as fish gills (Burggren and West, 1982), and in many larval or neotenic amphibian species branchial gas exchange (especially CO_2) is at least as important as pulmonary gas exchange. This is particularly true at lower temperatures at which, at least in aquatic or semiterrestrial forms, there is a physiological adjustment of gas exchange away from the lungs to alternative respiratory sites. Moreover, use of cutaneous gas exchange is ubiquitous in amphibians (see Feder and Burggren, 1985a,b; 1986) and, like the gills, can contribute heavily to gas exchange in both larvae and adults. Thus, gas exchange usually occurs across two or more distant respiratory sites, and frequently both air and water may be used as respiratory media.

It is essential, then, that pulmonary gas exchange in amphibians should be viewed as a part (sometimes a *small* part) of the animal's respiratory repertoire, rather than as the solo performer. This perspective is often not fully appreciated by mammalian physiologists. Thus, if to be considered in the biological context of the whole animal, future considerations of ventilatory control, acid-base bal-

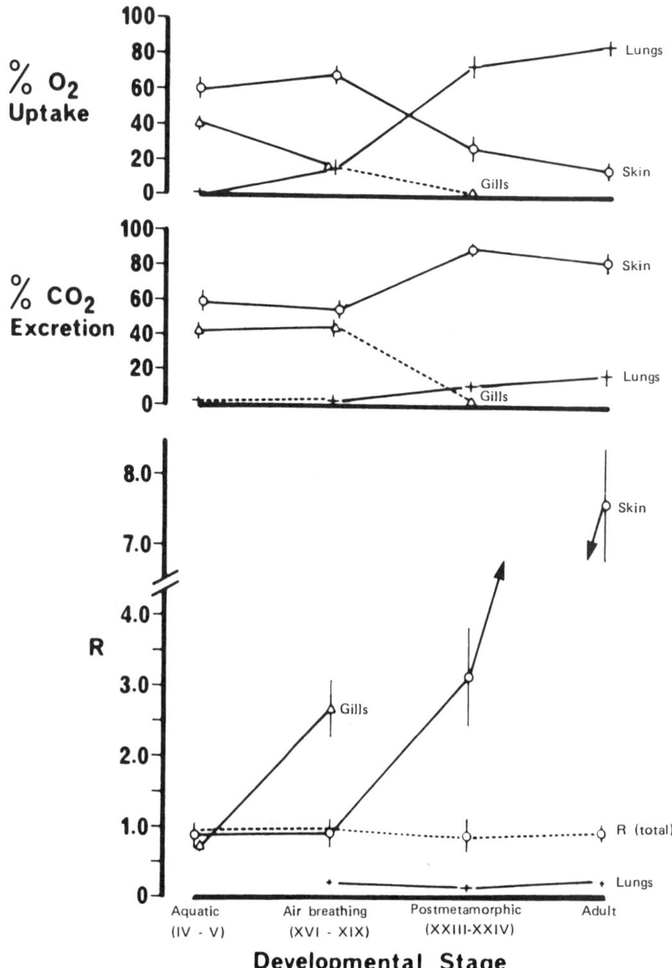

Figure 8 Oxygen and carbon dioxide exchange (expressed as percentage of total gas exchange) and R, the respiratory gas exchange ratio, for the gills, skin, and lungs of four different developmental stages of the bullfrog, *Rana catesbeiana*. (From Burggren and West, 1982.)

ance, and so forth, in amphibians must be expanded to incorporate the complex interactions of the lungs with the other respiratory organs. A complete respiratory analysis in such a situation obviously is much more complex than for the "simpler" case in higher vertebrates, which have only a single respiratory organ and use only a single respiratory medium. To date, few studies have attempted to meet such a challenge.

Finally, in addressing the question of "efficiency of amphibian lungs," it is noteworthy that because other highly effective gas exchange organs may be available to amphibians, there have been no strong selection pressures for the lungs to become highly alveolarized. Nonrespiratory functions (e.g., buoyancy, vocalization) have probably been at least as important in the evolutionary shaping of the lungs of extant amphibians. Because there are multiple competing demands upon the lungs of amphibians, it is perhaps unreasonable to expect that pulmonary function or structure in any given amphibian should show clear, nonequivocal evidence of specialization for a particular purpose. It is particularly unlikely that adaptions would occur along systematic lines.

B. Biochemistry-Metabolism of the Amphibian Lung

Numerous recent studies have revealed that the lungs of many higher vertebrates are the site of both production and secretion of materials for use in the lung and elsewhere, as well as potentially important sites of metabolism for anaerobic end products, particularly lactate (see Chap. 2). Teleogically, the lungs of amphibians might be expected to exhibit similar metabolic functions, given the common occurrence of apnea and the ability to sustain prolonged periods of primarily anaerobic metabolism (see Chaps. 22 and 24).

Unfortunately, extremely little is known about the metabolism of the amphibian lung, even though its importance in an evolutionary context is quite obvious. One of the few aspects of amphibian lung metabolism that has received considerable attention is the formation and subsequent action of surfactants or "surpellic" films. These substances, which are lipoprotein complexes, act to reduce surface tension in the lung alveoli. Lung surfactants are thought to help prevent alveolar collapse and reduce the mechanical work required to inflate the lungs.

The existence of surpellic lung films generally is demonstrated directly by examination of the properties of fluid washed from lungs or indirectly by electron microscopy. In the latter, evidence is sought for lamellated osmiophilic bodies (LOPBs), which are the intracellular storage sites of lung surfactants. According to these criteria, surpellic substances routinely have been identified in the lungs of anurans, including *Xenopus*, *Rana*, and *Bufo* (Bargmann and Knoop, 1956; Pattle and Hopkinson, 1963; Okada et al., 1962; Brooks, 1970; Pattle et al., 1977; Highes and Vergara, 1978). The lungs of the apodan *Ichthyophis* contain both LOPBs and surpellic film linings (Pattle et al., 1977), although other apodans have yet to be examined. Surfactant substances appear less consistently in urodeles. Surpellic films or LOPBs have been identified in *Ambysotma* (DeGroodt et al., 1960; Sorokin, 1963) and *Necturus* (Brooks, 1970). *Proteus* lacks both surpellic substances and LOPBs (Hughes, 1970, 1973). An intermediate situation apparently occurs in the genus *Triterus*, in which LOPBs are very infrequently observed (Okada et al., 1962; Pattle, 1976; Pattle et al., 1977), and the surfactant properties of lung washings are significant but low compared with other amphibians (Pattle et al., 1977).

It thus appears that pulmonary surpellic films are widely distributed among the extant amphibians, as indeed they are in reptiles and higher vertebrates (Pattle, 1976). Surpellic films (albeit with minor surfactant activities) or LOPBs are also found in the lungs of the Dipnoi (Hughes, 1967, 1973; Pattle, 1973) and in actinopterygian fishes (e.g., *Amia, Lepisosteus*) that use "lungs" or swimbladders for air breathing (Hughes, 1970, 1973). Lipoproteins with surpellic properties, stored in LOPBs, are thus widespread in phyletically ancient fishes and amphibians. This suggests that the capability for manufacturing these materials is a rather primitive characteristic, rather than a derived feature associated with the evolution of smaller alveoli in more complex lung structures.

Unfortunately, little information, other than for surfactants, is available for pulmonary biochemistry and metabolism. Further research is clearly warranted, particularly as interest in mammalian lung metabolism is growing (see Chap. 2).

C. Buoyancy

Putative pulmonary adaptations either for enhancement or reduction of buoyancy in amphibians have been alluded to by many authors (Goodrich, 1930; Noble, 1931; Guimond and Hutchison, 1976; Porter, 1976; to name but a few). Unfortunately, little experimental investigation has been carried out to back these contentions. For example, there have been no measurements, to my knowledge, of the specific density of various amphibians and how this relates to lung volume and habitat. However, the findings of a few recent studies are noteworthy. Wassersug and Feder (1983) studied the interactions of aquatic oxygen concentration, body size, and respiratory behavior on the stamina of anuran larvae. They concluded that the positive respiratory benefits of air breathing could be more than offset by the attendant increase in locomotor "costs" associated with increased buoyancy by air-filled lungs. High staminas were recorded in swimming larval *B. americanus*, which do not breathe air as larvae, compared with larvae of other species that do breathe air. Perhaps more convincingly, larval *X. laevis* when denied access to air actually had a greater stamina than those that were allowed to breathe air during swimming, presumably because of the increased locomotory costs incurred by increased buoyancy. Fishes actually have been demonstrated to modify buoyancy in response to changes in

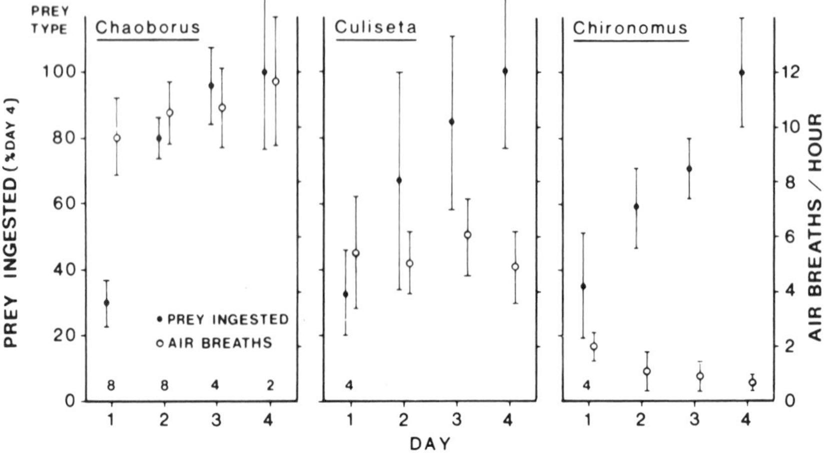

Figure 9 The relationship between air-breathing frequency, prey location in the water column, and prey ingestion in larvae of the salamander *Ambystoma tigrinum. Chaoborus, Culiseta*, and *Chironomus* represent prey items that are pelagic, mixed pelagic, and benthic, respectively. When only pelagic prey are available, air-breathing frequency of the larvae is high to maintain buoyancy. When only benthic prey are available, air-breathing frequency is low to maintain negative buoyancy. Presence of mixed benthic and pelagic prey results in an intermediate breathing-frequency. (From Lannoo and Bachmann, 1984.)

water current velocity (Gee, 1977). Collectively, all of these data suggest that, indeed, lung volume reduction might be adaptive in species inhabiting flowing water, particularly when pulmonary gas exchange can be supplanted by branchial or cutaneous exchange.

Lannoo and Backman (1984) have completed the only study, to my knowledge, that has concentrated specifically on the issue of buoyancy and lung structure-function in amphibians. These authors investigated air breathing in larvae of the salamander *Ambystoma tigrinum*, which regularly breathes air and achieves considerable gas exchange across the lungs (Whitford and Hutchison, 1965, 1966; Whitford and Sherman, 1968; Buggren and Wood, 1981). First, Lannoo and Backman (1984) demonstrated that buoyancy is highly correlated with air-breathing frequency in *Ambystoma* larvae and that surgical excision of the lungs (not such a radical procedure in amphibians that can breathe with skin and gills) eliminated the ability to float in the water column without constantly swimming.

They then examined the interactions of feeding, buoyancy, and air breathing in *Ambystoma*. These larvae feed on a mixture of pelagic and benthic prey, necessitating considerable movement through the water column. When feeding strictly on pelagic prey, the larvae float in the water column, apparently regulating lung volume to maintain neutral buoyancy. Independent of prey availability, the time spent floating in midwater is negatively correlated with illumination level—presumably this behavior reduces the risk of aerial predation. When only pelagic prey were made available, air-breathing frequency was highest (Fig. 9). When only benthic prey were available, air-breathing frequency was lowest, whereas mixed prey items produced an intermediate air-breathing frequency. These experiments clearly show that air-breathing frequency, the study of which is generally regarded as the "property" of respiratory physiologists, depends at least as much upon behaviors related to avoiding predators and securing prey items themselves as it does to respiratory requirements in the larvae of *Ambystoma*. Obviously, interpretation of lung structure and function in amphibians must take many widely ranging factors into consideration.

D. Vocalization

Anuran amphibians are renowned for making distinctive, highly audible vocalizations associated with intraspecific communication. To produce these sounds, the mouth and nares are actively kept closed while gas is driven back and forth between the buccal cavity and lungs through the open glottis. The qualities of the sound produced depend largely upon the properties of the resonating chamber formed by the buccal cavity. Many specializations of the buccal cavity of Anura are associated with various vocalization patterns (see Noble, 1931), and although a large lung volume might be imagined to enhance the sound level, adaptations of the lung for this purpose have not been described. In any event, sound production has been observed in lungless salamanders (Geyer, 1927; Noble, 1931).

E. Defense

When startled or otherwise disturbed, several anurans (particularly the family Bufonidae) will employ a series of rapid buccal compressions to grossly hyperinflate the lungs, after which the glottis is tightly closed. Not surprisingly, the apparent size of the animal increases, which no doubt tends to inhibit attack by predators. This behavior, reminiscent of that employed by some lizards to wedge themselves in rock cracks to avoid extrication, may have a significant impact upon pulmonary gas exchange. Although not quantified, intrapulmonary pressures during defensive inflation must be very much higher than during normal respiratory cycles, for the sides of the toad are stretched taut and the animal will resonate like a drum when struck. Under these conditions pulmonary capillary resistance must rise sharply owing to rising transmuran pressures. To what extent pulmonary blood flow is comprised during defensive inflation, and what the respiratory consequences are, have yet to be determined.

VI. Ontogenetic Changes in Lung Structure and Function

The ontogeny of pulmonary form and function represents a particularly interesting case study among the vertebrates. Before hatching or birth in higher vertebrates, all gas exchange is achieved through chorioallantoic (reptiles, birds) or placental (mammals) structures. The embryonic-fetal lungs effectively serve no apparent purpose until birth or hatching occurs. This situation is in sharp contrast with that in amphibian premetamorphic larvae in which, dependent to some extent upon species and environment, the lungs begin to be ventilated with air (and contribute to gas exchange) well before their morphological development is complete.

A. Morphology of the Developing Lung

In spite of an enormous literature on the developmental morphology of amphibians, surprisingly little attention has been paid to the ontogeny of the lungs, particularly in the context of its respiratory function. The most extensive quantitative accounts of pulmonary gross anatomy during amphibian ontogeny have been given by Strawinski (1956), by Czopek (1957, 1959, 1960) for *R. esculenta, A. mexicanum*, and *S. salamandra*, and by Atkinson and Just (1975) and Burggren and Mwalukoma (1983) for *R. catesbeiana*. Predictably, the lungs of very early larval stages examined soon after hatching are simple, nonseptate sacs with little vascularization and very small surface area. Almost all gas exchange occurs via the skin and gills at this time (see Fig. 8, Burggren and West, 1982). As development continues, primary septa (and secondary and tertiary septa in those species that possess them as adults) begin to form, sharply increasing the mass-specific pulmonary surface area. Lung compliance and the compliance-independent index for hysteresis for pressure-volume curves increase during larval development in *R. catesbeiana* (Dupre et al., 1985), resulting from increases in both lung structural complexity and increasing production of pulmonary surpellic films. Concomitant with increasing pulmonary septation, the vascularization of the lungs increases. Czopek (1965) and his colleagues have argued that the most effective measure of vascularization of a gas exchange organ is the cumulative length of the capillaries in that organ, a view endorsed by Hillman and Withers (1979). Figure 10 shows that, of the total length of respiratory capillaries from all sources (lungs, gills, skin, mouth) the percentage of total respiratory capillary length in the lungs increases steadily during development, particularly after the gills degenerate upon metamorphosis to the adult.

Interestingly, larval development represents a rather plastic developmental period in which environmental factors can modify pulmonary structure. Larval bullfrogs exposed to 30 days of moderate hypoxic exposure (P_{O_2} = 75 mm Hg) develop lungs with a significantly larger volume and a greater degree of internal

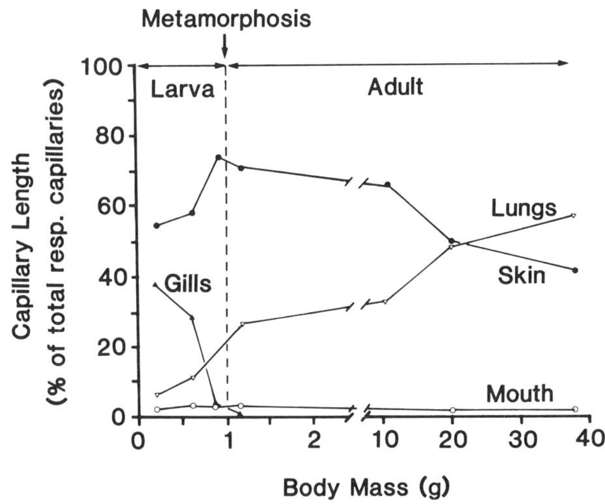

Figure 10 Development changes in cumulative capillary length in the skin, gills, lungs, and mouth (expressed as a percentage of the total cumulative length of all respiratory capillaries in these four tissues) in the salamander, *Salamandra salamandra*. (Data from Czopek, 1959b, 1960.)

septation than larvae raised under normoxic or hyperoxic conditions (Burggren and Mwalukoma, 1983). The blood-gas barrier remains unchanged, however. The lungs of adult bullfrogs subjected to the same experimental conditions of hypoxia show no morphological changes, but major adjustments in the respiratory properties of the blood were evident (Pinder and Burggren, 1983).

B. Respiratory Physiology of the Developing Lung

The contribution of the lungs to total gas exchange in amphibian larvae, and how it changes with metamorphosis to the adult, have been the object of several studies (see Burggren, 1984 for review). Ambystomatid salamanders and ranid frogs have been most extensively investigated. Under normoxic conditions (20°C), the lungs of resting, undisturbed larval bullfrogs are ventilated very infrequently, particularly at younger stages when air-breathing frequency may be less than 2 breaths an hour (West and Burggren, 1982; Burggren and Doyle, 1987). Consequently, the pulmonary contribution to total gas exchange, and carbon dioxide elimination in particular, is low (Fig. 8). As larval development proceeds, the gills degenerate and the lungs assume a progressively more important role in gas exchange, although the lungs must vie with the skin, which is an important site for both oxygen uptake and carbon dioxide elimination in almost all amphibians at all developmental stages (see Feder and Burggren, 1985a,b).

Some of the major arguments for the importance of the amphibian lung in buoyancy have been developed by observations on larvae rather than adults (Wassersug and Feder, 1983; Lannoo and Backman, 1984), and there is much circumstantial evidence of buoyancy regulation through fine adjustment in lung volume. Regulation of lung ventilation and volume, possibly mediated by chemosensitive mechanorecptors in the lungs, develops well before metamorphosis to the adult in *R. catesbeiana* (West and Burggren, 1983; Burggren and Doyle, 1987) and *A. tigrinum* (Heath, 1976; Burggren and Wood, 1981).

Thus many, if not all, of the functions attributable to the lungs in adult amphibians appear before metamorphosis, rather than as a result of this developmental process. All too often, however, the data on developing lung structure and function in amphibians are fragmentary. Only rarely is information available for a reasonably complete developmental series, as opposed to comparison of a single larval stage to the mature adult.

VII. Conclusions

The lungs of amphibians emerge as structurally simple organs relative to those of higher vertebrates. Part of this simplicity arises from the fact that amphibians, unlike most higher vertebrates, have both lower metabolic rates and an additional site, or sites, for respiratory gas exchange. Thus, the more complex lungs of reptiles and, particularly, birds and mammals, are simply not required in amphibians. Moreover, the nonrespiratory functions of the amphibian lung (most notably that of buoyancy) have clearly been a crucial factor in the pulmonary evolution of extant amphibians. Where multiple lung functions exist, extreme structural specialization for any one function (i.e., increased surface area for gas exchange) is less likely to develop.

In spite of this relative structural simplicity, the sophistication of pulmonary function in amphibians should not be underestimated. Effective gas exchange, regulated by mechanisms similar or identical to those in higher vertebrates, occurs in most amphibians. This performance might be viewed as all the more remarkable, given that amphibian lungs (1) must be regulated in concert with other gas exchange sites using a potentially different respiratory medium, (2) receive highly variable quantities of blood with variable amounts of oxygenated and deoxygenated blood admixture, (3) are subjected to high rates of plasma filtration, and (4) must coordinate competing demands for nonrespiratory functions. Perhaps the single most important area for future research on amphibian lungs lies in determining how these multifaceted competing pulmonary functions are regulated.

Acknowledgments

I thank Dr. Alan Pinder and Dr. Allan Smits for useful discussion during the manuscript preparation.

References

Andrzejewski, H. J., Czopek, J., Siankowa, L., Szarski, H. (1962). The vascularization of respiratory surfaces in amphibians reaching large body size (*Rana esculenta* L., *R. pipiens sphenocephal* Cope, and *R. grylio* Stejneger).

Andrzejewski, H. J., and Maciaszek, M. (1960). Unaczynienie powierzchni oddechowych u mlodych ookazow zaby trawnej (*Rana temporaria*), zaby moczorowej (*Rana terrestris* Andrz.) i rzekotki drzewnej (*Hyla arborea* L.). *Zesz. Nauk. Univ. Mikolaja Kopernika Biol. 5*:17-28.

Atkinson, B. G., and Just, J. J. (1975). Biochemical and histological changes in the respiratory system of *Rana catesbieana* larvae during normal and induced metamorphosis. *Dev. Biol. 45*:151-165.

Baer, J. G. (1937). L'appareil respiratoire des gymnophiones. *Rev. Suisse Zool. 44*:353-377.

Bargmann, W., and Knoop, A. (1956). Vergleichende elektronenmikroskopische Untersuchungen der Lungenkapillare. *Z. Zellforsch. Mikrosk. Anat. 44*: 263-281.

Bieniak, A., and Watka, R. (1962). Vascularization of respiratory surfaces in *Bufo cognatus* Say and *Bufo compactilis* Weigman. *Bull. Acad. Pol. Sci. II 10*:9-12.

Bonhoffer, K., and Kolatat, T. (1958). Druckvolumendiagramm und Dehungsrezeptoren der Froschlunge. *Pflugers Arch. 265*:477-484.

Boutilier, R. G., McDonald, D. G., and Toews, D. P. (1980). The effects of enforced activity on ventilation, circulation and blood acid-base balance in the aquatic gill-less urodele, *Cryptobranchus alleganiensis*: a comparison with the semi-terrestrial anuran, *Bufo marinus. J. Exp. Biol. 84*:289-302.

Brooks, R. E. (1970). Lung alveolar cytosomes: A consideration of their significance. *Z. Zellforsch. Mikrosk. Anat. 106*:484-497.

Browdowa, G. (1956). Unaczynienie powierzchni oddechowych traszki gorskiej (*Triturius alpestris* Laur.). *Stud. Soc. Sci. Torun. Sect. E (Zool.) 3*: 85-93.

Bruner, H. S. (1900). The heart of lungless salamanders. *J. Morphol. 16*:323-337.

Bruner, H. S. (1914). Pulmonary respiration amphibians. *Morphol. Jahrb. 48.* Cited in Goodrich (1930).

Burggren, W. W. (1985). Transition of respiratory processes during amphibian metamorphosis: From egg to adult. In *Respiration and Metabolism in embryonic Vertebrates*. Edited by R. S. Seymour. The Hague, Junk.

Burggren, W. W., and Doyle, M. E. (1987). Ontogeny of regulation of gill and lung ventilation in the bullfrog, *Rana catesbeiana. Respir. Physiol. 66*: 279-291.

Burggren, W. W., and Feder, M. E. (1986). Effect of experimental ventilation of the skin on cutaneous gas exchange in the bullfrog. *J. Exp. Biol. 121*: 445-450.

Burggren, W. W., and Moalli, R. (1984). 'Active' regulation of cutaneous gas exchange by capillary recruitment in amphibians: Experimental evidence and a revised model for skin respiration. *Respir. Physiol. 55*:379-392.

Burggren, W. W., and Mwalukoma, A. (1983). Respiration during chronic hypoxia and hyperoxia in larval and adult bullfrogs (*Rana catesbeiana*). I. Morphological responses of lungs, skin and gills. *J. Exp. Biol. 105*:191-203.

Burggren, W. W., and West, N. H. (1982). Changing respiratory importance of gills, lungs, and skin during metamorphosis in the bullfrog *Rana catesbeiana. Respir. Physiol. 47*:151-164.

Burggren, W. W., and Wood, S. C. (1981). Respiration and acid-base balance in the tiger salamander, *Ambystoma tigrinum*: Influence of temperature acclimation and metamorphosis. *J. Comp. Physiol. 144*:241-246.

Camerano, L. (1896). Ric. anat.-fisiol. i. a. Salamandrini apneumoni. *Anat. Anz. 12*. Cited in Goodrich (1930).

Campbell, G. (1971a). Autonomic innervation of the lung musculature of a toad (*Bufo marinus*). *Comp. Gen. Pharmacol. 2*:281-286.

Campbell, G. (1971b). Autonomic innervation of the pulmonary vasculature bed in a toad (*Bufo marinus*). *Comp. Gen. Pharmacol. 2*:287-294.

Campbell, G., and Duxson, M. J. (1978). The sympathetic innervation of lung muscle in the toad *Bufo marinus*: A revision and an explanation. *Comp. Biochem. Physiol. 60C*:65-73.

Campbell, G., Haller, C. J., and Rogers, D. C. (1978). Fine structural and cytochemical study of the innervation of smooth muscle in an amphibian (*Bufo marinus*) lung before and after denervation. *Cell Tissue Res. 194*: 419-432.

Carlson, A. J., and Luckhardt, A. B. (1920). Studies on the visceral sensory nervous system. I. Lung automatism and lung reflexes in the frog (*R. pipiens* and *R. catesbeiana*). *Am. J. Physiol. 54*:55-95.

Czopek, J. (1955a). The vascularisation of the respiratory surfaces of some *Salientia. Zool. Pol. 6*:101-134.

Czopek, J. (1955b). Vascularization of respiratory surfaces in *Leiopelma hochstetteri* Fitzinger and *Xenopus laevis* Daudin. *Acta Anat. 25*:346-360.

Czopek, J. (1957). The vascularization of respiratory surfaces in *Ambystoma mexicanum* (Cope) in ontogeny. *Zool. Pol. 8*:131-149.

Czopek, J. (1959a). Skin and lung capillaries in European common newts. *Copeia 1959*:91-96.

Czopek, J. (1959b). Vascularization of respiratory surfaces in *Salamandra Salamandra* L. in ontogeny. *Bull. Acad. Pol. Sci. Ser. Sci. Biol.* 7:473-478.

Czopek, J. (1962). Vascularization of respiratory surfaces of some *Caudata. Copeia 1962*:576-587.

Czopek, J. (1965). Quantitative studies on the morphology of respiratory surfaces in amphibians. *Acta Anat. 62*:296-323.

DeGroodt, M., Lagasse, A., and Sebruyns, M. (1960). Elektronemikroscopische Morphologie der Lungenalveolen des *Protopterus* and *Amblystoma. Proc. Int. Cong. Electron Micros*. Berlin, Springer-Verlag.

Downing, S. E., and Torrance, R. W. (1961). Vagal baroreceptors in the bullfrog. *J. Physiol. 156*:13P.

Dupre, R. K., Taylor, R. F., and Frazier, D. T. (1985). Static lung compliance during the development of the bullfrog, *Rana catesbeiana. Respir. Physiol. 59*:231-238.

Fedde, M. R., and Kuhlmann, W. D. (1978). Intrapulmonary carbon dioxide sensitive receptors: Amphibians to mammals. In *Respiratory Function in Birds, Adult and Embryonic*. Edited by J. Piiper. Berlin, Springer-Verlag.

Feder, M. E., and Burggren, W. W. (1985a). Cutaneous gas exchange in vertebrates: Design, patterns, control and implications. *Biol. Rev. 60*:1-45.

Feder, M. E., and Burggren, W. W. (1985b). Skin breathing in vertebrates. *Sci. Am. 253*:126-143.

Feder, M. E., and Burggren, W. W. (1986). The regulation of cutaneous gas exchange in vertebrates. In *Current Topics and Trends: Comparative Physiology and Biochemistry*. Vol. A: *Respiration, Circulation, Metabolism*. Edited by R. Gilles, Berlin, Springer-Verlag.

Fuhrmann, O. (1914). Le genre Typhlonecetes, *Neuchatel. Mem. Soc. Sci. Nat. 5*:112-138.

Gans, C. (1970). Respiration in early tetrapods–The frog is a red herring. *Evolution 24*:723-734.

Gaupp, E. (1904). Zur Lehre von dem Athmungsmechanismus beim Frosche. *Arch. Anat. Physiol. Anat. Abt.* 239-268.

Gaymer, R. (1971). Comparative studies on the caecilian amphibian *Hypogeophis rostratus*. Ph.D. thesis, University of Bristol.

Gee, J. H. (1977). Effects of size of fish, water temperature and water velocity on buoyancy alteration by fathead minnows, *Pimephales promelas. Comp. Biochem. Physiol. 56A*:503-508.

Geyer, H. (1927). Uber Lautausserungen der Molche. *Blatt Aquar. Terrar. Kde. 3*:27-28.

Goodrich, E. S. (1930). *Studies on the Structure and Development of Vertebrates*. London, MacMillan.

Guimond, R. W., and Hutchison, V. H. (1972). Pulmonary, branchial and cutaneous gas exchange in the mud puppy, *Necturus maculosus maculosus* (Rafinesque). *Comp. Biochem. Physiol. 42A*:367-392.

Guimond, R. W., and Hutchison, V. H. (1973). Trimodal gas exchange in the large aquatic salamander, *Siren lacertina* (Linnaeus). *Comp. Biochem. Physiol. 46A*:249-268.

Guimond, R. W., and Hutchison, V. H. (1974). Aerial and aquatic respiration in the congo eel *Amphiuma means means* (Garden). *Respir. Physiol. 20*: 147-159.

Guimond, R. W., and Hutchison, V. H. (1976). Gas exchange of the giant salamanders of North America. In *Respiration of Amphibious Vertebrates*. Edited by G. M. Hughes. New York, Academic Press.

Heath, A. G. (1976). Respiratory responses to hypoxia by *Ambystoma tigrinum* larvae, paedomorphs, and metamorphosed adults. *Comp. Biochem. Physiol. 55A*:45-49.

Hillman, S., and Withers, P. (1979). An analysis of respiratory surface area as a limit to activity metabolism in anurans. *Can. J. Zool. 57*:2100-2105.

Hoffman, T. (1875). Die Lungen-Lymphgefasse der *Rana temporaria*. Inaug-Dissert. Dorpat (quoted in Gaupp, 1904).

Holmgren, S., and Campbell, G. (1978). Adrenoceptors in the lung of the toad, *Bufo marinus*: Regional differences in response to amines and to sympathetic nerve stimulation. *Comp. Biochem. Physiol. 60C*:11-18.

Hopkins, G. S. (1896). The heart of some lungless salamanders. *Am. Nat.* 30.

Hughes, G. M. (1967). Evolution between air and water. In *Development of the Lung* (Ciba Foundation Symposium). Edited by A. S. deReuck and R. Porter. London, Churchill.

Hughes, G. M. (1970). Ultrastructure of the air-breathing organs of some lower vertebrates. *7th Int. Cong. Electron Microsc.* Paris, Soc. Franc. de Microsc. Electonique.

Hughes, G. M. (1973). Ultrastructure of the lung of *Neoceratodus* and *Lepidosiren* in relation to the lung of other vertebrates. *Folia Morphol. Prague 21*:155-161.

Hughes, G. M., and Vergara, G. A. (1978). Static pressure-volume curves for the lung of the frog (*Rana catesbeiana*). *J. Exp. Biol. 76*:149-165.

Hutchison, V. H., Haines, H. B., and Engbretson, G. (1976). Aquatic life at high altitude: Respiratory adaptations in the Lake Titicaca frog, *Telmatobius culeus. Resp. Physiol. 27*:115-129.

Hutchison, V. H. (1982). Physiological ecology of the telmatobid frogs of Lake Titicaca. *Natl. Geogr. Soc. Res. Reports 14*:357-361.

Jones, D. R., and Milsom, W. K. (1982). Peripheral receptors affecting breathing and cardiovascular function in no-mammalian vertebrates. *J. Exp. Biol. 100*:59-91.

Kampmeier, O. F. (1969). *Evolution and Comparative Morphology of the Lymphatic System*. Springfield, Ill., Charles C. Thomas.

Konigstein, H. (1903). Zur Morphologie und Physiologie des Gefasssystems am Respirationstract. *Z. Anat. Entwicklungsgesch. 1*:307-375.

Korgh, A. (1941). *The Comparative Physiology of Respiratory Mechanisms*. Philadelphia, University of Pennsylvania Press.

Kuhlmann, W. D., and Fedde, M. R. (1979). Intrapulmonary receptors in the bullfrog: Sensitivity to CO_2. *J. Comp. Physiol. 132A*:69-75.

Kuttner (1874). Contribution on the arrangement of the circulation in the frog lung. *Virchows Arch. 61*:21-43.

Lannoo, M. J., and Backman, M. D. (1984). On flotation and air breathing in *Ambystoma tigrinum* larvae: Stimuli for and the relationship between these behaviors. *Can. J. Zool. 62*:15-18.

Linnaeus, C. (1758). *10th Systema Naturae*.

Luckhardt, A. B., and Carlson, A. J. (1920). Studies on the visceral sensory system. II. Lung automatism and lung reflexes in the salamanders (*Necturus*, Axolotl). *Am. J. Physiol. 54*:122-137.

Luckhardt, A. B., and Carlson, A. J. (1921). Studies on the visceral sensory system; 6. Lung automatism and lung reflexes in *Cryptobranchus* with further notes on the physiology of the lung of *Necturus. Am. J. Physiol. 55*: 212-222.

Ludike, R. (1955). Uber den Respirationsapparat verschiedener Urodelen und seine Beziehungenzum Herzen. *Z. Morphol. Oekol. Tierre 43*:578-615.

Luhe, M. (1900). Lungenlose Urodelen. *Zool. Zentralbl. 7*. Cited in Goodrich (1930).

Macedo, H. de (1960). Vergleichende Untersuchungen an Arten Gattung *Telmatobium* (Amphibia, Anura). *Z. Wiss. Zool. 163*:35-396.

Malpighi, (1671). Anatomical observations, about the structure of the lungs of frogs, tortoises, and c. and perfecter animals; as also the texture of the spleen, and c. *Phil. Trans. R.Soc. 6*:2149-2150.

Marcus, H. (1908). Beitrage zur Kenntnis der Gymnophionen; VI. Uber den Ubergang von der Wasser- zur Luftatmung mit besonderer Berucksichtigung des Atemmechanismus von Hypogeophis. *Z. Anat. Entwicklungsgesch. 69*:328-343.

Marcus, H. (1922). Der Kehlkopf bei Hypogeophis. *Anat. Anz. Ergheft, 60*: 188-202.

Marcus, H. (1927). Lungenstudien. *Morphol. Jahrb. 58*:100-121.

Marcus, H. (1936). Uber die funktionelle und phylogenetische Bedeutung der Knorpelstacheln in der Lung von *Pipa. Anat. Anz. 81*:341-345.

McKean, T. (1969). A linear approximation of the transfer function of pulmonary mechanoreceptors in the frog. *J. Appl. Physiol. 27*:775-781.

McLean, J. R., and Burnstock, G. (1967). Innervation of the lung of the toad (*Bufo marinus*). II. Fluorescent histochemical localization of catecholamines. *Comp. Biochem. Physiol. 22*:767-773.

Meban, C. (1973). The pneumocytes in the lung of *Xenopus laevis. J. Anat. 114*:235-244.

Meekel, A. G. (1926). A pulmonary vestige in the lungless salamanders. *Anat. Rec. 34*:141.

Miller, D. A., and Bondurant, S. (1961). Surface characteristics of vertebrate lung extracts. *J. Appl. Physiol. 16*:1075-1077.

Milsom, W. K., and Jones, D. R. (1977). Carbon dioxide sensitivity of pulmonary receptors in the frog. *Experientia 33*:1167-1168.

Moalli, R., Meyers, R. S., Ultsch, G. R., and Jackson, D. C. (1981). Acid-base balance in a predominantly skin-breathing salamander, *Cryptobranchus alleganiensis. Respir. Physiol. 43*:1-12.

Mudge, G. P. (1898). An interesting case of connection between the lung and systemic circulatory system and of an abnormal hepatic blood supply in a frog (*Rana temporaria*). *J. Anat. Physiol. 33*:54-63.

Neil, E., Strom, L., and Zotterman, Y. (1950). Action potential studies of afferent fibres in the IXth and Xth cranial nerves of the frog. *Acta. Physiol. Scand. 20*:338-350.

Nilsson, S. (1985). *Autonomic Nerve Function in the Vertebrates*. Berlin, Springer-Verlag.

Noble, G. K. (1931). *The Biology of the Amphibia*. New York, McGraw-Hill Book Co.

Okada, Y., Ishiko, S., Daido, S., Kim, J., and Ikeda, S. (1962). Comparative morphology of the lung with special reference to the alveolar epithelial cells. a. Lung of the Amphibia. *Acta Tuberc. Jpn. 11*:63-72.

Pattle, R. E. (1973). Inter-species difference in surface properties of the lung. *Proc. R. Soc. Med. 66*:385-386.

Pattle, R. E. (1976). The lung surfactant in the evolutionary tree. In *Respiration in Amphibious Vertebrates*. Edited by G. M. Hughes. New York, Academic Press.

Pattle, R. E., and Hopkinson, D. A. W. (1963). Lung lining in bird, reptile, and amphibian. *Nature 200*:894.

Pattle, R. E., Schock, C., Creasey, J. M., and Hughes, G. M. (1977). Surpellic films, lung surfactant and their cellular origin in newt, ceacilian and frog. *J. Zool. (Long.) 182*:125-136.

Pinder, A. W., and Burggren, W. W. (1983). Respiration during chronic hypoxia and hyperoxia in larval and adult bullfrogs (*Rana catesbeiana*). II. Changes in respiratory properties of whole blood. *J. Exp. Biol. 105*:205-213.

Porter, K. R. (1972). *Herpetology*. Philadelphia, W. B. Saunders Co.

Price, J. A., and Pierce, J. A. (1963). The physical properties of the frog lung. *Proc. Soc. Exp. Biol. Med. 112*:538-541.

Romer, A. S. (1970). *The Vertebrate Body*, 4th ed. Philadelphia, W. B. Saunders Co.

Shelton, G. (1976). Gas exchange, pulmonary blood supply, and the partially divided amphibian heart. In *Perspectives in Experimental Biology*, Vol. 1. Zoology. Edited by P. Spencer-Davis. New York, Pergamon Press.

Shelton, G., and Boutilier, R. G. (1982). Apnoea in amphibians and reptiles. *J. Exp. Biol. 100*:245-273.

Shimada, K., and Kobayasi, S. (1966). Neural control of the pulmonary smooth muscle in the toad. *Acta Med. Biol. 13*:297-303.

Sorokin, S. P. (1963). Histochemistry in embryonic lungs. In *Neonatal Respiratory Adaptation*. Edited by T. K. Oliver, Jr. U.S. Public Health Publication No. 1432.

Smith, D. G., and Campbell, G. (1976). The anatomy of the pulmonary vascular bed in the toad *Bufo marinus*. *Cell Tissue Res. 165*:199-213.

Smith, D. G., and Rapson, L. (1977). Differences in pulmonary microvascular anatomy between *Bufo marinus* and *Xenopus laevis*. *Cell Tissue Res. 178*: 1-15.

Sprumont, P. (1969). Le relief intern du poumon de grenouille (*Rana ridibunda*). *Acta Anat. 73*:315.

Strawinski, S. (1956). Vascularization of respiratory surfaces in ontogeny of the edible frog, *Rana esculenta* L. *Zool. Pol. 7*:327-365.

Taglietta, V., and Casella, C. (1966). Stretch receptor stimulation in frog lungs. *Pflugers Arch. Gesamte Physiol. 292*:297-308.

Taglietta, V., and Casella, C. (1968). Deflation receptors in frog's lungs. *Pflugers Arch. Gesamte Physiol. 304*:81-89.

Tenney, S. M., and Tenney, J. B. (1970). Quantitative morphology of cold-blooded lungs: Amphibia and Reptilia. *Respir. Physiol. 9*:197-215.

Teski, I. (1978). In XIX Morphology Congress Symposium. Edited by E. Klika. Charles University, Prague.

Toews, D., and MacIntyre, D. (1978). Respiration and circulation in an apodan amphibian. *Can. J. Zool. 56*:998-1004.

Tsuchiya, S. (1959). Lung automatism in the Japanese toad. *J. Physiol. Soc. Jpn. 21*:272-279.

Warren, E. (1898). An abnormality in *Rana temporaria*. *Anat. Anz. 14*:551-552.

Warren, E. (1900). A further note on a variation in *Rana temporaria*. *Anat. Anz. 19*:442-443.

Wassersug, R. J., and Feder, M. E. (1983). The effects of aquatic oxygen concentration, body size and respiratory behaviors on the stamina of obligate aquatic (*Bufo americanus*) and facultative air breathing (*Xenopus laevis* and *Rana berlandieri*) anuran larvae. *J. Exp. Biol. 105*:173-190.

Watson, (1896). Abnormality in the arterial system of the frog. *Zool. Anz. 19*: 442-443.

West, N. H., and Burggren, W. W. (1982). Gill and lung ventilatory responses to steady-state aquatic hypoxia and hyperoxia in the bullfrog tadpole. *Respir. Physiol. 47*:165-176.

West, N. H., and Burggren, W. W. (1983). Reflex interactions between aerial and aquatic gas exchange organs in the larval bullfrog. *Am. J. Physiol. 244*: R770-R777.

Whitford, W., and Hutchison, V. H. (1965). Gas exchange in salamanders. *Physiol. Zool. 25*:228-242.

Whitford, W., and Hutchison, V. H. (1966). Cutaneous and pulmonary gas exchange in ambystomic salamanders. *Copeia 1966*:573-577.

Whitford, W., and Sherman, R. (1968). Aerial and aquatic respiration in Axolotl and transformed *Ambystoma tigrinum. Herpetology 24*:233-237.

Willnow, I., and Willnow, R. (1971). Anastomosen in Kaltbuterlungen. *Acta Anat. (Basel) 78*:127-135.

Wood, M. E., and Burnstock, G. (1967). Innervation of the lung of the toad (*Bufo marinus*). I. Physiology and pharmacology. *Comp. Biochem. Physiol. 22*:755-766.

7

Structure and Function of the Reptilian Respiratory System

STEVEN F. PERRY

Universität Oldenburg
Oldenburg, Federal Republic of Germany

I. Introduction

A reptile is like a unicorn: it does not exist, but everybody knows what it is. According to a recent cladistic analysis (Ax, 1984), amniotes consist of mammals and of a conglomerate made up of chelonians and their unnamed sister group, which contains birds and crocodilians, on the one hand, and lepidosaurs on the other. Thus, the only objective criterion that really unites reptiles is that they are amniotes that are neither mammals nor birds. Why, then, do they remain anatomically and physiologically identifiable?

The most important difference between reptiles and their mammalian and avian relatives is an interconnected array of characters related to the reputedly modest reptilian sustained metabolic rate. It ranges from one-thirtieth of that of equivalent-sized mammals in free-ranging lizards (Bennet and Nagy, 1977) to one-third of the resting mammalian oxygen consumption rate ($\dot{V}O_2$) in the

---

Financial support during this writing period was supplied by the Alberta Heritage Foundation for Medical Research, Grant 71-3806.

homoiothermic, loggerhead turtle (Lutcavage et al., 1985). Miniman and maximal $\dot{V}O_2$, of course, extend this range from zero (total anaerobiosis) to a $\dot{V}O_2$ similar to that of a resting mammal (Ultsch and Jackson, 1982; Wood et al., 1978).

If one trend can be identified as characteristic of the present research focus on the structure and function of the reptilian respiratory system, it is the tendency away from regarding reptiles as retarded mammals (1960s and before) and toward a recognition of the structure and function of the reptilian cardiorespiratory system as being correct for a reptile (1970s). Finally, an appreciation of the individual complexity and the noninterchangeability of data among different reptilian groups has emerged in the 1980s.

Recent years have seen a decline in reptilian respiratory studies. But at the same time, a number of integrative works have been published, that have combined morphology and physiology, and have provided new insight into the biology of respiration in reptiles.

The intent of the present review is not to provide a comprehensive account of all research concerning the structure or function of the respiratory system in reptiles because a number of such articles are already available (Bennett and Dawson, 1976; Duncker, 1978b, 1981; Glass and Wood, 1983; Hughes, 1977; Perry, 1987c; Shelton et al., 1986; Wood and Lenfant, 1976, 1979). Rather, I intend to point out some areas in which the integrative approach to understanding the respiratory strucure-function complex in reptiles has made significant advances in recent years. In addition, the most important background literature will be reviewed for comparative ontogeny of the reptilian lung with the hope of stimulating interest in this long-neglected discipline.

Expanding our knowledge of reptilian respiration helps not only to better understand reptiles: it should not be forgotten that our paleozoic ancestors were ectothermic, egg-laying reptiles. Each individual animal represents a unique combination of processes best suited to ensure the survival of the species. In some instances these processes can serve as models to increase our understanding of the origin and evolution of similar but now much more highly integrated processes in mammals.

II. Reptilian Lung Structure

A. Gross Anatomy and Terminology

Unfortunately there is to date no *Nomina Anatomica* for reptiles. Different investigators, thus, tend to refer to the same structures by different names or to use the same word (e.g., "air sac") to designate different structures.

Duncker's (1978b) nomenclature for structural types of lungs points a way out of this confusion (Fig. 1). He divides reptilian lung types into single-chambered (unicameral), few-chambered (paucicameral), and many-chambered (mulit-

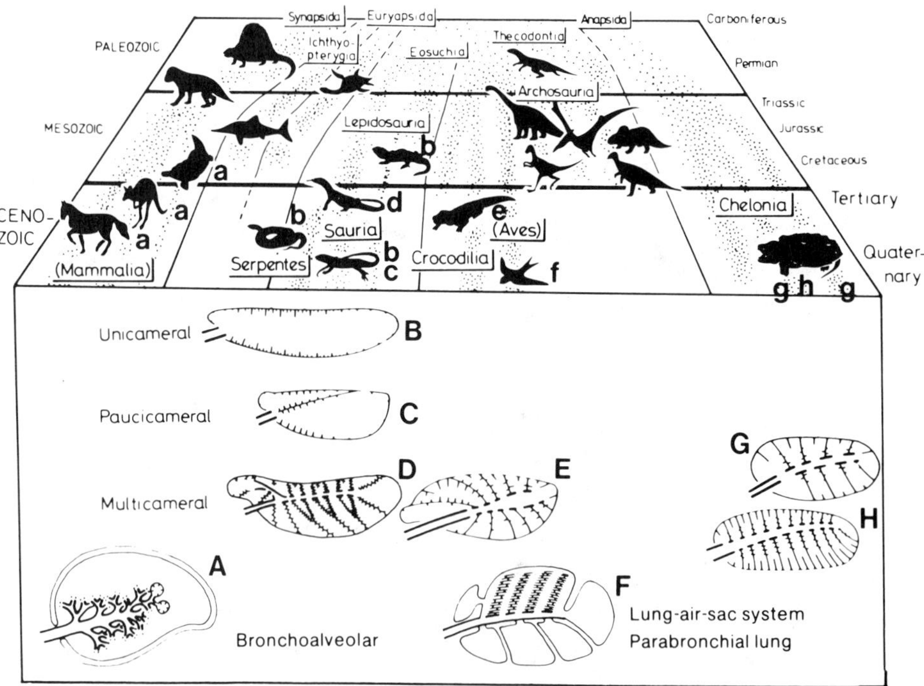

Figure 1 Phylogenetic tree of amniotes showing structural types of lungs of extant representatives. The bronchoalveolar lung (A) is present in all mammalian groups (a). Snakes (b), some lizards (b), and the tuatara (b) may possess unchambered, *unicameral* lungs (B). Other lizards, notably chaemeleontids, iguanids, and agamids (c), as well as nonvaranid platynotans, have *paucicameral* lungs (C), which are chambered but lack an intrapulmonary bronchus, whereas varanid lizards (d), crocodilians (e), as well as cryptodire (g, h) and pleurodire (g) chelonians possess multichambered, *multicameral* lungs (D, E, G, H). The avian lung-air sac system with its parabronchial lungs is unique to birds but can possibly be derived from the basic crocodilian plan. The lower-case letters on the animal profiles correspond to the upper-case letters on the lung schemata (After Perry, 1983).

cameral), much as did Milani (1894, 1897). Although this system of gross lung classification is not the only one found in the literature (see Marcus, 1937; Wolf, 1933), it provides the best basis for a modern reconsideration of structure-function analyses.

Proceeding from the gross anatomical to the histological level, we are concerned with the gas exchange regions (parenchyma) and their distribution relative to the large, central lumina of the unicameral lung or of lung chambers in paucicameral or multicameral types.

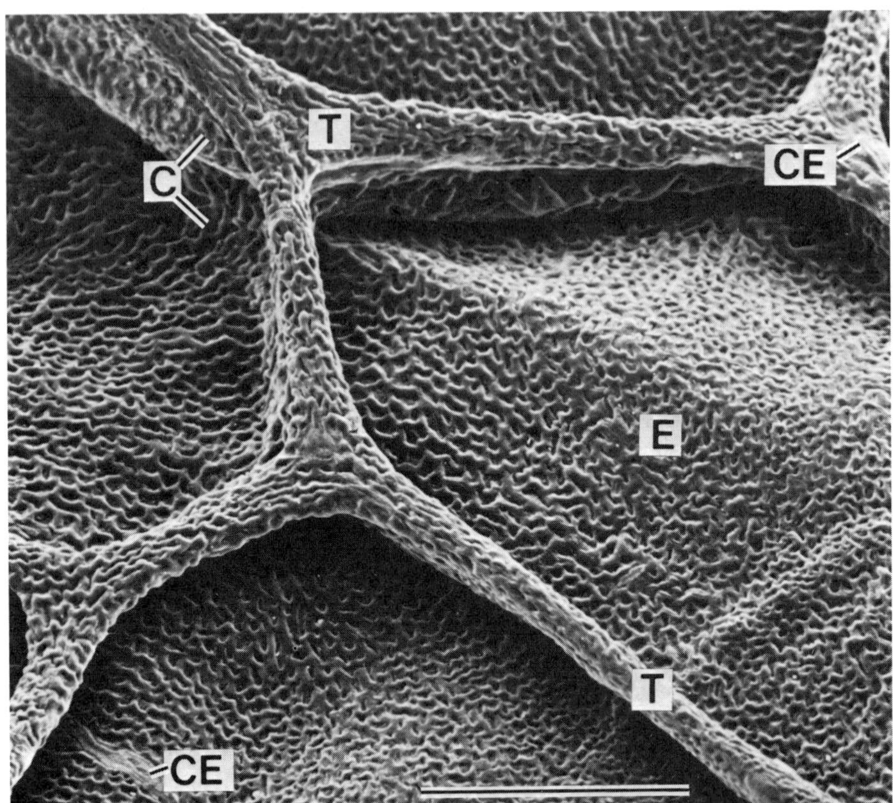

Figure 2 Scanning electron micrograph of a portion of the edicular parenchyma of a gecko lung, clearly showing trabeculae (T), shallow ediculae (E), and the network of capillaries (C). Each side of the interedicular speta has a separate capillary net. CE indicates avenues of ciliated epithelium on the trabeculae and occasionally on the edicular surface (scale line is 500 μm).

A typical unicameral lung consists of a tissue-free *central lumen* and a parenchymal layer, which contains gas exchange tissue and air spaces. The parenchyma forms a honeycomb-like system, the free ends of which are supported by *trabeculae* with a core of smooth muscle and elastic tissue. In the simplest parenchymal type, *trabecular parenchyma*, the trabeculae lie directly on the inner surface of the lung (Perry, 1983). Should the trabeculae be raised above the lung wall, they draw a double net of capillaries, as well as associated connective tissue, nerves, and smooth muscle, with them and, thus, form a network of polygonal cubicles (Fig. 2). Duncker (1978b) employes the word edicular (cubiclelike) if the parenchymal air spaces do not tend to be deeper than

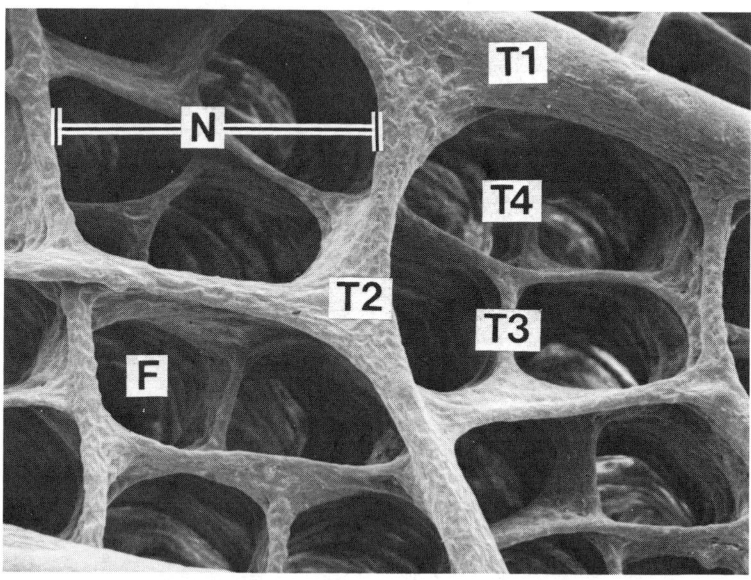

Figure 3 Scanning electron micrograph of a portion of the faveolar parenchyma of the teju lung. Trabeculae of first- (T1), second- (T2), third- (T3), and fourth-order (T4) are indicated. Ciliated epithelium (CE) is found primarily on first- and second-order trabeculae and is lacking on the faveolar surface. Faveolie (F) are grouped into niches (N), which are homologues of ediculae (see Fig. 2) (magnification is the same as in Fig. 2).

they are wide (Fig. 2), and faveolar (honeycomblike) if the air spaces form tubular structures (Fig. 3).

The termini *edicula(ae)* and *faveolus(i)* for the unit structure of the respective reptilian parenchymal types are deemed preferable to "air sac(s)" or "alveolus(i)." The latter designations should be reserved for the appropriate avian and mammalian structures, but unfortunately are still in use for reptilian lungs (Pohunkova and Hughes, 1985).

In addition, Perry (1983) has suggested a nomenclature that is compatible with that of Duncker (1978b) but is particularly well suited for describing changes within a given lung or within an ontogenetic or phylogenetic series. The parenchyma is first characterized as *heterogeneous* or *homogeneous* according to its distribution in the lung. Second, the "mesh" of the parenchyma is described as *sparse* or *dense*, and finally its height is given as *shallow* or *deep*. Thus, the lung of a typical colubrid snake would be described as unicameral with heterogeneously distributed, densely partitioned parenchyma, which is deep cranially and shallow caudally. This system combined with the characterization of uni-

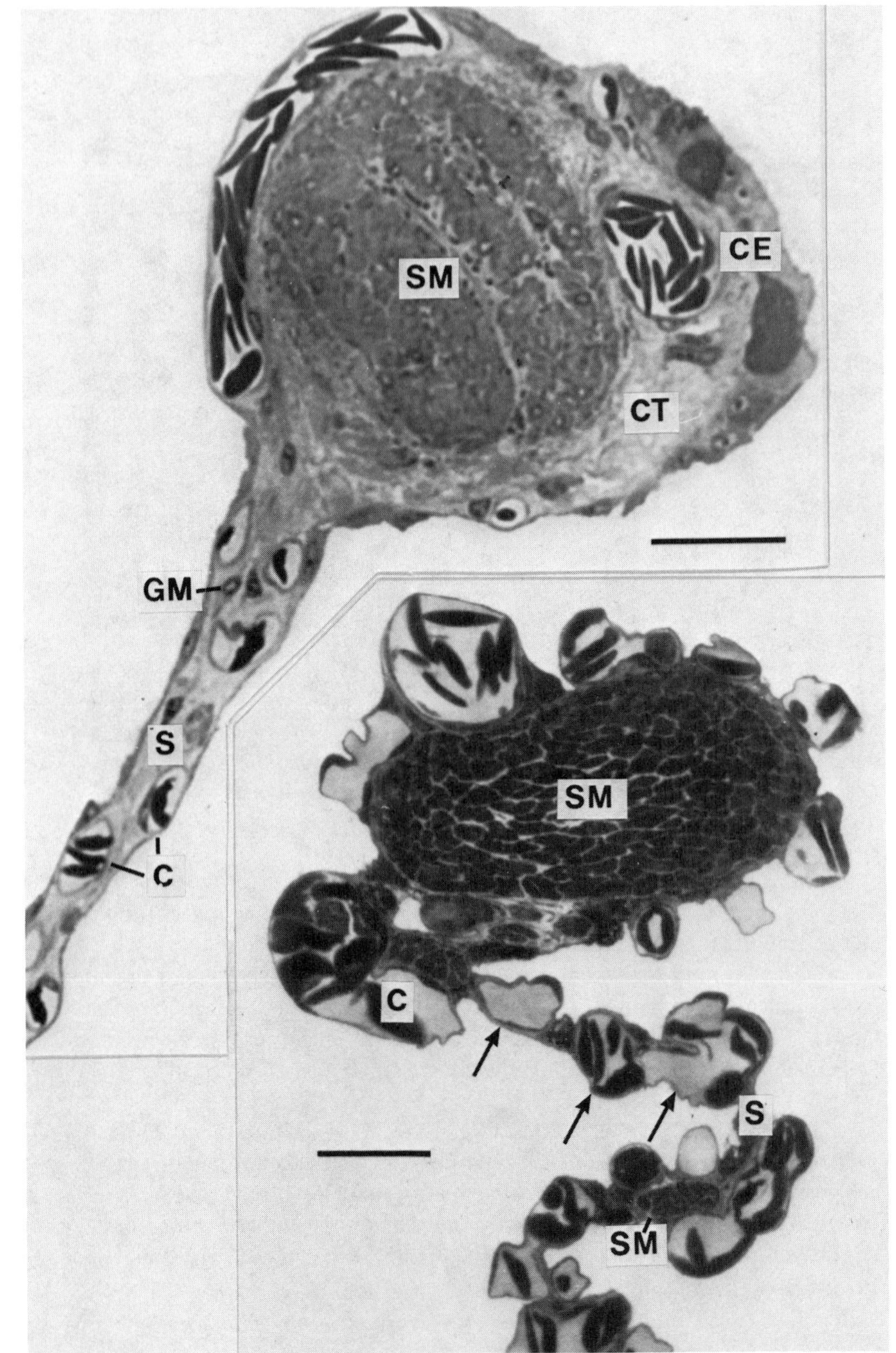
SM
CE
CT
GM
S
C
SM
C
S
SM

cameral, paucicameral, or multicameral lung type lends itself to graphic representation of all reptilian lungs (Perry, 1987c).

In paucicameral and multicameral lung types, Perry (1978, 1983) has referred to intercameral *septa* and to interfaveolar or interedicular *partitions*. Histologically, these septa and partitions are similar but ontogenetically they may differ (Hesser, 1906; Ogawa, 1920). Nevertheless, the usefulness of this distinction is disputable, because most modern investigators employ *septa* for both types of structures, and analogus terminology for mammalian lungs (e.g., interalveolar septa, interlobular septa) is in use.

Typically, each surface of the edicular or faveolar wall possesses its own capillary net (Figs. 2 and 4, top), which receives the deoxygenated blood from a branch of the pulmonary artery and delivers it to a subtrabecular vein or to branches of the pulmonary vein that lie in the lung wall. The *double* capillary net is best developed in lungs with edicular parenchyma (emydid turtles, crocodiles; see Fig. 4, top). In reptiles with faveolar parenchyma (e.g., the rattlesnake *Crotalus*, the emerald lizard *Lacerta*, and the teju *Tupinambis*), anastomoses across the interfaveolar septa are frequent, and the capillary net at these places is *single* (Cragg, 1975; Klemm et al., 1979; Luchtel and Kardong, 1981; Perry, 1983; see Fig. 4, bottom). In intermediate cases, e.g., the savanna monitor *Varanus exanthematicus*, capillary profiles may alternate across the interfaveolar septum, thus forming a *pseudo-single* network. In contrast to the single net condition, only one side of each capillary is developed to a thin air–blood exchange barrier (Duncker, 1978b, 1981; Hughes, 1978; Perry, 1983).

B. Lung Structure and Reptilian Phylogeny

Surprisingly, the oldest surviving reptilian groups (chelonians, crocodilians) have the most complex primary lung structure (Duncker, 1978b; Perry, 1983; see Fig. 1). But multicameral lungs are also typical of monitor lizards, which are not known earlier than the Cretaceous period (Romer, 1966). Thus, although primary lung structure is not of systematic significance at the subclass level, it increases in importance below the family level. Klaver (1973, 1977, 1979, 1980)

Figure 4 (Top) Cross section through a trabecula from a crocodile lung, showing the smooth muscular core (SM), the layer of submucosal connective tissue (CT), and clearance epithelium (CE). The interedicular septum (S) displays a double net of capillaries (C) and strands of smooth muscle (SM) (Toluidine blue; scale bar indicates 20 μm). (Bottom) Cross section through a trabecula of second- or third-order from the teju lung. Note the high degree of vascularity of the trabecula and of the interedicular septum (S). Arrows indicate respiratory capillaries (C) that show a thin air–blood barrier on both sides of the septum, thus, forming a single net (see text). Smooth-muscle (SM) bundles in the septum run parallel to the trabecula (Toluidine blue; scale bar indicates 20 μm). (Top photograph from Perry, 1986b, courtesy of the Company of Biologists.)

has successfully utilized lung gross anatomy in his recent revision of brooksians and chameleons within the family Chamaeleonidae. A similar study in the Varanidae is in progress (Becker et al., 1988).

As welcome as it is to see the lung successfully employed as a systematic index, it is, on the other hand, unfortunate. Thereby, lungs lose their innocence in the sense that phylogenetic trees and cladograms can no longer be used to help resolve the sequence in the development of lung structure without the danger of circular argumentation.

C. Lung Ontogeny

In preparation of this article, I was unable to find a single original publication on fetal lung development in reptiles more recent than 1942. The reasons include the eflux of German embryologists during World War II and the fact that the questions posed at the time appear to have been resolved.

The main questions during the nineteenth century concerned the mode of gross differentiation of lung chambers, of niches (groups of faveoli or ediculae), and of the faveoli and ediculae themselves:

1. Are chambers, niches, ediculae, and faveoli formed by bronchipetal encroachment of the septa into a primarily undivided central lumen, as maintained by Schulze (1871) or, rather, by bronchifugal budding of potential air spaces?
2. What are the formative (entwicklungsmechanische) influences in lung development that allow, in one group, the development of a multicameral and, in another group, of a unicameral lung?
3. What information can the developmental pattern in lungs give about the phylogenetic relationship of the animals studied?

Moser (1902) provides answers to all of these questions: (1) Lung differentiation is bronchifugal at all levels; (2) budding is accompanied by thickening of the epithelium at the bud tips; and (3) comparison of avian with crocodilian lung anlagen reveals striking similarities between these two groups.

These results were corroborated by later studies in the first quarter of the twentieth century (Miller, 1904; Hesser, 1906; Hochstetter, 1909; Reese, 1915), particularly on turtles and crocodilians. Heilmann's (1914) data on lizards and turtles, but not his discussion, also support Moser's (1902) contentions. Marcus (1937) and his coworker Hilber (1933), however, ignore the early work in favor of Marcus' own theories of spiral development and the putative influence of airflow on lung development. Broman retaliated quickly, at first in word (Broman, 1938), then in deed (Broman, 1939, 1940) using wax reconstructions to demonstrate that chamber development in the multicameral lungs of various crocodilians (*Caiman, Alligator*) and chelonians (*Thalassochelys Caretta, Chelonia, Der-*

mochelys, Emys) is both bronchifugal and monopodal. In crocodilians, the branching of the chambers themselves is also monopodal, whereas in the sea turtle it is dichotomous. Also, the chamber formation in the paucicameral chameleon lung (Broman, 1942) begins at a very early stage and is not formed by a later invagination of the intercameral septa. The fingerlike projections typical of many chameleon lungs (Klaver, 1977) are late developments. Such structures are not unique to chameleons, they are also seen in gekkonids of the genus *Uroplatus* (Werner, 1912) and in some varanids (Becker et al., 1988).

The role of fetal lung epithelial fluid secretion in chamber budding and in formation of the ediculae is stressed by both Hesser (1906) and Broman (1942). They also point out that the first pulmonary smooth muscle is visible in the anlagen of the trabeculae just when the ediculae begin to form, and they correlate this with the hydrostatic function of lung fluid. That this fluid is secreted by the lung itself is documented by the temporary spontaneous obliteration of the tracheal lumen just at the time of edicular formation in the gecko (*Tarentola*) lung (Hesser, 1906).

Developmental studies on reptiles since the end of World War II have been primarily directed toward ecological and endocrinological studies (for entrance to the literature see Fitch, 1970; Gans et al., 1985; Porter, 1972) or toward establishment of standard tables of development (Dufaure and Hubert, 1961; Pasteels, 1957; Yntema, 1968; Zehr, 1962). The use of reptiles in experimental embryology has been limited because of their seasonal parturition, to the reluctance of many species to lay eggs in captivity, and to the difficulty of successfully artificially incubating the eggs (Holder and Bellairs, 1962). The methods for in vitro organ culture, however, appear relatively uncomplicated compared with those for mammalian tissue (New, 1966). Improved techniques for egg incubation (Broer and Horn, 1985; Legler, 1956), coupled with technology transfer from standard avian tissue and organ culture methods, provide a virtually unexploited background for studies of reptilian lung development.

D. Histology and Ultrastructure

The descriptive microanatomy of reptilian lungs has attracted little attention during the past ten years, and the main focus of the few original studies has been the gas exchange epithelium (Bartels and Welsch, 1983, 1984; Hughes, 1978; Klemm et al., 1979; Luchtel and Kardong, 1981; Meban, 1977; 1978a,b; Pohunkova, 1978; Pohunkova and Hughes, 1985; Welsch, 1979; Welsch and Müller, 1980a,b).

These papers, as well as morphometrically oriented ones (Perry, 1978, 1983; Stinner, 1982) confirm the presence of two types of edicular/faveolar epithelial cells corresponding to the type I and type II pneumocytes of mammals and birds (Campiche, 1960; Petric, 1967). The published electron micrographs and observations suggest a qualitative difference in type II cells that corresponds to the type of parenchyma in which they occur (Welsch and Müller, 1980). Those from faveolar parenchyma (e.g., the "true" lizard *Lacerta*, the teju lizard *Tupinambis*, the rattlesnake *Crotalus*) tend to exhibit large, interconnected vacuoles (Klemm et al., 1979; Luchtel and Kardong, 1981; Meban, 1978a; Perry, 1983), whereas those from edicular parenchyma (e.g., the chelonians *Pseudemys, Testudo*; the crocodilians *Caiman, Crocodylus*; and the monitor lizard *Varanus*) appear compact, and their multilamellar bodies are either similar to those in mammalian lungs or are poorly differentiated (Meban, 1977; Perry, 1983; Perry, 1988a; Stratton, 1977; Welsch and Müller, 1980b). The type II cells of the sparsely partitioned, faveolar lungs of the slow worm, *Anguis fragilis*, show an intermediate structure (Meban, 1978b), whereas those of geckos (*Hemidactylus* and *Rhacodactylus*) are similar to lizards with more densely partitioned parenchyma or may lack multilamellar bodies altogether (Welsch and Müller, 1980; Perry et al., 1988b–see p. 236).

Respiratory epithelium tends to cover the small trabeculae (see Fig. 4, bottom) whereas clearance epithelium is found on large trabeculae (Fig. 5). In species with edicular parenchyma, exceptions are especially common: in the gecko (*Rhacodactylus*) large trabeculae may lack clearance epithelium, whereas patches of ciliated cells occur in the ediculae far from the nearest trabecula (see Fig. 2), whereas in the crocodile, even the smallest traveculae bear ciliated clearance epithelium (see Fig. 4, top).

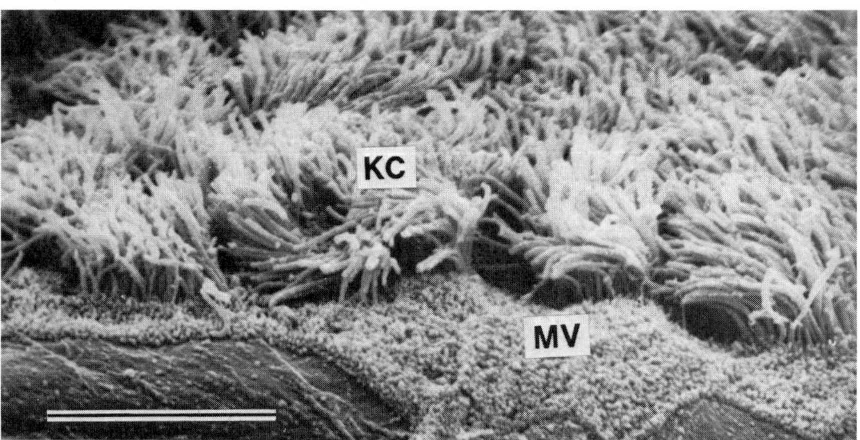

Figure 5 Scanning electron micrograph of ciliated, clearance epithelium on a first-order trabecula in the teju lung. Kinocilia (KC) as well as microvilli (MV) are clearly visible. Cells bordering the clearance epithelium form a microvillous hedge (scale bar indicates 10 μm).

The trabecular clearance epithelium in the species described in the recent literature (chelonians: *Carettocheyls, Erythmochelys, Chelonia, Trionyx, Testudo, Pseudemys*; crocodilians: *Caiman, Crocodylus*; lizards: *Hemidactylus, Agama, Chamaeleo, Tupinambis, Varanus*; snakes: *Thamnophis, Nerodia, Crotalus*) consists primarily of serous secretory cells and microvilli-rich ciliated cells (Klemm et al., 1979; Luchtel and Kardong, 1981; Perry, 1983; Pohunkova and Hughes, 1985; Welsch and Müller, 1980b; see Fig. 4, top). In addition to the serous secretory droplets and kinocilia that characterize the secretory cells and the ciliated cells, respectively, both cell types display a lateral labyrinth (Welsch and Müller, 1980a), and some authors suggest the possible role of these cells in resorption of lung fluid (Perry, 1987a; Scheuermann et al., 1983). This fluid presumably escapes from the pulmonary gas exchange capillaries (Burggren, 1982) and may be swept onto the trabeculae by ciliary action, as has been proposed for the amphibian lung (Kilburn, 1969). The secretory products of the serous cells may, as in invertebrate filter feeders, ensure the proper mechanical properties for ciliary transport of the semifluid film.

In addition to the serous and ciliated cells, small granule secretory cells and transitional cells, intermediate in structure between the serous secretory cells and type II pneumocytes, have been seen (Luchtel and Kardong, 1981; Perry, 1987a). In the basal region of the trabecular epithelium, endocrinelike cells are encountered (Luchtel and Kardong, 1981; Perry, 1988; Perry, unpublished observations; Scheuermann, 1987; Scheuermann et al., 1983). These cells, which are characterized by their predominantly basally located dense-core granules, may form organoid neuroepithelial bodies (*Pseudemys*) but may also occur in groups (*Crocodylus, Nerodia*) or singly (*Crocodylus, Caiman, Crotalus*) (Luchtel and Kardong, 1981; Perry, 1988a; Perry, unpublished observations; Scheuermann, 1987; Scheuermann et al., 1983, 1984). The putative function of these cells is discussed in Section III.D. The tracheal and extrapulmonary bronchial epithelium has been seldom studied in reptiles (Pastor et al., 1987; Tesik, 1984–see p. 236).

E. Functional Structure

Lung Statics and Dynamic Potential

The lungs of noncrodilian reptiles are not located in closed, pleural cavities, but together with the other viscera, they are, more or less, freely suspended in a common pleuroperitoneal space. The degree of "freedom" of suspension depends upon the development of the postpulmonary septum and the posthepatic septum, the cranial nephric fold (Broman, 1904, 1937; Duncker, 1978a,c; Goodrich, 1930). In general, however, heterogeneously partitioned lungs tend to be firmly attached to the body wall. This prevents the collapse of the densely partitioned regions into the more saclike, loosely and shallowly partitioned regions, which are exposed to the visceral cavity. Homogeneously partitioned lungs, on the other hand, can be freely suspended on delicate pulmonary ligaments (mesopneumonia) and still maintain their shape at any degree of inflation. Notwithstanding, attached homogeneously partitioned lungs (e.g., in sea turtles and soft-shelled turtles) are not uncommon.

In spite of the early description of smooth muscle and elastic tissue in reptilian lungs (Engel, 1962; Ogawa, 1920), the function is poorly known. A combined neurophysiological, pharmacological, and functional morphological study of the action of this musculature, such as that of Campbell and Duxson (1978) in the toad *Bufo marinus*, apparently has not been carried out for a reptile. In *Bufo*, epinephrine and norepinephrine both elicit contraction of the trabecular musculature and relaxation of the interedicular musculature, whereas sympathetic nerve stimulation cause contraction, then relaxation, of the entire lung. Acetylcholine brings about contraction of the trabecular musculature. Earlier studies in the skink, *Trachysaurus rugosus* (Burnstock and Wood, 1967), show that stimulation of the vagal sympathetic nerve trunks, as well as application of acetylcholine, causes contraction of the lung, but these authors do not differentiate between trabecular and interfaveolar musculature. Berger (1973) describes inhibitory noncholinergic, nonadrenergic innervation in the lungs of *Trachydosaurus*.

Welsch and Müller (1980a) studying six chelonian, one crocodilian, two lacertilian, and one ophidian species, employ the fine structure of varicosities to differentiate three types of nerves. Type 1 is characterized by electron-lucent vesicles 52-55 nm in diameter and by dense granules 80-90 nm in diameter. Type 2 (observed only in the garter snake *Thamnophis*) has oval, dense vesicles 250-350 nm in diameter, as well as some small, electron-lucent ones. Type 3 contains abundant small electron-lucent granules as well as two types of dense granules with diameters of 55-80 nm and 110-140 nm, respectively. Type 1 presumably represents cholinergic nerves and is found near smooth muscle. Types 2 and 3 are presumed to be purinergic/peptidergic and adrenergic, respectively, and both types may be inhibitory.

Nonvascular smooth muscle occupies between 8 and 14% of reptilian lung tissue (Perry, 1983; Perry, 1988a). In the Nile crocodile, approximately two-thirds of the pulmonary smooth muscle is located in the trabeculae. The remaining one-third is found in the central leaflet of the interedicular walls, where it is oriented perpendicular to the trabeculae (Perry, 1988a). Thus, these two muscle groups can act antagonistically, as demonstrated in the toad lung (Campbell and Duxson, 1978): contraction of the trabecular musculature around the concavity of the closed lung deepens the ediculae: contraction of the interedicular musculature lowers them.

In the teju (*Tupinambis nigropunctatus*), nonvascular smooth muscle makes up 9% of the total lung tissue volume and is equally distributed in the trabeculae and in the interfaveolar walls (Perry, 1983). In this species, however, the faveolar wall musculature is oriented parallel to that of the trabeculae. Its contraction throws the faveoli into accordian pleats, thus, effectively decreasing the height of the faveoli and acting antagonistically to the trabecular musculature (Perry et al., 1988a).

Morphometry

Reptilian lung morphometrics is an extremely time-consuming process. For the mammalian lung, Weibel and his coworkers have succeeded in perfecting and streamlining stereological methods for morphometry, thus enabling them to obtain measurements of morphometric-diffusing capacity in scores of experimental, domestic, and wild animals (see Weibel and Taylor, 1987). Fortunately, mammalian lung structure "conforms" reasonably well to the constraints of stereological morphmetry: the parenchyma is usually homogeneous and the alveolar surfaces approach random orientation in space.

Reptilian lungs, on the other hand, seem to be designed to confound the morphometrist. Because the parenchyma is usually heterogeneous and structurally different from part to part within the same lung, a large number of samples are necessary to obtain reliable measurements. To make matters worse, the structure of the ediculae and faveoli is often regionally so different (e.g., colubrid snakes, testudinid tortoises) that randomly oriented sections, which are unavoidable in one lung region, are unobtainable in adequate numbers for standard stereology in another. Thus, the lungs of only five reptilian species (*Lacerta* spp., *Pseudemys scripta, Varanus exanthematicus, Tupinambis nigropunctatus, Thamnophis siratis*) have now been morphometrically evaluated to date (Cragg, 1975; Perry, 1978, 1983; Stinner, 1982). Preliminary data for a sixth species (*Crododylus niloticus*) are also available (Perry, 1988b).

For interspecific comparison of the degree of specialization of the lung for gas exchange the following morphometric factors are of importance: the morphometrically determined standard lung volume at three-fourths total inflation (VL), parenchymal volume (VP), respiratory surface area—that portion of the lung surface underlain by capillaries (SAR), the harmonic mean thickness of the air-blood diffusion barrier across lung tissue (τ_{ht}), and the SAR/τ_{ht} ratio. The latter factor has been termed the anatomical diffusion factor (ADF; Perry, 1978). The ADF represents the anatomical component of the diffusing capacity of lung tissue (D_tO_2) exclusive of blood.

$$DtO_2 = KtO_2 \cdot SAR/\tau_{ht} = KtO_2 \cdot ADF \qquad (1)$$

where K_tO_2 is Krogh's constant of diffusion for oxygen in lung tissue.

A further indicator of lung function is the effective surface/volume ratio of the parenchyma (SAR/VP).

Inspection of Table 1 reveals the lungs of "a reptile" to be larger than those of a comparable mammal or bird but to have maximally 20% of the respiratory surface area of these homoiotherms. The main factor accounting for the low rep-

Table 1 Morphometry of the Lungs in Various Reptiles, Lungfish, Rat, and Pigeon

Indicator	Symbol	Units	Teju[a]	Lacerta[b]
Body weight	W	kg	0.72	0.02
Total lung volume	V_L	ml/kg	84.4	94.8
Parenchymal volume	%P	% of V_L	26.0	34.6
Parenchymal volume	V_P	ml/kg	22.0	32.8
Total parenchymal surface area	S_A	x 10^3 cm^2/kg	3.76	6.07
Resp. surface area	%AR	% of S_A	78.2	70.0
Resp. surface area	S_{AR}	x 10^3 cm^2/kg	2.94	4.25
Harmonic mean thickness of tissue barrier	τ_{ht}	x 10^{-4} cm (=μm)	0.46	0.53
Anat. diffusion factor	ADF	x 10^3 $cm^2 \cdot \mu m^{-1} \cdot kg^{-1}$ (x 10^7 cm/kg)	6.39	8.01
O_2 diffusing capacity of tissue barrier	D_tO_2	$ml \cdot min^{-1} \cdot kg^{-1} \cdot torr^{-1}$	1.9	2.5
Effective surface/volume ratio in parenchyma	S_{AR}/V_P	cm^2/cm^3	133.6	129.6

[a]Perry (1983).
[b]*Lacerta* ssp.; Cragg (1975).
[c]*Thamnophis sirtalis*; Stinner (1981).
[d]*Pseudemys scripta*; Perry (1978).
[e]*Crocodylus niloticus*; preliminary values from Perry (1988a).
[f]*Lepidosiren paradoxa*; Hughes and Weibel (1976).
[g]Young laboratory rats; Burri and Weibel (1971); numbers in parentheses indicate values assuming %AR = 100%.
[h]Domestic pigeon, *Columba livia*; Otten (1973); barrier thickness calculated by the author from electron micrographs generously provided by H.-R. Duncker. Numbers in parentheses indicate value for entire lung-air sac system.
[i]Calculated using KO_2 for rat lung tissue (Grote, 1967): at 30°C for reptiles and the lungfish and at 37°C for rat, K_{O_2} is 3.1 and 3.3 x 10^{-8} $cm^2 \cdot min^{-1} \cdot torr^{-1}$, respectively.
Source: After Perry (1983).

tilian lung surface area is the effective surface area/volume ratio in the parenchyma. This factor, in turn, depends upon the surface area/volume ratio of the parenchymal partitions themselves (S_A/V_P) and the vascularity (capillary density) of the partitions, expressed as percentage AR. These factors differ greatly among reptiles, ranging from S_A/V_P values of 21 cm^2/cm^3, with 83% vascularity in the turtle, and 30 cm^2/cm^3, with 50% vascularity in the crocodile, to 185, with 70% vascularity in *Lacerta*, and 171, with 78% vascularity in the teju.

Snake[c]	Monitor[a]	Turtle[d]	Crocodile[e]	Lungfish[f]	Rat[g]	Pigeon[h]	
1.00	0.44	1.0	4.11	0.5	0.14	0.45	
97.5	306.7	262.3	109.4	46.8	45.0	27.1	(178.7)
–	28.7	44.9	42.2	44.1	81.0	48.8	(7.4)
–	83.2	117.8	46.1	20.6	36.0	13.2	
2.00	6.13	2.49	1.37	0.88	(27.7)	–	
–	88.6	82.7	50.0	96.5	(100.0)	–	
–	5.43	2.06	0.69	0.85	27.7	40.3	
0.46	0.65	0.5	1.2	0.86	0.38	0.12	
4.4	8.35	4.12	0.57	0.88	72.89	335.83	
1.4	2.6	1.3	0.18	0.3	24.0	114.1	
101.0	65.3	18.0	15.0	41.2	750.0	3053.0	

The air-blood barrier (τ_{ht}) tends to be thicker in reptiles than in mammals and is 5 to 10 times thicker than in birds (Dubach, 1980; Gehr et al., 1981). Combining SAR and τ_{ht} according to Equation 1 we see that the anatomical diffusion factor (ADF) of reptilian lung tissue is 10 times lower than comparable mammalian and 50 times lower than comparable avian values.

Interestingly, among reptiles, the ADF does not depend upon the structural type of lung, as one might presume. *Lacerta* and the monitor arrive at almost identical D_tO_2 values by different avenus, or "strategies" (Perry, 1983; see Table 1). *Lacerta* has small unicameral lungs with a large surface area/volume ratio and a thin air-blood barrier, whereas the monitor has large, multicameral lungs with a moderately low surface area/volume ratio and a thicker air-blood barrier.

Comparison of reptilian with lungfish values in Table 1 reveals nothing that would allow one to distinguish between a lungfish and a reptile on the basis of these morphometric data alone. Only the lungfish lung volume is small by reptilian standards, but even this value is similar to that of a crocodile or sea turtle during diving (see Sec. IV of this chapter).

The study of factors regulating the pattern of differentiation in reptilian lung parenchyma relative to the maximal sustainable metabolic rate will occupy reptilian lung morphometrists in the future.

III. Reptilian Lung Function

Morphometrics represent only a static situation: physiology only a dynamic one. A combination of both methods is necessary to begin to understand lung function in an animal in which the lung parenchyma is movable, breathing occurs in episodes of variable length, and the quantity as well as the quality (degree of oxygen saturation) of the blood delivered to the lungs is instantaneously variable.

Faced with the large differences in reptilian lung structure, as previously described, it is natural for us to inquire into the physiological correlates: in other words, to ask why the lungs look the way they do. To begin to answer this question we need a set of criteria by which we can judge the degree of matching of anatomical and physiological variables. Four indicators of the effectivity of the lung as a gas exchange organ will be discussed: (1) diffusing capacity—comparison of morphometric and physiological values, (2) oxygen extraction, (3) ventilation–perfusion matching, and (4) breathing pattern optimization.

A. Diffusing Capacity

As attractive as the direct comparison of the same morphometrically and physiologically measured indicator appears, this procedure is fraught with difficulties. To begin with, the diffusing capacity of lung tissue given in Equation 1 represents a theoretical maximum that can never be attained by a living animal. In humans, for example, the erythrocytes (which are not even included in Eq. 1) provide a resistance to oxygen uptake that is at least as great as that of the lung tissues (Weibel, 1984). Unfortunately, the more factors that are introduced to make the morphometric diffusing capacity physiologically realistic, the more speculative the estimate becomes. Calculation of the entire diffusing capacity of the lung according to Equation 2

$$\frac{1}{DLO_2} = \frac{1}{D_tO_2} + \frac{1}{DPO_2} + \frac{1}{D_eO_2} \tag{2}$$

requires factors that are poorly known in reptiles, such as Θ, the rate of oxygen binding in erythrocytes (e), as well as measurements of diffusion distances within capillary blood plasma (P) based upon electron micrographs. The relationship of the latter to the reality of flowing blood is particularly questionable. Thus, one compares ADF directly to the physiologically measured diffusing capacity, using ADF/DO_2 as an index of relative efficiency. This index will have a value of somewhere between 3 and 8 (the lower value indicating the better matching of morphological and physiological indicators), and the units are those of $1/K$. Alternatively, one converts ADF to D_tO_2 using the factor $K_tO_2 = 3.1 \times 10^{-8}$ cm^2/min torr, which is Krogh's constant of diffusion for rat lung tissue at 30°C (Grote, 1967). The ratio of morphometrically determined D_tO_2 to the physio-

Table 2 Comparison of Morhometrically Determined D_tO_2 with Physiologically Determined DO_2 Values

	D_tO_2 ($ml \cdot min^{-1} \cdot kg^{-1} \cdot torr^{-1}$)	DO_2 ($ml \cdot min^{-1} \cdot kg^{-1} \cdot torr^{-1}$)	D_tO_2/DO_2
Turtle	1.18[a]	0.081[b]	14.6
Monitor	0.86[c]	0.073[d]	11.8
Teju	0.84[c]	0.049[d]	17.1
Dog	24.30[e]	0.96[f]	25.3
Man	9.05[g]	0.36[h]	25.1

[a]Perry (1978) for *Pseudemys scripta*, mean body weight 1.0 kg.
[b]Crawford et al. (1976) for *Pseudemys scripta*, mean body weight 1.5 kg.
[c]Perry (1983) for *Varanus exanthematicus* and *Tupinambis nigropunctatus*. Allometrically adjusted to 2.2 kg.
[d]Glass et al. (1981) for *Varanus exanthematicus* and *Tupinambis nigropunctatus* of 2.2 kg. DO_2 calculated as DCO × 1.23 (Foster, 1964).
[e]Siegwart et al. (1971).
[f]Haab et al. (1964).
[g]Gehr et al. (1981).
[h]Salorinne (1976).
All physiological values are for "resting", not maximally exercising specimens or subjects, because exercising values are not available for these reptiles.
Source: Perry (1983).

logically determined DO_2 is a unitless index of efficiency. Inspection of Table 2 shows these values to lie between 11 and 26.

The physiological measurement of DO_2 is not based upon Equations 1 or 2, because S and τ are physiologically inaccessible quantities. Instead, it is calculated according to Bohr's (1909) relationship:

$$\dot{V}O_2 = D_LO_2 \cdot \Delta\overline{PO}_2 \tag{3}$$

where $\Delta\overline{PO}_2$ is the mean partial pressure difference between "alveolar" air and fully arterialized blood. In reptiles, both of these factors are extremely variable. Most reptiles breathe intermittently (Glass and Wood, 1983), and numerous studies have demonstrated that pulmonary vascular perfusion is also intermittent, decreasing during breathing pauses (Burggren et al., 1977; Burggren and Shelton, 1979; Johansen et al., 1970, 1987; Shelton and Burggren, 1976; White, 1969; White and Ross, 1966). In addition, the degree of intracardiac shunting and, thus, the relative admixture of deoxygenated blood to the pulmonary circuit is also variable (Berger and Heisler, 1977; Mitchell et al., 1981; Shelton and Boutilier, 1982; White, 1976).

One further source of error lies in the fact that DO_2 is rarely determined directly, but rather it is calculated from DCO values. This conversion is open to criticism (Glass et al., 1981). Inspection of Table 2 reveals that as one progresses from reptiles with edicular parenchyma to the teju with faveolar parenchyma, and finally to the bronchoalveolar mammalian lung, the ratio of morphometrically determined D_tO_2 to the physiologically determined DO_2 tends to increase. The DO_2 measurements were obtained in resting animals; in exercising mammals, DO_2 increases by approximately a factor of 2 (Piiper et al., 1969; Turino et al., 1969).

Unfortunately, DO_2 appears not to have been measured in exercising reptiles, but values for the savanna monitor (*Varanus exanthematicus*) at various temperatures (Glass et al., 1981; Glass and Johnson,1982) indicate that DO_2 indeed rises with a thermally induced increase in $\dot{V}O_2$ in this species. Mitchell et al. (1981), however, studying PO_2 (see Eq. 3) in the resting and exercising savanna monitor and green iguana (*Iguana iguana*) have found an increase in the alveolar-arterial PO_2 gradient in both species during exercise.

It is thus possible that the mechanisms of meeting increased metabolic demand imposed by thermal stress involve acceleration of physical and chemical processes involved in Equations 1-3 and are fundamentally different from those regulating the response to isothermic exercise.

B. Oxygen Extraction

A second measure of lung efficiency is the pulmonary air convection requirement ($ACR = \dot{V}I/\dot{V}O_2$), or the more intuitively clear pulmonary oxygen extraction ($EO_2 = 1/CIO_2 \times 1/ACR$). EO_2 multiplied by 100 gives the percentage of EO_2, the percentage of oxygen extracted from inspired air.

It is interesting to note (Fig. 6) that the percentage of EO_2 for four marine and aquatic chelonian species (Glass and Wood, 1983) increases with increasing temperature to approximately 35°C. The terrestrial emydid, *Terrapene ornata*, shows both a low and high temperature maximum. At 30°C the EO_2 percentage values of all tested chelonians lie between approximately 15 and 25%.

Such high oxygen extraction values are unusual, and are matched in non-chelonians only by a 28% extraction in the primitive aquatic snake, *Acrochordis javonicus* (Glass and Johansen, 1976). In general, however, snakes show the lowest oxygen extraction, tending to lie between 6.5% and 10% of inspired oxygen at 30°C (Dean and Gratz, 1983; Dmi'el, 1972), although values as high 20% have been reported for the undisturbed garter snake, *Thamnophis elegans* (Hicks and Riedesel, 1983). Lizards tend to occupy an intermediate position between 10% and 15% oxygen extraction at 30°C (Ackerman and White, 1980; Bennett, 1972, 1973; Giordano and Jackson, 1973), with the lowest resting values near 7% being reported for *Lacerta* (Cragg, 1978a,b).

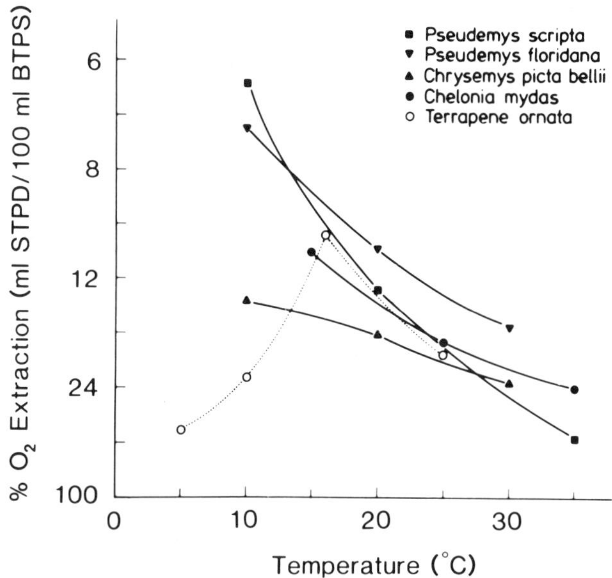

Figure 6 Oxygen extraction in five chelonian species as a function of ambient temperature. Relative hypoventilation at higher temperatures results in a greater oxygen extraction with increasing temperatures in all aquatic and marine species. The terrestrial box turtle (*T. ornata*) shows two extraction maxima. (After Glass and Wood, 1983, courtesy of the American Physiological Society.)

Most investigators report a decrease in Eo_2 percentage after exercise but an increase in Eo_2 percentage with increasing temperature within ecologically relevant bounds (see Hicks and Riedesel, 1983). In pilot experiments in which small numbers of snakes (*Nerodia sipedon*) and lizards (*I. iguana*) were exposed to nearly identical temperature stress and the respiratory values were recorded at various temperatures during the day, one notices a large scatter in breathing pattern and in the Eo_2. With increasing temperature (from 25 to 35°C) the scatter attenuates and Eo_2 percentage tends to increase in the iguana but not in the snake (Figs. 7 and 8).

Oxygen extraction may be related to breath-hold time (long breath holds increase the percentage Eo_2), to lung structure (edicular parenchyma may respond more rapidly to increased ventilation than does faveolar parenchyma), to central blood shunting mechanisms, or to any combination of these factors. To resolve this question, more experiments on minimally disturbed animals are necessary.

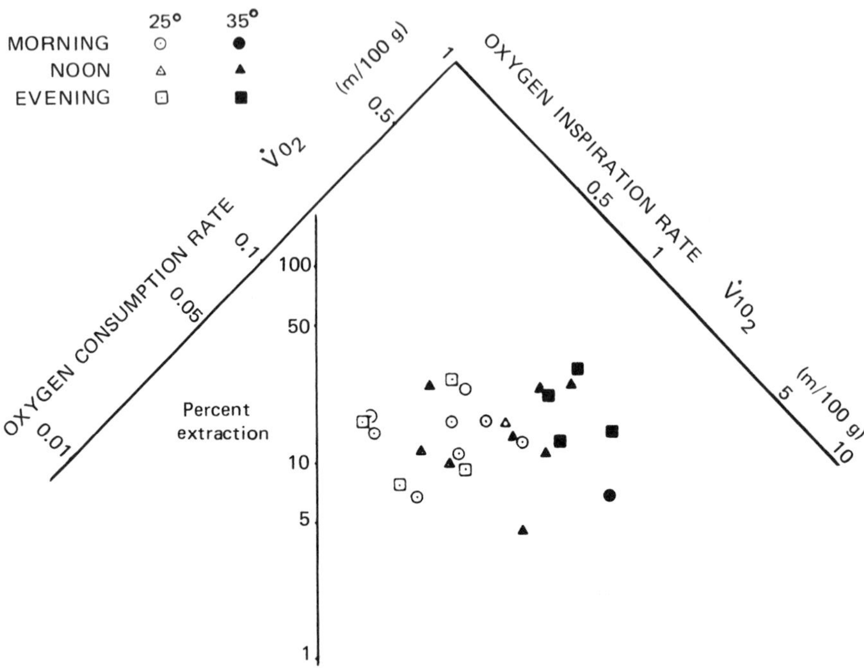

Figure 7 Double-logarithmic plot of $\dot{V}O_2$ and $\dot{V}IO_2$ in the northern water snake (*N. sipedon*). Data points represent individual experiments on four specimens. Each data point can be read off perpendicularly against each of three axes: $\dot{V}O_2$, $\dot{V}IO_2$, and $\dot{V}IO_2/\dot{V}O_2 \times 100 = \%$ extraction. (From S. F. Perry and R. M. Jones, unpublished.)

C. Ventilation-Perfusion Matching

Intuitively, we expect that in a perfectly tuned respiratory system the ventilation of gas exchange surfaces with fresh air and their perfusion with blood would be evenly matched: i.e., $\dot{V}A/\dot{Q}L = 1$, as it is in mammals. In fact, as recent reviews indicate (Glass and Wood, 1983; Shelton et al., 1986), representatives of all major reptilian groups do increase $\dot{V}E$ in response to metabolic stress (see Sect. III.D). Heart rate also increases in response to an exercise-induced increase in metabolic rate: on the average by 25% in lizards, 17% in snakes, and 13% in turtles and *Sphenodon* (Gatten, 1974). The presence of an unknown degree of blood mixing at the heart (Berger and Heisler, 1977; White, 1976) and gas mixing in the central lumen of the lung (Donnelly and Woolcock, 1977; Gratz et al., 1981; Spragg et al., 1980), however, invalidates any attempt to estimate ventilation–perfusion matching in reptiles on the basis of data summaries.

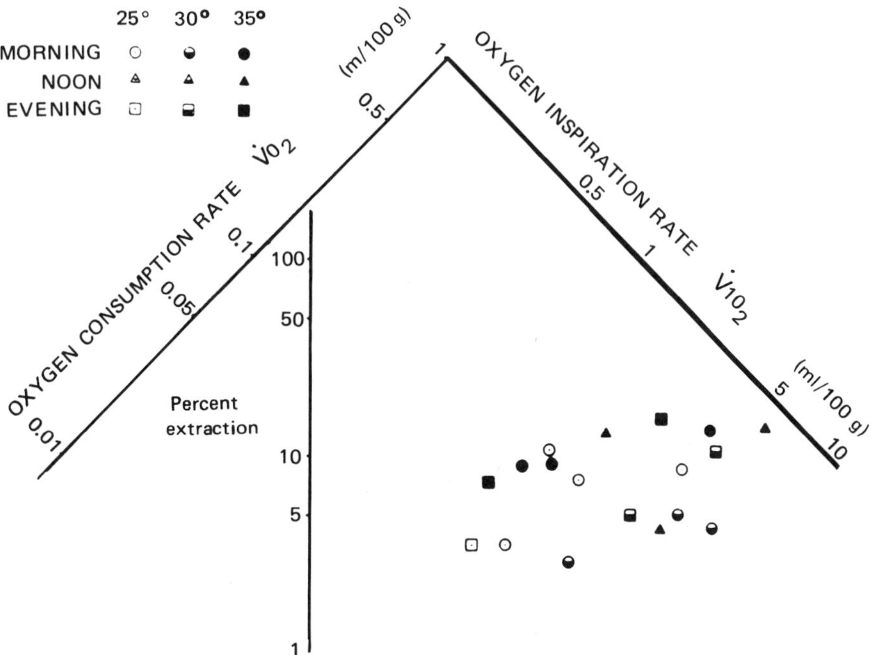

Figure 8 Double-logarithmic plot of $\dot{V}O_2$ and $\dot{V}IO_2$ in the green iguana (*I. iguana*). Data points represent individual experiments on four specimens. Each data point can be read off perpendicularly against three axes, as in Figure 7.

Glass and Wood (1983) conclude that a mammal-like $\dot{V}A/\dot{Q}L$ ratio is obtained only in the savanna monitor (*Varanus exanthematicus*) in which it is 1.2 over a wide temperature range. In the turtle (*Pseudemys floridiana*), unlike the monitor, $\dot{V}A/\dot{Q}L$ is 1.16 at low temperatures (10°C) but decreases to 0.65 at 35°C in keeping with the temperature-dependent increase in EO_2 percentage in this species (see Fig. 6; Kinney et al., 1977). In the anesthetized, artificially ventilated teju lizard (*Tupinambis nigropunctatus*) at 35°C, Hlastala et al. (1985) find ventilation-perfusion ratios ranging from 0.1 to 100, but centered between 5 and 10 (Fig. 9).

One measure of the effectiveness of ventilation-perfusion matching is the mean alveolar-arterial PO_2 gradient $(PA\text{-}Pa)O_2$, abbreviated $\Delta\overline{PO}_2$ in equation 3. In the face of a constant pulmonary diffusing capacity, $\dot{V}O_2$ varies directly with $\Delta\overline{PO}_2$. Thus, on the one hand, the capability of tolerating a large $\Delta\overline{PO}_2$ represents one possibility of supporting an increased $\dot{V}O_2$ in spite of a limited diffusing capacity. On the other hand, the resulting low PaO_2 may not be compatible

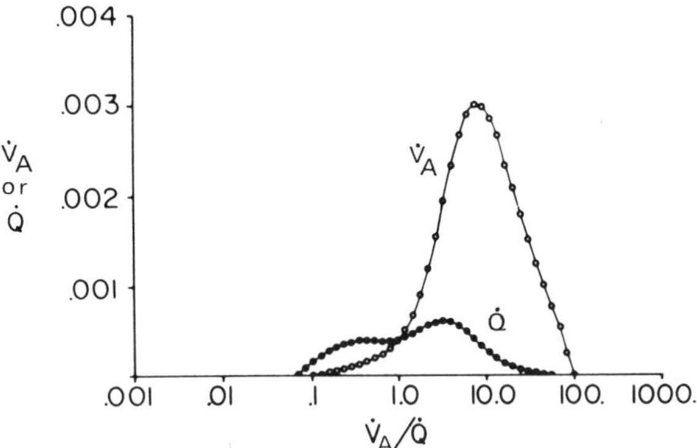

Figure 9 Semilogarithmic plot of faveolar ventilation or perfusion ($\dot{V}_A$ and $\dot{Q}$, respectively) as a function of the ventilation/perfusion ratio in the teju lizard, *Tupinambis nigropunctatus*. Ventilation/perfusion matching ($\dot{V}_A = \dot{Q}$) occurs at relatively low levels of $\dot{V}_A$ or $\dot{Q}$. Relative hypoventilation at very low $\dot{V}_A$ and $\dot{Q}$, and massive hyperventilation at high $\dot{V}_A$ and $\dot{Q}$ may explain poor O_2 extraction after exercise in species with faveolar parenchyma. (From Hlastala et al., 1986.)

with the increased metabolic demands. Certainly the more effective way of meeting increased aerobic demand is to first keep $\Delta\overline{PO_2}$ low, thereby increasing the diffusing capacity, and then to allow $\Delta\overline{PO_2}$ to rise when a further increase in ventilation is not longer feasible (see Chap. 13).

The anesthetized teju at 35°C shows a $\Delta\overline{PO_2}$ of 47.3 torr: a value reached in the green iguana (*I. iguana*) and the savanna monitor (*V. exanthematicus*) only after strenuous treadmill exercise (Hlastala et al., 1985; Mitchell et al., 1981). Resting values for the iguana and monitor are 18.6 and 13.6 torr, respectively (Mitchell et al., 1981). If we keep in mind the parenchymal anatomy of the species concerned, it appears that faveolar parenchyma limits convection, thus resulting in diffusion limitation. Interestingly, Hlastala et al. (1985) were not able to detect gas-phase diffusion limitation in the teju. It is possible that PAO_2 is leveled within the faveoli by a greater degree of oxygen extraction near the faveolar openings, where the convection is greatest. Morphometrically, approximately 60% of the diffusing capacity is located in the upper half of the faveoli. Here, 82% of the faveolar surface area lies over capillaries, as opposed to 77% in the lower half of the faveoli. In addition, the total capillary/faveolar surface area ratio is 10% greater in the upper half of the faveoli, indicating a tendency toward denser packing of capillaries there than in the lower half (Perry, 1983).

In the heterogeneously partitioned, multicameral lungs of the savanna monitor and the red-eared turtle a greater capillary density and thinner air–blood barrier in the regions nearest the intrapulmonary bronchus may also assure that

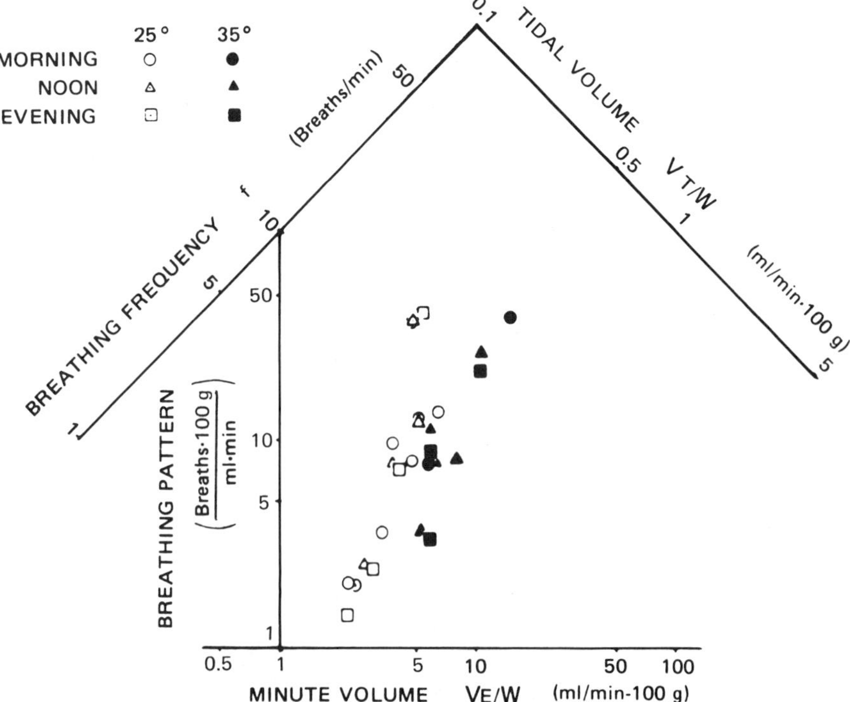

Figure 10 Double-logarithmic plot of breathing frequency (f) and tidal volume (VT) in the northern water snake (*N. sipedon*) at 25°C (open symbols) and 35°C (closed symbols). Data points of Figures 10 and 11 can be read off perpendicularly against each of four axes: f, $\dot{V}_T$, f/$\dot{V}_T$ = breathing pattern, and f x VT = $\dot{V}_E$. (From S. F. Perry and R. M. Jones, unpublished.)

those portions of the lung that are best ventilated also possess the best anatomical prerequisites for tissue-phase diffusion and perfusion (Perry, 1978, 1983). In the turtle, Spragg et al. (1980) have demonstrated by xenon gas resorption that the anatomical prerequisites are also physiologically exploited.

D. Breathing Pattern

Ventilation ($\dot{V}_E$) can be changed by altering breathing frequency (f), tidal volume (V_T) or both:

$$\dot{V}_E = f \cdot V_T \tag{4}$$

Figures 10 and 11 illustrate the interdependence of f and V_T, as well as the large degree of scatter, with no indication of central tendency often encoun-

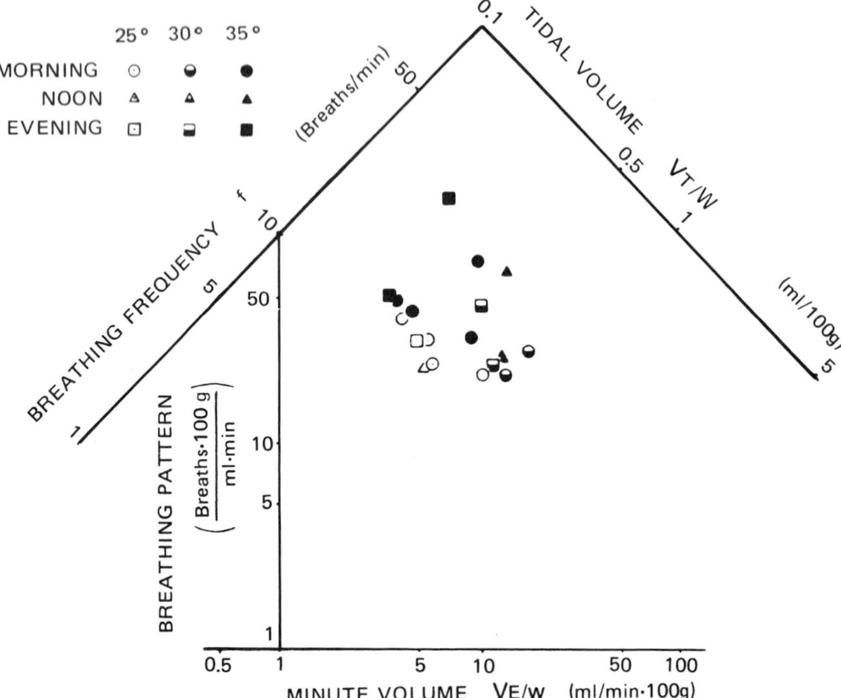

Figure 11 Double-logarithmic plot of breathing frequency (f) and tidal volume (VT) for the green iguana (*I. iguana*) at 25°C (open symbols), 30°C (half-closed symbols), and 35°C (closed symbols. Data points represent individual measurements on four specimens. (From S. F. Perry and R. M. Jones, unpublished.)

tered in measurements of breathing pattern in unrestrained reptiles. For the northern water snake, *Nerodia sipedon*, the index of breathing pattern, f/VT, in animals resting at 25° spans a 30-fold range. The distribution of f values is similar, whereas VT covers a range of only a factof of 2. The index of breathing pattern correlates positively with minute volume. Raising the temperature by 10°C focuses the f and VT within the range of existing values, but the combination of f and VT is such that $\dot{V}$E is increased (Perry and Jones, in preparation).

In the green iguana (*I. iguana*) the index of breathing pattern at 25° and 30°C is less scattered than in the snake, and raising the ambient temperature to 35°C clearly results in a tendency toward rapid, shallow breathing while the $\dot{V}$E remains unchanged.

Thus, it appears that there are species differences both in the degree of control of breathing pattern and in the type of response elicited by thermal stress. Differences in lung architecture and, thus, in a "gas exchange strategy" and blood gas constitution can provide some basis for the interpretation of the preceding data. The "choice" of breathing pattern that results in a particular $\dot{V}_E$, however, is not only a matter of optimization of blood P_{O_2}, P_{CO_2}, and pH. The respiratory muscles must also be considered.

The work of breathing per unit time ($\dot{W}$), also designated " minute work of breathing," increases in direct proportion to f but with the square of V_T.

$$\dot{W} = f/2C \cdot V_T^2 \tag{5}$$

In addition, the compliance of the respiratory system (C) is crucial. In reptiles static compliance is typically consistent over a wide range of volume for a given species (Perry and Duncker, 1980), but the dynamic compliance, particularly of the body wall, decreases with increasing breathing frequency (Milsom, 1984; Milson and Vitalis, 1984).

For mammals, the equivalent of Equation 5 contains two additional factors for airway resistance and plastic deformation. At least in the gecko (*Gekko gecko*) these appear to be insignificant (Milsom, 1984), but in the garter snake (*Thamnophis sirtalis*), extrapulmonary airway resistance may be of some importance (Bartlett et al., 1986).

In the gecko (*G. gecko*), the combination of f and V_T that yields minimum $\dot{W}$, is such that f lies between 30 and 60 breaths per minute (Fig. 12). In resting geckos, however, the overall f lies between 9 and 34 breaths per minute at 24° and 34°C, respectively (Milsom, 1984).

Like most reptiles (see Wood and Lenfant, 1976; Shelton et al., 1986), geckos breathe sporadically. During a breathing episode, f lies near 40 breaths per minute and is independent of temperature. The gecko thus maintains an energetically optimal breathing frequency during breathing episodes and regulates its long-term f by changing the length of the nonrespiratory pauses: 14 s at 24°C; 2 s at 34°C (Milsom, 1984). Experiments such as those just cited for the gecko are necessary in other species. Bartlett et al. (1986), for example, suggest that compliance is so high that it is unimportant in determining breathing pattern in the garter snake.

In response to exercise at a constant temperature, reptiles tend to increase V_T to a greater extent than f. A decrease in f has even been reported in Gould's monitor (*Varanus gouldii*) and the viper (*Vipera palestinae*) following stimulation to movement near preferred body temperatures (Bennett, 1973; Dmi'el, 1972).

Teleologically speaking it makes sense to "choose" an energetically cheap mode of compensation of responding to an environmental stimulus that is likely to elevate the metabolic rate for several hours (e.g., rise in temperature). The selective advantage of the relatively costly increase in V_T, coupled with exercise, is less clear. Strenuous exercise in reptiles is often coupled with fleeing from

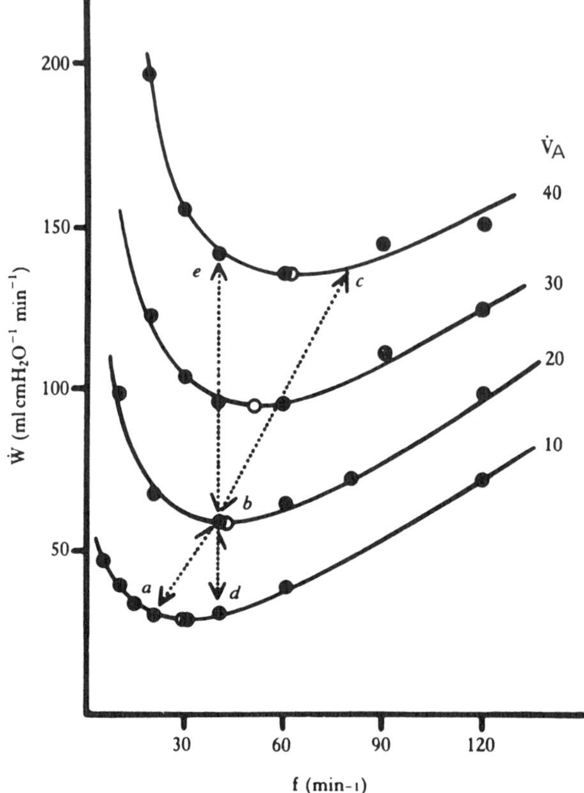

Figure 12 Relationship between minute work of breathing (Ẇ) and breathing frequency (f) at four levels of "alveolar" ventilation (V̇A). V̇A = f (VT – VD, where VD, dead space, is 0.50 ml/100 g. Note that the point of minimum work (open circles) lies between the intersection points of the line of constant frequency (*a b c*) and constant VT (*d b e*) with the experimentally determined work curves. The approximation of minimum work for each curve by maintaining constant VT and varying f is closer than by maintaining constant f and varying VT. (From Milsom and Vitalis, 1984, courtesy of the Company of Biologists.)

danger when energy-saving appears not to be as important as life-saving. In addition, rapid running or crawling, while at the same time trying to maintain a high breathing rate, is not compatible in lizards and snakes. Furthermore, after exercise, minimizing the frequency of flank movements by a low f may decrease the probability of being seen by the pursuer.

Physiologically speaking, the relative increase of VT at the expense of f would be expected to cause effective flushing of the central liminal dead space, and, thereby, ensure a high PO_2 and low PCO_2 in the ventilating air, thus, altering arterial pH. This hypothesis is not born out experimentally, however. Vagotomy, which causes increased VT and decreased f in snakes and turtles (Benchetrit and Dejours, 1980; Gratz, 1984), is not accompanied by any change in the arterial pH.

Changes in temperature and degree of activity are experienced by all reptiles. In contrast, hypercapnia and hypoxia may not be normally experienced except during periods of extended breath holding or confinement. Nevertheless, both stimuli influence the breathing pattern. The responses to either stimulus are varied: exposure to less than 4% CO_2 in inspired air shows nonreproducible, minor changes in breathing pattern. Above 4% inspired CO_2, snakes and lizards show an increased tidal volume and a decreased overall breathing frequency (prolonged breathing pauses), such that $\dot{V}E$ is reduced (Glass and Johansen, 1976; Gratz, 1979; Nielsen, 1961; Templeton and Dawson, 1963). In the turtle *Pseudemys scripta*, breathing carbon dioxide tends to increase both breathing frequency and tidal volume to about the same degree (Burggren et al., 1977; Glass et al., 1978; Jackson et al., 1974), whereas in the closely related *Chrysemys picta*, f increases about twice as much as does VT (Funk and Milsom, 1987; Glass et al., 1985; Milsom and Chan, 1986; Milsom and Jones, 1980; Silver and Jackson, 1985). Breathing frequency is increased primarily by closing the gaps between breathing episodes. The marine green turtle (*Chelonia mydas*), a breath holder by profession, shows an increase only in f in response to 6% inspired carbon dioxide (Jackson et al., 1979).

Short-term hypoxia produces little change in reptilian breathing patterns down to 10% oxygen. Below this level some species (e.g., chelonians, *Chelonia, Pseudemys, Chrysemys*; snake, *Acrochordus*) increase ventilation, others (e.g., turtle, *Chelydra*; lizard, *Dipsosaurus*; snake *Pituophis*) retain resting $\dot{V}E$ levels, whereas the lizards *Lacerta* and *Tarentola* decrease the ventilation rate (Boyer, 1966; Glass et al., 1983; Glass and Johansen, 1976; Jackson, 1973, 1985; Nielson, 1962). In those cases in which the ventilation rate remains unchanged or is reduced, the oxygen consumption rate is also reduced, and it is questionable if this condition can be maintained over the long term. The snake *Nerodia* (*Natrix*) *rhombifera* responds to even low levels of hypoxia, beginning at 15% oxygen, by a reduction in respiratory frequency and an increase in tidal volume, but $\dot{V}E$ remains constant until below 10% oxygen (Gratz, 1979). In *Chrysemys* the increase in $\dot{V}E$ elicited by severe hypoxia (3% O_2) is primarily due to an increase in the number of breaths in an episode, rather than to decreasing the respiratory pause duration as in hypercapnic exposure (Milsom and Chan, 1986).

E. Pulmonary Chemoreceptors and Mechanoreceptors

How does the reptilian brain know that the breathing pattern should be changed? This question is treated in detail in Part V of this volume. Here, we we shall address primarily the morphological side of the receptor question.

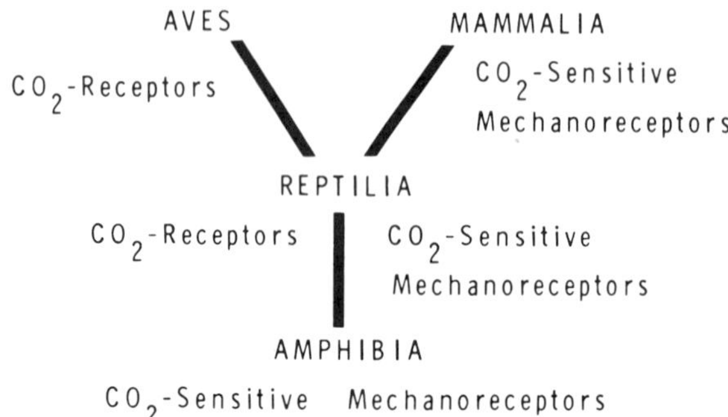

Figure 13 Schematic representation of intrapulmonary receptors in tetrapod lungs. (From Fedde and Kuhlmann, 1978.)

Fedde and Kuhlmann (1978) summarized the state of knowledge 10 years ago as shown in Figure 13. In the meantime, some dust has settled, but the general trends remain. Carbon dioxide-sensitive mechanoreceptors appear to be the stock from which both specific carbon dioxide receptors (in reptiles and birds) and mechanoreceptors, which are not devoid of carbon dioxide receptivity (reptiles and mammals), have been derived. Carbon dioxide-sensitive stretch receptors have been demonstrated in the teju lizard (*Tupinambis nigropunctatus*), in the painted turtle (*Chrysemys picta*), and are suspected in *Chelonia mydas*, the green turtle (Fedde et al., 1977; Gatz et al., 1975; Jackson et al., 1979; Jackson and Prange, 1977; Jones and Milsom, 1979; Milsom and Jones, 1976). In reptiles, both types of receptors appear to elicit the same type of response: sensory inhibition of the ventilatory response (Jones and Milsom, 1982; Milsom and Jones, 1980).

The carbon dioxide-sensitive stretch receptors have been localized to central regions of the intercameral septa in the painted turtle lung and appear to be sparsely distributed over widely separated regions of the lung wall in the unicameral teju lung (Fedde and Kuhlmann, 1978; Jones and Milsom, 1979). Morphologically, neuroepithelial bodies have been localized on the major trabeculae, and dense-core, granule-containing cells have been found in the interedicular septa of the red-eared turtle (*Pseudemys scripta elegans*), which is closely related to the painted turtle (Scheuermann, 1987; Scheuerman et al., 1983). In addition, the later type of endocrinelike cells have also been found in the faveolar walls of the teju lung (Perry and Aumann, 1987), but neuroepithelial bodies appear to be lacking in this species. In snakes and in crocodilians, however, endocrinelike cells are present either isolated or in groups in the trabecular epithelium (Luchtel and Kardong, 1983, shown in Figure but not mentioned in text; Perry, 1988a; Perry, unpublished).

In light of the importance of compliance and tidal volume in the work of breathing in reptiles, it may be significant that the activity of carbon dioxide-modulated *stretch* receptors directly affects the breathing pattern. The effect of lung stretching, of hypoxia, and of hypercapnia on the ultrastructure of neuroepithelial bodies in reptiles should be investigated.

IV. Crocodilian Reptiles

The gas exchange physiology and breathing patterns of many lizards and snakes have been studied (for references see reviews by Bennett, 1982; Bennett and Dawson, 1976; Glass and Wood, 1983; Shelton et al., 1986), and turtles are experiencing a resurgence in interest (Lutz, 1985). Studies on crocodilian respiration, however, remain so scattered and few that this subject deserves special attention here.

Although the general anatomy of crocodilian lungs has been known for 170 years (Meckel, 1818) and physiological studies of crocodilian respiration also date back to the nineteenth century (Krehl and Soetbeer, 1899), there are great gaps in our knowledge of the structure and function of crocodilian lungs. Some recent anatomical studies (Duncker, 1978a,b,c; 1981) provide a functional interpretation of early descriptive works (Broman, 1939; Hesser, 1906; Milani, 1897), whereas other investigations providing some descriptive and quantitative morphological information on crocodilian lungs are available (Perry, 1983; Perry, 1988a,b; Welsch and Müller, 1980b). Thorough morphometric and ultrastructural studies of individual species as well as comparative anatomical studies within the three major crocodilian subgroups (gavials, crocodiles, and alligators/caimans) are lacking.

Respiratory physiological investigations are limited to a small number of studies of, or including, metabolic rates (Anderson, 1961; Benedict, 1932; Buytendikjk, 1910; Boyer, 1966; Brown and Loveridge, 1981; Coulson and Hernandez, 1959, 1979, 1980; Davies, 1978; Krehl and Soetbeer, 1899; Hernandez and Coulson, 1952, 1980; Lewis and Gatten, 1985; Smith, 1975) and the control and nature of the breathing cycle (Davies et al., 1982; Gans and Clark, 1976; Gaunt and Gans, 1969; Glass and Johansen, 1979; Huggins et al., 1969; Naifeh et al., 1970a,b, 1971a,b,c). In addition, a number of papers concerning a special biochemical aspects of crocodilian metabolism as well as respiratory and acid-base status of crocodilian blood have been published. For entrance into this literature see Coulsen and Hernandez (1983) and Weber and White (1986).

Morphologically, the respiratory system of crocodilians is unique among reptiles in a number of ways. Not only are crocodilians the only reptiles to possess a total of intracardiac separation of systemic and pulmonary circulation (connected at the base of the pulmonary trunk and the left aorta by the foramen of Panizza; White, 1976), they also possess closed pleural cavities (Broman,

1904; Duncker, 1978a). In addition, special derivatives of the body wall musculature (Duncker, 1978c) form the longitudinally oriented diaphragmaticus muscle, which pulls the lungs and the fully encapsulated liver caudally during inspiration (Gans and Gaunt, 1976). Rib movement can, but must not, be involved in breathing.

Crocodilian lungs are tiny by reptilian standards. For submerged *Crocodylus porosus* the lung volume obeys the relationship $V_L = 0.0895\ W^{0.906}$. Thus a 1-kg specimen has a lung volume of only 46.8 ml, or similar to that of the loggerhead turtle, *Caretta caretta* (Milsom and Johansen, 1975), and approximately half that of a diving red-eared turtle (*Pseudemys scripta elegans*) or sea snake (*Pelamis platurus*) (Jackson, 1969, 1971; Graham et al., 1975; Wright and Kirschner, 1987). Anatomically, the lungs of crocodiles, caimans, and alligators (Duncker, 1978a; Milani, 1897; Perry, 1988b) demonstrate the most complicated, multicameral structure of any reptile. Three rows of arching tubular or sacular chambers radiate from the dorsal, lateral, and ventral aspects of the interpulmonary bronchus along the cranial half of its course. The intrapulmonary bronchus then loses its cartilage reinforcement and gives rise to a large number of primarily fingerlike chambers before ending in a terminal sac. Perforations allow extrabronchial communication particularly within chambers, but also between chambers (Perry, 1988b).

In contrast to their complicated primary structure, crocodilian lungs display a poorly specialized, edicular parenchyma with a low surface/volume ratio. The effective respiratory surface area in Nile crocodiles of approximately 4-kg body weight is only 700 cm^2/kg (Perry, 1988a), or 14% of that estimated by Marcus (1928) for an American alligator in the same weight range (Bennett and Dawson, 1976). By using the measured harmonic mean barrier thickness of 1.3 μm (Perry, 1987b), the morphometric diffusing capacity of the Nile crocodile is calculated at approximately one order of magnitude below that of a lizard or snake corrected allometically to the same weight range. These morphometric results are keeping with an oxygen consumption rate for Nile crocodiles of approximately 4 kg of 20% of the allometically adjusted $\dot{V}O_2$ for lizards at the same temperature (Bennett and Dawson, 1976; Brown and Loveridge, 1981), as well as with high PO_2 values in expired air of the Nile crocodile, ranging from 110 to 130 torr (Glass and Johansen, 1979), which imply a low gas exchange efficiency.

The allometrically corrected resting oxygen consumption in the alligator (*Alligator mississippiensis*), however, is some three times greater than that of the Nile crocodile and is not significantly lower than that of an equivalent lizard at the same temperature (Bennett and Dawson, 1976; Lewis and Gatten, 1985). Recent morphometric studies have not been conducted for the alligator, but Marcus (1928) estimates the pulmonary surface area of a 3.75-kg alligator to be 5000 cm^2/kg. Assuming the same capillary density as in the crocodile, the alligator would have an effective respiratory surface area of 2500 cm^2/kg, or 3.5 times that of the crocodile.

The alligator extracts 11% of the inspired oxygen at 15°C and 16% at 35°C (Davies et al., 1982). This efficiency drops drastically during carbon dioxide inhalation, the degree of this response being greater at lower temperatures. A similar increase in oxygen extraction with increasing temperature in the turtle *Chrysemys picta* has been explained as a temperature-dependent, relative hypoventilation (Funk and Milsom, 1987). In the turtle, however, the absolute effect of carbon dioxide is greater at high temperatures, but when corrected for the increased metabolic rate at high temperatures, remains constant.

The breathing cycle in crocodiles, alligators, and caimans consists typically of a series of breaths followed by a breathing pause, which varies from several minutes at low temperature to a few seconds at high temperature (Davies et al., 1982; Glass and Johnasen, 1979; Naifeh et al., 1970a). Bilateral vagotomy or medullar transection anterior to the nucleus laminaris causes an increase in tidal volume but does not abolish the episodal breathing pattern. Transection of the brain stem caudal to the nucleus laminaris, however, abolishes all breathing efforts (Naifeh et al., 1971a). Thus, breathing pattern appears to be established centrally. Within the lungs, isolated, innervated, endocrinelike cells are present within the trabecular epithelium (Perry, 1988b). More research is necessary to elucidate the role of central and peripheral mechanisms in controlling breathing pattern as well as the putative relationship of breathing pattern to the pH/pOH ratio in blood plasma in crocodilians.

V. Summary and Prognosis

Scattered descriptive morphological studies, morphometric data from three species of lizards, and one species each of snakes, turtles, and crocodiles, combined with physiological data concerning pulmonary diffusing capacity, oxygen consumption rate, oxygen extraction, and breathing patterns present an enticing but incomplete picture of respiration in reptiles. In recent years, some promising areas have crystallized out, in which concentrated effort could bring important advances, not only in the field of reptilian respiratory physiology, but also in respiratory physiology as a whole. These are (1) comparison of morphometrically and physiologically measured diffusing capacity; (2) study of gas exchange strategies: i.e., the correlation between the parenchymal structure and mechanism of ventilation of respiratory surfaces; (3) ventilation-perfusion matching; (4) dynamics of lung movement, including the structure and function of pulmonary smooth muscle; (5) control of breathing pattern; (6) pre- and posthatching lung development and the control of fluid excretion from the lung.

The latter field, especially, is in urgent need of reinvestigation. But all of these areas present a challenge for a multidisciplinary approach in which morphology, morphometry, developmental biology, physiology, and ecology, all play a part. In particular, in light of tightened animal protection and animal experimentation laws, as well as budgetary restrictions (which often channel work with "exotic" animals to low priority), innovative simple and effective noninvasive methods for measuring undisturbed reptiles (e.g., Bennett and Nagy, 1977; Porcell and Gonzalez, 1986) are urgently needed. In this way, the focus could be shifted from few measurements on many specimens to multiple measurements on few animals. Because lung morphometry can be performed on small sample sizes, the way would be opened to a new generation of multidisciplinary studies with a focus on case studies.

Particularly in the study of reptiles, the importance of the individual should not be forgotten. Although detailed study of a single individual cannot necessarily be generalized to this whole group, there is growing evidence that the group "reptile" is fictitious in any event. Although spoken 175 years ago, the following statement of Cuvier (1812) has lost none of its poignance: "Every [organism] is organized as a unit: a unique, closed system in which each of its parts corresponds mutually to one another."

Acknowledgments

The author gratefully acknowledges the patient and skillful assistance of Ms. Allena McSkimming in preparation of the manuscript as well as the critical review of the manuscript by Dr. J. E. Maloney.

References

Ackerman, R. A., and White, F. N. (1980). The effects of temperature on acid-base balance and ventilation of the marine iguana. *Respir. Physiol. 39*: 1337-147.

Anderson, H. T. (1961). Physiological adjustments to prolonged diving in the American alligator, *Alligator mississippiensis. Acta Physiol. Scand. 53*:23-25.

Ax, P. (1984). *Das Phylogenetische System*. Stuttgart, New York, G. Fischer.

Bartels, H., and Welsch U. (1983). Freeze fracture study of the turtle lung. I. Intercellular junctions in the air-blood barrier of *Pseudemys scripta. Cell Tissue Res. 231*:157-172.

Bartels, H., and Welsch, U. (1984). Freeze-fracture study of the turtle lung. 2. Rod-shaped particles in the plasma membrane of a mitochondria-rich pneumocyte in *Pseudemys (Chrysemys) scripta. Cell Tissue Res. 236*: 453-457.

Bartlett, D., Mortola, J. P., and Doll, E. J. (1986). Respiratory mechanics and control of the ventilatory cycle in the garter snake. *Respir. Physiol. 64*:13-27. 13-27.

Becker, H., Perry, S. F., and Böhme, W. (1988). Die Morphologie der Lungen der Gattung *Varanus* Merrum 1827 (Sauria: Varanidae) und ihre Bedentung für die Systematik der Varanidae. *Bonn. Zool. Beitr.* (in press).

Benchetrit, G., and Dejours, P. (1980). Ventilatory CO_2 drive in the tortoise, *Testudo horsfieldi. J. Exp. Biol. 87*:229-236.

Benedict, F. G. (1932). *The Physiology of Large Reptiles*. Washington, Carnegie Institution.

Bennett, A. F. (1982). The energetics of reptilian activity. In *Biology of the Reptilia*, Vol. 13, Physiology D, Physiological Ecology. Edited by C. Gans and F. H. Pugh. New York, Academic Press, pp. 155-199.

Bennett, A. F. (1972). The effect of activity on oxygen consumption, oxygen debt, and heart rate in the lizards *Varanus gouldii* and *Sauromalus hispidus. J. Comp. Physiol. 79*:259-280.

Bennett, A. F. (1973). Ventilation of two species of lizards during rest and activity. *Comp. Biochem. Physiol. 46A*:653-671.

Bennett, A. F., and Dawson, W. R. (1976). Metabolism. In *Biology of the Reptilia*. Vol. 5. Edited by C. Gans and W. R. Dawson. New York, Academic Press, pp. 127-223.

Bennett, A. F., and Nagy, K. (1977). Energy expenditure in free ranging lizards. *Ecology 58*:697-703.

Berger, P. J. (1973). Autonomic innervation of the visceral and vascular smooth muscle of the lizard lung. *Comp. Gen. Pharmacol. 4(13)*:1-10.

Berger, P. J., and Heisler, N. (1977). Estimation of shunting, systemic and pulmonary output of the heart, and regional blood flow distribution in unanaesthetized lizards (*Varanus exanthematicus*) by injection of radioactively labelled microspheres. *J. Exp. Biol. 71*:111-121.

Bohr, C. (1909). Über die spezifische Tätigkeit der Lungen bei der respiratorischen Gasaufnahme und ihr Verhalten zu der durch die Alveolenwand stattfindenden Gas-diffusion. *Skand. Arch. Physiol. 22*:221-280.

Boyer, D. R. (1966). Comparative effects of hypoxia on respiratory and cardiac function in reptiles. *Physiol. Zool. 39*:307-316.

Broer, W., and Horn, H.-G. (1985). Erfahrungen bei Verwendung eines Motorbruters zu Zeitigung von Reptilieneiern. *Salamandra 21*:304-310.

Broman, I. (1904). Die Entwicklungsgeschichte der Bursa omentalis und ähnlicher Recessusbildungen, *Entwicklungsgesch. Monogr.*, Wiesbaden.

Broman, I. (1937). Coelom. In *Handbuch der vergleichenden Anatomie der Wirbeltiere*. Vol. 3. Edited by L. Bolk, E. Göppert, E. Kallius, and W. Lubosch. Berlin, Urban and Schwarzenberg, pp. 989-1018.

Broman, I. (1938). Die Lehre von der "zentripetalen Lungenentwicklung"– eine wirklichkeitsfremde Spekulation. *Anat. Anz. 86*:225-226.

Broman, I. (1939a). Die Embryonalentwicklung der Lungen bei Krokodilen und Seeschildkröten. *Jahrb. Morphol. Mikrosk. Anat. 84*:244-306.

Broman, I. (1939b). Über die Embryonalentwicklung der Lungen bei den Sumpfschildkröten. *Jarhb. Morph. Mikrosk. Anat. 84*:541-584.

Broman, I. (1942). Über die Embryonalentwicklung der Chamaleonlunge. *Gegenbaurs Morphol. Jahrb. 87*:490-5324.

Brown, C. R., and Loveridge, J. P. (1981). The effect temperature on oxygen consumption and evaporative water loss in *Crocodylus niloticus. Comp. Bioch. Physiol. 69A*:51-57.

Burnstock, G., and Wood, M. J. (1967). Innervation of the lungs of the sleepy lizard (*Trachysaurus rugosus*). II. Physiology and pharmacology. *Comp. Biochem. Physiol. 22*:814-831.

Burggren, W. W. (1982). Pulmonary blood plasma filtration in reptiles: A "wet" vertebrate lung? *Science 215*:77-78.

Burggren, W. W., Glass, M., and Johnasen, K. (1977). Pulmonary ventilation: Perfusion relationships in terrestrial and aquatic chelonian reptiles. *Can. J. Zool. 55*:2024-2034.

Burggren, W. W., and Shelton, G. (1979). Gas exchange and transport during intermittent breathing in chelonian reptiles. *J. Exp. Biol. 82*:75-92.

Burri, P., and Weibel, E. R. (1971). Morphometric estimation of pulmonary diffusion capacity. II. Effect of PO_2 on the growing lung. Adaptation of the growing rat lung to hypoxia and hyperoxia. *Respir. Physiol. 11*:247-264.

Buytendijk, F. J. J. (1910). About exchange of gases in cold-blooded animals in connection with their size. *Proc. Sect. Sci. R. Acad. Sci. (Amsterdam) 13*: 48-53.

Campbell, G., and Duxson, M. J. (1978). The sympathetic innervation of lung muscle in the toad (*Bufo marinus*): A revision and an explanation. *Comp. Biochem. Physiol. 60C*:65-73.

Campiche, M. (1960). Les inclusions lamellaiares des cellules alveolaires dans le poumon du raton. Relations entre l'ultrastructure et la fixation. *J. Ultrastruct. Res. 3*:302-312.

Coulson, R. A., and Hernandez, T. (1959). Source and function of urinary ammonia in the alligator. *Am. J. Physiol. 197*:873-879.

Coulson, R. A., and Hernandez, T. (1979). Increase in metabolic rate of the alligator fed proteins or amino acids. *J. Nutr. 109*:538-550.

Coulson, R. A., and Hernandez, T. (1980). Oxygen debt in reptiles: Relationship between the time required for repayment and metabolic rate. *Comp. Biochem. Physiol. 65A*:453-457.

Coulson, R. A., and Hernandez, T. (1983). Alligator metabolism. Studies on chemical reactions in vivo. *Comp. Biochem. Physiol. 74B*:1-182.

Cragg, P. (1975). Respiration and Body Weight in the Reptilian Genus, *Lacerta*: A Physiological, Anatomical and Morphometric Study. Ph.D. thesis, Bristol University.

Cragg, P. (1978a). Oxygen consumption in the lizard genus *Lacerta* in relation to diel variation, maximum activity and body weight. *J. Exp. Biol. 77*:33-56.

Cragg, P. (1978b). Ventilatory patterns and variables in rest and activity in the lizard, *Lacerta. Comp. Biochem. Physiol. 60A*:399-410.

Crawford, E. C. Jr., Gatz, R. N., Magnussen, H., Perry, S. F., and Piiper, J. (1976). Lung volumes, pulmonary blood flow and carbon monoxide diffusing capacity of turtles. *J. Comp. Physiol. 107*:169-178.

Cuvier, G. (1812). Recherches sur les ossements fossiles de quadrupèdes. Paris, Deterville.

Davies, D. G., Thomas, J. L., and Smith, E. N. (1982). Effect of body temperature on ventilatory control in the alligator. *J. Appl. Physiol. Respir. Environ. Exercise Physiol. 52*:114-118.

Dean, J. B., and Gratz, R. K. (1983). The effect of body temperature and CO_2 breathing on ventilation and acid-base status in the northern water snake *Nerodia spiedon. Physiol. Zool. 56*:290-301.

Dmi'el, R. (1972). Effect of activity and temperature on metabolism and water loss in snakes. *Am. J. Physiol. 223*:510-516.

Donnelly, P. M., and Woolcock, A. J. (1977). Ventilation and gas exchange in the carpet python, *Morelia spilotes variegata. J. Comp. Physiol. 122*:403-418.

Dubach, M. B. (1980). Quantitative Analyse des Atemapparates von Haussperling, Wellensittich und Veilchenohrkolibri. Ph.D. dissertation, University of Zurich.

Dufaure, J. P., and J. Hubert. (1961). Table de développement du lézard vivipare: *Lacerta* (Zootoca) *vivipara*. Jacquin. *Arch. Anat. Microsc. Morphol. Exp. 50*:309-328.

Duncker, H.-R. (1978a). Coelom-gliederung der Wirbeltiere–funktionelle Aspekte. *Verh. Anat. Ges. 72*:91-112.

Duncker, H.-R. (1978b). General morphological principles of amniotic lungs. In *Respiratory Function in Birds, Adult and Embryonic*. Edited by J. Piiper. Heidelberg, Springer-Verlag, pp. 2-15.

Duncker, H.-R. (1978c). Funktionsmorphologie des Atemapparates und Coelomgliederung bei Reptilien, Vögeln und Säugern. *Verh. Dtsch. Zool. Ges. 1978*:99-132.

Duncker, H.-R. (1981). Stammesgeschichte der Struktur- und Fuktionsprinzipien der Wirbeltierlungen. *Verh. Anat. Ges. 75*:279-303.

Engel, S. (1962). *Lung Structure*. Springfield, Ill., C. C. Thomas, pp. 243-271.

Fedde, M. R., Kuhlmann, W. D., and Scheid, P. (1977). Intrapulmonary receptors in the tegu lizard. I. Sensitivity to CO_2. *Respir. Physiol. 29*:35-48.

Fedde, M. R., and Kuhlmann, W. D. (1978). Intrapulmonary carbon dioxide sensitive receptors: Amphibians to mammals. In *Respiratory Function in Birds, Adult and Embryonic*. Edited by J. Piiper, Heidelberg, Springer-Verlag, pp. 33-50.

Fitch, H. S. (1970). Reproductive cycles of lizards and snakes. *Univ. Kans. Publ. Mus. Nat. Hist. 52*:1-247.

Funk, G. D., and Milsom, W. K. (1987). Changes in ventilation and breathing pattern produced by changing body temperature and inspired CO_2 concentration in turtles. *Respir. Physiol. 67*:37-51.

Gans, C., Billett, F., and Maderson, P. (1985). *Biology of the Reptilia*. Vol. 14. Development. New York, John Wiley & Sons.

Gans, C., and Clark, B. (1976). Studies on ventilation of *Caiman crocodilus. Respir. Physiol. 26*:285-301.

Gaunt, A. S., and Gans, C. (1969). Diving bradycardia and withdrawal bradycardia in *Caiman crocodilus. Nature 223*:207-208.

Gaunt, A. S., and Gans, C. (1969). Mechanics of respiration in the snapping turtle, *Chelydra serpentina* (Linne). *J. Morphol. 128*:195-228.

Gehr, P., Mwangi, D. K., Ammann, A., Maloiy, G. M. O., Taylor, C. R., and Weibel, E. R. (1981). Design of the mammalian respiratory system. V. Scaling morphometric pulmonary diffusing capacity to body mass: Wild and domestic mammals. *Respir. Physiol. 44*:61-86.

Giordano, R. V., and Jackson, D. C. (1973). The effect of temperature on ventilation in the green iguana (*Iguana iguana*). *Comp. Biochem. Physiol. A45*:235-238.

Gatten, R. E., Jr. (1974). Percentage contribution of increased heart rate to increased oxygen transport during activity in *Pseudemys scripta, Terrapene ornata* and othe reptiles. *Comp. Biochem. Physiol. 48A*:649-652.

Gatz, R. N., Fedde, M. R., and Crawford, E. C. (1975). Lizard lungs: CO_2 receptors in *Tupinambis nigropunctatus. Experienta 31*:455-456.

Glass, M. L., Boutilier, R. G., and Heisler, N. (1985). Effects of body temperature on respiration, blood gases and acid-base status in the turtle *Chrysemys picta bellii. J. Exp. Biol. 114*:37-51.

Glass, M. L., Boutilier, R. G., and Heisler, N. (1983). Ventilatory control of arterial Po_2 in the turtle *Chrysems picta bellii*: Effects of temperature and hypoxia. *J. Comp. Physiol. 151*:145-153.

Glass, M. L., Burggren, W. W., and Johnasen, K. (1978). Ventilation in an aquatic and in a terrestrial chelonian reptile. *J. Exp. Biol. 72*:165-179.

Glass, M. L., and Johansen, K. (1979). Periodic breathing in the crocodile *Crocodylus niloticus*: Consequences for the gas exchange ratio and control of breathing. *J. Exp. Zool. 208*:379-326.

Glass, M. L., and Johansen, K. (1982). Pulmonary oxygen diffusing capacity of the lizard *Tupinambis teguixin. J. Exp. Zool. 249*:385-388.

Glass, M., and Johansen, K. (1976). Control of breathing in *Acrochordus javanicus*, an aquatic snake. *Physiol. Zool. 49*:328-340.

Glass, M. L., Johansen, K., and Abe, A. S. (1981). Pulmonary diffusing capacity in reptiles (relations to temperature and O_2-uptake). *J. Comp. Physiol. 211*:1-6.

Glass, M. L., and Wood, S. C. (1983). Gas exchange and control of breathing in reptiles. *Physiol. Rev. 63*:232-259.

Goodrich, E. S. (1930). *Studies on the Structure and Development of Vertebrates*. London, Macmillan.

Graham, J. B., Gee, J. H., and Robison, F. S. (1975). Hydrostatic and gas exchange functions of the lung of the sea snake *Pelamis platurus. Comp. Biochem. Physiol. A50*:477-482.

Gratz, R. K. (1984). Effect of bilateral vagotomy on the ventilatory responses of the water snake. *Am. J. Physiol. 246*:R221-227.

Gratz, R. K. (1979). Ventilatory response of the diamondback water snake, *Natrix rhombifera*, to hypoxia, hypercapnia and oxygen demand. *J. Comp. Physiol. 129*:105-110.

Gratz, R. K., Ar, A., and Geiser, J. (1981). Gas tension profile of the lung of the viper, *Vipera xanthina palestinae. Respir. Physiol. 44*:165-176.

Grote, J. (1967). Die Sauerstoffdiffusionskonstanten im Lungengewebe und Wasser und ihre Temperaturabhängigkeit. *Pflügers Arch. 295*:245-254.

Hernandez, T., and Coulson, R. A. (1952). Hibernation in the alligator. *Proc. Soc. Exp. Biol. Med. 79*:145-149.

Hernandez, G., and Coulson, R. A. (1980). Anaerobic glycolysis and replacement of oxygen debt in the alligator. *Comp. Biochem. Physiol. 67A*:283-286.

Hesser, C. (1906). Über die Entwicklung der Reptilienlunge. *Anat. Hefte 29*: 277-308.

Hicks, J. W., and Riedesel, M. L. (1983). Diurnal ventilatory patterns in the garter snake, *Thamnophis elegans. J. Comp. Physiol. 149*:503-510.

Hilber, H. (1933). Der formative Einfluss der Luft auf die Atemorgane. (Vergleichende Untersuchung über Bau und Entwicklung von Reptilien-und Säugerlungen). *Morphol. Jahrb. 71*:184-265.

Hlastala, M. P., Standaert, T. A., Pierson, D. J., and Luchtel, D. L. (1985). The matching of ventilation and perfusion in the lung of the tegu lizard, *Tupinambis nigropunctatus. Respir. Physiol. 60*:277-294.

Hochstetter, F. (1909). Beiträge zur Entwicklungsgeschichte der europäischen Sumpfschildkröte (*Emys lutaria* Marsili). 2. Die ersten Entwicklungsstadien der Lungen und die Bildung der sogenannten Nebengekröse. *Denkschr. Akad. Wiss. 84*:111-159.

Holder, L. A., and Bellairs, A. d'A. (1962). The use of reptiles in experimental embryology. *Br. J. Herpetol. 3*:54-61.

Huggins, S. E., Hoff, H. E., and Pena, R. V. (1969). Heart and respiratory rates in crocodilian reptiles under conditions of minimal stimulation. *Physiol. Zool. 42*:320-333.

Hughes, G. M. (1977). Dimensions and the respiration of lower vertebrates. In *Scale Effects in Animal Locomotion*. Edited by P. J. Pedley. New York, Academic Press, pp. 57-81.

Hughes, G. M. (1978). A morphological and ultrastructural comparison of some vertebrate lungs. In *XIX Morphological Congress Symposia*. Edited by E. Klika. Prague, Charles University, pp. 393-405.

Jackson, D. C. (1969). Buoyancy control in the freshwater turtle, *Pseudemys scripta elegans. Science 166*:1649-1657.

Jackson, D. C. (1971). Mechanical basis for lung volume variability in the turtle *Pseudemys scripta elegans. Am. J. Physiol. 220*:754-758.

Jackson, D. C. (1973). Ventilatory response to hypoxia in turtles at various temeratures. *Respir. Physiol. 18*:178-187.

Jackson, D. C. (1985). Respiration and respiratory control in the green turtle *Chelonia mydas. Copeia* 664-671.

Jackson, D. C., Kraus, D. R., and Prange, H. D. (1979). Ventilatory response to inspired CO_2 in the sea turtle: Effects of body size and temperature. *Respir. Physiol. 38*:71-81.

Jackson, D. C., Palmer, S. E., and Meadow, W. L. (1974). The effects of temperatures and carbon dioxide breathing on ventilation and acid-base status of turtles. *Respir. Physiol. 20*:131-146.

Jackson, D. C., and Prange, H. D. (1979). Ventilation and gas exchange during rest and exercise in adult green sea turtles. *J. Comp. Physiol. 134*:315-319.

Johansen, K., Abe, A. S., and Andresen, J. H. (1987). Intracardiac shunting revealed by angiocardiography in the lizard, *Tupinambis teguixin. J. Exp. Biol. 130*:1-12.

Johansen, K., Lenfant, C., and Hanson, D. (1970). Phylogenetic development of pulmonary circulation. *Fed. Proc. Biol. 29*:1124-1129.

Jones, D. R., and Milsom, W. K. (1979). Functional characteristics of slowly adapting pulmonary stretch receptors in the turtle (*Chrysemys picta*). *J. Physiol (Lond.) 291*:37-49.

Jones, D. R., and Milsom, W. K. (1982). Peripheral receptors affecting breathing and cardiovascular function in non-mammalian vertebrates. *J. Exp. Biol. 100*:59-91.

Kilburn, K. H. (1969). Alveolar clearance of particles. A bullfrog lung model. *Arch. Environ. Health 18*:556-63.

Kinney, J. L., Matsuura, D. T., and White, F. N. (1977). Cardiorespiratory effects of temperature in the turtle, *Pseudemys floridana. Respir. Physiol. 31*:309-325.

Klemm, R. D., Gatz, R. N., Westfall, J. A., and Fedde, M. R. (1979). Microanatomy of the lung parenchyma of a tegu lizard, *Tupinambis nigropunctantus. J. Morphol. 161*:257-280.

Klaver, C. J. J. (1973). Lung anatomy: Aid in chameleon taxonomy. *Beaufortia 269*:155-177.

Klaver, C. J. J. (1977). Comparative lung morphology in the genus *Chamaeleo* Laurenti, 1768 (Sauria: Chamaeleonidae) with a discussion of taxonimic and zoogeographic implications. *Beaufortia 327*:167-199.

Klaver, C. (1979). A review of *Brookesia* systematics with a special reference to lung-morphology (Reptilia: Sauria:Chamaeleonidae). *Bonn. Zool. Beitr. 30*:162-175.

Klaver, C. (1980). Lung-morphology in the Chamaeleonidae (Sauria) and its bearing upon phylogeny, systematics and zoogeography. *Z. Zool. Syst. Eveolutionsforsch. 19*:36-58.

Krehl, L., and Soetbeer, F. (1899). Untersuchungen über die Wärmeökonomie der poikilothermen Wirbelthiere. *Pflügers Arch. Gesamte Physiol. 77*: 611-638.

Legler, J. M. (1956). A simple and practical method of artificially incubating reptile eggs. *Herpetologica 12*:290.

Lewis,L. Y., and Gatten, R. E. (1985). Aerobic metabolism of American alligators, *Alligator mississippiensis*, under standard conditions and during voluntary activity. *Comp. Biochem. Physiol. 80A*:441-447.

Luchtel, D. L., and Kardong, K. V. (1981). Ultrastructure of the lung of the rattlesnake, *Crotalus viridis oreganus. J. Morphol. 169*:29-47.

Lutcavage, M., Baier, H., and Lutz, P. L. (1985). Pulmonary gas transport in the loggerhead sea turtle. *Physiologist 28*:283 (abstr.).

Lutz, P. (1985). The regulatory biology of sea turtles. *Copeia 1985*:662-663.

Marcus, H. (1928). Lungenstudie V. Vergleichende Untersuchung über die respiratorische Oberfläche und ihr Verhältnis zum Körpergewicht. *Morphol. Jahrb. 59*:561-566.

Marcus, H. (1937). Lungen. In *Handbuch der vergleichenden Anatomie der Wirbeltiere, III*. Edited by L. Bolk, E. Goppert, E. Kallius, and W. Lubosch. Berlin, Urban and Schwarzenberg, pp. 909-988.

Meban, C. (1977). Ultrastructure of the respiratory epithelium in the lungs of the tortoise, *Testudo graeca. Cell Tissue Res. 181*:267-275.

Meban, C. (1978a). Functional anatomy of the lungs of the greeen lizard, *Lacerta viridis. J. Anat. 125*:421-431.

Meban, C. (1978b). The respiratory epithelium in the lungs of the slow-worm, *Anguis fragilis. Cell Tissue Res. 190*:337-347.

Meckel, J. F. (1818). Ueber das Respirationssystem der Reptilien. *Arch. Physiol. 4*:60-69.

Milani, A. (1894). Beiträge zur Kenntnis der Reptilienlunge. I. Lacertilia. *Zool. Jahrb, Abt. Anat. Ont. 7*:545-592.

Milani, A. (1897). Beiträge zur Kenntnis der Reptilienlunge. II. *Zool. Jahrb. Abt. Anat. Ont. 10*:93-153.

Miller, W. S. (1904). The development of the lung of *Chrysemys picta. Am. J. Anat. 3*:15-16.

Milsom, W. K. (1984). The interrelationship between pulmonary mechanics and spontaneous breathing in the tokay lizard, *Gekko gecko*. *J. Exp. Biol.* *113*:203-214.

Milsom, W. K., and Chan, P. (1986). The relationship between lung volume, respiratory drive and breathing pattern in the turtle, *Chrysemys picta*. *J. Exp. Biol.* *120*:233-247.

Milsom, W. K., and Johansen, K. (1975). The effect of buoyancy induced lung volume changes on respiratory frequency in a chelonian (*Caretta caretta*). *J. Comp. Physiol.* *98*:157-160.

Milsom, W. K., and Jones, D. R. (1976). Are reptilian pulmonary receptors mechano- or chemoreceptive? *Nature* *261*:327-328.

Milsom, W. K., and Jones, D. R. (1980). The role of vagal afferent information and hypercapnia in control of breathing pattern in chelonia. *J. Exp. Biol.* *87*:53-63.

Milsom, W. K., and Vitalis, T. Z. (1984). Pulmonary mechanics and work of breathing in the lizard *Gekko gecko*. *J. Exp. Biol.* *113*:187-202.

Mitchell, G. S., Gleeson, T. T., and Bennett, A. F. (1981). Pulmonary oxygen transport during activity in lizards. *Respir. Physiol.* *43*:365-375.

Moser, F. (1902). Beiträge zur vergleichenden Entwicklungsgeschichte der Wirbeltierlunge. (Ampibien, Reptilien, Vögel, Säuger). *Arch. Mikrosk. Anat. Entw.* *60*:587-668.

Naifeh, K. H., Huggins, S. E., and Hoff, H. E. (1970). The nature of the ventilatory period in crocodilian respiration. *Respir. Physiol.* *10*:338-348.

Naifeh, K. H., Huggins, S. E., and Hoff, H. E. (1971). The nature of the nonventilatory period in crocodilian respiration. *Respir. Physiol.* *11*:178-185.

Naifeh, K. H., Huggins, S. E., and Hoff, H. E. (1971). Study of the control of crocodilian respiration by anesthetic dissection. *Respir. Physiol.* *13*:186-197.

Naifeh, K. H., Huggins, S. E., and Hoff, H. E. (1971). Effects of brain stem section on respiratory patterns of crocodilian reptiles. *Respir. Physiol.* *13*: 186-197.

Naifeh, K. H., Huggins, S. E., Hoff, H. E., Hugg, T. W., and Norton, R. E. (1970). Respiratory patterns in crocodilian reptiles. *Respir. Physiol.* *9*:31-42.

New, D. A. T. (1966). *The Culture of Vertebrate Embryos*. London, Academic Press, pp. 99-118.

Nielsen, B. (1961). On the regulation of respiration in reptiles. I. The effect of temperature and CO_2 on the respiration of lizards (*Lacerta*). *J. Exp. Biol.* *38*:301-314.

Nielsen, B. (1962). On the regulation of respiration in reptiles. II. The effect of hypoxia with and without moderate hypercapnia on the respiration and metabolism of lizards. *J. Exp. Biol.* *39*:107-117.

Ogawa, C. (1920). Contributions to the histology of the respiratory spaces of the vertebrate lungs. *Am. J. Anat.* *27*:333-393.

Pasteels, J. (1957). Une table analytique du developpement des reptiles. I. Stades de gastrulation chez les cheloniens et les lacertiliens. *Ann. Soc. R. Zool. Belg. 87*:217-241.

Perry, S. F. (1978). Quantitative anatomy of the lungs of the red-eared turtle, *Pseudemys scripta elegans. Respir. Physiol. 35*:245-262.

Perry, S. F. (1983). Reptilian lungs. Functional anatomy and evolution. *Adv. Anat. Embryol. Cell Biol. 79*:1-81.

Perry, S. F. (1988a). Functional morphology of the lungs of the Nile crocodile. *Crocodylus niloticus* (Laurenti). Nonrespiratory paremters. *J. Exp. Biol. 134*:99-117.

Perry, S. F. (1988b). Quantitative morphology of the crocodile lung. *Fortschr. Zool.* (in press).

Perry, S. F. (1988c). Mainstreams in the evolution of vertebrate respiratory structures. In *Form and Function in Birds*. Edited by A. S. King and J. McLelland. Vol. 4, Ch. 1. London, Academic Press.

Perry, S. F., and Duncker, H.-R. (1980). Interrelationship of static mechanical factors and anatomical structure in lung evolution. *J. Comp. Physiol. 138*: 321-334.

Perry, S. F., and Duncker, H.-R. (1978). Lung architecture, volume and static mechanics in five species of lizards. *Respir. Physiol. 34*:61-81.

Perry, S. F., and Jones, R. M. (in preparation). Effect of ambient temperature on breathing pattern in the green iguana, *Iguana iguana*, and the northern water snake, *Nerodia spiedon*.

Perry, S. F., Aumann, U., and Maloney, J. E. (1988a). Intrinsic lung musculature and associated ganglion cells in a teiid lizard, *Tupinambis nigropunctatus* Spix. *Herpetologica* (in press).

Petrik, P. (1967). The ultrastructure of the chicken lung in the final stages of embryonic development. *Folia Morphol. 15*:176-186.

Piiper, J., Huch, A., Kötter, D., and Herbst, R. (1969). Pulmonary diffusing capacity at basal and increased O_2 uptake levels in anesthetized dogs. *Respir. Physiol. 6*:219-232.

Pohunkova, H. (1978). Ultrastructure and cytochemistry of respiratory epithelium of amphibians and reptiles. In *XIX Morphological Congress Symposia*. Edited by E. Klika. Prague, Charles University, pp. 407-415.

Pohunkova, H., and Hughes, G. M. (1985). Ultrastructure of the lungs of the garter snake. *Folia Morphol. 33*:254-258.

Porcell, L. de V., and Gonzales, J. G. (1986). Effect of body temperature on the ventilatory responses in the lizard *Gallotia galloti. Respir. Physiol. 65*:29-37.

Porter, K. R. (1972). *Herpetology*. Philadelphia, W. B. Saunders.

Reese, A. M. (1915). The development of the lungs of the alligator. *Smithson. Misc. Collect. 65*(2):1-11.

Romer, A. S. (1966). *Vertebrate Paleontology*, 3rd ed. Chicago, University of Chicago Press.

Scheuermann, D. W. (1987). Morphology and cytochemistry of the endocrine epithelial system in the lung. *Int. Rev. Cytol. 106*:35-88.

Scheuermann, D. W., de-Groodt-Lasseel, M. H. A., Stilman, C., and Meisters, M. L. (1983). A correlative light-, fluorescence- and electron-microscopic study of neuroepithelial bodies in the lung of the red-eared turtle, *Pseudemys scripta elegans. Cell Tissue Res. 234*:249-269.

Scheuermann, D. W., de Groodt-Lasseel, M. H. A., and Stilman, C. (1984). A light and fluorescence cytochemical and electron microscopic study of granule-containing cells in the intrapulmonary ganglia of *Pseudemys scripta elegans. Am. J. Anat. 171*:377-399.

Schulze, F. E. (1871). Die Lungen. In *Strickers Handbuch der Lehre von den Geweben*, Vol. I. Leipzig, pp. 480-484.

Shelton, G., and Burggren, W. (1976). Cardiovascular dynamics of the chelonia during apnoea and lung ventilation. *J. Exp. Biol. 64*:323-343.

Shelton, G., Jones, D. R., and Milsom, W. K. (1986). Control of breathing in ectothermic vertebrates. In *Handbook of Physiology*. Sect. 3. The Respiratory System, Vol. 2. Control of Breathing. Part 2. Edtied by A. P. Fishman, N. S. Cherniac, J. G. Widdicombe, and S. R. Geiger. Washington, American Physiological Society, pp. 857-909.

Smith, E. N. (1975). Oxygen consumption, ventilation and oxygen pulse of the American alligator during heating and cooling. *Physiol. Zool. 48*:326-327.

Silver, R. B., and Jackson, D. C. (1985). Ventilatory and acid-base responses to long-term hypercapnia in the freshwater turtle, *Chrysemys picta bellii. J. Exp. Biol. 114*:662-672.

Spragg, R. G., Ackermann, R., and White, F. N. (1980). Distribution of ventilation in the turtle *Pseudemys scripta. Respir. Physiol. 42*:73-86.

Stinner, J. N. (1982). Functional anatomy of the lung of the snake, *Pituophis melanoleucus. Am. J. Physiol. 243*:R251-R257.

Taylor, C. R., Karas, R. H., Weibel, E. R., and Hoppeler, H. (1987). Adaptive variation in the mammalian respiratory system in relation to energetic demand. *Respir. Physiol. 69*:1-127.

Templeton, J. R., and Dawson, W. R. (1963). Respiration in the lizard *Crotaphytus collaris. Physiol. Zool. 36*:104-121.

Turino, G. M., Bergofsky, E. H., Goldring, R. M., and Fishman, A. P. (1969). Effect of exercise on pulmonary diffusing capacity. *J. Appl. Physiol. 18*: 447-456.

Ultsch, G. R., and Jackson, D. C. (1982). Long-term submergence at 3°C of the turtle, *Chrysemys picta bellii*, in normoxic and severely hypoxic water. I. Survival, gas exchange and acid-base status. *J. Exp. Biol. 96*:11-28.

Weber, R. E., and White, F. N. (1986). Oxygen binding in alligator blood related to temperature, diving, and "alkaline tide." *Am. J. Physiol. 251* (Regulatory Comp. Physiol. *20*:R901-908.

Weibel, E. R. (1984). *The Pathway for Oxygen. Structure and Function in the Mammalian Respiratory System*. Cambridge, Mass., Harvard University Press.

Weibel, E. R., and Taylor, C. R. (1981). The design of the mammalian respiratory system. *Respir. Physiol. 44*:1-164.

Welsch, U. (1979). *Die Stellung der Reptilienlunge in der Phyogenese nach licht- und elektronen-mikroskopischen Untersuchungen am Alveolarepithel, am Bindegewebe und an der Innervation*. Inauguraldissertation zur Erlangung der Doktorwurde der Med. Fakultat der Universitat Kiel.

Welsch, U., and Müller, W. (1980a). Elektronenmikroskopische Beobachtungen zur Innervation der Reptilienlunge. *Z. Mikrosk. Anat. Forsch. (Lepiz.) 94*: 435-444.

Welsch, U., and Müller, W. (1980b). Feinstrukturelle Beobachtungen am Alveolarepithel von Reptilien unterschiedlicher Lebensweise. *Z. Mikrosk. Anat. Forsch. (Leipz.) 94*:479-503.

Werner, F. (1912). Beiträge zur Anatomie Seltener Reptilien mit besonderer Berüchsichtigung der Atmungsorgane. *Arb. Zool. Inst. Wien. 19*:373-424.

White, F. N. (1976). Circulation. In *Biology of the Reptilia*, V. Physiology A. Edited by C. Gans and W. R. Dawson. New York, Academic Press, pp. 275-334.

White, F. N. (1969). Redistribution of cardiac output in the diving alligator. *Copeia 1969*:567-570.

White, F. N., and Ross, G. (1966). Circulatory changes during diving in the turtle. *Am. J. Physiol. 211*:15-18.

Wolf, S. (1933). Zur Kenntnis von Bau and Funktion der Reptilienlunge. *Zool. Jahrb. Abt. Anat. Ont. 57*:139-190.

Wood, S. C., and Lenfant, C. (eds.) (1979). *Evolution of Respiratory Processes. A Comparative Approach*. New York, Marcel Dekker.

Wood, S. C., and Lenfant, C. (1976). Respiration: Mechanics, control and gas exchange. In *Biology of the Reptilia*. V. Physiology. Edited by A. C. Gans and W. R. Dawson. New York, Academic Press, pp. 225-274.

Wood, S. C., Johansen, K., and Gatz, R. K. (1977). Pulmonary blood flow, ventilation/perfusion ratio, and oxygen transport in a varanid lizard. *Am. J. Physiol. 233*:R89-R93.

Wood, S. C., Johansen, K., Glass, M. L., and Maloiy, G. M. O. (1978). Aerobic metabolism of the lizard *Varanus exanthematicus*: Effects of activity, temperature and size. *J. Comp. Physiol. 127*:331-336.

Wright, J. C., and Kirschner, D. S. (1987). Allometry of lung volume during voluntary submergence in the saltwater crocodile *Crocodylus porosus. J. Exp. Biol. 130*:433-436.

Yntema, C. L. (1968). A series of stages in the embryonic development of *Chelydra serpentina. J. Morphol. 125*:219-252.

Zehr, D. R. (1962). Stages in the normal development of the common garter snake, *Thamnophis sirtalis sirtalis. Copeia 1962*:322-329.

References Added in Proof

Pastor, L. M., Ballesta, J., Hernandez, F., Perez-Tomas, R., Zuasti, A., and Ferrer, C. (1987). A microscopic study of the tracheal epithelium of *Testudo graeca* and *Pseudemys scripta elegans. J. Anat. 153*:171-183.

Perry, S. F., Bauer, A. M., Russell, A. P., Alston, J. T., and Maloney, J. E. (1988b). The lungs of the gecko *Rhacodactylus leachianus* (Reptilia: Gekkonidae): a correlative gross anatomical, light- and electron microscopic study. *J. Morphol.* (in press).

Tesik, I. (1984). The ultrastructure of the tracheal epithelium in European common lizard (*Lacerta agilis* L.) and in sand lizard (*Lacerta vivipara* Jacq.). *Anat. Anzeiger 155*:329-340.

8

Lung Structure and Function
Birds

FRANK L. POWELL

University of California at San Diego
La Jolla, California

I. Introduction

The structure of the avian respiratory system suggests a very efficient model of gas exchange (reviewed by Powell and Scheid, 1988). Birds have nine large air sacs that function primarily as bellows to ventilate the lungs where most gas exchange occurs. Gas exchange occurs in parabronchi, which are open-ended, tube-like structures that do not change volume. They are ventilated in a flow-through manner and perfused with mixed venous blood along their entire length by the pulmonary circulation. Thus, ventilation and pulmonary blood flow can be considered as occurring perpendicular to one another, and avian gas exchange can be described by a crosscurrent model. The efficacy of crosscurrent gas exchange is potentially greater than cocurrent (or alveolar) gas exchange, but less than countercurrent gas exchange (see Chap. 13).

In ideal crosscurrent gas exchange, arterial PO_2 is predicted to be greater than expired PO_2 and arterial PCO_2 is predicted to be less than expired PCO_2. Such observations have been made for CO_2 in birds under a variety of conditions but is seldom reported for O_2, except in extreme hypoxia (Powell and Scheid, 1988). Factors that limit avian gas exchange from achieving ideal crosscurrent levels include ventilatory and perfusive shunts, functional inhomogeneities, and diffusion resistances. Recent advances in our understanding of the physiology of these limitations and progress toward a quantitative explanation of pulmonary O_2 and CO_2 exchange in birds are reviewed in this chapter.

II. Dead Space Ventilation

A. Background

A quantitative description of gas exchange in birds requires a measure of the effective ventilation of the lung. By analogy with alveolar ventilation ($\dot{V}_A$) in mammals, this will be referred to as parabronchial ventilation ($\dot{V}_P$) and it differs from total inspired or expired ventilation ($\dot{V}_I$ or $\dot{V}_E$) because of the dead space ventilation ($\dot{V}_D$). The $\dot{V}_D$ in birds not only includes ventilation of upper airways but may result from ventilatory shunts in which airflow may bypass the parabronchi. Scheid and Piiper (1988) recently reviewed the current literature and concluded that ventilatory shunts do not occur in resting birds (Fig. 1). However recent studies (Hastings and Powell, 1986) suggest that this pattern may not always apply and that some expiratory gas from caudal air sacs may flow directly out the primary bronchus. Also, inspriatory gas may enter cranial secondary bronchi (medioventrales) and the cranial air sacs directly from the primary bronchus (see Fig. 1). Both of these shunts involve a breakdown in the aerodynamic valving mechanism that rectifies flow in the avian lung. Also, there is recent evidence (Hempleman and Powell, 1985) suggesting that both inspiratory and expiratory flows are not caudal to cranial (i.e., unidirectional) in all paleopulmonic parabronchi. However, this topic is better considered as functional inhomogeneity in a later section (see under Sect. IV.C).

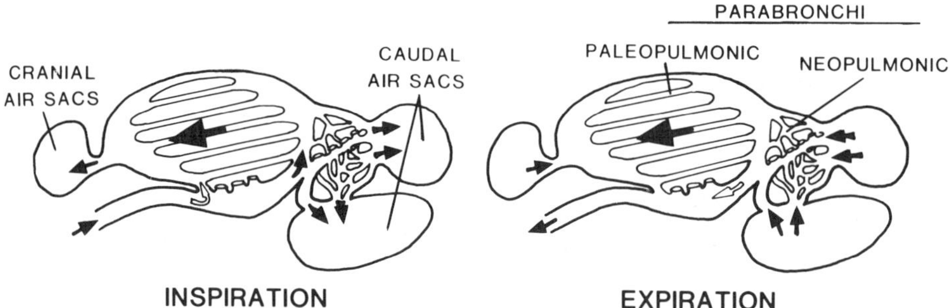

Figure 1 Pathways of airflow in the avian respiratory system during inspiration and expiration. Filled arrows show the generally accepted pathway and open arrows show possible ventilatory shunts. The expiratory shunt is referred to as the mesobronchial shunt.

B. Measures of Dead Space

Anatomical Dead Space Volume

With tidal ventilation, the volume of the airways proximal to gas exchange sites will always be dead space. Such dead space is termed *serial* or *anatomical* dead space. Hinds and Calder (1971) measured tracheal volume on 27 species of birds and found in situ volume (ml) was related to body mass (kg) as:

$$\text{Vtr} = 3.7\ M_b^{1.09}$$

This equation is reasonably accurate for most, but not all commonly studied birds. It underestimates measured values of the anatomical dead space volume (VDa) in Pekin ducks (Bech et al., 1984; Hastings and Powell, 1986a) and domestic pigeons (Hinds and Calder, 1971) by $\leq$ 20% However, it overestimates VDa in domestic fowl (Hinds and Calder, 1971) by as much as 100% Thus, VDa should be measured or allometric predictions confirmed on the species in question for quantitative studies of gas exchange.

Unfortunately, the usual physiological method for measuring anatomic dead space, the Fowler method, is not always valid in birds (cf. Hastings and Powell, 1986b). This technique analyzes a CO_2 expirogram (a plot of expired P_{CO_2} versus cumulative expired volume) assuming that the terminal plateau of the expirogram is only gas expired from the lung. In anesthetized, artificially ventilated ducks there is evidence against the terminal plateau being pure end-parabronchial gas (Hastings and Powell, 1986b). This results in the Fowler VDa changing with tidal volume, which is inconsistent with the rigid upper airways of birds. Thus, use of the Fowler technique to estimate VDa is not justified in birds (unless assumptions can be validated under the specific conditions being studied), and morphometric measurements are the only current means of accurately measuring VDa.

Physiological Dead Space Volume

Physiological dead space volume ($V_{D_{phys}}$) includes VDa and dead space within the lung, known as parabronchial dead space (VDP) in birds (Scheid and Piiper, 1987). The $V_{D_{phys}}$ is an "as if" volume calculated by assuming the bird lung consists of an ideal (i.e., no diffusion limitations, homogeneous) crosscurrent gas exchange compartment and a ventilated unperfused dead space compartment. In terms of flow (volumes times respiratory frequency), $\dot{V}_{D_{phys}}$ is the difference between measured expired ventilation ($\dot{V}_E$) and ventilation of the ideal parabronchial compartment ($\dot{V}_P$):

$$\dot{V}_{D_{phys}} = \dot{V}_E - \dot{V}_P$$

The $\dot{V}_P$ is calculated assuming that mixed-expired P_{CO_2} ($P_{\bar{E}CO_2}$) is a flow-weighted average from dead space P_{CO_2} and the ideal compartment P_{CO_2} (P_{EiCO_2}). If $P_{ICO_2} = 0$. then:

$$\dot{V}P/\dot{V}E = 1 - ((PEiCO_2 - P\bar{E}CO_2)/PEiCO_2)$$

The $P\bar{E}CO_2$ is measured and $PEiCO_2$ is determined from a crosscurrent O_2-CO_2 diagram (Fig. 2).

Although the Bohr equation, substituting end-expired PCO_2 for $PEiCO_2$, and the Enghoff modification of the equation, substituting arterial PCO_2 for $PEiCO_2$, are frequently used to estimate VD_{phys} in mammals, they are not applicable to birds. Figure 2 shows that arterial blood and end-parabronchial gas are not in equilibrium in crosscurrent lungs, and VD_{phys} that is calculated from the Enghoff modification underestimates true VD_{phys} (cf. Hastings and Powell, 1986a). Also, end-expired and end-parabronchial PCO_2 are not always in equilibrium for reasons to be discussed under Section II. The calculation of VD_{phys} for birds, therefore, is not simple. It requires knowledge of O_2 and CO_2 blood equilibrium curves and a quantitative–usually computer–model of crosscurrent gas exchange. However, the only experimental measurements necessary to calculate VD_{phys} are ventilation, mixed venous blood, and mixed expired gas, which can be made under relatively normal conditions on awake animals.

In anesthetized, artifically ventilated Pekin ducks (3.14-kg body mass), VD_{phys} averaged 46.5 ml compared with an anatomic plus instrument dead space of 36.6 ml (Hastings and Powell, 1986a). This additional 9.9 ml of dead

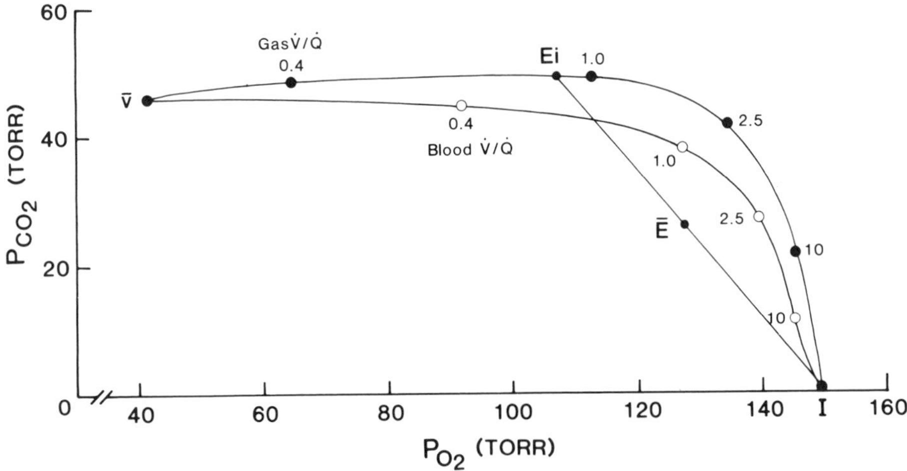

Figure 2 Crosscurrent O_2–CO_2 diagram showing the separate blood and gas $\dot{V}/\dot{Q}$ lines running between the mixed venous ($\bar{v}$) and inspired (I) points. Arterial blood and expired gas are not in equilibrium for most $\dot{V}/\dot{Q}$. Ei and E represent ideal and mixed expired gas points, respectively. The line connecting measured PI and $P\bar{E}$ points intersects the modeled gas $\dot{V}/\dot{Q}$ line at PEi.

space, V_{DP}, is not necessarily an actual ventilated unperfused volume in the lung but, rather, a measure of nonideal CO_2 elimination, including functional inhomogeneities and ventilatory shunts. To put the magnitude of these limitations in perspective, consider that the natural V_{Da} (i.e., without instrument dead space) in these ducks was only 15 ml. In other words, limitations resulting in V_{DP} are two-thirds as large as the limitations from rebreathing anatomical dead space and, therefore, are very significant.

C. Ventilatory Shunts

Mesobronchial Shunt Flow

Most of the gas expired from caudal air sacs passes through the parabronchi contributing to $\dot{V}_P$ (see Fig. 1). However, the mechanisms directing flow through the parabronchi may not always be 100% effective, and some gas may be shunted past exchange tissue through the mesobronchus (mesobranchial shunt flow; $\dot{V}_M$). Studies on ducks with flow probes showed that during panting there was a "small" expiratory flow in the mesobronchus (Bretz and Schmidt-Nielsen, 1971). Unfortunately the methods used were not quantitative but it has been generally assumed that mesobronchial shunting is not significant.

Measurements of P_{O_2} and P_{CO_2} with a low-suction rate mass spectrometer in the lungs of spontaneously breathing, anesthetized ducks revealed that end-expired P_{CO_2} was less than end-parabronchial P_{CO_2} (Powell et al., 1981). These results were consistent with a mesobronchial shunt equaling 12% of expiratory flow ($\dot{V}_M/\dot{V}_E = 0.12$). That same paper analyzed earlier studies in the literature and found evidence for a $\dot{V}_M/\dot{V}_E$ equaling 10 to 25% in domestic fowl. However, these calculations of $\dot{V}_M/\dot{V}_E$ apply to only the *end* of expiration. Also, they assume the shunt source P_{CO_2} is equal to caudal air sac or caudal secondary bronchial (mediodorsales) P_{CO_2}; if shunt P_{CO_2} is actually greater, the mesobronchial shunt fraction is underestimated, and vice versa.

A more recent study of anesthetized, artificially ventilated ducks indicates the mesobronchial shunt fraction may be much greater than previously estimated, especially at the beginning of expiration (Hastings and Powell, 1986b). Here V_M/V_T was calculated by rearranging a mixing equation describing $P\bar{E}_{CO_2}$ as a flow-weighted average of end-parabronchial P_{CO_2} (Pe_{CO_2}) and shunt P_{CO_2} (Ps_{CO_2}). If $P_{ICO_2} = 0$:

$$V_T \cdot P\bar{E}_{CO_2} = (V_T - V_{Da} - V_M) \cdot Pe_{CO_2} + V_M \cdot Ps_{CO_2}$$

Maximal expired P_{CO_2} and estimates of caudal air sac P_{CO_2} were used for Pe_{CO_2} and Ps_{CO_2}, respectively. Table 1 summarizes the changes in V_M with changes in V_T and the method of artifical ventilation. The effect of V_T on V_M was different with the two methods of artificial ventilation; V_M increased with V_T when the Harvard respirator was used, but it was constant, with changing V_T when the constant-flow ventilator was used. The difference in mesobronchial

Table 1 Effect of Tidal Volume (V_T) and Method of Artificial Ventilation on Mesobronchial Shunt (V_M) in Anesthetized Ducks[a]

	V_T	V_M	V_T	V_M
Harvard respirator	83.4 ±3.4 (8)	18.6 ±5.2 (5)	173.3 ±14.3 (8)	41.0 ±5.2 (8)
Constant-flow ventilator	103.2 ±7.2 (10)	19.2 ±4.8 (8)	212.7 ±11.7 (10)	22.1 ±2.1 (10)

[a]Values in ml ± S.E.M. n (in parentheses) is less for V_M than for V_T if V_M was calculated to be < 0 ml.

shunting resulting from the method of artificial ventilation probably represents the sensitivity of shunts to expiratory flow *rate* pattern.

It was possible to analyze constant-flow ventilator data for temporal changes in $\dot{V}_M/\dot{V}_E$. The CO_2 expirograms were distorted and terminal plateaus were not usually found, except at high tidal volumes. The results were best explained by a variable mesobronchial shunt, which may cause a temporal functional inhomogeneity (see under Sect. IV.C). The $\dot{V}_M$ was estimated as 75 to 100% of $\dot{V}_E$ at the start of expiration and decreased to 0% near the midpoint of expiration with a large V_T and the constant-flow ventilator (see Fig. 4 in Hastings and Powell, 1986b). This temporal pattern of $\dot{V}_M$ is qualitatively consistent with theoretical predictions (see under Sect. II.C).

The magnitude of $\dot{V}_M$ estimated by Hastings and Powell (1986b) was considerable. Because the mode of ventilation was unnatural and $\dot{V}_M$ was sensitive to the method of ventilation, experiments should be repeated on spontaneously breathing birds under different conditions. In addition to CO_2 expirograms, necessary measurements include estimates of V_{Da}, P_{eCO_2}, and P_{SCO_2}; cranial and caudal air sac P_{CO_2} would be good measures of P_{eCO_2} and P_{SCO_2}, respectively.

Aerodynamic Valving

Aerodynamic valving is the mechanism that determines airflow patterns in the avian lung (reviewed by Scheid and Piiper, 1987). If aerodynamic valving "fails," then there can be a ventilatory shunt. For example, inspiratory aerodynamic valve failure at the cranial secondary bronchial (medioventrales) openings into the primary bronchus results in fresh air entering cranial air sacs as a shunt (see Fig. 1). It is only recently that a quantitative theory of aerodynamic valving in avian lungs has been developed and tested experimentally (Banzett et al., 1987; Barnas et al., 1985).

Simply stated, the theory predicts that aerodynamic valving is sensitive to gas density and velocity. Airflow with sufficient momentum will follow the "valved" pathway. Momentum was experimentally decreased both by substituting 80% helium:20% O_2 for 80% argon:20% O_2 and decreasing respiratory frequency at constant VT in anesthetized geese. Tracer gas measurements indicated that the inspiratory aerodynamic valve failed at least partially at all flows with the He:O_2 mixture and failed only partially at long respiratory periods with Ar:O_2. The expiratory aerodynamic valve has not yet been studied from this viewpoint.

The physiological significance of these results deserves further investigation. The change in gas density with He:O_2 is comparable to ascending to an altitude near the summit of Mount Everest. More modest changes in density corresponding to more common altitudes of bird flight would also be of interest. Studying the effects of flow by different breathing patterns, not just different breathing rates, would also be of interest. For example, one could ask if gas velocity could be maintained sufficiently in panting to preserve valving or if accelerative forces become limiting.

D. Physiological Changes

The possibility of ventilatory shunts in birds has led to much speculation about their role in ventilatory adjustments to activity and the environment. However, there have been few studies in which changes in the ventilatory flow pattern can be conclusively demonstrated. Direct measurements of flow pattern do show changes with panting (see Scheid and Piiper, 1988), and VM has been shown to change with the method of artificial ventilation, as noted earlier. Studies focusing on extraction of blood gases or oxygen are often suggestive but, usually, are not conclusive on their own.

Bech et al. (1984) calculated parabronchial O_2 extraction for thermoneutral and cold ducks as:

$$EPO_2 = (\dot{V}O_2 \cdot 100)/\dot{V}P \cdot 0.2095)$$

where VP was estimated from the difference between VT and VDa measured morphometrically. Cold exposure (-20°C) increased O_2 consumption 42%, and EPO_2 increased from 31 to 41%. The investigators calculated that 79% of this change must be a change in parabronchial O_2 extraction and the remainder could be explained by changes in ventilation frequency–tidal volume relationships. One possible explanation of increased EPO_2 is a decreased ventilatory shunt, but changes in lung-diffusing capacity, with the reported increased cardiac output, or the effects of ventilation–perfusion mismatch, with reported changes in mixed venous blood gases, could also be involved. Similar qualifications apply to other studies of E_{O_2} in birds (e.g., Bouverot et al., 1974, 1979; Brent et al., 1983, 1984; Bucher, 1985).

One of the most convincing arguments for a change in aerodynamic valving and ventilatory shunting is the ostrich during thermal panting. Schmidt-Nielsen et al. (1969) first noted the constancy of arterial P_{CO_2} in these birds during heat stress; this contrasted with the hypocapnia found in most panting birds (Calder and Schmidt-Nielsen, 1968). Jones (1982) studied the distribution of pulmonary blood flow with microspheres in thermoneutral and heat-stressed ostriches and concluded that changes in the distributions were not sufficient to explain Pa_{CO_2} homeostasis when air sac ventilation increased 16-fold. He concluded that a change in ventilatory shunting was the most likely explanation.

Comparisons of arterial blood gases and ventilation in ducks exposed to hypobaric and isobaric hypoxia indicate that hypobaria may increase ventilatory shunting, consistent with theoretical predictions of the effect of gas density in aerodynamic valving (see under Sect. II.C). Powell et al. (1986) showed that ventilation was significantly greater in ducks exposed to simulated altitudes of 7750 m in a hypobaric chamber compared with the same level of hypoxia induced by lowering F_{IO_2} at sea level. However, Pa_{O_2} and Pa_{CO_2} were not significantly different, and the results cannot be explained by changes in frequency–tidal volume relationships. Because cardiac output and pulmonary blood flow distribution are not expected to be affected by barometric pressure and because expected changes in diffusion limitations are only consistent with larger changes in ventilatory shunts, these experiments are strong evidence that ventilatory shunts are sensitive to altitude. However, direct measurement of V_M or inspiratory valve failure should be made to resolve this issue.

III. Blood Flow Shunts

Shunts of pulmonary blood flow past effective gas exchange tissue in avian lungs are very small. Abdalla and King (1976) found no evidence for pulmonary arteriovenous anastomoses in chickens using 10- to 33-μm diameter spores and microspheres. Inert gas studies measured perfusion of unventilated gas exchange tissue in the lungs of anesthetized pump-ventilated geese at less than 1% of the cardiac output (Powell and Wagner, 1982b). Burger et al. (1979) found that venous admixtures equaled 2.7% of cardiac output in anesthetized, unidirectionally ventilated ducks but, as discussed later, this may include extrapulmonary shunts.

Bickler et al. (1986) compared shunts measured in anesthetized, pump-ventilated ducks by inert gas and O_2 methods. Extrapulmonary shunts, such as bronchial or thebesian venous drainage into pulmonary venous blood, reduce Pa_{O_2} just as does an intrapulmonary shunt. Hence, an O_2 shunt that is calculated from the difference in arterial and predicted end-capillary O_2 content during 100% O_2 breathing includes intrapulmonary and extrapulmonary shunts. By contrast, inert gases are not metabolized by bronchial or cardiac tissues, thus inert gases measure only an intrapulmonary shunt. Inert gas shunts average 1.3% of cardiac output, whereas an O_2 shunt averaged 6.3 to 8%. This indicates an extrapulmonary shunt of at least 5%, which is larger than expected. A possible explanation is the vertebral venous-pulmonary circulatory connections, which have been described for chickens by Burger and Estavillo (1977) and which apparently also exist in ducks (Bickler et al., 1986).

The quantitative effects of extra- or intrapulmonary shunts on physiological gas exchange depend upon the shape of the blood-O_2 equilibrium curve (O_2 EC). Maginniss (1985) pointed out the advantage of sparrow O_2 EC being steeper than humans over the physiological range for loading O_2 in hypoxic conditions. Similarly, shunts will reduce Pa_{O_2} less if the upper O_2 EC is steep. Generally, an O_2 EC can be considered steep in its upper range if the Hill coefficient exceeds 2.5 at high saturations. Most birds studied show nonlinear Hill plots and steep O_2 EC at high P_{O_2} (Lutz et al., 1974; Scheipers et al., 1975; Lapennas and Reeves, 1983; Maginniss, personal communication). It is still not clear if the large extrapulmonary shunts measured by Bickler et al. (1986) are "normal" or not but the shape of the avian O_2 EC reduces their consequences for O_2 exchange.

IV. Functional Inhomogeneities

A. Background

Gas exchange in an ideal homogeneous lung depends upon ventilatory, perfusive and diffusive conductances (G_{vent}, G_{perf}, and G_{diff}; see Chap. 13. In reality, lungs are not homogeneous. West et al. (1977) hypothesize that only three to five parabronchial atria may form the functional unit of pulmonary blood flow in birds, and ventilation could certainly vary between parabronchi. Differences in conductance matching between functional gas exchange units reduces gas exchange efficacy by increasing expired-arterial P_{O_2} differences. Conductance mismatch can occur spatially, e.g., G_{vent}/G_{perf} between parabronchi or G_{diff}/G_{perf} along a parabronchus, or temporally, e.g., changes in G_{vent} during a breath.

B. Spatial Inhomogeneities

Series Inhomogeneity

Several microsphere studies have shown that blood flow is not uniform along parabronchi but is relatively greater at the inspiratory end (reviewed by Powell and Scheid, 1988). However, as Holle et al. (1978) pointed out, such serial inhomogeneity does not affect gas exchange unless the gas is diffusion limited or, more specifically, there is G_{diff}/G_{perf} inhomogeneity along the parabronchus. It is not known exactly how G_{diff} is distributed along a parabronchus, but even if it was perfectly uniform and G_{perf} was distributed according to the microsphere data, the effects on O_2 are predicted to be extremely small (Holle et al., 1978).

Parallel Inhomogeneities

The crosscurrent O_2-CO_2 diagram (see Fig. 2) showed that even small changes in $\dot{V}/\dot{Q}$ can change PaO_2 tens of torr. Thus, *mixed* arterial PO_2 from several crosscurrent exchange units in a real bird lung will be depressed by low $\dot{V}/\dot{Q}$ units given parallel G_{vent}/G_{perf} inhomogeneity. Parallel $\dot{V}/\dot{Q}$ inequality has been measured in birds by three methods, and all agree that it is greater than serial $\dot{Q}$ inhomogeneity and that its effect on physiological gas exchange will be correspondingly greater.

Hempleman et al. (1983) used a seven-compartment model of $\dot{V}/\dot{Q}$ inequality in a study of unanesthetized ducks unidirectionally ventilated with a mesobronchial-blocking catheter. There is no possibility for ventilatory shunting or temporal variations in $\dot{V}_P$ with this preparation. They were able to predict the measure values of arterial and mixed end-parabronchial PO_2 and PCO_2 within 0.5 torr using a log-normal $\dot{V}/\dot{Q}$ distribution and 3 to 5% blood shunt.

Another approach at estimating parallel inhomogeneity is to assume that CO_2 is not diffusion limited and that deviations in its behavior from ideal crosscurrent predictions are caused by inhomogeneity. Burger et al. (1979) applied this method to anesthetized, unidirectionally ventilated hypoxic ducks. After correcting for ventilatory and perfusive shunts, they calculated that the $\dot{V}/\dot{Q}$ ratios in a two-compartment model differed from each other by an average factor of 2.6. This is less than predicted from the multiple inert gas elimination technique, but the difference may be explained by lack of temporal inhomogeneities in the preparation. Also, they may have overestimated shunts, thereby underestimating $\dot{V}/\dot{Q}$ mismatch. The perfusive shunt was calculated by the O_2 method (i.e., venous admixture in hyperoxia, see Sect. III) which may include low $\dot{V}/\dot{Q}$ inhomogeneity. The ventilatory shunt was calculated from uptake of the soluble gas chloroform. In this preparation with a mesobronchial-blocking catheter the large measured ventilatory shunt of 9.4 ± 4.7% of $\dot{V}_I$ must represent inhomogeneity measured as high $\dot{V}/\dot{Q}$ by other methods (see later discussion). Hempleman and Powell (1986) applied the CO_2 technique to assess $\dot{V}/\dot{Q}$ inhomogeneity without correcting for shunts and determined $\dot{V}/\dot{Q}$ would differ in a two-compartment model by an average factor of 5.8. This is larger than the average factor of 2.6 determined by Burger and coworkers (1979), presumably, because of shunts; Hempleman and Powell did not use mesobranchial-blocking catheters.

The most complete description of parallel inhomogeneity in bird lungs, to date, comes from application of the multiple inert gas elimination technique (Powell and Wagner, 1982a). Essentially, continuous distribution of $\dot{V}/\dot{Q}$ including perfusive shunt ($\dot{V}/\dot{Q} < 0.01$) and deadspace ($\dot{V}/\dot{Q} > 1000$) can be obtained from tidally ventilated animals. In anesthetized pump-ventilated geese (Powell and Wagner, 1982b), the perfusive shunt averaged less than 1% of cardiac output and dead space was approximately that predicted from anatomic and instrument dead space. Distributions were bimodal with a high $\dot{V}/\dot{Q}$ mode averaging 17% of nondeadspace $\dot{V}$ and 0.3% of cardiac output.

For O_2 and CO_2, the high $\dot{V}/\dot{Q}$ mode is functionally dead space and could account for 40% of measured $\dot{V}_{D\,phys}$ (see Sect. II.B). Thus, the fact that such gas exchange units are perfused at all may be of no physiological significance because they affect arterial P_{O_2} and P_{CO_2} very little. The $\dot{V}/\dot{Q}$ inhomogeneity centered around the overall ratio has a more significant effect on physiological gas exchange. If the main mode of the $\dot{Q}$ versus $\dot{V}/\dot{Q}$ distribution is considered log normal, then it has a standard deviation of 0.56. This is slightly higher than in healthy humans or dogs.

A more meaningful perspective may be to consider how much of the difference between measured P_{aO_2} and that predicted for crosscurrent lungs is caused by parallel inhomogeneity. Preliminary results indicate over one-half of this 25 torr P_{O_2} difference can be explained by measured $\dot{V}/\dot{Q}$ inequality in geese (Powell, 1982). All of the nonideal behavior for CO_2 exchange can be explained by measured $\dot{V}/\dot{Q}$ distributions (Powell and Scheid, 1988), which is consistent with the 40% unexplained O_2 deficit being a diffusion limitation (see Sect. V.A). However, postpulmonary shunts (see Sect. III) and temporal inhomogeneities (see Sect. IV.C) have not been included in quantitative models of phyisological gas exchange with $\dot{V}/\dot{Q}$ inhomogeneity, and they could also be involved.

Mechanisms determining $\dot{V}/\dot{Q}$ distributions in birds are just starting to be studied with the multiple inert gas elimination technique. The high $\dot{V}/\dot{Q}$ mode observed in geese was not affected by changes in blood volume or cardiac output (Powell and Wagner, 1982b). A high $\dot{V}/\dot{Q}$ mode is also observed in emus (Baudinette, Love, and McEvoy, personal communications), but it is not consistently observed in ducks (Bickler et al., 1986). Emus have purely paleopulmonic lungs, thereby supporting Powell and Wagner's (1982b) contention that bimodal $\dot{V}/\dot{Q}$ distributions could not represent a simple paleopulmonic–neopulmonic difference. The difference between geese and ducks has not been explained, but recall that this difference is not significant for O_2 and CO_2 exchange.

The $\dot{V}/\dot{Q}$ distributions in anesthetized, artificially ventilated ducks are apparently insensitive to acute change in inspired P_{O_2}. Hyperoxia (Bickler et al., 1986) or hypoxia corresponding to 9000-m altitude (Powell and Hastings, 1983) did not significantly change log standard deviations of $\dot{Q}$ versus $\dot{V}/\dot{Q}$ distribu-

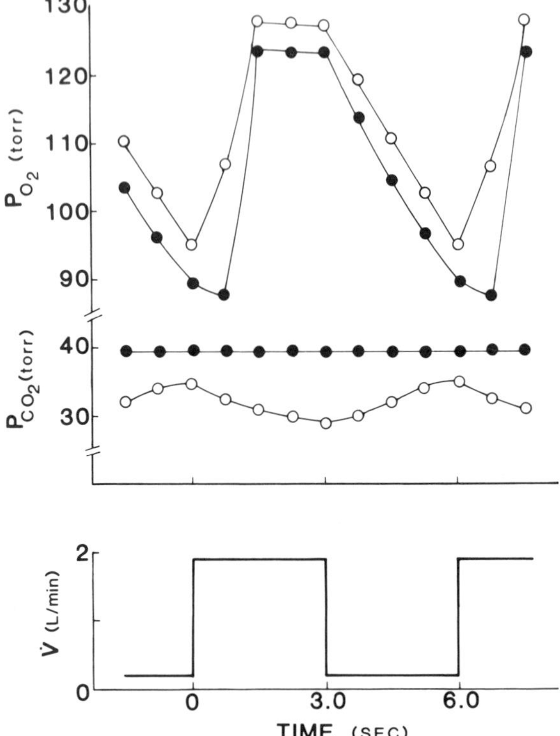

Figure 3 Effect of temporal changes in ventilation on expired gas (closed symbols) and arterial blood (open symbols) when cardiac output is constant (1.2 L/min). $P\bar{v}O_2$ = 57 torr, $P\bar{v}CO_2$ = 40 torr, PIO_2 = 145 torr, $PICO_2$ = 0.2 torr, hematocrit = 35.

tions. However, this may not be the best variable to test for changes in $\dot{V}/\dot{Q}$ distributions, and alternative measures have not yet been applied. If diffusion limitations are not dominant, O_2 exchange efficacy can improve in hypoxia if inhomogeneity is constant because hypoxia changes effective blood solubility for O_2 (βbO_2). This affects G_{vent}/G_{perf} which is the important variable (Burger et al., 1979; Powell and Scheid, 1988). The effects of chronic hypoxia and breathing pattern also have not yet been investigated.

C. Temporal Inhomogeneities

Changes in the Magnitude of Parabronchial Ventilation

Variations in $\dot{V}P$ during the ventilatory cycle will lead to temporal changes in $\dot{V}/\dot{Q}$ if pulmonary blood flow is relatively constant, as is expected. Hastings

Table 2 Modeled Effects of Temporal Inhomogeneities on Crosscurrent O_2 Exchange[a]

Ventilation	Inspired tensions	PaO_2 (torr)	$\dot{M}O_2$ (mmol/min)
Constant	Constant	116.1	1.89
Constant	Variable	114.4	1.87
Stepped	Constant	109.2	1.83
Stepped	Variable	110.0	1.84
Physiological	Variable	106.5	1.80

[a]Ventilation was constant at 1 L/min, stepped between 0.2 and 1.8 L/min at 3-s intervals or modeled after a physiological flow pattern with time averaged $\dot{V}$ of 1 L/min at 10 breaths/min. Inspired gas tensions were constant or variable as described in text. $P\bar{v}O_2$ = 56.8 torr, $\dot{Q}$ = 1.2 L/min, and other values were typical for Pekin ducks.
Source: Hastings (1985).

(1985) modeled the effect of such temporal variations on inert and physiological gases for an otherwise ideal crosscurrent lung. Arterial blood gases were affected more than expired gases because arterial partial pressures responded to changes occurring anywhere along a parabronchus, but expired gases reflect only changes reaching the expiratory end of a parabronchus. As expected, the effect depended on blood-gas solubility or G_{vent}/G_{perf}. With square-wave changes in $\dot{V}P$, CO_2 exchange was not significantly affected, but O_2 was (Fig. 3).

Table 2 shows the effects of changes in ventilatory flow and gas tensions entering the parabronchi during the ventilatory cycle on O_2 exchange. Changes in gas tensions consider that, upon inspiration, dead space gas enters the parabronchi first, then fresh air enters, and during expiration, that from the caudal air sac enters. Changes in $\dot{V}P$ seem more important than PI under the conditions simulated. In reality, O_2 consumption would not decrease 5% as indicated, but other physiological variables (e.g., $P\bar{v}$, $\dot{V}P$, and $\dot{Q}$) would change to maintain the metabolic rate.

The measurable effects predicted here contrast with an earlier experimental study (Scheid et al., 1977). They found no significant differences between apparent DLO_2 measured during continuous and periodic unidirectional ventilation of anesthetized ducks. Hastings' model predicts that significant changes ($\geq$10%) should have occurred for a nondiffusion-limited gas with solubility similar to that for O_2 during the hypoxic conditions in Scheid and associates' experimental study. Reasons for this disagreement are not clear.

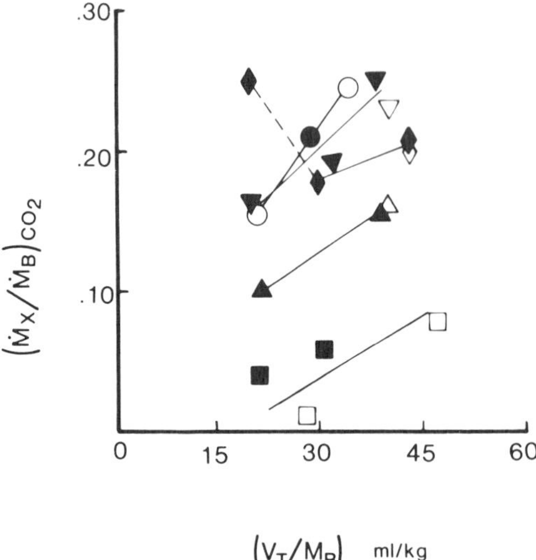

Figure 4 Nondeadspace CO_2 sources in caudal air sacs of five penguins ($\dot{M}XCO_2$) relative to total body CO_2 production ($\dot{M}BCO_2$). Different-shaped symbols represent different birds; open vs. filled symbols represent different instrument dead spaces. $(\dot{M}X/MB)CO_2$ increases with mass-specific tidal volume (VT/VB) in all but one case, suggesting that part of tidal volume is ventilating parabronchi before entering caudal air sacs. Because penguins have purely paleopulmonic lungs, this implies flow reversal during inspiration versus expiration in some parabronchi.

Reversal of Parabronchial Ventilation

Piiper and Scheid (1973) pointed out that a parabronchial flow reversal during the ventilatory cycle would create a functional breathhold. Thus, flow reversal can be considered a type of temporal inhomogeneity. Although methods are available to model this problem (e.g., Hastings, 1985), the specific effects of flow reversal have not been studied. Piiper and Scheid (1973) did predict that drops in PO_2 could be intolerably high. However, given recent evidence for flow reversal, this must not be the case.

Evidence for flow reversal comes from a study on the source of CO_2 in caudal air sacs of penguins (Powell and Hempleman, 1985). Three additional penguins have been studied since that publication, and the results are shown in Figure 4. There is a CO_2 source to the caudal air sacs equaling 4 to 22% of total body CO_2 production that cannot be explained by reinhaled dead space and that increases with tidal volume. Penguins have no neopulmonic parabronchi (Duncker, 1971); thus, fresh air should not traverse exchange areas on its way to caudal air sacs unless flow reverses in the paleopulmonic parabronchi. Air sac wall gas exchange and the Hazelhoff loop (see Scheid and Piiper, 1988) could account for less than one-half of the nondead space source. There was no evidence for air sac stratification which also could act as a CO_2 source. It was concluded that the most likely explanation was a flow reversal in the paleopulmonic parabronchi connected to the laterobronchi or fourth ventrobronchus; these have no direct air sac connections (Duncker, 1971). The contribution of such flow reversal to measurements of parallel $\dot{V}/\dot{Q}$ distributions and, in fact, to the general relationships of spatial and temporal inhomogeneities in birds' lungs, remain to be determined.

V. Membrane Diffusion Limitations

A. Physiological Measurements

Recent studies show that a bird lung's diffusing capacity for O_2 (DLO_2) increases with O_2 consumption (Geiser et al., 1984; Hempleman and Powell, 1986; Kiley et al., 1985). The mechanism of increased DLO_2 is unclear. In the study of Kiley et al. (1985) on awake running ducks, the calculated increase may just reflect the assumptions of the calculations (see Powell and Scheid, 1987) being better satisfied, i.e., an "apparent" increase. Geiser et al. (1984) and Hempleman and Powell (1985) both used the metabolic uncoupler 2,4-dinitrophenol to increase O_2 consumption, and the results were comparable with those in exercising ducks. Although Geiser and coworkers studied birds mostly in normoxia, which violates some assumptions necessary to measure DLO_2, the results of these two studies are similar. Neither study could account for the apparent increase in DLO_2 by ventilation-perfusion inhomogeneity changes (although the CO_2 method used underestimates inhomogeneity, see under Sect. IV.B, and some changes may not have been detected). Changes in air capillary diffusion resistance are probably not involved because they are already predicted to be negligible in resting birds (Scheid, 1978).

Hempleman and Powell (1985) also found an increase in DLO_2 when O_2 flow to one lung was increased by temporarily ligating the pulmonary artery to the other lung. Linear regressions showed DLO_2 was tightly coupled with pulmonary blood flow. In alveolar lungs, it is generally held that increased DLO_2 with exercise is the result of capillary recruitment and distension so DLO_2 and pulmonary blood flow are expected to be coupled in mammals. However, it is not clear that pulmonary blood capillaries are recruited or distended with pulmonary blood flow in avian lungs. Pulmonary vascular resistance calculated for one lung does not change with a doubling of pulmonary blood flow in ducks, sugesting minimal changes in capillary dimensions (Powell et al., 1985). On the other hand, Powell and Mazzone (1983) reported blood capillary folds and pleats in electron micrographs from rapidly frozen goose lungs, which is suggestive of a capacity for recruitment and for distension. Thus, the mechanism by which blood flow affects DLO_2 remains controversial. It may involve improved G_{diff}/G_{perf} matching (see under Sect. IV.B).

B. Morphometric Measurements

There are several recent morphometric studies of avian lungs and, in general, they indicate more favorable conditions for diffusive transfer of gases than in nonflying mammals of comparable size (see Maina and King, 1984). However, as Abdalla et al. (1982) point out, the physiological significance of morphometric estimates of DLO_2 is not easily evaluated. The magnitude of a diffusion limitation for a given DLO_2 depends upon the *model* of a gas exchange with all else equal (see Chap. 13). It is possible that the serial multicapillary design of the parabronchus requires a greater diffusing capacity to maintain O_2 uptake at the expiratory end where PO_2 is low. Preliminary model results (Hempleman and Powell, 1983; and unpublished) indicate that diffusion disequilibrium can occur at the expiratory end of a parabronchus with modest decreases in diffusing capacity.

Given all of these considerations, it is still interesting to note that morphometric and physiological estimates of DLO_2 in birds overlap (Powell and Scheid, 1987) in contrast to mammals (Crapo and Crapo, 1983; Weibel, 1984). Determining reasons for this avian-mammalian difference should help define mechanisms of the physiological-morphometric DLO_2 difference and the physiological significance of a generally large DLO_2 in birds.

VI. Summary

The difference between ideal crosscurrent predictions and experimental measurements of PaO_2 in birds remains to be quantitatively explained. The best estimates of diffusing capacities underestimate the role of ventilation-perfusion inhomogeneities, and the best estimates of ventilation-perfusion inhomogeneities have not been used in a model that also considers diffusion limitations. Difference between PaO_2 measurements and predictions that include best estimates of ventilation-perfusion mismatch presumably include extrapulmonary shunts, diffusion resistances, and other functional inhomogeneities, such as serial G_{diff}/G_{perf} mismatch and temporal $\dot{V}/\dot{Q}$ mismatch. However, these other functional inhomogeneities may also cause errors in estimates of parallel $\dot{V}/\dot{Q}$ mismatch; hence, interactions of inhomogeneities need to be systematically and formally explored. Finally, quantitative experiments need to be conducted on birds under conditions more normal than those encountered in most respiratory physiology laboratories to understand the differences and similarities of respiration in birds and other animals in a broad comparative sense.

References

Abdalla, M. A., Maina, J. N., King, A. S., King, D. Z., and Henry, J. (1982). Morphometrics of the avian lung. 1. The domestic fowl (*Gallus gallus* variant *domesticus*). *Respir. Physiol. 47*:267-278.

Abdalla, M. A., and King, A. S. (1976). Pulmonary arteriovenous anastomoses in the avian lung: Do they exist? *Respir. Physiol. 27*:187-191.

Banzett, R. B., Butler, J. P., and Fredberg, J. F. (1987). Proposed mechanism for aerodynamic valving of inspiratory flow in birds. *Fed. Proc. 46*:792.

Barnas, G. M., Banzett, R. B., Jones, J., and Butler, J. P. (1985). Direct test of aerodynamic valving in the avian lung. *Fed. Proc. 44*:1384.

Bech, C., Johansen, K., Brent, R., and Nicol, S. (1984). Ventilatory and circulatory changes during cold exposure in the Pekin duck *Anas platyrhynchos*. *Respir. Physiol. 57*:103-112.

Bickler, P. E., Maginniss, L. A., and Powell, F. L. (1986). Intrapulmonary and extrapulmonary shunt in ducks. *Respir. Physiol. 63*:151-160.

Bouverot, P., Douguet, D., and Sébert, P. (1979). Role of the arterial chemoreceptors in ventilatory and circulatory adjustments to hypoxia in awake Pekin ducks. *J. Comp. Physiol. 133*:177-186.

Bouverot, P., Hildwein, G., and LeGoff, D. (1974). Evaporative water loss, respiratory pattern, gas exchange and acid-base balance during thermal panting in Pekin ducks exposed to moderate heat. *Respir. Physiol. 21*:255-269.

Brent, R., Pedersen, P. F., Bech, C., and Johansen, K. (1984). Lung ventilation and temperature regulation in the European coot *Fulica atra*. *Physiol. Zool. 57*:19-25.

Brent, R., Rasmussen, J. G., Bech, C., and Martini, S. (1983). Temperature dependence of ventilation and O_2-extraction in the kittiwake, *Rissa tridactyla*. *Experientia 39*:1092-1093.

Bretz, W. L., and Schmidt-Nielsen, K. (1971). Bird respirations: Flow patterns in the duck lung. *J. Exp. Biol. 54*:103-118.

Bucher, T. L. (1985). Ventilation and oxygen consumption in *Amazona viridigenalis*. *J. Comp. Physiol. 155*:269-276.

Burger, R. E., Meyer, M., Graf, W., and Scheid, P. (1979). Gas exchange in the parabronchial lung of birds: Experiments in unidirectionally ventilated ducks. *Respir. Physiol. 36*:19-37.

Burger, R. E., and Estavillo, J. A. (1977). Pulmonary circulation–vertebral venous interconnection in the chicken. *Anat. Rec. 188*:39-44.

Calder, W. A., and Schmidt-Nielsen, K. (1968). Panting and blood carbon dioxide in birds. *Am. J. Physiol. 215*:477-482.

Crapo, J. D., and Crapo, R. O. (1983). Comparison of total lung diffusion capacity and the membrane component of diffusion capacity as determined by physiologic and morphometric techniques. *Respir. Physiol. 51*:183-194.

Duncker, H.-R. (1971). The lung air sac system of birds. A contribution to the functional anatomy of the respiratory apparatus. *Adv. Anat. Embryol. Cell Biol. 45*:1-171.

Geiser, J., Gratz, R. K., Hiramoto, T., and Scheid, P. (1984). Effects of increasing metabolism by 2,4-dinitrophenol on respiration and pulmonary gas exchange in the duck. *Respir. Physiol. 57*:1-14.

Hastings, R. H., and Powell, F. L. (1986a). Physiological dead space and effective parabronchial ventilation in ducks. *J. Appl. Physiol. 60*:85-91.

Hastings, R. H., and Powell, F. L. (1986b). Single breath CO_2 measurements of deadspace in ducks. *Respir. Physiol. 63*:139-149.

Hastings, R. H. (1985). Effective ventilation in ducks. Ph.D. dissertation, Univ. of Calif., San Diego.

Hempleman, S. C., and Powell, F. L. (1983). The course of P_{O_2} and P_{CO_2} changes in avian pulmonary capillaries. *Fed. Proc. 42*:993.

Hempleman, S. C., and Powell, F. L. (1986). Influence of pulmonary blood flow and O_2 flux on D_{O_2} in avian lungs. *Respir. Physiol. 63*:285-292.

Hempleman, S. C., Adamson, T. P., and Burger, R. E. (1983). A model of regional ventilation-perfusion inhomogeneity in the avian lung–implications for gas exchange and intrapulmonary chemoreceptor microenvironment. *Comp. Prog. Biomed.* 7:11-18.

Hinds, D. S., and Calder, W. A. (1971). Tracheal dead space in the respiration of birds. *Evolution 25*:429-440.

Holle, J. P., Heisler, N., and Scheid, P. (1978). Blood flow distribution in the duck lung and its control by respiratory gases. *Am. J. Physiol. 234*:R146-R154.

Jones, J. H. (1982). Pulmonary blood flow distribution in panting ostriches. *J. Appl. Physiol. Respir. Environ. Exercise Physiol. 53*:1411-1417.

Kiley, J. P., Faraci, F. M., and Fedde, M. R. (1985). Gas exchange during exercise in hypoxic ducks. *Respir. Physiol. 59*:105-115.

Lapennas, G. N., and Reeves, R. B. (1983). Oxygen affinity of blood of adult domestic chicken and red jungle fowl. *Respir. Physiol. 52*:27-39.

Lutz, P. L., Longmuir, B., and Schmidt-Nielsen, K. (1974). Oxygen affinity of bird blood. *Respir. Physiol. 20*:325-350.

Maginniss, L. A. (1985). Blood oxygen transport in the house sparrow *Passer domesticus. J. Comp. Physiol. B 155*:277-283.

Maina, J. W., and King, A. S. (1984). Correlations between structure and function in the design of the bat lung: A morphometric study. *J. Exp. Biol. 111*:43-61.

Piiper, J., and Scheid, P. (1973). Gas exchange in avian lungs: Models and experimental evidence. In *Comparative Physiology*. Edited by L. Bolis, K. Schmidt-Nielsen, and S. H. P. Maddrell. Amsterdam, North-Holland Publishing, pp. 161-185.

Powell, F. L., and Scheid, P. (1988). Physiology of gas exchange in the avian system. In *Form and Function in Birds*, Vol. 4. Edited by A. S. King and J. McLelland. London, Academic Press (in press).

Powell, F. L., Shams, H., and Hempleman, S. C. (1986). Effect of hypobaric and isobaric hypoxia on ventilation and arterial blood-gases in ducks. *Physiologist 29*:178.

Powell, F. L., Hastings, R. H., and Mazzone, R. W. (1985). Pulmonary vascular resistance during unilateral pulmonary arterial occlusion in ducks. *Am. J. Physiol. 249*:R39-R43.

Powell, F. L., and Hempleman, S. C. (1985). Sources of carbon dioxide in penguin air sacs. *Am. J. Physiol. 248*:R748-R752.

Powell, F. L., and Hastings, R. H. (1983). Effects of hypoxia on ventilation-perfusion matching in birds. *Physiologist 26*:A-50.

Powell, F. L., and Mazzone, R. W. (1983). Morphometrics of rapidly frozen goose lung. *Resp. Physiol. 51*:319-332.

Powell, F. L. (1982). Diffusion in avian lungs. *Fed. Proc. 41*:2131-2133.

Powell, F. L., and Wagner, P. D. (1982a). Measurement of continuous distributions of ventilation-perfusion in non-alveolar lungs. *Respir. Physiol. 48*: 219-232.

Powell, F. L., and Wagner, P. D. (1982b). Ventilation-perfusion inequality in avian lungs. *Respir. Physiol. 48*:233-241.

Powell, F. L., Geiser, J., Gratz, R. K., and Scheid, P. (1981). Airflow in the avian respirtory tract: Variations of O_2 and CO_2 concentrations in the bronchi of the duck. *Respir. Physiol. 44*:195-213.

Scheid, P., and Piiper, J. (1988). Respiratory mechanics and air flow in birds. In *Form and Function in Birds*, Vol. 4. Edited by A. S. King and J. McLelland. London, Academic Press (in press).

Scheid, P. (1978) Analysis of gas exchange between air capillaries and blood capillaries in avian lungs. *Respir. Physiol. 32*:27-49.

Scheid, P., Worth, H., Holle, J. P., and Meyer, M. (1977). Effects of oscillating and intermittent ventilatory flow on efficacy of pulmonary O_2 transfer in the duck. *Respir. Physiol. 31*:251-258.

Scheipers, G., Kawashiro, T., and Scheid, P. (1975). Oxygen and carbon dioxide dissociation of duck blood. *Respir. Physiol. 24*:1-13.

West, N. H., Bamford, O. S., and Jones, D. R. (1977). A scanning electron microscope study of the microvasculature of the avian lung. *Cell Tissue Res. 176*:553-564.

Schmidt-Nielsen, K., Kanwisher, J., Lasiewski, R. C., Cohn, J. E., and Bretz, W. L. (1969). Temperature regulation and respiration in the ostrich. *Condor 71*:341-352.

Weibel, E. R. (1984). *The Pathway for Oxygen–Structure and Function in the Mammalian Respiratory System*. Cambridge, Harvard University Press, pp. 359-363.

Part Three

Gas Exchange and Transport

9

Ontogeny of Respiration
Mammals

JAMES METCALFE and MICHAEL K. STOCK

Oregon Health Sciences University
and Portland Veterans Administration Medical Center
Portland, Oregon

I. Introduction

Respiration encompasses all of the processes involved in the passage of the respiratory gases between the exchange surface and the interior of the cells. Because of space limitations and our own interest, this chapter will be concerned mainly with oxygen transport. In terms of oxygen exchange with the environment, the ontogeny of respiration in viviparous mammals may be divided into three phases. During the preplacental phase, transport of oxygen to embryonic tissues occurs by diffusion from the local environment (oviduct, uterine lumen) without the aid of an organ for respiratory exchange with maternal blood, and in the very early stages, without the aid of a vascular system in the embryo. As the embryo increases in size the effectiveness of this arrangement rapidly diminishes. The second phase of respiratory development is characterized by maternal–fetal gas exchange by diffusion across the placenta. Finally, at parturition, the transition is made to pulmonary respiration.

In this chapter we will first consider briefly the oxygen environment and metabolism of the embryo before establishment of placental exchange. We will then examine the factors that regulate the growth and respiratory function of the placenta. Prenatal development of the lung, the subject of an earlier volume in this series (Hodson, 1977), and the transition from placental to pulmonary respiration are currently active areas of investigation (Jones and Nathanielsz, 1985; Perelman et al., 1985; Rooney, 1985; Burri, 1984), but limited space precludes discussing them here. The bibliography is not exhaustive; we have given preference to recent references and to those that serve as points of entry into the literature.

II. Preplacental Respiration

A. Synopsis of Preplacental Development

The duration of the preplacental period varies markedly among species, ranging from a few days to many months in some cases of embryonic diapause or "delayed implantation" (Renfree, 1982). In the human, this period lasts approximately 2 to 3 weeks. Fertilization typically occurs in the ampulla of the oviduct (Moore, 1977) within 24 h of ovulation. The zygote enters the uterus at the morula stage about 3 days after fertilization. Implantation begins about 2 days later with attachment of the blastocyst to the endometrial epithelium; usually in the upper part of the uterus, slightly more frequently on the posterior than on the anterior wall. During the next week, the blastocyst actively invades the uterine endometrium and the trophoblast differentiates into cytotrophoblast and syncytiotrophoblast. Isolated cavities (lacunae) appear in the syncytiotrophoblast and soon fill with maternal blood from ruptured capillaries and secretions from eroded endometrial glands; constituents of this nutrient fluid diffuse to the embryonic disk. When uterine vessels join with the trophoblastic lacunae 11 to 12 days after fertilization the uteroplacental circulation begins. Primary chorionic villi appear as outgrowths of the trophoblast during the next several days; they become secondary villi as they acquire a mesenchymal core. By the end of the third postfertilization week embryonic blood is circulating through the capillaries of what are now tertiary villi, and physiological exchange between the mother and the embryo is established. A similar series of events occurs in other mammals, although important differences exist in the precise timing of the various stages, the extent to which embryonic gas exchange may rely upon accessory structures (e.g., the yolk sac or allantois), and the structure and growth pattern of the placenta (see Battaglia and Meschia, 1986; Hearn, 1986; Faber and Thornburg, 1983; Renfree, 1982).

B. Early Oxygen Environment

Little is known of the oxygen environment of the early mammalian embryo; the location and small size of the organism make in situ metabolic studies extremely difficult. Failure of embryos flushed from the reproductive tract to grow in culture at a rate comparable with that achieved in vivo (Fischer, 1987; Papaioannou and Ebert, 1986) attests to the importance of the maternal environment for nurturing development before implantation. The chemical constituents of oviductal and uterine fluids and variations in their composition induced by changes in hormonal status have been studied (Roblero and Riffo, 1986; Mastroianni, 1982; Biggers and Borland, 1976), but the critical components of the maternal environment have not been identified. In particular, the influence of luminal oxygen tension (PO_2) on growth and metabolism of the preimplantation embryo has not been systematically investigated.

The potential for exchange between the embryo and its environment depends upon its stage of development and its location (Biggers and Borland, 1976). The mammalian egg is small compared with those of other vertebrates, but large (0.1 mm diameter) relative to other maternal cells (McLaren, 1982). The volume of the preimplantation embryo, which is a major determinant of the efficacy of oxygen and carbon dioxide exchange by simple diffusion, remains unchanged or declines during the initial cleavage divisions. In the human blastocyst at implantation there are fewer than 100 cells, the average size of which is similar to that of adult cells.

The metabolic rate of the unfertilized mammalian ovum is very low, similar to that of a relatively inert tissue such as bone. Oxygen consumption increases very little in the early cleavage stages, but it rises exponentially between the morula and the blastocyst stage in the mouse and rabbit (McLaren, 1982; Mills and Brinster, 1967). The metabolic rate of the blastocyst is as high as that of most active tissues and its energy is derived primarily from oxidative phosphorylation. Dry weight and total protein content of the embryo decline during cleavage in some species; therefore, weight-specific oxygen consumption increases. There is a marked shift in substrate requirements and metabolism in the very early stages of development, which may be related to a change in mitochondrial structure (Magnusson et al., 1986; Biggers and Borland, 1976). Because the maturing blastocyst displays a high rate of oxidative metabolism (Magnusson et al., 1986; Fridhandler et al., 1956), the availability of oxygen may be important in sustaining normal development before the establishment of placental exchange.

The oxygen tension within the female reproductive tract depends upon the species, the site, and the physiological state of the maternal organism. Values for the uterus and oviduct range from less than 10 torr to approximately 60 torr in the rat (Yochim and Mitchell, 1968), rabbit (Mastroianni and Jones, 1965), guinea pig (Garris and Whitehead, 1981), and rhesus monkey (Maas et al., 1976). Intraluminal PO_2 is apparently determined by uterine vasodynamic and metabolic activity under the control of ovarian steroid hormones. This concept is supported by the close temporal correlation reported between plasma estradiol concentration, uterine blood flow, and intrauterine PO_2, all of which peak at the time of implantation in the normal pregnant guinea pig (Garris and Whitehead, 1981) and by the observation that intraluminal PO_2 is markedly reduced by acutely decreasing uterine blood flow (Garris and Whitehead, 1981; Hammer et al., 1981). In the species examined to date, the intraluminal PO_2 at the time of ovulation and implantation is comparable with the optimum PO_2 established in vitro for a variety of early developmental processes, including maturation of ovarian oocytes (Gwatkin and Haidri, 1974), fertilization (Brackett and Williams, 1968), cleavage of early embryos (Papaioannou and Ebert, 1986), and blastocyst development (Daniel, 1968). The frequency of reproductive loss during the peri-implantation period, which normally accounts for a substantial fraction of gestational failures, may be increased by maternal hypoxia (Ingalls et al., 1952; Atland, 1949). The normal increase in luminal oxygen availability during the peri-implantation period may serve as a stimulus for biochemical and metabolic changes in the progestational uterus (Simpson and Mitchell, 1983; Yochim and Mitchell, 1968). The regional specificity of implantation in a number of species, and the presence of local hyperemia at the implantation sites, strongly suggest a hemotropic effect. The possibility that oxygen is the critical blood-borne factor in this interaction cannot be dismissed (Garris and Whitehead, 1981; Yochim and Mitchell, 1968).

III. Placental Respiration

A. Placental Structure

Placental structure varies widely among mammals, and several classification schemes have been advanced (see Battaglia and Meschia, 1986; Faber and Thornburg, 1983). Important differences occur in gross morphology [diffuse vs. compact (cotyledonary, zonary, discoidal)], the number of histological layers separating maternal blood from the fetal chorion (epitheliochorial, endotheliochorial, hemochorial), and the relative geometry of maternal and fetal placental vascular beds (parallel vs. nonparallel vessels, concurrent vs. countercurrent flows).

The human placenta is of the compact (discoidal), hemochorial type and comprises tissues of both maternal (decidua basalis) and fetal origin (chorionic plate and villi). Maternal arterial blood is ejected from spiral, terminal branches of the uterine arteries into the intervillous space where it bathes the chorionic villi containing the fetal capillaries. Oxygen diffuses from maternal erythrocytes in the intervillous space across the villous membrane and fetal capillary endothelium to the fetal red cells; carbon dioxide and other metabolic wastes follow a similar path in reverse. Maternal blood drains from the intervillous space through the uterine veins to reenter the systemic circulation. On the fetal side, relatively deoxygenated blood enters the placenta by way of the paired umbilical arteries. It passes through the closed villous microcirculation where it is reoxygenated and returns to the fetus through a single umbilical vein.

B. Placental Growth

The placenta normally increases in size until term in the human (Sands and Dobbing, 1985) and in the rhesus monkey (Hill, 1975). The cotyledonary placenta of the sheep, on the other hand, ceases to increase in weight at the end of the second trimester (Kulhanek et al., 1974). Molteni and coworkers (1978) examined placental growth for human infants with different intrauterine growth patterns. The weight of placentas from infants whose birth weight was appropriate or large for gestational age increased linearly from 23 weeks to term. In contrast, the weight of the placentas from infants who were small for gestational age plateaued at approximately 36 weeks of gestation. Early in pregnancy the placenta is large relative to the fetus. Subsequent placental growth fails to keep pace with that of the fetus, thus the placental/fetal weight ratio declines during pregnancy. In the human this ratio reaches unity at about 105 days of gestation (Gellén and Györi, 1969).

Winick and Noble (1966) observed that the weight, protein, and RNA contents of the rat placenta increased linearly on days 14 to 19 of pregnancy, then declined until term (day 21), whereas the DNA content did not change after day 17. Measurements of thymidine and leucine incorporation corroborated the interpretation that DNA synthesis ceased on day 17, whereas protein synthesis continued through day 19. More recently, Soares (1987) has reported that the DNA content increased significantly from day 19 to day 21 in the junctional, but not in the labyrinthine, zone of the rat placenta; protein content of both zones increased until term.

Winick and associates (1967) concluded that the terminal phase of placental growth in the human was also characterized by cell enlargement (hypertrophy) without cell division. Placental weight, protein, and RNA content increased linearly until term, whereas DNA content leveled off at a placental weight of about 300 g (35-36 weeks gestation). Weinberg and his associates (1970) found decreased uptake of tritiated thymidine with advancing gestational age in the human placenta, with slightly different rates obtaining for the trophoblast and mesenchymal core of the villus. Other investigators, however, have challenged this pattern of placental growth. The DNA content in the hemochorial placenta of the rhesus monkey increases linearly through 160 days of gestation (term = 165 days) (Hill, 1975). Similarly, Sands and Dobbing (1985) observed no sign of a late gestational plateau in human placental DNA content. Iversen and Farsund (1985), using flow cytometry, measured 6.4% of the cells in S-phase (DNA syntheses) in normal human placentas at term. Three-dimensional reconstruction of serial thin sections and scanning electron microscopy of vessel casts from human placentas also indicate that fetal capillary proliferation in the terminal villi continues until parturition (Kaufmann et al., 1985).

In the sheep, fetal growth during the last third of gestation takes place without any increase in placental weight or DNA content; nonetheless, urea permeability increases fivefold between 90 days and term (Kulhanek et al., 1974). Thus, it appears that a period of cellular growth is followed by a period of functional maturation. Additional evidence for this feature of placental development derives from other species as well. Diffusing capacity for carbon monoxide in the guinea pig placenta increases more than fourfold during the last trimester of pregnancy (Bissonnette and Wickham, 1977). The increase parallels the change in fetal weight but is not related to placental weight. If pregnancy is prolonged in the rabbit by maternal administration of chorionic gonadotropin, fetal weight increases markedly with no significant change in placental weight (Harding, 1970), suggesting that the term placenta has the capacity to support further fetal growth. In the study by Kulhanek and coworkers (1974), sheep placentas that were undergrown displayed reduced DNA content and no compensatory increase in urea permeability per gram of DNA compared with placentas of normal size and comparable age. Functional maturation, defined as urea permeability per unit weight of fetus, was limited near term in growth-retarded placentas.

Regulation of placental growth is poorly understood. There is a good linear correlation between fetal birthweight and placental weight during the last third of gestation in humans (Adair and Thelander, 1925; Aherne, 1966) and in the rhesus monkey (Hill, 1975; Kerr et al., 1971); nonetheless, the relationship between placental and fetal growth is not well defined. It is not clear whether the two are independently controlled or subject to a single regulatory mechanism. Some investigators have suggested that placental growth (functional development) is dictated by the increasing demands of the fetus for oxygen and nutrients. Others contend that fetal growth is constrained by the size (functional capacity) of the placenta.

Recent descriptive studies make clear the potential for a humoral contribution to the control of placental as well as fetal growth (see D'Ercole and Underwood, 1986; Fisher, 1986; Simpson and MacDonald, 1981). Unfortunately, nowhere is the complexity of maternal-placental-fetal interaction more apparent than in prenatal endocrine regulation and function. The situation is complicated by our lack of knowledge concerning the nature and extent of chemical "traffic" among these three components, the capacity of the placenta to alter substances presented to it by mother or fetus, the interaction among classic hormones and growth factors, the ontogeny of receptor function in the fetus and placenta, and the inevitable differences among species in the endocrine, paracrine, and autocrine requirements for normal placental and fetal growth.

The placenta is an important source of polypeptide hormones, several of which are unique to pregnancy, including chorionic gonadotropin (CG) and chorionic somatomammotropin (CS, placental lactogen). A number of traditional hypothalamic neuropeptides have also been identified in the placenta, including gonadotropin-releasing hormone (GnRH, or leuteinizing hormone-releasing hormone), thyrotropin-releasing hormone (TRH), somatotropin release-inhibiting factor (SRIF, or somatostatin), corticotropin-releasing factor (CRF), and growth hormone-releasing factor (GRF). Because synthetic GnRH increases the in vitro production of CG, progesterone, and estrogens from placental explants, placental GnRH has been hypothesized to have a paracrine role in regulating CG and steroid hormone production and release. Similarly, the observations that SRIF-containing cytotrophoblastic cells disappear as gestation advances and that CS production increases progressively during the last half of pregnancy support the speculation that syncytiotrophoblastic production of CS is also under paracrine control (Fisher, 1986). Isolation of a biologically active growth hormone-releasing factor from near-term rat placenta is consistent with this scheme (Baird et al., 1985). Recent evidence emphasizes the heterogeneity of the placenta as an endocrine organ. The CS content of the two morphologically and functionally distinct zones of the rat placenta (junctional and labyrinthine) exhibit reciprocal changes during gestation (Soares, 1987). The labyrinthine zone, which is in direct contact with the developing embryo, contributes negligibly to total placental CS content on day 13 of pregnancy, but it is the predominant source at term. Soares postulates that CS-secreting cells in the labyrinthine region may be more responsive to "signals" from the fetus and have greater access to, and influence on, the fetus.

Placental growth has been shown to be sensitive to steroid hormones. Synthesis of DNA in the terminal portions of the mesometrial arteries in the guinea pig, as indicated by incorporation of tritiated thymidine, increases 40-fold with the onset of pregnancy; this event can be mimicked by exogenous estradiol administration (Makinoda and Moll, 1986). Estradiol may thus contribute to regulation of vasoproliferation and placental blood flow during gestation.

Growth factors are also potential regulators of placental growth, presumably by an autocrine or paracrine mechanism or by mediating the actions of classic hormones. Placental explants and cultured fibroblasts derived from preterm and term human placentas have been shown to secrete insulinlike growth factors I and II (IGF-I, IGF-II) (Fant et al., 1986). Specific placental receptors have been reported for IGF-I (Fujita-Yamaguchi et al., 1986), as well as for triiodothyronine (T_3; Banovac et al., 1986), and epidermal growth factor (EGF; Smith and Talamantes, 1986). The density of EGF receptors in the mouse placenta rises and falls during gestation (Smith and Talamantes, 1986), although the significance of this relative to the action (if any) of EGF on the placenta is unknown. An angiogenic and mitogenic factor has been isolated from the human placenta and extraembryonic membranes and has been partially characterized (Burgos, 1986; Fuchs et al., 1985).

Several studies suggest that unidentified fetal factors influence placental growth. If the rhesus monkey fetus is removed by cesarean section, the placenta is retained past term, but the normal increase in size with gestation is arrested (Lanman et al., 1975). Despite degenerative changes in the stroma, the trophoblast persists and there is even evidence of cytotrophoblastic hypertrophy and hyperplasia, indicating that factors of nonfetal origin are also operational. An immunological component is suggested by the observation that placentas from mouse fetuses that are genetically dissimilar to their mother grow significantly larger than those of fetuses whose parents are of the same strain (Beer et al., 1975). The observation that mean placental (and fetal) weight is reduced in allogenic pregnancies by removal of the maternal spleen or para-aortic lymph nodes suggests that the increase in placental weight is due to a maternal reaction against fetal tissue histocompatibility antigens. Finally, "maturation" of the human placenta, as determined by ultrasonic grading, is accelerated in twin compared with singleton pregnancies (Ohel et al., 1987); the physiological significance of the presumed structural differences is unknown.

C. Placental Gas Exchange

Diffusion through tissue is described by Fick's law. When applied to the placenta, this states that the rate of transfer of oxygen is directly proportional to the exchange area and the difference in mean partial pressure of oxygen between maternal and fetal blood and is inversely proportional to the barrier thickness. Diffusion is also dependent upon the physical properties of the exchange barrier and the solubility and diffusivity of oxygen in the tissue.

The quantity of oxygen diffusing across the placenta per unit time per unit oxygen partial pressure difference is the placental diffusing capacity for oxygen (DO_2). The DO_2 is difficult to determine with any degree of precision because oxygen is consumed by the placenta and because the mean PO_2 difference cannot be measured directly. Therefore, DO_2 is calculated from measurements of the diffusing capacity for carbon monoxide (DCO). Species differences in carbon monoxide-diffusing capacity are large and apparently unrelated to the morphological classification of the placenta. Theoretical calculations indicate that the wide variation arises, in part, from differences in exchange area and, in part, from differences in barrier thickness (Faber and Thornburg, 1983).

Diffusion of oxygen actually occurs through multiple compartments. Thus, the total resistance to diffusion (the inverse of total diffusing capacity) may be thought of as the sum of the series resistances of the individual compartments. In the placenta, this sum includes the resistance of the maternal blood, maternal tissue, fetal tissue, and fetal blood. Diffusing capacity of the blood is influenced by the rate of reaction of oxygen with hemoglobin.

The concept that physiological maturation of the placenta may be dissociated from growth of the organ per se is important relative to its respiratory function. Factors that could account for an increase in the diffusing capacity of the placenta include (1) increased maternal placental blood flow (for flow-limited substances); (2) increased surface area for exchange, or (3) decreased thickness of the placental barrier (for diffusion-limited substances); and (4) increased facilitated or active transport (for substances that depend upon nondiffusional transfer). The role of placental blood flow will be considered in Section III.D. Changes affecting nondiffusional transport will not be addressed. Although an oxygen carrier has been postulated in the placenta, the evidence for it is not compelling (Faber and Thornburg, 1983).

Several groups of workers have made morphometric analyses of the histological composition of the human placenta at term (Teasdale and Jean-Jacques, 1985; Boyd, 1984; Mayhew et al., 1984; Laga et al., 1973; Aherne and Dunnill, 1966). The most recent of these morphometric studies was based on the placentas of 14 healthy women born and raised in Santa Cruz, Bolivia at an altitude of 400 m (Mayhew et al., 1986). The physical dimensions of the components of resistance in the human placenta are presented in Table 1. From these dimensions the diffusing capacity of each component in the pathway of oxygen diffusion was calculated together with the total diffusing capacity of the placental membrane. The latter averaged 3 $cm^3 \cdot min^{-1} \cdot torr^{-1}$ of oxygen, a value at the lower end of the range (3-6 $cm^3 \cdot min^{-1} \cdot torr^{-1}$ of O_2) presented by other groups, but at the upper end of physiological estimates of placental diffusing capacity (1-3 $cm^3 \cdot min^{-1} \cdot torr^{-1}$ of O_2). The systematic difference between morphometric and physiological estimates may be rationally explained by the presence of vascular shunts, oxygen consumption by the placenta itself, and regional heterogeneity in perfusion/diffusion and perfusion/perfusion ratios (Metcalfe et al., 1967).

Morphometric and physiological analyses of placental diffusing capacity agree in attributing most of the resistance to oxygen diffusion to the "placental membrane." According to the study of Mayhew and colleagues (1986), 89% of the total resistance to oxygen diffusion between maternal and fetal blood can be explained by the resistance in the villous membrane (the trophoblast, fetal basal lamina, and fetal capillary endothelium). As might be predicted, changes in the thickness or surface area of the villous membrane exert a significant influence on the calculated diffusing capacity; a 40% decrease in the surface area of either the chorionic villi or the fetal capillaries resulted in a decrement of diffusing capacity that was similar in magnitude to that induced by a 40% increase in the harmonic mean thickness of the villous membrane. Changes in the total surface area of either maternal erythrocytes or fetal erythrocytes, secondary to changes in

Table 1 Stereological Estimates of the Physical Dimensions of the Components of the Human Placenta at Term[a]

Volume (cm^3)	
intervillous space	173 ± 10.3
fetal capillary bed	43.5 ± 4.70
Surface area (m^2)	
maternal erythrocytes (mean only)	82.4
chorionic villi	7.0 ± 0.59
fetal capillaries	5.4 ± 0.56
fetal erythrocytes (mean only)	28.0
Harmonic mean distances (μm)	
maternal plasma	1.9 ± 0.17
villous membrane	4.9 ± 0.25
fetal plasma	0.6 ± 0.03

[a]Mean ± standard deviation.
Source: Mayhew et al. (1986).

hematocrit, had relatively little influence on total placental diffusing capacity. During gestation, fetal capillary volume, capillary surface area, and villous surface area increase, whereas villous membrane thickness decreases (Boyd, 1984; Aherne and Dunnill, 1966). Morphometric estimates also agree with physiological estimates in showing that the diffusing capacity of the placenta and fetal weight are positively correlated (Mayhew et al., 1984; Longo et al., 1969).

The harmonic mean thickness of the placental villous membrane from women who were born and raised at high altitudes in La Paz, Bolivia (3600 m; Jackson et al., 1985) was 25% less (3.6 vs. 4.9 μm) than that of lowlanders residing in Santa Cruz (400 m; Mahew et al., 1986), suggesting placental adaptation to chronic relative hypoxia. Gilbert and coworkers (1979) found that the physiological diffusing capacity of the guinea pig placenta increased in response to chronic hypoxia resulting from maternal exposure to 12% O_2; however, subsequent studies from the same laboratory have failed to consistently confirm this observation (Bacon et al., 1984). Conversely, the adverse effect on birth weight of maternal cigarette smoking during pregnancy (Stein and Kline, 1983), in part, may be due to a decrease in the diffusing capacity of the placenta. Van der Velde and his associates (1985) observed a 50% increase in the thickness of the basal laminae of the trophoblast and the fetal capillaries in the placentas of heavy smokers. They also noted more frequent duplication of the capillary basal lamina in the smokers' placentas and a decrease in the diameter of the villous capillaries.

Placental involvement has long been noted in several complications of pregnancy. A morphometric study compared the histology of the placentas of five women with severe preeclampsia, who gave birth to growth-retarded term infants, with the placentas of a group of normal women (Teasdale, 1985); no difference was found in the weight of the placentas or in the fractional volume of the placenta containing the structures or compartments concerned with metabolic exchange between mother and fetus. The villous and capillary surface densities and areas were similar in the two groups. Unfortunately, no measurement was made of the distance between maternal and fetal capillary blood. The placental/fetal weight ratio was increased in preeclamptic pregnancies. Significant increases were also demonstrated in the number of syncytiotrophoblastic nuclei per unit volume of peripheral villous tissue and in the intervillous space volume per unit total villous tissue volume, presumably a result of loss of villous connective tissue and reduced size of the villi. These changes were interpreted by the author as compensatory for the primary defect in toxemia of pregnancy. However, Teasdale's findings (1985) are at variance with those of previous investigators who showed a significant reduction in the total placental volume, parenchymal volume, and surface area of the villi (Boyd and Scott, 1985; Clavero-Nuñez et al., 1971; Aherne and Dunnill, 1966). Boyd and Scott (1985) reported a significant increase in the volume fraction occupied by fetal capillaries in the placentas of preeclamptic women, whereas Aherne and Dunnill (1966) and Clavero-Nuêz and associates (1971) observed decreases in fetal capillary surface area. In idiopathic fetal growth retardation, Teasdale (1984) found a significant decrease in placental size and a slight, but not statistically significant, increase in the placental/fetal weight ratio. The placentas were characterized by marked reductions in parenchymal tissue and in the surface areas of exchange (capillary and villous surface areas). These differences disappeared, however, when placental volumes and surface areas were normalized to fetal weight. Lee and Yeh (1986) examined the fetal vasculature of six placentas from infants who were small for gestational age following pregnancies complicated by oligohydramnios, hypertension, or severe preeclampsia. The principal changes observed were less branching of arteries and veins, capillaries with variable diameter, numerous budlike capillary projections, and H-shaped capillary anastomoses. The latter two features were interpreted as indicative of compensatory capillary neovascularization.

D. Control of Placental Respiration

Considerable progress has been made in understanding the developmental physiology of the mechanisms regulating pulmonary respiration (Jones and Nathanielsz, 1985; Haddad and Mellins, 1984; Harding, 1984; Read and Henderson-Smart, 1984; Rigatto, 1984; Walker, 1984). Our knowledge of the physiological regulation of prenatal respiration is more uncertain.

Transport of oxygen from the atmosphere to fetal tissues occurs by a complex chain of events involving bulk transport and simple diffusion (see Battaglia and Meschia, 1986) and is ultimately dependent upon the physiology of the mother, the placenta, and the fetus. Placental oxygen transfer is dependent upon uterine and umbilical arterial oxygen tensions, the relative geometry of the maternal and fetal placental vascular beds, the rates of maternal and fetal placental blood flow, placental oxygen consumption, and the placental diffusing capacity for oxygen. Although it may be naive to speak of the "control" of prenatal respiration, it is instructive to consider the physiological adaptations that facilitate maternal-fetal oxygen transport.

Pregnancy induces a number of changes in maternal cardiovascular and respiratory physiology (see Metcalfe et al., 1988) that help insure adequate oxygen delivery to the conceptus. Relative hyperventilation, which occurs during the progestational phase of each menstrual cycle, persists with pregnancy and inceases progressively as gestation proceeds. The increase in minute ventilation during human pregnancy is due to increased tidal volume; respiratory frequency does not change. The magnitude of the decline in arterial PCO_2 is correlated with the plasma progesterone concentration; however, the mechanism of this respiratory stimulation is unknown. Additional evidence for pregnancy-induced alterations in maternal respiratory control derives from the increase in the magnitude of the ventilatory response to hypoxia and to inhaled CO_2. The fall in maternal arterial PCO_2 facilitates diffusion of carbon dioxide from fetal blood in the placenta and allows the fetus to develop at a PCO_2 and pH comparable with those experienced postnatally.

Maternal blood oxygen affinity, which is subject to the opposing forces of respiratory alkalosis (secondary to hyperventilation) and an increased erythrocytic 2,3-diphosphoglycerate concentration (secondary to the alkalosis), decreases slightly during pregnancy (Bauer et al., 1969). Failure of the normal decline in hemoglobin-oxygen affinity has been associated with intrauterine growth retardation (Ortner et al., 1983).

Maternal cardiovascular changes are also important during the normal course of pregnancy. Maternal blood volume and cardiac output increase with gestation in the human, guinea pig, and sheep; although the magnitude and temporal pattern of the change differs significantly among species (see Metcalfe et al., 1988). The regional distribution of maternal cardiac output is altered during pregnancy; blood flow to the uterus increases progressively with gestation. There is also a redistribution of blood flow within the uterus. In the nonpregnant ovine uterus, for example, blood flows to the myometrium, the endometrium, and the prospective sites of implantation are roughly equal. When pregnancy occurs, the placental cotyledons are increasingly favored; approximately 88% of the total uterine blood flow at term is directed to the cotyledons. From the standpoint of fetal respiration, it is important to remember that a substantial fraction of the uterine blood flow does not supply the placenta and is, therefore, not available for exchange. A similar situation occurs on the fetal side; approximately 6% of the ovine umbilical blood flow near term perfuses the intercotyledonary chorion. The actual "shunt" flow may be even greater if additional shunts exist within the placenta. Factors that interfere with maternal placental blood flow (e.g., hypotension, hypertension, uterine contractions, decreased cardiac output) or maternal blood oxygenation (e.g., cigarette smoking, anemia, methadone addiction) may adversely affect oxygen delivery to the conceptus.

In general, the growing demand of the fetus for oxygen outpaces the increase in uterine blood flow; therefore, oxygen extraction from blood in the uteroplacental circulation increases with gestation. Marked species differences appear to be related to differences in placental strucure and uterine perfusion (Murray et al., 1985). Fetal systemic oxygen delivery is the product of the umbilical venoarterial oxygen content difference and umbilical blood flow. Umbilical oxygen uptake is influenced by umbilical arterial oxygen tension and the affinity of fetal hemoglobin for oxygen.

The mammalian fetus develops normally and is able to grow rapidly with an arterialized blood oxygen tension that is extremely hypoxic by adult standards (i.e., 20-25 torr). Several fetal adaptations contribute to adequate tissue oxygenation. In a number of species, but not all, the fetal hemoglobin has a greater affinity for oxygen than that of the mother (see Table 4.1 in Faber and Thornburg, 1983). Fetal P_{50}, the oxygen tension at which half of the hemoglobin is saturated, is approximately 4 torr less than maternal P_{50} in humans and rabbits, 11 torr less in the guinea pig, and 17 torr less in the sheep. Narrowing of the P_{50} difference between mother and fetus produces fetal growth retardation and placental enlargement in the rat (Hebbel et al., 1980). A second important fetal adaptation is a relatively high level of tissue perfusion; fetal cardiac output per unit body weight is high relative to that of the adult, and tissue vascular resistance is very low.

IV. Conclusions

The ontogeny of respiration in eutherian mammals provides an example of the careful orchestration and complex integration of maternal and fetal physiology that is the hallmark of successful viviparity. Diffusional transport of oxygen from the local maternal environment during the earliest stages of development gives way gradually to respiratory exchange between adjacent maternal and fetal vascular beds in the placenta. At birth, placental exchange is abruptly terminated with the expulsion of this organ, and survival of the neonate is dependent upon an immediate transition to pulmonary ventilation.

Our understanding of perinatal respiration would be enhanced by a more detailed description of the oxygen environment during gestation, especially in the early stages that have traditionally defied close scrutiny. We lack quantitative information concerning the range of values for oxygen supply that are compatible with normal fetal growth and development.

It should be emphasized that our present concepts of prenatal respiration in mammals are derived from experiments on only a small number of species. Additional comparative studies, both anatomical and physiological, will undoubtedly reveal diverse maternal and fetal adaptations that facilitate respiratory exchange; the understanding of these adaptations will help clarify unifying biological principles.

References

Adair, F. L., and Thelander, H. (1925). A study of the weight and dimensions of the human placenta in its relation to the weight of the newborn infant. *Am. J. Obstet. Gynecol. 10*:172-205.

Aherne, W. (1966). A weight relationship between the human foetus and placenta. *Biol. Neon. 10*:113-118.

Aherne, W., and Dunnill, M. S. (1966). Quantitative aspects of placental structure. *J. Pathol. Bacteriol. 91*:123-139.

Atland, P. D. (1949). Breeding performance of rats exposed repeatedly to 18,000 feet simulated altitude. *Physiol. Zool. 22*:235-246.

Bacon, B. J., Gilbert, R. D., Kaufmann, P., Smith, A. D., Trevino, F. T., and Longo, L. D. (1984). Placental anatomy and diffusing capacity in guinea pigs following long-term maternal hypoxia. *Placenta 5*:475-488.

Baird, A., Wehrenberg, W. B., Böhlen, P., and Ling, N. (1985). Immunoreactive and biologically active growth hormone-releasing factor in the rat placenta. *Endocrinology 117*:1598-1601.

Banovac, K., Ryan, E. A., and O'Sullivan, M. J. (1986). Triiodothyronine (T_3) nuclear binding sites in human placenta and decidua. *Placenta 7*:543-549.

Battaglia, F. C., and Meschia, G. (1986). *An Introduction to Fetal Physiology*. New York, Academic Press.

Bauer, C., Ludwig, M., Ludwig, I., and Bartels, H. (1969). Factors governing the oxygen affinity of human adult and foetal blood. *Respir. Physiol. 7*:271-277.

Beer, A. E., Billingham, R. E., and Scott, J. R. (1975). Immunogenetic aspects of implantation, placentation and feto-placental growth rates. *Biol. Reprod. 12*:176-189.

Biggers, J. D., and Borland, R. M. (1976). Physiological aspects of growth and development of the preimplantation mammalian embryo. *Annu. Rev. Physiol. 38*:95-119.

Bissonnette, J. M., and Wickham, W. K. (1977). Placental diffusing capacity for carbon monoxide in unanesthetized guinea pigs. *Respir. Physiol. 31*:161-168.

Boyd, P. A. (1984). Quantitative structure of the normal human placenta from 10 weeks of gestation to term. *Early Hum. Dev. 9*:297-307.

Boyd, P. A., and Scott, A. (1985). Quantitative structural studies on human placentas associated with pre-eclampsia, essential hypertension and intrauterine growth retardation. *Br. J. Obstet. Gynaecol. 92*:714-721.

Brackett, B. G., and Williams, W. L. (1968). Fertilization of rabbit ova in a defined medium. *Fertil. Steril. 19*:144-155.

Burgos, H. (1986). Angiogenic factor from human term placenta. Purification and partial characterization. *Eur. J. Clin. Invest. 16*:486-493.

Burri, P. H. (1984). Fetal and postnatal development of the lung. *Annu. Rev. Physiol. 46*:617-628.

Clavero-Nuêz, J. A., Negueruela, J., and Botella-Llusia, J. (1971). Placental morphometry and placental circulometry. *J. Reprod. Med. 6*:209-217.

Daniel, J. C., Jr. (1968). Oxygen concentrations for culture of rabbit blastocysts. *J. Reprod. Fertil. 17*:187-190.

D'Ercole, A. J., and Underwood, L. E. (1986). Regulation of fetal growth by hormones and growth factors. In *Human Growth*, 2nd ed., Vol. 1, Developmental Biology Prenatal Growth. Edited by F. Falkner and J. M. Tanner. New York, Plenum Press, pp. 327-338.

Faber, J. J., and Thornburg, K. L. (1983). *Placental Physiology: Structure and Function of Fetomaternal Exchange*. New York, Raven Press.

Fant, M., Munro, H., and Moses, A. C. (1986). An autocrine/paracrine role for insulin-like growth factors in the regulation of human placental growth. *J. Clin. Endocrinol. Metab. 63*:499-505.

Fischer, B. (1987). Development retardation in cultured preimplantation rabbit embryos. *J. Reprod. Fertil. 79*:115-123.

Fisher, D. A. (1986). The unique endocrine milieu of the fetus. *J. Clin. Invest. 78*:603-611.

Fridhandler, L., Hafez, E. S. E., and Pincus, G. (1956). Respiratory metabolism of mammalian eggs. *Proc. Soc. Exp. Biol. Med. 92*:127-129.

Fuchs, A., Lindenbaum, E., and Marcoudas, N. G. (1985). Location of the angiogenic activity in the pregnant human uterus. *Acta Anat. 124*:241-244.

Fujita-Yamaguchi, Y., LeBon, T. R., Tsubokawa, M., Henzel, W., Kathuria, S., Koyal, D., and Ramachandran, J. (1986). Comparison of insulin-like growth factor I receptor and insulin receptor purified from human placental membranes. *J. Biol. Chem. 261*:16727-16731.

Garris, D. R., and Whitehead, D. S. (1981). Uterine blood blow and timing of blastocyst implantation in the guinea pig. *Am. J. Physiol. 241*:E142-E145.

Gellén, J., and Györi, I. (1969). The weight increase of the placenta and embryo in early human pregnancy. *J. Obstet. Gynecol. Br. Commonw. 76*:990-992.

Gilbert, R. D., Cummings, L. A., Juchau, M. R., and Longo, L. D. (1979). Placental diffusing capacity and fetal development in exercising or hypoxic guinea pigs. *J. Appl. Physiol. 46*:828-834.

Gwatkin, R. B. L., and Haidri, A. A. (1974). Oxygen requirements for the maturation of hamster oocytes. *J. Reprod. Fertil. 37*:127-129.

Haddad, G. G., and Mellins, R. B. (1984). Hypoxia and respiratory control in early life. *Annu. Rev. Physiol. 46*:629-643.

Hammer, R. E., Goldman, H., and Mitchell, J. A. (1981). Effects of nicotine on uterine blood flow and intrauterine oxygen tension in the rat. *J. Reprod. Fertil. 63*:163-168.

Harding, P. G. R. (1970). Chronic placental insufficiency. An experimental model. *Am. J. Obstet. Gynecol. 106*:857-864.

Harding, R. (1984). Function of the larynx in the fetus and newborn. *Annu. Rev. Physiol. 46*:645-659.

Hearn, J. P. (1986). The embryo-maternal dialogue during early pregnancy in primates. *J. Reprod. Fertil. 76*:809-819.

Hebbel, R. P., Berger, E. M., and Eaton, J. W. (1980). Effect of increased maternal hemoglobin oxygen affinity on fetal growth in the rat. *Blood 55*:969-974.

Hill, D. E. (1975). Cellular growth of the rhesus monkey placenta. In *Fetal and Postnatal Cellular Growth*. Edited by D. B. Cheek, New York, John Wiley & Sons, pp. 283-288.

Hodson, W. A., ed. (1977). *Development of the Lung. Lung Biology in Health and Disease*, Vol. 6. New York, Marcel Dekker.

Ingalls, T. H., Curley, F. J., and Prindle, R. A. (1952). Experimental production of congenital anomalies. Timing and degree of anoxia as factors causing fetal deaths and congenital anomalies in the mouse. *N. Engl. J. Med. 247*:758-768.

Iversen, O. E., and Farsund, T. (1985). Flow cytometry in the assessment of human placental growth. *Acta Obstet. Gynecol. Scand. 64*:605-607.

Jackson, M. R., Joy, C. F., Mayhew, T. M., and Haas, J. D. (1985). Stereological studies on the true thickness of the villous membrane in human term placentae: A study of placentae from high-altitude pregnancies. *Placenta 6*:249-258.

Jones, C. T., and Nathanielsz, P. W. eds. (1985). *The Physiological Development of the Fetus and Newborn*. London, Academic Press.

Kaufmann, P., Bruns, U., Leiser, R., Luckhardt, M., and Winterhager, E. (1985). The fetal vascularisation of term human placental villi. II. Intermediate and terminal villi. *Anat. Embryol. 173*:203-214.

Kerr, G. R., Campbell, J. A., Helmuth, A. C., and Waisman, H. A. (1971). Growth and development of the fetal rhesus monkey (*Macaca mulatta*). II. Total nitrogen, protein, lipid, glycogen, and water composition of major organs. *Pediatr. Res. 5*:151-158.

Kulhanek, J. F., Meschia, G., Makowski, E. L., and Battaglia, F. C. (1974). Changes in DNA content and urea permeability of the sheep placenta. *Am. J. Physiol. 226*:1257-1263.

Laga, E. M., Driscoll, S. G., and Munro, H. N. (1973). Quantitative studies of human placenta. I. Morphometry. *Biol. Neonate 23*:231-259.

Lanman, J. T., Mitsudo, S. M., Brinson, A. O., and Thau, R. B. (1975). Fetectomy in monkeys (*Macaca mulatta*): Retention of the placenta past normal term. *Biol. Reprod. 12*:522-525.

Lee, M. M. L., and Yeh, M. (1986). Fetal microcirculation of abnormal human placenta. I. Scanning electron microscopy of placental vascular casts from small for gestational age fetus. *Am. J. Obstet. Gynecol. 154*:1133-1139.

Longo, L. D., Power, G. G., and Forster, R. E. II (1969). Placental diffusing capacity for carbon monoxide at varying partial pressures of oxygen. *J. Appl. Physiol. 26*:360-370.

Maas, D. H. A., Storey, B. T., and Mastroianni, L., Jr. (1976). Oxygen tension in the oviduct of the rhesus monkey (*Macaca mulatta*). *Fertil. Steril. 27*: 1312-1317.

Magnusson, C., Einarsson, B., and Nilsson, B. O. (1986). Oxygen consumption by the mouse blastocyst at activation for implantation. *Acta Physiol. Scand. 127*:215-221.

Makinoda, S., and Moll, W. (1986). Deoxyribonucleic acid synthesis in mesometrial arteries of guinea pigs during oestrous cycle, pregnancy and treatment with oestradiol benzoate. *Placenta 7*:189-198.

Mastroianni, L. (1982). Physiological basis for human in vitro fertilization. In *Embryonic Development*, Part B: Cellular Aspects. Edited by M. M. Burger and R. Weber. New York, Alan R. Liss, p. 55-68.

Mastroianni, L., Jr., and Jones, R. (1965). Oxygen tension within the rabbit fallopian tube. *J. Reprod. Fertil. 9*:99-102.

Mayhew, T. M., Jackson, M. R., and Haas, J. D. (1986). Microscopical morphology of the human placenta and its effects on oxygen diffusion: A morphometric model. *Placenta 7*:121-131.

Mayhew, T. M., Joy, C. F., and Haas, J. D. (1984). Structure-function correlation in the human placenta: The morphometric diffusing capacity for oxygen at full term. *J. Anat. 139*:691-708.

McLaren, A. (1982). The embryo. In *Reproduction in Mammals*, 2nd ed. Vol. 2, Embryonic and Fetal Development. Edited by C. R. Austin and R. V. Short. Cambridge, Cambridge University Press, pp. 1-25.

Metcalfe, J., Bartels, H., and Moll, W. (1967). Gas exchange in the pregnant uterus. *Physiol. Rev. 47*:782-838.

Metcalfe, J., Stock, M. K., and Barron, D. H. (1988). Maternal physiology during gestation. In *Physiology of Reproduction*. Edited by E. Knobil and J. D. Neill. New York, Raven Press, pp. 2145-2176.

Mills, R. M., Jr., and Brinster, R. L. (1967). Oxygen consumption of preimplantation mouse embryos. *Exp. Cell Res. 47*:337-344.

Molteni, R. A., Stys, S. J., and Battaglia, F. C. (1978). Relationship of fetal and placental weight in human beings: Fetal/placental weight ratios at various gestational ages and birth weight distributions. *J. Reprod. Med. 21*:327-334.

Moore, K. L. (1977). *The Developing Human*, 2nd ed. Philadelphia, W. B. Saunders.

Murray, R. D., Jones, R. O., Johnson, R., Meschia, G., and Battaglia, F. C. (1985). Uterine and whole body oxygen extractions in the pregnant rabbit under chronic steady-state conditions. *Am. J. Obstet, Gynecol. 152*:709-715.

Ohel, G., Granat, M., Zeevi, D., Golan, A., Wexler, S., David, M. P., and Schenker, J. G. (1987). Advanced ultrasonic placental maturation in twin pregnancies. *Am. J. Obstet. Gynecol. 156*:76-78.

Ortner, A., Zech, H., Humpeler, E., and Mairbaeurl, H. (1983). May high oxygen affinity of maternal hemoglobin cause fetal growth retardation? *Arch. Gynecol. 234*:79-85.

Papaioannou, V. E., and Ebert, K. M. (1986). Development of fertilized embryos transferred to oviducts of immature mice. *J. Reprod. Fertil. 76*:603-608.

Perelman, R. H., Farrell, P. M., Engle, M. J., and Kemnitz, J. W. (1985). Developmental aspects of lung lipids. *Annu. Rev. Physiol. 47*:803-822.

Read, D. J. C., and Henderson-Smart, D. J. (1984). Regulation of breathing in the newborn during different behavioral states. *Annu. Rev. Physiol. 46*: 675-685.

Renfree, M. B. (1982). Implantation and placentation. In *Reproduction in Mammals*, 2nd ed. Vol. 2, Embryonic and Fetal Development. Edited by C. R. Austin and R. V. Short. Cambridge, Cambridge University Press, pp. 26-69.

Rigatto, H. (1984). Control of ventilation in the newborn. *Annu. Rev. Physiol. 46*:661-674.

Roblero, L. S., and Riffo, M. D. (1986). High potassium concentration improves preimplantation development of mouse embryos in vitro. *Fertil. Steril. 45*: 412-416.

Rooney, S. A. (1985). The surfactant system and lung phospholipid biochemistry. *Am. Rev. Respir. Dis. 131*:439-460.

Sands, J., and Dobbing, J. (1985). Continuing growth and development of the third-trimester human placenta. *Placenta 6*:13-22.

Simpson, D. A., and Mitchell, J. A. (1983). Temporal correlation between intrauterine oxygen tension and endometrial H4-lactic dehydrogenase in the guinea pig. In *Oxygen Transport to Tissue IV*. Edited by H. I. Bicher and D. F. Bruley. New York, Plenum Press, pp. 587-591.

Simpson, E. R., and MacDonald, P. C. (1981). Endocrine physiology of the placenta. *Annu. Rev. Physiol. 43*:163-188.

Smith, W. C., and Talamantes, F. (1986). Characterization of the mouse placental epidermal growth factor receptor: Changes in receptor number with day of gestation. *Placenta* 7:511-522.

Soares, M. J. (1987). Developmental changes in the intraplacental distribution of placental lactogen and alkaline phosphatase in the rat. *J. Reprod. Fertil. 79*:93-98.

Stein, Z., and Kline, J. (1983). Smoking, alcohol and reproduction. *Am. J. Public Health 73*:1154-1156.

Teasdale, F. (1985). Histomorphometry of the human placenta in maternal preeclampsia. *Am. J. Obstet. Gynecol. 152*:25-31.

Teasdale, F. (1984). Idiopathic intrauterine growth retardation: Histomorphometry of the human placenta. *Placenta 5*:83-92.

Teasdale, F., and Jean-Jacques, G. (1985). Morphometric evaluation of the microvillous surface enlargement factor in the human placenta from midgestation to term. *Placenta 6*:375-381.

Van der Velde, W. J., Copius Peereboom-Stegeman, J. H. J., Treffers, P. E., and James, J. (1985). Basal lamina thickening in the placentae of smoking mothers. *Placenta 6*:329-340.

Walker, D. W. (1984). Peripheral and central chemoreceptors in the fetus and newborn. *Annu. Rev. Physiol. 46*:687-703.

Weinberg, P. C., Cameron, I. L., Parmley, T., Jeter, J. R., and Pauerstein, C. J. (1970). Gestational age and placental cellular replication. *Obstet. Gynecol. 36*:692-696.

Winick, M., and Noble, A. (1966). Quantitative changes in ribonucleic acids and protein during normal growth of rat placenta. *Nature 212*:34-35.

Winick, M., Coscia, A., and Noble, A. (1967). Cellular growth in human placenta. I. Normal placental growth. *Pediatrics 39*:248-251.

Yochim, J. M., and Mitchell, J. A. (1968). Intrauterine oxygen tension in the rat during progestation: Its possible relation to carbohydrate metabolism and the regulation of nidation. *Endocrinology 83*:706-713.

10

Hemoglobin Structure and Function

ROY E. WEBER*

Odense University
Odense, Denmark

RUFUS M. G. WELLS

University of Auckland
Auckland, New Zealand

I. Introduction and Aims

The transfer of oxygen from the gas exchange surfaces of the gills or lungs to the metabolizing tissues of animals is vital to aerobic life. As expressed by Fick in 1870, the rate of O_2 transfer is the product of the blood flow rate and the difference in O_2 concentrations in arterial and mixed venous blood, i.e., $\dot{V}O_2 = \dot{Q}(CaO_2 - C\bar{v}O_2)$. Hemoglobin (Hb) increases the O_2-carrying capacity of blood (about 40-fold in humans) increasing the efficiency of the energy-costly cardiac output. The Hb molecule is, moreover, exquisitely engineered to optimize the capacitance (i.e., the $CaO_2 - C\bar{v}_2$ difference for a given decrease in PO_2; see β in Fig. 1) through oxygenation-linked binding of allosteric cofactors (i.e., ligands other than O_2 which bind at sites remote from the prosthetic heme group but modulate its affinity through changes in protein conformation).

Hemoglobin bridges wide and independent variations in O_2 tension at the sites of loading and unloading and shows adaptations both to environmental

**Present affiliation*: University of Aarhus, Aarhus, Denmark.

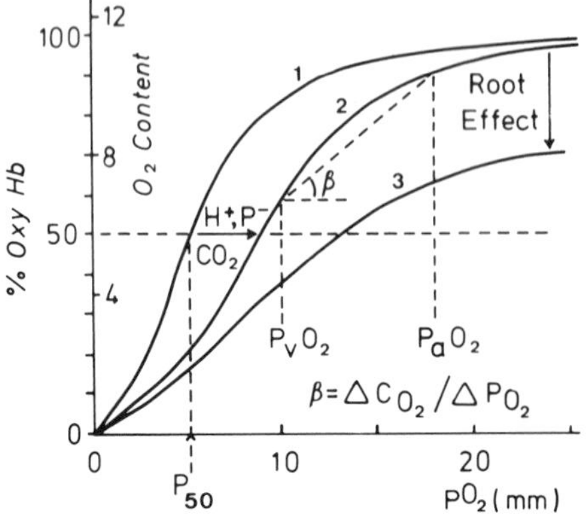

Figure 1a Generalized O_2 equilibrium curve, illustrating half-saturation O_2 tension (P_{50}), the decreases in O_2 affinity (increases in P_{50}) associated with the Bohr effect (H^+), anionic organic phosphate binding (P^-) and CO_2 binding, the Root effect (decreased O_2-carrying capacity at low pH), and the blood O_2 capacitance (β, the fall in blood O_2 content for a given arteriovenous O_2 tension decrease).

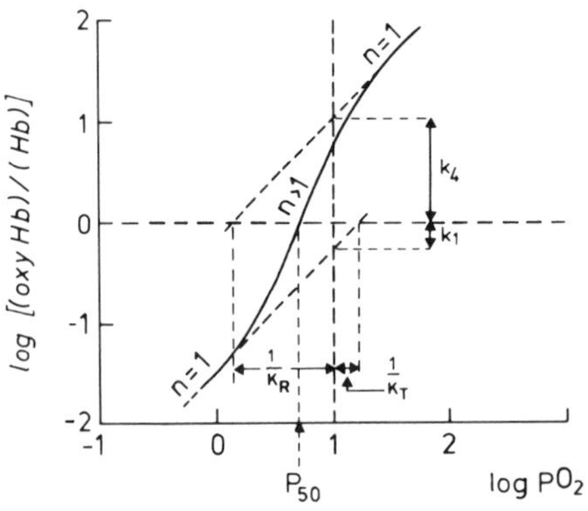

Figure 1b Hill plot of O_2 equilibrium data, illustrating the Hill coefficient, ($n > 1$ reflecting cooperative O_2 binding), and graphical evaluation of KT and KR (the association equilibrium constants for O_2 binding to Hb in the deoxygenated and oxygenated states, respectively) and k_1 and k_4 (the association constants for binding the first and last O_2 molecules to tetrameric Hbs).

conditions and to metabolic requirements, which govern O_2 availability and transport to the tissues. The adaptations may involve quantitative changes (in the total Hb concentration), which will largely be omitted in this review, or qualitative changes (in Hb-O_2-binding properties) and may be inter- or intraspecific. Interspecific adaptations that have evolved during species differentiation are manifested as differences in the structure or the intrinsic oxygenation properties of Hbs from different species. Intraspecific adaptations occur within individual animals and, generally, involve changes in third factors that influence Hb's functional properties within the erythrocytic microenvironment. Stereochemical structural studies of vertebrate hemoglobins indicate that the functionally important species differences have evolved by only a few amino acid substitutions in key positions, whereas most of the substitutions that distinguish species have little if any influence on functional properties (Perutz, 1983).

Most vertebrates have multiple genes that code for several globin types. This results in different "isohemoglobins," the number and proportions of which may vary from species to species. Specific Hbs may also arise during development when embryonic and fetal components are replaced by adult Hbs. Different individuals of the same species (representing subspecific taxa) may, moreover, have alternative Hbs, referred to as *allohemoglobins* or *polymorphism*. Functional heterogeneity of multiple Hbs provides a rich source of material for studies on structure-function relationships in Hbs in particular, and proteins in general.

The best known allosteric interaction is the classic Bohr effect* that first was described as the suppressing effect of CO_2 on blood O_2 affinity (Bohr et al., 1904) and now is known to result from inhibiting, heterotropic interactions between proton and CO_2-binding sites on the one hand, and the O_2-binding heme groups on the other, promoting O_2 delivery to the relatively acid and hypercapnic tissues. The Hb-O_2 affinity is also decreased by chloride and certain erythrocytic organic phosphates, such as 2,3-diphosphoglycerate (DPG), inositol pentaphosphate (IPP), and ATP, that occur commonly in red cells of mammals, birds, and ectothermic vertebrates, respectively, and by bicarbonate that binds to crocodilian Hbs (Benesch and Benesch, 1967; Gillen and Riggs, 1971; Weber et al., 1975a; Bauer et al., 1981; Perutz and Brunori, 1982). In some fish, ATP coexists with other nucleoside triphosphates (NTP), chiefly guanosine triphosphate (GTP). Other factors that may modulate Hb-O_2 affinity are lactate (Guesnon et al., 1979), urea found at high levels in the blood of elasmobranchs and estivating animals (Weber et al., 1983), and nicotinamide dinucleotides (Cashon et al., 1986).

In this chapter we plan to review current concepts about (1) the major structural and functional characteristics of Hbs of different vertebrate taxa (species adaptations), and (2) the major functional adaptations to different environmental conditions, metabolic requirements, and modes of life.

II. Phenomenological Structural and Functional Properties

In reviewing Hb structure-function relationships in Hbs, the human Hb A molecule can conveniently be used as a basis for comparison, without implying that man is the animal kingdom's model of perfection, but because it is the most intensively studied protein whose behavior can be described in terms of the basic stereochemical reactions.

*($\theta = \Delta \log P_{50}/\Delta pH$).

Human Hb is tetrameric, consisting of two α- and two β-chains, each of which carries one heme. Isohemoglobin, Hb A, makes up about 92% of the adult Hb system. The α- and β-chains contain 141 and 146 amino acid residues and seven and eight helical segments, respectively (designated A–H), that are separated by nonhelical segments (AB, BC, etc.) and preceded by and followed by others (NA and HC). Oxygen binding is associated with small changes in the tertiary structure of segments near the heme, and a large shift in quaternary structure, from the T(ense) to the R(elaxed) state, as one $\alpha\beta$ dimer rotates relative to the other (see Perutz, 1983). Heterotropic ligands (such as protons, CO_2, and organic phosphates, which decrease O_2 affinity of vertebrate Hb) bind preferentially to the deoxygenated Hb, forming salt bridges within and between the chains that stabilize the T-structure, lowering its O_2 affinity and resulting in cooperative O_2 binding (see Fig. 1).

Substantial advances have been made in identifying the binding sites of heterotropic factors (Perutz, 1983). For instance, *DPG* binds to seven cationic amino acid residues in the cavity between the β-chains of human Hb, namely Val-1, His-2, and His-143 of both β-chains, and Lys-82 of one β-chain (Fig. 2). In "stripped" (phosphate-free) Hb, *protons* bind to α1-Val and β146-His (which account for about 30 and 40%, respectively, of the alkaline Bohr effect; Kilmartin, 1977), and to β82-Lys. In the presence of organic phosphates, protons also bind to the β2- and β143-His residues. At low pH the latter residue, moreover, contributes to the reversed acid Bohr effect (increase in affinity with proton binding). *Carbon dioxide* undergoes oxygenation-linked binding with the NH_2-terminal α1- and β1-Val (forming carbamino compounds that account for about 7% of CO_2 transport from the tissues to the lungs), whereas *chloride* binds to α1-Val and β82-Lys. Different ligands may thus compete for the same sites.

A. Cyclostomes

The Hbs of these primitive, jawless vertebrates stand apart from those of other vertebrates, in that they are monomeric when oxygenated and contain only one kind of chain. Although this quaternary structure should preclude allosteric and cooperative effects (Bauer et al., 1975; Wells et al., 1986), hagfish Hb exhibits a cooperativity that can be attributed to subunit assembly and decreased affinity when deoxygenated (Briehl, 1963). The influence of factors, such as pH and temperature (but not ATP), on quaternary structure thus provides a unique mechanism for control of Hb function.

B. Fish

Salient features of fish Hbs are that they have NTP (mainly ATP, sometimes GTP, occastionally UTP) as organic phosphate effectors, although some species

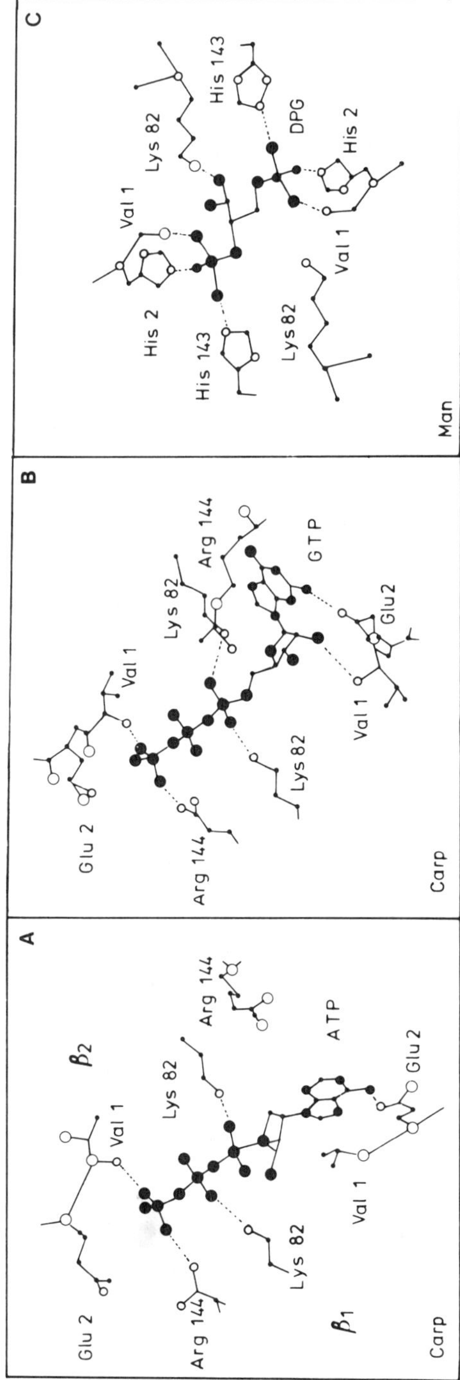

Figure 2 The binding sites of (A) ATP and (B) GTP to carp Hb, and (C) DPG to human Hb. (Modified after Gronenborn et al., 1984, and Arnone, 1972. Permission granted by Academic Press, London, for Figs. 2A and B and by Macmillan Journals Limited for Fig. 2C.)

additionally use DPG or IPP (reviewed by Weber, 1982) and that they may exhibit Root effects. Fish Hbs have either glutamic or aspartic acids at $\beta 2$ and arginine at $\beta 144$, which in deoxygenated Hb creates a constellation of charged groups that is stereochemically complementary to strain-free ATP or GTP (Perutz and Brunori, 1982). The O_2 affinity of eel and carp Hbs is depressed by GTP about twice as much as by ATP, predicting a greater capacity of GTP for hydrogen bonding with the protein than for ATP (Weber et al., 1975, 1976a; Weber and Lykkeboe, 1978). Modeling confirms this, indicating that ATP forms five H bonds with carp Hb (involving β_2 1-Val, β_1 2-Glu, and β_1 144-Arg and with β_{1+2} 82-Lys, whereas GTP will form a unique *additional* bond with β_1 1-Val, when it is rotated about 180° about its long axis compared with ATP (Gronenborn et al., 1984; see also Fig. 2).

The Root effect, which lowers O_2-carrying capacity at low pH, may be considered an enhanced version of the Bohr effect. It is believed to be responsible for the secretion of O_2 into the swim bladder and eye, where the lactic acid level increases by countercurrent concentration in elaborate capillary networks. Recent evidence suggests that simple "salting out" may be the major mechanism for gas secretion in the swim bladder and that CO_2 has a specific effect on the Root effect (Ingerman and Terwilliger, 1982; Bridges et al., 1983). Perutz's molecular model suggests that the Root effect can be explained by the presence of a single residue, $\beta 93$-Ser (cysteine in mammals), which stabilizes the COOH-terminal salt bridges in the T structure, reducing its O_2 association constant K_T. Hemoglobins from deep-sea fish possessing swim bladders have two approximately equal populations of heme groups which may represent α- and β-subunits, respectively, one of which exhibits a Root effect (Noble et al., 1986).

Fish Hbs display striking *multiplicity*. Seventy-seven genera of Amazonian fish examined by Fyhn et al. (1979) showed a mean of 4.0 electrophoretic components per phenotype but no clear correlation between Hb heterogeneity and habitat preference or mode of life. Three major functional categories may be distinguished (Weber et al., 1976b); class I comprises species with single Hbs or multiple Hbs that exhibit similar pH and temperature dependence in their O_2 affinities (e.g., carp, plaice, and flounder); class II comprises multiple Hbs that exhibit significantly mutual differences in functional properties (often electrophoretically anodal components with normal pH and temperature sensitivities and cathodal Hbs with reduced effects, e.g., trout and eel), and class III in which the Hbs show pH effects but no temperature sensitivity (e.g., warm-bodied tuna and some lamnid sharks). The Hbs of class II vary in organic phosphate interaction. In eels the cathodal Hb exhibits a reversed Bohr effect and much greater ATP and GTP sensitivity than in anodal components (Weber et al., 1975, 1976a); in trout, however, the cathodal Hbs lack significant heterotropic phenomena, whereas the anodal Hb IV responds strongly to phosphates and pH (Brunori et al., 1975, Weber et al., 1976c). In the cathodal Hbs of the catfish, *Catostomus clarkii*, which are insensitive to pH and phosphates, the polar amino acids involved in proton and phosphate binding are replaced by neutral ones (Powers, 1972; Perutz, 1983).

C. Amphibians

Hemoglobin polymorphism and multiplicity are both widespread among larval and adult amphibians. Predominantly aquatic amphibians and tadpoles have Hbs of high affinity, cooperativity of $n \sim 2$, and small Bohr and phosphate effects (Boutillier and Toews, 1981; Lima et al., 1985; Weber et al., 1985), despite appreciable concentrations of erythrocytic ATP and DPG (Hazard and Hutchison, 1982).

Stripped amphibian Hbs appear to exhibit a dichotomy, showing normal Bohr effects in adult anurans and reversed ones in anuran tadpoles and premetamorphosed urodeles, such as *Amphiuma*, although the aquatic neotenic salamander, *Necturus*, shows a pronounced ϕ-value of -0.6 (Watt and Riggs, 1975, Bonaventura et al., 1977; Jokumsen and Weber, 1980; Weber et al., 1985). In the tadpole of *Rana catesbeiana* the pH insensitivity is explained by acetylation of the NH_2-terminal α-chain amino acid residues (which account for about 30% of ϕ in humans), and the replacement of residue β94 (that in humans forms an H-bond with β146, which accounts for a further 40% of ϕ) with asparagine, whereas β143-His, which is responsible for the reversed acid Bohr effect, is retained (Maruyama et al., 1980; Watt et al., 1980). The β-chains, however, have the same phosphate-binding sites as humans, whereby a normal Bohr effect is found in the presence of ATP (see Perutz 1983). In the adult bullfrog the β-chains lack an NH_2-terminal segment of six residues, explaining the low phosphate effects (Tam et al., 1986). In *R. temporaria* blood, Hb polymerization is indicated by n-values much greater than 4 (the maximum for tetrameric Hb) at high O_2 saturation (Lykkeboe and Johansen, 1978).

D. Noncrocodilian Reptiles

Detailed structural studies of these Hbs are lacking, although these promise to be rewarding in view of distinctive functional properties and significant degrees of multiplicity. The two major Hbs of the freshwater turtle, *Phrynops hilarii*, exhibit pronounced differences in O_2 affinity and Bohr effects, and only one is sensitive to phosphates and CO_2 effectors (Reischl et al., 1984b). Hemoglobin from *Sphenodon*, the sole survivor of the relict Order Rhynchocephalia, which dominated in the Triassic Period, poses a problem in being almost noncooperative but having a large ATP effect (Wells et al., 1983; Perutz, 1983). Loggerhead and green turtle (*Caretta caretta* and *Chelonia mydas*) Hbs show heterogeneous Hill plots (with n = 1 and insensitivity to pH, CO_2, and phosphates at low saturation but not at high saturation; Lutz and Lapennas, 1982). It is not known whether the structural basis is Hb heterogeneity or a feature of individual components.

The burrowing reptile, *Amphisbaena alba*, the land snake, *Boa constrictor*, and the seasnake, *Pelamis platurus*, exhibit high intrinsic Hb-O_2 affinities, small Bohr factors in the absence of phosphates, and large ATP sensitivities (Schwantes et al., 1976; Johansen et al., 1980a; Weber, unpublished) reflecting a large regulatory capacity for P_{50} in squamate reptiles compared with other vertebrates.

E. Crocodilians

Oxygen affinities of crocodilian Hbs are insensitive to organic phosphates but strongly suppressed by CO_2 (Bauer and Jelkmann, 1977; Grigg and Cairncross, 1980) because of oxygen-linked binding of two bicarbonate ions per Hb tetramer at low pH (Bauer et al., 1981) which raises the blood "carbon dioxide Bohr effect" to more than four times the "fixed acid" value (Weber and White, 1986). Stereochemical considerations show that the binding site is created by the NH_2-terminal β-chain residues (namely, serine in caiman and acetylated alanine in the Nile and Mississippi crocodiles compared with valine in humans), and by the adjacent (β2) amino acid residues (proline, serine, and serine, respectively) that force the crocodilian polypeptide termini to bend toward the bicarbonate ion (Perutz et al., 1981; Perutz, 1983). These β2 differences together with serine at β143 (compared with phosphate-binding histidine in teleosts and humans) explain the loss of phosphate sensitivity.

Crocodilians appear to have only one tetrameric Hb, which may polymerize to octamers (Jelkmann and Bauer, 1980). Polymers and tetramers from *Alligator* do not show significantly different affinities, Bohr and Cl^- effects (Weber, unpublished).

F. Birds

The phosphate effector in bird erythrocytes is IPP which is presumed to bind in the cavity between β-chains (as known for DPG and IHP in human Hb). In chicken Hb this cavity is lined by two basic residues, β135-Arg and β139-His in addition to the four DPG sites retained in humans, except that position 143 now is occupied by arginine, indicating 12 possible IPP attachment points (see Perutz, 1983; Gersonde and Ganguly, 1986). Hemoglobin from the bar-headed goose, which crosses the Himalayas at 9000 m, differs from that of the plain-dwelling grey lag goose by only four amino acid substitutions, one of which (α119-Pro →Ala; Oberthur et al., 1982; Perutz, 1983) is basic to a small increase in intrinsic O_2 affinity, which is greatly amplified in life by IPP interaction (Rollema and Bauer, 1979).

Characteristically birds have two isoHbs, a minor Hb D (also labeled Hb_1) comprising 10 to 40% of the total, and a major Hb A (Hb_2), although some species have only a single component. The two components share the same β-chain, but their α-chains differ significantly in primary structure, causing a slightly higher O_2 affinity and a greater IHP effect in Hb A (see Schnek et al., 1984). The observation that IHP and Hb A increase the solubility of Hb D suggests a novel role for organis phosphates (Baumann et al., 1984) and functionally important interaction between the isoHbs.

G. Mammals

On the basis of Hb properties, mammals can be divided into two categories, a few with low intrinsic O_2 affinity and little or no DPG sensitivity (ruminants, cats, and a lemur), and the majority, in which O_2 affinities are high but strongly decreased by DPG (Bunn, 1971). The different affinities may be attributed to β2 substitutions, with the high-affinity Hbs having hydrophilic residues and the low-affinity Hbs having hydrophobic residues, which stabilize the low-affinity T structure through intramolecular interactions (Perutz and Imai, 1980). In the white rhinoceros the substitution of β2 histidine for glutamic acid nearly abolishes the DPG and CO_2 effects, leaving Cl^- and protons as major effectors controlling O_2 affinity.

The molecular strategies in mammals vary greatly as illustrated by high-altitude ruminants. Llamas have a high blood-O_2 affinity, despite a relatively low intrinsic Hb-O_2 affinity, resulting from substitution of β2 histidine for neutral asparagine, which reduces DPG binding (Bartels et al., 1963; Bauer et al., 1980). High-altitude adaptation thus seems to have evolved at the expense of the reserve of allosteric control. Although *Llama vicugna* and *L. pacos* Hbs share the same β-chains, they have different affinities, demonstrating an influence of the α-chains (Kleinschmidt et al., 1986). In striking contrast to the llama, yak blood O_2 affinity is similar to lowland mammals despite its significantly higher intrinsic Hb-O_2 affinity; yak, moreover, differ from most other mammals in having two or more major adult Hbs as well as two major fetal Hbs, which coexist in calves, exhibiting cascaded O_2 affinities (Bartels et al., 1963; Weber, Lalthantluanga, and Braunitzer, unpublished).

In addition to the normal, high-affinity DPG-binding site between the two β-chains, dromedary Hb appears to have a second, low-affinity DPG site at the NH_2-termini of the α-chains (Amiconi et al., 1985). The biological significance appears to be unknown.

III. Functional Adaptations

Within the frames set by molecular structure (reviewed in Sect. II), Hb function displays remarkable plasticity in adapting to specific environmental conditions, metabolic processes, and modes of life. These adaptations, which primarily involve modification of the conditions under which Hb operates within the erythrocytic microenvironment, will be briefly reviewed in terms of the factors eliciting the responses and the regulatory mechanisms and will be illustrated with selected examples.

A. Hypoxia and Hypercapnia

Ambient O_2 and CO_2 tensions may vary greatly because of organismal respiration and photosynthesis, particulary in aquatic and subterranean habitats, and O_2 tensions also fall with altitude. Hypoxia and hypercapnia are induced internally by the corresponding ambient conditions and also, by inefficient gas exchange and transport as well as factors, such as activity and temperature, that increase aerobic metabolism. The most general response to ambient hypoxia in vertebrates seems to be hyperventilation, which raises Hb-O_2 affinity and O_2 loading through lowered CO_2 tension and increased blood pH.

Aquatic Habitats

Hypoxia

Fish exposed to low ambient O_2 tensions characteristically show decreased erythrocytic concentrations of NTP, which increase Hb-O_2 affinity directly through decreased allosteric interaction and, indirectly, through an altered Donnan distribution of protons across the red cell membranes, resulting in increased red cell pH and O_2 affinity (Wood and Johansen, 1972, 1973; Weber and Lykkeboe, 1978; Soivio et al., 1980). The responses are important in aquatic habitats, where limiting O_2 availability places a premium on O_2 loading.

Where substantial amounts of both NTPs are present, GTP plays a larger role in regulating blood O_2 affinity, freeing ATP for "more primitive" commitments as a vehicle for transfer of bond energy. This follows from a greater effect of GTP on O_2 affinity and the greater concentrational changes seen more generally in GTP than in ATP (Weber et al., 1975a). Accordingly, GTP competes more effectively than does ATP against CO_2 for common binding sites (the NH_2-termini of the β-chains) as demonstrated in Hb of the lungfish, *Protopterus amphibius*, which experiences pronounced hypercapnia during estivation (Fig. 3). Also, the modulator effectivity of GTP is less impeded by the presence of divalent cations, such as Mg^{2+}, despite similar GTP-Mg^{2+} and ATP-Mg^{2+} stability constants (Weber and Lykkeboe, 1978).

Analysis of precise O_2 equilibria of tench Hb (in terms of the Monod-Wyman-Changeux two-state model; see Fig. 1) that encompasses extremely high and low O_2 saturation sheds light on the differential ATP and GTP control mechanisms. Although both autochthonous phosphates decrease O_2 affinity by reducing K_T and delaying the T/R conformation shift at low NTP/Hb ratios and

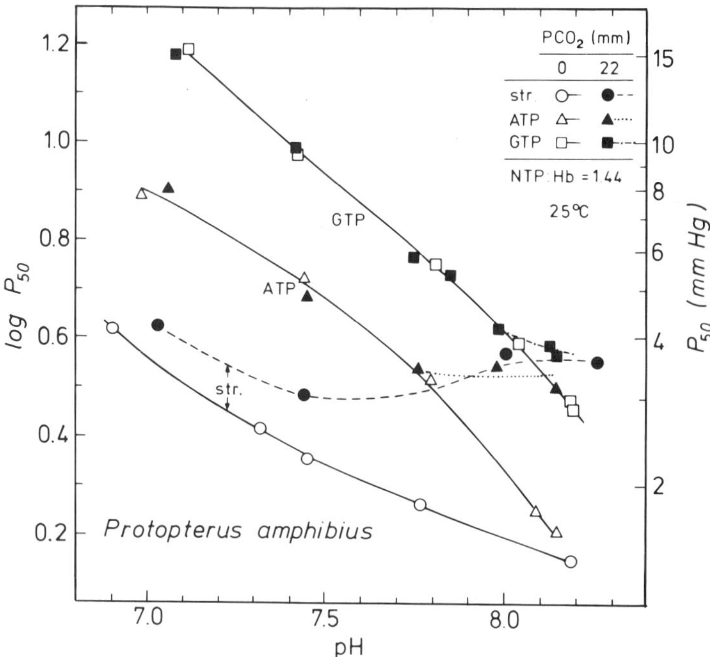

Figure 3 pH dependence of P_{50} values of stripped lungfish (*Protopterus amphibius*) Hb measured at 25°C in TrisCl buffer of constant ionic strength (0.06) in the absence of NTP (open and closed circles) and in the presence of ATP (open and closed triangles) and GTP (open and closed squares) at NTP/Hb tetramer ratios of 1.44 and in the absence (open symbols) and presence (closed symbols) of carbon dioxide at a partial pressure of 22 mm Hg.

by reducing the KR, at high NTP/Hb ratios, GTP exerts a greater effect at both levels (Weber et al., 1987a).

The cellular mechanisms that reduce NTP under hypoxia remain unresolved. That it simply results from decreased oxidative phosphorylation in the erythrocytes is unlikely because killifish and tench erythrocytes incubated in vitro show reduced NTP concentrations only under complete anoxia (Greaney and Powers, 1978; Jensen and Weber, 1985a), which is not achieved in the short transit time of the blood in tissue capillaries. This indicates that other, organismic mechanism may be involved (Tetens and Lykkeboe, 1981). That ATP ⟷ GTP conversion may be implicated in adaptive modulation of allosteric effectivity in vivo follows from the presence of nucleoside diphosphokinases and guanosine monophosphokinases in carp and eel erythrocytes (see Weber, 1982).

Hypoxic acclimation increases the Mg^{2+}/NTP ratio in carp red cells (0.86 compared with 0.52 in normoxia; Weber and Lykkeboe, 1978), which may contribute to decrease NTP modulator capacity through increased Mg^{2+}-NTP complexing. In trout, the Mg^{2+}/NTP ratio similarly appears to decline with increasing acclimation temperature (Houston and Koss, 1984).

Adaptive increases in fish blood O_2 affinity may also be mediated by erythrocyte swelling that tends to reduce the Hb and NTP concentrations (Weber et al., 1976c). Swelling occurs in trout exposed to hypoxia, activity, handling stress, and temperature increase, and appears to be astonishingly rapid (within 10-30 s of stress initiation) and to be under adrenergic control (Soivio and Nikinmaa, 1981; Nikinmaa, 1982). In trout erythrocytes, epinephrine activates a Na^+-in/H^+-out exchange, raising intracellular pH and HCO_3^-; the HCO_3^- is then partly exchanged for extracellular Cl^-. In vitro epinephrine administration additionally decreases ATP in trout red cells (Nikinmaa, 1983). The Na^+-H^+ exchange in fish differs from birds, in which the volume increase is associated with inward Na^+-K^+-Cl^- cotransport (reviewed by Nikinmaa, 1986). In tench, red cell pH shows a strong, inverse dependence on Hb oxygenation above half-saturation (Jensen, 1986). The low red cell-buffering capacity, the large Bohr-Haldane effect (Jensen, 1986), and the uptake-release of most Bohr protons at high O_2 saturations (Weber et al., 1987a) contribute to higher arterial red cell pH values in the hypoxic than in the normoxic tench (Jensen and Weber, 1985b, 1987a).

In the lamprey, *Lampreta fluviatilis*, in which the Hb is insensitive to organic phosphates, blood oxygen affinity increases under hypoxia because of red cell swelling and active cellular pH regulation (Nikinmaa and Weber, 1983; Nikinmaa et al., 1986).

The qualitative nature of the response depends upon the severity of the hypoxic stimulus as evidenced in trout, in which mild hypoxia (PO_2 = 60 mm Hg) results in an increased red cell pH that is partly catecholamine-induced, whereas deep hypoxia (35 mm Hg) decreases the NTP/Hb ratios, and very deep hypoxia (30 mm Hg) results in increased O_2-carrying capacity and acidosis followed by partial pH recovery (Tetens and Lykkeboe, 1985).

Hypercapnia

Hypercapnic water decreases fish blood pH, which, subsequently, is almost completely compensated for by HCO_3^- accumulation (Heisler, 1984). In tench, intraerythrocytic pH decreases transiently under hypoxia-hypercapnia but is then raised to values exceeding the preexposure level, in parallel with red cell swelling, reduced red cell GTP, and recovery of plasma pH, which promote O_2 loading (Jensen and Weber, 1985b).

Carbon dioxide and phosphates bind to uncharged $-NH_2$ and protonated $-NH_3^+$ groups of the Hb chains, respectively, and thus, have opposite influences on the Bohr effect (see Fig. 3). Carbon dioxide has only small effects on fish Hbs (Weber and Lykkeboe, 1978; Farmer et al., 1979), presumably, a result of acetylation of NH_2-termini of the α-chains.

Acid Water

Environmental acidification of freshwater systems may impose stresses on the O_2 transporting functions of blood. A low pH solubilizes soil aluminium, and Al-containing acid water causes branchial secretion of mucus which increases the water-blood diffusion barrier, as indicated by ensuing internal hypoxia (Muniz and Leivestad, 1980; Malte, 1986; Jensen and Weber, 1987a). In tench, in hard water, this induces a selective reduction in GTP and an increase in red cell pH (mainly as a result of a decrease in O_2 saturation above 50%; Jensen and Weber, 1987a).

Isohemoglobins

The occurrence of cathodal Hbs with high, pH-independent O_2 affinities in class II teleosts (see p. 284) may represent a preadaptation that safeguards O_2 transport over a broad range of O_2 tensions and activity-induced blood acidoses. The blood affinity increase seen in eels in hypoxic conditions is largely attributable to the high sensitivity of the cathodal Hbs to GTP (Weber et al., 1976a). That changes in Hb componentry may contribute to intraspecific adaptation follows from the differential effects of hypoxia and temperature on the concentrations of the individual isoHbs of trout (Tun and Houston, 1986).

Water-Air Transitions

Fish

Aquatic animals switching to air breathing owing to anoxic conditions in the water, to droughts, or to metamorphosis, experience significant increases in internal P_{CO_2} resulting from the higher aerial O_2 availability and the reduced ventilation of the gas exchange surfaces. This, however, does not apply to fish that use auxillary organs for O_2 uptake but retain the gills for CO_2 excretion. In the gut-breathing Amazonian teleost, *Plecostomus*, an NTP-induced increase in blood O_2 affinity during facultative air breathing suggests improved O_2 extraction from swallowed air, and blood HCO_3^- concentration is increased to counter the negative effects of the respiratory acidosis on O_2 loading (Weber et al., 1979; Wood et al., 1979).

Air-breathing fish faced with permanently increased O_2 availability frequently appear to have organic phosphates other than ATP (GTP and IPP; see Bartlett, 1978) that exert greater depressant effects on Hb-O_2 affinity. The NTP-correlated increase in blood O_2 affinity seen in the estivating African lungfish, *Protopterus amphibius*, (Johansen et al., 1976a) might not be adaptive to improved O_2 loading as in water breathers but, rather, to a reduction in O_2 unloading and, hence, metabolic rate, enabling the lungfish to tide over year-long periods of suspended animation. The toad, *Xenopus laevis*, when induced to estivate by water deprivation, similarly shows increased blood urea levels that raise Hb-O_2 affinity (Jokumsen and Weber, 1980).

Amphibians

Amphibians illustrate diverse strategies for aquatic-terrestrial transition that may overlap with metamorphic transformation. In the adult salamander, *Dicamptodon ensatus*, the ATP-induced decrease in blood O_2 affinity correlates with the greater O_2 availability and energy demands for activity compared with those of the aquatic neotenes (Wood, 1971). In contrast, the higher NTP, DPG, and IPP concentrations, as well as Hb with a higher Hb-phosphate affinity in the tadpole bullfrog than in the adults (see Hazard and Hutchison, 1978) might reflect a need to preserve regulatory ability in the face of uncertain O_2 availability in the aquatic environment. In bullfrog tadpoles the two isoHbs that are most abundant in earliest development have higher O_2 affinities than the two other components that dominate in later stages (Watt and Riggs, 1975).

The salamanders *Necturus* and *Amphiuma*, and the bullfrog, form a series with decreasing blood O_2 affinities and higher Bohr factors with increasing O_2 availability and the dependence on air as a respiratory medium (Lenfant and Johansen, 1967). Some frogs are known to overwinter at the bottom of ponds, but possible adaptations in the blood apparently have not been investigated.

Diving Reptiles

The concept that large Bohr factors may be adaptive to efficient utilization of O_2 reserves during diving does not hold for snakes, turtles, and lizards (Wood and Lenfant, 1976; Seymour, 1976; Burggren et al., 1977; Palomeque et al., 1977).

The strikingly heterogeneous Hill plots of blood and Hbs from the aquatic green and loggerhead turtles (showing coöperativity and pH, CO_2, and phosphate effects only at high saturations) appear to be well suited to diving by providing efficient O_2 unloading when respiration is aerobic and by conserving O_2 through the diminishing Bohr effect and cooperativity as internal pressures fall (Maginniss et al., 1980; Lutz and Lapennas, 1982). In *Chrysemys picta bellii* submerged for several months at 3°C and a PO_2 of 1-5 mm Hg, blood O_2 approaches zero and lactate increases to 200 mmol (Ultsch and Jackson, 1982).

Terrestrial Habitats

Altitudinal Hypoxia

The Titicaca frog, living at high altitude, has Hb with a high affinity and cooperativity and low Bohr effect, as is typical of aquatic amphibia; its altitude adaptations are a high Hb concentration and a large skin surface area (Hutchison et al., 1976).

Most available data on altitude adaptations in Hb function concern birds and mammals. The key (α119-Pro → Ala) amino acid substitution, which appears basic to the ability of the bar-headed goose to load O_2 at Himalayan altitudes, provides a splendid example of molecular adaptation. That Ruppel's vulture has a considerably lower intrinsic Hb-O_2 affinity than does human Hb A, but it can fly at 11,000 m where O_2 tensions in the vapor-saturated lung air will be below 30 mm Hg, (Heibl, Weber, and Braunitzer, unpublished) poses tantalizing questions concerning the physiological mechanisms of tissue O_2 supply under low O_2 availability and high systemic O_2 demand. Altitude simulations provide possible answers. Pigeons acclimated to 9150 m, show remarkably high blood pH and low P_{CO_2} values (7.85 and 10.6 mm Hg, respectively; Lutz and Schmidt-Nielsen, 1977) both of which will directly favor O_2 loading by allosteric interaction and indirectly by reducing the effect of IPP. Also, when anaerobic energy metabolism may become important, as shown by lactate accumulation, the O_2 supply to the brain may be protected by increased cerebral blood flow (Faraci et al., 1984); O_2 uptake and CO_2 loss in the opthalmic retial heat exchangers, which cool the blood (Bernstein et al., 1984); and by the temperature-dependence of affinity.

Only scanty information appears available for the intraspecific adaptations of bird Hb function at altitude. Pionetti and Bouverot (1977) found that a 3-week sojourn of pigeons at 400 m in an altitude chamber, raised the cellular Hb concentration, without compromising blood P_{50} possibly a result of decreased IPP concentration.

In humans the response to altitude depends upon the severity of the hypoxic stimulus. Sudden subjection to mild hypoxia increases blood DPG concentration and P_{50}, which raises conductance (see Fig. 1) by bringing the steep part of the O_2 equilibrium curve into range with the prevailing arterial-venous P_{O_2} difference. Severe hypoxia, on the other hand, lowers DPG and P_{50}, which again increases capacitance at the lower, in vivo O_2 tensions (see Turek et al., 1973). The latter change is consistent with the finding that artificially increasing the O_2 affinity of rat blood by Hb carbamoylation prevented suffocation at an ambient P_{O_2} of about 45 mm Hg, a pressure at which control animals died (Eaton, 1974).

Rather than modulating the chemical environment of the Hb, sheep overcome altitude acclimation in a unique way, synthesizing high-affinity Hb C (see Maginniss et al., 1986). The fact that Hb C is also formed in severe anemia indicates that tissue hypoxia triggers the response. The inverse relationship in mice between erythrocyte life-span and altitude suggests that adaptational responses include replacement of existing red cells with those that have a higher Hb content, thus increasing O_2 capacity without parallel increases in blood viscosity (Abbrecht and Littel, 1972), and that have isoHbs better suited to prevailing conditions.

Intraspecific adaptations may be genetically coded. Thus, when acclimated to the same altitude, specimens of the deer mouse, *Peromyscus maniculatus*, representing 35 populations and 10 nominal subspecies, reveal an inverse relationship between blood P_{50} and native altitude that, as a rule, persists in their progenies (Snyder et al., 1982).

Hemoglobins from large mammals have higher intrinsic O_2 affinities that contribute to lower metabolic rates (by O_2 delivery at a lower tension, than that of small mammals). This may be advantageous to larg animals at high altitude, and a historical implication is found in Hannibal's successful crossing of the Alps in the year 218 B.C. with the help of elephants (Heibl, 1987).

Burrow and Cave Conditions

Oxygen and CO_2 concentrations in sealed burrows and caves can deviate strongly from those in normal air (attaining 10.0 and 10.8%, respectively, in golden hampster burrows; Kuhnen, 1986).

In the primitive apodan caecilian, high blood and Hb affinities and small Bohr and ATP effects are seen as adaptive to its hypoxic-hypercapnic fossorial habit (Wood et al., 1975). The Hb of the burrowing reptile, *Amphisbaena alba*, has high O_2 affinity combined with high ATP sensitivity (Johansen et al., 1981), indicating a large scope for allosteric modulation to variable ambient O_2 tensions.

Burrowing mammals generally have relatively high blood O_2 affinities that are based on different molecular mechanisms. The African mole rat, *Heterocephalus glaber*, has a high intrinsic Hb-O_2 affinity and high DPG levels (Johansen et al., 1976b). In the mole, *Talpa europea*, and the pangolin, *Manis pentadactyla*, the intrinsic affinities are similar to other animals, but the Hb of the mole shows low DPG sensitivity and no CO_2 effect in the presence of DPG, whereas erythrocytes of the pangolin have low DPG levels (Jelkman et al., 1981; Weber et al., 1986). In the mole rat, *Splanax ehrenbergi*, hypoxic-hypercapnic acclimation reduces the blood DPG/Hb ratio suggesting an adaptive increase in O_2 loading (Ar et al., 1977). Hemoglobin of the bat, *Tadarida braziliensis*, which frequents hypercapnic caves, has a lower intrinsic affinity than does human Hb, that appears compensated for by a smaller CO_2 effect (Kleinschmidt et al., 1987).

B. Temperature

The oxygenation reaction of Hb is exothermic. Evaluated as $R \cdot \Delta \ln P_{50} (1/T_1 - 1/T_2)^{-1}$, where R = the gas constant and T_1 and T_2 = absolute temperatures, the overall heat of reaction (ΔH^{obs}), which reflects the magnitude of the temperature effect, encompasses the intrinsic heat of reaction (ΔH^{intr}), the heat of solution of O_2 ($\Delta H^{sol} = \sim 13\ kJ \cdot mol^{-1}$), and contributions from oxygenation-linked reactions, such as the heats of proton and phosphate displacement.

$$\text{Thus } \Delta H^{obs} = \Delta H^{inter} + \Delta H^{sol} + \sum_A \Delta X^A \cdot \Delta H^A$$

where ΔX^A = the number of effector ions A (protons or anions) displaced and ΔH^A = the heat of displacement (see also Imai, 1982). At high pH where there is no proton binding ($\phi = 0$) and in the absence of other allosteric effectors, ΔH^{intr} approximates -45 to 55 $kJ \cdot mol^{-1}$.

Increasing temperature, however, also decreases O_2 affinity indirectly by the Bohr effect because of the pH decrease associated with maintenance of constant relative alkalinity. In the alligator, in which significant temperature shifts attend basking and submergence, ΔH at the in vivo pH values associated with each temperature is almost twice that at constant pH (-47 and -24 kJ · mol^{-1}, respectively; Weber and White, 1986). The indirect temperature effect may be even greater when based on the intracellular Bohr effect ($\phi_i = \Delta \log P_{50}/\Delta pH_i$) and $\Delta pH_i/\Delta t$ relationship, which may exceed the corresponding values based on whole blood pH (see Wells and Weber, 1985; Reischl et al., 1984b). In *Necturus* Hb, the pH-dependent increase in ΔH reflects a heat of proton dissociation that is intermediate between those for histidine and α-amino acid residues (where most of the Bohr protons bind in humans), and the ATP-induced decrease in ΔH indicates a heat of ATP displacement of + 80 kJ · $(mol\ ATP)^{-1}$ at pH 7.5 (Weber et al., 1985), agreeing well with the value of + 74 kJ obtained by direct measurement on carp Hb at pH 7.55 (Greaney et al., 1980).

Although the reduced O_2 affinity at higher temperatures increases O_2 delivery in parallel with O_2 consumption, it may also hamper O_2 loading, particularly in aquatic environments. Thus, when the ambient temperature increases to 23°C, arterial O_2 content in trout starts to decline and venous blood becomes completely deoxygenated (Heath and Hughes, 1973). Blood temperature sensitivity accordingly is almost zero (ΔH^{obs} = -4kJ · mol^{-1}) in the tree frog, *Chiromantis petersi*, whose preferred body temperature is 40°C (Johansen et al., 1980b). A reduced ΔH^{obs} value is also seen in reptilians experiencing large variations in body temperature, and it may allow reptiles diving into cold water to maintain a low-affinity/high-capacitance equilibrium curve (see Wood and Lenfant, 1976).

The quantitative and qualitative nature of intraspecific thermoacclimatory responses of poikilothermic vertebrates differ, showing no clear relationship to the respiratory medium. Whereas warm acclimation decreases blood P_{50} and NTP in the teleosts brown bullhead, killifish, carp, and Antarctic cod, and in the pancake tortoise (Grigg, 1969; Greaney and Powers, 1978; Wood et al., 1978; Albers et al., 1983), it increases P_{50} in Australian blackfish, European eel, the Antarctic fish, *Pagothenia borchgrevinki*, neotenic *Ambystoma tigrinum* salamanders, and in the snake, *Vipera berus* (Johansen and Lykkeboe, 1979; Dobson and Baldwin, 1982; Wood et al., 1982; Tetens et al., 1984; Laursen et al., 1985). Carp blood O_2 affinity is nearly independent of acclimation temperature despite a pronounced acute temperature effect, owing to decreases both in ATP and in oxy-labile carbamate formation at higher temperatures (Alber et al., 1983).

Hemoglobin also transports heat, because heat absorbed upon deoxygenation in the tissues is released in the lungs or gills. A blood ΔH of -42 kJ · mol^{-1} and the fact that glucose catabolism consumes six O_2 molecules and produces

2885 kJ (see Coates, 1975), accordingly, indicates that 252 kJ, or about 9% of the heat produced is transported by Hb. Tuna and some lamnid sharks that have warm bodies lack a normal temperature effect whereby heat transport is eliminated (or reversed when ΔH is positive). This helps to conserve body heat and prevents premature O_2 release to the venous circulation (Cech et al., 1984) and gas emboly as cold, branchially efferent blood is warmed. That this mechanism does not make an important contribution to body heterothermia is indicated by the fact that the blue marlin is not warm-bodied although its Hb shows temperature-insensitive O_2 binding in the presence of ATP (Weber, Wood, and Daxboeck, unpublished).

Low-temperature effects, such as those found in cathodal teleost Hbs, may protect O_2 loading at high temperature. In bluefin tuna Hb I, the temperature-independence of P_{50} is explained by normal temperature dependence at low saturation, which reverses at high saturation because of endothermic dissociation of a large number of Bohr protons late in the oxygenation process (at the third and fourth oxygenation steps; Ikedo-Saito et al., 1983). In contrast, in trout Hb I, carbon monoxide binding is exothermic at high saturation but endothermic at low saturation because of the endothermic conformational changes conditioned to the subunit in the T-state (Wyman et al., 1977; Fig. 4), and this also is seen for O_2-binding in cutthroat trout Hb F3 (Southard et al., 1986). Although the overall oxygenation reaction is normal in tench Hb, binding of the third O_2 molecule is endothermic in the presence of ATP because of the heat of displacement of the phosphate (Jensen and Weber, 1978b; Fig. 4).

Mammals of low body temperature (TB) show reduced blood temperature effects that favor maintenance of a high tissue O_2 diffusion gradient at low TB, but this does not apply invariably. In the fossorial African and Middle Eastern mole rats and the hibernating hedgehog, $\Delta \log P_{50}/\Delta°C = 0.013, 0.015$, and 0.017, respectively (Clausen and Ersland, 1968; Johansen et al., 1976; Ar et al.,1977), compared with 0.22 in humans and the fossorial Chinese pangolin, which also has low body temperature, and with 0.016 in the pig (Weber et al., 1986; Willford and Hill, 1986).

Thermal acclimation may modulate O_2 transport through alteration in specific Hb components as illustrated by cold and warm acclimated goldfish, which have two and three isoHbs, respectively. This modification also occurs in cell-free conditions suggesting that altered subunit combinations rather than de novo Hb synthesis is involved (Houston, 1980). Thermoacclimatory changes observed in isoHbs, which have no direct effect on O_2 binding (as seen in trout; Weber et al., 1976b), may alter function via changes in the distribution of protons and other charges across the red cell membrane.

C. Activity

Active fish are characterized by large Bohr factors ($\phi = -1.2$ and -1.0 in albacore tuna and blue marlin, respectively; Cech et al., 1984; Dobson et al., 1986),

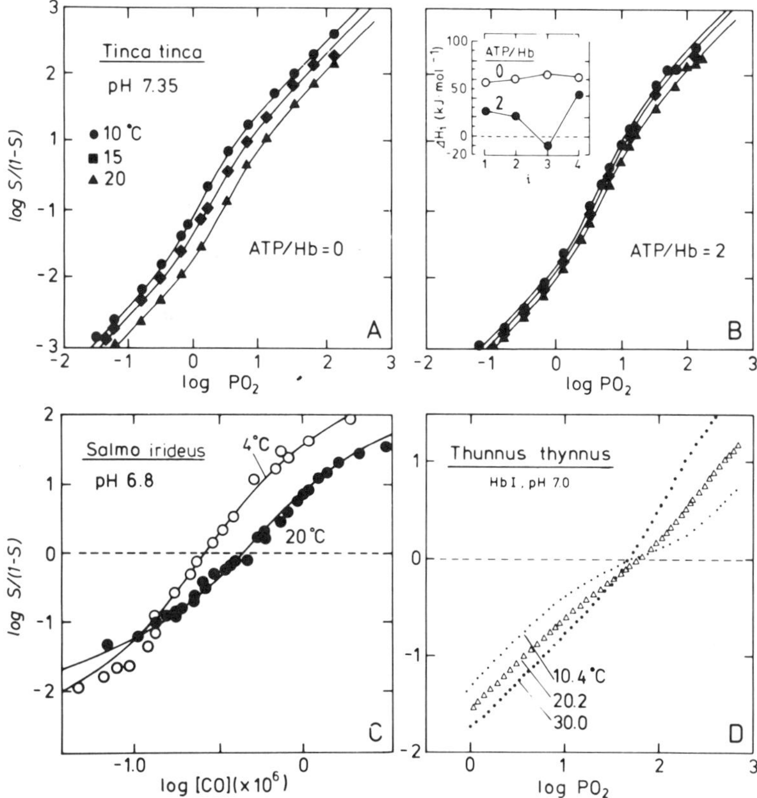

Figure 4 Hill plots of tench Hb at 10, 15, and 20°C, (A) in the absence of ATP, (B) at an ATP/Hb tetramer ratio of 2, and (inset) the heats of oxygenation of the four hemes (i = 1 to 4) in the absence and presence of ATP. Hill plots of (C) trout Hb I, and (D) tuna Hb I, showing opposite temperature effects at high and low ligand saturations. (Modified after Jensen and Weber, 1987b; Wyman et al., 1977; Ikeda-Saito et al., 1983. Permission for reproducing Figs. 4C and D granted by Academic Press, London.)

which may be expected to increase O_2 delivery during activity when tissue pH falls and O_2 demand increases. This concept is, however, complicated by the fact that Hbs with large Bohr factors have high capacities for buffering protons (high Haldane effects). In active fish with a high blood-buffering capacity, large Bohr effects may safeguard O_2 unloading in the face of small changes in blood pH (Dobson et al., 1986).

The release of red cells from the spleen of exercising fish boosts the O_2-carrying capacity (Yamamoto et al., 1980) but may also increase O_2 affinity, given the decrease in red cell NTP during hypoxia and possible hypoxic splenic packing.

In crocodilians, in which slow movements are rapidly punctuated by violent activity during predation and escape, resulting in blood pH values as low as 6.6, the fixed acid Bohr effect is low, limiting O_2 affinity decrease, and lactate production might even favor an increase in affinity by driving off HCO_3^-, which is responsible for the large CO_2 Bohr effect (Grigg and Cairncross, 1980; Weber and White, 1986).

Sustained swimming for up to 200 days does not alter the O_2 affinity or ATP/Hb ratio in trout blood (Davie et al., 1986). In humans, physical training increases blood DPG concentration without decreasing O_2 affinity owing to a concomitant decrease in corpuscular Hb concentration (Shappel et al., 1971). An opposite response is seen in standard-bred racehorses (decreased blood DPG and increased O_2 affinity), which may relate to the release of red cells stored in the spleen at low pH, which stimulates DPG-splitting enzyme activity (Lykkeboe et al., 1977).

D. Adaptations to Vivipary

Internal ontogenetic development requires specific Hb adaptations to secure the transfer of O_2 from the maternal to the embryonic or fetal organism. In mammals, O_2 transfer across the placental membranes is facilitated by higher fetal blood oxygen affinities which, in turn, may be attributable to (1) unique fetal Hbs with higher intrinsic O_2 affinity (as in sheep and goats), or a lower sensitivity to DPG (as in primates); or (2) to lower fetal DPG concentrations (as in dogs, horses, and pigs). The diversity of Hbs that characterize mammalian development, with multiple embryonic Hbs replaced by fetal and adult components, has been reviewed (Brittain and Wells, 1983). The systems of mouse and pig have been characterized in some detail (Purdie et al., 1983; Weber et al., 1987b). In embryonic pigs (Fig. 5) in which five different polypeptide chains form four embryonic Hbs and adult Hb A (see Fig. 5), the earliest Hbs have lowest cooperativities, highest affinities, and lowest Bohr effects, i.e., properties that may compensate for the weak development of anatomical structures for gas exchange. These Hbs are gradually replaced by ones of lower affinity and greater cooperativity and Bohr effects as the gas exchange structures develop and the placental diffusion barriers are reduced.

Lower vertebrates show diverse strategies for maternal–fetal O_2 transfer, reflecting a polyphyletic origin of viviparity. The dogfish, *Squalus acanthias*, has specific fetal Hb and higher O_2 affinity in fetal hemolysates (Manwell, 1963). In the sea perch, *Embiotoca lateralis*, the fetal Hb has a higher intrinsic O_2 affinity, and the fetal red cells additionally have lower NTP and Hb concentrations than in the adult (Ingermann and Terwilliger, 1981). The blenny, *Zoarces viviparus*, which in contrast to sea perches is an ovarian breeder that lacks anatom-

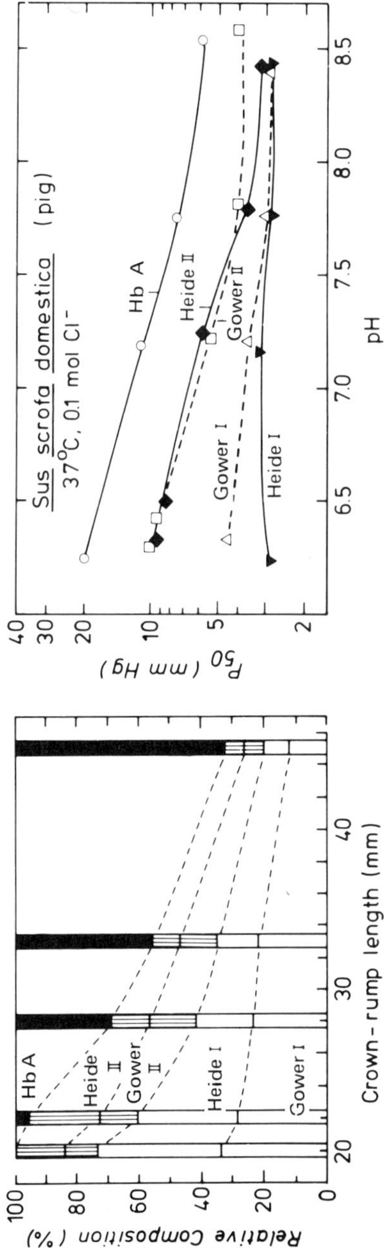

Figure 5 Changes in concentrations of the embryonic Hbs Hb Gower I, Hb Heide I, Hb Gower II and Hb Heide II, and adult Hb A, in early pig embryos (20–50 mm crown–rump length) and the O_2 affinities and Bohr effects of these Hbs. (Data from Weber et al., 1987b.)

ical maternal-fetal connections, exhibits much higher O_2 affinity in fetal than in the adult blood (P_{50} = 9 and 23 mm Hg at pH 7.5 and 10°C) that is specifically due to intrinsic Hb differences, whereas there are no significant differences in NTP concentrations and ATP sensitivity (Weber and Hartvig, 1984). In the apodan amphibian, *Typhlonectes compressicauda*, the skink, *Sphenomorphus quoyii* (which has a well developed placenta), and the snake, *Agkistrodon piscivorous* (which is born within egg membranes), the fetal and maternal Hbs appear to be identical, indicating different phosphate concentrations (Garlick et al., 1979; Grigg and Harlow, 1981; Birchard et al., 1984). Although the Hb systems of the fetal and adult garter snake, *Thamnophis sirtalis*, are electrophoretically distinct, their intrinsic O_2 affinities are the same, and the higher blood affinity in the fetus is attributable to higher metHb concentrations than in the adult (Pough, 1977).

References

Abbrecht, P. H., and Littel, J. D. (1972). Erythrocyte life-span in mice acclimated to different degrees of hypoxia. *J. Appl. Physiol. 32*:443-445.

Albers, C., Goetz, K.-H., and Hughes, G. M. (1983). Effect of acclimation temperatures on intraerythrocytic acid-base balance and nucleoside triphosphates in the carp, *Cyrpinus carpio. Respir. Physiol. 54*:145-149.

Amiconi, G., Bertollini, A., Bellelli, A., Coletta, M., Condo, S. G., and Brunori, M. (1985). Evidence for two oxygen-linked binding sites for polyanions in dromedary hemoglobin. *Eur. J. Biochem. 150*:387-393.

Ar, A., Arielli, R., and Shkolnik, A. (1977). Blood gas properties and function in the fossorial mole rat under normal and hypoxic-hypercapnic atmospheric conditions. *Respir. Physiol. 30*:201-218.

Arnone, A. (1972). X-ray diffraction study of binding of 2,3-diphosphoglycerate to human deoxyhemoglobin. *Nature 237*:146-149.

Bartels, H., Hilpert, P., Barbey, K., Betke, K., Riegel, K., Lang, E. M., and Metcalfe, J. (1963). Respiratory functions of blood of the yak, llama, camel, Dybowski deer, and African elephant. *Am. J. Physiol. 205*:331-336.

Bartlett, G. R. (1978). Water soluble phosphates of red cells. *Can. J. Zool. 56*: 870-877.

Bauer, C., Engels, U., and Paleus, S. (1975). Oxygen binding to haemoglobins of the primitive vertebrate *Myxine glutinosa. Nature 256*:66-68.

Bauer, C., Forster, M., Gros, G., Mosca, A., Perrella, M., Rollema, S., and Vogel, D. (1981). Analysis of bicarbonate binding to crocodilian hemoglobin. *J. Biol. Chem. 256*:8429-8435.

Bauer, C., and Jelkmann, W. (1977). Carbon dioxide governs the oxygen affinity of crocodile blood. *Nature 269*:825-827.

Bauer, C., Rollema, H. S., Till, H. W., and Braunitzer, G. (1980). Phosphate binding by llama and camel hemoglobin. *J. Comp. Physiol. 136*:67-70.

Baumann, R., Goldbach, E., Haller, E.-A., and Wright, P. G. (1984). Organic phosphates increase the solubility of avain haemoglobin D and embryonic chicken haemoglobin. *Biochem. J. 217*:767-771.

Benesch, R., and Benesch, R. E. (1967). The effect of organic phosphates from the human erythrocyte on the allosteric properties of hemoglobin. *Biochem. Biophys. Res. Comm. 26*:162-167.

Bernstein, M. H., Duran, H. L., and Pinshow, B. (1984). Extrapulmonary gas exchange enhances brain oxygen in pigeons. *Science 226*:564-566.

Birchard, G. F., Black, C. P., Schuett, G. W., and Black, V. (1984). Fetal maternal blood respiratory properties of an ovoviviparous snake the cottonmouth, *Agkistrodon piscivorous. J. Exp. Biol. 108*:247-255.

Bohr, C., Hasselbalch, K., and Krogh, A. (1904). Uber einen in biologischer Beziehung wichtigen Einfluss, den die Kohlensaurespannung des Blutes auf desen Sauerstoffbindung. *Skand. Arch. Physiol. 16*:402-412.

Bonaventura, C., Sullivan, B., Bonaventura, J., and Bourne, S. (1977). Anion modulation of the negative Bohr effect of the haemoglobin from a primitive amphibian. *Nature 265*:474-476.

Boutilier, R. G., and Toews, D. P. (1981). Respiratory properties of blood in a strictly aquatic and predominantly skin-breathing urodele, *Cryptobranchus alleganiensis. Respir. Physiol. 46*:161-167.

Bridges, C. R., Hlastala, M. P., Riepl, G., and Scheid, P. (1983). Root effect induced by CO_2 and fixed acid in the blood of the eel, *Anguilla anguilla. Respir. Physiol. 51*:275-286.

Briehl, R. W. (1963). The relation between oxygen equilibrium and aggregation of subunits in lamprey hemoglobin. *J. Biol. Chem. 238*:2361-2366.

Brittain, T., and Wells, R. M. G. (1983). Oxygen transport in early mammalian development: Molecular physiology of embryonic hemoglobins. In *Development of Mammals*, Vol. 5. Edited by M. H. Johnson. Amsterdam. Elsevier Publishing, pp. 135-154.

Brunori, M., Falcioni, G., Fortuna, G., and Giardina, B. (1975). Effect of anions on the oxygen binding properties of the hemoglobin components from trout (*Salmo irideus*). *Arch. Biochem. Biophys. 168*:512-519.

Bunn, H. F. (1971). Differences in the interaction of 2,3-diphosphoglycerate with certain mammalian hemoglobins. *Science 172*:1049-1050.

Burggren, W., Hahn, C. E. W., and Foex, P. (1977). Properties of blood oxygen transport in the turtle *Pseudemys scripta* and the tortoise *Testudo graeca*: Effects of temperature, CO_2 and pH. *Respir. Physiol. 31*:39-50.

Cashon, R., Bonaventura, C., and Bonaventura, J. (1986). The nicotinamide adenine dinucleotides as allosteric effectors of human hemoglobin. *J. Biol. Chem. 261*:12700-12705.

Cech, J. J., Laurs, R. M., and Graham, J. B. (1984). Temperature induced changes in blood gas equilibria in the albacore, *Thunnus alalunga*, a warm-bodied tuna. *J. Exp. Biol. 109*:21-34.

Clausen, G. A., and Ersland, A. (1968). The respiratory properties of the blood of the hibernating hedgehog. *Respir. Physiol. 5*:221-233.

Coates, M. (1975). Hemoglobin function in the vertebrates. An evolutionary model. *J. Mol. Evol. 6*:285-307.

Davie, P. S., Wells, R. M. G., and Tetens, V. (1986). Effects of sustained swimming on rainbow trout muscle structure, blood oxygen transport and lactate dehydrogenase isoenzymes: Evidence for increased aerobic capacity of white muscle. *J. Exp. Zool. 237*:159-171.

Dobson, G. P., and Baldwin, J. (1982). Regulation of blood oxygen affinity in the Australian blackfish *Gadopsis marmoratus*. II. Thermal acclimation. *J. Exp. Biol. 99*:245-254.

Dobson, G. P., Wood, S. C., Daxboeck, C., and Perry, S. F. (1986). Intracellular buffering and oxygen transport in the Pacific blue marlin (*Makaira nigricans*): Adaptations to high-speed swimming. *Physiol. Zool. 59*:150-156.

Eaton, J. D., Skelton, T. D., and Berger, E. (1974). Survival at extreme altitude: Protective effect of increased hemoglobin-oxygen affinity. *Science 183*: 743-745.

Faraci, F. M., Kilgore, D. L., and Fedde, M. R. (1984). Oxygen delivery to the heart and brain during hypoxia: Pekin duck vs. bar-headed goose. *Am. J. Physiol. 247*:R69-R75.

Farmer, M. (1979). The transition from water to air breathing: Effects of CO_2 on hemoglobin function. *Comp. Biochem. Physiol. 62A*:109-114.

Fick, A. (1870). Uber die Messung des Blutquantums in den Herzventrikeln. *Sitzber. Physik. Med. Ges. Würzburg* XVI.

Fyhn, U. E. H., Fyhn, H. J., Davis, B. J., Powers, D. A., Fink, W. L., and Garlick, R. L. (1979). Hemoglobin heterogeneity in Amazonian fishes. *Comp. Physiol. Biochem. 62A*:39-66.

Garlick, R. L., Davis, B. J., Farmer, M., Fyhn, H. J., Fyhn, U. E. H., Noble, R. W., Powers, D. A., Riggs, A. F., and Weber, R. E. (1979). A fetal-maternal shift in the oxygen equilibrium of hemoglobin from the viviparous caecilian, *Typhlonectes compressicaudus. Comp. Biochem. Physiol. 62A*:239-244.

Gillen, R. G., and Riggs, A. (1971). The hemoglobins of a fresh water teleost, *Cichlasoma cyanoguttatum* (Baird and Girard). I. The effects of phosphorylated organic compounds upon the oxygen equilibria. *Comp. Biochem. Physiol. 38B*:585-595.

Gersonde, K., and Ganguly, T. (1986). Inositol phosphates as modulators of oxygen affinity in hemoglogin. In *Phytic Acid: Chemistry and Applications*. Edited by E. Graf. Minneapolis, Pilatus Press, pp. 195-248.

Greaney, G. S., Hobish, M. K., and Powers, D. A. (1980). The effects of temperature and pH on the bonding of ATP to carp (*Cyprinus carpio*) deoxyhemoglobin. *J. Biol. Chem. 255*:445-453.

Greaney, G. S., and Powers, D. A. (1978). Allosteric modifiers of fish hemoglobins: In vitro and in vivo studies of the effect of ambient oxygen and pH on erythrocyte ATP concentrations. *J. Exp. Zool. 203*:339-350.

Grigg, G. C. (1979). Temperature induced changes in the oxygen equilibrium curve of the blood of the brown bulhead *Ictalurus nebulosus. Comp. Biochem. Physiol. 29*:1203-1223.

Grigg, E. C., and Cairncross, M. (1980). Respiratory properties of the blood of *Crocodylus porosus. Respir. Physiol. 41*:367-380.

Grigg, G. C., and Harlow, P. (1981). A fetal-maternal shift of blood oxygen affinity in an Australian viviparous lizard, *Spenomorphus quoyii* (Reptilia, Scincidae). *J. Comp. Physiol. 142*:495-499.

Gronenborn, A. G., Clore, G. M., Brunori, M., Giardina, B., Falcioni, G., and Perutz, M. (1984). Stereochemistry of ATP and GTP bound to fish haemoglobins. *J. Mol. Biol. 178*:731-742.

Guesnon, P., Poyart, C., Bursaux, E., and Bohn, B. (1979). The binding of lactate and chloride ions to human adult hemoglobin. *Respir. Physiol. 38*: 115-129.

Hazard, E. S., and Hutchison, V. H. (1982). Distribution of acid-soluble phosphates in the erythrocytes of selected species of amphibians. *Comp. Biochem. Physiol. 73A*:111-124.

Heath, A. G., and Hughes, G. M. (1973). Cardiovascular and respiratory changes during heat stress in rainbow trout (*Salmo gairdneri*). *J. Exp. Biol. 59*: 323-338.

Heibl, I. (1987). Hannibals Alpenubergang aus molekular-biologisher Sicht. *Naturwiss. Rundsch. 1*:14-15.

Heisler, N. (1984). Acid-base regulation in fishes. In *Fish Physiology*, Vol. XA. New York, Academic Press, pp. 315-401.

Houston, A. H. (1980). Components of the hematological response of fishes to environmental temperature change: A review. In *Environmental Physiology of Fishes*. Edited by A. Ali, New York, Plenum Publishing, pp. 241-298.

Houston, A. H., and Koss, T. F. (1984). Plasma and red cell ionic composition in rainbow trout exposed to progressive temperature increases. *J. Exp. Biol. 110*:53-67.

Hutchison, V. H., Haines, H. B., and Engbretson, G. (1976). Respiratory adaptation in the Lake Titicaca frog, *Telmatobius culeus. Respir. Physiol. 27*: 115-129.

Ikeda-Saito, M., Yonetani, T., and Gibson, Q. H. (1983). Oxygen equilibrium studies on hemoglobin from the bluefin tuna (*Thunnus thynnus*). *J. Mol. Biol. 168*:673-686.

Imai, K. (1982). *Allosteric effects in Hemoglobins.* Cambridge, Cambridge University Press, pp. xvi; 1-275.

Ingerman, R. I., and Terwilliger, R. C. (1981). Intraerythrocytic organic phosphates of fetal and adult seaperch (*Embiotoca lateralis*): Their role in maternal-fetal oxygen transport. *J. Comp. Physiol. 144*:253-259.

Ingermann, R. I., and Terwilliger, R. C. (1982). Presence and possible functional significance of Root effect hemoglobins in fishes lacking functional swim bladders. *J. Exp. Zool. 220*:171-177.

Jelkmann, W., and Bauer, C. (1980). Oxygen binding properties of caiman blood in the absence and presence of carbon dioxide. *Comp. Physiol. Biochem. 65A*:331-336.

Jelkmann, W., Oberthur, W., Kleinschmidt, T., and Braunitzer, G. (1980). Adaptation of hemoglobin function to subterranean life in the mole, *Talpa europea. Respir. Physiol. 46*:7-16.

Jensen, F. B. (1986). Pronounced influence of Hb-O_2 saturation on red cell pH in tench blood in vivo and in vitro. *J. Exp. Zool. 238*:119-124.

Jensen, F. B., and Weber, R. E. (1985a). Kinetics of the acclimational response of tench to combined hypoxia and hypercapnia. I. Respiratory responses. *J. Comp. Physiol. 156B*:197-203.

Jensen, F. B., and Weber, R. E. (1985b). Kinetics of the acclimational response of tench to combined hypoxia and hypercapnia. II. Extra- and intracellular acid-base status in the blood. *J. Comp. Physiol. 156B*:205-211.

Jensen, F. B., and Weber, R. E. (1987a). Internal hypoxia-hyperoxia in tench exposed to aluminium in acid water. Effects on blood gas transport, acid-base status and electrolyte composition in arterial blood. *J. Exp. Biol. 127*:427-442.

Jensen, F. B., and Weber, R. E. (1987b). Thermodynamic analysis of precisely measured oxygen equilibria of tench hemoglobin and their dependence on ATP and protons. *J. Comp. Physiol. 157*:137-143.

Johansen, K., Abe, A. S., and Weber, R. E. (1980a). Respiratory properties of whole blood and hemoglobin from the burrowing reptile, *Amphisbaena alba. J. Exp. Zool. 214*:71-77.

Johansen, K., and Lykkeboe, G. (1979). Thermal acclimation of aerobic metabolism and O_2-Hb binding in the snake, *Vipera berus. J. Comp. Physiol. 130*: 293-300.

Johansen, K., Lykkeboe, G., Kornerup, S., and Maloiy, G. M. O. (1980b). Temperature insensitive O_2 binding in blood of the tree frog *Chiromantis petersi. J. Comp. Physiol. 136*:71-76.

Johansen, K., Lykkeboe, G., Weber, R. E., and Maloiy, G. M. O. (1976a). Respiratory properties of lungfish blood in awake and estivating lungfish, *Protopterus amphibius. Respir. Physiol. 27*:335-345.

Johansen, K., Lykkeboe, G., Weber, R. E., and Maloiy, G. M. O. (1976b). Blood respiratory properties in a mammal of low body temperature, the naked mole rat, *Heterocephalus glaber. Respir. Physiol. 28*:303-314.

Jokumsen, A., and Weber, R. E. (1980). Hemoglobin-oxygen binding properties in the blood of *Xenopus laevis*, with special reference to the influences of estivation and salinity and temperature acclimation. *J. Exp. Biol. 80*:19-37.

Kilmartin, J. V. (1977). The Bohr effect of human hemoglobin. *TIBS* Nov. 1977:247-249.

Kleinschmidt, T., Marz, J., Jurgens, K. D., and Braunitzer, G. (1986). Interaction of allosteric effectors with α-globin chains. The primary structure of two Tylopoda hemoglobins with high oxygen affinity; vicuna (*Lama vicugna*) and alpaca (*Lama pacos*). *Biol; Chem. Hoppe-Seyler 367*:153-160.

Kleinschmidt, T., Rucknagel, P., Weber, R. E., and Braunitzer, G. (1987). The primary structure and functional properties of the hemoglobin from the free-tailed bat *Tadarida brasiliensis* (Chiroptera). Samll effect of carbon dioxide on oxygen affinity. *Biol. Chem. Hoppe-Seyler 368*:681-690.

Kuhnen, G. (1986). O_2 and CO_2 concentrations in burrows of euthermic and hibernating golden hamsters. *Comp. Biochem. Physiol. 84A*:517-522.

Laursen, J. S., Andersen, N. A., and Lykkeboe, G. (1985). Temperature acclimation and oxygen binding properties of blood of the European eel, *Anguilla anguilla. Comp. Biochem. Physiol. 81A*:79-86.

Lenfant, C., and Johansen, K. (1967). Respiratory adaptations in selected amphibians. *Respir. Physiol. 2*:247-260.

Lima, A. A. M., Meirelles, N. C., Airoldi, L. P. S., and Focesi, A. (1985). Allosteric effect of protons and adenosine triphosphate on hemoglobins from aquatic amphibia. *J. Comp. Physiol. 155*:353-355.

Lutz, P. L., and Lapennas, G. N. (1982). Effects of pH, CO_2 and organic phosphates on oxygen affinity of sea turtle hemoglobins. *Respir. Physiol. 48*: 75-87.

Lutz, P., and Schmidt-Nielsen, K. (1977). Effect of simulated altitude on blood gas transport in the pigeon. *Respir. Physiol. 30*:383-388.

Lykkeboe, G., and Johansen, K. (1978). An O_2-Hb "paradox" in frog blood? (n-values exceeding 4.0). *Respir. Physiol. 35*:119-127.

Lykkeboe, G., Schougaard, H., and Johansen, K. (1977). Training and exercise change respiratory properties of blood in racehorses. *Respir. Physiol. 29*: 315-325.

Maginnis, L. A., Olszowka, A. J., and Reeves, R. B. (1986). Oxygen equilibrium curve shape and allohemoglobin interaction in sheep whole blood. *Am. J. Physiol. 250*:R298-R305.

Maginnis, J. B., Song, Y. K., and Reeves, R. B. (1980). Oxygen equilibria of ectotherm blood containing multiple hemoglobins. *Respir. Physiol. 42*: 329-343.

Malte, H. (1986). Effects of aluminium in hard, acid water on metabolic rate, blood gas tensions and ionic status in the rainbow trout. *J. Fish Biol. 29*: 187-198.

Manwell, C. (1968). Fetal and adult hemoglobins in the spiny dogfish *Squalus suckleyi. Arch. Biochem. Biophys. 101*:504-511.

Maruyama, T., Watt, K. W. K., and Riggs, A. (1980). Hemoglobins of the tadpole of the bullfrog, *Rana catesbeiana*. Amino acid sequence of the α chain of a major component. *J. Biol. Chem. 255*:3285-3293.

Muniz, I. P., and Leivestad, H. (1980). Toxic effects of aluminium on the brown trout, *Salmo trutta* L. In *Ecological Impact of Acid Precipitation*. Edited by D. Draplos and A. Tollan. Norway, Johs Grefslie Press, pp. 320-321.

Nikinmaa, M. (1983). Adrenergic regulation of haemoglobin oxygen affinity in rainbow trout red cells. *J. Comp. Physiol. 152*:67-72.

Nikinmaa, M. (1986). Control of red cell pH in teleost fishes. *Ann. Zool. Fennici 23*:223-235.

Nikinmaa, M., Kunnamo-Ojala, T., and Railo, E. (1986). Mechanisms of pH regulation in lamprey (*Lampetra fluviatilis*) red blood cells. *J. Exp. Biol. 122*: 355-367.

Nikinmaa, M., and Weber, R. E. (1983). Hypoxic acclimation in the lamprey, *Lampetra fluviatilis*: Organic and erythrocytic responses. *J. Exp. Biol. 109*:109-119.

Noble, R. W., Kwiatkowski, L. D., De Young, A., Davis, B. J., Haedrich, R. L., Tam, L.-T., and Riggs, A. (1986). Functional properties of hemoglobins from deep-sea fish: correlations with depth distribution and presence of a swimbladder. *Biochim. Biophys. Acta 870*:552-563.

Oberthur, W., Braunitzer, G., and Wurdinger, I. (1982). Hamoglobine, XLVII. Das hamoglobin der Streifengans. Primarstruktur und Physiologie der Atmung, Systematik und Evolution. *Hoppe-Seyler's Z. Physiol. Chem. 363*: 581-590.

Palomeque, J., Sese, P., and Planas, J. (1977). Respiratory properties of the blood of turtles. *Comp. Physiol. Biochem. 57A*:479-483.

Perutz, M. F. (1983). Species adaptation in a protein molecule. *Mol. Biol. Evol. 1*:1-28.

Perutz, M. F., and Brunori, M. (1982). Stereochemistry of cooperative effects in fish and amphibian hemoglobins. *Nature 299*:421-426.

Perutz, M. F., Bauer, C., Gros, G., Leclercq, F., Vandecasserie, C., Schnek, A. G., Braunitzer, G., Friday, A. E., and Joysey, K. A. (1981). Allosteric regulation of crocodilian hemoglobin. *Nature 291*:682-684.

Perutz, M., and Imai, K. (1980). Regulation of oxygen affinity of mammalian haemoglobins. *J. Mol. Biol. 136*:183-191.

Pionetti, J.-M., and Bouverot, P. (1977). Effects of acclimation to altitude on oxygen affinity and organic phosphate concentrations in pigeon blood. *Life Sci. 20*:1207-1212.

Pough, F. H. (1977). Ontogenetic change in molecular and functional properties of blood of garter snakes, *Thamnophilis sirtalis*. *J. Exp. Zool.* *201*:47-56.

Powers, D. A. (1972). Hemoglobin adaptation for fast and slow water habitats in sympatric catastomid fishes. *Science 177*:360-362.

Purdie, A., Wells, R. M. G., and Brittain, T. (1983). Molecular aspects of embryonic mouse haemoglobin ontogeny. *Biochem. J. 215*:377-383.

Reischl, E., Hohn, M., Jaenicke, R., and Bauer, C. (1984a). Bohr effect, electron spin resonance, and subunit dissociation of the hemoglobin components from the turtle *Phrynops hilarii*. *Comp. Biochem. Physiol. 78B*:251-257.

Reischl, E., Jelkmann, W., Gotz, K. H., Albers, C., and Bauer, C. (1984b). Oxygen binding and acid base status of the blood from the freshwater turtle, *Phrynops hilarii*. *Comp. Biochem. Physiol. 78B*:443-446.

Rollema, H. S., and Bauer, C. (1979). The interaction of inositol pentaphosphate with the hemoglobin of the highland and the lowland geese. *J. Biol. Chem. 254*:12038-12043.

Schappel, S. D., Murray, J. A., Bellingham, A. J., Woodson, R. D., Detter, J. C., and Lenfant, C. (1971). Adaptation to exercise: Role of hemoglobin affinity for oxygen and 2,3-diphosphoglycerate. *J. Appl. Physiol. 30*:827-832.

Schnek, A. G., Paul, C., and Leonis, J. (1984). Evolution and adaptation of avian and crocodilian hemoglobins. In *Respiratory Pigments in Animals. Relation Structure-Function*. Edited by J. Lamy, J. P. Truchot, and R. Gilles. Heidelberg, Springer-Verlag, pp. 141-158.

Schwantes, A., Schwantes, M. L., Bonaventura, C., Sullivan, B., and Bonaventura, J. (1976). Hemoglobins of *Boa constrictor amarali*. *Comp. Biochem. Physiol. 54B*:447-450.

Seymour, R. S. (1976). Blood respiratory properties in a sea snake and a land snake. *Austr. J. Zool. 24*:313-320.

Snyder, L. E., Born, S., and Lechner, A. J. (1982). Blood oxygen affinity in high- and low-altitude populations of the deer mouse. *Respir. Physiol. 48*:89-105.

Soivio, A., and Nikinmaa, M. (1981). The swelling of the erythrocytes in relation to the oxygen affinity of the blood in rainbow trout. In *Stress in Fish*. Edited by A. D. Pickering. London, Academic Press, pp. 103-119.

Soivio, A., Nikinmaa, M., and Westman, K. (1980). The blood oxygen binding properties of hypoxic *Salmo gairdneri*. *J. Comp. Physiol. 136*:83-87.

Southard, J. N., Berry, C. R., and Farley, T. M. (1986). Multiple hemoglobins of the cutthroat trout, *Salmo clarki*. *J. Exp. Zool. 239*:7-16.

Tam, L.-L., Gray, G. P., and Riggs, A. F. (1986). The hemoglobins of the bullfrog *Rana catesbeiana*. *J. Biol. Chem. 261*:8290-8294.

Tetens, V., and Lykkeboe, G. (1981). Blood respiratory properties of rainbow trout, *Salmo gairdneri*: Responses to hypoxia acclimation and anoxic incubation of blood in vitro. *J. Comp. Physiol. 145*:117-125.

Tetens, V., and Lykkeboe, G. (1985). Acute exposure of rainbow trout to mild and deep hypoxia: O_2 affinity and O_2 capacitance of arterial blood. *Resp. Physiol. 61*:221-225.

Tetens, V., Wells, R. M. G., and DeVries, A. L. (1984). Antarctic fish blood: Respiratory properties and the effects of thermal acclimation. *J. Exp. Biol. 109*:265-279.

Tun, N., and Houston, A. H. (1986). Temperature, oxygen, photoperiod, and the hemoglobin system of the rainbow trout, *Salmo gairdneri. Can. J. Zool. 64*:1883-1888.

Turek, Z., Kreuzer, F., and Hoofd, L. J. C. (1973). Advantage or disadvantage of a decrease of blood oxygen affinity for tissue oxygen supply at hypoxia. A theoretical study comparing man and rat. *Pflügers Arch. 342*:185-197.

Ultsch, G. R., and Jackson, D. C. (1982). Long-term submergence at 3°C of the turtle *Chrysemys picta bellii*, in normoxic and severely hypoxic water. I. Survival, gas exchange and acid-base status. *J. Exp. Biol. 96*:11-28.

Watt, K. W. K., and Riggs, A. (1975). Hemoglobins of the tadpole of the bullfrog, *Rana catesbiana*. Structure and function of the isolated components. *J. Biol. Chem. 250*:5934-5944.

Watt, K. W. K., Maruyama, T., and Riggs, A. (1980). Hemoglobins of the tadpole of the bullfrog, *Rana cateisbeiana*. Amino acid sequence of the β chain of a major component. *J. Biol. Chem. 255*:3294-3301.

Weber, R. E. (1982). Intraspectific adaptation of hemoglobin function in fish to environmental oxygen availability. In *Exogenous and Endogenous Influences on Metabolic and Neuron Control*, Vol. 1. Biochemistry. Edited by A. D. F. Addink and N. Spronk. Oxford, Pergamon Press, pp. 87-102.

Weber, R. E., and Hartvig, M. (1984). Specific fetal hemoglobin underlies the fetal-maternal difference in blood O_2 affinity in a viviparous teleost. *Mol. Physiol. 6*:27-32.

Weber, R. E., Heath, M. E., and White, F. N. (1986). Oxygen binding functions of blood and hemoglobin from the Chinese pangolin, *Manis pentadactyla*: Possible implications of burrowing and low body temperature. *Respir. Physiol. 64*:103-113.

Weber, R. E., Jensen, F. B., and Cox, R. P. (1987a). Analysis of teleost hemoglobin by Adair and Monod-Wyman-Changeux models. Effects of nucleoside triphosphates and pH on oxygenation of tench hemoglobin. *J. Comp. Physiol. 157*:145-157.

Weber, R. E., Kleinschmidt, T., and Braunitzer, G. (1987b). Embryonic pig hemoglobins Gower I ($\zeta_2\epsilon_2$), Gower II ($\alpha_2\epsilon_2$), Heide I ($\zeta_2\theta_2$) and Heide II ($\alpha_2\theta_2$): Oxygen-binding functions related to structure and embryonic oxygen supply. *Respir. Physiol. 69*:347-357.

Weber, R. E., and Lykkeboe, G. (1978). Respiratory adaptations in carp blood. Influence of hypoxia, red cell organic phosphates, divalent cations and CO_2 on hemoglobin-oxygen affinity. *J. Comp. Physiol. 128*:127-137.

Weber, R. E., Lykkeboe, G., and Johansen, K. (1975). Biochemical aspects of the adaptation of hemoglobin-oxygen affinity in eels to hypoxia. *Life Sci. 17*:1345-1350.

Weber, R. E., Lykkeboe, G., and Johansen, K. (1976a). Physiological properties of eel hemoglobin: Hypoxic acclimation, phosphate effects and multiplicity. *J. Exp. Biol. 64*:75-88.

Weber, R. E., Sullivan, B., Bonaventura, J., and Bonaventura, C. (1976b). The hemoglobin system of the primitive fish *Amia calva*. Isolation and functional characterization of the individual hemoglobin components. *Biochim. Biophys. Acta 434*:18-31.

Weber, R. E., Wells, R. M. G., and Rossetti, J. E. (1983). Allosteric interactions governing oxygen equilibria in the hemoglobin system of the dogfish, *Squalus acanthias. J. Exp. Biol. 103*:109-120.

Weber, R. E., Wells, R. M. G., and Rossetti, J. E. (1985). Adaptations to neoteny in the salamander, *Necturus maculosus*. Blood respiratory properties and interactive effects of pH, temperature and ATP on hemoglobin oxygenation. *Comp. Biochem. Physiol. 80A*:495-501.

Weber, R. E., and White, F. N. (1986). Oxygen binding in alligator blood related to temperature, diving and "alkaline tide." *Am. J. Physiol. Regul. Integrat. Comp. Physiol. 20*:R901-R908.

Weber, R. E., Wood, S. C., and Davis, B. J. (1979). Acclimation to hypoxic water in facultative air-breathing fish: Blood oxygen affinity and allosteric effectors. *Comp. Biochem. Physiol. 62A*:125-129.

Weber, R. E., Wood, S. C., and Lomholt, J. P. (1976c). Temperature acclimation and oxygen-binding properties of blood and multiple haemoglobins of rainbow trout. *J. Exp. Biol. 65*:333-345.

Wells, R. M. G., Forster, M. E., Davison, W., Taylor, H. H., Davie, P. S., and Satchell, G. H. (1986). Blood oxygen transport in free-swimming hagfish, *Eptatretus cirrhatus. J. Exp. Biol. 123*:43-53.

Wells, R. M. G., Tetens, V., and Brittain, T. (1983). Absence of cooperative haemoglobin-oxygen binding in *Sphenodon*, a reptilian relic from the Triassic. *Nature 306*:500-502.

Wells, R. M. G., and Weber, R. E. (1985). Fixed acid and carbon dioxide Bohr effects as functions of hemoglobin-oxygen saturation and intra-erythrocytic pH in the blood of the frog, *Rana temporaria. Pflügers Arch. Eur. J. Physiol. 403*:7-12.

Willford, D. C., and Hill, E. P. (1986). Modest effect of temperature on the porcine oxygen dissociation curve. *Respir. Physiol. 64*:113-123.

Wood, S. C. (1971). Effects of metamorphosis on blood respiratory properties and erythrocyte adenosine triphosphate level of the salamander *Dicamptodon ensatus* (Eschscholtz). *Respir. Physiol. 12*:53-65.

Wood, S. C., Hoyt, R. W., and Burggren, W. W. (1982). Control of hemoglobin function in the salamander, *Ambystoma tigrinum. Mol. Physiol. 2*:263-272.

Wood, S. C., and Johansen, K. (1972). Adaptation to hypoxia by increased HbO_2 affinity and decreased red cell ATP concentration. *Nature 237*: 278-279.

Wood, S. C., and Johansen, K. (1973). Organic phosphate metabolism in nucleated red cells. Influence of hypoxia on eel Hb-O_2 affinity. *Neth. J. Sea Res.* 7:328-338.

Wood, S. C., and Lenfant, C. J. M. (1976). Respiration: Mechanics, control and gas exchange. In *Biology of the Reptilia.* Edited by C. Gans and W. R. Dawson. New York, Academic Press, pp. 225-274.

Wood, S. C., Lykkeboe, G., Johansen, K., Weber, R. E., and Maloiy, G. M. O. (1978). Temperature acclimation in the pancake tortoise *Malacochersus tornieri*: Metabolic rate, blood pH, oxygen affinity and red cell organic phosphates. *Comp. Biochem. Physiol. 59A*:155-160.

Wood, S. C., Weber, R. E., and Davis, B. J. (1979). Effects of air-breathing on acid-base balance in the catfish *Hypostomus* spp. *Comp. Biochem. Physiol. 62A*:185-187.

Wood, S. C., Weber, R. E., Maloiy, G. M. O., and Johansen, K. (1975). Oxygen uptake and blood respiratory properties of the caecilian *Boulengerula taitanus. Respir. Physiol. 24*:355-363.

Wyman, J., Gill, S. J., Noll, L., Giardina, B., Colosimo, A., and Brunori, M. (1977). The balance sheet of a hemoglobin. Thermodynamics of CO binding by hemoglobin trout I. *J.Mol. Biol. 109*:195-205.

Yamamoto, K.-I., Itazawa, Y., and Kobayashi, H. (1980). Supply of erythrocytes into the circulating blood from the spleen of exercised fish. *Comp. Biochem. Physiol. 65A*:5-11.

11

Oxygen Homeostasis in Lower Vertebrates
The Impact of External and Internal Hypoxia

JAMES W. HICKS*

Scripps Institution of Oceanography
University of California at San Diego
La Jolla, California

STEPHEN C. WOOD

Lovelace Medical Foundation
Albuquerque, New Mexico

I. Introduction

Vertebrates meet their long-term energy needs by aerobic metabolism. This dictates a continuous and adequate amount of oxygen. The movement of O_2 from the ambient medium to the tissues and of CO_2 in the reverse direction is maintained through the coordinated interactions of the four transfer processes illustrated in Figure 1. These are (1) ventilation (convection); (2) alveolar gas to pulmonary capillary (diffusion); (3) circulation (convection); and (4) capillaries to the cellular sites of utilization (diffusion).

These transfer processes are taxed when there is an increase in metabolic demand (exercise or temperature) or a reduction in the availability of O_2 (hy-

**Present affiliation*: Creighton University School of Medicine, Omaha, Nebraska.

This work was supported by an NIH Training Grant (HL07212), a grant from the Flinn Foundation, Phoenix, Arizona, and a grant from the National Science Foundation (PCM300472).

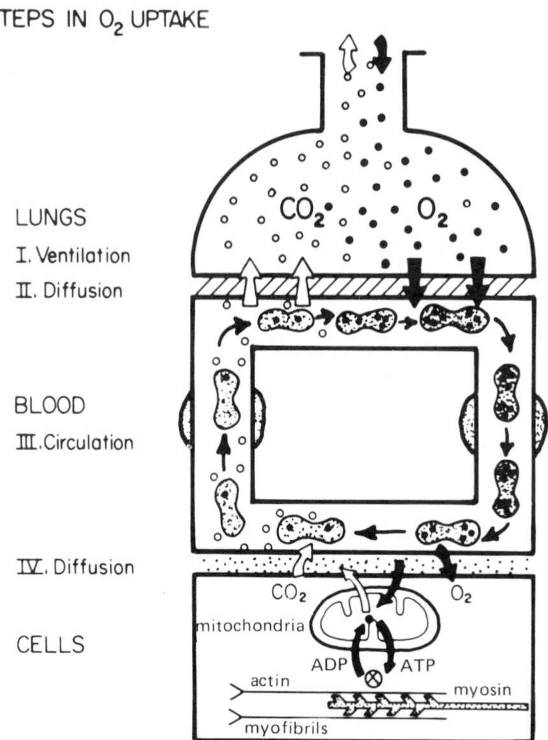

Figure 1 Schematic diagram of the various steps involved in gas exchange. (From Wood, 1981b.)

poxia). Animals may experience periods of reduced O_2 availability resulting from either external hypoxia (lowered alveolar PO_2 because of high altitude or hypoventilation) or internal hypoxia (lowered arterial O_2 content because of anatomical or physiological shunts or a reduced O_2-carrying capacity).

For most ectothermic vertebrates, stress caused by external hypoxia is amplified by the presence of central vascular or intracardiac shunts (internal hypoxia) that also lower arterial saturation. The purpose of this chapter is to provide an integrative account of the interactions of external and internal hypoxia and the resulting impact on O_2 homeostasis. We hope to identify and stimulate areas of future research. We are not comprehensively reviewing adaptations to hypoxia, control of breathing, or heart structure and function.

In addition, we will discuss previous models of O_2 transport in the presence of central vascular or intracardiac shunts and present a new model that describes the impact of differential shunting patterns between the dual aortic arch system present in reptilian vertebrates. These models will provide a framework with which to interpret experimental data by showing the anatomical and hemodynamic basis of the interactions between O_2 affinity and arterial PO_2 in terms of O_2 transport and circulation.

II. The Oxygen Cascade

The simplified diagram in Figure 1 pertains to lung breathing, but the basic principles are the same for all gas exchange organs of vertebrates (Piiper and Scheid, Ch. 13). The transfer rate of O2 ($\dot{M}O_2$) from medium to tissue can be represented by a series of equations (Table 1). At each step, the parameters that define the transfer rate ($\dot{M}O_2$) are determined by a number of variables (see Table 1). Each variable is potentially adjustable in terms of increases in O_2 demand or when O_2 supply is limited.

As O_2 flows from the ambient medium to the cells, a significant drop of PO_2 occurs at the major sites of resistance: ventilation, diffusion across the gas exchanger from medium to blood, circulation, and diffusion into the cells. The drop in PO_2 from the gas exchange surface to mixed pulmonary venous blood is usually not significant unless disease (diffusion impairment) is present or physiological shunting ($\dot{V}/\dot{Q}$ inequalities) is significant. These drops in PO_2 have classically been referred to as the *oxygen cascade* (Otis, 1987).

Table 1 Variables at Each Step in O_2 Transport

Process	Transfer equation	Modifying variables
Lung ventilation	$\dot{M}O_2 = \dot{V}air\ (C_iO_2 - C_eO_2)$	Frequency, tidal volume, dead space
Blood-gas barrier	$\dot{M}O_2 = DL\ (PAO_2 - P_cO_2)$	Surface area, capillary volume, thickness of alveolar wall, hemoglobin concentration
Blood circulation	$\dot{M}O_2 = \dot{V}_b\ (C_aO_2 - C_vO_2)$	Heart rate, stroke volume O_2EC, 2,3-DPG, [Hb], distribution blood flow
Blood-cell barrier	$\dot{M}O_2 = DT\ (PCO_2 - P_tO_2)$	Surface area of muscle cells, mitochondrial density, capillary volume and density, enzyme concentration

In birds and mammals, the circulatory system is normally divided into systemic and pulmonary circuits that are connected in series. The blood leaving the gas exchange organ ("arterialized") represents the O_2 supply to the tissues. Therefore, O_2 homeostasis of "higher" vertebrates is achieved by the matching of ventilation and perfusion in the gas exchange organ and by the distribution of arterialized blood in the peripheral circulation.

In lower vertebrates, the systemic and pulmonary circulations are not complete in series but are also connected by various parallel pathways. Consequently, the definition of arterialized blood and O_2 homeostasis is more complicated. For example, in reptiles the anatomical configuration of the heart results in the potential for differential outputs to both the systemic and pulmonary vasculatures (White, 1976). Systemic venous blood, bypassing the lungs, represents a right-to-left shunt (R–L), while recirculation of oxygenated blood through the lungs is termed a left-to-right shunt (L–R). The mixing of venous and arterial blood has an impact on both the PO_2, through changes in O_2 content and affinity, and on PCO_2 through the Haldane effect. In these vertebrates, the variable and selective distribution of both oxygenated and deoxygenated blood is a major factor in O_2 homeostasis.

III. External Hypoxia

A. Ventilatory Response

Most reptiles rely exclusively on aerial respiration to meet gas exchange requirements. As in most "lower" vertebrates, reptiles are usually periodic breathers in which short periods of active ventilation are interspersed with longer periods of breath holding (Glass and Wood, 1983; Shelton et al., 1986). These periodic patterns in ventilation are reflected in the perfusion of the gas exchange organ, with increased perfusion during ventilation followed by a decreased perfusion during apnea (Johansen and Burggren, 1980).

The ventilatory response to hypoxia has been reviewed in detail (Glass and Wood, 1983; Shelton et al., 1986; Jackson, Chap. 20). In general, exposure to aerial hypoxia results in increased ventilation, with the threshold inspired PO_2 (PIO_2) depending on species and body temperature (Table 2). Glass et al. (1983) studied the hypoxic ventilatory response of the turtle, *Chrysemys picta belli* as a function of body temperature. When the critical arterial PO_2 was plotted on the appropriate in vivo O_2 dissociation curve, it appeared that the ventilatory response occurred at roughly the same saturation (about 50%). The mechanism of this phenomenon remains to be determined. However, the sensitivity of the ventilatory system to arterial saturation observed in reptiles may also occur in fish, (Randall, 1982) and has been suggested in mammals (Lahiri and Gelfand, 1981). Although the ventilatory response to hypoxia is well docu-

Table 2 The Impact of Temperature on Critical Inspired PO_2 in Reptiles

Species	Temp (°C)	Critical inspired PO_2 (mm Hg)	Ref.
Turtle			
Chrysemys picata	11	12	
	20	16	Glass et al. (1983)
	30	32	
Pseudemys scripta	10	23	
	20	ca. 50	Jackson (1973)
	30	71	
Lizards			
Ctenosaura pectinata	25	39	
	30	52	Dupre et al. (1984)
	35	66	
Sauromalus obesus	30	15	
	35	38	Boyer (1967)
	40	72	

mented for reptiles, the distribution of systemic and venous blood into pulmonary and systemic circuits (e.g., shunt levels) in response to hypoxia remains relatively unknown and provides a worthwhile area of investigation.

B. Metabolic Depression and Temperature Regulation

Depression of metabolic demand may be one of the most potent of the numerous physiological and biochemical "strategies" of adaptation to hypoxia (Hochachka and Dunn, 1983; Hochachka, Chap. 2). Metabolic depression has been documented in a number of invertebrates and vertebrates, but the biochemical mechanism(s) of this response remains uncertain. A potential mechanism to lower metabolic demands is through the Q_{10} effect, whereby a decrease of body temperature results in a reduction of metabolic rate (for a Q_{10} of 2.5, the depression of metabolic rate is about 11%/°C). For example, survival of near-drownings in children submerged up to 45 min has been attributed to metabolic depression caused by a decrease in body temperature (Siebke et al., 1975).

Most ectotherms exist in a thermal mosaic. They manipulate this mosaic through both behavioral and physiological mechanisms to achieve and maintain body temperatures different from ambient. When provided with a thermal choice, ectotherms spend most of the time at a single temperature or range of

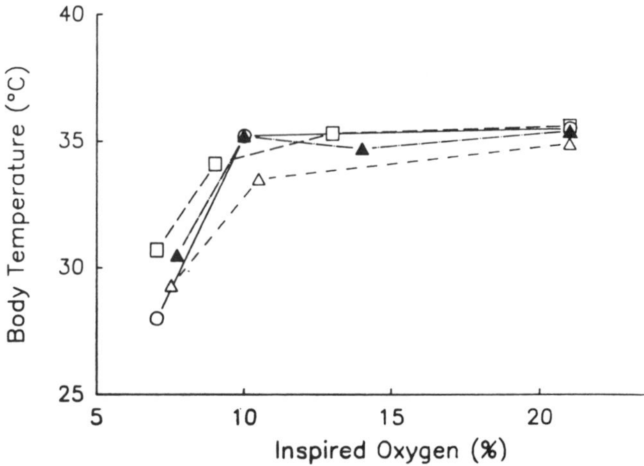

Figure 2 The impact of inspired oxygen on preferred body temperature in four species of lizards. Open circle, *Iguana iguana*; open triangle, *Varanus exanthematicus*; closed triangle, *Ctenosauria pectinata*; open square, *Varanus varius*. (Data from Hicks and Wood, 1985.)

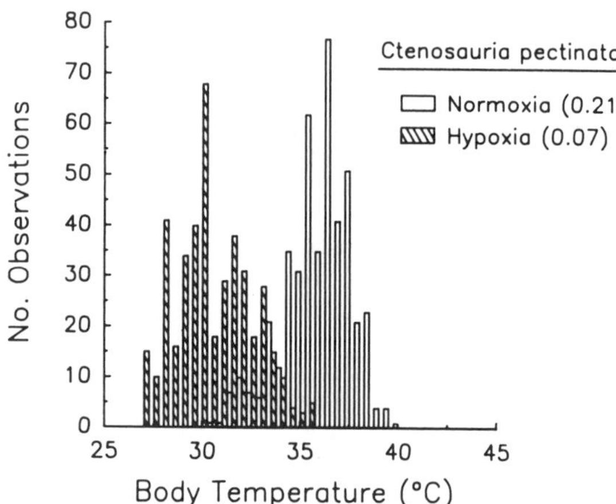

Figure 3 The impact of hypoxia (FIO_2 = 0.07) on the distribution of body temperatures in a linear thermal gradient in the lizard *C. pectinata*. (Data from Hicks, 1984.)

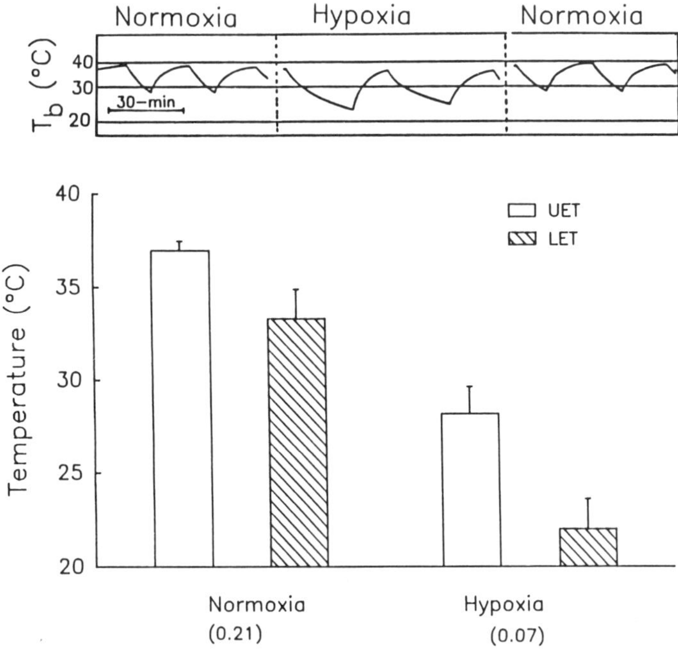

Figure 4 Upper panel; shuttling in the green iguana, *I. iguana* during normoxia, exposure to hypoxia, and return to normoxia. Lower panel; summary of changes in upper exit temperature (UET) and lower exit temperature (LET) during normoxia and hypoxia in *I. iguana*. (Data from Hicks, 1984; Hicks and Wood, 1985.)

temperatures, often referred to as *preferred* or *mean selected* body temperature (Tb) (Pough and Gans, 1982).

An analysis of O_2 transport in lower vertebrates led to the hypothesis that ectotherms challenged with hypoxia would behaviorally lower their preferred temperature (Wood, 1984). Experimental confirmation of this hypothesis was subsequently obtained for various species. Hicks and Woods (1985) observed that exposure to hypoxic gas mixtures resulted in significant reductions in the preferred body temperature of four species of lizards (Fig. 2). As shown in Figure 2, the thermoregulatory response to hypoxia was not graded by exhibited a threshold between 7 and 10% O_2. During hypoxic exposure, lizards exhibited two basic patterns of behavior responses. Common to both patterns was the avoidance of the warmer sections of the thermal gradient within 5 to 15 min folllwing hypoxic exposure. Following this initial response animals would either tend to exhibit little variation in body temperature or would continue to select a broad range of body temperatures lower than prehypoxic levels (Fig. 3).

Table 3 The Impact of External Hypoxia on Preferred Body Temperature in Ectotherms

Species	Selected T_b	Selected T_b	Ref.
Crustacean			
Procambarus	22.1	17.6	Dupre et al. (1985)
Fish			
Carassius auratus	23.0	20.9	Dupre et al. (1985)
Amphibian			
Ambystoma tigrinum	18.8	16.2	Dupre et al. (1985)
Reptile			
Iguana iguana	35.4	28.1	Hicks and Wood (1985)
Ctenosaura pectinata	35.5	30.6	Hicks and Wood (1985)
Varanus exanthematicus	34.9	29.2	Hicks and Wood (1985)
V. varius	35.6	30.6	Hicks and Wood (1985)

Another index of thermoregulatory behavior in ectotherms is *shuttling*. Lizards shuttle between two thermal environments when forced to select temperatures above or below their normal preferred range (Heath, 1970). The temperature at which the animal exits the warm environment is the upper exit temperature (UET). The temperature at which the animal leaves the cool environment is the lower exit temperature (LET). In *Iguana*, hypoxic levels of 7% O_2 resulted in reductions of the UET from 37° to 33.6°C and the LET decreased from 28° to 22°C (Fig. 4). Similar results have also been observed in *Ctenosaura* and *Varanus* (Hicks, 1984).

Reptiles have the physiological capacity to control the rate of change of body temperature during constant environmental conditions. This results in a hysteresis in the rates of heating and cooling, with heating rates being faster than cooling rates (Bartholomew, 1982). Healing and cooling rates in *Iguana* and *C. pectinata* were also influenced by hypoxia, so that rates of heating and cooling no longer differed. Restrictions of appendage blood flow produces similar results in heating and cooling in the American alligator (Turner and Tracy, 1983), suggesting that hypoxia produces peripheral vascular constriction.

Recent data from a variety of animals (both invertebrate and vertebrates) indicate that the behavioral reduction of body temperature may be a general response to hypoxia among ectotherms (Table 3). However, the stimulus that triggers the behavioral hypothermia is not yet known. Acute exposure to external hypoxia reduces both PO_2 and O_2 content of arterial blood. However, a reduction in preferred temperature is also observed during anemic hypoxia (reduction in hematocrit (Hct) with normal arterial PO_2). Hicks and Wood (1985) reported that a 50% reduction in Hct resulted in a 4 to 8°C decrease in the preferred body temperature of *Iguana iguana, Ctenosaura pectinata*, and *Varanus exanthematicus*. Additional experiments showed that body temperatures return to control values following reinfusion of red blood cells (Fig. 5). The absence of a graded response to inspired PO_2 makes it difficult to differentiate between hypoxia per se and the consequences of hypoxia, i.e., transient acid-base disturbances resulting from lactic acid production or hyperventilation.

For endotherms, hypoxia may induce a decrease in metabolic heat production that promotes the associated hypothermia (Hill, 1959; Horstman and Banderet, 1977). Therefore, it is often assumed that the hypoxic hypothermia results from diminished capacity of the thermoregulatory system (Moore, 1959). An alternative explanation is that hypoxia, or the consequences of hypoxia, promotes a resetting of the thermal regulatory set-point(s) (Hicks, 1984; Dupre et al., 1986). A reduction in thermal set-points is supported by the shuttling experiments in lizards (Hicks and Wood, 1985). Additionally, a common index of thermal set-points is the temperature at which evaporative cooling mechanisms, such as panting or sweating, are initiated. Dupre et al. (1986) have reported in both the basilisk, *Basiliscus vittatus* and the green iguana, *I. iguana*, a reduction in both skin and core temperatures at the onset of gaping (an evaporative cooling mechanism) with exposure to 7% O_2 (Fig. 6).

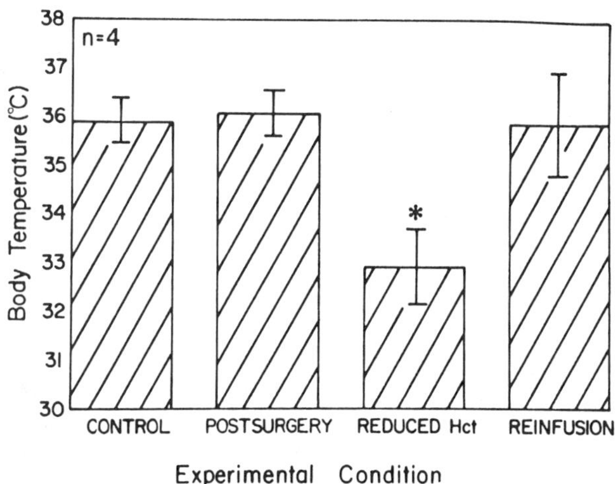

Figure 5 The effects of anemic hypoxia followed by reinfusion of packed RBCs on mean body temperature of *Varanus exanthematicus* in a linear thermal gradient. (Data from Hicks, 1984.)

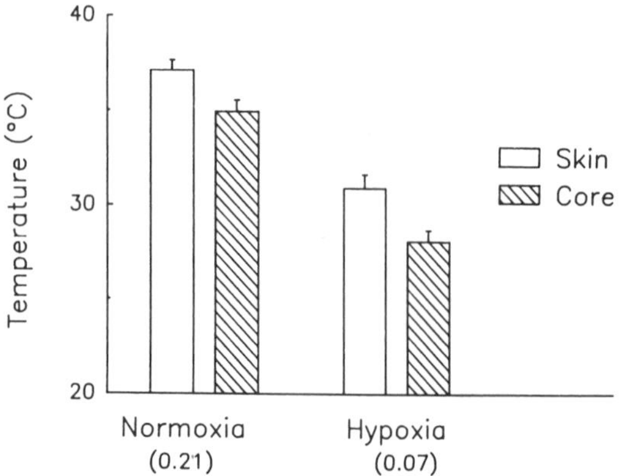

Figure 6. The impact of hypoxia on the gaping threshold in *B. vittatus*. Gaping threshold is defined as the temperature required to elicit the gaping thermoregulatory behavior (evaporative cooling mechanism; see text). Note both skin and core temperatures at which gaping occurs decreased with hypoxia. (Data from Dupre et al., 1986.)

The concept of changes in thermal set-point(s) is not novel. Indeed, a corollary to the hypoxic thermal response would be the well-documented response of fever, which is an elevated thermoregulatory set-point occurring in all vertebrates yet studied. The fever occurs in response to infection with appropriate pathogens and has several adaptive advantages (Kluger, 1979). It is not surprising that nonthermal inputs have a dramatic influence on thermoregulatory behavior in ectotherms. Environmental conditions, such as the presence of predators or competitors and availability of sunlight, may alter set-points or cause the animal to abandon thermoregulation altogether (Huey, 1982). In addition, various physiological cues, such as reproductive state or hydration state, may influence thermoregulatory behavior (Garrick, 1974; Dupre and Crawford, 1985).

The lowering of body temperature during hypoxic exposure is an adaptive response. As mentioned earlier, the thermal sensitivity of metabolism is described by the temperature coefficient (Q_{10}) or change in metabolic rate per 10°C change in temperature (Prosser, 1973). The general formula for Q_{10} is

$$Q_{10} = (k_1/k_2)^{10/(t_1 - t_2)} \tag{1}$$

where k_1[1] and k_2 are the metabolic rates at temperatures t_1 and t_2, respectively. For most ectotherms, the Q_{10} of metabolism ranges from 1.5 to 3.0 (Bennett and Dawson, 1976). Obviously, any lowering of body temperature will have a positive impact on the tolerance to hypoxia by reducing metabolic demands. For example, assuming a Q_{10} of 2, a reduction in body temperature of 5°C would produce a 50% reduction in O_2 demand.

An additional benefit of hypothermia during hypoxia is a decreased reliance on anaerobiosis. The maintenance of aerobic metabolism during progressive

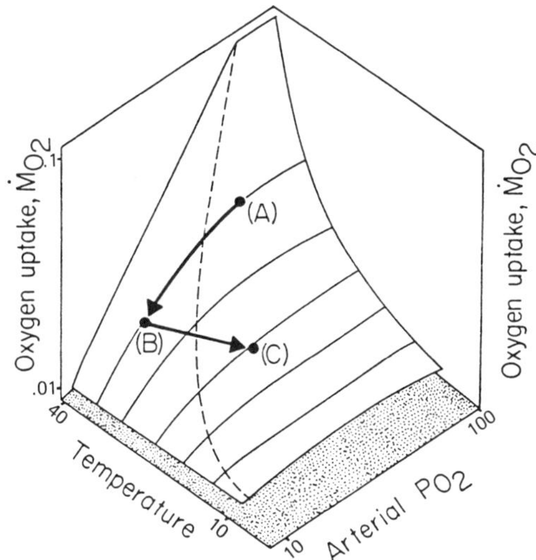

Figure 7 Three-dimensional plot of O_2 uptake ($\dot{M}O_2$) as a function of temperature and arterial O_2 tension (PaO_2). The dashed line represents the critical PO_2. Solid arrows connecting points (A), (B), and (C) represent the response of ectotherms during exposure to hypoxic conditions (see text for discussion). (From Hicks, 1984.)

hypoxia requires a sufficient driving pressure for diffusion of O_2. As PO_2 decreases below a critical value, the rate of oxidative metabolism decreases and lactic acid is generated. The PO_2 value at which the normal rate of oxidative metabolism cannot be maintained is termed the *critical* PO_2. Among ectotherms, the critical PO_2 may be directly correlated with the O_2 affinity (P_{50}) of blood (Wood and Hicks, 1985), for both inter- and intraspecies comparisons. The reduction in critical PO_2 during hypothermia is evident within the context of Fick's law of diffusion.

$$\dot{M}O_2 = D \times (\text{Pcap } O_2 - \text{Pcell } O_2) \qquad (2)$$

where a lower O_2 requirement during hypothermia requires a lower driving pressure for the diffusion of O_2 into the tissues. A reduction in critical PO_2 with a lowering of body temperature has been observed in fish (Fry and Hart, 1948), turtles (Glass et al., 1983; White and Somero, 1982), dogs (Warley and Gutierrez, 1984), and pigs (Willford et al., 1986).

The physiological consequences of lowering body temperature in response to hypoxia are summarized graphically in Figure 7, a three-dimensional representation of the effects of arterial O_2 tension (x axis), on metabolic rate ($\dot{M}O_2$, y axis) at different body temperatures (z axis). At each temperature, there is a curve (solid line) that describes the influence of progressive hypoxia on metabolic rate. The inflection point of each one of these curves represents the critical PO_2 (P_cO_2) and are connected by the dashed line. Point A represents the O_2 uptake and the corresponding arterial O_2 tension at the preferred body temperature. As the animal experiences progressive levels of hypoxia, the critical PO_2 will eventually be reached, at which point the O_2 uptake will decrease (bold line A–B). If the animal maintains its preferred temperature at the same level, its ATP requirements will have to be met through anaerobic pathways. At this point, the animal has a number of physiological options: (1) increase ventilation, (2) optimize ventilation-perfusion matching, (3) increase cardiac output, (4) decrease the level of R–L shunt and possibly increase L–R shunt, (5) redistribute blood in the periphery, and (6) rely heavily on anaerobic pathways. Ectotherms lower their preferred temperature (bold line B-C), resulting in the following potential physiological benefits: (1) raising the arterial content by left-shifting the O_2EC, (2) decreasing the overall energy requirements by the Q_{10} effect, and (3) decreasing the critical PO_2 and the reliance on anaerobic pathways.

C. Biological Relevance

It is clear that the thermoregulatory responses to hypoxia occur at PO_2 levels not normally experienced in nature, prompting the question: Is this response biologically relevant? Various studies have reported significant decreases in mean selected temperature, panting threshold, and critical thermal maximum with altitude in both amphibians and reptiles (Bradford, 1984; Hertz, 1979; Hertz and Huey, 1981; Hertz et al., 1979). However, no general patterns of altitudinal differences in thermoregulation can presently be made (Huey, 1982).

The decrease in body temperature with anemia may have adaptive importance. A variety of parasitic infestations may affect reptilian red blood cells (Saint-Girons, 1970). For example, 25% of the natural population of the western fence lizard, *Sceloporus occidentalis* is parasitized by *Plasmodium mexicanum* (Schall et al., 1982). Such animals are anemic in that 1 to 30% of the RBCs are immature, and blood hemoglobin concentrations are decreased by 25%. It would be of interest to study the thermal biology of these animals in response to their parasitic infestation. Finally, the biological relevance of this response must be put into a broader phylogenetic context. First, what is relevant or significant is "flavored" by our present day stable environment. However, over geologic time the environment has been extremely variable. Evidence suggests that the Devonian (the period in which lung breathing began to appear) was associated with extreme hypoxic conditions. On the basis of analysis of phytoplanktonic fossil records and by using variations in abundance, distribution, and diversification through geologic time, Tappan (1967) has suggested that Devonian O_2 levels were only 10% of present day levels. Viewed in these terms, a lowering of thermal set-points may have been very important in terms of survivability during this period. Second, the area generally thought to be involved in integration of thermal information is the hypothalamus, which is a phylogenetically conservative area of the vertebrate brain (Bligh, 1973; Kluger, 1979).

Hypoxic mammals become hypothermic, but this has usually been conceived as a failure of the thermoregulatory system. Recent data suggest that the thermoregulatory centers in the mammalian brain also respond to hypoxia in a controlled manner. In a heterothermic mammal (ground squirrel) a reduction of set-point for temperature regulation occurs during hypoxia (Wood et al., 1985). In this study, exposure to hypoxia (10% O_2) reduced body temperature by 6°C. When inspired O_2 was returned to 21%, the animals immediately began to shiver and body temperature increased. Additionally, Dupre et al. (1987) have reported that exposure to 10% O_2 results in both a broadening and a reduction of the upper and lower critical temperatures of the thermoneutral zone of Wistar rats. Is an hypoxic-induced reduction in thermal set-points relevant for man? For example, in neonates, congenital heart malformations combined with pulmonary distress can result in severe hypoxemia. Under these conditions, are the thermal set-points lowered? Would there be a decrease in mortality if the body temperature were allowed to decrease? Clearly, many more detailed experiments into the thermal biology of all vertebrates are required before answers to such questions are provided.

IV. Internal Hypoxia

A. Cardiovascular Anatomy and Shunts

A detailed description of the anatomy and function of the reptilian heart is beyond the scope of this chapter but has been reviewed elsewhere (White, 1976; Johansen and Burggren, 1980; Burggren, 1985; Van Mierop and Kutsche, 1985). Nonetheless, before addressing the impact of intracardiac shunts on O_2 homeostasis, a general review of heart structure and function is required. Basically, the noncrocodilian heart consists of two atrial chambers and a ventricle which is subdivided into three anatomically interconnected cava. A distinctive feature of the reptilian ventricular anatomy is the presence of a septumlike structure, often referred to as the horizontal septum or *Muskelleiste*, which develops from the ventral wall of the ventricle. This septum divides the ventricle into a smaller cavum pulmonale and larger cavum dorsale. An incomplete vertical septum within the cavum dorsale further subdivides this cavity into cavum arteriosum and cavum venosum. The pulmonary artery originates from the cavum pulmonale and the right aortic (RA_O) and left aortic (LA_O) arches arise from the cavum venosum. In chelonians, a third systemic arch (brachiocephalic) has been reported emerging from the cavum venosum (Shelton and Burggren, 1976; Burggren, 1985). However, in most studies of the reptilian cardiovascular system (Griel, 1903; O'Donoghue, 1918; Goodrich, 1916, 1919; Rau, 1924; Mathur, 1946; Khalil and Zaki, 1964; White, 1959, 1968; Van Mierop and Kutsche, 1985) a third systemic arch emerging separately from the ventricle has never been reported. A third systemic arch probably depicts a rare condition that is not representative of the general anatomical design.

Observations of the reptilian heart led anatomists (Goodrich, 1919; Rau, 1924) to propose a scheme of blood flow through the reptilian ventricle that has remained essentially unchanged. During diastole, the cavum arteriosum is filled with oxygenated pulmonary venous blood, while deoxygenated systemic venous blood flows from the right atrium through the cavum venosum to the cavum pulmonale. During systole, blood is ejected from the cavum pulmonale into the pulmonary circuit, while the cavum arteriosum blood is ejected through the cavum venosum and into the left and right aortic arches. Simultaneous pressure measurements in all three cava and outflow tracts of chelonian and squamates indicate a functional patency between the cava during both isometric and isotonic phases of systole (Johansen, 1959; Burggren, 1977a, 1977b; Shelton and Burggren, 1976). One extensively studied group of reptiles, the varanid lizards (genus: *Varanus*), may be unique among noncrocodilian reptiles in that a highly developed muscular ridge results in a mammalianlike dual-pressure pump during systole.

These general anatomical features of the reptilian cardiovascular system result in the potential for differential outflow to both the pulmonary and systemic circuits (e.g., intracardiac shunts). Numerous methods have been used to estimate the direction and magnitude of these shunts including application of the Fick principle for O_2 levels of the inflowing and outflowing blood of the ventricle (Baker and White, 1970; White et al., 1986); angiocardiography (Prakash, 1952; Foxon et al., 1953; Johansen et al., 1987), simultaneous pressure or flow measurements in the major outflow vessels and ventricular cava (Millen et al., 1964; White and Ross, 1966; Millard and Johansen, 1973; Shelton and Burggren, 1976; Burggren and Johansen, 1982), and the simultaneous injection of radioactively labeled microspheres into the left and right atrium (Berger and Heisler, 1977; Heisler et al., 1983; Heisler and Glass, 1985; White et al., 1986). Results from studies employing simultaneous pressure measurments, flow measurements, angiocardiographic techniques, and blood gas measurements have suggested that the magnitudes of R-L and L-R shunting are variable and dependent on the physiological state of the animal. For example, in turtles during lung ventilation, levels of R-L shunt are small (20-30%) and increase with apnea (60-70%) (White and Ross, 1966; Shelton and Burggren, 1976; White et al., 1986).

The variation of shunt magnitude with ventilatory state has been recently questioned. Simultaneous injections of radioactively labeled microspheres into the central circulation of the monitor lizard, *Varanus exanthematicus* indicated R-L shunt levels of 30% and L-R shunt values of 11%, with shunt levels remaining constant during ventilation and apnea. By utilizing the same method in the turtle, *Chrysemys picta belli*, Heisler and Glass (1985) exhibited both R-L and L-R shunts that were independent of ventilatory state at 15° and 30°C. Inherent technical problems with earlier methods were suggested to explain the apparent discrepancy between the reported results and the results of former studies (Heisler and Glass, 1985).

Recently, White et al. (1986) reexamined the impact of ventilatory state on the magnitude of intracardiac shunting in the turtle *P. scripta* utilizing both blood gas analysis and radiolabeled microspheres. On the basis of blood gas analysis of right and left atria and the three outflow tracts of the heart, *P. scripta* exhibited simultaneously occurring R-L and L-R shunts during both ventilation and apnea. During ventilation, the R-L shunt was small (between 20 and 30%) and significantly increased during apnea (between 50 and 90%). The exact level of R-L shunt could not be determined from blood gases because of the potential for O_2 differences between left and right aortic arches (see Sect. IV.D). Interestingly, determinations of R-L shunt by both blood gas analysis and microspheres were in good agreement during apnea and diverged only during ventilation. The accuracy of microspheres in determining R-L shunt during ventilation may be influenced by the interactions of three factors: (1) timing of microsphere injections relative to a ventilatory period, (2) the latency of washout from the ventricle, and (3) the rate of R-L shunt development following a ventilatory period.

The mechanisms of intracardiac shunts and their variability are presently controversial and have been reviewed in detail (White, 1976; Heisler and Glass, 1985; Burggren, 1985). Basically the functional patency of the three cava results in the distribution of cardiac output to the pulmonary and systemic circuits being influenced by adjustments in the peripheral resistance of these two circuits (White, 1976; Burggren, 1985). In addition, vagally induced changes in the elctrical and mechanical events in the heart may also influence the distribution of the cardiac output into the pulmonary and systemic circuits (Burggren, 1978). In varanid lizards, the well-developed horizontal septum may reduce the influences of peripheral resistances on intracardiac shunt levels. On the basis of the distribution of microspheres and on postmortem anatomical observations, Heisler et al. (1983) have suggested that during systole tight depression of the horizontal septum prevents translocation of mixed venous blood from cavum venosum to cavum pulmonale from occurring. Thus, during systole the degree of R-L shunting depends on the cavum arteriosum/cavum venosum volume ratio. In addition, the degree of L-R shunt should be dependent on the end-systolic volume of the cavum venosum. Heisler and colleagues have termed this mechanism the *washout* model and have concluded that changes in peripheral resistances play a minor role in determining the distribution of cardiac output into the pulmonary and systemic circuits.

Before fully understanding the mechanisms responsible for intracardiac shunts in reptiles, more detailed information about the dynamic intracardiac events must be determined. For example, what is the cavum venosum volume? Should it be consider a static volume (volume at end-diastole), or is it a dynamic volume (e.g., is there translocation of mixed venous blood into cavum pulmonale during early systole)? Is there a reproducible correlation between the

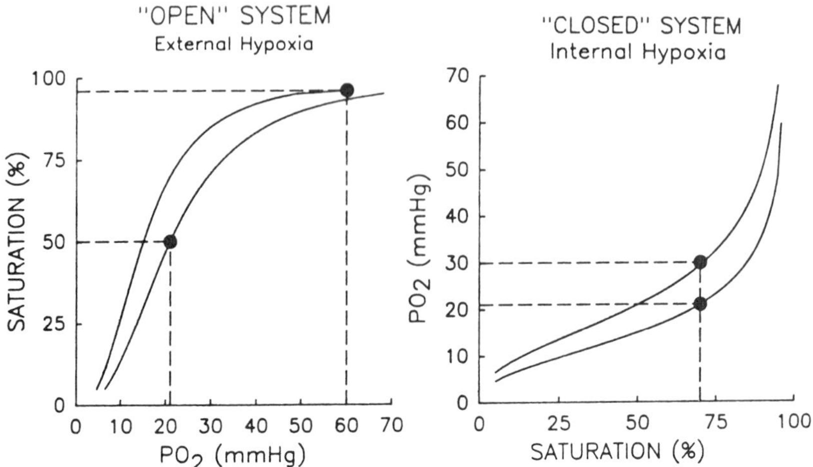

Figure 8 The relationship between PO_2 and hemoglobin saturation in both an "open" (gas exchange organ) and "closed" (shunt) system. In the open system PO_2 is the independent variable. During exposure to hypoxia a right shift in the O_2EC results in a decrease in saturation. In the closed system PO_2 becomes the dependent variable. Under consitions of internal hypoxia an "up-shift in the O_2EC is always advantageous as it increases PO_2.

cavum venosum volume and the percentage of R-L shunt for both an intra- and interspecies comparison? What is the end-systolic volume of the cavum venosum, and how is it correlated with L-R shunt? What impact do changes in peripheral resistances have on end-systolic and end-diastolic volumes in the cava? There are now no clear answers and, clearly, more research into mechanisms of intracardiac shunts and the impact of physiological states on shunts is needed.

B. Cardiovascular Shunts and Blood Gases

The presence of cardiovascular shunts have an important impact on O_2 homeostasis of lower vertebrates. Obviously, intracardiac shunts lower the hypoxic reserve through desaturation of pulmonary venous blood. Additionally, the potential for modulation provides an alternative mechanism for altering PO_2 independently of ventilation. Therefore, to fully understand the impact of shunts on O_2 homeostasis, it is important to provide a framework in which to conceptualized the interactions of shunts on the arterial and venous blood gases.

Recently, it has been emphasized that in the presence of cardiovascular shunting, the PO_2 of arterial and venous bloods become independent variables of the O_2 content (determined by degree and distribution of mixed venous blood) and the O_2 affinity in both theory (Rossoff et al., 1980; Turek and Kreuzer,

1981) and practice (Wood, 1981a). This extended the theory of in vitro "mixing method" for measuring O_2 affinity (Haab et al., 1960) to an in vivo condition.

In mammalian and avian physiology the association between O_2 affinity and PO_2 is relatively unimportant, except in pathological conditions (i.e., congenital heart disease, diffusion impairment, or severe $\dot{V}/\dot{Q}$ inhomogeneity). However, in ectothermic vertebrates, temperature-induced changes in O_2 affinity may routinely have an impact on both the arterial and venous PO_2.

Theoretical considerations of the interactions of shunts on blood gases have been previously detailed (Rosoff et al., 1980; Turek and Kreuzer, 1981; Wood, 1984; Wood and Hicks, 1985). Normally, in respiratory physiology, the relationship between PO_2 and blood O_2 content is treated in terms of an "open" system, i.e., the PO_2 is an independent variable in which the blood comes into equilibrium (Fig. 8). Treating the lung as an ideal gas exchanger, end-capillary PO_2 is assumed to be in equilibrium with the lung gas and, thus, for this "perfect" compartment, the O_2 content of end-capillary blood is a function of lung PO_2 (P_AO_2), O_2 affinity (P_{50}) and hemoglobin concentration, [Hb]. Under conditions of external hypoxia, a right shift in the O_2EC will be disadvantageous because of the lowering of O_2 content.

Any quantity of blood that lowers the saturation from the perfect value is referred to as the *shunt* compartment and includes anatomical shunting, physiological shunting, diffusion limitations, and $\dot{V}/\dot{Q}$ mismatching. In terms of shunting, the arterial content is determined by rearranging the shunt equation of Berggren (1942):

$$Q_s/Q_t = (C_pO_2 - C_aO_2/(C_pO_2 - C_vO_2) \quad (3)$$

where C_pO_2 = perfect compartment O_2 content, C_aO2 = systemic arterial O_2 content, and C_vO_2 = mixed venous O_2 content. Defining nonshunt fraction as $Q_{ns}/Q_t = 1 - Q_s/Q_t$ and solving for C_aO_2 results in:

$$C_aO_2 = Q_s/Q_t\,(C_vO_2) + Q_{ns}/Q_t(C_pO_2) \quad (4)$$

Under conditions of shunt, relationship between O_2 content and PO_2 is treated as a closed system, in which the PO_2 becomes the dependent variable and is a function of P_{50}, [Hb], and the C_aO_2 (see Fig. 8). Under conditions of internal hypoxia an "up-shift" in the O_2EC is always advantageous as it increases PO_2. A summary of the two-compartment model and its equations are shown in Figure 9.

The relationships outlined above also apply to CO_2. The change in saturation of mixed blood will impact the PCO_2 through the Haldane effect. Desaturation of pulmonary venous blood owing to shunting will shift the CO_2 dissociation curve to the left and upward. Depending on the resulting CO_2 content, the magnitude of Haldane effect, and the shape of the CO_2 dissociation curve, the

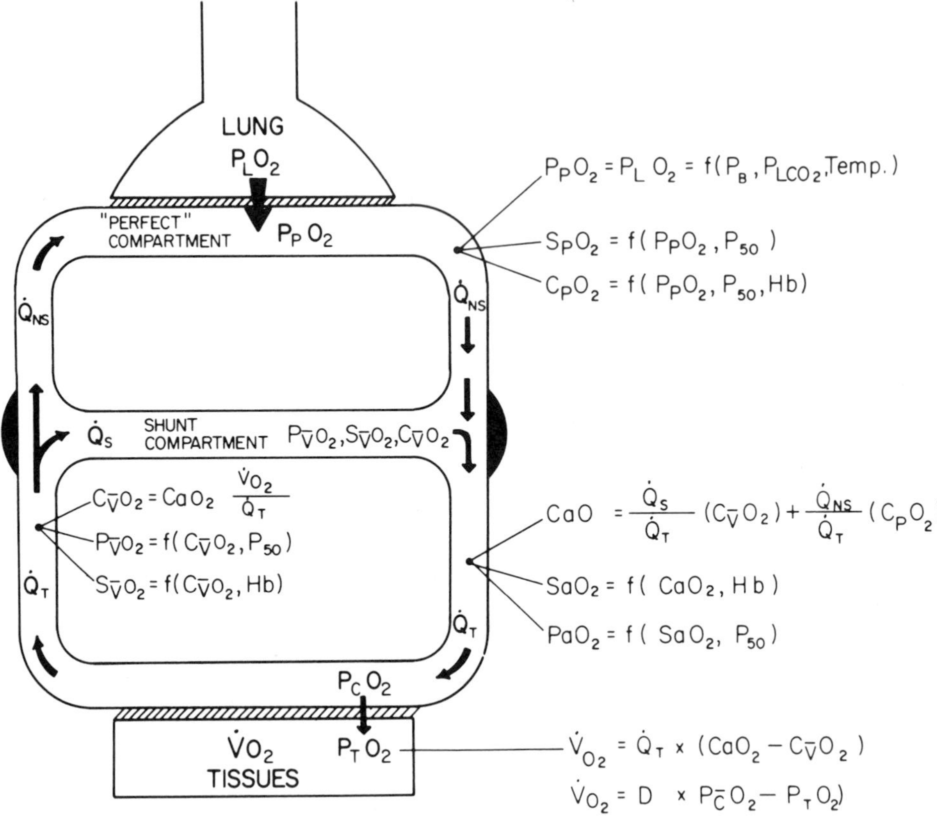

Figure 9 The two-compartment O_2 transport model in animals with intracardiac shunts. The equations represents the relationships of the O_2 transport parameters that make up the various compartments. Model is adapted from Rosoff et al. (1980). (Reprinted from Wood, 1984.)

PCO_2 of systemic arterial blood can be lower, equal to, or higher than P_pCO_2. The potential impact of shunts on CO_2 are discussed by White (Chap. 15).

C. Predictions of a Two-Compartment Model

The two-compartment model provides a concise, integrated framework in which to interpret experimental findings. On the basis of computer analysis of this model, (Wood, 1984; Hicks, 1984; Wood and Hicks, 1985) the impact of O_2 affinity on arterial and venous blood gases and their relationship with respiratory gases have been made.

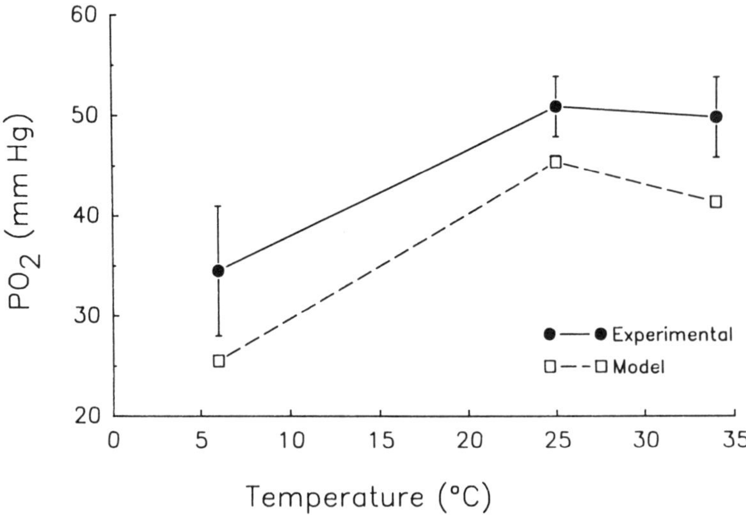

Figure 10 Computer predictions and experimental data for the systemic PO_2 of *Pseudemys scripta* at various body temperatures. (Data from Wood, 1984.)

A central prediction of the two-compartment model is that any right shift in the O_2EC, resulting from temperature or pH, will produce an increase in the arterial PO_2. This has been confirmed in amphibians, in reptiles, and in mammals with artificial shunts (Wood, 1982). However, the increase in PaO_2 is not indeterminant but reaches a "breaking point" where further decreases in O_2 affinity produce a plateau, then a decrease in PaO_2. The breaking point results from a combination of a reduction in pulmonary capillary $[O_2]$ as the lung PO_2 decreases and the O_2EC is right-shifted at higher temperatures. The relationship of the breaking point to body temperature is dependent on the temperature sensitivity of Hb, the magnitude of the Bohr effect, and the degree of R-L shunting. The breaking point has been confirmed experimentally in turtles (Wood, 1984) and exhibits good agreement within the defined limits of the computer analysis (Fig. 10). A functional analysis of gas transport in turtles (White and Bickler, 1987) has reported a similar trend in both arterial and venous PO_2. In the lizard, *Varanus exanthematicus* the arterial PO_2 exhibits no breaking point over a temperature range of 15° to 40°C, resulting from the maintenance of high pulmonary PO_2s, low temperature sensitivity of blood, and the relatively small magnitude of shunts.

Desaturation of arterial blood caused by shunting results in the uncoupling of alveolar (lung PO_2) and arterial PO_2, such that the (PAO_2 - PaO_2) differences

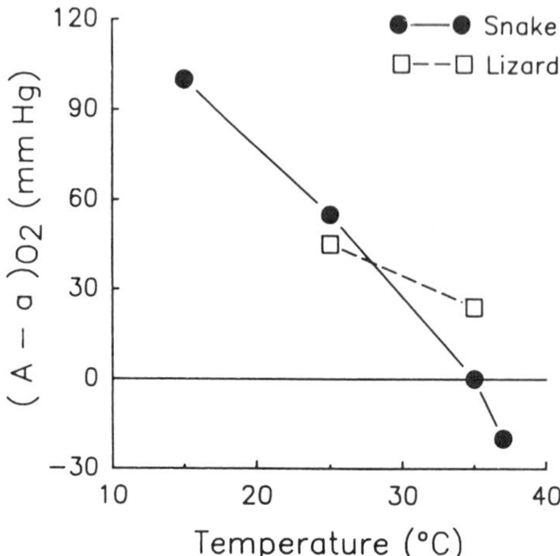

Figure 11 The $(A\text{-}a)O_2$ at various temperatures in a snake, *Pituophis melanolucus*, and lizard, *Varanus niloticus*. Note that at high body temperatures the $(A\text{-}a)O_2$ reverses as predicted by Wood (1984). (Data for snake from Stinner, 1987; for lizard from Hicks, Ishimatsu, and Heisler, unpublished observation.)

increases as body temperature decreases. This trend has been observed in lizards (Wood et al., 1977; Hicks, Ishimatsu, and Heisler, unpublished observations) and snakes (Stinner, 1987; Fig. 11). The increasing $(A\text{-}a)O_2$ gradient at lower temperatures results from an increase in P_{AO_2}, the presence of shunt and the decrease in Pa_{O_2} caused by a left shift in the O_2EC. A similar impact of O_2 affinity on $(A\text{-}a)O_2$ has been reported when desaturation of pulmonary venous blood resulting from $\dot{V}/\dot{Q}$ inhomogeneities exist (Turek and Kruezer, 1981). The relationship between P_{AO_2} and arterial P_{O_2} can be theoretically extrapolated to conditions in which the O_2EC of systemic blood has a lower affinity than pulmonary capillary blood and consequently Pa_{O_2} will exceed P_{AO_2} (Wood, 1984). This has been experimentally confirmed in snakes at high body temperatures (see Fig. 11).

D. Limitations of the Two-Compartment Analysis

The two-compartment analysis provides a broad and general framework in which to interpret the interactions of shunts on arterial and venous blood gases. However, like all models, it is limited in its application by the assumptions that it is built upon. First, the approach used is applicable to only steady-state gas exchange and can predict only "time-averaged" trends in blood gases. Lower vertebrates are rarely if every in a steady state. In fact, periodic breathing, periodic pulmonary perfusion, variable shunt magnitude, all make steady state an uncommon condition. Second, the two-compartment approach cannot distinguish the type of shunt. Desaturation of arterial blood from ideal levels may result from increases in R-L shunts, diffusion limitations, heterogeneous distribution of V/Q, or a combination of any, or all, of these. Therefore, as a framework for

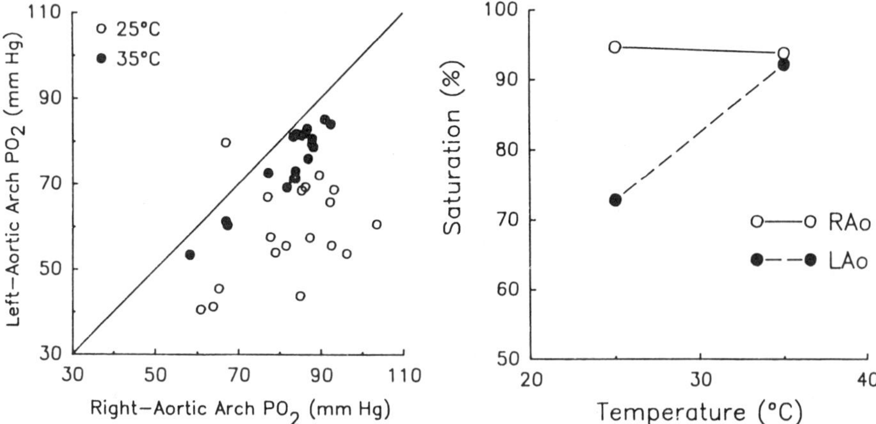

Figure 12 PO_2 and saturation differences between two aortic arches of the Nile monitor lizard, *Varanus niloticus* at 25° and 35°C. (Data from Ishimatsu et al., 1988.)

interpreting experimental data, the two-compartment model can point to only potential causes for desaturation of arterial blood but not to specific causes. Finally, the two-compartment analysis utilizes the standard shunt equation (Eq. 4) that implies no significant difference in blood gas levels between the right and left aortic blood. However, the potential for a differential distribution of O_2 between the left and right arch does exist in lower vertebrates and substantially alters interpretations of overall levels of R-L shunt.

Oxygen Distribution in the Systemic Arches

Few studies have examined the O_2 distribution between the two aortic arches in reptiles. In the turtle, *Chelydra serpentina*, no difference was found in the O_2 saturation levels of right and left aortic arches (Steggerda and Essex, 1957). Similarly, White (1959) reported no significant difference in right or left aortic $[O_2]$ in the snake *Coluber constrictor* and the lizard, *I. iguana*. In contrast, Khalil and Zaki (1964) found consistently higher O_2 levels in the right aorta than in the left aorta in snakes (*Zamenis diadema*), turtles (*Testudo leithii*), and crocodilians (*Crocodylus niloticus*). In the monitor lizard, *Varanus exanthematicus*, Burggren and Johansen (1982) reported higher PO_2 and O_2 contents in the right aorta than the left aortic arch. However, these studies were under the short-term experimental conditions of heart exposure, anesthesia, artificial ventilation, and supine position, and they should not be taken as representative of normal intracardiac patterns.

Few studies have examined the O_2 levels from different arterial sites under extended conditions. Tucker (1966) compared the O_2 content of right or left aortic arch with dorsal aortic blood in *I. iguana*. Of the 10 animals studied, three exhibited higher $[O_2]$ in the right aortic arch and two exhibited lower $[O_2]$ in the left aortic arch when compared with dorsal aortic blood. The remaining animals showed no significant difference in $[O_2]$ from the three vascular sites. Baker and White (1970) analyzed blood from the carotid artery and dorsal aorta in *I. iguana*. They showed that during heating $[O_2]$ in the carotid artery (direct branch of right aorta) was higher than in the dorsal aorta. No difference in $[O_2]$ from these two sites was observed in temperature-acclimated animals. Recently, Ishimatsu et al. (1988) studied the distribution of O_2 in the outflow vessels of permanently annulated, fully recovered, freely moving monitor lizards, *Varanus niloticus*, at 25° and 35°C. These studies reported higher values for O_2 in the right aortic blood compared with left aortic blood, with the difference increasing at 25°C (Fig. 12). The difference in aortic blood must result from a differential-shunting pattern between the two arches. This difference in shunt is evident when examining the effects of temperature on O_2 saturation from the two arches. For LA_O blood the saturation increased as temperature increased, in contrast to RA_O saturation that remained constant (see Fig. 12).

Three-Vessel Analysis

The existence of significant O_2 differences between the two aortic arches prevents the use of the standard shunt equation to describe the partitioning of oxygenated and deoxygenated blood into the systemic circuit. This is appreciated by examining the conventional shunt equation in terms of the flow model on which it is based. The standard shunt equation relies on two inflows and two outflows with four possible flow directions for the two types of incoming blood (Fig. 13). However, for noncrocodilian reptiles, the anatomy can be represented by a three-vessel model (see Fig. 13) in which there are three instead of two outflow vessels and there are six instead of four possible flow directions. These flows are y and x, the fraction of mixed venous blood entering the right and left aortic arch respectively (R-L shunt), α which is the fraction of pulmonary venous blood recirculating into the pulmonary circulation (L-R), β, and $(1 - \beta)$ the fraction of pulmonary venous blood entering left and right aortic arches, respectively, and finally $(1 - x - y)$ the fraction of systemic venous return entering the pulmonary circulation. Solution of the three-vessel model depends on blood O_2 measurements from five sites (PA, pulmonary artery; LA, left atrium; RA, right atrium; LA_O, left aortic arch; and RA_O, right aortic arch), as well as additional blood O_2 data from three additional sites, or independent determination of total R-L shunt level. Ishimatsu et al. (1988) have derived the equations and techniques necessary to describe the various flow patterns in the presence of three outflow vessels. Recently, Tazawa and Johansen (1987) have reported

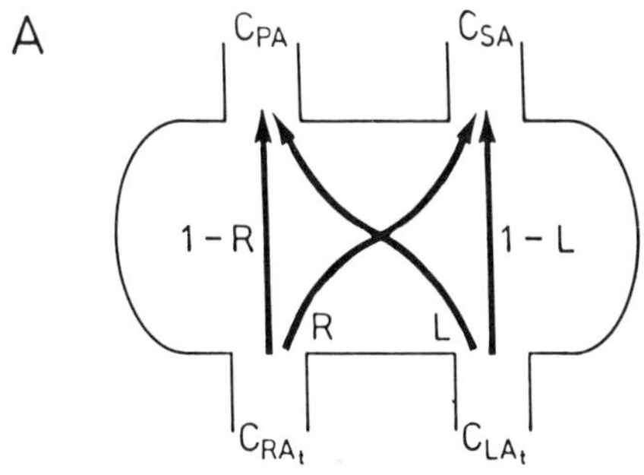

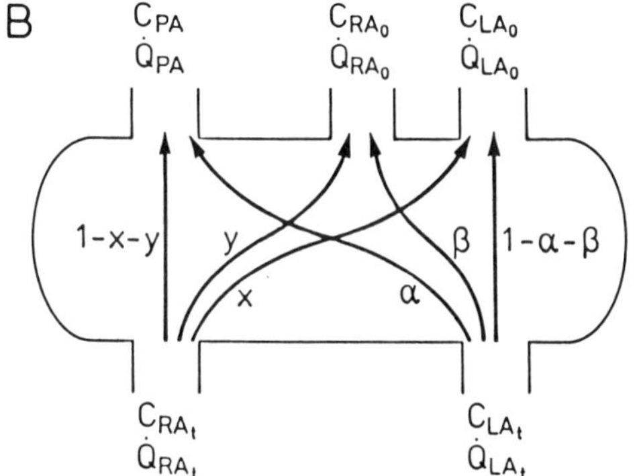

FUNDAMENTAL EQUATIONS

1 $\dot{Q}_{PA} = \dot{Q}_{LA_t} = (1-x-y)\cdot\dot{Q}_{RA_t} + \alpha\cdot\dot{Q}_{LA_t}$

2 $\dot{Q}_{RA_0} = y\cdot\dot{Q}_{RA_t} + \beta\cdot\dot{Q}_{LA_t}$

3 $\dot{Q}_{LA_0} = x\cdot\dot{Q}_{RA_t} + (1-\alpha-\beta)\cdot\dot{Q}_{LA_t}$

Figure 13 (A) The two-vessel model (two inflows and two outflows) on which the standard shunt equation is based. PA, pulmonary artery; SA, systemic artery, RA_t, right atrium; and LA_t, left atrium. For all vessels C = O_2 concentration. Intercardiac shunts are described by R, right-left shunt; and L, left-right shunt. (B) The three-vessel model (two inflows and three outflows) that describes intracardiac flow patterns in the presence of dual aortic arches. RA_o, right aortic arch; LA_o, left aortic arch. The fundamental Equations (1, 2, and 3) that describe the various flows in this model are shown. See text for a detailed description the three-vessel model. (Adapted from Ishimatsu et al., 1988.)

solutions for calculation of overall shunting patterns in the incomplete double circulation of air-breathing fishes, lung fishes, amphibians, reptiles, and embryonic birds and mammals. Their solution to the noncrocodilian cardiovascular system suggest that the various shunting fractions can be calculated from blood O_2 measurements from five central sites and the additional blood analysis from a single systemic site (dorsal aorta or femoral artery).

In the presence of differential shunting between the two aortic arches, the calculation of total R-L shunt from a single arch or its direct branch will be

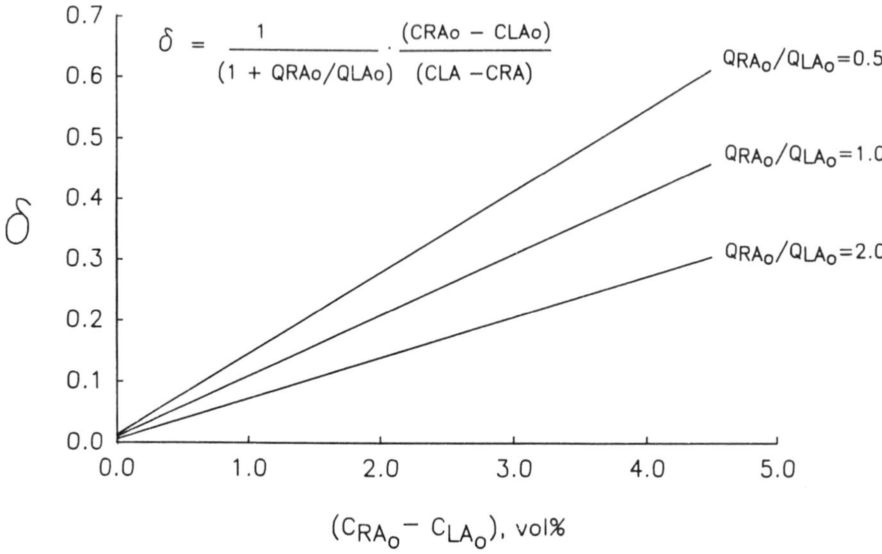

Figure 14 The difference between the actual shunt in a three-vessel system and the shunt calculated from a single aortic arch (δ), as a function of O_2 difference between the arches ($CRA_0 - CLA_0$) and the flow ratio between the arches (QRA_0/QLA_0). Note as ($CRA_0 - CLA_0$) increases resulting error increases. In addition the magnitude of this error is influenced by QRA_0/QLA_0.

in error. By using the fundamental equations presented by Ishimatsu et al. (1988), equations that determine the difference between the shunt in a three-outflow vessel system and the shunt calculated from a single arch can be derived. Designating the ratio of right aortic flow to left aortic flow (QRA_0/QLA_0) as r, and applying the conventional shunt equation to a three outflow system results in the following two equations:

$$\delta = r/(1 + r) \cdot (CLA_0 - CRA_0)/CLA - CRA) \tag{5}$$

where C = O_2 concentration, and δ = the difference between the actual shunt (three-vessel) and the shunt calcuated from CLA_0 only.

$$\delta' = 1/(1 + r) \cdot (CRA_0 - CLA_0)/CLA - CRA) \tag{6}$$

where δ' = the difference between the actual shunt and the shunt calculated from CRA_0 only.

It is apparent from Equations 5 and 6, and as shown in Figure 14, that the magnitude of error depends on the ($CRA_0 - CLA_0$) and QRA_0/QLA_0. In addition, when $CRA_0 > CLA_0$ then $\delta <$ and $\delta' > 0$ and thus the total R-L shunt must be between the values calculated from Equation 4 using either CLA_0 or CRA_0.

Under these stated conditions of differential shunting to the two systemic arches, interpretation of blood gas data in terms of overall shunting is dramatically altered. For example, in the Nile monitor lizard, *V. niloticus* no significant difference in the PO_2 or saturation of right aortic arch blood was found as temperature increased from 25° to 35°C. Given only this sampled site would have led to the erroneous conclusion that the total level of R-L shunt did not change as temperature increased. However, this study also showed that both PO_2 and saturation of left aortic blood increased as temperature increased. In the context of the three-vessel analysis, the total R-L shunt at 25°C was larger with most of the outflow directed into the LA_0. At 35°C the total shunt decreased, with the LA_0 continuing to receive most of the mixed venous blood (Ishimatsu et al., 1988).

Clearly, the existence of dual aortic arches requires the investigator to establish the degree of separation between the two arches or design the experiment such that O_2 samples from either arch will be taken. Conclusions about total R-L shunt that are based on a single arch cannot be made. Finally, the presence of differential outflow to the aortic arch system begs the questions: What is the systemic arterial PO_2 in reptiles? and What is the impact of various physiological states (e.g,, diving, ventilation, exercise) on the distribution of blood between the two arches?

V. Conclusions

The existence of vascular shunting provides an additional mechanism in the regulation of O_2 homeostasis, where the PO_2 is regulated by the matching of ventilation and blood flow to the respiratory organ as well as the magnitude and distribution of shunts. Among the reptiles, the magnitude of the R-L and L-R shunts are variable and are dependent on physiological states. The variable distribution of O_2 into the two aortic arches makes the cardiovascular system of lower vertebrates increasingly complex. The diversity of physiological requirements, habitats, and adaptations makes it difficult to draw general conclusions concerning the adaptability of intracardiac shunts. However, the potential for impact on both O_2 and CO_2 homeostasis provides exciting areas for future research in comparative physiology.

References

Baker, L. A., and White, F. N. (1970). Redistribution of cardiac output in response to heating in *Iguana iguana. Comp. Biochem. Physiol. 35*:253-262.

Bartholomew, G. H. (1982). Physiological control of body temperature. In *Biology of the Reptilia*, Vol. 12. Edited by C. Gans and F. H. Pough. New York, Academic Press, pp. 17-24.

Bennett, A. F., and Dawson, W. R. (1976). Metabolism. In *Biology of the Reptilia*, Vol. 5. Edited by C. Gans and W. R. Dawson. New York, Academic Press, pp. 127-223.

Berger, P. J., and Heisler, N. (1977). Estimation of shunting, systemic and pulmonary output of the heart, and regional blood flow distribution in unanesthetized lizards (*Varanus exanthematicus*) by injection of radioactively labelled microspheres. *J. Exp. Biol. 71*:11-121.

Berggren, S. (1942). The oxygen deficit of arterial blood caused by nonventilating parts of the lung. *Acta Physiol. Scand. Suppl. 4*:5-91.

Bligh, J. (1973). *Temperature Regulation in Mammals and Other Vertebrates.* Amsterdam, North-Holland.

Bradford, D. F. (1984). Temperature modulation in high elevation amphibian *Rana mucosa. Copeia* 1984, 966-976.

Burggren, W. W. (1977a). The pulmonary circulation of the chelonian reptile: Morphology, pharmacology and hemodynamics. *J. Comp. Physiol. 116*: 303-324.

Burggren, W. W. (1977b). Circulation during intermittent lung ventilation in the garter snake, *Thamnophis. Can. J. Zool. 55*:720-725.

Burggren, W. W. (1978). Influence of intermittent breathing on ventricular depolarization patterns in chelonian reptiles. *J. Physiol. 378*:349-364.

Burggren, W. W. (1985). Hemodynamics and regulation of central cardiovascular shunts in reptiles. In *Cardiovascular Shunts: Phylogenetic, Ontogenetic and Clinical Aspects.* Edited by K. Johansen and W. Burggren. Copenhagen, Munksgaard, pp. 121-142.

Burggren, W. W., and Johansen, K. (1982). Ventricular hemodynamics in the monitor lizard, *Varanus exanthematicus*: Pulmonary and systemic pressure separation. *J. Exp. Biol. 96*:343-354.

Dupre, R. K., and Crawford, E. (1985). Behavioral thermoregulation during dehydration and osmotic loading of the desert iguana. *Physiol. Zool. 58*: 357-363.

Dupre, R. K., Hicks, J. W., and Wood, S. C. (1984). Ventilatory responses of the Mexican black iguana to hypoxia and hypercapnia at different body temperatures. *Physiologist 27*:285.

Dupre, R. K., Martinez, M. J., and Wood, S. C. (1985). Temperature selection during hypoxia: Aquatic organisms. *Fed. Proc. 44*:999.

Dupre, R. K., Hicks, J. W., and Wood, S. C. (1986). The effect of hypoxia on evaporative cooling thresholds of lizards. *J. Therm. Biol. 11*:223-227.

Dupre, R. K., Romero, A. M., and Wood, S. C. (1988). Thermoregulation and oxygen uptake in hypoxic animals. In *Oxygen Transfer from Atmos-*

phere to Tissues. Edited by N. C. Gonzales and M. R. Fedde, New York Plenum Press (in press).

Foxon, G. E. H., Griffith, J., and Price, M. (1953). Circulation in *Lacerta viridis. Nature 172*:312.

Fry, F. E. J., and Hart, J. S. (1948). The relation of temperature to oxygen consumption in the goldfish. *Biol. Bull. 94*:66-77.

Garrick, L. D. (1974). Reproductive influences on behavioral thermoregulation in the lizard, *Scleoporus occidentalis. Physiol. Behav. 12*:85-91.

Glass, M. L., Boutilier, R. G., and Heisler, N. (1983). Ventilatory control of arterial PO_2 in the turtle *Chrysemys picta bellii*: Effects of temperature and hypoxia. *J. Comp. Physiol. 151*:145-153.

Glass, M. L., and Wood, S. C. (1983). Gas exchange and control of breathing in reptiles. *Physiol. Rev. 63*:232-260.

Goodrich, E. S. (1916). On the classification of the Reptilia. *Proc. R. Soc. Lond. 89*:261-276.

Goodrich, E. S. (1919). Note on the reptilian heart. *J. Anat. (Lond.) 53*:289.

Griel, A. (1902). Beiträge zur vergleichenden Anatomie und Entwicklungsgeschicte des Herzens und des Truncus arteriosis der Wirbelthiere. *Morphol. Jarhb. 31*:123-310.

Haab, P. E., Piiper, J., and Rahn, H. (1960). Simple method for rapid determination of an O_2 dissociation curve of the blood. *J. Appl. Physiol. 15*:1148-1149.

Heath, J. E. (1970). Behavioral regulation of body temperature in poikilotherms. *Physiologist 13*:339-410.

Heisler, N., Neumann, P., and Maloiy, G. M. O. (1983). The mechanism of intracardiac shunting in the lizard *Varanus exanthematicus. J. Exp. Biol. 105*: 15-31.

Heisler, N., and Glass, M. L. (1985). Mechanisms and regulation of central vascular shunts in reptiles. In *Cardiovascular Shunts: Phylogenetic, Ontogenetic, and Clinical Aspects*. Edited by K. Johansen and W. Burggren. Copenhagen, Munksgaard, pp. 334-353.

Hertz, P. E. (1979). Sensitivity to high temperature in three West Indian grass anoles (Sauria, Iguanidae), with a review of heat sensitivity in the genus. *Comp. Biochem. Physiol. 53A*:217-222.

Hertz, P. E., and Huey, R. B. (1981). Compensation for altitudinal changes in ther thermal environment by some *Anolis* lizards on Hispaniola. *Ecology 62*:515-521.

Hertz, P. E., Arce-Hernandez, A., Ramirez-Vasquez, J., Tirado-Rivera, W., and Vasquez-Vives, L. (1979). Geographical variation of heat sensitivity and water loss rates in the tropical lizard, *Anolis gundlachi. Comp. Biochem. Physiol. 62A*:947-953.

Hicks, J. W. (1984). Oxygen Homeostasis and Temperature Regulation in Lizards. Ph.D. dissertation. University of New Mexico.

Hicks, J. W., and Wood, S. C. (1985). Temperature regulation in lizards: effects of hypoxia. *Am. J. Physiol. 248*:R595-R600.

Hill, J. R. (1959). The oxygen consumption of newborn and adult mammals. Its dependence on the oxygen tension in the inspired air and on the environmental temperature. *J. Physiol. (Lond.) 149*:346-373.

Hochachka, P. W., and Dunn, J. F. (1983). Metabolic arrest: The most effective means of protecting tissues against hypoxia. In *Hypoxia, Exercise and Altitude: Proceedings of the Third Banff International Hypoxia Symposium*. New York, Alan R. Liss, pp. 297-303.

Horstman, D. H., and Banderet, L. E. (1977). Hypoxia-induced metabolic and core temperature changes in the squirrel monkey. *J. Appl. Physiol. 42*: 273-278.

Huey, R. B. (1982). Temperature, physiology and ecology of reptiles. In *Biology of the Reptilia*, Vol. 12. Edited by C. Gans and F. H. Pough. New York, Academic Press, pp. 25-91.

Ishimatsu, A., Hicks, J. W., and Heisler, N. (1988). Analysis of intracardiac shunting in the lizard, *Varanus niloticus*: A new model based on blood oxygen levels and microsphere distribution. *Respir. Physiol. 71*:83-100.

Jackson, D. C. (1973). Ventilatory responses to hypoxia in turtles at various temperatures. *Respir. Physiol. 12*:131-140.

Johansen, K. (1959). Circulation in the three chambered snake heart. *Circ. Res.* 7:828-832.

Johansen, K., and Burggren, W. W. (1980). Cardiovascular function in lower vertebrates. In *Hearts and Heart-Like Organs*. New York, Academic Press, pp. 61-117.

Johansen, K., Abe, A. S., and Andersen, J. H. (1987). Intracardiac shunts revealed by angiocardiography in the lizard *Tupinambis teguixin*. *J. Exp. Biol.* 1-12.

Khalil, F., and Zaki, K. (1964). Distribution of blood in the ventricle and aortic arches in Reptilia. *Z. Vgl. Physiol. 48*:663-689.

Kluger, M. J. (1980). Fever in ectotherms: Evolutionary implications. *Am. Zool. 19*:295-304.

Lahiri, S., and Gelfand, R. (1981). Mechanisms of acute ventilatory responses. In *Regulation of Breathing*, Vol. II. Edited by T. F. Hornbein. New York, Marcel Dekker, pp. 773-821.

Mathur, P. N. (1946). The anatomy of the reptilian heart. Part II. Serpentes, Testudinata and Loricata. *Proc. Indian Acad. Sci. B20*:1-29.

Millen, J. E., Murdaugh, H. V., Bauer, C. B., and Robin, D. (1964). Circulatory adaptation to diving in the freshwater turtle. *Science 145*:591-593.

Millard, R. W., and Johansen, K. (1973). Ventricular outflow dynamics in the lizard, *Varanus niloticus*: Responses to hypoxia, hypercarbia and diving. *J. Exp. Biol. 60*:871-880.

Moore, R. E. (1959). Oxygen consumption and body temperature in newborn kittens subjected to hypoxia and reoxygenation. *J. Physiol. (Lond.) 149*: 500-518.

O'Donoghue, C. H. (1918). The heart of the leathery turtle, *Dermochelys (Sphargis) coriacea.* With a note on the septum ventriculorum in the Reptilia. *J. Anat. 52*:823-890.

Otis, A. B. (1987). An overview of gas exchange. In *Handbook or Physiology*, Sect. 3. The Respiratory System, Vol. IV. Edited by L. E. Fahri and S. M. Tenney. Washington, American Physiological Society, pp. 1-11.

Pough, F. H. (1980). Blood oxygen transport and delivery in reptiles. *Am. Zool. 20*:173-185.

Pough, F. H., and Gans, C. (1982). The vocabulary of reptilian thermoregulation. In *Biology of the Reptilia*, Vol. 12. Edited by C. Gans and F. H. Pough. New York, Academic Press, pp. 17-24.

Prakash, R. (1952). The radiographic demonstration of the mode of action of the heart of a lizard *Uromastix hardwickii* Gray. *Indian J. Radiol. 6*:126-128.

Rau, A. S. (1924). Observations of the anatomy of the heart of *Tiliqua scincoides* and *Eunectes murinus. J. Anat. 59*:60-71.

Rosoff, L., Zeldin, R., Hew, E., and Aberman, A. (1980). Changes in blood P_{50}: effects on oxygen delivery when arterial hypoxemia is due to shunting. *Chest 77*:142-146.

Saint-Girons, M. (1970). Morphology of the circulating blood cells. In *Biology of the Reptilia*, Vol. 3. Edited by C. Gans and T. Parsons. London, Academic Press, pp. 73-91.

Schall, J. J., Bennett, A. F., and Putnam, R. F. (1982). Lizards infected with malaria: Physiological and behavioral consequences. *Science 217*:1057-1058.

Shelton, G., and Burggren, W. W. (1976). Cardiovascular dynamics of the Chelonia during apnea and lung ventilation. *J. Exp. Biol. 64*:323-343.

Shelton, G., Jones, D. R., and Milsom, W. K. (1986). Control of breathing in ectothermic vertebrates. In *Handbook of Physiology, Sect. 3: The Respiratory System*, Vol. II, Bethesda, American Physiological Society, pp. 857-909.

Siebke, H., Rod, T., Breivik, H., and Lind, B. (1975). Survival after 40 minutes submersion without cerebral sequelae. *Lancet* June 7:1275-1277.

Steggerda, F. R., and Essex, H. E. (1957). Circulation and blood pressure in the vessels and heart of the turtle *Chelydra serpentina. Am. J. Physiol. 190*: 320-326.

Stinner, J. N. (1987). Thermal dependence of air convection requirement and blood gases in the snake *Coluber constrictor. Am. Zool. 27*:41-47.

Tappan, H. (1967). Primary production, iosotopes, extinctions and the atmosphere. *Paleogeogr. Paleoclimatol. Paleoecol. 4*:187-210.

Tazawa, H., and Johansen, K. (1987). Comparative model analysis of central shunts in vertebrate cardiovascular systems. *Comp. Biochem. Physiol. 86A*:595-607.

Tucker, V. A. (1966). Oxygen transport by the circulatory system of the green iguana (*Iguana*) at different body temperatures. *J. Exp. Biol. 44*:77-92.

Turek, Z., and Kreuzer, F. (1981). Effects of shifts of the O_2 dissociation curve upon alveolar-arterial O_2 gradients in computer models of the lung with ventilation-perfusion mismatching. *Respir. Physiol. 45*:133-139.

Turner, J. S., and Tracy, C. R. (1983). Blood flow to appendages and the control of heat exchange in American alligators. *Physiol. Zool. 56*:195-200.

Van Mierop, L. H. S., and Kutsche, L. M. (1985). Some aspects of comparative anatomy of the heart. In *Cardiovascular Shunts: Phylogenetic, Ontogenetic and Clinical Aspects*. Edited by K. Johansen and W. Burggren. Copenhagen, Munksgaard, pp. 38-56.

Warley, A., and Gutierrez, G. (1984). Oxygen delivery in hypothermia. *Physiologist 27*:251.

White, F. N. (1959). Circulation in the reptilian heart (Squamata) *Anat. Rec. 135*:129-134.

White, F. N. (1968). Functional anatomy of the heart of reptiles. *Am. Zool. 8*: 211-219.

White, F. N. (1976). Circulation. In *Biology of the Reptilia*. Vol. 5. Edited by C. Gans and W. R. Dawson. New York, Academic Press, pp. 275-334.

White, F. N., and Ross, G. (1966). Circulatory changes during experimental diving in the turtle. *Am. J. Physiol. 211*:15-18.

White, F. N., and Bickler, P. E. (1987). Gas exchange in the turtle: A model analysis. *Am. Zool. 27*:31-39.

White, F. N., and Somero, G. (1982). Acid-base regulation and phospholipid adaptations to temperature: Time courses and physiological significance of modifying the milieu for protein function. *Physiol. Rev. 62*:40-90.

White, F. N., Hicks, J. W., and Ishimatsu, A. (1986). The influence of ventilatory state on intracardiac shunting in the trutle, *Pseudemys scripta. Physiologist 29*:178.

Willford, D. C., Hill, E. P., White, F. C., and Moores, W. Y. (1986). Decreased critical mixed venous oxygen tension and critical oxygen transport during induced hypothermia in pigs. *J. Clin. Monit. 2*:155-168.

Wood, S. C. (1981a). The effect of oxygen affinity on arterial P_{O_2} in animals with vascular shunts. *J. Appl. Physiol. 53*:1360-1364.

Wood, S. C. (1981b). Oxygen transport during exercise at sea level and high altitude. In *Sports Medicine*. Edited by O. Appenzeller and R. Atkinson. Baltimore, Urban and Schwarzenber, pp. 223-244.

Wood, S. C. (1984). Cardiovascular shunts and oxygen transport in lower vertebrates. *Am. J. Physiol. 247*:R3-R14.

Wood, S. C., and Hicks, J. W. (1985). Oxygen homeostasis in vertebrates with cardiovascular shunts. In *Cardiovascular Shunts: Phylogenetic, Ontogenetic and Clinical Aspects.* Edited by K. Johansen and W. Burggren. Copenhagen, Munksgaard, pp. 354-362.

Wood, S. C., Dupre, R. K., and Hicks, J. W. (1985). Hypothermia: An adaptive response to hypoxia. *Proc. 4th Int. Hypoxia Symp.* p. 12.

12

Temperature and Oxygen Supply in the Avian Brain

MARVIN H. BERNSTEIN

New Mexico State University
Las Cruces, New Mexico

I. Introduction

When they fly or encounter hot environments, birds often become hyperthermic, sometimes developing body temperatures of 44°C or higher. In flying birds, this reflects the large increase in the use of metabolic energy, most of which is internally converted to heat, and the storage of some of this heat. Hudson and Bernstein (1981) have calculated that a white-necked raven that raises body temperature by 1.3°C in 5 min of flight stores 30% of its total heat production. In this respect, birds are like many mammals that also store heat and elevate body temperature during exercise. Controlled heat storage helps birds by increasing the thermal gradient for radiative and convective heat loss to the environment or by decreasing the thermal gradient for heat gain when the environment is hotter than the body. Hyperthermia also reduces the need for evaporative cooling and forestalls the need to drink until the animal alights, perhaps at a source

---

Preparation of this chapter supported in part by NSF grant PCM-8402659.

of drinking water, or until the environmental temperature becomes cooler. Finally, muscle function may be more efficient at higher temperatures.

In both birds and mammals, tolerance of even brief bouts of extreme hyperthermia evidently requires concomitant protection for the brain because in many species the brain is regulated at a lower temperature than the body core. This is achieved by the cooling of cerebral arterial blood within a vascular network, or rete, where arterial blood flows countercurrent to cooler venous blood. The latter arrives at the rete after perfusing the moist surfaces lining the buccopharyngeal and nasal cavities and the eyes, where it is cooled by evaporation of water. A single rete (the carotid rete) occurs in some mammal species; it is located centrally below the base of the brain. (see Baker, 1982, for review). In birds the ophthalmic rete (OR) is paired and situated within or overlying each temporal bone between the eye and ear. Its arterial component seems to supply the orbit as well as the brain.

It has been suggested (Bernstein et al., 1984) that water vapor might not be the only gas transferred between blood and air in the heads of birds. The dense networks of blood vessels close to the evaporative surfaces and the large partial pressure gradients across them suggest that O_2 and CO_2 might also move across tissue and plasma barriers, enriching venous O_2 and depleting venous CO_2. By flowing countercurrent to arterial blood in the OR, venous blood might then pass O_2 to arterial blood while taking up arterial CO_2. This would benefit the brain by enhancing arterial P_{O_2}. The benefit during exercise, when cardiac output is accelerated and a large proportion of it is allocated to flight muscles, would be especially important. The well-known tolerance of birds to high altitude, it has been reasoned, might also be explained, in part, by such a cephalic gas transfer mechanism.

This chapter is then a review of the available information on the physiological properties of the OR and a more detailed description of the available evidence about air-blood and arteriovenous gas exchanges in the heads of birds.

II. Brain Temperature

A. Brain Cooling

The first measurements of brain temperature (T_B) in birds were made in domestic fowl (Richards, 1970; Scott et al., 1970), in which the brain was cooler than the body core. Richards (1970) was the first to attribute brain cooling to heat exchange in the OR. Brain temperature was investigated further in the large (31-kg) ratite, *Rhea americana*, by Kilgore et al. (1973). They selected rheas because, like some of the mammals that had been studied previously and shown to regulate T_B independently (Taylor and Lyman, 1972), they move about by running, and they do so in hot environments, and also because it was thought, at first, that cooling in its long (ca. 80-cm) neck might also affect brain cooling.

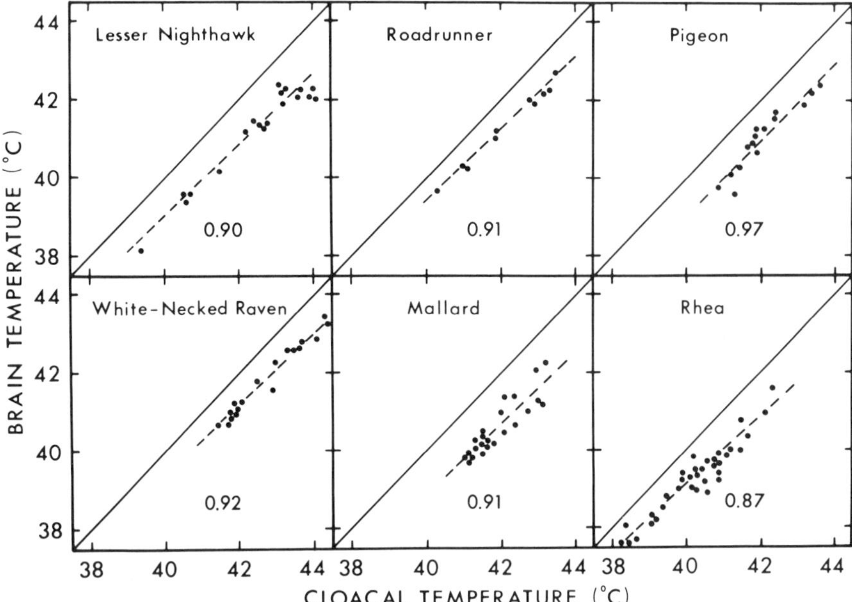

Figure 1 Relationship of brain (hypothalamic) temperature to cloacal temperature in six species of birds. Solid lines pass through isothermal points. Dashed lines are least-squares regression lines fitted to the data, with slopes as shown. In all measurements the brain was cooler than the cloaca, and brain temperature increased with cloacal temperature. (From Kilgore et al., 1976. Data for rhea from Kilgore et al., 1973.)

Insulated thermocouples were implanted in the brain (anterior hypothalamus or neostriatum), in anterior and posterior positions within the carotid artery, and in the cloaca, and continuous temperature recordings were made from the conscious animals during ambient heat exposure. Over the range of air temperature (T_A) from 31 to 47°C and of cloacal temperatures (T_C) from 38 to 42°C, the brain was always approximately 1°C cooler than the cloaca, although the difference between T_C and T_B (ΔT) increased slightly at higher body temperatures. No temperature difference was observed between brain thermocouple sites, suggesting nearly uniform distribution of cooled arterial blood. From the carotid's origin at the aorta to its entry into the brain case, blood temperature was constant, indicating that arterial blood was not cooled in the neck.

To provide additional information on the phylogenetic distribution of the phenomenon, Kilgore et al. (1976) measured T_B in five more species of birds, representing different orders, sizes, flight patterns, and environments. These included the 47-g lesser nighthawk (*Chordeiles acutipennis*), the 251-g roadrunner

(*Geococcyx californianus*), the 361-g pigeon (*Columba livia*), the 385-g white-necked raven (*Corvus cyrptoleucus*), and the 1156-g mallard (*Anas platyrhynchos*). As shown in Figure 1, all showed mean ΔT values between 0.8 and 1.3°C, over a T_C range of several degrees. The authors pointed out that ΔT probably reflects the effectiveness of heat exchange in the OR and that this in turn depends upon arteriovenous temperature differences, vascular dimension, and blood flow in the OR.

Additional T_B data have been provided by Bernstein et al. (1979a) for the American kestrel (*Falco sparverius*), by Crowe and Withers (1979) for helmeted guinea fowl (*Numida meleagris*), by Kilgore et al. (1981) for bobwhite quail (*Colinus virginianus*), by Bech and Midtgård (1981) for the zebra finch (*Poephila guttata*), and by Kleinhaus et al. (1985) for the sand partridge (*Ammoperdix heyi*) and the chukar (*Alectoris chukar sinaica*). In all of these species T_B was lower than T_C. In domestic fowl (Arad et al., 1984a), sand partridges, and chukars (Kleinhaus et al., 1985) hypohydration caused a decrease in ΔT during heat stress. However, when T_C had risen high enough for panting to begin in these species, ΔT increased again, in direct proportion to T_C. Eventually ΔT reached the level observed in normally hydrated birds.

The cooling of the avian brain has special significance during exercise, when heat production may exceed resting levels by an order of magnitude or more. Measurements have, therefore, been performed in both flying and running birds. During flights at a speed of 10 m/s and a T_A of 23°C in a wind tunnel, American kestrels (*Falco sparverius*) increased their T_C for the first 5 min, then reached a steady state. Brain temperature rose for only 1 min, however, so ΔT nearly doubled (Bernstein et al., 1979a). Unlike flying kestrels, bobwhite running on a treadmill at a T_A of 20°C decreased ΔT. When the quail ran at a T_A of 30°C, however, ΔT increased (Kilgore et al., 1981). Thus, at least some birds appear to store heat during exercise, allowing T_C to rise, but they regulate T_B over a narrow range. The increase in ΔT with exercise is exacerbated by hot environments, and this implies that the OR improves its heat transfer effectiveness during heat stress.

B. Role of the Ophthalmic Rete

Both morphological and physiological information is now available implicating the OR in cooling the avian brain. Richards (1967, 1968, 1970) described the anatomy of this structure and its associated vasculature. Its arterial component forms from the external ophthalmic artery, an extracranial branch of the internal carotid artery, whereas the venous component derives from the same sources as does the intracranial cavernous sinus, that is, from branches of the facial, maxillary, and mandibular veins. The anatomy suggests that blood flows to the brain either directly through the internal carotids or through the OR. Experiments in which selected arteries were occluded led Richards and Sykes

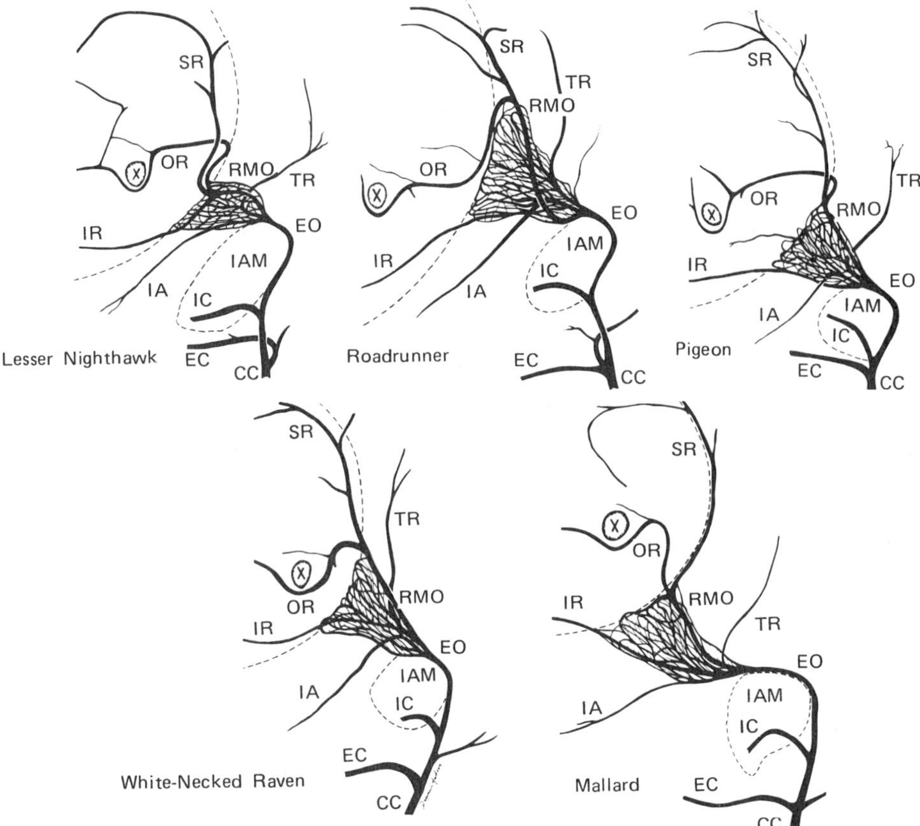

Figure 2 Diagram of a portion of the cephalic arteries and the arterial component of the ophthalmic rete in five species of birds. Drawn from latex-injected specimens. Dashed lines show outlines of orbit and internal auditory meatus. Abbreviations: CC, common carotid; EC, external carotid; EO, external ophthalmic; IA, inferior alveolar; IAM, internal auditory meatus; IC, internal carotid; IR, infraorbital ramus; OR, ophthalmic ramus; RMO, ophthalmic rete; SR, supraorbital ramus; TR, temporal ramus; X, optic nerve. (From Kilgore et al., 1976.)

(1967) to conclude that either route could supply the entire blood flow requirements of the brain, although it is still not yet known how blood flow is allocated among the cerebral arteries.

As part of their comparative study, Kilgore et al. (1976) presented diagrams of the arterial component of the OR in five bird species, as reproduced in Figure 2, based on dissections of latex-injected specimens. They concurred with Richard's description of the arterial and venous origins of the OR. They also noted that the arteries draining the OR curve intracranially and merge with branches of the internal carotid carrying blood to the brain.

Midtgård (1985) has pointed out that the external ophthalmic artery continues through the body of the OR as a shunt vessel. The thick, smooth-muscle coating of this vessel is richly supplied with adrenergic neurons. The other retial arteries, and even the veins, are similarly innervated, and it is reasonable to suggest that venous blood flowing from anterior cephalic mucosa can be directed by sphincteric veins through the OR (Midtgård, 1984a). Thus, proportioning of OR blood flow between shunt and exchange vessels, the total flow of cooled venous blood through the OR and, therefore, the control of blood temperature in the excurrent arteries, all seem to be under sympathetic control.

Additional information on OR anatomy and other aspects of the cephalic vasculature in several avian species has been supplied by numerous investigators, beginning with Ottley (1879), and has been briefly summarized by Midtgård (1984c). The details have been made available through the anatomical investigations of Bech and Midtgård (1981), Midtgård (1983, 1984a, 1984c, 1985), Midtgård et al. (1983), Arad and Midtgård (1984), and Arad et al. (1987).

Interspecific variation in OR structure has been summarized by Midtgård (1983) in the form of an allometric analysis of OR morphometry for 40 species of birds spanning a 20,000-fold range of body mass. In this study the numbers of arteries in the OR were counted, and their lengths, luminal diameters, and wall thicknesses were measured. The data were used to calculate the luminal cross-sectional areas and the maximum arterial surface area available for heat exchange. The results were presented in equations of the form $Y = a \cdot M^b$, where Y is one of the morphometric parameters, a is the coefficient, and b the exponent of the body mass (M) in grams. Values of a and b for each parameter, in passerine and nonpasserine birds, are given in Table 1.

By assuming that blood flow through the large arteries in birds scales according to that in mammals, Midtgård (1983) also estimated that arterial blood flow in OR arteries ($\dot{V}a$, L/s) can be expressed as:

$$\dot{V}a = 1.5 \times 10^{-7} \cdot M^{0.74} \tag{1}$$

Because 0.74 is also the exponent for the numbers of arteries in the OR of passerine birds (see Table 1), OR flow and the number of OR arteries evidently increase in direct proportion.

Inspection of Table 1 reveals that small passerines ($M < 62$ g) have fewer OR arteries than nonpasserines of equal mass, whereas the opposite is true for passerines weighing more than this. Despite this, arterial length is about the same in passerines and nonpasserines of similar size, and the same can be stated for luminal diameter. Table 1 also shows that luminal cross-sectional area and total exchange surface scale nearly directly with body mass in passerines, but approximately with the square root of body mass in nonpasserines. Thus, nonpasserines

Table 1 Allometric Expressions for Arterial Numbers and Dimensions in the Ophthalmic Retia of Passerine and Nonpasserine Birds Having Body Mass M (g)

Y	a	b	r
Passerines			
maximum number of arteries	1.6	0.74	0.90
length of arteries (m)	1.1×10^{-3}	0.27	0.92
diameter of arterial lumen (m)	1.9×10^{-5}	0.18	0.76
total cross-sectional area of arterial lumina (m^2)	0.4×10^{-9}	1.09	0.96
total arterial exchange surface (m^2)	1.2×10^{-7}	1.09	0.98
Nonpasserines			
maximum number of arteries	16.1	0.18	0.30
length of arteries (m)	0.9×10^{-3}	0.26	0.79
diameter of arterial lumen (m)	1.9×10^{-5}	0.17	0.80
total cross-sectional area of arterial lumina (m^2)	4.7×10^{-9}	0.52	0.72
total arterial exchange surface (m^2)	8.3×10^{-7}	0.59	0.75

a and b are coefficient and exponent, respectively, for the expression $Y = a M^b$, where Y is the morphometric parameter indicated, and r is the correlation coefficient.
Source: Data from Midtgård (1983).

weighing less than 75 g have arteries with greater total cross-sectional areas than passerines of similar size. Most interestingly for OR heat exchange, the crossover body mass for maximum arterial exchange surface is 48 g; nonpasserines weighing less than this have greater exchange surfaces than similar-sized passerines, and conversely for birds weighing more than 48 g. It can, therefore, be predicted that, if other factors are equal, large passerine species have more effective brain-cooling systems than nonpasserines of similar size.

The possibility that OR dimensions are correlated with the effectiveness of the OR in cooling arterial blood has been explored in domestic fowl and mallards. In fowl, Midtgård et al. (1983) confirmed that brain-cooling ability is correlated with maximal arterial exchange area in the OR. Furthermore, among breeds of fowl, those well-adapted to desert conditions possessed ophthalmic retia with greater arterial exchange surfaces (Arad and Midtgård, 1984). In growing mallards, arterial exchange surface increased with body mass from hatching to adulthood (Arad et al., 1987) in a manner indistinguishable from that for adults of multiple species (see Table 1). Furthermore, the increase in arterial exchange surface was correlated with increased brain cooling during growth (Arad et al., 1984b). These results further implicate the OR in brain cooling.

Additional evidence for the brain-cooling role of the OR has been provided by Kilgore et al. (1979) who succeeded in occluding blood flow in the arterial supply to the OR in pigeons. Their results clearly demonstrate the importance of the OR in maintaining brain-cooling ability, for when the arterial flow was completely halted, ΔT reversed; the brain became warmer than the body core by 0.4°C. This result was not obtained in nonoperated or sham-operated controls, or in birds in which the arteries were only partially blocked. In these birds ΔT was not significantly different from that measured previously by Kilgore et al. (1976).

In birds with completely occluded OR arteries, all arterial blood to the brain must have passed through the intracranial branches of the internal carotid. These lie close to the cavernous sinus, which conveys some of the venous blood from cephalic evaporative cooling surfaces. Despite this, Kilgore et al. (1979) observed no brain cooling when OR flow was halted, suggesting that countercurrent cooling of cerebral carotid blood is not likely in intact birds. The authors interpreted the ΔT reversal in OR-occluded birds to reflect heightened endogenous heat production by the brain at the site of measurement. They interpreted a maintained ΔT of 1°C or greater in intact controls exposed to hot air to indicate that a large fraction of cerebral blood flow passes through the OR during heat stress.

C. Role of Cephalic Heat Loss

As necessary as the OR is to brain cooling, it cannot function unless its venous blood is first cooled while perfusing anterior cephalic surfaces. Information is now available that implicates the nasal and buccal mucosa and the eyes in this process. In addition, Hagan and Heath (1980) have demonstrated the ability of the bill in mallards to dissipate large fractions of metabolic heat; this region may also contribute to cooling venous blood flowing to the OR.

Morphological information on mucosal heat loss tissue is available principally from the work of Midtgård (1984a) on mallards. In these birds the vasculature of the oral, nasal, and ocular integument was found to include extensive networks of arteriovenous anastomoses (AVAs) and venous plexuses, as well as capillary beds. Representative densities of AVAs are 350 cm^{-2} in the lower eyelid, 220 cm^{-2} in the middle nasal concha, 170 cm^{-2} at the tip of the bill, 75 cm^{-2} in the palate, 7 cm^{-2} in the lateral nasal wall, and zero in the caudal nasal concha. The density of AVAs is thus higher in regions thought to be associated with heat loss. This, along with data on cephalic blood flow during heat stress (Bęch and Johansen, 1980), suggest that surface blood flow during panting and gular flutter increases greatly and changes rapidly.

Physiological evidence for the role of cephalic evaporation in brain cooling comes from the experiments of Bernstein et al. (1979b), who caused pigeons exposed to moderate and severe heat stress (T_A 30-54°C), to breathe through tracheostomies so that respiratory ventilation bypassed the anterior airways. The procedure did not inhibit gular flutter and both T_C and T_B remained unchanged, suggesting that evaporative cooling must have continued. Nasopharyngeal evaporation could be completely prevented, while normal respiratory ventilation continued, by blocking the nares and sealing the beak. This was followed by a reduction of ΔT from 1.1 to 0.4°C. When the eyes were closed and sealed as well ΔT reversed, T_B rising above T_C by 0.4°C just as in pigeons with occluded retial arteries (Kilgore et al., 1979). Bernstein et al. (1979b) interpreted these results to mean that anterior cephalic evaporation is required to cool the venous blood in the OR. They agreed with Kilgore et al. (1979) that the reversal in ΔT may reflect brain metabolism, but added that at a T_A exceeding head temperature, the high surface area/volume ratio at the head compared with the rest of the body might permit more rapid heat gain.

The observation of limited brain cooling, even when buccopharyngeal evaporation was prevented, and the complete abolition of brain cooling when the eyes were covered suggested an important role for ocular evaporation in the cooling of retial venous blood (Bernstein et al., 1979b). This was explored by Pinshow et al. (1982) who simultaneously measured intraocular, hypothalamic, and colonic temperatures in conscious pigeons exposed to various thermal regimens. They showed that selective ventilation of the corneas with air at 25°C quickly reduced T_B by 1.1°C, whereas cessation of ocular ventilation or prevention of corneal evaporation increased T_B. Body temperature remained unchanged in all experiments. These results have been confirmed by Midtgård (1984b) in pigeons and mallards.

Pinshow et al. (1982) also pointed out that the irises in pigeons are richly supplied by looping blood vessels that become engorged during heat stress. When a vasoconstrictor (phenylephrine) was topically applied to the eye, these vessels visibly constricted and eye temperatures decreased almost immediately. Brain temperature was unaffected by this procedure, however, suggesting compensation by evaporative cooling elsewhere. Pinshow et al. (1982) concluded that venous return from the various cephalic cooling surfaces may flow in parallel to the OR. Vasomotor adjustments may independently control heat loss at each of these surfaces to regulate the temperature in the venous blood of the OR and, thereby, to finely tune arterial cooling.

Midtgård (1983) has called attention to the close anatomical relationship between the arteries draining the OR and the eyes, and Frost et al. (1975) and Midtgård (1983, 1984b) have suggested that the OR may serve to cool the eyes as well as the brain. Indeed, Midtgård (1984b) has recorded central ocular temperatures as much as 3.5°C below T_C. In cold climates or while diving, birds may benefit from this by cooling the arterial blood flowing to the eyes, thus conserving the body heat (Schmidt and Simon, 1979). In hot environments or bright light, eye cooling would prevent overheating of the retina.

Thus, a scenario has evolved in which (1) the eye helps cool the OR's venous blood, and (2) cooling of the OR's arterial blood controls eye temperature. This intriguingly implies that the anterior portion of the eye provides cooling for the posterior portion through the indirect intermediary of the OR. Additional information about actual blood flow pathways and allocations must be obtained before final conclusions on this point can be drawn.

D. Models of Brain Cooling

The availability of information about vascular dimensions in the OR (Midtgård, 1983) made it possible to apply heat transfer theory to evaluate the OR's effectiveness as a countercurrent heat exchanger and its potential for brain cooling. To do this Midtgård (1983) first assumed that the OR is an ideal heat exchanger, implying that it is completely insulated, that its surface area for arteriovenous heat transfer is equally distributed throughout, and that its heat transfer coefficient is constant throughout the exchange area. It was also assumed that blood flow in the arterial and venous components of the system were equal and that the specific heat of blood was constant everywhere. These assumptions imply that the differences between mean arterial and mean venous temperatures are constant at all points in the OR. The validity of some of these assumptions may be questionable, but they permitted construction of a simple model of heat transfer that probably predicts, to a close approximation, the change in temperature of arterial blood during its traverse of the OR.

In this model, the cooling of arterial blood varies inversely with the heat transfer coefficient (U) for OR arteries. Midtgård (1983) derived an expression for U by assuming that this parameter expresses total heat conductance from arteries to veins. Because heat conductance is the inverse of resistance to heat transfer and because the total of this resistance is the sum of the individual resistances of arterial and venous blood and of the tissue separating them, the expression for total resistance for heat transfer (1/U) is:

$$1/U = 1/ha + E/k + 1/hv \qquad (2)$$

where ha and hv are heat transfer coefficients for arterial and venous blood (assumed to be equal), k is the thermal conductivity of arterial walls, and E is arterial wall thickness. Midtgård (1983) calculated h as Nu k/Z, where Nu (the Nusselt number) is a dimensionless constant equal to 3.66, and Z is the luminal diameter of the arteries. Thus, by substitution,

$$1/U = (0.55\ Z + t)/k \qquad (3)$$

Using the allometric information in Table 1 for the terms in Equation 3, Midtgård found that U scaled as $4.6 \times 10^4 M^{-0.18}$ for passerine birds and as $4.6 \times 10^4 M^{-0.17}$ for nonpasserines, where U is in $W/(m^2 °C)$ and M is body mass in grams.

On this basis, Midtgård (1983) calculated that the change in arterial blood temperature along the length of the OR was nearly independent of body size, averaging between 3 and 4°C in both passerines and nonpasserines. This was true despite considerable variability in the measured values of ΔT, and, as Table 1 indicates, significant variation with body size in OR morphometry.

Additional analysis of OR function was carried out by Clair (1985) who applied a model for countercurrent heat exchange, which was developed by Mitchell and Myers (1968) and was based on conservation of energy between arterial and venous blood, to measurements of OR dimensions and temperatures in double-crested cormorants (*Phalacrocorax auritus*). A number of assumptions also are inherent in this analysis, including constant blood thermal conductances throughout the system and equal arterial and venous flows. Some of the conclusions from this analysis are that blood can flow from the OR to the brain and eye at a temperature nearly as low as that of the evaporative surfaces. Thus, in agreement with Midtgård (1983), arteriovenous heat exchange in the OR appears to occur in nearly perfect concordance with ideal heat exchange theory. Clair (1985) also found that the blood-cooling capacity of the OR was independent of OR dimensions; it appeared as if the effective heat exchange area might be greater than necessary to achieve maximum arterial cooling. Several assumptions remain untested in both models (Midtgård, 1983; Clair, 1985). More information about vascular dimensions–particularly in the OR veins–and about arterial and venous blood flow will be required before the validity of the assumptions and the calculations based on them can be tested further.

In summary, the mechanisms employed by birds for independent regulation of brain temperature appear to include the following components:

1. Regulation of blood temperature in OR veins by modulating ventilation and perfusion of evaporative surfaces
2. Regulation of blood flow in OR veins by venoconstriction and venodilation
3. Proportioning cephalic arterial blood flow between the external ophthalmic and the intracephalic carotid routes by arterioconstriction and arteriodilation in the OR
4. Proportioning arterial blood flow between heat exchange vessels and shunt vessels in the OR by arterioconstriction and arteriodilation in these two vessel types

III. Brain Oxygen Supply

Because a large fraction of cerebral blood flow appears to pass through the OR, and because a decrease in arterial blood temperature of several degrees can occur there, the question arose as to whether or not there is an effect on arterial O_2 transport. Decreased temperature increases O_2 affinity in mammalian blood; it was therefore anticipated that cooling of the brain's arterial supply in birds might significantly reduce its O_2 tension. To investigate this possibility Bernstein et al. (1984) measured cerebral PO_2 in pigeons, and Pinshow et al. (1985) measured the effects of temperature on oxyhemoglobin equilibrium in pigeon blood.

A. Cerebral PO_2

Bernstein et al. (1984) reasoned that to quantify the effect of OR cooling, blood gases should be measured in arterial blood both before entering and after leaving the OR. Retial afferent blood was, therefore, sampled in pigeons from the cervical region of the carotid artery. However, technical problems precluded sampling of blood from any of the retial efferent arteries. Instead, simultaneous with carotid sampling, the authors took cerebrospinal fluid (CSF) from a lateral brain ventricle using a glass cannula, in a modification of the technique of Brakkee et al. (1979), and measured gas tensions in these samples as well. This was done on the assumption that because the site of sampling was within 1 mm of the choroid plexus where CSF is formed, the PO_2 at the sampling site would nearly equal that of the blood perfusing the plexus which, in turn, would represent the admixture of arterial blood arising from the OR and the intracephalic carotid.

It was anticipated that $PcsfO_2$ would be lower than PaO_2 because of arterial cooling. Instead, the $PcsfO_2$ exceeded the PaO_2. For example, when PaO_2 was 82 torr, $PcsfO_2$ was 114 torr, a 39% increase. Similarly, $PcsfCO_2$ (23 torr) was found to be significantly lower, by 26%, than $PaCO_2$ (31 torr). A possible explanation for these results is that the carbonic anhydrase reaction in the ependymal cells of the choroid plexus might add bicarbonate to CSF and H^+ to choroid blood plasma. According to a mechanism proposed by Jankowska and Grieb (1979), bicarbonate from the erythrocytes would then move into the plasma, maintaining charge balance, and combine with H^+ to produce CO_2. Moving into the erythrocytes, this CO_2 would provide the source for new erythrocytic bicarbonate and H^+. The latter would facilitate oxyhemoglobin dissociation and cause the observed elevation in $PcsfO_2$.

To test if this accounts for the results, Bernstein et al. (1984) performed experiments in pigeons, similar to those described by Bernstein et al. (1979b) in which respiratory ventilation was rerouted to avoid airflow over the anterior cephalic evaporative surfaces. Tracheostomized pigeons were fitted with brain and carotid cannulae for CSF and arterial blood sampling as in the previous experiment. When the beak and nares were sealed, arterial blood gases were unaf-

Table 2 Mean PO_2 ± 1 SD in Cerebrospinal Fluid (CSF)[a] and Arterial Blood[b], and Mean of Differences ± 1 SD Between Individual $Pcsf_{O_2}$ and Pa_{O_2} Determinations in Control and Tracheostomized Pigeons[c]

	Cerebrospinal fluid	Arterial blood	Difference	P
Control (11)	113.6 ± 2.6	82.0 ± 3.3	31.6 ± 4.2	$<10^{-9}$
ARB (10)	91.9 ± 1.8	82.4 ± 2.0	9.5 ± 2.6	$<10^{-6}$
ARB, eyes sealed (9)	82.5 ± 1.8	83.1 ± 2.1	-0.6 ± 2.0	<0.25

[a]CSF sampled anaerobically via a glass cannula in the lateral ventricle near the choroid plexus. Gas tension measured by a calibrated electrode at body temperature.

[b]Blood sampled anaerobically via a polyethylene cannula in the cervical segment of the internal carotid. Gas tension measured by a calibrated electrode at body temperature.

[c]In pigeons, contact was prevented between air and heat loss surfaces of oral and nasal cavities (anterior respiratory bypass; ARB), or ARB was accompanied by preventing contact between air and ocular surfaces (eyes sealed). P is the significance of the mean difference between PO_2 in CSF and blood. Number in parentheses is the number of individual experiments. The null hypothesis was rejected at $P < 0.01$. All gas tensions are given in torr.

Source: Data from Duran (1982) and Bernstein et al. (1984).

fected, but PO_2 and PCO_2 in CSF decreased and increased, respectively, compared with controls. However $Pcsf_{O_2}$ was still higher than Pa_{O_2}. When the eyes along with the beak and nares were closed and sealed against contact with air, $Pcsf_{O_2}$ decreased further, becoming indistinguishable from the unchanged Pa_{O_2}. Table 2 gives the results of the PO_2 measurements.

The authors concluded that acid-base changes in the ependymal cells could not be the only principle at work in evincing the PO_2 difference between CSF and arterial blood, because if it were, preventing contact between cephalic evaporative surfaces and air would not have abolished the PO_2 difference. To explain all the experimental results, Bernstein et al. (1984) proposed the hypothesis summarized in Section I: that in intact birds, O_2 and CO_2 are exchanged between air and the blood perfusing the mucosa in contact with air, increasing Pv_{O_2} and decreasing Pv_{CO_2} in the OR, so that the veins act as an O_2 source and a CO_2 sink for arterial blood. This compensates for the tendency of Pa_{O_2} to fall because of the leftward shift in the oxyhemoglobin equilibrium curve (OEC) in response to cooling. Indeed, the authors estimated that, if arteriovenous gas exchange in the OR is complete, Pa_{O_2} and arterial oxygen saturation (Sa_{O_2}) could actually increase, to the advantage of the animal.

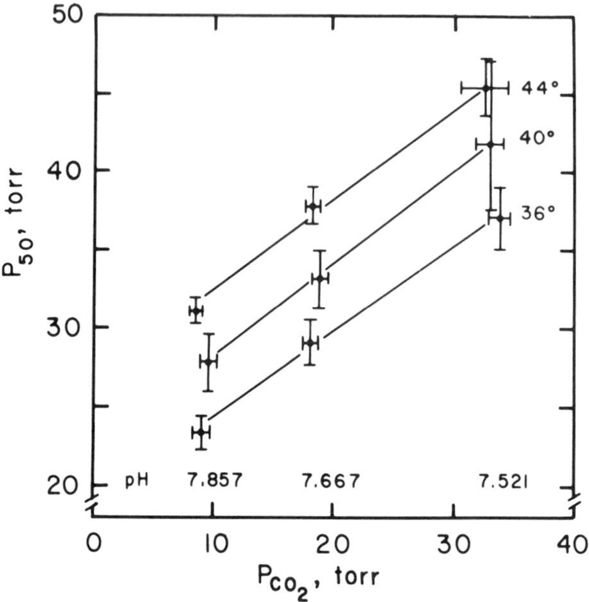

Figure 3 Oxygen tension at half-saturation of hemoglobin (P_{50}) in relation to CO_2 tension (PCO_2) and temperature in tonometered samples of pigeon blood. Means of blood pH measured after tonometry are also indicated. The relationship of pH to PCO_2 is given by Equation 4 in text. Points are means of duplicate determinations from six birds. Horizontal and vertical bars include ± 1 SD. Diagonal lines represent least-squares linear regression lines for data at each temperature (36, 40, and 44°C). Data are described by Equation 5 in text. (From Pinshow et al., 1985.)

B. Role of Oxyhemoglobin Equilibrium

Evaluation of this hypothesis required quantitative information about the effects of temperature and the CO_2 Bohr effect on the OEC. Pinshow et al. (1985) therefore measured P_{50} in pigeon blood in relation to temperature and PCO_2. Figure 3 summarizes the results. As expected, P_{50} increased with both temperature and PCO_2. The authors noted the dependence of pH on PCO_2, as described by:

$$pH = 8.423 - 0.595 \log PCO_2 \tag{4}$$

However, the data did not allow the separation of the indirect effects of CO_2 on P_{50}, through changes in pH, from the direct effects. To describe the data in Figure 3, therefore, Pinshow et al. (1985) presented the following equation relating P_{50}, temperature, and PCO_2:

$$P_{50} = 1.049\,T + 0.573\,P_{CO_2} - 19.444 \tag{5}$$

They then wrote the following expression relating the O_2 tension to the percentages of O_2-saturated blood (SO_2):

$$\ln P_{O_2} = a + b \ln [SO_2/(100 - SO_2)] + c \ln [SO_2/(100 - SO_2)]^2 \tag{6}$$

where a is the constant for the polynomial and b and c are the first- and second-order coefficients. Because at P_{50} $\ln [SO_2/(100 - SO_2)]$ is zero, a = $\ln P_{50}$. Therefore in analyzing the potential role of blood in exchanging gases at the anterior cephalic mucosa and the OR, Pinshow et al. (1985) used Equation 5 to provide values for a in Equation 6 corresponding to the temperature and P_{CO_2} values expected at the putative gas exchange sites. Throughout the analysis they used values for b and c in Equation 6 determined for the pigeon blood data of Hirsowitz et al. (1977) (0.3645 and -0.0163, respectively). This was based on the independent finding that the shape of the OEC in pigeons does not change with P_{50} (Maginniss, Bernstein, and Pinshow, in preparation). In this fashion the authors generated families of OECs to estimate the P_{O_2} and SO_2 in arterial blood draining the OR and flowing to the brain.

When venous blood was assumed to flow from the cephalic mucosa to the OR at reduced P_{O_2} and temperature and at elevated P_{CO_2}, as would be expected if blood gases were exchanged only between mucosal blood and tissue, the arterial blood was calculated to undergo a 10-torr reduction in P_{O_2} because of cooling in the OR. In another scenario, however, Pinshow et al. (1985) calculated the consequences of gas exchange both across cephalic mucosal surfaces between the blood and air, and between the arteries and veins in the OR. Figure 4 shows the family of OECs used for this analysis in normoxic pigeons, with curves calculated for blood P_{CO_2} of 33 torr (curves 1, 2) or 18 torr (curves 3, 4) and for blood temperature of 41°C (curves 1, 3) or 36°C (curves 2, 4).

It was assumed that arterial blood arrives at both the evaporative surfaces and the OR under the conditions represented by point a. Cooling at those sites displaces the OEC, so arterial blood resides at point b. If, because of the 33-torr P_{CO_2} difference between blood and air, CO_2 is lost to the atmosphere at the mucosa, the OEC would move further (curve 4), and if, because of a P_{O_2} difference exceeding 100 torr, O_2 diffuses from the atmosphere to the blood, the resulting P_{O_2} would be 73 torr and the SO_2 would be 95% (point d). These, then, are the approximate conditions proposed by these authors to exist in *venous* blood arriving at the OR.

Within the OR this venous blood now takes up heat and CO_2 from arterial blood, moving the OEC back to curve 1, so the P_{VO_2} becomes 108 torr (point f). Meanwhile, the loss of CO_2 and heat displaces the arterial OEC to curve 4 (point c). The resulting AV P_{O_2} difference is thus − 54 torr. Assuming that countercurrent exchange of gases is complete, as it is for heat (Midtgård, 1983, Clair,

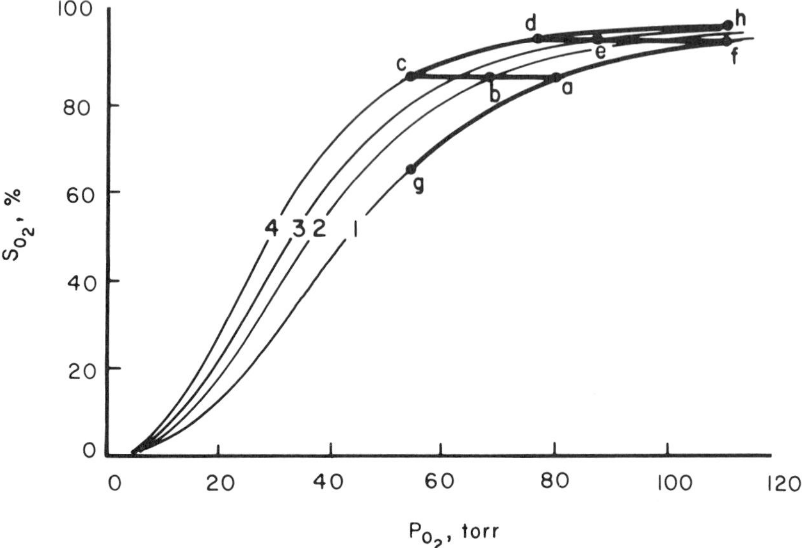

Figure 4 Oxygen equilibrium curves for pigeon blood calculated by Equations 5 and 6 in text. Curves are for blood PCO_2 of 33 (curves 1, 2) or 18 torr (curves 3, 4) and for blood temperature of 41 (curves 1, 3) or 36°C (curves 2, 4). Heavy lines and lettered points illustrate changes in PO_2 and O_2 saturation (SO_2) hypothesized to occur at various sites within cephalic circulation as blood is cooled at mucosal surfaces of head and within ophthalmic retia (OR), and as O_2 and CO_2 are exchanged between mucosal blood and air and between arterial and venous blood in the OR. Details and definitions of points a through h are given in text. (Redrawn from Pinshow et al., 1985.)

1985). The venous blood moves down curve 1 to point g, whereas arterial blood moves up curve 4 to point h.

The results of this analysis suggest that if arterial blood enters the OR at 41°C with a PO_2 of 80 torr, a PCO_2 of 33 torr, and an SO_2 of 87%, it could flow to the brain at 36°C with a PO_2 of 108 torr, a PCO_2 of 18 torr, and an SO_2 near 100%. The O_2-combining properties of pigeon blood are thus consistent with the possibility that mucosal and retial gas exchange supplements the brain's O_2 supply.

Pinshow et al. (1985) repeated the calculations for hypoxic pigeons at a simulated altitude of 7000 m above sea level, where arterial blood entering the OR at 39.5°C would be expected to have a PO_2 of 26 torr, a PCO_2 of 14 torr, and an SO_2 of 40% (Weinstein et al., 1985). The results showed that if arterial blood were cooled to 36°C in the OR, it could flow to the brain at a PO_2 of 54 torr and an SO_2 of 95%, representing a doubling of both these parameters over systemic arterial values. The authors suggested that this could provide normal cerebral O_2 delivery with little or no increase in cerebral blood flow. The advantage in a bird flying at high altitude, in addition to assuring cerebral oxygenation, would be to permit a larger fraction of the cardiac output to be allocated to flight muscle, perhaps lessening the total cardiac effort required.

C. A Nonsystemic Pathway from Atmosphere to Brain

In view of the suggestive results from the $Pcsf_{O_2}$ measurements and the OEC analysis just summarized, it seemed necessary to establish as directly as possible the existence of an exclusively cephalic gas pathway from air to brian. Pierce et al. (in preparation) therefore carried out experiments using H_2 as a physiologically inert, easily detectable marker. For measurement of relative H_2 concentrations, platinum electrodes were implanted in the hypothalamus and in an internal carotid artery, together with silver–silver chloride reference electrodes. Thermocouples were also placed in the brain and colon for determination of ΔT. Halothane-anesthetized birds were tracheally intubated through the glottis to separate the ventilatory gases from oral, nasal, and ocular surfaces.

When H_2 was introduced into inspired air, it appeared rapidly in carotid blood and almost simultaneously in brain. When H_2 flow was halted, carotid H_2 disappeared immediately and brain H_2 washed out in characteristic exponential fashion. The response depended on H_2 concentration; stepwise increases in inspired H_2 concentration gave stepwise increases in carotid and brain electrode currents. Sample traces of electrode currents recorded during these experiments are shown in Figure 5.

Figure 5 also shows the result of a sample experiment in which H_2 was introduced into the nasal passages alone, rather than into the inspired air. Here, only the electrode current in the brain increased. The augmentation was as great as when H_2 was introduced through the respiratory tract. Increases in nasal H_2 flow, however, elicited little or no further increase in brain H_2.The increase in carotid H_2 was delayed and slight, a small fraction of the response to respiratory H_2. The results suggest that H_2 reached the brain by a nonsystemic route, and was then washed into the venous circulation. The rise in carotid H_2 occurred secondary to that in brain and probably reflects recirculated H_2 that was not removed in the first pass through the lungs.

To investigate further the route followed to the brain by H_2 introduced into the nasal passages, Pierce et al. (in preparation) manipulated the effective vascular exchange surfaces in both the nasal mucosa and the OR. The effective exchange area in the mucosa was functionally modified by use of a vasodilator (phenoxybenzamine) or a vasoconstrictor (phenylephrine) applied topically in halothane-anesthetized pigeons with implanted brain and arterial H_2-sensing electrodes. The results of a typical experiment are shown in Figure 6. When H_2

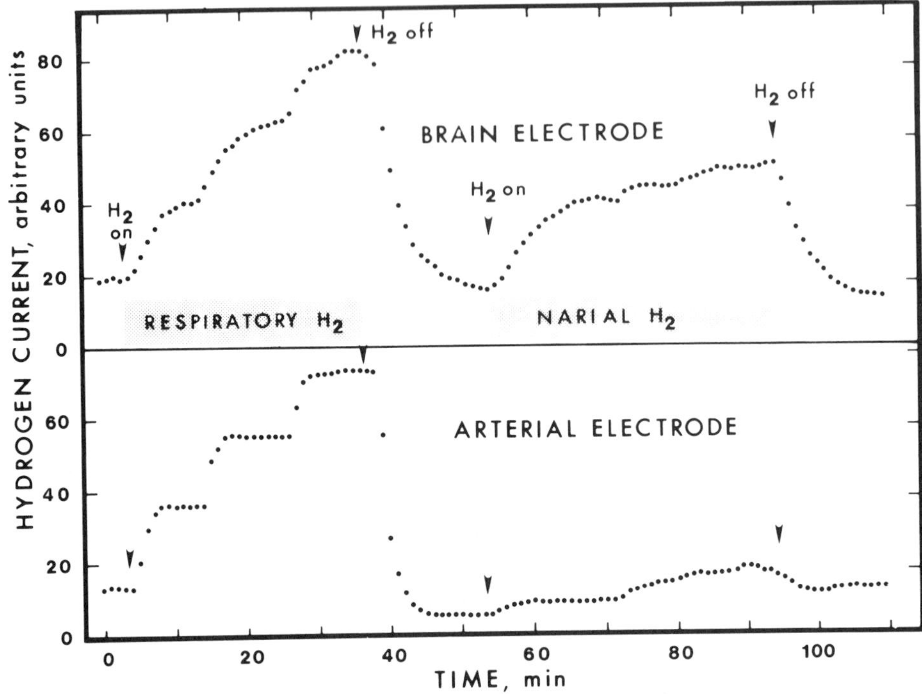

Figure 5 Sample recordings of current in H_2-sensing electrodes implanted in brain (hypothalamus) and in cervical region of a carotid artery in a pigeon. Tracings show effects of introducing H_2 (arrows) into the respiratory tract (3–37 min) or into the external nares (53–94 min). Hydrogen introduced into the lungs alone, at flows increasing stepwise, caused rapid corresponding increases in the H_2 concentrations of both arterial blood and brain. Hydrogen flowing into the nasal cavity alone caused a similar increase in the brain's H_2 concentration but little change in the arterial H_2 concentration. The results suggest that the H_2 absorbed in the lungs was transported to the brain through pulmonary and systemic pathways, whereas the H_2 absorbed across the nasal epithelium moved to the brain by an exclusively cephalic route. (Data from Pierce, Bernstein, and Pinshow, in preparation.)

was introduced exclusively into the nasal passages, brain electrode current rose to a plateau as observed previously. Vasodilation was accompanied by an additional rise in brain H_2. Vasoconstriction elicited reversal of the response, brain H_2 washing out nearly to baseline, despite the continued flow of H_2 through the nasal passages. These results were interpreted to indicate that final H_2 concentration in the brain depends, in part, on the effective vascular exchange surface in the nasal mucosa.

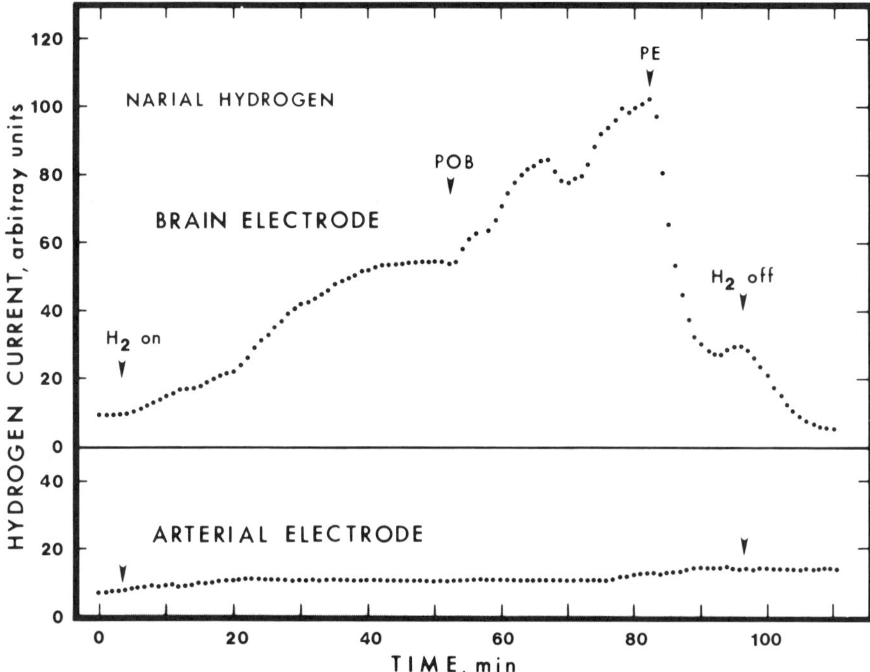

Figure 6 Sample recordings of current in H_2-sensing electrodes implanted in brain (hypothalamus) and in cervical regions of a carotid artery in a pigeon. Tracings show effects of introducing H_2 (arrows) into the external nares. Brain electrode current increased as in Figure 5, attaining a steady state in 40 min. When phenoxybenzamine (POB), a vasodilator, was applied to the nasal mucosa at 51 min, brain H_2 concentration rapidly increased. When phenylephrine (PE), a vasoconstrictor, was applied to the nasal mucosa at 82 min, brain H_2 concentration decreased. All data were obtained at constant H_2 flow and pressure. The results suggest that the movement of H_2 from nasal membranes to the brain depends on mean vascular diameter and, thus, on the exchange area in the mucosa, and perhaps on mucosal blood flow as well. (Data from Pierce, Bernstein, and Pinshow, in preparation.)

The effective vascular exchange surface in the OR was modified by altering ΔT in halothane-anesthetized pigeons. This was achieved by subjecting the animals to exogenous heat loads that raised T_C (Pierce et al., in preparation). It was assumed, in concert with studies described in Section II, that changes in ΔT were proportional to effective heat exchange surface in the OR. As previously, the pigeons had H_2-sensing electrodes and themocouples implanted in the brain and the carotid artery, and H_2 gas flowing through the nasal passages. As ΔT increased so did peak brain H_2 current, and conversely. This was taken as evidence favoring the participation of the OR in the transfer of H_2 to brain. It was also concluded that the effectiveness of this transfer depends, in part, on the availability of exchange surface in the OR.

A potential criticism of this work is that H_2, a small molecule, is more diffusible in tissue than O_2 or CO_2. Indeed, on the basis of molecular weights alone Graham's law predicts that H_2 diffuses four times faster than O_2, whereas the Chapman-Enskog equation, which takes temperature and pressure into account, predicts that the diffusion coefficient for H_2 is 7.5 times that for O_2 at 41°C and 1 atm. On this basis, experimental results confirming a nonsystemic H_2 route from nasal passages to brain would not necessarily imply an exclusively cephalic mechanism for the transfer of O_2. However, Kawashiro et al. (1975a) have shown that molecular diameter is a better predictor of the diffusion coefficient than molecular mass. The ratio of their H_2 and O_2 diffusion coefficients is only about 1.5, suggesting that the diffusion rates of the two gases in similar tissues under similar conditions is much closer than would be expected from the difference between their molecular masses.

The diffusion coefficient for a gas diffusing in a liquid can be defined as the ratio of Krogh's diffusion constant (K) for the gas to its solubility (α) (Dejours, 1982). Therefore, the values of these two parameters for H_2 and O_2 are also similar, helping to justify further the use of H_2. For example, the solubility of H_2 in water at 40°C is 71% of O_2 solubility, and a similar ratio would be expected for plasma. Moreover, H_2 solubility in vertebrate skeletal muscle at 37°C is 1.13×10^{-6} mmol/(cm^3 · torr) (Campos Carles et al., 1975), compared to 1.38×10^{-6} mmol/cm^3 · torr) for O_2 (Bartels, 1971). In rat skeletal muscle K_{O_2} at 37°C is 2.18×10^{-11} mmol/(cm · s · torr) (Kawashiro et al., 1975b), compared to a K_{H_2} in the same tissue at the same temperature of 2.78×10^{-11} mmol/(cm · s · torr) (Kawashiro et al., 1975a). Thus, in view of the similarities in the properties of H_2 and O_2, it seems reasonable to use H_2 as an O_2 analogue in the experiments, as described.

D. Diffusibility

In evaluating the hypothesis under discussion it is instructive to consider the O_2 diffusion capacity (D_{O_2}) in the vessels of the OR. Estimation of D_{O_2} in arteries and veins requires morphometric information for each vessel type. Unfortunately, such information is available for OR arteries only, as summarized in Table 1. On the basis of qualitative histological examination (Midtgård et al., 1983; Arad and Midtgård, 1984; Arad et al., 1987), it is highly unlikely that the numbers and dimensions of OR veins and arteries are similar. It is, therefore, unlikely that the maximum venous exchange surface, for example, is similar to the corresponding value for arteries, and it would be difficult to estimate even the order of magnitude by which they differ.

The information about arterial dimensions, however, allows the estimation of DO_2 for this type of vessel (DaO_2). The DaO_2 is the inverse of total diffusion resistance, which is, in turn, the sum of the diffusion resistances in the arterial plasma ($1/DpO_2$) and in the arterial walls ($1/DwO_2$). Because in the hypothesis under examination, 80% or more of the hemoglobin is saturated in normoxic birds, facilitated O_2 diffusion can be considered negligible, hence, diffusion resistance in the erythrocytes and plasma are indistinguishable.

If we consider the mean diffusion distance in plasma to be half the mean luminal radius, or one-fourth the mean luminal diameter (Z), then DpO_2 in mmol/(s · torr) is given by 4 KpO_2 Ap/Z, where KpO_2 is the Krogh diffusion constant in plasma in mmol/(s · cm · torr) and Ap is maximum plasma exchange surface in cm^2. The latter equals the total inner surface area of the artery walls, and is given by:

$$Ap = \pi Z \cdot L \cdot N \tag{7}$$

In Equation 7 L is the mean artery length in cm and N is the total number of arteries in the OR.

For the arterial walls the mean diffusion distance is the mean wall thickness (E) in cm. DwO_2 is then given by KwO_2 Aw/E, where KwO_2 is the Krogh diffusion constant for arterial walls and Aw is the maximum wall exchange surface in cm^2. Aw is equivalent to the total outer surface area of the artery walls and, thus, to the total arterial exchange surface determined by Midtgård (1983) (see Table 1). The expression for $1/DaO_2$ thus becomes:

$$1/DaO_2 = Z/(4\,KpO_2\,Ap) + E/(KwO_2\,Aw) \tag{8}$$

Combining Equations 7 and 8:

$$1/DaO_2 = 1/(4\,\pi\,KpO_2\,L\,N) + E/(KwO_2\,Aw) \tag{9}$$

This shows that the total arterial diffusion resistance, as would be expected, is directly proportional to wall thickness and inversely proportional to the area of the exchange surface, to the mean length and number of arteries, and to the diffusional properties of O_2 in plasma and arterial walls.

Equation 9 can be solved for DaO_2 in a bird of known body mass by substituting values obtained from the applicable expressions in Table 1. It is also necessary to assume, with Midtgård (1983), that E = 0.2 Z, based on measurements in OR arteries after perfusion with fixative at physiological pressures. As a sample calculation of DaO_2 I have chosen a 400-g nonpasserine bird, to correspond to a pigeon; have assumed KpO_2 to be the same as that for water, 4.6×10^{-11} mmol/(s · cm · torr); and have assumed KwO_2 to be the same as that for vertebrate skeletal muscle, 2.2×10^{-11} mmol/(s · cm · torr) (Kawashiro et al., 1975b). The Krogh constants are also assumed to be independent of temperature (Dejours, 1981). The calculated value for DaO_2 is then 3.9×10^{-9} mmol/

(s · torr). For comparison, estimates of minimum DO_2 in human lung are nearly 4×10^6 times greater than this (Weibel, 1984).

E. Evaluation of the Hypothesis

For any longitudinal segment dL of the OR, the total rate of molar O_2 flux across arterial walls ($\dot{M}aO_2$, mmol/s) can be written:

$$\dot{M}aO_2 = D_{dL}O_2 \, (P_{dL}aO_2 - P_{dL}vO_2) \qquad (10)$$

where $D_{dL}O_2$ is the O_2 diffusing capacity, and $P_{dL}aO_2$ and $P_{dL}vO_2$ are the respective arterial and venous PO_2, all for segment dL. Assuming for simplicity that exchange surfaces are evenly distributed along the length of the OR, then for dL = 0.1 L, $D_{dL}O_2$ is about 10^{-10} mmol/(s · torr). At the blood flow calculated for the retial arteries in a 400-g bird by Midtgård (1983) allometric estimate (see Eq. 1), the net increase in arterial O_2 content within the segment, when $P_{dL}aO_2$ is 80 torr and $P_{dL}vO_2$ is 115 torr, is about 8×10^{-5} mmol/L. Because the O_2 content of arterial blood entering the OR in normoxic pigeons is greater than 6 mmol/L (Weinstein et al., 1985), the increase calculated here, even if sustained for all segments throughout the length of the OR, would be insignificantly small.

From this it seems that either (1) no significant O_2 flux can occur across arterial walls at any reasonable local AV difference in PO_2, precluding the enhancement of O_2 in arterial blood flowing to the brain; (2) assumptions made in the derivation of DaO_2 are invalid; (3) factors that significantly enhance O_2 diffusing capacity in OR arteries have been neglected in the above analysis; or (4) the dimensions of and blood flow in OR arteries in pigeons are greatly different from those calculated by the expressions in Table 1.

At the moment, it is not possible to determine with certainty which of these conclusions separately or in combination may be valid. However, the experimental results of Bernstein et al. (1984), showing an elevation of $PcsfO_2$ over PaO_2 in pigeons and its abolition by prevention of contact between air and cephalic evaporative surfaces, are difficult to reconcile with the calculation of DaO_2. So are the results of the experiments by Pierce et al. (in preparation) using H_2 as an inert gas tracer. The discrepancies between the experimental and theoretical results so far available make it seem premature to accept conclusion (1). Additional data on PO_2 in brain and CSF are clearly required. It is obvious, too, that actual morphometric data should be used for calculating DaO_2, rather than values obtained by solving allometric equations. Ultimately, the measurement of gases in arterial blood flowing into and out of the OR will be decisive. Should an increase in PaO_2 and a decrease in $PaCO_2$ be observed, there will be little doubt that the OR plays a role in brain O_2 supply. Meanwhile, however, final judgment must be held in abeyance.

References

Arad, Z., and Midtgård, U. (1984). Differences in the structure of the rete ophthalmicum among three breeds of domestic fowls, *Gallus gallus* f. *domesticus* (Aves). *Zoomorphology 104*:184-187.

Arad, Z., Midtgård, U., and Bernstein, M. H. (1987). Post-hatching development of the rete ophthalmicum in relation to brain temperature of mallard ducks (*Anas platyrhynchos*). *Am. J. Anat. 179*:137-142.

Arad, Z., Midtgård, U., and Skadhauge, E. (1984a). Effect of dehydration on body-to-brain temperature difference in heat-stressed fowl (*Gallus domesticus*). *J. Comp. Physiol. B 154*:295-300.

Arad, Z., Toledo, C. S., and Bernstein, M. H. (1984b). Development of brain temperature regulation in the hatchling mallard duck *Anas platyrhynchos*. *Physiol. Zool. 57*:493-499.

Baker, M. A. (1982). Brain cooling in endotherms in heat and exercise. *Annu. Rev. Physiol. 44*:85-96.

Bartels, H. (1971). Diffusion coefficients and Krogh's diffusion constants. Table 14 in *Respiration and Circulation*. Edited by P. L. Altman and D. S. Dittmer, Bethesda, Federation of American Societies for Experimental Biology, pp. 21-23.

Bech, C., and Johansen, K. (1980). Blood flow changes in the duck during thermal panting. *Acta Physiol. Scand. 110*:351-355.

Bech, C., and Midtgård, U. (1981). Brain temperature and the rete mirabile ophthalmicum in the zebra finch (*Poephila guttata*). *J. Comp. Physiol. 145*: 89-93.

Bernstein, M. H., Curtis, M. B., and Hudson, D. M. (1979a). Independence of brain and body temperatures in flying American kestrels, *Falco sparverius*. *Am. J. Physiol. 237*:R58-R62.

Bernstein, M. H., Duran, H. L., and Pinshow, B. (1984). Extrapulmonary gas exchange enhances brain oxygen in pigeons. *Science 226*:564-566.

Bernstein, M. H., Sandoval, I., Curtis, M. B., and Hudson, D. M. (1979b). Brain temperature in pigeons: Effects of anterior respiratory bypass. *J. Comp. Physiol. 129*:115-118.

Brakkee, J. H., Wiegant, V. M., and Gispen, W. H. (1979). A simple technique for rapid implantation of a permanent cannula into the rat brain ventricular system. *Lab. Anim. Sci. 29*:78-81.

Campos Carles, A., Kawashiro, T., and Piiper, J. (1975). Solubility of various inert gases in rat skeletal muscle. *Pflügers Arch. 359*:209-218.

Clair, P. M. (1985). The rete mirabile ophthalmicum of the double-crested cormorant (*Phalacrocorax auritus*): Its form and function. M.S. Thesis, New Mexico State University.

Crowe, T. M., and Withers, P. C. (1979). Brain temperature regulation in helmeted guineafowl. *S. Afr. J. Sci. 75*:362-365.

Dejours, P. (1981). *Principles of Comparative Respiratory Physiology*. Amsterdam, Elsevier/North-Holland Biomedical Press.

Duran, H. L. (1982). Gas tensions and acid-base status in arterial blood and cerebrospinal fluid of pigeons, *Columba livia*: Relation to countercurrent exchange in the rete mirabile ophthalmicum. M.S. thesis. New Mexico State University.

Frost, P. G. H., Siegfried, W. R., and Greenwood, P. J. (1975). Arteriovenous heat exchange systems in the jackass penguin *Spheniscus demersus. J. Zool. 175*:231-241.

Hagan, A. A., and Heath, J. E. (1980). Regulation of heat loss in the duck by vasomotion in the bill. *J. Therm. Biol. 5*:95-101.

Hirsowitz, L. A., Fell, K., and Torrance, J. D. (1977). Oxygen affinity of avian blood. *Respir. Physiol. 31*:51-62.

Hudson, D. M., and Bernstein, M. H. (1981). Temperature regulation and heat balance in flying white-necked ravens, *Corvus cryptoleucus. J. Exp. Biol. 90*:267-281.

Janowska, L., and Grieb, P. (1979). Relationship between arterial and cisternal CSF oxygen tension in rabbits. *Am. J. Physiol. 236*:F220-F225.

Kawashiro, T., Campos Carles, A., Perry, S. F., and Piiper, J. (1975a). Diffusivity of various inert gases in rat skeletal muscle. *Pflügers Arch. 359*:219-230.

Kawashiro, T., Nüsse, W., and Scheid, P. (1975b). Determination of diffusivity of oxygen and carbon dioxide in respiring tissue: Results in rat skeletal muscle. *Pflügers Arch. 359*:231-251.

Kilgore, D. L., Jr., Bernstein, M. H., and Hudson, D. M. (1979). Brain temperatures in birds. *J. Comp. Physiol. 110*:209-215.

Kilgore, D. L., Jr., Birchard, G. F., and Boggs, D. F. (1981). Brain temperatures in running quail. *J. Appl. Physiol. 50*:1277-1281.

Kilgore, D. L., Jr., Boggs, D. F., and Birchard, G. F. (1979). Role of the rete mirabile ophthalmicum in maintaining the body-to-brain temperature difference in pigeons. *J. Comp. Physiol. 129*:119-122.

Kilgore, D. L., Bernstein, M. H., and Schmidt-Nielsen, K. (1973). Brain temperature in a large bird, the rhea. *Am. J. Physiol. 225*:739-742.

Kleinhaus, S., Pinshow, B., Bernstein, M. H., and Degen, A. A. (1985). Brain temperature in heat-stressed, water-deprived desert phasianids: Sand partridge (*Ammoperdix heyi*) and chukar (*Alectoris chukar sinaica*). *Physiol. Zool. 58*:105-116.

Midtgård, U. (1983). Scaling of the brain and the eye cooling system in birds: A morphometric analysis of the rete ophthalmicum. *J. Exp. Zool. 225*: 197-207.

Midtgård, U. (1984a). Blood vessels and the occurrence of arteriovenous anastomoses in cephalic heat loss areas of mallards, *Anas platyrhynchos* (Aves). *Zoomorphology 104*:323-335.

Midtgård, U. (1984b). Eye temperature in birds and the significance of the rete ophthalmicum. *Vidensk. Medd. Dans. Naturhist. Foren. 145*:173-181.

Midtgård, U. (1984c). The blood vascular system in the head of the herring gull *(Larus argentatus). J. Morphol. 179*:135-152.

Midtgård, U. (1985). Innervation of the avian ophthalmic rete. *Fortsch. Zool. 30*:401-404.

Midtgård, U., Arad, Z., and Skadhauge, E. (1983). The rete ophthalmicum and the relation of its size to the body-to-brain temperature difference in the fowl *(Gallus domesticus). J. Comp. Physiol. 153*:241-246.

Mitchell, J. W., and Myers, G. E. (1968). An analytical model of the countercurrent heat exchange phenomena. *Biophys. J. 8*:897-911.

Ottley, W. (1879). A description of the vessels of the neck and head in the ground hornbill *Bucorvus abyssinicus. Proc. Zool. Soc. 30*:461.

Pinshow, B., Bernstein, M. H., and Arad, Z. (1985). Effects of temperature and P_{CO_2} on O_2 affinity of pigeon blood: Implications for brain O_2 supply. *Am. J. Physiol. 249*:R758-R764.

Pinshow, B., Bernstein, M. H., Lopez, G. E., and Kleinhaus, S. (1982). Regulation of brain temperature in pigeons: Effects of corneal convection. *Am. J. Physiol. 242*:R577-R581.

Richards, S. A. (1967). Anatomy of the arteries of the head in the domestic fowl. *J. Zool. 152*:221-234.

Richards, S. A. (1968). Anatomy of the veins of the head in the domestic fowl. *J. Zool. 154*:223-234.

Richards, S. A. (1970). Brain temperature and the cerebral circulation in the chicken. *Brain Res. 23*:265-268.

Richards, S. A., and Sykes, A. H. (1967). Response of the domestic fowl (*Gallus domesticus*) to occlusion of the cervical arteries and veins. *Comp. Biochem. Physiol. 21*:39-50.

Schmidt, I., and Simon, E. (1979). Temperature changes of the hypothalamus and body core in ducks feeding in cold water. *Pflügers Arch. 378*:227-230.

Scott, N. R., Johnson, A. T., and van Tienhoven, A. (1970). Measurement of hypothalamic temperature and heart rate of poultry. *Trans. ASAE 13*:342-347.

Taylor, C. R., and Lyman, C. P. (1972). Heat storage in running antelopes: Independence of brain and body temperatures. *Am. J. Physiol. 222*:114-117.

Weibel, E. R. (1984). *The Pathway for Oxygen: Structure and Function in the Mammalian Respiratory System*. Cambridge, Harvard University Press.

Weinstein, Y., Bernstein, M. H., Bickler, P. E., Gonzales, D. V., Samaniego, F. C., and Escobedo, M. A. (1985). Blood respiratory properties in pigeons at high altitudes: Effects of acclimation. *Am. J. Physiol. 249*:R765-R775.

13

Gas Exchange
Theory, Models, and Experimental Data

JOHANNES PIIPER

Max Planck Institute for Experimental Medicine
Göttingen, Federal Republic of Germany

PETER SCHEID

Ruhr-Universität
Bochum, Federal Republic of Germany

I. Introduction

The aim of this short review chapter is to describe and discuss some models that are being used to analyze the performance of vertebrate gas exchange organs. These models can be traced down to a small number of prototypes, which will first be presented and then briefly characterized (Sect. II).

Three component processes typically determine the functional properties of gas exchange organs: convective transport by flowing medium (water or air), diffusional exchange between medium and blood (and chemical reactions in blood), and convective transport by blood flow. Because gas exchange in most species, namely, in mammals and birds, is limited inappreciably by diffusion, it is, at first, convenient to treat the gas transfer properties by considering only ventilation and perfusion, neglecting diffusion limitation (Sect. III).

Diffusion is then introduced (in Sect. IV) by incorporating a diffusion barrier into the widely applicable diffusion-perfusion model. Resistances to diffusion, however are not limited to the tissue barrier separating blood from medium but typically also occur in the medium and in blood. Two examples of such diffusion limitation in the medium will be presented: diffusion resistance offered by alveolar gas in mammalian lungs (Sect. V) and diffusion in the interlamellar water of fish gills (Sect. VI). The interaction of all three component processes (ventilation, diffusion, and perfusion) will be shown in gas exchange models for fish gills (Sect. VII).

When considering real gas exchange organs, an important functional aspect must be dealt with, which is the functional inhomogeneity, meaning that ventilation, perfusion, and the diffusing properties are not equally allotted to the multitude of parallel units within a gas exchange organ. The effects of such inhomogeneity will be exemplified by the best-studied and probably most important inhomogeneity: the unequal distribution of ventilation to perfusion (Sect. VIII).

Our review is restricted to an analysis of gas exchange models. Many important properties and aspects of the gas exchange systems, although, in principle, amenable to study by models, will be totally excluded. These include (1) water versus air as gas exchange medium; (2) chemical binding of O_2 and CO_2 by blood with its kinetics; (3) interactions with mechanics of breathing and energy cost of breathing; (4) analysis of nervous and humoral regulatory mechanisms; (5) special adjustments, such as air-breathing organs of fishes, multiple gas exchange organs, and bimodal breathing. Most of these areas are covered in other chapters of this book.

A. Symbols

It proved to be impractical to use a completely unified system of definitions and symbols, particularly for the partial pressures of gases (P). For general compari-

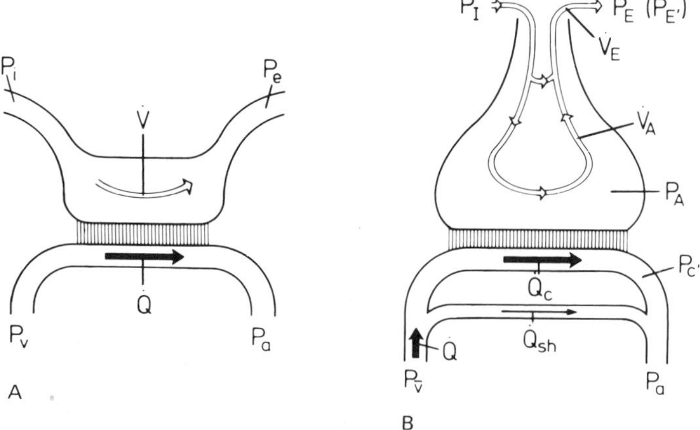

Figure 1 Illustration of the more important symbols used in this article. (A) Generalized symbols, used for general modeling, fish gills, and bird lungs. (B) Mammalian symbols, used for mammalian lungs.

sons of models and for fish gills, a "generalized" set of symbols was used, but for mammals' lungs it was appropriate to adopt the generally accepted "mammalian" symbols. The more important symbols are shown in Figure 1.

Medium

In the generalized set m refers to medium; i and e denote medium entering and exiting from the gas exchange area, respectively. For mammalian lungs the symbols are: A (alveolar), E (expired), E′ (end-expired), I (inspired).

Blood

For the generalized models the symbols are: b, blood; v (venous), and a (arterialized), blood entering and leaving the gas exchange area, respectively. For mammalian lungs, the symbols used are: $\bar{v}$, mixed venous; a, arterial; c, capillary, c′, end-capillary.

Ventilation

$\dot{V}$ is the generalize symbol for ventilation. For mammals, the ventilation effective in gas exchange is the alveolar ventilation, $\dot{V}_A$, the total ventilation (measured as expired gas) being $\dot{V}_E$ (the difference $\dot{V}_E - \dot{V}_A$ is the dead space ventilation).

Perfusion

The symbol for gas exchange organ perfusion is $\dot{Q}$. In mammalian lungs a capillary flow, $\dot{Q}c$, and a shunt flow, $\dot{Q}sh$, may be differentiated.

II. The Various Models for Vertebrate Gas Exchange Organs

The four models of Figure 2 have been proposed to describe the gas exchange behavior of the main types of respiratory organs in vertebrates (Piiper and Scheid, 1972, 1975, 1977, 1982): (A) countercurrent model for fish gills; (B) crosscurrent model for parabronchial lungs of birds; (C) ventilated or mixed pool model for the alveolar lungs of mammals; and (D) open model for amphibian skin. We will describe the characteristic features of these models in the following text.

A. Countercurrent Model for Fish Gills

The countercurrent flow of water and blood in the secondary lamellar sieve results from the gill anatomy in both teleost and elasmobranch fish. The counter-

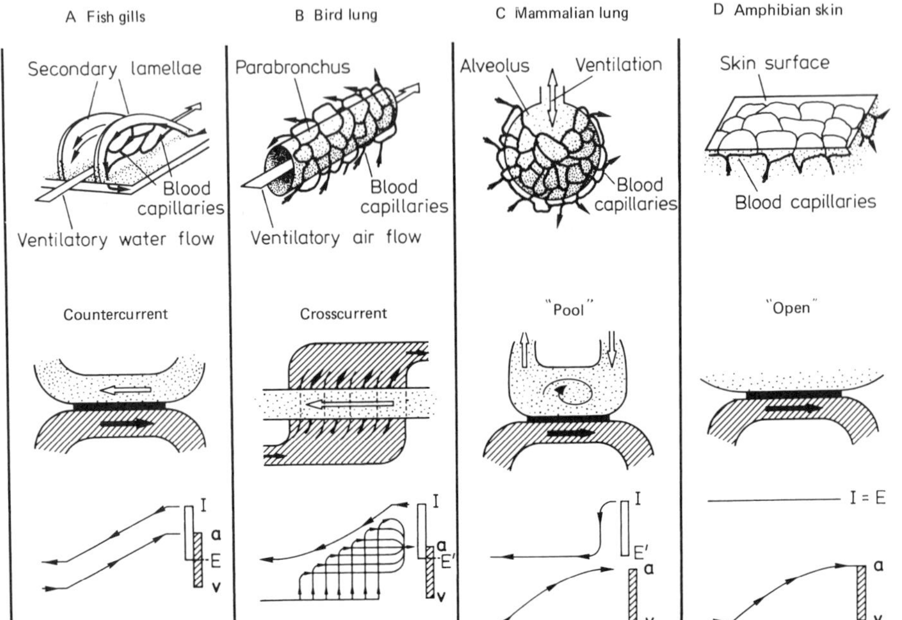

Figure 2 Basic structural and functional models for analysis of external gas exchange in vertebrates. Upper row, schema of anatomy. Lower row, models and profiles of partial pressures (PO_2) increases, PCO_2 decreases from bottom to top). (After Piiper and Scheid, 1982.)

current model, which is appropriate for this flow arrangement, offers the highest inherent gas transfer efficiency of all gas exchangers because the outflowing blood (a, in Fig. 2) approaches equilibrium with the inflowing medium (i) and the outflowing medium (e), with the inflowing blood (v) (Hughes and Shelton, 1962; Piiper and Scheid, 1982, 1983b, 1984). Hence, gas partial pressure Pa may be equal to Pi, and Pe equal to $P\bar{v}$.

This condition of perfect or near-perfect equilibrium has, however, never been found in fish. Usually not even a "crossing over" of blood and water partial pressures is observed (i.e., PaO_2, PeO_2, and $PaCO_2 < PeCO_2$). This impaired efficiency must be attributed to diffusion limitation or to functional inhomogeneities (unequal distribution of water to blood flow, water shunt, blood shunt, or to all). A comprehensive analysis of O_2 transfer has been performed based on experimental results in the rainbow trout (Randall et al., 1967), in the carp (Itazawa and Takeda, 1978), and in the dogfish, *Scyliorhinus canicula* (Short et al., 1979) and *S. stellaris* (Piiper and Baumgarten-Schumann, 1968b; Scheid and Piiper, 1976; Piiper et al., 1986).

B. Crosscurrent Model for Parabronchial Lungs of Birds

The appropriateness of the crosscurrent, or serial-multicapillary, model for analysis of gas transfer in avian lungs is supported not only by the anatomical arrangement of pulmonary blood vessels (Duncker, 1974) but also by the experimental observation that reversal of gas flow in parabronchi does not alter the efficiency of air–blood gas transfer (Scheid and Piiper, 1972).

As for maximum inherent efficiency, the crosscurrent model is inferior to the countercurrent model, although a crossing over of partial pressure (i.e., $PaO_2 > PeO_2$, and $PaCO_2 < PeCO_2$; see Fig. 2B) does occur in this as in the countercurrent model (see Scheid, 1979). For CO_2 exchange the crosscurrent model can, moreover, achieve an unexpectedly high efficiency as a result of the Haldane effect, whereby end-expired PCO_2 can exceed not only arterial but even mixed venous PCO_2 (Meyer et al., 1976).

Measurements in various birds have generally found arterial PO_2 to be lower than end-expired PO_2, although the ideal crosscurrent model would predict the reverse. Apparently, diffusion limitation and functional inhomogeneities reduce the overall gas exchange efficiency in the parabronchial lung, and more so for O_2 than for CO_2 (Scheid, 1978, 1979).

C. Mixed Pool Model for Alveolar Lungs

Because of the importance of the mixed pool model for mammalian and, in particular, for human lungs, it has become the most extensively studied model (for review see Piiper and Scheid, 1980). Its intrinsic maximum efficiency is lower than that of either the countercurrent or the crosscurrent models: in the mixed pool model PO_2 in arterial blood can be only lower or equal to alveolar PO_2, but not higher.

In mammalian lungs the gas exchange is usually only slightly limited by diffusion. The observed partial pressure differences between alveolar gas and arterial blood are predominantly due to functional inhomogeneities (ventilation–perfusion inequality, shunt).

D. Open Model for Amphibian Skin

Cutaneous gas exchange is important in all amphibians and is the sole mode of respiration in lungless salamanders (in all plethodontids and in some representatives of other groups). Cutaneous respiration, moreover, plays a varying role in many reptiles and fishes.

The model for cutaneous respiration, a blood capillary equilibrating across a tissue layer with a medium of constant composition, is the same as that used for analysis of gas exchange in mammalian lungs (where alveolar gas is substituted for the environmental medium). A detailed analysis of cutaneous gas exchange in the lungless salamander, *Desmognathus fuscus*, (Piiper et al., 1976) led to the conclusion that both O_2 uptake and CO_2 output were limited mainly by diffusion. The marked decrease of O_2 uptake observed in hypoxia in this animal appeared to be a necessary consequence of diffusion limitation.

In most amphibians, cutaneous gas exchange occurs in addition to pulmonary gas exchange. The respiratory quotient (R) of skin gas exchange is, in these animals, considerably higher than that of pulmonary gas exchange (Rahn and Howell, 1976), which is due to differences in the gas transfer conductances of both routes. Thus, because cutaneous gas exchange is predominantly limited by tissue (and water) diffusion, for which the conductance is considerably higher for CO_2 than for O_2, it contributes substantially more to CO_2 excretion than to O_2 uptake. In the lung, on the other hand, ventilation limitation predominates, which does not favor either gas. This behavior is independent of the medium surrounding the skin, air, or water.

E. Limitations to the Applicability of the Models

The models have been analyzed on the basis of simplfying assumptions (Piiper and Scheid, 1972, 1975, 1977, 1982). When these simple models are applied to experimental gas exchange data, one usually finds a much lower efficiency than expected. This may result from strong diffusion limitation, but it may also be due to a number of complicating factors listed and assessed in the following:

1. The simplified models are applicable to steady-state gas exchange only; whereas ventilation, in reality, is always cyclic, as is cardiac output. In spite of this, in animals breathing regularly and not too slowly (mammals, birds, fish in many cases), ventilation and blood flow may be considered as continuous with sufficient accuracy. In amphibians and reptiles, however, very slow or periodic breathing (several consecutive breaths preceded and followed by apneic periods) is common (for review see Glass and Wood, 1983). In these cases of unsteady states, more elaborate models containing capacitances for O_2 an CO_2 must be used for analysis of gas exchange and transport (Piiper, 1982a). In all diving air breathers, capacitances attain prominent importance as measures for the availability of O_2 and for CO_2 stores.

2. All gas exchange organs consist of numerous units (secondary lamellae in fish gills, alveoli in mammalian lungs, parabronchi in avian lungs) arranged, essentially, in parallel. It generally can be stated that if any two of the variables influencing the conductances (e.g., ventilation, blood flow, or diffusive conductance) are distributed differently among the units (functional inhomogeneity), the total gas exchange efficiency of the system is reduced compared with equal distribution (functional homogeneity). Identification and quantitative assessment of the effects of inhomogeneities (unequal distribution of ventilation or diffusing capacity to blood flow) are usually difficult tasks. If the inhomo-

geneities are neglected, or if their extent is underestimated, the diffusive conductance may be undervalued by a large factor.

3. Lungs are connected to the external body surface by conducting airways in which little or no gas exchange takes place and which, therefore, constitutes a respiratory dead space. In mammals, the effect of this anatomical dead space on pulmonary gas exchange is usually taken into account by using alveolar partial pressure (P_A) and by defining an effective or alveolar ventilation, calculated as total ventilation minus dead space ventilation (in reality, ventilation of the alveolar space is nearly equal to total ventilation, but part of it is ineffective as it represents reinspiration of dead space gas). Thus $\dot{V}$ and Pe of the generalized models (see Fig. 1) are replaced by their alveolar counterparts, $\dot{V}_A$ and P_A.

Because there is no mixing pool in bird lungs comparable with the mammalian alveolar space, application of the concept of dead space and alveloar gas is problematic (Scheid et al., 1987). Fish are sometimes said to have the advantage of having no dead space because their ventilation is unidirectional. But water flow bypassing the interlamellar spaces would functionally correspond to dead space ventilation, and water moving fast in the central stream through the interlamellar spaces may contribute little to gas exchange and, thus, act as dead space ventilation. Here, as well as in many other instances, there is a transition from *diffusion limitation* to *dead space ventilation*.

4. According to the general arrangement of the circulatory system and to its connection with the respiratory organ, in fish, birds, and mammals can it be expected that systemic arterial blood is essentially identical in composition with the blood leaving the respiratory organ and that respiratory organ perfusion is close to body perfusion (cardiac output). In amphibians and reptiles, central (intracardiac and extracardiac) blood mixing may lead to considerable deviations from these conditions and, even in fish, there is anatomical and functional evidence for several kinds of accessory vascular pathways, some of which act as shunts (reviewed by Laurent, 1984).

In reptiles and amphibians, with their incomplete separation of right and left hearts, shunting is always expected to occur and to reduce arterial P_{O_2}. Further complications arise in amphibians because part of the skin is supplied with arterialized blood from systemic arterial branches and part by venous blood through the pulmocutaneous artery. Arterialized skin blood enters through the venous system. In the lungless plethodontids, in which skin (and buccal mucosa) is the only site of gas exchange, the circulatory system is secondarily simplified into a system in which the gas exchange organ is in parallel to the systemic capillaries (in contrast to fish, birds, and mammals) and in which all organs, including skin, receive blood of the same composition (mixed cardiac blood) (Gatz et al., 1975).

5. As we will show in the following discussion, applicability of the models rests on the experimental data for gas partial pressure entering and leaving the gas exchange area. Although sampling of gas or water entering or leaving the animal, as well as sampling of blood in larger vessels, is relatively easy, the relationship of the partial pressures thus obtained to those at the gas exchange area depends on structural and functional factors. With reference to the medium side in Figure 1A, Pi and Pe in fish are close to inspited (P_I) and expired (P_E) values. Similarly, for mammals (Fig. 1B) in which Pi is taken to be P_I and Pe is set equal to alveolar partial pressure, P_A, obtained from expired air (after dead space exhalation and with precautions for breath-holding effects). For birds, however, the relation of Pi and Pe to P_I and P_E is complex and depends on the airflow pattern in the lung. According to direct sampling (Powell et al., 1981), Pe is close to P in end-expired gas or in clavicular air sac gas, but proper use of Pi is more complex. Caudal air sac gas or a mixture calculated from inspired and reinhaled dead space gas may be used, but the effect of neopulmonic gas exchange remains a problem, to different degrees in different avian species.

For blood, Pv in mammals and birds is equal to mixed venous partial pressure, $P\bar{v}$, sampled in the right ventricle or in the pulmonary artery; for fish, it is the P in cardiac blood. Partial pressure in blood leaving the gas exchange area (Fig. 1) may differ from Pa in systemic arteries because of shunt, and this is true for all systems. For reptiles and amphibians, obtaining Pv and Pa may be more complex, depending upon the circulatory system, and there is little to generalize.

In the following sections of the model properties, we will use the symbols referring to the gas exchange area (Fig. 1A), except for the mammalian lung in which we use the customary quantities and symbols (Fig. 1B).

III. Ventilation and Perfusion

Ventilation and perfusion are, many times, the processes limiting gas transfer, whereas diffusion is less important as a limiting factor (mammalian lungs, avian lungs). Moreover, it is in the absence of diffusion limitation that the functional differences between the different models (countercurrent, crosscurrent, mixed pool) are most marked. We will first compare the models without diffusion impairment.

A. Mixed Pool Model (Alveolar Lungs)

In the absence of diffusion limitation and of inhomogeneities, a continuously ventilated and perfused model will evidence equality of alveolar and arterial partial pressures. Thus, mass transport in steady state by ventilation and by circulation is given by the mass balance equation:

$$\dot{V} = (f \cdot C_I - C_A) = \dot{Q} \cdot (Ca - C\bar{v}) \tag{1}$$

where C denotes concentrations (amount of substance per volume) for both air and blood. The factor f (in steady state equal to P_{AN_2}/P_{IN_2}) is the correction factor when the gas exchange ratio, R = CO_2 output/O_2 uptake, does not equal unity and accounts for the fact that expired $\dot{V}$ is unequal to inspired $\dot{V}$ (for water ventilation, f = 1.0 for all R).

Concentration, C, is conveniently replaced by partial pressure, P, using the capacitance coefficient or effective solubility, β, (Piiper et al., 1971). In air, β is constant for all (ideal) gases at 1/RT (R, gas constant; T, absolute temperature); for O_2 (and inert gases) in water, β is the physical solubility (α); for CO_2 in carbonated water at low P_{CO_2}, β is increased over α by CO_2-bicarbonate-carbonate buffering (Dejours et al., 1968; Piiper and Baumgarten-Schumann, 1968a; Truchot et al., 1980). For blood, β results from the slope of the dissociation curves and is generally strongly dependent on the partial pressure. For convenience we will refer to β in gas as β_g and to β in water as β_W, whereas for blood we will use β without any subscript.

The following relationship is obtained from Equation 1 (when β is not constant it designates the slope of the line crossing the dissociation curve at Pa and $P\bar{v}$):

$$\frac{Pa - P\bar{v}}{f \cdot P_I - Pa} = \frac{\dot{V}_A \cdot \beta_g}{\dot{Q} \cdot \beta} \tag{2}$$

Equation 2 shows that Pa (= P_A) relative to $P\bar{v}$ and P_I is determined by the ratio ($\dot{V}_A \cdot \beta_g/(\dot{Q} \cdot \beta)$, i.e., by the ratio of ventilation conductance to perfusion conductance: the higher the ratio, the closer is P_A (= Pa) to P_I (Fig. 3A).

The relationship of Equation 2 has been introduced by Farhi (1967) to describe elemination of inert gases of different partition coefficients, $\lambda = \beta/\beta_g$. When these gases are not contained in inspired gas (P_I = 0), Equation 2 simplifies to

$$\frac{Pa}{P\bar{v}} = \frac{\lambda}{\lambda + \dot{V}_A/\dot{Q}} \tag{3}$$

which is the fundamental relationship for analysis of $\dot{V}_A/\dot{Q}$ inequalities in lungs using multiple inert gases of differing λ (Farhi, 1967; see the following discussion).

To avoid confusion and ambiguity, recall that alveolar and arterial P_{O_2} and P_{CO_2} in a homogeneous lung at steady state are exclusively determined by the alveolar ventilation, $\dot{V}_A$, and the metabolic rates, $\dot{M}_{O_2}$ and $\dot{M}_{CO_2}$:

$$Pa_{O_2} = f \cdot P_{IO_2} - \frac{\dot{M}_{CO_2}}{\dot{V}_A \cdot \beta_g} \tag{4a}$$

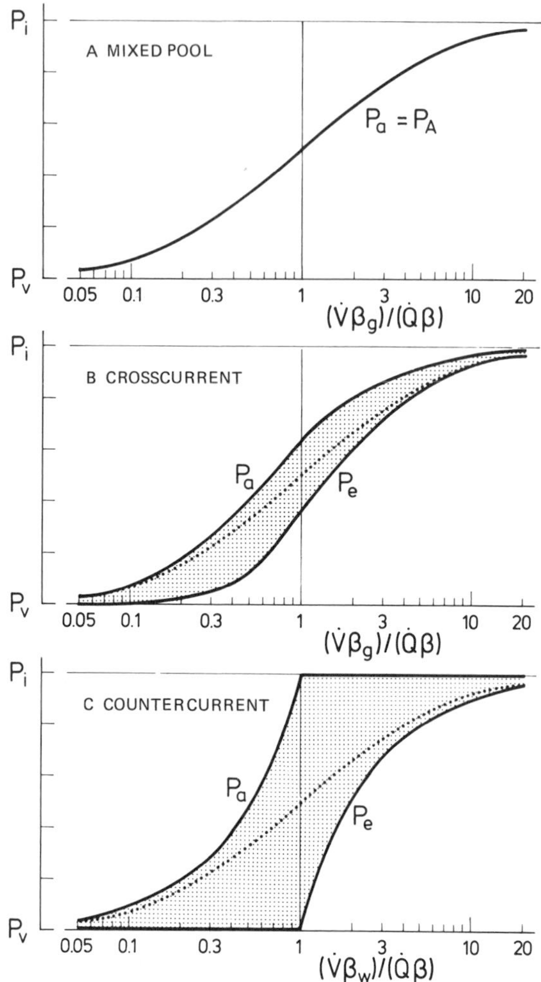

Figure 3 Partial pressures in gas (expired, Pe, or alveolar, PA, respectively) and blood (arterialized or arterial, Pa) leaving the gas exchange area, relative to the gas (Pi and blood Pv) entering the gas exchange area, as functions of the ventilatory/perfusive conductance ratio, $(\dot{V} \cdot \beta_g)/(\dot{Q} \cdot \beta)$ or $(\dot{V} \cdot \beta_w)/(\dot{Q} \cdot \beta)$, for three models. In (B) and (C), the dotted line marks the curve for model (A), and the shaded area, the blood–gas overlap region where the ratio (Pe – Pa)/(Pi – Pv) is negative. (After Piiper and Scheid, 1972.)

$$PaCO_2 = f \cdot PICO_2 + \frac{\dot{M}CO_2}{\dot{V}A \cdot \beta_g} \tag{4b}$$

Equations 4a and 4b determine the absolute value of Pa, whereas Equations 2 and 3 define the relative value of Pa in relation to PI and $P\bar{v}$. Thus, for given values of $\dot{V}A$, $\dot{Q}$, $\dot{M}$, and PI, Pa follows from Equation 4, and $P\bar{v}$ then from Equation 2 or 3.

B. Countercurrent and Crosscurrent Models

In crosscurrent and countercurrent models without diffusion limitation (and heterogeneity) an "overlap" of gas and blood partial pressures occurs (see Fig. 3) such that for a gas taken up (O_2) the order is $Pi > Pa > Pe > Pv$, and $Pi < Pa < Pe < Pv$ for a gas eliminated (i.e., CO_2). A negative ratio (Pe - Pa/(Pa - Pv) is the quantitative expression for the medium-blood overlap (Piiper and Scheid, 1972), illustrated in Figure 3B by the stippled areas. For the ideal mixed pool model, (Pe - Pa)/(Pi - Pv) = 0.

It is evident that for the countercurrent and crosscurrent model $PaO_2 = PeO_2$, or $PaCO_2 = PeCO_2$ indicates reduced gas exchange efficiency (by diffusion limitation or by functional inhomogeneity), whereas for the alveolar lung Pa = PA means the presence of ideal gas exchange conditions.

C. Mismatch Shunt in Countercurrent Model (Fish Gills)

The enhanced gas exchange efficiency (i.e., the relative overlap) of the countercurrent model and, to a lesser extent, of the crosscurrent model, strongly depends upon the value of the $(\dot{V} \cdot \beta_W)/(\dot{Q} \cdot \beta)$ ratio (Fig. 3C). Complete blood-gas equlibration, i.e., Pe = Pv and at the same time Pa = Pi, is achieved only when $(\dot{V} \cdot \beta_W)/(\dot{Q} \cdot \beta) = 1$. When there is excess perfusion conductance and, hence, $(\dot{V} \cdot \beta_W)/(\dot{Q} \cdot \beta) < 1$, Pe = Pv but Pa < Pi, despite the absence of diffusion limitation. This may be termed a *mismatch blood shunt* because the same result of partial pressures is obtained in a model in which the blood flow constituting the excess perfusive conductance is diverted from the gas exchange zone to pass through a blood shunt (Fig. 4A). By analogy, excess ventilatory conductance, resulting in $(\dot{V} \cdot \beta_W)/(\dot{Q} \cdot \beta) > 1$, is equivalent to a *mismatch water shunt* (Fig. 4C).

It follows from these considerations of the mismatch shunts that, starting from the ideal match, i.e., $(\dot{V} \cdot \beta_W)/(\dot{Q} \cdot \beta) = 1$, an increase in either water or blood flow does not increase the rates of gas transfer in the system. In particular, when ventilation is increased, increasing $(\dot{V} \cdot \beta_W/(\dot{Q} \cdot \beta)$ from unity to above unity, blood oxygenation remains unaffected. If, on the other hand, blood flow is increased, diminishing $(\dot{V} \cdot \beta_W)/(\dot{Q} \cdot \beta)$ from unity to below unity, arterial oxygenation is diminished, but the total O_2 supplied by the increased flow of arterial blood remains unaffected. It is possible that the marked variations in ar-

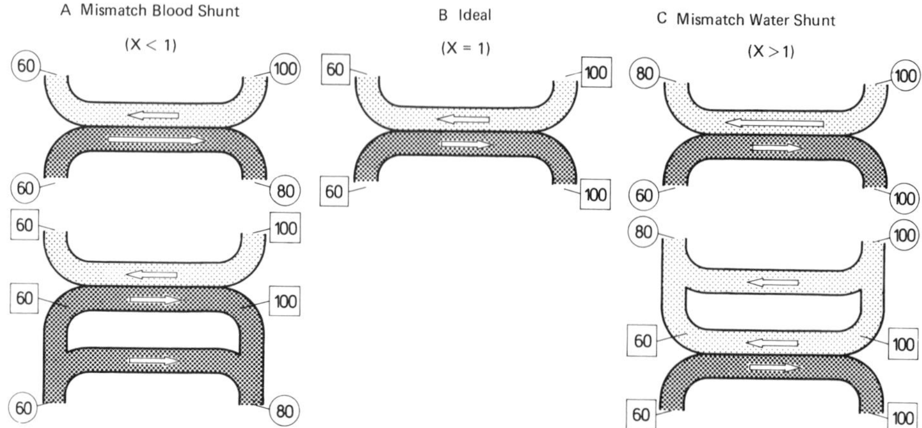

Figure 4 Equivalence between the effects of conductance mismatch and shunt in the countercurrent system, assuming Pi = 100 and Pv = 60 units. In (B), the ideal system with $X = (\dot{V} \cdot \beta_W)/(\dot{Q} \cdot \beta) = 1$. In (A) (upper figure), mismatch is produced by doubling perfusive conductance which leads to $(\dot{V} \cdot \beta_W)/(\dot{Q} \cdot \beta) < 1$ and lowers Pa to 80. The same effect is obtained when the extra blood flow is channeled through a blood shunt, whereby ideal matching conditions in the gas exchange compartment are restored (A, lower figure). In (C), a mismatch is created by doubling water flow conductance, whereby $(\dot{V} \cdot \beta_W)/\dot{Q} \cdot \beta) > 1$ and Pe = 80. The same effect is produced by a water shunt. (After Piiper and Scheid, 1984.)

terial PO_2 observed in fish with rather constant ventilation (Piiper and Schumann, 1967) are, in part, attributable to changes in mismatch shunts caused by transitory changes in the cardiac output.

Mismatch shunts are specific for the countercurrent model (Piiper and Scheid, 1983b). In the ventilated pool model of alveolar lungs, increased ventilation always increases arterial PO_2 (and decreases PCO_2), and increased cardiac output means little change in arterial PO_2 (provided there is no important diffusion limitation) but improved oxygen supply to the tissues, as evidenced from increased $P\bar{v}O_2$. Parabronchial lungs behave similarly to alveolar lungs.

IV. Diffusion and Perfusion

A. Alveolar Lungs

Diffusive Equilibration and Equilibration Coefficient

Many times, gases are transferred between a medium of (relatively) constant composition and blood through a tissue barrier. Examples are gas exchange in mammalian lungs, cutaneous gas exchange in amphibians, and gas absorption from gas cavities in the body. Although in every particular case a large number of factors are involved in this exchange, a very simple model, which contains the basic variables and demonstrates their interaction, may be used for the basic understanding and evaluation. We will develop the model for a homogeneous alveolar lung.

The model is composed of a uniform alveolar space that is separated from a blood stream of uniform velocity by a homogeneous flat diffusion barrier, the diffusive conductance of diffusing capacity, D, of which is defined as rate of diffusive transfer per effective partial pressure difference (Fig. 5).

We will assume that transfer by diffusion is perpendicular across the barrier, and that there is instantaneous mixing within a cross-sectional element of blood, and that transport by blood is by square-front bulk flow with negligible axial diffusion. The diffusive and convective transport rates in steady state equal each other and, with the assumptions, can be described by the following equation:

$$\dot{Q} \cdot \beta \cdot dP_c = (P_A - P_c) \cdot dD \tag{5}$$

[$\dot{Q}$, blood flow; β, (effective) solubility in blood; dP_c, partial pressure difference between inflow and outflow of the blood element corresponding to the element of diffusing capacity, dD; P_A, alveolar gas partial pressure; P_c, partial pressure in blood in the element considered.

Integration of Equation 5 from the venous end ($\bar{v}$) to a point, x, along the capillary of length xo yields:

$$\frac{P_A - P_c(x)}{P_A - P_{\bar{v}}} = \exp\left[-\frac{D}{\dot{Q} \cdot \beta} \cdot \frac{x}{x_0}\right] \tag{6}$$

This equation shows the exponential time course of equilibration along the capillary, the exponent being proportional to $D/(\dot{Q} \cdot \beta)$. For the equilibration reached at the end of the capillary ($x = x_0$), one obtains:

$$\frac{P_A - P_a}{P_A - P_{\bar{v}}} = \exp\left[-\frac{D}{\dot{Q} \cdot \beta}\right] \tag{7}$$

The relationship shows that the extent of alveolar-capillary equilibration is determined by the ratio $D/(\dot{Q} \cdot \beta)$, the equilibration coefficient (see Scheid and Piiper, 1987). The higher the value of $D/(\dot{Q} \cdot \beta)$, the more complete is the equilibration reached, and it is unimportant whether a high $D/(\dot{Q} \cdot \beta)$ is achieved by high D, or by low $\dot{Q}$, or low β, or by their combinations.

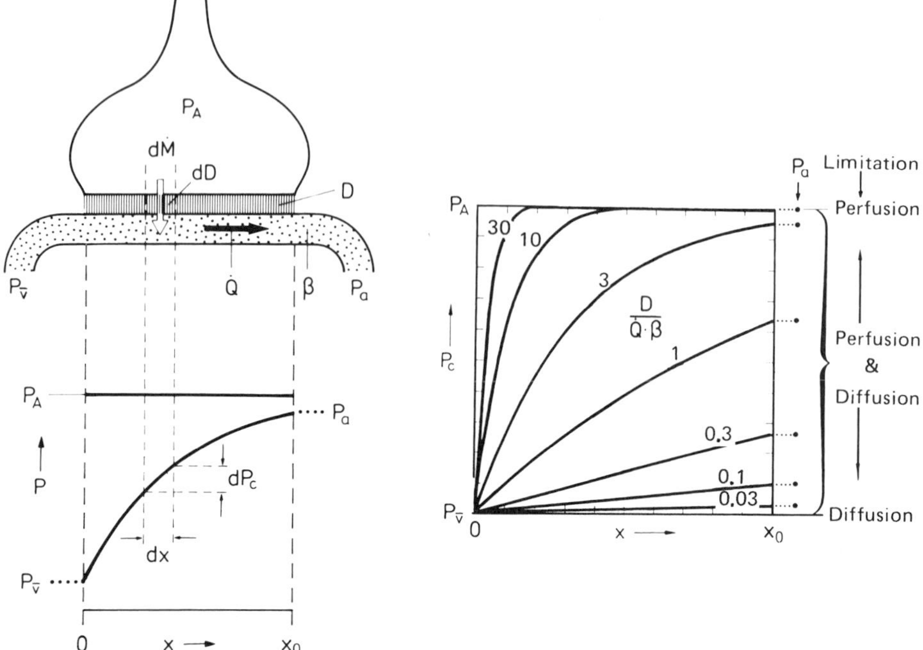

Figure 5 The perfusion–diffusion model. Left, a model and partial pressure profile in blood. An arbitrary differential element is bounded by broken lines for illustration of Equation 5. Right, partial pressure profiles and end-capillary partial pressure (Pa), relative to the alveolar (PA) and mixed venous values ($P\bar{v}$), according to Equations 6 and 7. The transition from predominant diffusion limitation to predominant perfusion limitation is indicated. (After Piiper and Scheid, 1981.)

Overall Conductance and Component Conductances

Gas conductance (G) is generally defined as transfer rate, $\dot{M}$, divided by the effective partial pressure difference, $P_1 - P_2$,

$$G = \dot{M}/(P_1 - P_2) \tag{8}$$

The total conductance for alveolar gas exchange, G_{tot}, may thus be defined by the relationship,

$$G_{tot} = \dot{M}/(P_A - P\bar{v}) \tag{9}$$

Its components are the diffusive conductance, which is equal to the diffusing capacity, D, and the perfusive conductance, which by definition is equal to $\dot{Q} \cdot \beta$:

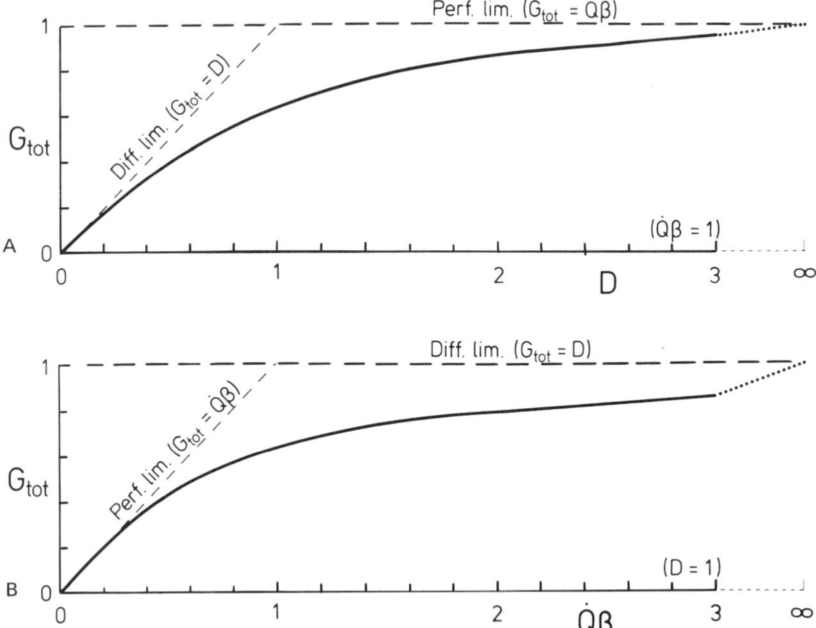

Figure 6 Total conductance, G_{tot}, as function of diffusive conductance, D (top), and perfusive conductance, $\dot{Q} \cdot \beta$ (bottom). The limiting cases of pure perfusion and diffusion limitation are marked by broken lines. (After Piiper and Scheid, 1981.)

$$\dot{Q} \cdot \beta = \dot{M}/(Pa - P\bar{v}) \qquad (10)$$

Combination of Equations 7, 9, and 10 yields:

$$G_{tot} = \dot{Q} \cdot \beta \cdot \left\{ 1 - \exp\left[-D/(\dot{Q} \cdot \beta)\right] \right\} \qquad (11)$$

It is evident that for $D \to \infty$, $G_{tot} = \dot{Q} \cdot \beta$ (perfusion limitation) and for $\dot{Q} \cdot \beta \to \infty$, $G_{tot} = D$ (diffusion limitation). In Figure 6 the change of G_{tot} is shown (1) for varying D at constant $\dot{Q} \cdot \beta$ and (2) for varying $(\dot{Q} \cdot \beta)$ at constant D. The following is evident:

1. At very low values of D, $G_{tot} = D$ (diffusion limitation, Fig. 6A), but when D is increased, G_{tot} increases less than D (combined diffusion and perfusion limitation), and at very high D, G_{tot} becomes independent of D (perfusion limitation).

Table 1 Parameters for Diffusion and Perfusion Limitation

$$L_{diff} = 1 - \frac{G_{tot}}{G_{tot}(D \rightarrow \infty)} = \exp\left[-\frac{D}{\dot{Q}\cdot\beta}\right]$$

$$L_{perf} = 1 - \frac{G_{tot}}{G_{tot}(\dot{Q}\beta \rightarrow \infty)} = 1 - \frac{1 - \exp\left[-\frac{D}{\dot{Q}\cdot\beta}\right]}{\left[\frac{D}{\dot{Q}\cdot\beta}\right]}$$

$$J_{diff} = \frac{\partial G_{tot}}{\partial D} = \exp\left[-\frac{D}{\dot{Q}\cdot\beta}\right]$$

$$J_{perf} = \frac{\partial G_{tot}}{\partial(\dot{Q}\cdot\beta)} = 1 - \left[1 + \frac{D}{\dot{Q}\cdot\beta}\right]\cdot\exp\left[-\frac{D}{\dot{Q}\cdot\beta}\right]$$

$$K_{diff} = \frac{\partial G_{tot}/G_{tot}}{\partial D/D} = \frac{\frac{D}{\dot{Q}\cdot\beta}}{\exp\left[\frac{D}{\dot{Q}\cdot\beta}\right] - 1}$$

$$K_{perf} = \frac{\partial G_{tot}/G_{tot}}{\partial(\dot{Q}\cdot\beta)/(\dot{Q}\cdot\beta)} = 1 - K_{diff}$$

2. At very low $\dot{Q} . \beta$, $G_{tot} = \dot{Q}\cdot\beta$ (perfusion limitation; Fig. 6B). When $\dot{Q}\cdot\beta$ is increased, G_{tot} increases less than $\dot{Q}\cdot\beta$ (combined perfusion and diffusion limitation), and at very high $\dot{Q}\cdot\beta$, G_{tot} is independent of $\dot{Q}\cdot\beta$ and is determined solely by D (diffusion limitation).

Several parameters may be used to describe diffusion and perfusion limitation in quantitative terms. The definitions and equations for these parameters are listed in Table 1.

1. The *extent of limitation*, L denotes the relative reduction in G_{tot} from the limiting value it would attain without the respective limitation to its actual value (Piiper and Scheid, 1981).

2. The *sensitivity coefficients*, J, of diffusion and perfusion dependence are defined as the differential increase of G_{tot} produced by a differential increase of diffusion or perfusion conductance (Piiper and Scheid, 1983a).

3. The *relative sensitivity coefficients*, K, are defined as the relative differential increase in G_{tot} brought about by a relative differential increase of diffusion or perfusion conductance (Piiper and Scheid, 1983a).

Diffusion–Perfusion Limitation for Various Gases

The pulmonary diffusing capacity, D, is determined, according to Fick's diffusion law, by the following properties of the diffusion barrier: diffucion coefficient (d), solubility (α), surface area (F), and thickness (h),

$$D = d \cdot \alpha \cdot F/h \tag{12}$$

For the $D/(\dot{Q} \cdot \beta)$ ratio one obtains,

$$\frac{D}{\dot{Q} \cdot \beta} = \frac{d \cdot \alpha}{\beta} \cdot \frac{F}{h \cdot \dot{Q}} \tag{13}$$

This relationship reveals that it is not the diffusion coefficient (d) but the product $d \cdot \alpha/\beta$ that determines the diffusion-perfusion behavior of gases for given geometry (F/h) and blood flow ($\dot{Q}$).

The diffusion coefficient, d, for gases in tissues or water is approximately inversely proportional to the square root of the molecular mass of the gas (Graham's law; see Kawashiro et al., 1975). Thus the d values for very light gases (like H_2) and very heavy gases (like SF_6) should differ by a factor of about 8.

The α/β ratio should be near unity for all inert gases (except for highly lipid-soluble gases, for which α/β may be above unity; see Meyer et al., 1980). For gases chemically bonded in blood, the β value may be greatly increased over its physical solubility in blood, β_{phys}. With appropriate Pa and $P\bar{v}$ and blood dissociation curves, one obtains the following approximate values for the β/β_{phys} ratio $[= (Ca - C\bar{v}) \cdot (Pa - P\bar{v})^{-1} \cdot (\beta_{phys})^{-1}]$: CO_2, 10; O_2 in normoxia, 30; O_2 in hypoxia, 170; CO in hypoxia, 40,000. Accordingly, the α/β ratio shows a much greater variability among gases than the diffusivity, d.

For the exchange of gases that are chemically bonded in blood, the reaction rate of chemical bonding may be limiting. In first approximation, this could be taken into account by reducing the diffusivity, d, by a (dimensionless) coefficient, r (< 1), to an apparent diffusivity, d_{app}:

$$d_{app} = d \cdot r \tag{14}$$

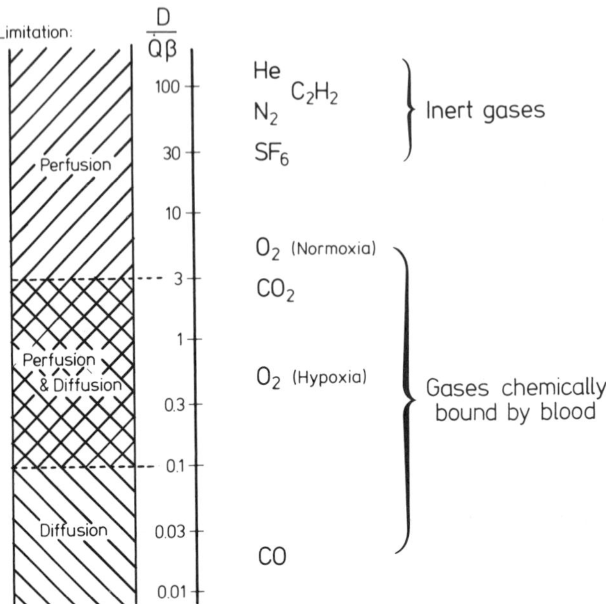

Figure 7 Diffusion–perfusion limitation in alveolar–capillary transfer of various gases. Center: the $D/(\dot{Q} \cdot \beta)$ ratio on logarithmic scale. Left: the perfusion and diffusion limitation areas are marked by different hatching; end of limitation area is taken at $L = 0.05$ (see Table 1). Right: approximate location of inert and chemically bonded gases for alveolar–capillary transfer in normal human lungs in resting conditions. (After Piiper and Scheid, 1981.)

Thus, the effective $D/(\dot{Q} \cdot \beta)$ for chemically bonded gases may be further reduced compared with inert gases.

In Figure 7 the equilibration coefficient, $D/(\dot{Q} \cdot \beta)$, of alveolar–capillary transfer is estimated for various gases in human lungs. The basis for this estimate is $D_{O_2} = 60$ ml · min^{-1} · torr^{-1} (Meyer et al., 1981), $D_{CO_2} = 200$ ml · min^{-1} · torr^{-1} (Piiper et al., 1980), and approximate relative α, β, and d values. The main features are the following:

1. The transfer of all inert gases, practically, is not diffusion limited.
2. Oxygen and CO_2 transfer extends from a predominantly perfusion limitation to the range of combined diffusion and perfusion limitation.
3. Carbon monoxide transfer is almost exclusively diffusion (and reaction) limited.

Table 2 Measured and Estimated Data on O_2 Uptake and Transport at High Altitude[a]

Quantity	Units	Rest	Max. exercise
O_2 uptake	$l \cdot min^{-1}$	0.3[b]	2.26
$\dot{Q}$	$l \cdot min^{-1}$	6[b]	25
$(Ca - C\bar{v})O_2$	$ml \cdot l^{-1}$	50	89
PaO_2	torr	43	39
$P\bar{v}O_2$	torr	31	24
βO_2	$ml \cdot l^{-1} \cdot torr^{-1}$	4.2	5.9
DO_2	$ml \cdot min^{-1} \cdot torr^{-1}$	54	65
$[D/(\dot{Q} \cdot \beta)]O_2$		2.1	0.44
$L_{diff}\,O_2$		0.12	0.64
$L_{perf}\,O_2$		0.59	0.19
$[K_{diff}/K_{perf}]O_2$		0.40	3.9

[a]5350 m; barometric pressure = 390 torr; inspired PO_2 (H_2O saturated at 37°C) = 72 torr.
[b]Estimated.
Source: After Cerretelli (1976). DO_2, after Meyer et al. (1981).

Application to Oxygen Uptake in High-Altitude Hypoxia

It follows from the preceding analysis that the alveolar–capillary equilibration deficit in the physiologically interesting situation of deep hypoxia, when pulmonary O_2 uptake is limited by both perfusion and diffusion, can be particularly well analyzed using the $D/(\dot{Q} \cdot \beta)$ concept. This is because (1) β, the slope of the O_2 dissociation curve, is large, thus producing a small $D/(\dot{Q} \cdot \beta)$ and, therefore, pronounced effects of diffusion limitation; (2) β is relatively independent of PO_2 (the blood O_2 dissociation curve between Pa and $P\bar{v}$ is nearly linear); (3) the disturbing effects of functional inhomogeneities are of reduced importance.

Cerretelli (1976) has reported measurements of O_2 transport variables on members of the 1973 Italian Mount Everest expedition in the base camp (altitude 5350 m). The values required for our analysis are presented in Table 2 and lead to the following conclusions.

1. Both at rest and during exercise there is considerable diffusion limitation as shown by the L_{diff} values.

2. In resting conditions, the limiting role of perfusion is quantitatively more important than that of diffusion. But in heavy exercise, diffusion limitation clearly predominates ($L_{diff} > L_{perf}$). The ratio K_{diff}/K_{perf} of 4 indicates that a given relative increase of D is four times more effective in increasing G_{tot} for O_2 (i.e., in increasing $\dot{M}O_2$ for constant $(PA - P\bar{v})O_2$) than the same relative increase of the cardiac output, $\dot{Q}$.

B. *Cutaneous Gas Exchange in Amphibians*

Cutaneous gas exchange, aside from pulmonary or branchial gas exchange, occurs, to a certain extent, in all vertebrates but is of particular importance in amphibians (see Feder and Burggren, 1985). It is best studied in lungless salamanders in which all gas transfer takes place through the body skin and the buccopharyngeal mucosa.

To estimate cutaneous diffusing capacity and cutaneous blood flow as well as cardiac output in an exclusively skin-breathing salamander (*Desmognathus fuscus*), the equilibration kinetics of soluble inert gases (mainly freon-22) were measured and compared in living and dead animals (Gatz et al., 1975). The estimated $D/(\dot{Q} \cdot \beta)$ ratio for cutaneous transfer of freon-22 averaged 0.42 to 0.63, showing combined diffusion and perfusion limitation. Estimation of the $D/(\dot{Q} \cdot \beta)$ ratio for O_2 and CO_2 yielded ranges, 0.03 to 0.05 for O_2 and 0.06 to 0.09 for CO_2, showing predominant diffusion limitation of cutaneous exchange of these gases. The dependence of O_2 uptake upon the ambient PO_2 was in agreement with the diffusion-limited nature of O_2 transfer. Moreover, the estimated DO_2 was in reasonable agreement with the DO_2 derived from morphometric measurements (Piiper et al., 1976).

More recently it has been shown that plethodontid salamanders are capable of increasing their O_2 uptake during exercise several times above the resting level (Withers, 1980; Feder, 1985; Full, 1985). This is difficult to explain without the assumption of a substantial increase in D. Similarly, studies by Burggren and Moalli (1984) and Malvin and Hlastala (1986) have shown that, in frogs, the skin conductance for gases can be changed, apparently by regulation of the number of perfused capillaries.

V. Diffusion in Medium

A. Diffusion Limitation in the Alveolar Space of Mammalian Lungs

Incomplete Intrapulmonary Gas Mixing (Stratification)

In mammalian lungs, inspired gas is not expected to achieve direct contact with the surface of the alveolar epithelium because the considerable end-expired lung

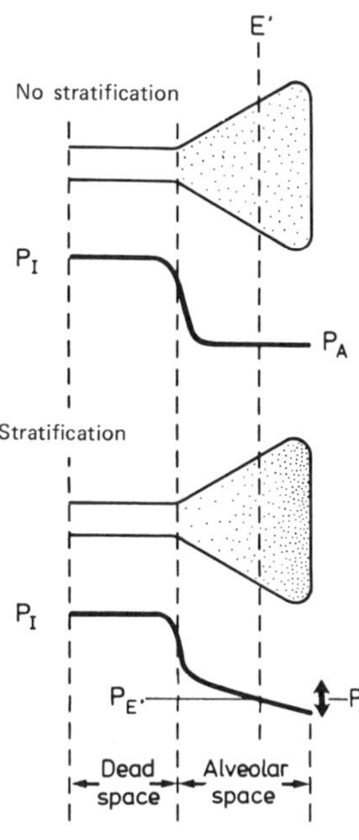

Figure 8 Schematic representation of stratification. Density of stippling in lung models visualizes partial pressure (or concentration) of a gas (e.g., CO_2). The concentration profile of a gas with inspired value highest (e.g., O_2) is also shown. E′ denotes end-expired gas. (After Scheid and Piiper, 1980.)

volume is interposed. This gas volume is spread out as a layer of no more than a few millimeters thickness, owing to the enormous increase of the cross-sectional area of the airways from the trachea to the alveolar ducts. Nonetheless, it may constitute a barrier to exchange of gases between inspired gas and pulmonary capillary blood. The process by which this barrier is overcome may be viewed as a mixing process, leading to homogenization of lung gas during the respiratory cycle. Both diffusive and convective mixing (particularly that resulting from the mechanical action of the heart beat) are involved within a complex lung structure with a complex flow regimen (for review, Scheid and Piiper, 1980). The result of incomplete intrapulmonary gas mixing is generally termed *stratification*, i.e., persistence of axial concentration differences in (peripheral) lung airways during the respiratory cycle.

Evidently, intrapulmonary gas mixing is never complete under physiological conditions and, even after extremely prolonged breath holding, there remains a nonmixing space in the proximal airways, termed (anatomical or series) *dead space*. In this sense, dead space is a stratificational phenomenon, and a very marked one. Stratification proper, however, refers to persistence of significant axial concentration (or partial pressure) gradients inside the gas-exchanging airways of the alveolar space (Fig. 8).

The separation line of dead space and alveolar space cannot be regarded as a sharp boundary because anatomically there is the "transition zone" (Weibel,

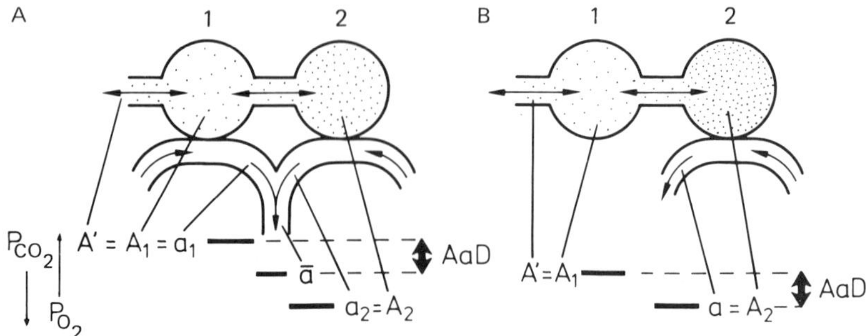

Figure 9 Models to show the origin of alveolar–arterial differences for CO_2 and O_2 (AaD) in lungs with incomplete gas mixing in alveolar space. Gas–blood diffusion is assumed to be nonlimiting. Density of stippling marks concentration of CO_2. (A) Model with two compartments ventilated in series. The AaD is due to the fact that end-expired gas (A′) originates in the proximal compartment (1) only, whereas arterial blood is a mixture. (B), Like (A), but only the distal compartment (2) is perfused. An AaD arises because end-expired gas (A′) is derived from the proximal compartment (1) and arterial blood, from the distal compartment (2). (After Scheid and Piiper, 1980.)

1963), and functionally there is a gradual change of expired gas concentration, plotted against time or volume, from the inspired to the end-expired value. The delimitation of stratification in alveolar space from concentration gradients related to dead space is difficult and may, occasionally, remain unsolved.

Effects on Efficiency of Alveolar Gas Exchange

The important consequence of stratified inhomogeneity is to reduce the efficiency of alveolar gas exchange by creating partial pressure differences for O_2 and CO_2 between end-expired (alveolar) gas and arterial (end-capillary) blood, i.e., alveolar–arterial differences (AaD) (Fig. 9). Thus, the effects of stratification (stratified inhomogeneity) are basically similar to those of unequal distribution of ventilation to perfusion (parallel inhomogeneity).

Stratified inhomogeneity, resulting from incomplete mixing along the axis of peripheral airways, can produce the same patterns of AaD for O_2 and CO_2 as ventilation-perfusion inequality, particularly of the alveolar dead space type. Therefore, it is difficult to determine which part of AaD is attributable to stratification, particularly because there may exist combined or transitional forms of series and parallel inhomogeneity (discussed later).

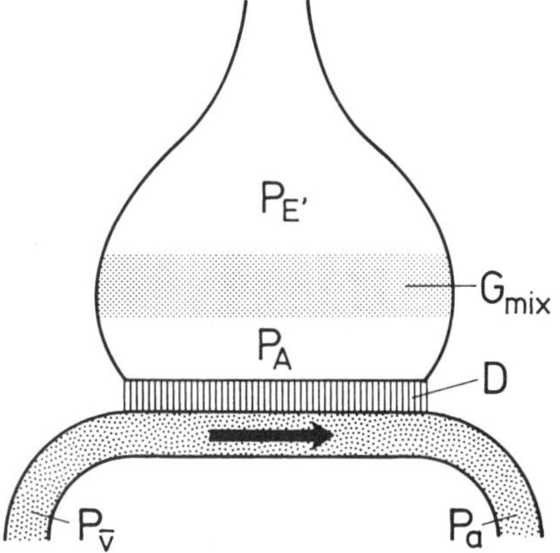

Figure 10 Simplified lung model for analysis of incomplete intrapulmonary gas mixing (stratification). Analogous to model (B) of Figure 9. The partial pressure difference PE' – PA is due to finite G_{mix} (Eq. 15), the difference PA – Pa, to finite D (Eq. 7).

Experimental Methods and Results

Whereas sloping alveolar plateaus (see Fig. 8) may occur in the presence of stratification, they are of limited value in its estimation because other effects produce alveolar slopes as well (see Scheid and Piiper, 1980). In particular, breath holding and functional heterogeneities with sequential emptying produce alveolar slopes in the steady state and in single breath.

Given the application of inert gases with low solubility and widely differing diffusivity (Georg et al., 1965; Cumming et al., 1967), we have performed several studies designed to estimate the extent of stratification (reviewed by Piiper, 1979; Scheid and Piiper, 1980).

To arrive at quantitative evaluation, an extremely simplified lung model of "lumped parameter" type was employed. In the model, all resistance to intrapulmonary mixing was concentrated into a uniform "gas-filled membrane" dividing the alveolar space into a proximal and a distal compartment (Fig. 10). The permeability of the barrier was characterized by the *mixing conductance*, G_{mix},

$$G_{mix} = \dot{M}/(P_{E'} - P_A) \tag{15}$$

where PA refers to distal alveolar gas in contact with blood, PE', to end-expired gas or to gas at an earlier part of the alveolar plateau.

Three experimental approaches were used for estimating G_{mix} (see Scheid and Piiper, 1980). In the first, G_{mix} was estimated by comparing the wash out of He with the simultaneous wash out of SF_6 in excised dog lung lobes. In the second approach, intrapulmonary mixing for He, Ar, and SF_6 was measured during breath holding in man. In the third series, simultaneous wash out of He and SF_6 was studied in man. In all approaches, G_{mix} was quantitatively estimated for the test gas and for O_2 and was compared with values of the lung diffusing

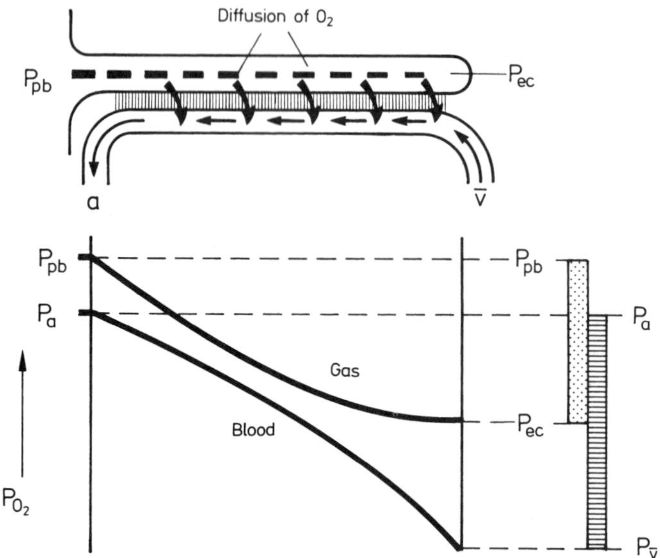

Figure 11 Partial pressure profiles of O_2 in avian air capillary model. In spite of considerable fall of PO_2 along the air capillary, arterial PO_2 (Pa) is close to parabronchial PO_2 (Ppb) because of the distal-to-proximal direction of capillary blood flow along the air capillary. The countercurrent-like behavior is illustrated by the gas–blood PO_2 overlap.

capacity for O_2, DO_2. The ratio $(D/G_{mix})O_2$ was in the range of 0.1 to 0.6, suggesting that about 10 to 40% of the total resistance to O_2 uptake ($1/D + 1/G_{mix}$) from gas inspired into the alveolar space down to pulmonary capillary blood was attributable to incomplete gas mixing in the alveolar gas (stratification). Although the results of these studies must be considered with reservations because of both modeling problems and limited experimental accuracy, they appear to indicate that stratification exerts a measurable limitation on alveolar gas exchange in mammalian lungs.

These results and interpretations are not in agreement with theoretical studies on lung models based on the symmetrical Weibel lung model (Scheid and Piiper, 1980). These calculations yield practically no sloping alveolar plateau, i.e., no stratification (Paiva, 1973). There is anatomical and functional evidence, however, for asymmetry, meaning unequal distribution of G_{mix} to VA and $\dot{V}A$, and for sequential expiration. A coupling of sequential ventilation to incomplete gas mixing may greatly increase the slope of alveolar plateau. There is, thus, probably an unequal distribution of G_{mix}, meaning coexistence in lungs of parallel compartments with very little and with strong stratification, the strongly stratified compartments expiring last (Meyer et al., 1983; Hook et al., 1985).

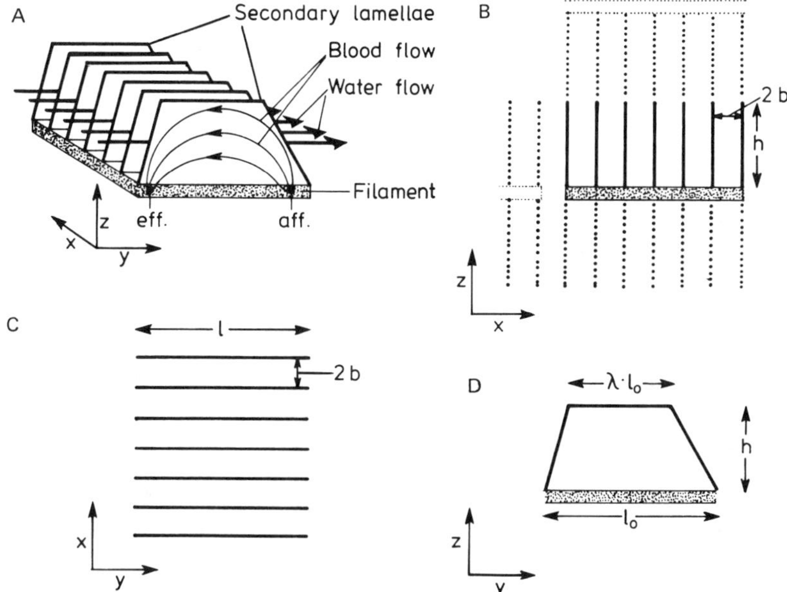

Figure 12 Fish gill model and characteristic measurements. (A) Model for a row of secondary lamellae on a gill filament. The spatial axes x, y, and z serve for orientation of the cross sections in the other quadrants. (B) A cross section of the secondary lamellae parallel to the filament surface. (C) A cross section of the secondary lamellae along the filament length. The secondary lamellae of adjacent filaments are shown by broken lines. (D) The trapezoidal lamella. (After Piiper, 1982b.)

B. Stratification in Air Capillaries of Bird Lungs

Diffusion is the only mechanism by which respired gases are transported within the air capillaries between the parabronchial lumen and the gas-blood-separating membrane (Fig. 11). The anatomical situation may be compared with the radial diffusion of gases from the conducting airways into the alveoli of the alveolar lung, except for the generally longer pathways into the air capillaries. Analysis of gas exchange between blood capillaries and air capillaries (Scheid, 1978) shows that significant concentration gradients exist along the gas phase of the air capillaries. The effect of this stratified resistance is restricted, however, owing to the arrangement of capillary blood flow in the air capillary from peripheral to proximal (see Fig. 11). In fact, in this countercurrent-like arrangement gas can exchange with blood at proximal parts of the air capillary, whereby the (stratified) diffusion resistance offered by the air capillaries does not have to be passed by all gas exchanged with the blood.

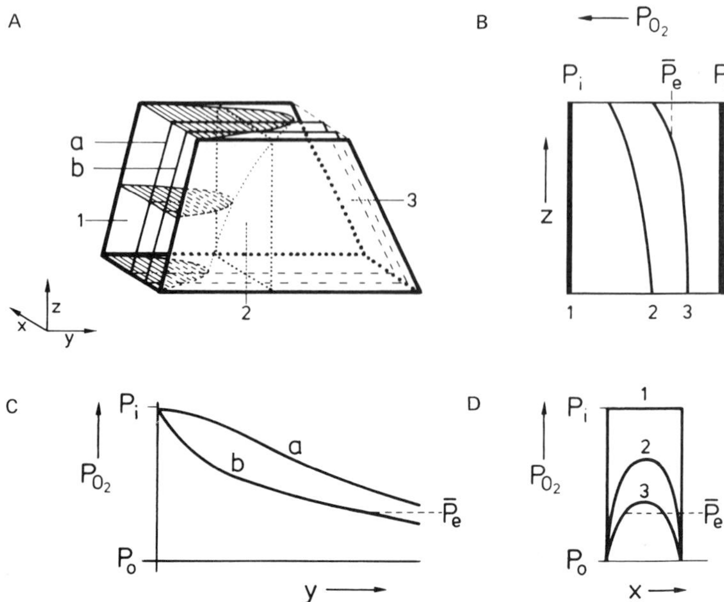

Figure 13 Water velocity and PO_2 profiles in model for interlamellar space. PO, PO_2 on plate surface; Pi, PO_2 of inspired water; $\bar{P}$e, PO_2 of mixed expired water. (A) Model showing parabolic velocity profiles (marked by hatching) for base, middle plane, and top. Three transverse sections (1, entry; 2, middle; 3, exit) are indicated. a and b refer to vertical sections in the y–z plane, in the middle, and toward one side, respectively. (B) Longitudinal (y direction) PO_2 profiles in planes a and b (at a fixed z value). (C) Vertical (z direction) PO_2 profiles in planes 1, 2, and 3 (at a fixed x value). (D) Transverse (x direction) PO_2 profiles in planes 1, 2, and 3 (at a fixed z value). (After Piiper, 1982b.)

C. Diffusion Limitation in the Interlamellar Water of Fish Gills

The fish gill apparatus consists of gill arches, each of which carries a double row of gill filaments. The filaments with a row of secondary lamellae on each side form a fine sieve for respiratory water flow with slitlike, elongate pores (Fig. 12). The blood lacunae of the secondary lamellae are perfused by venous blood. Oxygen has to diffuse through interlamellar water to reach the secondary lamellar surface and the intralamellar blood. Because the diffusivity of O_2 in water is much lower than in air (air/water ratio for the Krogh diffusion constant is about 3×10^4), considerable diffusion limitation is expected, and its effect on gas exchange has been estimated on the basis of models.

Model

To assess the role of diffusion limitation within the interlamellar water, use is made of a simplified gill model (Fig. 13) in which the O_2 partial pressure at the secondary lamellar surface, Po, is assumed to be constant throughout the secondary lamella (in reality, the PO_2 at secondary lamellar increases from the venous inflow to the arterialized outflow end). Water flow is assumed to be laminar (with parabolic velocity profile) and to be inversely proportional to slit length, which decreases from the base to the free edge because of the trapezoidal shape of the secondary lamella. Thus, there are velocity gradients in both x and z directions (Fig. 13). Oxygen is assumed to diffuse in the x direction only, i.e., perpendicularly to the secondary lamellar surface (Scheid and Piiper, 1971; Piiper, 1982b; Piiper and Scheid, 1984).

The PO_2 profiles in the interlamellar water of the model can be calculated from the differential equation ($P = PO_2$) for combined diffusional (x direction) and convectional (y direction) transport,

$$\frac{\partial P}{\partial y} = \frac{d}{v} \cdot \frac{\partial^2 P}{\partial x^2} \tag{16}$$

in which d is the diffusion coefficient of O_2 in water and v is the linear water velocity (varying with x and z). The equation, which is derived from Fick's second law of diffusion, can be numerically integrated for the appropriate boundary and initial conditions (Scheid and Piiper, 1971).

The resulting PO_2 profiles, schematically shown in Fig. 13, display PO_2 gradients in all three spacial dimensions: (1) $\partial P/\partial y$, reflecting the progressive O_2 depletion by uptake across the lamellar surface; (2) $\partial P/\partial x$, resulting from resistance to diffusion; (3) $\partial P/\partial z$, resulting from the base-to-apex velocity gradient. Because of the gradients (2) and (3), PO_2 in outflowing water (Pe) varies considerably across the cross section. The decisive variable for the overall O_2 uptake is the PO_2 in the (flow-weighted) mixed expired water ($\overline{P}e$ obtained by double integration of Pe with respect to x and z.

The resulting $\overline{P}e$ allows calculation of a parameter, ϵ, which designates the inefficiency of O_2 equilibration and is equivalent to a functional water shunt (see the following):

$$\epsilon = \frac{\overline{P}e - Po}{Pi - Po} \tag{17}$$

Po is the constant PO_2 of the secondary lamellar surface (see earlier). It has been shown (Scheid and Piiper, 1971) that ϵ is determined by the (dimensionless) parameter φ,

$$\varphi = \frac{b^2 \cdot \overline{v}}{lo \cdot d} \tag{18}$$

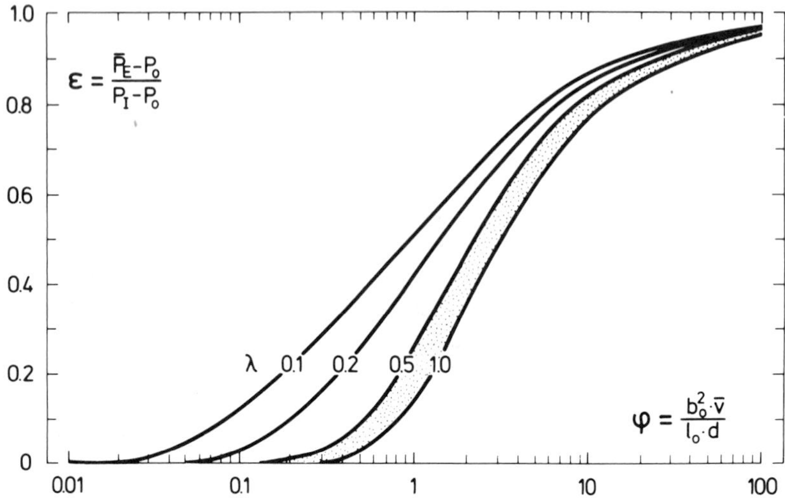

Figure 14 Inefficiency of O_2 equilibration (ϵ) as a function of φ for selected values of tapering (λ). Stippled area: range of estimated λ values. (After Piiper, 1982b.)

and by the tapering factor λ (ratio of top/base length of lamella). The parameter contains two geometric dimensions, the half-width of the interlamllar space, b, and its base length, 1_O, the mean water flow velocity, $\bar{v}$, and the diffusion coefficient of O_2 in water, d. For the same geometry (and diffusivity), φ is proportional to mean water velocity $\bar{v}$ and, thereby, to the water flow or ventilation, $\dot{V}$. With increasing φ (and decreasing λ), the inefficiency of ϵ increases (Fig. 14).

Application and Results

Estimates using experimental values for ventilation and morphometric data for teleost fish gills yield values for O_2 equilibration ranging from 0.02 to about 10 (Scheid and Piiper, 1971). The corresponding ϵ values (for $1 > \gamma > 0.5$) range from close to zero to about 80%, typical values for basal resting conditions being 0–5%; for increased ventilation due to hypoxia, they are around 10–50%.

These estimates of the O_2 equilibration inefficiency, obtained on the basis of the present model, must be considered as minimum estimates for several reasons: 1) Particularly with enhanced respiratory movements, water shunts are likely to occur due to the spreading apart of secondary lamellar rows; 2) water irrigating nonperfused or little-perfused secondary lamellae would act as a water shunt; and 3) the pulsatile nature of water flow is predicted to reduce the O_2 extraction efficiency.

The inefficiency parameter, ϵ, has the meaning of a fractional effective water shunt: It defines what fraction of the respiratory water may be considered as shunted (with unchanged P_{O_2} value) when the remainder is assumed to equilibrate completely with the secondary lamellae. On the other hand, since the inefficiency derives from diffusion limitation, it is more appropriate to use ϵ for calculating an apparent or effective diffusing capacity of interlamellar water, Dw. In the equivalent model used for this analysis, the continuously distributed water velocity of the laminar flow model is replaced by a model with a stagnant water layer lining the secondary lamellar surface and separating it from a central core of mixed flow. In this model the central core equilibrates with the wall according to the equation:

$$\epsilon = \exp[-D_W/(\dot{V} \cdot \alpha)], \tag{19}$$

where $\dot{V}$ is ventilation (water flow) and the α solubility of O_2 in water. Transformation yields:

$$D_W = \dot{V} \cdot \alpha \cdot \ln(1/\epsilon). \tag{20}$$

In the following section the D_W values will be viewed in connection with other variables determining efficiency of gas exchange in fish gills.

VI. Ventilation, Diffusion, and Perfusion

In general, ventilation, diffusion, and perfusion determine gas exchange in the gas exchange organs, and their interplay is described below.

A. The Various Models

For the mixed-pool system of alveolar lungs, the ventilation/diffusion/perfusion system may be considered as the sum of the ventilation and diffusion-perfusion systems, whereby the resistance corresponding to the total inspired-to-mixed venous conductance, $1/G_{tot}$, is the sum of the ventilatory resistance (inverse of the ventilatory conductance, $\dot{V} \cdot \beta_g$) and the total diffusion-perfusion resistance (inverse of the conductance of Equation 11):

$$\frac{1}{G_{tot}} = \frac{1}{\dot{V}_A \cdot \beta_g} + \frac{1}{\dot{Q} \cdot \beta \cdot [1 - \exp[-D/(\dot{Q} \cdot \beta)]]} \tag{21}$$

No such separation can be applied to the crosscurrent or the countercurrent models. The equation for G_{tot} for the crosscurrent model is

$$G_{tot} = \dot{V} \cdot \beta_g \cdot \left\{1 - \exp\left[-\frac{\dot{Q} \cdot \beta}{\dot{V} \cdot \beta_g} \left\langle 1 - \exp[-D/(\dot{Q} \cdot \beta)] \right\rangle \right]\right\} \tag{22}$$

and for the countercurrent system,

$$G_{tot} = \dot{V} \cdot \beta_w \cdot \frac{1 - \exp[D/(\dot{V} \cdot \beta_w) - D/(\dot{Q} \cdot \beta)]}{(\dot{V} \cdot \beta_w)/(\dot{Q} \cdot \beta) - \exp[D/(\dot{V} \cdot \beta_w) - D/(\dot{Q} \cdot \beta)]} \tag{23}$$

Only in the particular case of $\dot{V} \cdot \beta_g = \dot{Q} \cdot \beta$ is such separation possible for the countercurrent model:

$$\frac{1}{G_{tot}} = \frac{1}{D} + \frac{1}{\dot{Q} \cdot \beta} = \frac{1}{D} + \frac{1}{\dot{V} \cdot \beta_w} \tag{24}$$

B. Diffusion-Limited Countercurrent Exchange in Fish Gills

The application of the model to fish gills is of particular interest for two reasons. First, the three conductances, $\dot{V} \cdot \beta_W$, D, and $\dot{Q} \cdot \beta$, appear to be of similar magnitude both for O_2 and CO_2; hence, none of them can be neglected. (In mammalian and avian lungs, under many conditions it may be assumed that $D \to \infty$; in salamander skin in air, that $\dot{V} \cdot \beta_g \to \infty$, meaning absence of stratification in air surrounding the animal.) Second, because of the high diffusion resistance in water, D consists of a membrane and a water component, and their separation is complex.

In the following, two model variants and their application to the analysis of experimental data in the elasmobranch fish, *Scyliorhinus stellaris*, will be summarized.

The Additive Model

In the simplest approximation to consider both diffusion resistances in water (diffusing capacity, D_W) and in the water-blood barrier (diffusing capacity, D_m) are assumed to be additive:

$$\frac{1}{D_{m+w}} = \frac{1}{D_w} + \frac{1}{D_m} \tag{25}$$

in which D_W is obtained from gill ventilation according to Equation 20 and D_m from morphometry. Mean values for the elasmobranch *S. stellaris* (Piiper et al., 1986) are presented in Table 3 and show the following:

1. D_W increases with $\dot{V}$, and this is due to the decrease of the mean diffusion distance for O_2 in the interlamellar water with decreasing extent of water–lamellar surface equilibration, which is equivalent to decreasing thickness of the effective "stagnant layer."

2. The ratio D_m/D_W is higher than unity, meaning that resistance to diffusion in interlamellar water is more important than that of the water–blood tissue barrier. This feature may vary according to fish species.

Table 3 Comparison of Diffusing Capacities for O_2 (D)[a] in the Dogfish *Scyliorhinus stellaris*

	Resting		
	Quiescent	Alert	Swimming
Water temperature (°C)	17	18.3	18.3
Body mass (kg)	2.18	2.53	2.53
Ventilation ($ml \cdot min^{-1}$)	425	810	2320
O_2 uptake ($\mu mol \cdot min^{-1}$)	62	124	218
Physiological, D_{eff}	0.83	1.62	1.95
Membrane, D_m	3.87	4.42	4.42
Water, D_w	2.10	2.63	3.00
Additive, D_{m+w}	1.36	1.65	1.79
D_m/D_w	1.84	1.68	1.47
D_{m+w}/D_{eff}	1.64	1.02	0.92

[a]D in $\mu mol \cdot min^{-1} \cdot torr^{-1}$.
Source: After Piiper et al., 1986.

The Integrated Model

In the additive model of gill gas transfer, conductances (resistances) were segregated into an interlamellar water component and a tissue barrier component. The water component was calculated assuming constant P_{O_2} on the lamellar surface. This is true only when $\dot{Q} \cdot \beta \rightarrow \infty$. In real gills, $\dot{Q} \cdot \beta$ is finite, and the arteriovenous P_{O_2} difference is considerable. To assess the consequences of this deficiency of the additive model, the more realistic, integrated model was developed (Scheid et al., 1986).

In this model, both water and tissue resistances to O_2 diffusion are incorporated, and P_{O_2} is allowed to change both in water and blood (Fig. 15). Oxygen transport by convection and diffusion is determined by three simultaneous equations describing (1) the P_{O_2} gradient in interlamellar water, which is determined by simultaneous forward water flow and transversal O_2 diffusion; (2) the O_2 flux across the tissue barrier, which is equal to the O_2 flux at the water-barrier interface; and (3) the O_2 flux across the barrier, which is equal to O_2 transport by blood. Two diffusing capacities were calculated on the basis of this model and compared with a reference diffusing capacity.

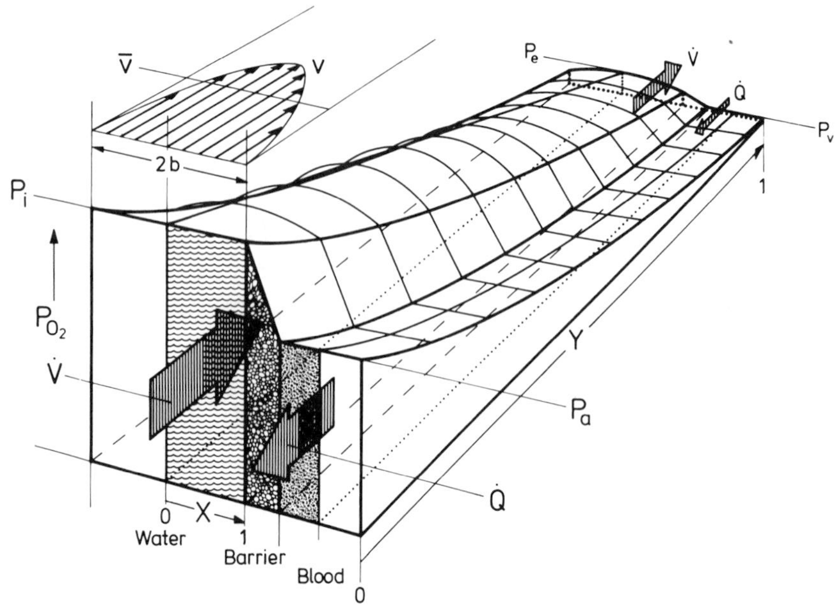

Figure 15 Integrated model for analysis of water–blood O_2 transfer in fish gills. The exchange unit comprises the water–blood tissue barrier with one-half of the interlamellar water flow and of the intralamellar blood flow. Axial extension (Y) is from water inflow and blood outflow at Y = 0 to water outflow and blood inflow at Y = 1. Water flow is with parabolic transversal flow profile (X direction), whereas blood is axially mixed. The PO_2 profiles are schematically shown. (After Scheid et al., 1986.)

1. The integrated diffusing capacity, D_{int}, was calculated from Pi, Pe, Pa, and Pv and the rate of O_2 transfer ($\dot{M}$) on the basis of the countercurrent model, assuming resistance to diffusion to reside in a barrier separating water flow from blood flow (Piiper and Scheid, 1984):

$$D_{int} = \frac{\dot{M}}{(Pi - Pe) - (Pa - Pv)} \cdot \left[\ln \frac{Pi - Pa}{Pe - Pv} \right] \tag{26}$$

2. The O_2 diffusing capacity for interlamellar water, D_w, was obtained from calculated ϵ according to Equation (20) and was combined with D_m, according to Equation 25 to yield D_{m+w}.

3. Because for full equilibration the mean diffusion path-length is one-fourth the interlamellar distance, the D for this water layer is $\tilde{D}_w$. The corresponding additive D is the reference diffusing capacity D_{add},

$$\frac{1}{D_{add}} = \frac{1}{\tilde{D}_w} + \frac{1}{D_m} \tag{27}$$

which is determined by the assumed geometrical dimensions and physical constants only.

Calculations showed that D_{int} was always higher than D_{m+w}, and increased with increase in $\dot{V} \cdot \beta_W$ and $\dot{Q} \cdot \beta$. However, most important was the finding that in the physiological range (as measured in *S. stellaris*) the differences between all D values were less than 10%. Thus, D_{m+w} also appears to be a reasonable approximation to the effective diffusing capacity, in spite of the simplifying assumptions.

A linear blood O_2 equilibrium curve was assumed in the model. The computer model by Malte and Weber (1985) takes the actual curvatures of blood O_2 equilibrium curves into account.

Experimental Values and Models

The mean experimental D values, D_{eff}, determined for the elasmobranch, *S. stellaris*, in various conditions are presented in Table 3. The D_{eff} is seen to increase with the O_2 uptake. The ratio D_{m+w}/D_{eff} is > 1 in resting quiescent fish, but in resting alert and in swimming fish, the ratio is close to unity.

The effective or physiological D is quite regularly found to be smaller than the morphometric D in mammalian lungs, and the difference may be attributed to functional inhomogeneities such as ventilation–perfusion inequality and shunt. The agreement between the morphometric and the physiological D values in resting alert and swimming fish is remarkable. If it is not due to artifacts, this agreement indicates that little functional inhomogeneity was present.

VII. Unequal Distribution of Ventilation to Perfusion

A lung model in which ventilation ($\dot{V}A$) is unequally distributed to blood flow ($\dot{Q}$), whereby different parallel regions have different ratios of $\dot{V}A/\dot{Q}$, has reduced gas exchange efficiency and, thus, yields alveolar–arterial differences for O_2 and CO_2 (AaD). The basic mechanism for generation of AaD is the absence of diffusion limitation. The higher the $\dot{V}A/\dot{Q}$ ratio in a given unit, the higher PO_2 and the lower PCO_2 in alveolar gas and arterialized blood of this region, and vice versa for lower $\dot{V}A/\dot{Q}$. The "mixed" alveolar gas is biased to regions with high $\dot{V}A/\dot{Q}$ and, thus, with high PO_2 and low PCO_2, because it constitutes a ventilation-weighted average. Conversely, mixed arterial blood is biased to regions with low $\dot{V}A/\dot{Q}$ and, thus, with low PO_2 and high PCO_2, because of perfusion-weighted mixing. The result is a higher PO_2 and a lower PCO_2 in expired

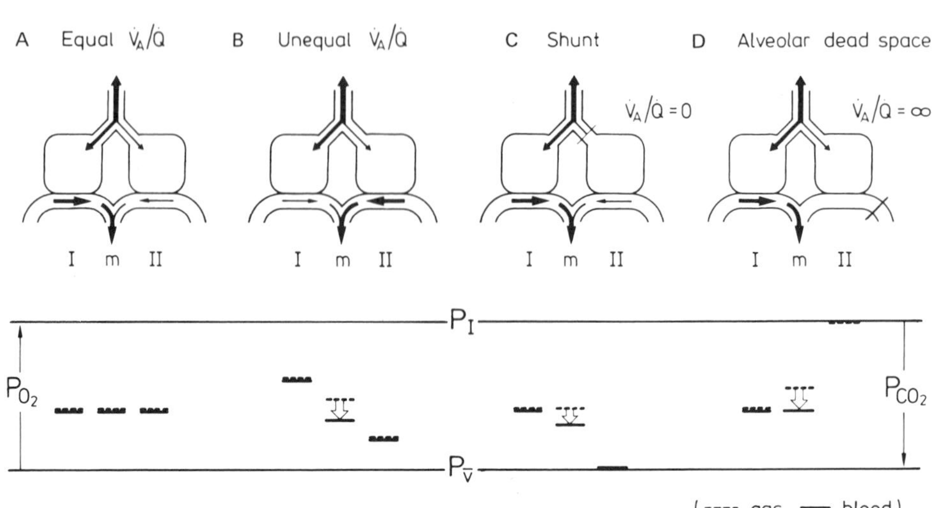

Figure 16 Schematic explanation of alveolar–arterial differences (AaD) caused by unequal distribution of $\dot{V}_A$ to $\dot{Q}$. Indicated are compartments I and II with their gas and blood partial pressures (below) as well as the P values in mixed gas and blood (m). The AaD, visualized by open arrows, are qualitatively similar but quantitatively different for O_2 and CO_2. (A) Equal distribution, no AaD. (B) Unequal $\dot{V}_A/\dot{Q}$ distribution, AaD because of different flow-weighting of gas and blood. (C) Shunt. Compartment II has no ventilation, its exiting blood is unchanged mixed venous blood. (D) Alveolar dead space; compartment II has no blood flow, its ventilation is alveolar dead space ventilation, adding unchanged inspired gas expired from compartment I.

alveolar gas than in exiting arterial blood (Fig. 16B), although P_{CO_2} and P_{O_2} in alveolar gas and arterialized blood are equal in every lung region and also for the volume-averaged whole lung.

Extreme cases of $\dot{V}_A/\dot{Q}$ inequality are (1) compartment with zero $\dot{V}_A/\dot{Q}$ whose perfusion is venous admixture or shunt (Fig. 16C); (2) compartment with infinite $\dot{V}_A/\dot{Q}$ whose ventilation is alveolar dead space ventilation (Fig. 16D).

A. The Conventional Three-Compartment Lung Model

Although the alveolar–arterial P_{O_2} and P_{CO_2} differences are the important consequences and measures of $\dot{V}_A/\dot{Q}$ inequality, there are problems in obtaining alveolar gas that will satisfy the analytical, simplified lung model (continuous ventilation). The end-tidal gas, as measure for (average) alveolar gas, becomes questionable and of limited value when (1) there is a large regional variation of P_{CO_2} and P_{O_2} (as in diseased human lungs); (2) there is no clear alveolar

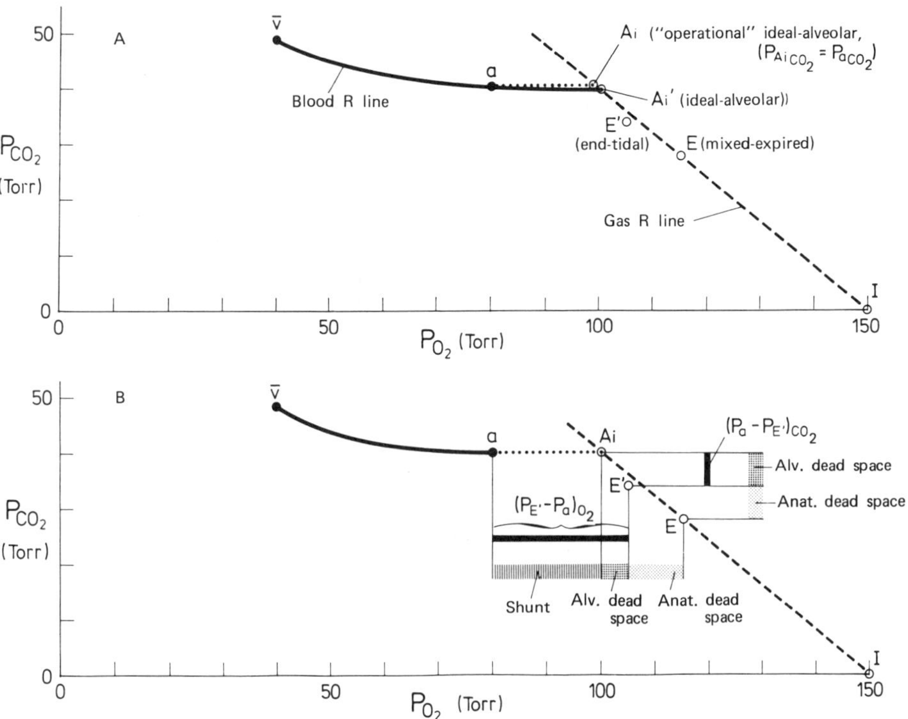

Figure 17 Analysis of the effects of unequal distribution of $\dot{V}A$ to $\dot{Q}$ upon alveolar gas exchange in the PO_2–PCO_2 diagram. In (A), blood and gas R lines and various gas and blood PCO_2/PO_2 values are shown. The end-tidal point (E′) is slightly below the gas R line (see text). In (B), the alveolar–arterial PO_2 and PCO_2 differences and their splitting into their components, "shuntlike" effect and "alveolar–dead space-like" effect, are shown, along with the effect of anatomical dead space.

plateau, but PCO_2 rises and PO_2 falls during the expiration; (3) there is sequential emptying, i.e., some lung regions, usually with high PCO_2 and low PO_2, expire last; (4) the breathing frequency is very high (problems in recording) or very low (effects of continuing gas exchange, see previous discussion).

In all such cases an "ideal alveolar" gas composition can be indirectly obtained (Riley and Cournand, 1949, 1951; Rahn, 1949). The ideal alveolar gas is the alveolar gas that an ideal lung would have with the same alveolar ventilation ($\dot{V}A$), blood flow ($\dot{Q}$), inspired gas ($PICO_2$, PIO_2) and mixed-venous blood ($P\bar{v}CO_2$, $P\bar{v}O_2$). It can be derived from a plot of blood and gas R lines in the O_2-CO_2 diagram (Fig. 17). The ideal alveolar point (Ai) is the intersection of the blood R line, starting from the mixed venous point ($\bar{v}$), with the gas R line, starting from the inspired point (I). Because the blood CO_2 dissociation curve is much steeper than the blood O_2 dissociation curve, i.e., $\beta CO_2/\beta O_2$ ratio is high, the slope of the blood R line near Ai is small, permitting one to approximate $P_{Ai}CO_2$ by P_aCO_2. By this approximation, an "operational" ideal alveolar point is determined. (The approximation is acceptable in normoxia and hyperoxia, less so in hypoxia, and fails in hypercapnic hypoxia when $\beta CO_2/\beta O_2$ is close to unity.)

Algebraically, the slope of the gas R line is obtained from the inspired-expired differences for PCO_2 and PO_2, and the ideal alveolar PO_2 ($P_{Ai}O_2$) is given by P_aCO_2 on it:

$$P_{Ai}CO_2 = P_aCO_2 \tag{28}$$

$$P_{Ai}O_2 = P_IO_2 - (P_aCO_2 - P_ICO_2) \cdot \frac{P_IO_2 - P_EO_2}{P_ECO_2 - P_ICO_2} \tag{29}$$

The ideal alveolar-to-arterial PO_2 difference, $P_{Ai}O_2 - P_aO_2$, is due to admixture of blood from lung areas with low $\dot{V}_A/\dot{Q}$ ratio (shuntlike effect). It can be simulated by admixture of venous blood according to the relationship:

$$\frac{\dot{Q}_{sh}}{\dot{Q}} = \frac{C_{Ai}O_2 - C_aO_2}{C_{Ai}O_2 - C_{\bar{v}}O_2} \tag{30}$$

where $\dot{Q}_{sh}/\dot{Q}$ is the fractional venous admixture and $C_{Ai}O_2$ is the O_2 content of blood equilibrated with ideal alveolar gas.

The PO_2 (and PCO_2) difference between P_{Ai} and P_E defines the physiological or effective dead space ventilation, $\dot{V}_{D_{phys}}$:

$$\frac{\dot{V}_{D_{phys}}}{\dot{V}_E} = \frac{P_aCO_2 - P_ECO_2}{P_aCO_2 - P_ICO_2} = \frac{P_EO_2 - P_{Ai}O_2}{P_IO_2 - P_{Ai}O_2} \tag{31}$$

With the end-tidal gas (E′) the difference between P_{Ai} and P_E is subdivided into two components, the difference $P_{E'} - P_E$ being attributable to the "anatomic" dead space ventilation ($\dot{V}_{D_{ana}}$), the difference $P_{Ai} - P_{E'}$, to alveolar dead space ($\dot{V}_{D_{alv}}$) ventilation, resulting from ventilation of underperfused up to nonperfused lung regions. For CO_2 ($P_{Ai}CO_2 = P_aCO_2$), one obtains:

$$\frac{\dot{V}_{D_{ana}}}{\dot{V}_E} = \frac{P_{E'}CO_2 - P_ECO_2}{P_{E'}CO_2 - P_ICO_2} \tag{32}$$

$$\frac{\dot{V}_{D_{alv}}}{\dot{V}_A} = \frac{P_aCO_2 - P_{E'}CO_2}{P_aCO_2 - P_ICO_2} \tag{33}$$

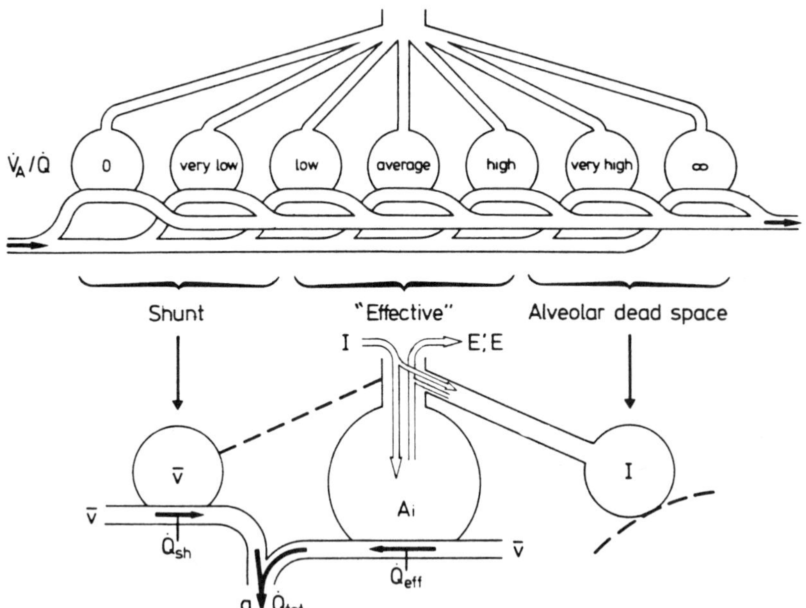

Figure 18 Unequal distribution of alveolar ventilation ($\dot{V}A$) to blood flow ($\dot{Q}$). Top, multicompartment model approaching continuous $\dot{V}A/\dot{Q}$ distribution. Bottom, three-comparment model with potentially same O_2 and CO_2 exchange efficiency as the multicomparment model. The perfusion of compartments with very low to zero $\dot{V}A/\dot{Q}$ acts as shunt. The alveolar ventilation of compartments with very high to infinite $\dot{V}A/\dot{Q}$ is functionally equivalent to alveolar dead space ventilation.

The end-expired point, E′ is usually below the gas R line (see Fig. 17), and this may be attributable to the breath-holding effect of expiration. Hence, the values for $\dot{V}D_{ana}$ and $\dot{V}D_{alv}$ are different for O_2 and CO_2.

This analysis yields a functional (analogous) three-compartment model (Fig. 18, bottom), composed of (1) a compartment effective in gas exchange, with complete gas-blood equilibration; (2) a shunt compartment representing the venous admixture, which is equivalent to perfusion of underventilated lung regions and produces the $PAiO_2 - PaO_2$ difference; (3) an alveolar dead space compartment whose ventilation has the same effect as ventilation of underperfused lung regions, engendering the $PE'O_2 - PAiO_2$ difference.

The results of a representative analysis using values measured in anesthetized dogs are shown in Table 4.

The analysis is applicable to reptiles and amphibians as far as their lungs can be visualized as a mixed pool system, and their inhomogeneity as $\dot{V}/\dot{Q}$ in-

Table 4 Analysis of Alveolar Gas Exchange in Anesthetized Supine Dogs[a]

$PaCO_2$	41.2	$(Pa - PE')CO_2$	5.4
PaO_2	81.3	$(PE' - Pa)O_2$	24.3
$PAiO_2$	98.8	$(PAi - Pa)O_2$	17.5
	$\dot{V}D_{phys}/\dot{V}E$	0.40[b]	
	$\dot{V}D_{ana}/\dot{V}E$	0.31[b]	
	$\dot{V}D_{alv}/\dot{V}A$	0.13	
	$\dot{Q}_{sh}/\dot{Q}$	0.10	

[a]Mean body weight, 27 kg. Spontaneous breathing. Mean values of 23 measurements in seven dogs. Partial pressures, P, in torr. $PIO_2 \sim 146$ torr.
[b]Apparatus dead space not subtracted.
Source: After Aoyagi et al., 1965.

homogeneity. The effect of a true intracardiac right-to-left shunt should be separated from effects arising in the lungs. But a relatively regular breathing is a prerequisite.

In birds, whose lungs operate on the basis of the crosscurrent system, it must be considered that in ideal conditions (homogeneous lungs) there is a negative $PE'O_2 - PaO_2$ and a negative $PaCO_2 - PE'CO_2$, so that identical PE′ and Pa may indicate some inhomogeneity effect. An analysis of $\dot{V}/\dot{Q}$ maldistribution using a two-compartment model has been performed in the duck by Burger et al. (1979).

B. Detection of Continuous Distributions of $\dot{V}A$ to $\dot{Q}$

Distinction between low $\dot{V}A/\dot{Q}$ and shunt, and between high $\dot{V}A/\dot{Q}$ and alveolar dead space ventilation, and estimation of the real extent of $\dot{V}A/\dot{Q}$ inhomogeneity have been made possible by use of multiple inert gases of different solubility in blood (Farhi, 1967). The gases are best infused intravenously, whereby a steady state is achieved (Wagner et al., 1974a,b; see Hlastala, 1984).

The method is based on inert gas elimination by an ideal lung, which can be described by Equation 3, and shows the inert gas retention, $Pa/P\bar{v}$, to depend only on the partition coefficient, λ, and on $\dot{V}A/\dot{Q}$. This means that (1) a gas of given λ is the more efficiently eliminated (less retained: $Pa/P\bar{v}$ smaller) the higher the $\dot{V}A/\dot{Q}$ ratio; (2) at a certain $\dot{V}A/\dot{Q}$ ratio, the gas with higher λ is less efficiently eliminated (more retained). It follows for use of several gases of different λ:

1. For an ideal lung with given $\dot{V}A/\dot{Q}$, Pa (= PA) for gases of different λ will follow the curve determined by Eqauation 3 (Fig. 19A).

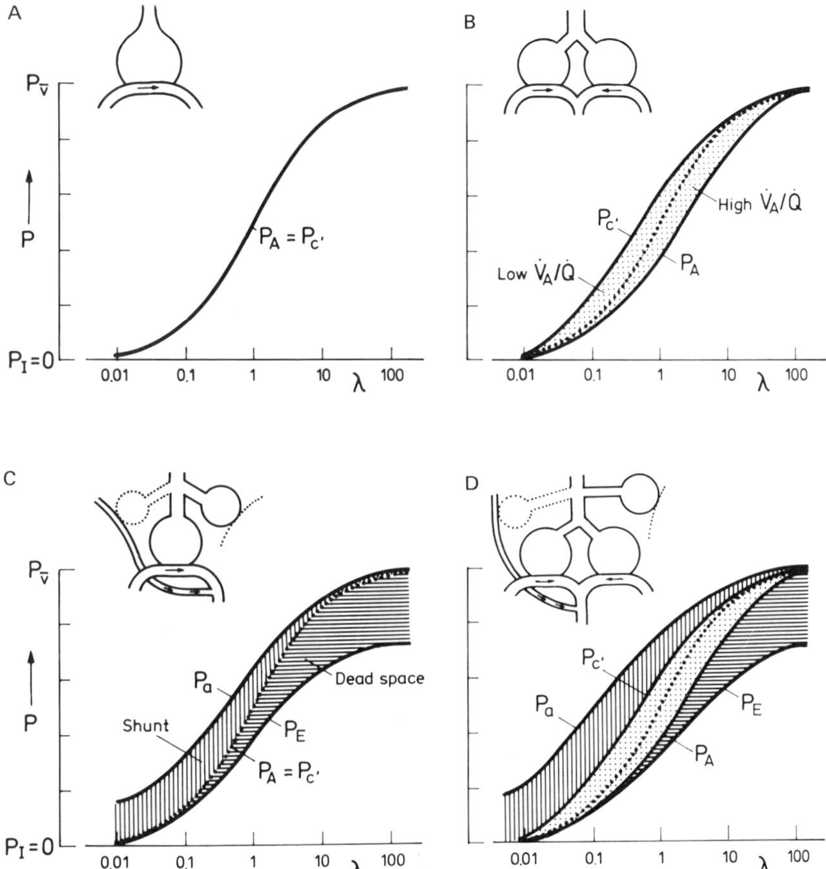

Figure 19 Inert gas elimination by lungs with $\dot{V}A/\dot{Q}$ inhomogeneity as function of the partition coefficient λ (= β/β_g). (A) Homogeneous lung model. The curve PA = Pc′ corresponds to Equation 3. The same curve is inscribed in B, C, and D as dotted line. (B) Lung model with $\dot{V}A/\dot{Q}$ inhomogeneity, symbolized by two comparments with differing $\dot{V}A/\dot{Q}$ ratio. (C) Lung model with shunt and (physiological) dead space ventilation. (D) Lung model combining models B and C.

2. For a lung with $\dot{V}A/\dot{Q}$ inhomogeneity (Fig. 19B), the Pa curve will be displaced to the left (mainly as effect of low $\dot{V}A/\dot{Q}$), PA will be displaced to the right (effect of high $\dot{V}A/\dot{Q}$), and the slopes of both will be flattened relative to that of the ideal lung. From these deviations the extent and pattern of $\dot{V}A/\dot{Q}$ inhomogeneity may be estimated.

3. In a lung with (anatomical) shunt and (anatomical and alveolar) dead space ventilation but no further $\dot{V}A/\dot{Q}$ heterogeneity (Fig. 19C), gas and blood

values in the gas-exchanging compartment are equal, $P_A = Pc'$ and the following are found:

a. The shunt reduces the $P\bar{v} - Pc'$ difference for all gases by a constant factor:

$$\frac{\dot{Q}_{sh}}{\dot{Q}} = \frac{Pa - Pc'}{P\bar{v} - Pc'} \tag{34}$$

For very low λ, when $Pc' = 0$ (= P_I), the fractional shunt becomes identical with the retention, $Pa/P\bar{v}$.

b. Dead space ventilation reduces the P_A values for all gases by a constant factor:

$$\frac{\dot{V}_{D\,phys}}{\dot{V}_E} = \frac{P_A - P_E}{P_A} \tag{35}$$

in which $\dot{V}_{D\,phys}$ is the physiologic dead space ventilation. For very high λ, when $P_A = P\bar{v}$, the fractional dead space ventilation is obtained from the relationship:

$$\frac{\dot{V}_{D\,phys}}{\dot{V}_E} = 1 - \frac{P_E}{P\bar{v}} \tag{36}$$

4. Combination of the cases B and C yields the general case with shunt, dead space ventilation, and $\dot{V}_A/\dot{Q}$ inequality (Fig. 19D). From the experimentally determined curves of Pa and P_E vs. λ, first the Pc' (c′ denotes blood flow-weighted mean end-capillary blood) curve is constructed according to Equation 34; second, the P_A (A denotes ventilation-weighted mean alveolar gas) curve is derived according to Equation 35. The remaining difference between the P_A and Pc' curves is due to $\dot{V}_A/\dot{Q}$ inequality, the extent and pattern of which can be derived therefrom.

By use of six gases of suitable λ (from < 0.01, SF_6, to > 100, acetone) and applying particular numerical procedures, continuous $\dot{V}_A$ to $\dot{Q}$ distributions have been determined in laboratory animals and in normal and diseased humans, as exemplified by Figure 20 (reviewed by West, 1977; Hlastala, 1984). The technique is laborious and difficult, and a very high accuracy is required particularly in measuring Pa and $P\bar{v}$. Nevertheless, the uniqueness of recovered $\dot{V}_A/\dot{Q}$ distributions must remain questionable, because it is derived only from the data of four gases (the extreme λ gases being used for determination of shunt and dead space). In spite of these problems, the method is now successfully applied in physiological and clinical pulmonary function laboratories.

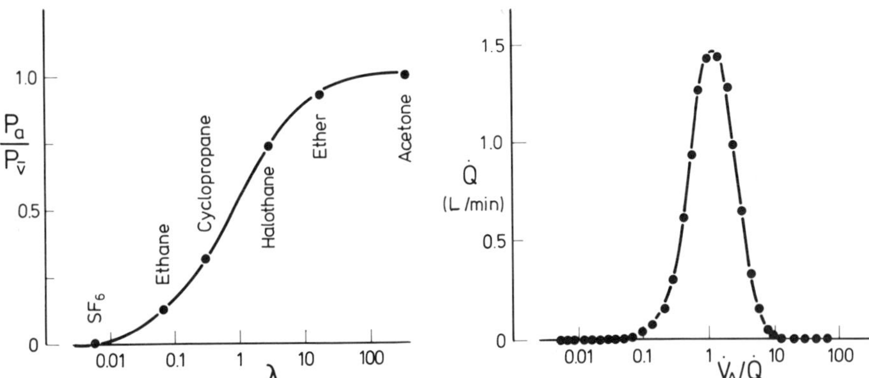

Figure 20 Left, example of a plot of retention ($Pa/P\bar{v}$) as function of the blood–gas partition coefficient (λ), measured in man by the multiple inert gas infusion technique. Right, the $\dot{V}A/\dot{Q}$ inhomogeneity derived from the left example in terms of (continuous) distribution of blood flow to compartments with differing $\dot{V}A/\dot{Q}$ ratios. (After West, 1977.)

The method has recently been applied to the domestic duck with remarkable success. Here the evaluation must be based on a (nondiffusion-limited) crosscurrent model (Powell and Wagner, 1982a,b). It should be noted that the method is not applicable in water breathing because here inert gases covering a wide range in the blood–water partition coefficient, rather than the blood–gas partition coefficient, must be used, but they are unavailable.

VIII. Unequal Distribution of Diffusing Capacity

An unequal distribution of diffusing capacity (diffusive conductance) has received relatively little attention in the analysis of the function of gas exchange organs. In the following, two examples relating to gas exchange in mammalian lungs will be presented.

A. Inequality of the Equilibration Coefficient

It was shown previously that the equilibration coefficient $D/(\dot{Q} \cdot \beta)$ determines the extent of equilibration of pulmonary capillary blood with alveolar gas in mammalian lungs. There is a number of factors that are expected to produce some local variability of this ratio.

1. Capillary length may vary considerably among parallel lung units. A short capillary is bound to have low D, high $\dot{Q}$ (because of reduced re-

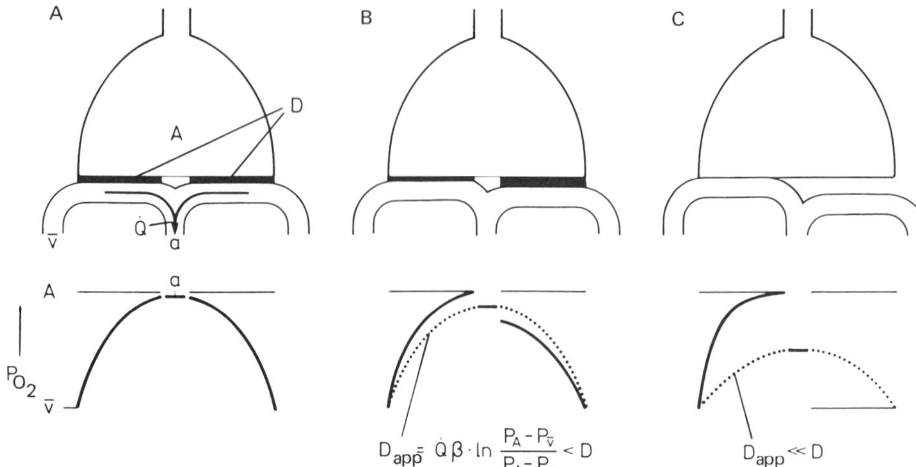

Figure 21 Gas transfer efficiency of lung models with $D/\dot{Q}$ or $D/(\dot{Q} \cdot \beta)$ inhomogeneity. Lower row: PO_2 profiles in capillary blood of the two compartments and PO_2 in mixed arterial (end-capillary) blood. (A) Homogeneous model. (B) Same total D as in (A) but unequally distributed to $\dot{Q}$; AaD is increased. (C) All D is allotted to the left compartment, blood flow to the right compartment acting as shunt flow.

sistance to flow), and a short transit time (discussed earlier). In the extreme case this unit may act as a shunt.

2. The thickness of the gas–blood barrier may vary, particularly with incipient alveolar edema.
3. Pulmonary capillary blood flow varies regionally because of variable distension by hydrostatic pressure.
4. Variations of hematocrit are known to occur in microcirculation, the branch that has less resistance and higher flow receives disproportionately more red blood cells and, thus, has a higher β.
5. In relatively hypoventilated lung areas (low $\dot{V}A/\dot{Q}$ ratio), the effective β is increased owing to the shape of the blood O_2 dissociation curve, leading to increased diffusion limitation.

The effect of unequal $D/(\dot{Q} \cdot \beta)$ is to reduce the overall gas transfer, because a decrease of $D/(\dot{Q} \cdot \beta)$ diminishes gas transfer more than an increase of the ratio enhances it. The extreme example of $D/(\dot{Q} \cdot \beta) = 0$ leads to shunt (Piiper, 1961a; Fig. 21).

An evaluation of the alveolar gas exchange inefficiency in terms of $D/\dot{Q}$ inequality was attempted in anesthetized dogs when the alveolar-arterial differences appeared not to fit the expectation for $\dot{V}A/\dot{Q}$ inequality (Piiper et al., 1961).

Generally, there may be both $\dot{V}A/\dot{Q}$ and $D/(\dot{Q} \cdot \beta)$ inequality in lungs. In this case, the gas exchange behavior of lungs may be analyzed in terms of a two-dimensional $\dot{V}A/\dot{Q}$ and $D/(\dot{Q} \cdot \beta)$ "field" (Piiper, 1961b). In this field, three edges, $D/(\dot{Q} \cdot \beta) = 0$ (shunt), $\dot{V}A/\dot{Q} = 0$ (shunt, but not when breathing 100% O_2), $\dot{V}A/\dot{Q} \rightarrow \infty$ (alveolar dead space ventilation), mark the absence of gas exchange and the "ideal point" is represented by $D/(\dot{Q} \cdot \beta) = \infty$ and a normal $\dot{V}A/\dot{Q}$.

B. Unequal Distribution of Gas-Phase Conductance

In recent years asymmetrical lung airway models, i.e., with asymmetric pattern of branching and highly varying lengths of the airway branches, have received attention to explain the slope of the alveolar plateau for inert, low-soluble test gases (see previous discussion) (DeVries et al., 1981; Bowes et al., 1982; Paiva and Engel, 1984). In terms of function, this means essentially local variation of diffusion resistance. The simplest analogue model for unequally distributed airways diffusion resistance is a two-compartment model with varied G_{mix}/VA ratio.

Indeed, such a model has been devised to explain the experimental results of anesthetized dogs in which the sloping alveolar plateau was measured for several insoluble inert gases of different diffusivity (Meyer et al., 1983; Hook et al., 1985). The experimental data could be simulated by a two-compartment model in which low $\dot{V}A/VA$ was associated with low G_{mix}/VA and delayed emptying during expiration.

References

Aoyagi, K., Piiper, J., and May, F. (1965). Alveolärer Gasaustausch und Kreislauf am narkotisierten Hund bei Spontanatmung und bei künstlicher Beatmung. *Pflügers Arch. 286*:311-316.

Bowes, C., Cumming, G., Horsfield, K., Loughhead, J., and Preston, S. (1982). Gas mixing in a model of pulmonary acinus with asymmetrical alveolar ducts. *J. Appl. Physiol. 52*:624-633.

Burger, R. E., Meyer, M., Graf, W., and Scheid, P. (1979). Gas exchange in the parabronchial lung of birds: Experiments in unidirectionally ventilated ducks. *Respir. Physiol. 36*:19-37.

Burggren, W. W., and Moalli, R. (1984). "Active" regulation of cutaneous gas exchange by capillary recruitment in amphibians: Experimental evidence and a revised model for skin respiration. *Respir. Physiol. 55*:379-392.

Cerretelli, P. (1976). Limiting factors to oxygen transport on Mount Everest. *J. Appl. Physiol. 40*:658-667.

Cumming, G., Horsfield, K., Jones, J. G., and Muir, D. C. F. (1967). The influence of gaseous diffusion on the alveolar plateau at different lung volumes, *Respir. Physiol. 2*:386-398.

Dejours, P., Armand, J., and Verriest, G. (1968). Carbon dioxide dissociation curves of water and gas exchange of water-breathers. *Respir. Physiol. 5*: 23-33.

DeVries, W. R., Luijendijk, S. C. M., and Zwart, A. (1981). Helium and sulfur hexafluoride washout in asymmetric lung models. *J. Appl. Physiol. 51*: 1122-1130.

Duncker, H.-R. (1974). Structure of the avian respiratory tract. *Respir. Physiol. 22*:1-19.

Farhi, L. E. (1967). Elimination of inert gas by the lung. *Respir. Physiol. 3*:1-11.

Feder, M. E. (1985). Effects of thermal acclimation on locomotor energetics and locomotor performance in a lungless salamander. *Physiologist 28*:342.

Feder, M. E., and Burggren, W. W. (1985). Cutaneous gas exchange in vertebrates: Design, patterns, control, and implications. *Biol. Rev. 60*:1-45.

Full, R. J. (1985). Exercising without lungs: Energetics and endurance in a lungless salamander. *Plethodon jordani. Physiologist 28*:342.

Gatz, R. N., Crawford, E. C., Jr., and Piiper, J. (1975). Kinetics of inert gas equilibration in an exclusively skin-breathing salamanders, *Desmognathus fuscus. Respir. Physiol. 24*:15-29.

Georg, J., Lassen, N. A., Mellemgaard, K., and Vinther, A. (1965). Diffusion in the gas phase of the lungs in normal and emphysematous subjects. *Clin. Sci. 29*:525-532.

Glass, M. L., and Wood, S. C. (1983). Gas exchange and control of breathing in reptiles. *Physiol. Rev. 63*:232-260.

Hlastala, M. P. (1984). Multiple inert gas elimination technique. *J. Appl. Physiol. 56*:1-7.

Hook, C., Meyer, M., and Piiper, J. (1985). Model simulation of single-breath washout of insoluble gases from dog lung. *J. Appl. Physiol. 58*:802-811.

Hughes, G. M., and Shelton, G. (1962). Respiratory mechanisms and their nervous control in fish. *Adv. Comp. Physiol. Biochem. 1*:275-364.

Itazawa, Y., and Takeda, T. (1978). Gas exchange in the carp gills in normoxic and hypoxic conditions. *Respir. Physiol. 35*:263-269.

Kawashiro, T., Charles, A. C., and Piiper, J. (1975). Diffusivity of various inert gases in rat skeletal muscle. *Pflügers Arch. 359*:219-230.

Laurent, P. (1984). Gill internal morphology. In *Fish Physiology*, Vol. XA. Edited by W. S. Hoar and D. J. Randall. Orlando Academic Press, pp. 73-183.

Malte, H., and Weber, R. E. (1985). A mathematical model for gas exchange in the fish gill based on non-linear blood gas equilibrium curves. *Respir. Physiol. 62*:359-374.

Malvin, G. M., and Hlastala, M. P. (1986). Regulation of cutaneous gas exchange by environmental O_2 and CO_2 in the frog. *Respir. Physiol. 65*:99-111.

Meyer, M., Worth, H., and Scheid, P. (1976). Gas-blood CO_2 equilibration in parabronchial lungs of birds. *J. Appl. Physiol. 41*:302-309.

Meyer, M., Tebbe, U., and Piiper, J. (1980). Solubility of inert gases in dog blood and skeletal muscle. *Pflügers Arch. 384*:131-134.

Meyer, M., Scheid, P., Riepl, G., Wagner, H. J., and Piiper, J. (1981). Pulmonary diffusing capacities for O_2 and CO measured by a rebreathing technique. *J. Appl. Physiol. 51*:1643-1650.

Meyer, M., Hook, C., Rieke, H., and Piiper, J. (1983). Gas mixing in dog lungs studied by single-breath washout of He and SF_6. *J. Appl. Physiol. 55*: 1795-1802.

Paiva, M. (1973). Gas transport in the human lung. *J. Appl. Physiol. 35*:401-410.

Paiva, M., and Engel, L. A. (1984). Model analysis of gas distribution within human lung acinus. *J. Appl. Physiol. 56*:418-425.

Piiper, J. (1961a). Unequal distribution of pulmonary diffusing capacity and the alveolar-arterial P_{O_2} differences: Theory. *J. Appl. Physiol. 16*:493-498.

Piiper, J. (1961b). Variations of ventilation and diffusing capacity to perfusion determining the alveolar-arterial O_2 difference: Theory. *J. Appl. Physiol. 16*:507-510.

Piiper, J. (1979). Series ventilation, diffusion in airways and stratified inhomogeneity. *Fed. Proc. 38*:17-21.

Piiper, J. (1982a). Respiratory gas exchange at lungs, gills and tissues: Mechanisms and adjustments. *J. Exp. Biol. 100*:5-22.

Piiper, J. (1982b). Diffusion in the interlamellar water of fish gills. *Fed. Proc. 41*:2140-2142.

Piiper, J., and Baumgarten-Schumann, D. (1968a). Transport of O_2 and CO_2 by water and blood in gas exchange of the dogfish (*Scyliorhinus stellaris*). *Respir. Physiol. 5*:326-337.

Piiper, J., and Baumgarten-Schumann, D. (1968b). Effectiveness of O_2 and CO_2 exchange in the gills of the dogfish (*Scyliorhinus stellaris*). *Respir. Physiol. 5*:338-349.

Piiper, J., and Scheid, P. (1972). Maximum gas transfer efficacy of models for fish gills, avian lungs and mammalian lungs. *Respir. Physiol. 14*:115-124.

Piiper, J., and Scheid, P. (1975). Gas transport efficacy of gills, lungs and skin: Theory and experimental data. *Respir. Physiol. 23*:209-221.

Piiper, J., and Scheid, P. (1977). Comparative physiology of respiration: Functional analysis of gas exchange organs in vertebrates. In *Respiration Physiology II*. Int. Rev. Physiol. Ser. Vol. XIV. Edited by J. G. Widdicombe. Baltimore, Univ. Park, pp. 219-253.

Piiper, J., and Scheid, P. (1980). Blood-gas equilibration in lungs. In *Pulmonary Gas Exchange*. Edited by J. B. West. New York, Academic Press, pp. 131-171.

Piiper, J., and Scheid, P. (1981). Model for capillary-alveolar equilibration with special reference to O_2 uptake in hypoxia. *Respir. Physiol. 46*:193-208.

Piiper, J., and Scheid, P. (1982). Models for a comparative functional analysis of gas exchange organs in vertebrates. *J. Appl. Physiol. 53*:1321-1329.

Piiper, J., and Scheid, P. (1983a). Comparison of diffusion and perfusion limitations in alveolar gas exchange. *Respir. Physiol. 51*:287-290.

Piiper, J., and Scheid, P. (1983b). Physical principles of gas exchange in fish gills. In *Gills*. Edited by D. F. Houlihan, J. C. Rankin, and T. J. Shuttleworth. London and New York, Cambridge University Press, pp. 45-62.

Piiper, J., and Scheid, P. (1984). Model analysis of gas transfer in fish gills, In *Fish Physiology*, Vol. XA. Edited by W. S. Hoar and D. J. Randall. Orlando, Academic Press, pp. 229-262.

Piiper, J., and Schumann, D. (1967). Efficiency of O_2 exchange in the gills of the dogfish, *Scyliorhinus stellaris. Respir. Physiol. 2*:135-148.

Piiper, J., Haab, P., and Rahn, H. (1961). Unequal distribution of pulmonary diffusing capacity in the anesthetized dog. *J. Appl. Physiol. 16*:491-506.

Piiper, J., Dejours, P., Haab, P., and Rahn, H. (1971). Concepts and basic quantities in gas exchange physiology. *Respir. Physiol. 13*:292-304.

Piiper, J., Gatz, R. N., and Crawford, E. C., Jr. (1976). Gas transport characteristics in an exclusively skin-breathing salamander, *Desmognathus fuscus* (Plethodontidae). In *Respiration of Amphibious Vertebrates*. Edited by G. M. Hughes. New York, Academic Press, pp. 339-356.

Piiper, J., Meyer, M., Marconi, C., and Scheid, P. (1980). Alveolar-capillary equilibration kinetics of $^{13}CO_2$ in human lungs studied by rebreathing. *Respir. Physiol. 42*:29-41.

Piiper, J., Scheid, P., Perry, S. F., and Hughes, G. M. (1986). Effective and morphometric oxygen-diffusing capacity of the gills of the elasmobranch *Scyliorhinus stellaris. J. Exp. Biol. 123*:27-41.

Powell, F. L., and Wagner, P. D. (1982a). Measurement of continuous distributions of ventilation-perfusion in non-alveolar lungs. *Respir. Physiol. 48*: 219-232.

Powell, F. L., and Wagner, P. D. (1982b). Ventilation-perfusion inequality in avian lungs. *Respir. Physiol. 48*:233-241.

Powell, F. L., Geiser, J., Gratz, R. K., and Scheid, P. (1981). Airflow in the avian respiratory tract: Variations of O_2 and CO_2 concentrations in the bronchi of the duck. *Respir. Physiol. 44*:195-213.

Rahn, H. (1949). A concept of mean alveolar air and the ventilation-blood flow relationships during pulmonary gas exchange. *Am. J. Physiol. 158*:21-30.

Rahn, H., and Howell, B. J. (1976). Bimodal gas exchange. In *Respiration of Amphibious Vertebrates*. Edited by G. M. Hughes. New York, Academic Press, pp. 271-285.

Randall, D. J., Holeton, G. F., and Stevens, E. D. (1967). The exchange of oxygen and carbon dioxide across the gills of rainbow trout. *J. Exp. Biol. 46*: 339-348.

Riley, R. L., and Cournand, A. (1949). "Ideal" alveolar air and the analysis of ventilation-perfusion relationships in the lungs. *J. Appl. Physiol. 1*:825-847.

Riley, R. L., and Cournand, A. (1951). Analysis of factors affecting partial pressures of oxygen and carbon dioxide in gas and blood of the lungs: Theory. *J. Appl. Physiol. 4*:77-101.

Scheid, P. (1978). Analysis of gas exchange between air capillaries and blood capillaries in avian lungs. *Respir. Physiol. 32*:27-49.

Scheid, P. (1979). Mechanisms of gas exchange in bird lungs. *Rev. Physiol. Biochem. Pharmacol. 86*:137-186.

Scheid, P., and Piiper, J. (1971). Theoretical analysis of respiratory gas equilibration in water passing through fish gills. *Respir. Physiol. 13*:305-318.

Scheid, P., and Piiper, J. (1972). Cross-current gas exchange in avian lungs: Effects of reversed parabronchial air flow in ducks. *Respir. Physiol. 16*:304-312.

Scheid, P., and Piiper, J. (1976). Quantitative functional analysis of branchial gas transfer: Theory and application to *Scyliorhinus stellaris* (Elasmobranchii). In *Respiration of Amphibious Vertebrates*. Edited by G. M. Hughes. London, Academic Press, pp. 17-38.

Scheid, P., and Piiper, J. (1980). Intrapulmonary gas mixing and stratification. In *Pulmonary Gas Exchange*. Edited by J. B. West. New York, Academic Press, pp. 87-130.

Scheid, P., and Piiper, J. (1987). Blood-gas equilibration in lungs and pulmonary diffusing capacity. In *A Quantitative Approach to Respiratory Physiology*. Edited by H. K. Chang and M. Paiva. (Lung Biology in Health and Disease. Edited by C. Lenfant). New York, Marcel Dekker (submitted).

Scheid, P., Hook, C., and Piiper, J. (1986). Model for analysis of counter-current gas transfer in fish gills. *Respir. Physiol. 64*:365-374.

Scheid, P., Fedde, M. R., and Piiper, J. (1988). Gas exchange and air sac composition in the unanesthetized domestic goose. *J. Exp. Biol.* (in press).

Short, S., Taylor, E. W., and Butler, P. J. (1979). The effectiveness of oxygen transfer during normoxia and hypoxia in the dogfish (*Scyliorhinus canicula* L.) before and after cardiac vagotomy. *J. Comp. Physiol. 132*:289-295.

Truchot, J. P., Toulmond, A., and Dejours, P. (1980). Blood acid-base balance as a function of water oxygenation: A study at two different ambient CO_2 levels in the dogfish, *Scyliorhinus canicula. Respir. Physiol. 41*:13-28.

Wagner, P. D., Laravuso, R. B., Uhl, R. R., and West, J. B. (1974a). Continuous distributions of ventilation-perfusion ratios in normal subjects breathing air and 100% O_2. *J. Clin. Invest. 54*:54-68.

Wagner, P. D., Saltzman, H. A., and West, J. B. (1974b). Measurement of continuous distributions of ventilation-perfusion ratios: Theory. *J. Appl. Physiol. 36*:588-599.

Weibel, E. R. (1963). *Morphometry of the Human Lung*. Berlin and New York, Springer-Verlag.

West, J. B. (1977). Ventilation-perfusion relationships. *Am. Rev. Respir. Dis. 116*:919-943.

Withers, P. C. (1980). Oxygen consumption of plethodontid salamanders during rest, activity, and recovery. *Copeia 1980*: 781-786.

14

Diffusing Capacity

MOGENS L. GLASS*

University of Aarhus
Aarhus, Denmark

I. Introduction

This chapter deals with physiologically determined diffusing capacity (D), which is discussed in a comparative context. The aim is to provide a broad overview of differences between vertebrate classes. In addition, the effects of environmental changes or exercise on D are emphasized. The chapter will focus on DO_2 and DCO, because comparative data on DCO_2 are scarce. Gas exchange models are not presented because they are discussed in Chapter 13 by Piiper and Scheid. Likewise, other chapters will represent the comparative morphology of vertebrate gas exchange systems. As a further limitation, the conditions are discussed only for adult animals.

The comparative aspects of diffusive transport have been reviewed (Piiper, 1982; Scheid, 1982) and mammalian values discussed in detail (Forster and

---

**Present affiliation*: Max Planck Institute for Experimental Medicine, Göttingen, Federal Republic of Germany.

Support was provided by the Danish Natural Science Research Council and the Alexander von Humboldt-Stiftung.

Crandall, 1976). It is recommended that the reader consult these publications for additional information.

II. Physiological Estimation of DL: Basic Concepts

Bohr (1909) proposed an equation, which defines pulmonary diffusing capacity (DL),

$$D_{L}x = \frac{\dot{V}_X}{(P_A - P_{\bar{c}})_X} \quad (\text{ml STPD} \cdot \text{min}^{-1} \cdot \text{torr}^{-1})$$

where $\dot{V}_X$ represents the amount of the gas species x that diffuses, per unit time, through the membrane that separates alveolar gas and pulmonary blood; PA denotes the alveolar partial pressure of the gas, and $P\bar{c}$ the mean partial pressure in the pulmonary capillary blood. DL represents a gas conductance (G) because respiratory conductance equations are of the general form,

$$G_X = \frac{\dot{V}_X}{\Delta P_X}$$

(see Chap. 13).

The study by Bohr (1909) addressed the question of whether pulmonary O_2 uptake can be described exclusively as a diffusive process or if an active transport must be assumed to account for total O_2 uptake. Bohr devised an integration technique for calculation of $(P_A - P\bar{c})O_2$, while taking the shape of O_2 dissociation curve into account (Bohr integration). In spite of that, he estimated $D_{L}O_2$ indirectly based on the few available data for the uptake kinetics of CO from the alveolar gas. The choice of CO rather than O_2 can be motivated by the high capacitance coefficient for CO, implying that the CO backpressure in the pulmonary capillaries will be negligible, provided that low CO concentrations are applied (although see Piiper et al., 1969). Bohr assumed that a conversion from DLCO to $D_{L}O_2$ could be obtained from the relative solubilities and molecular weights of the gases, which would result in: $D_{L}O_2 = 1.23 \cdot D_{L}CO$. Applying these estimates for $D_{L}O_2$ to data for gas exchange at rest and during exercise Bohr concluded that O_2 uptake, in part, occurred by active transport.

Soon after publication, the conclusions advanced by Bohr were criticized by Krogh and Krogh (1910) who had developed a manometric method for measurement of CO at low concentrations. Applying this technique they measured PACO and CO uptake taking point samples seconds apart. The authors reassessed DLCO for humans and concluded that the values were large enough to account for gas exchange, and an active O_2 transport was not to be assumed, which soon became the accepted view (see also Krogh, 1910). Thus, Bohr's final conclusion did not hold, but he should certainly be credited for his pioneering analysis.

Although the basic approach is still the same, the methods for measurement and calculation of DLCO and DLO_2 have greatly improved since 1909. A method that is frequently applied is based on continuous monitoring of alveolar CO concentration during a short rebreathing maneuver (Kruhøffer, 1954). During the past decade this method has benefited from the development of respiratory mass spectrometers, which allow simultaneous monitoring of several gases including $C^{18}O$. By this technique DL can be measured along with lung volumes (by He dilution) and pulmonary perfusion calculated from uptake kinetics for a blood-soluble gas (acetylene, N_2O, freon, etc.). The theory of these rebreathing methods has been reviewed by Hook and Meyer (1982), who also provide a careful evaluation of potential methodological problems. The rebreathing method is widely applied, although alternative approaches are possible including a "steady-state" method (see Forster and Crandall, 1976) and a single-breath technique (see Takezawa et al., 1980).

A fundamental problem concerns conversion from DLCO to DLO_2 or to $DLCO_2$. Bohr (1909) applied simple calculations, which are valid if the gas transport depends exclusively on diffusion. This assumption was questioned by Kruhøffer (1954), who reported a reduced DLCO when the alveolar PO_2 was elevated to hyperoxic levels. This indicated that CO competed with O_2 for reaction sites with hemoglobin, i.e., DLCO is both diffusion and reaction dependent. Reaction rates between erythrocytes and CO were measured by Roughton and Forster (1957), who concluded that the rates were too slow to allow simple diffusion-based equations for DL. Adding diffusing resistances in series they proposed the equation,

$$1/DL = 1/DM + 1/Vc \cdot \theta$$

where DM represents the diffusing capacity of the pulmonary membrane; θ = reaction rate between whole blood and CO or O2, and Vc = pulmonary capillary volume. The reaction rate between gas and whole blood includes transport within pulmonary capillary plasma, passage of the erythrocyte membrane, transport within cell plasma, and the reaction between gas and the hemoglobin molecule. The equation by Roughton and Forster precludes any simple conversion from DLCO to DLO_2. Fortunately, methods are also available for direct determination of DLO_2 (see Adaro et al., 1976; Hook and Meyer, 1982). One recently developed approach is based on rebreathing of the stable isotope $^{18}O_2$ at low concentrations (see Meyer et al., 1981). Applying respiratory mass spectrometry Meyer et al. (1981) performed simultaneous measurements of DL for CO and O_2 in man. Values for the ratio DLO_2/DLCO were close to 1.2 both during rest and exercise. This can be interpreted as evidence that DL is diffusion-dependent, implying that the conversion factor is determined by the

the ratio of the Krogh diffusion coefficient of the gases, KO_2/KCO. Nevertheless, Meyer et al. (1981) caution that an alternative interpretation is possible. The ratio of 1.2 might result from $\theta O_2/\theta CO$, because the literature is inconsistent for these reaction rates predicting $1 < \theta O_2/\theta CO < 3.3$ (Meyer et al., 1981).

A recent study has provided important information on the relative roles of diffusion and reaction in O_2 uptake by human erythrocytes (Yamaguchi et al., 1985). The data suggested that θO_2 may be greatly underestimated in reaction experiments because of diffusion resistance within the medium for the reaction. This result strongly suggest diffusion as the predominant process. It should, however, be pointed out that this has only been established for mammalian conditions and may not apply to gas exchange in other vertebrate classes (see Abdalla et al., 1982).

III. Comparative Aspects

Krogh (1910) published a paper on gas exchange in the tortoise, in which he stated the exclusive diffusion-dependence of $DLCO$, and he later published an excellent book on comparative respiratory physiology (Krogh, 1941). Nevertheless, more than half a century would pass between the pioneering studies on diffusing capacity and the early studies on nonmammalian gas exchange organs. Thus, many of these studies are comparatively recent. Selected data for the diffusing capacities of vertebrate gas exchange organs are compiled in Table 1, which also includes information on O_2 uptake and perfusion. The individual vertebrate gas exchangers will be discussed in the following sections.

A. Fish Gills

The gills are the major site of O_2 uptake in fish, although uptake through the skin can not be neglected (see Randall, 1985). As described in Chapter 4, by Laurent, the secondary lamellae are the gas exchange surfaces of the gills, and the smallest gas exchange unit is the space between adjacent lamellae. Moreover, the gills are characterized by countercurrent water and blood flow. These basic arrangements are found both in teleost and elasmobranch fish (Scheid and Piiper, 1976; Piiper and Scheid, 1984).

The diffusing capacity of fish gills is often referred to as the transfer factor, TO_2. Formally, this term may be more correct than DO_2, because, as mentioned, the O_2 uptake of gills and lungs may, to some degree, depend on reaction rates and not exclusively on diffusive transport. A simple approach to the calculation of TO_2 is based on arithmetic mean values for PO_2,

$$TO_2 = \dot{V}O_2 \; / \left[\left(\frac{PI + PE}{2}\right) - \left(\frac{Pa + P\bar{v}}{2}\right) \right]$$

Table 1 Oxygen Uptake, Perfusion, and Diffusing Capacity of Vertebrate Gas Exchangers

	W (kg)	TB (°C)	$\dot{V}O_2$ (ml STPD · kg^{-1} · min^{-1})	$\dot{Q}$ (ml · kg^{-1} · min^{-1})	DO_2 (ml STPD · kg^{-1} · min^{-1} · $torr^{-1}$)	Remarks on determination	Ref.
Selachian larger spotted dogfish *Scyliorhinus stellaris*	2.18[a]	17[a]	0.64[a]	22[a]	0.019[b]	Modified Bohr integration; animal quiescent	[a]Bauman-Schumann and Piiper, 1968 [b]Piiper et al., 1986
Teleost fish trout *Salmo gairdneri*	0.35	10	1.1	–	0.017	Simple equation, Randall et al., 1967	Bath and Eddy, 1979
Amphibian bullfrog *Rana catesbeiana*	0.26	20	0.49	25	0.027	CO rebreathing; conversion assuming $DO_2 = 1.23 \cdot DCO$	Glass et al., 1981b [c]Glass et al., 1981a
Reptile Tegu lizard *Tupinambis teguixin*	1.3–4.1	25	1.2[c]	25	0.032[d]	O_2 rebreathing method, Adaro et al., 1979	[d]Glass and Johansen, 1982
Mammal, nonspecific	1.6	38	8.8[e]	171[c]	1.06[f]	DO_2 corrected to body mass of 1.6 kg	[e]Calculated from allometric equations (Dejours, 1975) [f]Scheid, 1979
Bird, domestic duck *Cairina moschata*	1.8	41	10.3	206	1.27	Calculated from equation by Scheid and Piiper, 1970	Burger et al., 1979

where I denotes inspired; E, expired; a, arterial; and $\bar{v}$ mixed venous blood (Randall et al., 1967). Scheid and Piiper (1976) critically evaluated this simplified approach and recommended application of a theoretically more accurate formula. From studies on the gill function of the larger spotted dogfish, *Scyliorhinus steallaris*, Piiper et al. (1977) calculated TO_2 by both the simple and the alternative formula. The comparison also included a third equation, which was based on the Bohr integration technique (Bohr, 1909) as modified for a countercurrent gas exchanger. Surprisingly, the three different approaches resulted in highly consistent values. This is fortunate, considering that the simple approach had been applied in several studies. According to an analysis by Scheid and Piiper (1976), the error caused by the simple approach is less when the conductances for gill ventilation and perfusion are well matched ($G_{vent} \cong G_{perf}$). Consequently, the consistent values for TO_2 in *Scyliorhinus* indicate a close matching of these conductances. One of the studies on *Scyliorhinus* presents data for the diffusive/perfusive conductance ratio for the branchial O_2 transfer (Piiper et al., 1977). This ratio (G_{diff}/G_{perf}) was 0.8 at rest and 0.6 during moderate exercise, which indicates the presence of a strong diffusion limitation, in particular during exercise (see Chap. 13).

Data for the TO_2 of various species have been compiled and reviewed by Johansen (1982). In most species the values for TO_2 are of the same order of magnitude, but lightly lower, than those for DLO_2 of reptiles of similar body weights and at the same temperature. An extraordinarily high TO_2 is characteristic of one group of teleost fish, the tunas. The skipjack tuna (*Katsuwonus pelamis*) has a very high TO_2 ($0.12 \text{ ml } O_2 \cdot kg^{-1} \cdot min^{-1} \cdot torr^{-1}$), which is considerably larger than for other teleost fish (Stevens, 1972). The high TO_2 of the tuna correlates with a "standard" O_2 uptake two to three times larger than that for most similar-sized fish. This O_2 demand is accompanied by a low tolerance to hypoxia and, consequently, when exposed to hypoxic water, the skipjack tuna will increase swimming speed in an attempt to escape (Gooding et al., 1981).

Values for TO_2 are determined not only by the structure and functional status of the secondary lamellar tissue but also by diffusion within the interlamellar water spaces. The importance of this additional component is that the diffusion coefficient for O_2 is 10^4 times larger in air than in water (see Scheid and Piiper, 1971). The components of the resistance to branchial O_2-transfer have been analyzed in *Scyliorhinus* (Scheid and Piiper, 1971, 1976; Piiper et al., 1986). Within its secondary lamellae, the maximum pathway for diffusion is considerably larger than the thickness of the tissue barrier separating water and blood (Piiper et al., 1986). The combined water and membrane resistance (D_{m+w}) to branchial O_2 transfer in *Scyliorhinus* was estimated (Scheid and Piiper, 1977; Piiper et al., 1986) based on calculations from a model for the diffusion resistance within the interlamellar water (see Scheid and Piiper, 1971) and on morphological data. The recent calculations by Piiper et al. (1986) indicated that diffusion resistance is greater across the water compartment than across the water–blood barrier, in particular when the dogfish was at rest. At rest, the measured values for To_2 were also lower than those estimated for D_{m+w}, whereas $To_2 \cong D_{m+w}$ for alert or swimming fish. As an interesting consequence, this close agreement indicates that nondiffusive components are unimportant during exercise. One of the possible explanations for the better agreement between To_2 and D_{m+w} during activity will be discussed later (see Booth, 1979).

In considering the major role of the interlamellar resistance to diffusion, it seems relevant to mention briefly some recent data concerning the muscular control of the positions of adjacent filaments on a gill arch. These positions are controlled mainly by striated adductor and abductor muscles (see Laurent, 1984), but adrenergically innervated smooth muscles have recently been discovered in the perch, *Perca fluviatilis* (Duval-Erb and Laurent, cited in Laurent, 1984) and also in the cod, *Gadus morhua*, in which activation of this musculature increases the angle between adjacent filaments (Nilsson, 1985). Thus, the mechanisms for adjustment of filament position are more complex than previously believed, and further groups of smooth muscle may be involved (Nilsson, 1985).

An increase in To_2 occurs during exercise as well as during exposure to environmental hypoxia and increase of body temperature (Randall et al., 1967; Johansen, 1982). Mechanisms that may account for such increases have most often been studied in relation to hypoxia. Studying the rainbow trout, *Salmo gairdneri*, Booth (1979) reported that only 58% of the secondary lamellae are perfused at rest under normoxic conditions. This proportion increased to 71% during hypoxia. Such a recruitment of secondary lamellae represents a parallel to pulmonary capillary recruitment in air-breathing vertebrates (see Sect. III.C). As an additional effect of hypoxia the lamellae of the rainbow trout are distended, which results in a larger area for diffusion and a significant decrease of the mean harmonic distance between water and blood (Soivio and Tuurala, 1981). The distension is caused by an increased afferent lamellar pressure during hypoxia (Petterson and Johansen, 1982).

Several studies have focused on the effects of catecholamine release on respiratory functions, in particular during exercise (Butler et al., 1986). Treatment with epinephrine caused a substantial increase in the number of perfused secondary lamellae in the rainbow trout (Booth, 1979), but a recent study reported that repeated burst swimming was required to attain catecholamine levels that could cause significant vascular effects (Butler et al., 1986). By contrast, catecholamines released during spontaneous swimming in the lesser spotted dogfish, *S. canicula*, exert considerable effects on the branchial vasculature (Butler et al., 1986).

A large value for To_2 is not beneficial in all environments that fish may encounter. As pointed out by Bath and Eddy (1979), the gas exchange functions of the gills may conflict with their role in ion exchange. They studied gas exchange and ionic regulation in rainbow trout, which were rapidly transferred from fresh to salt water. This transition temporarily caused a reduction of O_2 uptake to two-thirds of the previous value. Concomitantly, arterial PO_2 decreased from 110 to 80 torr, whereas TO_2 was decreased to 69% of the value in fresh water. This "shut down" could be interpreted as an active regulation, serving to reduce ionic and osmotic stress. As an alternative, also studied by Bath and Eddy, the decrease of TO_2 may result from water losses from the gills to seawater, which causes shrinkage and decrease of the secondary lamellar surfaces.

Strongly reduced branchial O_2-conductance in air-breathing fish may occur under some circumstances. The theoretical possibility exists, that O_2 obtained by air breathing is lost from the skin and the gills when these fish are exposed to anoxic or hypoxic water (see Johansen, 1968). Recently, this aspect was studied in the South American lungfish, *Lepidosiren paradoxa*, which is an obligatory air breather with reduced gills, and in the bichir, *Polypterus sp.*, which possesses well-developed gills and can survive without air breathing when in well-aerated water (Babiker, 1984). When these fish were exposed to near-anoxic water an adequate O_2 uptake was maintained by air breathing, and O_2 losses from the fish to the water were absent or, at least, undetectably small (Lomholt and Glass, 1987). It is not known how this spectacular shut down in achieved. As a possible explanation the functional respiratory surface area may be reduced to a minimum by shunting of blood away from the gills (Johansen, 1968; Fishman et al., 1985; Randall, 1985).

B. Diffusing Capacity of the Amphibian Skin

Cutaneous gas exchange is of variable importance in amphibians and may also occur in aquatic reptiles (Glass and Wood, 1983). Salamanders of the North American family Plethodontidae predominantly depend on skin breathing because lungs or gills are absent (Gatz et al., 1974; Piiper et al., 1976). These lungless salamanders are small, i.e., body weight about 6 g for *Desmognathus fuscus*, and they often inhabit cold mountain streams. Clearly, the implications of size and preferred habitat are a high surface/volume ratio and a low O_2 consumption. These characteristics are understandable on the basis of studies on DO_2 for skin breathing in *D. fuscus* (Piiper et al., 1976). The DO_2 was estimated by various methods including inert gas equilibration, calculation based on O_2 uptake and arterial PO_2, and calculation from morphometric data. These estimates were consistent, although morphometrically calculated DO_2 accounted for the highest value. The values for DO_2 indicated a strong diffusion limitation to the cutaneous O_2 uptake, and a PO_2 gradient of no less than 100 torr occurred between atmospheric air and arterial blood (Piiper et al., 1976).

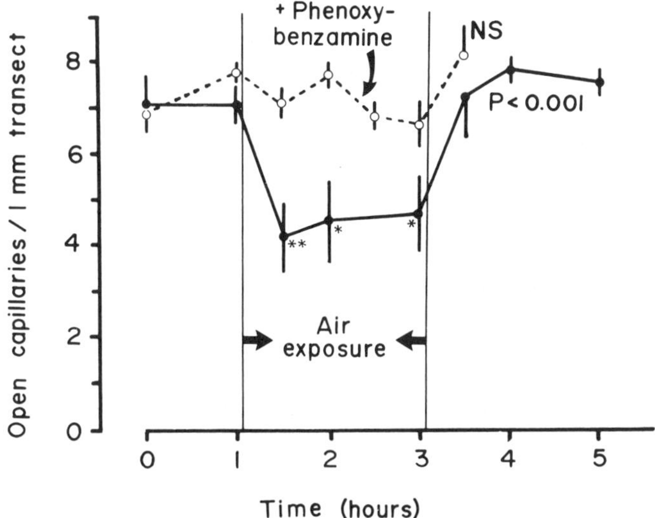

Figure 1 The number of perfused capillaries in the hind foot web of *Rana catesbeiana* decreases during air exposure. This effect is abolished by treatment with phenoxybenzamine, which prevents vasoconstriction of the skin. (After Burggren and Moalli, 1984. Reproduced with permission from *Respiration Physiology*.)

The diffusing capacity for cutaneous gas exchange has also been studied in the bullfrog, *Rana catesbeiana*, in which about 20% of the total O_2 uptake and 80% of the CO_2 elimination depend on skin breathing (Burggren and Moalli, 1984). Jackson (1978) has provided evidence for a predominant diffusion dependence of cutaneous CO_2 elimination in the bullfrog, because measured values for DCO_2 changed little with temperature, as would be expected based on a low Q_{10} for KCO_2. Recently, however, Burggren and Moalli (1984) measured the number of open capillaries in portions of the hind foot web of the bullfrog and found that significantly more were perfused when the bullfrog was in water than when out of water (Fig. 1). The capillary recruitment caused increases in cutaneous blood flow and surface area for gas exchange, and thereby in DO_2. Thus, skin breathing may be more regulated and dependent on perfusion patterns than previously assumed.

The importance of the regulation of perfusion to cutaneous gas exchange is also suggested by other recent studies. For example, Boutilier et al. (1986) measured the distribution of the output from the pulmocutaneous artery, which branches to supply the lung and part of the skin in the bullfrog. The skin received 20% of the pulmocutaneous blood flow during normoxia, whereas blood flow to the skin was strongly reduced during exposure to aquatic hypoxia. Conversely, the perfusion of the skin increased relative to normoxic values, if the intrapulmonary PO_2 was lowered while the water was normoxic.

C. Vertebrate Lungs

The O_2 uptake of an ectothermic vertebrate is only about 20% of the value for a similar-sized mammal or bird when resting (standard) values are compared, and the body temperature of the ectothermic animal is high (see Glass and Wood, 1983). This difference correlates well with the values for pulmonary ventilation and perfusion (Table 1). As an example, the minute ventilation of a resting lizard may increase with temperature but only to reach about 20% of the value for a similar-sized mammal (Glass and Wood, 1983). The different O_2 demand is also reflected on a tissue level. Thus, the mitochondrial volume density and surface area is much larger in a mammal than in a reptile (Else and Hulbert, 1981). Correspondingly, Pough (1980) estimates that the capillary surface area per unit muscle weight of a reptile is about 20% of the value for a mammal of similar body mass.

With this background, it is not surprising when classes are compared that a close correlation is evident between a high O_2 demand and a large D_L. This matching is also evident from morphological estimates of D_L, in which the relatively simple reptilian lung has been compared with the lungs of mammals and birds (see Perry, 1978; and Chap. 7). Thus, the morphological and physiological approaches agree for the general trend, but it should be pointed out, that morphometrically estimated D_{LO_2} values often considerably exceed those obtained for reptiles and mammals by means of physiological methods. As an example, the values obtained differ by a factor of 16 for the turtle *Pseudemys scripta* and the discrepancy may be even wider in mammals (see Perry, 1978). Part of the difference may be due to inhomogeneities such as nonuniform distribution of ventilation, perfusion, and D_L, leading to local mismatching, and cardiovascular shunts could also contribute to the problem (Chap. 13). The apparent values for D_{LO_2} will increase, if inhomogeneities and shunts are reduced and approach "true" values (Piiper, 1969). Consequently, physiological methods may underestimate D_{LO_2}, but it remains, nevertheless, problematic to identify morphological estimates with true values, because calculation of these requires assumptions about the conditions in the live animal (Weibel, 1971). The classes of pulmonary airbreathers will be discussed in the following section.

Amphibians and Reptiles

The simplest amphibian or reptilian lung consists of paired saclike organs, although multicameral lungs are found in some groups of reptiles. The gas exchange surfaces are honeycomblike extensions of the pulmonary wall—the

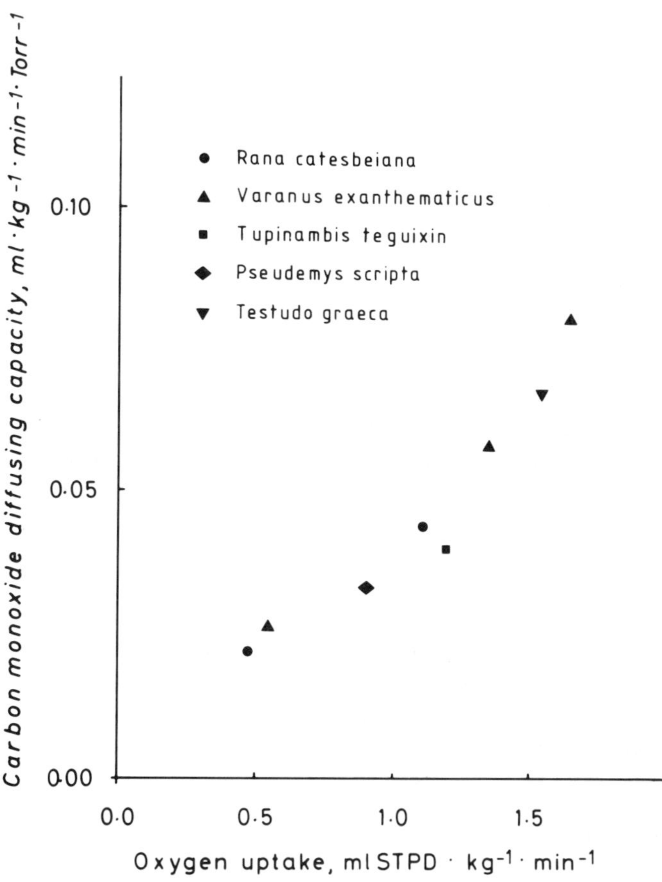

Figure 2 Relationship between DLCO and $\dot{V}O_2$ in ectothermic airbreathers. Note increase of DL with rising temperature. *Pseudemys scripta*, 1.6 kg, and *Testudo graeca*, 1.0 kg, 20–23°C (Crawford et al., 1976). *Tupinambis teguixin*, 2.2 kg, 25–27°C, *Varanus exanthematicus*, 2.2 kg, 18, 26, and 36°C (Glass et al., 1981b). *Rana catesbeiana*, 0.26 kg, 20 and 30°C (Glass et al., 1981a). (Reproduced with permission from *Acta Physiol. Scand.*)

faveoli (Duncker, 1978; Perry, 1978). Several recent studies on the function of these lungs report DLCO or DLO_2, $\dot{V}O_2$, and pulmonary perfusion for reptiles including chelonians and lizards (Crawford et al., 1976; Glass et al., 1981a; Glass and Johansen, 1982; Gatz et al., 1987). In addition, one amphibian, the bullfrog, *Rana catesbeiana*, has been studied (Glass et al., 1981b). The weight-specific values for DLCO of the bullfrog were in the same range as those for reptiles.

A close correlation between DLCO and $\dot{V}O_2$ is evident, when data for amphibians and reptiles are presented, as in Figure 2. Apparently, this relationship implies that DLCO is matched to the species-specific "standard" O_2 uptake, and also that DLCO increases along with $\dot{V}O_2$ as a result of activity or increased body temperature. The effects of activity on DL in reptiles have not been studied, whereas data are available for DL at different temperatures. A Q_{10} value of 2.0 was measured for DLCO of the bullfrog, *R. catesbeiana* (Glass et al., 1981b); Q_{10} = 2.8 was reported for the monitor lizard, *Varanus exanthematicus* (Glass et al., 1981b. A Q_{10} value of as high as 3.0 was measured for DLO_2 in the Tegu lizard, *Tupinambis teguixin* (Glass and Johansen, 1982). These results may seem surprising, considering that the Krogh diffusion constants in aqueous media change only slightly with temperature (Q_{10} for $KO_2 \cong$ 1.1; see Bartels, 1971). Dependence of DL on reaction rates and not exclusively on diffusion could, in part, explain this discrepancy (see Power et al., 1971). The increases of DL values with rising temperature could also result from recruitment of a larger number of pulmonary capillaries (see Forster and Crandall,1976). It should also be pointed out that functional inhomogeneities may cause an underestimation of DLO_2 at low temperature when $\dot{V}O_2$ is reduced (Piiper, 1969).

A simple proportional conversion from DLCO to the physiologically more relevant DLO_2 is problematic. This motivated direct measurements of DLO_2 in the Tegu lizard, *Tupinambis teguixin* (Glass and Johansen, 1982). By comparing those data with values for DLCO in *Tupinambis* (Glass et al., 1981b), a ratio of DLO_2/DLCO $\cong$ 1.6 is suggested. The direct measurement of DLO_2 permitted application of models to quantify diffusion and perfusion limitations to gas transport (see Chap. 13). Such calculations indicated that the pulmonary O_2 uptake of the lizard is limited both by perfusion and by diffusive transport (Glass and Johansen, 1982).

Important to gas transport in amphibians and reptiles are central vascular right-to-left shunts, i.e., part of the systemic venous return is shunted into pulmonary venous blood. Except in crocodilians, the anatomical basis for these shunts is continuity between ventricular chambers (for details see Burggren, 1984; Heisler and Glass, 1984). Systemic venous admixture may greatly decrease PaO_2 and arterial saturation relative to pulmonary venous values. Therefore, the values for PaO_2 may depend more on central-shunting patterns than on pulmonary gas exchange (see Wood, 1984). Very large PA - Pa O_2 gradients (100 torr) may occur in this situation, in particular at low temperature (Fig. 3). In this context Seymour (1978) studied $(PA - Pa)O_2$ in the sea snake, *Laticauda colubrina*. A large PO_2 gradient between alveolar gas and arterial blood persisted despite inspiration of hyperoxic gas mixtures. This indicates that the gradients predominantly result from shunting of systemic venous blood into the arteries.

Clearly, the pulmonary diffusing capacity of a reptile is adequate relative to its gas exchange. This conclusion is of particular interest in the context of a

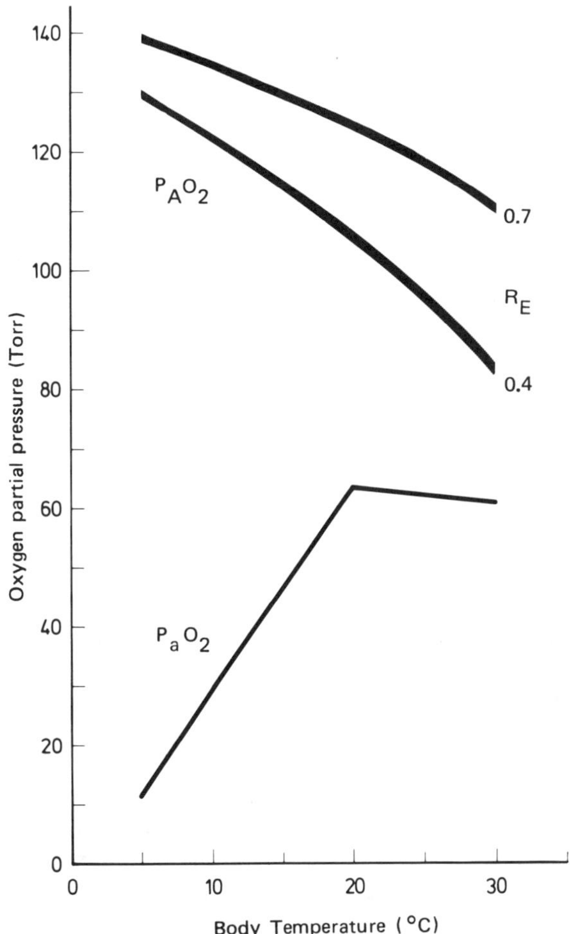

Figure 3 Large PO_2 differences may occur between alveolar gas and arterial blood in reptiles, here the turtle *Chrysemys picta bellii*. Alveolar PO_2 calculated assuming $PACO_2 \cong PaCO_2$. (Based on Glass et al., 1985.)

study on blood plasma filtration in reptiles (Burggren, 1981). As a consequence of the undivided ventricle, the pulmonary arterial blood pressure of a typical reptile is close to the systemic arterial pressures. Thereby, the reptilian lung is often perfused at high pressure relative to values for mammalian lungs (see also Burggren, 1984). Burggren (1981) reported that the net loss of plasma into the lung is an order of magnitude larger than in mammals and suggested that the concept of the lungs as a dry organ may not apply to reptiles.

Mammals

More studies exist for D_L of the alveolar mammalian lung than for any other vertebrate gas exchanger. Therefore, it is only possible to discuss some specific points.

The D_{LO_2} as well as D_{LCO} may increase with exercise in mammals, although usually less than twofold (Stokes et al., 1981; Meyer et al., 1981; Ichinose et al., 1986). Likewise, increases of D_{LCO} occur during exposure to hypoxia or hypercapnia. Recently, Ichinose et al. (1986) studied the separate and combined effects of exercise, hypoxia, and hypercapnia in dogs. Interestingly, the highest values for D_{LCO} (2.5 $ml \cdot kg^{-1} \cdot min^{-1} \cdot torr^{-1}$) exceeded those obtained in earlier studies and were in the same range as the morphometric estimates (Weibel et al., 1983). This is a unique and promising situation for D_L estimates in mammals.

An important question is, whether the increases of D_L are only apparent (see earlier section) or are real. The most unequivocal data concerning this question have been obtained in hypoxia experiments, which indicate that part of the increase is real and can be attributed to pulmonary capillary recruitment (Capen and Wagner, 1982; Ichinose et al., 1986). The exposure of dogs to hypoxia caused an increase of pulmonary vascular resistance with a concomitant redistribution of pulmonary perfusion which, in turn, augmented the surface area for gas exchange resulting from recruitment (Capen and Wagner, 1982).

As evident from other chapters of this book the morphometric estimation of D_L in mammals is often related to allometric considerations. The physiological data for D_{LCO} in mammals are also sufficiently extensive to allow estimation of the dependence on body mass. Takezawa et al. (1980) measured D_{LCO} in mammals ranging from 40 to 4000 g. They calculated a mass exponent of 0.74 both for inter- and intraspecific scaling within the studied mass range. However, Takezawa et al. also analyzed their data in relation to those for larger mammals, and this comparison suggested an interspecies mass exponent of 0.98. This value is highly consistent with an interspecies exponent of 0.95 for the morphometrically measured D_{LO_2} in mammals (Weibel, 1982). The apparently almost linear scaling of D_L with body mass implies that small mammals have a relatively smaller $D_L/\dot{M}O_2$ ratio than larger species. This invites the question of whether or not pulmonary O_2 uptake in mammals can be diffusion limited under certain conditions, in particular for species of small body mass (Weibel, 1982). One of the most frequently studied mammals—man—will be discussed first.

Diffusion limitation is not determined by D_L alone, but by the diffusive/perfusive conductance ratio. $D/\beta\dot{Q}$, where β is the capacitance coefficient and $\dot{Q}$ is the perfusion (see Chap. 13). Therefore, diffusion limitation may develop despite increases of D_L in situations such as exposure to hypoxia. By applying the equation, $G_{diff}/G_{perf} = D/\beta\dot{Q}$, to human gas exchange at rest, Piiper and Scheid (1981) calculated a ratio exceeding 3, which implies a predominant perfusion limitation to pulmonary O_2 uptake. In addition, they analyzed the situation at high altitude, i.e., 5000 m or more. The analysis indicated that diffusion limitation becomes important at these altitudes and even predominant during exercise. These predictions have recently been confirmed in exercise experiments with humans at sea level or at simulated altitudes up to more than 4500 m (Torre-Bueno et al., 1985). Diffusion limitation was absent at sea level and moderate altitude (1500 m), but it became evident at higher altitudes, even during relatively light exercise. A decrease of Pa_{O_2} to values within the steep portion of the O_2 dissociation curve, whereby β increased, contributed to this effect.

As an overall conclusion, extreme conditions are required before diffusion limitation becomes important in humans. The question remains: Is diffusion limitation significant in small mammals? On the basis of morphometrically determined D_{LO_2}, Weibel (1982) calculated that diffusive resistance is insignificant in small mammals at rest. Considering $\dot{V}O_2$ during maximal exercise, however, he estimated that $P_A - P\bar{c})O_2$ may reach 30 torr in a 500-g mammal. Physiologically determined D_{LCO} values for a 500-g mammal are about seven times smaller than those measured morphometrically (compare Takezawa et al., 1980; Gehr et al., 1981). This may suggest that diffusion limitation is important in small exercising mammals.

Birds

The structure and function of the parabronchial avian lung is described in detail in the Chapter 8; for other reviews see Scheid (1979) and Fedde (1986). Some morphological characteristics will briefly be pointed out in the present context. Although the total surface area of the compact avian lung may be smaller than in the mammal (Scheid, 1979), the respiratory surface area per unit volume is considerably larger when comparing species of the same body mass (Abdalla et al., 1982). The increased surface area results from the avian air capillaries, the gas exchange zone surrounding the parabronchi, being much smaller than mammalian alveoli. The diffusion distance from the gas phase to blood is also shorter in the avian lung. Thus, a mean harmonic thickness of only 0.31 μm was measured in the domestic fowl (Abdalla et al., 1982). In addition, physiological measurements indicate that diffusion resistance within air capillaries is negligible (Burger et al., 1979).

Physiological estimates for D_L are available for two species of birds: the domestic fowl, *Gallus gallus* (Piiper et al., 1969; Scheid and Piiper, 1970) and the domestic form of the moscovy duck, *Cairina moschata* (see Burger et al., 1979). It should be emphasized that these are domestic birds and their respiratory surface area is considerably smaller than for free-living species (Scheid, 1979). The value for D_{LCO} measured in the domestic fowl was 0.57 ml · kg^{-1} · min^{-1} · $torr^{-1}$, which is 44% larger than D_{LCO} for a domestic mammal with similar body mass, the white rabbit (Takezawa et al., 1980).

The DLO_2 has repeatedly been assessed in the moscovy duck (Scheid and Piiper, 1970; Scheid et al., 1978; Burger et al., 1979) and was estimated to be 1.3 ml · kg^{-1} · min^{-1} · $torr^{-1}$ when shunts and inhomogeneities were corrected for (see Table 1). This is larger than the mammalian value and, in addition, Scheid and Piiper (1970) pointed out that for an equal overall DLO_2, the parabronchial lung is a more efficient gas exchanger than the alveolar lung. This is due to its crosscurrent arrangement of gas and blood flows (see Chap. 8), which allows PaO_2 to exceed end-parabronchial PO_2. Thus, the arterialization is most efficient in the bird for a given DLO_2 and ventilation. How impressively the avian gas exchange system may perform is documented by high-altitude migrations, such as those of the barheaded geese, *Anser indicus*, which regularly fly over the Himalayan mountains at altitudes exceeding 8800 m. Tolerance of hypoxia was studied in this species, which maintained a PaO_2 of 22 torr with an inspired PO_2 of 23 torr, corresponding to an altitude of 11,580 m (Black and Tenney, 1980).

As emphasized by Piiper et al. (1969) the early values obtained for DL in birds seemed too low to account for the performance during exercise, during which time O_2 uptake may increase 25 times. Moreover, an underestimation is indicated by the hypoxia experiments. It may be pointed out that the early experiments were performed under strenuous experimental conditions. Studying unrestrained and unanesthetized domestic fowl in deep hypoxia. Shams and Scheid (personal communication) recently measured DLO_2 to 3 times larger than the values reported by Burger et al. (1979). This may indicate that DLO_2 was underestimated in earlier studies or, alternatively, that birds possess a large potential for increase of DLO_2. The recent data may solve some problems, but the values for DLO_2 measured by Burger et al. (1979) were in excellent agreement with morphometric calculations (Abdalla et al., 1982) which, consequently, also underestimate DLO_2. As a possible explanation θO_2 values assumed for the bird blood may have been too low, which would lead to an overestimation of the intracapillary resistance to O_2 transport.

IV. General Conclusion

As pointed out by Forster and Crandall (1976), recent studies on DL are abundant, although the scientific novelty of the concept has worn off. It is, however, obviously important to understand a major step in vertebrate gas exchange. In addition, a number of major challenges currently exist in the field. Some of these are (1) to account for the discrepancies between morphological and physiological estimates for DLO_2; (2) to assess the relative importance of diffusion and reaction limitation to O_2 transport in different vertebrate gas exchangers; (3) to account for increases of DLO_2, when O_2 uptake is augmented. A particular problem is to explain increases of DL with rising body temperature.

Recently, progress has been made toward solutions to these questions, but much research is still needed before complete pictures are obtained for the different vertebrate classes.

Acknowledgment

I thank Dr. T. B. Bentley for comments on the manuscript.

References

Abdalla, M. A., Maina, J. N., King, A. S., King, D. Z., and Henry, J. (1982). Morphometrics of the avian lung. 1. The domestic fowl (*Gallus gallus* variant *domesticus*). *Respir. Physiol. 47*:267-278.

Adaro, F., Scheid, P., Teichmann, J., and Piiper, J. (1979). A rebreathing method for estimation of pulmonary DO_2: Theory and measurement in dog lungs. *Respir. Physiol. 18*:43-63.

Babiker, M. M. (1984). Development of dependence on aerial respiration in *Polypterus senegalus* (Cuvier). *Hydrobiologica 110*:351-363.

Bartels, H. (1971). Diffusion coefficients and Krogh's diffusion constants. Diffusion coefficients of gases in water. In *Respiration and Circulation*. Edited by P. L. Altman and D. S. Ditmer. Bethesda, Federation of the American Societies of Experimental Biology, pp. 21-24.

Bath, R. N., and Eddy, F. B. (1979). Ionic and respiratory regulation in rainbow trout during rapid transfer to sea water. *J. Comp. Physiol. 134*:351-357.

Baumgarten-Schumann, D., and Piiper, J. (1968). Gas exchange in the gills of resting unanesthetized dogfish (*Scyliorhinus stellaris*). *Respir. Physiol. 5*: 317-325.

Black, C. P., and Tenney, S. M. (1980). Oxygen transport during progressive hypoxia in high-altitude and sea level water fowl. *Respir. Physiol. 39*:217-239.

Bohr, C. (1909). Über die spezifische Tätigkeit der Lungen bei der respiratorischen Gasaufnahme. *Scand. Arch. Physiol. 22*:221-280.

Booth, J. H. (1979). The effects of oxygen supply, epinephrine and acetylcholine on the distribution of blood flow in trout gills. *J. Exp. Biol. 83*:31-39.

Boutilier, R. G., Glass, M. L., and Heisler, N. (1986). The relative distribution of pulmocutaneous blood flow in *Rana catesbeiana*: Effects of pulmonary or cutaneous hypoxia. *J. Exp. Biol. 126*:33-39.

Burger, R. E., Meyer, M., Graf, W., and Scheid, P. (1979). Gas exchange in the parabronchial lung of birds: Experiments in unidirectional ventilated ducks. *Respir. Physiol. 36*:19-37.

Burggren, W. W. (1982). Pulmonary plasma filtration in a turtle: A wet vertebrate lung? *Science 215*:77-78.

Burggren, W. W. (1985). Hemodynamics and regulation of central cardiovascular shunts in reptiles. In *Cardiovascular Shunts*. Edited by K. Johansen and W. W. Burggren. Alfred Benzon Symposium 21. Copenhagen, Munksgaard, pp. 121-136.

Burggren, W. W., and Moalli, R. (1984). "Active" regulation of cutaneous gas exchange by capillary recruitment in amphibians: Experimental evidence and a revised model for skin respiration. *Respir. Physiol. 55*:379-392.

Butler, P. J., Metcalfe, J. D., and Ginley, S. A. (1986). Plasma catecholamines in the lesser spotted dogfish and the rainbow trout at rest and during different levels of exercise. *J. Exp. Biol. 123*:409-421.

Capen, R. L., and Wagner, W. W., Jr. (1982). Intrapulmonary blood flow redistribution during hypoxia increases gas exchange surface area. *J. Appl. Physiol. 52*:1575-1581.

Crawford, E. C., Jr., Gatz, R. N., Magnussen, H., Perry, S. F., and Piiper, J. (1976). Lung volumes, pulmonary blood flow and carbon monoxide diffusing capacity of turtles. *J. Comp. Physiol. 107*:167-178.

Dejours, P. (1975). *Principles of Comparative Respiratory Physiology*. Amsterdam, New York, Oxford, North-Holland/American Elsevier.

Duncker, H.-R. (1978). General morphological principles of amniotic lungs. In *Respiratory Function in Birds, Adult and Embryonic*. Edited by J. Piiper. Berlin, Heidelberg, New York, Springer-Verlag, pp. 2-15.

Else, P. L., and Hulbert, A. J. (1981). Comparison of the "mammal machine" and the "reptile machine": Energy production. *Am. J. Physiol. 240*: R3-R9.

Fedde, M. R. (1986). Respiration. In *Avian Physiology*, 4th ed. Edited by P. D. Sturkie. New York, Berlin, Heidelberg, Tokyo, Springer-Verlag, pp. 191-220.

Fishman, A. P., DeLaney, R. G., Laurent, P., and Szidon, J. P. (1985). Blood shunting in lungfish and humans. In *Cardiovascular Shunts*. Edited by K. Johansen and W. W. Burggren. Alfred Benzon Symposium 21. Copenhagen, Munksgaard, pp. 88-95.

Forster, R. E., and Crandall, E. D. (1976). Pulmonary gas exchange. *Annu. Rev. Physiol. 38*:69-95.

Gatz, R. N., Crawford, E. C., Jr., and Piiper, J. (1974). Respiratory properties of the blood of a lungless salamander *Desmognathus fuscus*. *Respir. Physiol. 20*:33-41.

Gatz, R. N., Glass, M. L., and Wood, S. C. (1987). Pulmonary function of the green sea turtle, *Chelonia mydas*. *J. Appl. Physiol. 62*:459-463.

Gehr, P., Alwanyi, D. K., Ammann, A., Maloiy, G. M. O., Taylor, C. R., and Weibel, E. R. (1981). Design of the mammalian respiratory system. V. Scaling and morphometric pulmonary diffusing capacity to body mass: Wild and domestic mammals. *Respir. Physiol. 44*:61-86.

Glass, M. L., and Johansen, K. (1982). Pulmonary oxygen diffusing capacity of the lizard *Tupinambis teguixin*. *J. Exp. Zool.* *219*:385-388.

Glass, M. L., and Wood, S. C. (1983). Gas exchange and control of breathing in reptiles. *Physiol. Rev.* *63*:232-261.

Glass, M. L., Abe, A. S., and Johansen, K. (1981a). Pulmonary diffusing capacity in reptiles (relations to temperature and O_2-uptake). *J. Comp. Physiol.* *142*:509-514.

Glass, M. L., Burggren, W. W., and Johansen, K. (1981b). Pulmonary diffusing capacity of the bullfrog (*Rana catesbeiana*). *Acta Physiol. Scand.* *113*: 485-490.

Glass, M. L., Boutilier, R. G., and Heisler, N. (1985). The effects of body temperature on respiration, blood gases and acid-base status in the turtle *Chrysemys picta bellii*. *J. Exp. Biol.* *114*:37-51.

Gooding, R. M., Neill, W. H., and Dizon, A. E. (1981). Respiration rates and low-oxygen tolerance limits in skipjack tuna, *Katsuwonus pelamis*. *Fish. Bull.* *79*:31-48.

Heisler, N., and Glass, M. L. (1985). Mechanisms and regulation of central vascular shunts in reptiles. In *Cardiovascular Shunts*. Edited by K. Johansen and W. W. Burggren. Alfred Benzon Symposium 21. Copenhagen, Munksgaard, pp. 334-354.

Hook, C., and Meyer, M. (1982). Pulmonary blood flow, diffusing capacity and tissue volume by rebreathing: Theory. *Respir. physiol.* *48*:255-279.

Ichinose, Y., Scotto, P., Meyer, M., and Piiper, J. (1986). Pulmonary diffusing capacity for carbon monoxide in awake dogs. *Respiration* *50*:279-285.

Jackson, D. C. (1978). Respiratory control and CO_2 conductance: Temperature effects in a turtle and a frog. *Respir. Physiol.* *33*:103-114.

Johansen, K. (1968). Air-breathing fishes. *Sci. Am.* *219*:102-111.

Johansen, K. (1982). Respiratory gas exchange of vertebrate gills. In *Gills*. Edited by D. F. Houlihan, J. C. Rankin, and T. J. Shuttleworth. Soc. Exp. Biol. Series 16. Cambridge, Cambridge University Press, pp. 99-128.

Krogh, A. (1910). On the mechanism of gas exchange in the lungs. *Scand. Arch. Physiol.* *23*:248-278.

Krogh, A. (1941). *The Comparative Physiology of Respiratory Mechanisms*. Philadelphia, University of Pennsylvania Press.

Krogh, A., and Krogh, M. (1910). Rate of diffusion of CO into lungs of man. *Skand. Arch. Physiol.* *23*:236-247.

Kruhøffer, P. (1954). Studies on the lung diffusion coefficient for carbon monoxide in normal human subjects by means of $C^{14}O$. *Acta Physiol. Scand.* *32*:106-123.

Laurent, P. (1984). Gill internal anatomy. In *Fish Physiology*, Vol. XA. Edited by W. S. Hoar and D. J. Randall. Orlando, Academic Press, pp. 73-183.

Lomholt, J. P., and Glass, M. L. (1987). Gas exchange of air-breathing fishes in near-anoxic water. *Acta Physiol. Scand. 129*:45A.

Meyer, M., Scheid, P., Riepl, G., Wagner, H.-J., and Piiper, J. (1981). Pulmonary diffusing capacities for O_2 and CO measured by a rebreathing technique. *J. Appl. Physiol. 51*:1643-1650.

Nilsson, S. (1985). Filament position in fish gills is influenced by a smooth muscle innervated by adrenergic nerves. *J. Exp. Biol. 118*:433-438.

Perry, S. F. (1978). Quantitative anatomy of the lungs of the red-eared turtle, *Pseudemys scripta elegans. Respir. Physiol. 35*:245-280.

Petterson, K., and Johansen, K. (1982). Hypoxic vasoconstriction and the effects of adrenaline on gas exchange efficiency in fish gills. *J. Exp. Biol. 97*:263-272.

Piiper, J. (1969). Apparent increase of the O_2 diffusing capacity with increased O_2 uptake in inhomogeneous lungs: Theory. *Respir. Physiol. 6*:209-218.

Piiper, J. (1982). A model for evaluating diffusion limitation in gas-exchange organs of vertebrates. In *A Companion to Animal Physiology*. Edited by C. R. Taylor, K. Johansen, and L. Bolis. Cambridge, Cambridge University Press, pp. 49-64.

Piiper, J., and Scheid, P. (1981). Model for capillary-alveolar equilibration with special reference to O_2 uptake in hypoxia. *Respir. Physiol. 46*:193-208.

Piiper, J., and Scheid, P. (1984). Model analysis of gas transfer in fish gills. In *Fish Physiology*, Vol. XA. Edited by W. S. Hoar and D. J. Randall. Orlando, Academic Press, pp. 229-262.

Piiper, J., Pfeifer, K., and Scheid, P. (1969). Carbon monoxide diffusing capacity of the respiratory system in the domestic fowl. *Respir. Physiol. 6*:309-317.

Piiper, J., Gatz, R. N., and Crawford, E. C., Jr. (1976). Gas transport characteristics in an exclusively skin-breathing salamander *Desmognathus fuscus* (Plethodontidae). In *Respiration of Amphibious Vertebrates*. Edited by G. M. Hughes. London, Academic Press, pp. 339-356.

Piiper, J., Meyer, M., Worth, H., and Willmer, H. (1977). Respiration and circulation during swimming activity in the dogfish *Scyliorhinus stellaris. Respir. Physiol. 30*:221-239.

Piiper, J., Scheid, P., Perry, S. F., and Hughes, G. M. (1986). Effective and morphometric oxygen-diffusing capacity of the gills of the elasmobranch *Scyliorhinus stellaris. J. Exp. Biol. 123*:27-41.

Pough, F. H. (1980). Blood oxygen transport and delivery in reptiles. *Am. Zool. 20*:173-185.

Power, G. G., Aoki, V. S., Lawson, W. H., Jr., and Gregg, J. B. (1971). Diffusion characteristics of pulmonary blood-gas barrier at low temperatures. *J. Appl. Physiol. 31*:438-446.

Randall, D. (1985). Shunts in fish gills. In *Cardiovascular Shunts.* Edited by K. Johansen and W. W. Burggren. Alfred Benzon Symposium 21, Copenhagen, Munksgaard, pp. 71-82.

Randall, D. J., Baumgarten, D., and Malyusz, M. (1972). The relationships between gas and ion transfer across the gills of fishes. *Comp. Biochem. Physiol. 41A*:629-637.

Randall, D. J., Holeton, G. F., and Stevens, E. D. (1967). The exchange of oxygen and carbon dioxide across the gills of rainbow trout. *J. Exp. Biol. 6*:339-348.

Roughton, F. J. W., and Forster, R. E. (1957). Relative importance of diffusion and chemical rates in determining rate of exchange of gases in the human lung, with special reference to true diffusing capacity of the pulmonary membrane and volume of blood in lung capillaries. *J. Appl. Physiol. 11*: 290-302.

Scheid, P. (1979). Mechanisms of gas exchange in bird lungs. *Rev. Physiol. Biochem. Pharmacol. 86*:137-186.

Scheid, P. (1982). Diffusion in gas exchange of vertebrates. In *Exogenous and Endogenous Influences on Metabolic and Neural Control.* Edited by A. D. F. Addink and N. Spronk. Oxford, New York, Pergamon Press, pp. 115-125.

Scheid, P., and Piiper, J. (1970). Analysis of gas exchange in the avian lung: Theory and experiments in the domestic fowl. *Respir. Physiol. 9*:246-262.

Scheid, P., and Piiper, J. (1971). Theoretical analysis of respiratory gas equilibration in water passing through fish gills. *Respir. Physiol. 13*:305-318.

Scheid, P., and Piiper, J. (1976). Quantitative functional analysis of branchial gas transfer: Theory and application to *Scyliorhinus stellaris* (Elasmobranchii). In *Respiration of Amphibious Vertebrates.* Edited by G. M. Hughes. London, New York, Academic Press, pp. 17-38.

Scheid, P., Burger, R. E., Meyer, M., and Graf, W. (1978). Diffusion in avian pulmonary gas exchange: Role of diffusion resistance of the blood-gas barrier and the air capillaries. In *Respiratory Function in Birds, Adult and Embryonic.* Edited by J. Piiper. Berlin, Heidelberg, New York, Springer-Verlag, pp. 136-141.

Seymour, R. S. (1978). Gas tensions and blood distribution in sea snakes at surface pressure and at stimulated depth. *Physiol. Zool. 51*:388-407.

Soivio, A., and Tuurala, H. (1981). Structural and circulatory responses to hypoxia in the secondary lamellae of *Salmo gairdneri* gills at two temperatures. *J. Comp. Physiol. 145*:37-43.

Stevens, E. D. (1972). Some aspects of gas exchange in tuna. *J. Exp. Biol. 56*: 809-823.

Stokes, D. L., MacIntyre, N. R., and Nadel, J. A. (1981). Nonlinear increases in diffusing capacity during exercise by seated and supine subjects. *J. Appl. Physiol. 51*:858-863.

Takezawa, J., Miller, F. J., and O'Neill, J. J. (1980). Single-breath diffusing capacity and lung volumes in small laboratory mammals. *J. Appl. Physiol. 48*:1052-1059.

Torre-Bueno, J. R., Wagner, P. D., Saltzman, H. A., Gale, G. E., and Moon, R. E. (1985). Diffusion limitation in normal humans during exercise at sea level and at simulated altitude. *J. Appl. Physiol. 58*:989-995.

Weibel, E. R. (1970/71). Morphometric estimation of pulmonary diffusing capacity. I. Model and method. *Respir. Physiol. 11*:54-75.

Weibel, E. R. (1982). The pathway for oxygen: Lung to mitochondria. In *A Companion to Animal Physiology.* Edited by C. R. Taylor, K. Johansen, and L. Bolis. Cambridge, Cambridge University Press, pp. 31-48.

Weibel, E. R., Taylor, C. R., O'Neil, J. J., Leith, D. E., Gehr, P., Hoppeler, H., Langman, V., and Baudinette, R. V. (1983). Maximal oxygen consumption and pulmonary diffusing capacity: A direct comparison of physiologic and morphometric measurements in canids. *Respir. Physiol. 54*:173-188.

Wood, S. C. (1984). Cardiovascular shunts and oxygen transport in lower vertebrates. *Am. J. Physiol. 16*:3-14.

Yamaguchi, K., Nguyen-Phu, D., Scheid, P., and Piiper, J. (1985). Kinetics of O_2 uptake and release by human erythrocytes studied by a stopped-flow technique. *J. Appl. Physiol. 58*:1215-1224.

15

Carbon Dioxide Homeostasis

FRED N. WHITE

Scripps Institution of Oceanography
University of California at San Diego
La Jolla, California

I. Introduction

Carbon dioxide is a ubiquitous product of oxidative metabolism which, by virtue of its interaction with water, produces carbonic acid, bicarbonate ions, and protons. Of these products, protons exert profound effects on numerous biochemical reactions, either stimulating, slowing, or blocking them (White and Somero, 1982). The defense of a constant pH, by respiratory control or renal compensation, is a central theme of mammalian acid-base regulation and human therapeutics. There is some sense of urgency concerning acid-base balance and, hence, CO_2 regulation, in the famous monograph of Peters and Van Slyke (1931): "During more than a half century it has been recognized that for the maintenance in the organism of a state compatible with life the reaction of the inner fluids must be slightly to the alkaline side of the neutral point, and that

Part of the work discussed in this chapter was supported by National Institutes of Health Grant HL 17731 and National Science Foundation Grant PCM 8204545.

much deviation from this physiological reaction is disastrous." The role of CO_2 as a respiratory stimulant is closely tied to the maintenance of a balance between CO_2 production and excretion, with the net effect of a stable reaction (pH) which is "slightly to the alkaline side of the neutral point."

Peters and Van Slyke were speaking about acid-base and CO_2 regulations in humans where the conditions surrounding regulations are thermally clamped around 37°C. Unlike most mammals, ectothermic vertebrates exist in media (air, water) which differ in physical and chemical characteristics. Organs of gas exchange (gills, lungs) differ in structure, and changing thermal conditions of the environment may produce large variations in body temperature, metabolism, solubility of gases, and shifts in positions of both O_2 and CO_2 dissociation curves. Although the paleontological record provides evidence for the taxonomic pathways leading from aquatic to terrestrial transitions and to mammals and birds, we must look to contemporary lower vertebrates for clues to the functional pathways that accompanied vertebrate evolution. An important element in the radiation of vertebrates has been the development of mechanisms that served the need of O_2 acquisition to fuel the metabolic fire while, at the same time, coping with the "smoke" of that fire, carbon dioxide.

II. The Pathway from Water to Air Breathing

The pioneers that transcended the interface between water and air were fish. The fossil record suggests that the pathway leading to primitive amphibians originated from sarcopterygian stock through crossopterygians. Present day lung fishes represent a continuum of a side branch of the line leading to amphibians and, thus, may offer the only extant clues to those early transitions that led to the adoption of lung breathing by early amphibians.

The transitional forms leading to reptiles are possibly represented by the seymouriamorphs, reptilelike amphibians of the Permian period. Romer (1972) contended that the presence of a well-developed rib cage and dermal scales in these animals indicates that they exhibited near or complete dependence on the lung for total gas exchange. No contemporary amphibian meets this condition because modern forms are highly dependent on cutaneous gas exchange, especially for CO_2 excretion. Among extant ectotherms, it is only among reptiles that complete dependence on lungs for both O_2 and CO_2 exchange is observed.

A. Similarities and Differences in Gas Exchange: Lungfish, Amphibians, Reptiles

The patterns of ventilation and perfusion of the gas exchanger of lower vertebrates have a profound influence on the temporal fluxes of the respiratory gases. Additionally, when extrapulmonary gas exchange (skin, gills) is involved, differential fluxes of the respiratory gases across these routes may occur.

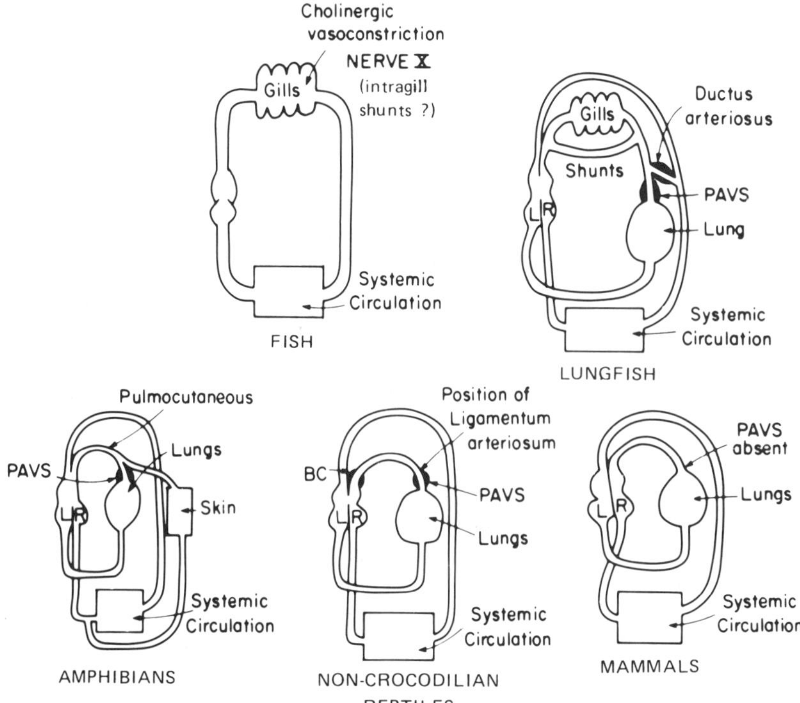

Figure 1 Occurrence of a cholinergic vasoconstrictor system (nerve 10) innervating the gas exchanger. For lungfish, amphibians, and noncrocodilian reptiles, the innervation supplies the afferent vascular supply to the lungs (PAVS; pulmonary arterial vasoconstrictor segment). The bulbus chordis (BC) may also contract under vagal cholinergic influence. Contraction of PAVS increases pulmonary arterial resistance and may cause redistribution of venous blood (shunt).

The pattern of ventilation in the lungfish (*Protopterus*), lunged amphibians, and most reptiles is periodic, several breaths being followed by breath-holding periods of variable lengths. During ventilation, heart rate and pulmonary blood flow are elevated relative to the breath-holding period (Johansen, 1972, 1984; Shelton and Boutilier, 1982; White, 1976). The reduction of pulmonary blood flow during breath holding has been ascribed to a fall in the ratio of systemic to pulmonary vascular resistance. The presence of an incompletely divided ventricle (except in crocodilians), results in right-to-left intracardiac shunting owing to the rise in pulmonary vascular resistance. There persists in all of these groups a cholinergic vasoconstrictor innervation of the pulmonary artery (Fig. 1). In *Protopterus* the pulmonary arterial vasoconstrictor area originates near the junction of the patent ductus arteriosus (Fishman et al., 1984). The situation is similar in amphibians and reptiles, the constrictor zone commencing near the hilus of the lung immediately distal to the ductus remnant (ligamentum arteriosum). This cholinergic vasoconstrictor system may be considered as a long-standing homologue among these phylogenetically distinct groups.

Amphibians and reptiles maintain a low respiratory exchange ratio in the lung gas during breath holding. All contemporary lunged amphibians exhibit bimodal respiration, exchanging gas across both the lungs and skin. Dependency on these avenues for O_2 and CO_2 exchange is not evenly distributed, the R values of the skin system being uniformly high, whereas those for pulmonary exchange are low. Low pulmonary R values have been attributed to cutaneous CO_2 exchange in amphibians (Shelton and Boutilier, 1982). However, in the turtle, *Psuedemys scripta*, the low R of breath hold is followed by recovery of the expected R during the brief ventilatory periods that occupy about 15% of the breathing cycle time. This "bursting" of CO_2 across the blood–lung interface has been called cyclic CO_2 exchange (Ackerman and White, 1979). According to Rahn and Howell (1976): "It is the handling of carbon dioxide by the lung system that appears to have been the greatest obstacle in the transition from water-breathing to the modern lung, which is first encountered in our present-day reptiles." This assessment can be recast for the necessity of modern amphibians, which Romer (1972) considered to be degenerate and specialized, to remain tied to high humidity or aqueous environments to conserve water losses across the skin. Arid environments, occupied by many reptiles, require the presence of a water-conserving integument that is ill adapted to gas exchange. Exploitation of the terrestrial environment, in one sense, shifted the burden of O_2 acquisition and CO_2 elimination to the lung.

B. Breathing Air and Water: Influences on Carbon Dioxide Homeostasis

The physical and chemical properties of air and water offer differing challenges to animals that depend on these media for gas exchange. Fish gills, a flow-through system, are grossly overventilated in comparison with lung breathers. The water convection requirement (liters of water ventilated per millimole O_2 consumed) is much greater than the air convection requirement of lung breathers.

A high water flow rate is required to support the metabolism because of the relatively low concentration of O_2 in water compared with air. The concentration of a gas, C_g, is the product of the partial pressure, P_g, and the capacitance coefficient, β_g, where β is defined as the increment in C_g per increment in P_g. At 20°C, β_{water}, is 1.8×10^{-3} mmol $\cdot$ L^{-1} $\cdot$ $torr^{-1}$, whereas β_{air} is 5.47×10^{-2}, an approximately 30-fold difference. Thus, water equilibrated with air contains one-thirtieth the amount of O_2 as an equivalent volume of air. At this temperature βCO_2 is similar for both media. Higher affinity hemoglobin in fishes and countercurrent circulation in the gills appear to be mechanisms for improving O_2 extraction from water. Yet, water convection requirements appear to exceed air convection requirements for lung breathers by around 15 times (Dejours et al., 1970; Dejours, 1972). This high water convection requirement coupled with high relative gill blood flow results in near equilibrium of CO_2 in blood and water. Gill-breathing fish typically exhibit an arterial P_{CO_2} of only a few torr. The nature of gill ventilation, high H_2O flow requirements to support oxidative metabolism, and the low range of P_{CO_2} in blood combine to make alterations in gill ventilation an ineffective method of regulating the acid-base state. Consequently, fish faced with requirements to regulate acid-base condition, as during temperature transients, rely on active transport of ions which ultimately institute pH corrections via alterations in $[HCO_3^-]$. In contrast, lung breathers, by adjusting the ventilation/CO_2 production ratio, are equipped with a mechanism for rapidly responding to conditions that would otherwise compromise acid-base balance.

III. Carbon Dioxide and Acid-Base Homeostasis

Ectothermic animals may experience a wide range of body temperatures on daily or seasonal time scales. Although we think of humans, and other endotherms, as essentially temperature stable, this is not strictly true. The tissues of exercising humans, or humans in the cold, may exhibit considerable thermal heterogeneity. If we consider that the arterialized blood entering the arterial tree is at a constant CO_2 content, at say 37°C, this content will remain unchanged as blood enters the small arterial and precapillary system of a warmer tissue (exercising muscle) or one that is cool (skin in the cold). Thus, regional blood temperature is subject to change. This thermal instability has an important impact on P_{CO_2} and pH of the blood, which fact can be appreciated when a sample of blood is kept air-tight (at constant CO_2 content) while the P_{CO_2} and pH are measured at various temperatures (Fig. 2). As Rosenthal (1948) noted, in vitro blood exhibits a direct relationship between temperature and P_{CO_2}, whereas the pH is altered at -0.0147 units/°C. The slope of the pH change is essentially parallel to the neutral pH of water (pNH_2O). One can conclude that the criterion of a blood reaction "slightly to the alkaline side of the neutral point," which was emphasized by Peters and Van Slyke (1931) for 37°C is, in fact, manifest by blood of constant CO_2 content at differing temperatures because a constant alkalinity relative to neutral water is maintained. Albery and Lloyd (1967) postulated that this behavior must be attributable to a dominant protein buffer, the pK of which must resemble that of neutral water. He specified for this buffer a pK near 7 and a heat of enthalpy of 7 kcal/mol. Reeves (1972), in searching for this buffer

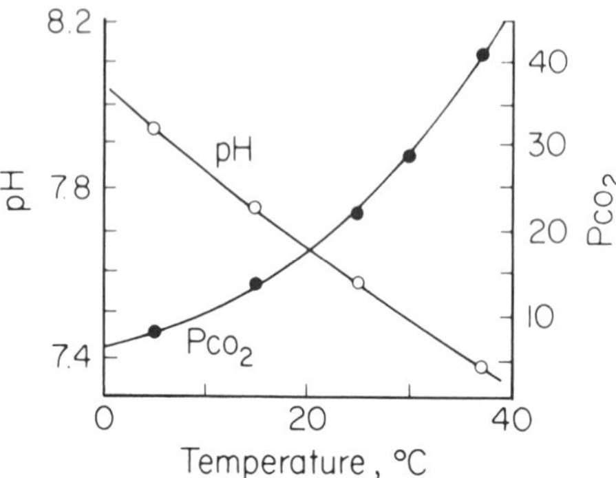

Figure 2 Behavior of in vitro blood at constant CO_2 content as a function of temperature. (Based on Rosenthal, 1948. Reprinted from White, F. N. In *Pediatric Cardiology*, Vol. 6. Edited by C. Marcelletti, R. Anderson, A. Becker, A. Carno, D. diCarlo and E. Mazzera. Edinburgh, Churchill Livingstone, 1986, with permission of the publisher.)

system, has identified the peptide-linked histidyl imidazole group as the only component that appears in sufficient concentration and that has an appropriate pK. He further demonstrated that the addition of imidazole to simple aqueous solutions would result in a pH-temperature relationship characteristic of blood when the CO_2 content was held constant. This system results in an invariable fraction of total histidine imidazoles in the unprotonated form, i.e., the ratio of unprotonated to protonated imidazole moieties (α) remains constant. Reeves (1972) has called this alphastat regulation, a condition resulting in stability of the net protein charge.

Studies of the effect of acclimation temperature on the arterial pH of a fish (Randall and Cameron, 1973), frogs, turtles (Howell et al., 1970; Jackson et al., 1974; Kinney et al.,1977), and alligators (Davies et al., 1982) have revealed that these animals, although in vivo open systems, exchanging gases with the environment, exhibit arterial ΔpHs that closely resemble those of in vitro blood held at a constant CO_2 content.

The similarity among many vertebrates in their maintenance of an "alphastat" pattern of acid-base regulation has important implications for the biochemical integrity of the organism (White and Somero, 1982; Somero and White, 1985) and the electrical stability of the hypothermic mammalian heart (Swain et al., 1984; Kroncke et al., 1986). The regulation of a constant CO_2 level in the organism through ventilatory control is a prerequisite for alphastat regulation in lung-breathing vertebrates.

IV. Cardiopulmonary Regulation of Carbon Dioxide by Lung-Breathing Vertebrates

Studies of the effect of body temperature on ventilation in several species of reptiles (alligators: Davies et al., 1982; turtles: Jackson et al., 1974; Kinney et al., 1977) indicate that the air convection requirement (ACR = liters of gas ven-

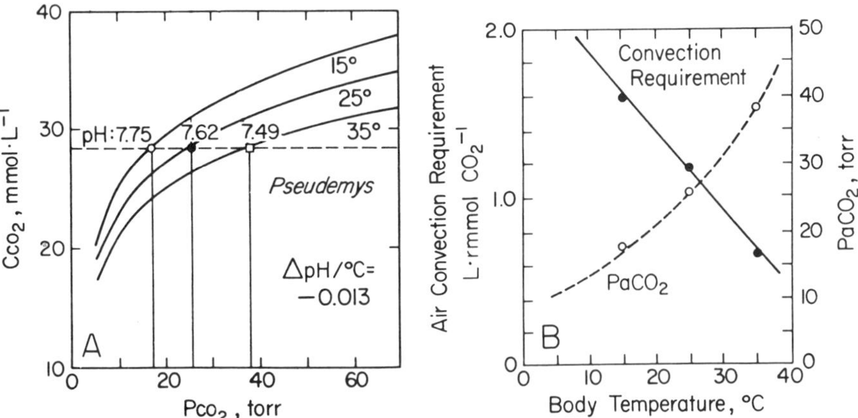

Figure 3 The inverse relationship between air convection requirement and body temperature in a turtle is responsible for the direct relationship of $PaCO_2$ and temperature (panel B). When the observed $PaCO_2$s are related to the oxygenated CO_2 dissociation curve, an essentially constant CO_2 content, at various temperatures, is observed (dashed line). The resultant ΔpH/°C is similar to that observed in in vitro blood (see Fig. 2). (Based on Kinney et al., 1977; CO_2 dissociation curves based on Weinstein et al., 1986.)

tilated per millimole O_2 or CO_2 consumed or produced) varies inversely with body temperature. This pattern of relative underventilation at higher temperatures and metabolic rates seems paradoxical in comparison with the mammalian pattern of pacing ventilation in proportion to O_2 consumption during exercise, i.e., the ACR remains stable within a broad range of metabolic demands. However, ACR remains stable in turtles at various levels of metabolism *at a given body temperature* (Jackson, 1971). There is a specific ACR for each temperature.

The effect of this temperature-ventilation pattern is exemplified in Figure 3B for the turtle, in which ACR is related to body temperature and arterial PCO_2. These findings indicate that the relative hypoventilation associated with higher temperatures is responsible for the direct relationship of $PaCO_2$ to temperature. This pattern resembles that of in vitro blood at constant CO_2 content. When the observed PCO_2s are related to the oxygenated CO_2 dissociation curve, it is seen that an essentially constant CO_2 content prevails (Fig. 3A). A ΔpH/°C of -0.013 is not far removed from that expected for alphastat regulation.

A comparison of distantly related ectothermic and endothermic species at common body temperature points out fundamental similarities in the respiratory poise of air-breathing vertebrates for CO_2 homeostasis (White and Bickler, 1987). Figure 4A displays data relating air convection requirements and associ-

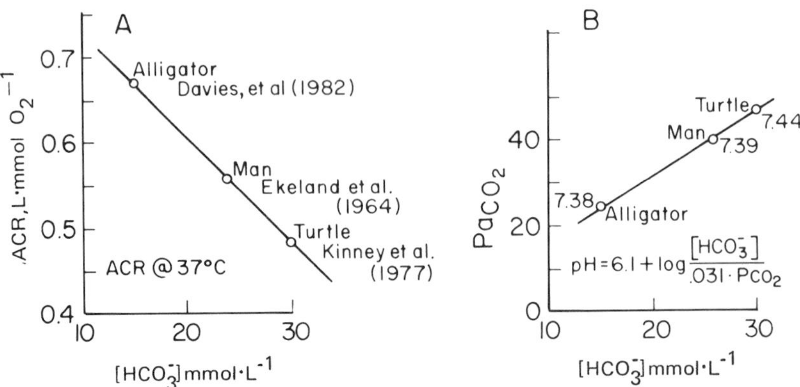

Figure 4 (A) Relationship of air convection requirement to blood $[HCO_3^-]$s in three vertebrate species. All values are adjusted to 37°C. (B) Relationship of arterial PCO_2 to blood $[HCO_3^-]$s. The corresponding arterial pH values, calculated at 37°C from the Henderson-Hasselbach relationship, are shown. (Reprinted from White, F. N. and Bickler, P. E., *Am. Zool. 27*:31–39, 1987, with permission of the Am. Soc. of Zoologists.)

ated arterial $[HCO_3^-]$s for turtle, alligator, and humans, all at 37°C. The graph simply says that the species possessing high $[HCO_3^-]$s have lower ACRs. Because lower ACR represents a relative hypoventilation we can anticipate that animals characterized by low ACR will exhibit higher PCO_2s in arterialized blood. Figure 4B displays an interspecific PCO_2-$[HCO_3^-]$ diagram for the comparison species along with the calculated pHs. Convergence among these species at similar pHs indicates that each animal adjusts respiratory intensity such that the PCO_2-$[HCO_3^-]$ relationship results in a similar pH. Such a finding has regulatory implications that conceivably place regulation of O_2 transport in conflict with the regulation of CO_2 and raises the question: In what manner do the components of cardiorespiratory gas exchange interact to achieve effective gas transport of both O_2 and CO_2 as an ectothermic lung breather experiences a wide range of body temperatures, metabolic intensity, ventilatory and perfusive requirements, and thermally induced alterations in blood gas transport properties (shifts in O_2 and CO_2 dissociation curves)?

Figure 5 displays the components of cardiopulmonary gas exchange for a vertebrate lung, the so-called ventilated pool system (Piiper and Scheid, 1977). Two convective components (ventilation, perfusion) are separated by a diffusion barrier. The convective processes are displayed through an expanded form of the Fick equation. For the convective processes, the equation incorporates gas flux ($\dot{M}$), a flow ($\dot{V}$), the capacitance coefficient β, for the gas in question, and the gas partial pressure differences across the component process (PiO_2–PeO_2

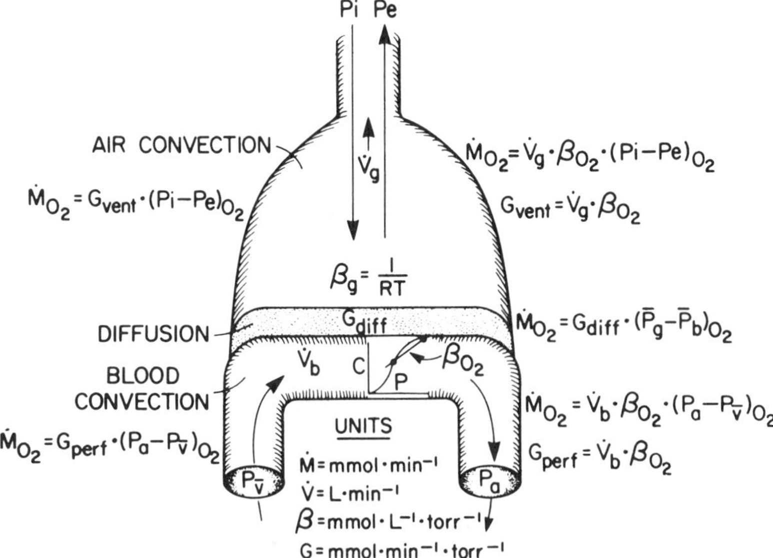

Figure 5 Pulmonary gas exchange model showing the serial relationships between ventilation, diffusion, and perfusion. Expansion of the Fick equation allows the recognition of conductances (G values) for the processes of exchange for each gas. The total conductance for the system is defined as the ratio of gas consumption to the greatest partial pressure difference across the system, i.e., $G_{tot}, O_2 = \dot{M}O_2/(P_i - P_v)O_2$. (Reprinted from White, F. N., and Bickler, P. E., *Am. Zool. 27*:31-39, 1987, with permission of the American Society of Zoologists.)

for ventilation; $PaO_2 - PvO_2$ for perfusion). It should be noted that β is the same value (1/RT) for both gases in the gas phase, whereas for β in blood, β is derived from the slopes of lines connecting arterial and venous points for O_2 and CO_2 referenced to the respective dissociation curves with due consideration of both Bohr and Haldane effects. The product of $\dot{V}$ and β for a gas has the property of a conductance ($G = \dot{V} \cdot \beta$). Although ventilatory conductance (G_{vent}) is the same for both O_2 and CO_2, the perfusive conductances (G_{perf}) for the two gases are expected to differ widely owing to large differences in β values. The total conductance across the system is the ratio of $\dot{M}_{gas}$ to the maximum partial pressure differences across the gas exchanger, thus,

$$G_{tot}\ O_2 = \dot{M}O_2/(P_i - P_v)O_2;\ G_{tot}\ CO_2 = \dot{M}CO_2/(P_v - P_i)CO_2$$

For the ventilated pool model the arrangement of the components of gas exchange (ventilation, diffusion, perfusion) may be considered to be an "in series"

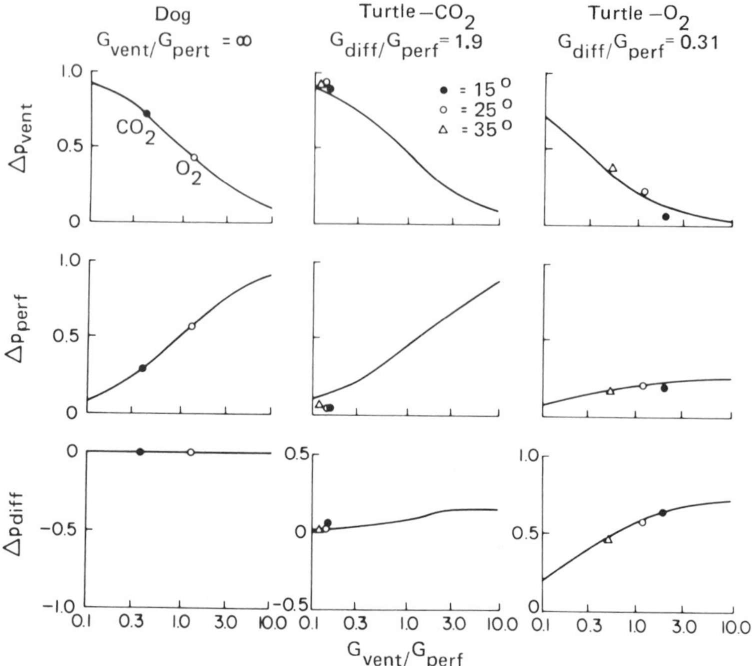

Figure 6 Relative resistances (Δp values) as functions of G_{vent}/G_{perf} for O_2 and CO_2. Solid curves are theoretical values. Data points for turtle are based on experimental values. Note the tight grouping of points related to CO_2 exchange. Data for the dog are derived from G_{vent}/G_{perf} values which are referenced to theoretical curves (dog values based on Aoyagi et al., 1965). (Reprinted from White, F. N., and Bickler, P. E., *Am. Zool.* 27:31–39, 1987, with permission of the American Society of Zoologists.)

system, analagous to an electrical circuit. Thus, resistances attributable to the component processes may be appreciated from knowledge of conductances: $1/G_{tot} = 1/G_{vent} + 1/G_{diff} + 1/G_{perf}$. Of the conductances (or, resistances) G_{tot}, G_{vent}, and G_{perf} are subject to measurement. Knowledge of these values allows calculation of G_{diff}, although it is important to realize that calculated values of G_{diff} may be influenced by factors that are not strictly diffusive (ventilation-perfusion inequalities, shunt). From such assessments of resistance distributions a relative resistance for each process may be assigned (fraction of the total resistance attributable to the process).

The $\dot{V}/\dot{Q}$ concept of mammalian physiology is inappropriate when making comparisons of transport of gases that differ greatly in β values (O_2 and CO_2 in

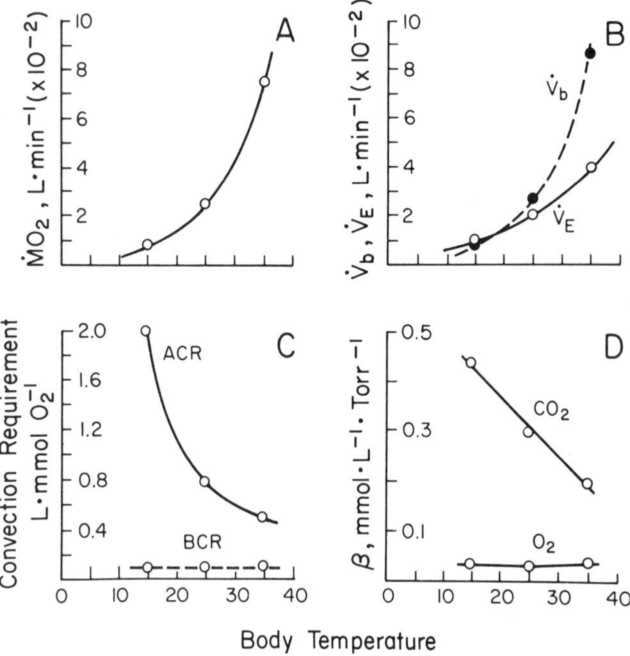

Figure 7 Gas exchange parameters as functions of body temperature in the turtle. $\dot{V}b$ = pulmonary blood flow; $\dot{V}E$ = ventilation; ACR = air convection requirement; BCR = blood convection requirement; β = blood capacitance coefficient. (Data from White and Bickler, 1987.)

blood). Due consideration of these differences in transport characteristics is incorporated in G_{vent}/G_{perf} values. The G_{vent}/G_{perf} values, for differing body temperatures may be related to relative resistances of the processes of gas exchange to gain a picture of how the gas exchange system is poised in regard to both O_2 and CO_2 transport. At any given G_{perf}/G_{diff} value for a gas, theoretical curves, based on equations developed by Piiper and Scheid (1977), may be constructed where relative resistances of the processes of gas exchange are plotted as functions of G_{vent}/G_{perf} values. In Figure 6 the solid lines are theoretical curves based on G_{perf}/G_{diff} values derived from data of White and Bickler (1987). At the three temperatures studied, G_{perf}/G_{diff} values for O_2 and CO_2 varied little and their mean values are utilized for heuristic reasons. The data points shown are derived from experimental studies, and relative resistances for the processes are calculated from the assumption that the reciprocal of the total conductance of a gas is equal to the sum of the reciprocals of the individual conductances, i.e., the data points exhibited are derived independently from the theoretically determined curves. These points exhibit a generally strong correlation with the theoretical curves. Of special interest is the close clustering, at all temperatures, of G_{vent}/G_{perf} and relative resistances for CO_2, i.e., these values appear to be essentially fixed across a range of temperature, metabolism, and shifts in positions of the dissociation curves. Essential to this finding is the marked decline in β values for CO_2 with increasing temperature, a relatively constant blood convection requirement, and an inverse relationship between air convection requirement and body temperature. The trends are shown in Figure 7. In great contrast to CO_2, the blood β values for O_2 are uniformly low and stable. Primarily because of a shift to the right of the O_2 dissociation curve and the fall in ACR with rising BT, at temperatures above approximately 30°C, there was a large fall in hemoglobin (Hb) saturation of arterial blood, due to underventilation as reflected in the trend of G_{vent}/G_{perf} for O_2 (see Fig. 6). Due to stability of G_{vent}/G_{perf} for CO_2, the CO_2 content of blood was maintained at an essentially constant level across the temperature range.

Is there an optimal overall $\dot{V}/\dot{Q}$ for this animal? For CO_2 the answer is clearly, no. However, there are optimal $\dot{V}/\dot{Q}$s for CO_2 *at each BT*, i.e., those $\dot{V}/\dot{Q}$s that correlate with the observed constant G_{vent}/G_{perf} of about 0.15 (Fig. 8). The result is near constancy in CO_2 content of the organism. For O_2 transport, a $\dot{V}/\dot{Q}$of 0.7 correlates with the preferred temperature of the animal, 29°C (Brattstrom, 1965). Below this temperature Hb saturation remains in a narrow zone of 90 to 95% saturated and the continual rise in $\dot{V}/\dot{Q}$ does little to alter O_2 content of arterial blood. However, the decline in $\dot{V}/\dot{Q}$ at higher temperatures is associated with plummeting Hb saturation values. In other words, above 29°C the lungs are underventilated insofar as O_2 transport is concerned; below this temperature the lungs are progressively overventilated. If an ideal $\dot{V}/\dot{Q}$ exists for O_2 transport, it is the ratio (~ 0.7) that is found at 29°C, the behaviorally regulated "preferred" temperature. The G_{vent}/G_{perf} O_2 of 1, at this temperature, represents an exact matching of ventilatory and perfusive conductances. All $\dot{V}/\dot{Q}$s above or below that at 29°C are "nonideal" insofar as O_2 transport is concerned; however, each is "ideal" for CO_2 transport if maintenance of a constant CO_2 content of the organism is considered a regulatory "goal."

Correlates of gas transport properties with ventilatory level strongly suggest that CO_2 is the controlled variable. Figure 9A displays data relating observed mean ventilation levels and G_{perf} CO_2 at various temperatures. The G_{perf} $CO_2/\dot{V}_E$ is narrowly constrained in the range of 0.37 to 0.42. No close relationship was found between G_{perf} O_2 and $\dot{V}_E$. Figure 9B illustrates the relationship between air convection requirement and blood βCO_2 at the three temperatures studied. Here a constant β/ACR of 0.3 is observed, whereas a 2.2-fold increase in β between 35 and 15°C is associated with a 2.28-fold increase in ACR. Although these correlations between blood transport properties of CO_2 and ventilatory parameters are suggestive of variables that influence ventilation, experimental linkage with the receptor systems controlling ventilation are

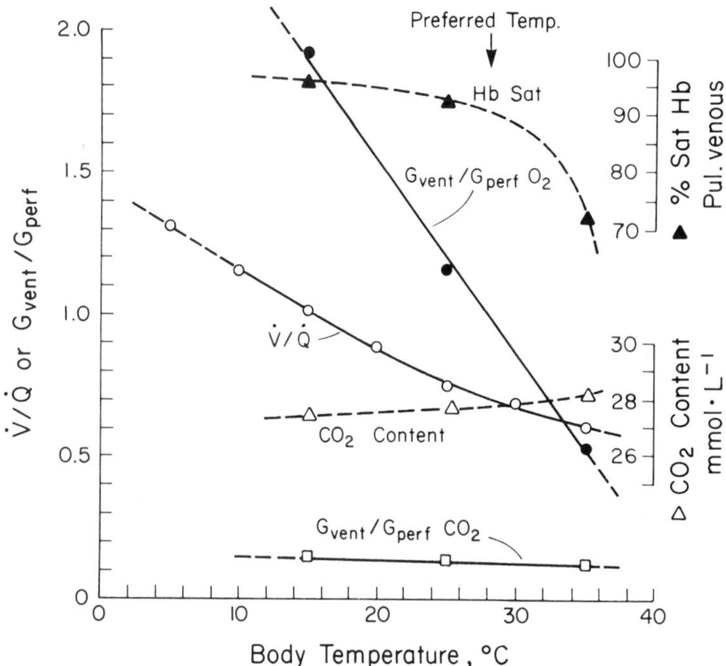

Figure 8 Relationship of body temperature of the turtle to overall ventilation/perfusion ratio ($\dot{V}/\dot{Q}$) and to the ventilation/perfusion conductance ratios for the two gases (G_{vent}/G_{perf}). Above the preferred temperature the sharp fall in Hb saturation is associated with low $\dot{V}/\dot{Q}$ and G_{vent}/G_{perf} for O_2. Relative stability of blood CO_2 content is a result of the stability in G_{vent}/G_{perf} for CO_2. (Based on data from White and Bickler, 1987.)

largely lacking. A model analysis of blood and cerebrospinal fluid (CSF) acid-base characteristics, in which the observed blood CO_2 conductances for the whole body and observed $\dot{V}$Es were applied, indicates that the resulting ΔpH/°C for CSF is -0.012, near the observed ΔpH/°C of blood of -0.013 (White et al., 1985).

A hypothetical model, in which the temperature-dependent blood transport properties of CO_2 are viewed as a determinant of the rates of proton binding to receptors exposed to a CSF environment is shown in Figure 10. The model envisions the perfusive conductance of CO_2 as a primary determinant of CO_2 transport across the CSF-blood diffusion interface. The level of protonization of the chemoreceptors oscillates between a subthreshold state (Zsth) to threshold (Zth) at a time constant (dZ/dt) that depends on the rate of CO_2 transport from source to sink. The inverse relationship between blood βCO_2 and body temperature is viewed as a primary modulator of the CO_2 to CSF

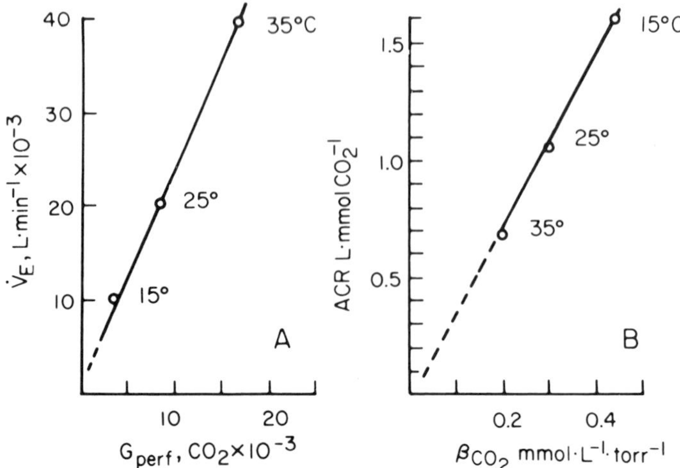

Figure 9 (A) Ventilation as a function of perfusive conductance (G_{perf}) for CO_2. (B) Air convection requirement (ACR) as a function of the blood effective capacitance coefficient (β) for CO_2. (Reprinted from White, F. N. and Bickler, P. E., 1987), with permission of the American Society of Zoologists.)

flux rate relative to the rate of CO_2 production at each body temperature. Thus, the β component of G_{perf} CO_2, which declines with increasing temperature, may modulate the rates of proton activation of central chemoreceptor activity such that the air convection requirement is inverse to body temperature.

Reeves (1972), on the basis of the role of histidine-linked imidazole in dominating the charge state of proteins under conditions in which pH varies with the pK′ of imidazole as temperature is altered, advanced the hypothesis that the receptor system dominating ventilatory responses to CO_2, or proton disturbances, may involve imidazole. In other words, if the protonated/unprotonated imidazole ratio (α) is considered a regulated parameter, the neural sensor of CO_2-linked perturbations in proton concentration may itself involve imidazole.

Hitzig and Jackson (1978) directly perfused the CSF of the turtle with artificial CSF and gained evidence for the presence of CSF receptors sensitive to protons. The receptors are largely temperature-insensitive, the ventilatory responses to a given perturbation in CSF being essentially similar at differing temperatures.

Hitzig (1982) altered pH in turtles by changing body temperature and changing strong ion difference in artifical CSF perfusing the ventricles of intact

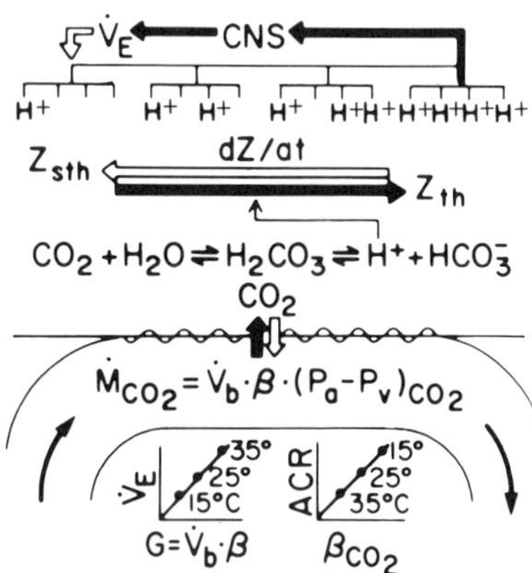

Figure 10 Hypothetical model in which CO_2 blood transport properties are related to the behavior of proton-activated respiratory receptors that are influenced by the acid–base status of the cerebrospinal fluid. The perfusive conductance of CO_2 (G) is viewed as a determinant of the rate of change in protonization of respiratory receptors (dZ/dt). The inverse relationship between body temperature and air convection requirement (ACR) is related to the blood capacitance coefficient (β) for CO_2. The rate of alteration between a subthreshold level of protonization of the receptor (Zsth) and its threshold (Zth) is depicted as being governed by dZ/dt. (Based on White et al., 1985.)

turtles. The calculated CSF α-imidazole correlated with ventilation in both cases, leading to the conclusion that the alphastat hypothesis for ventilatory control was correct, i.e., that the central neural receptors involved imidazole as the immediate receptor mechanism affected by protons. However, Burton (1986) has pointed out that calculation of α-imidazole involves an estimate of the pK′ which may be variable in magnitude depending on the location and microenvironment of the imidazole moiety within various proteins. Nattie (1986) has also argued that Hitzig's (1982) interpretations suffer from this weakness, i.e., a calculated α-imidazole based on a value for the pK′ of imidazole that may not apply in vivo. Thus, he states "These indirect evaluations of the alphastat hypothesis cannot be conclusive."

A more direct approach to testing the hypothesis that imidazole participates as a receptor site for proton-mediated ventilatory control has been undertaken by Nattie (1986a,b). He utilized diethyl pyrocarbonate (DEPC), an agent known to bind to imidazole groups (Lundbald and Noyes, 1984). Reversal of DEPC effects by hydroxylamine (HDA) indicates a high probability that the reactant with DEPC was imidazole. Nattie (1986b), using conscious rabbits, administered DEPC through the cisterna magna and observed a dose-dependent resting hypoventilation and inhibition of ventilatory responses to CO_2 in glomectomized animals and in response to acidic artificial CSF. The latter response was prevented by administration of HDA following DEPC. In a subsequent paper Nattie (1986a) presents evidence that DEPC, applied to the rostral chemosensitive zone of the ventrolateral medulla increased the threshold and decreased the slope of the respiratory response to CO_2 as judged by phrenic nerve activity. Treatment of this area of the medulla with HDA immediately after DEPC prevented these effects, a result that indicates that imidazole was the DEPC reactant. Nattie concluded that the results are consistent with the hypothesis, which was originally advanced by Reeves (1972), that histidine-imidazole is involved in the mechanism of central chemoreception, and that only the rostral area of the ventrolateral zone of the medulla of the cat utilizes a DEPC-inhibitable mechanism. These studies by Nattie offer a promising approach to the study of central chemoreceptors as they relate to ventilatory control. They also represent the first direct attempts to test the specific hypothesis that imidazole participates as a primary reactant in mediating central neural ventilatory responses to CSF acid-base perturbations. However, Nattie (1986b) is "uneasy about chemical specificity of the DEPC effect for imidazole as studied in vivo. Other confirmatory evidence is needed." His results, on the other hand, seem to increase the probability that the receptor system described in Figure 10 is a membrane-associated imidazole site that is sensitive to protons, and that the regulatory response (increase or decrease in ventilatory drive) oscillates around some fixed α of imidazole. This is clearly an area deserving more intense investigation in both ectothermic and endothermic vertebrates.

V. Unsteady States and Carbon Dioxide Homeostasis

The preceding analysis of gas exchange, which follows the assumptions implicit in the work of Piiper and Scheid (1977), incorporates the assumption of steady-state conditions. Although unsteady states are abhorrent to physiologists, they represent the reality of living systems. In what follows, considerations of natural breath holding and ventilation, hibernation, and diurnal rhythms in metabolism, all of which involve alterations in CO_2 homeostasis, will be examined.

A. Natural Breath Holding and Ventilation

Most reptiles exhibit intermittent ventilation, i.e., a pattern of brief ventilatory bouts interrupted by breath-hold periods of variable duration. In turtles, the distribution and magnitude of the cardiac output vary in relation to respiratory state. Heart rate and output decline during breath holding, and a sizable right-to-left intracardiac shunt of 60 to 70% of the cardiac output develops; a left-to-right shunt of about 20 to 30% occurs during ventilation (White and Ross, 1966). Right-to-left shunts during natural breath holding are also reported for crocodilians (White, 1969), amphibians (Shelton and Boutilier, 1982), and lungfish (Fishman et al., 1985). The direction and magnitude of shunt is importantly influenced by neurogenic control of the systemic/pulmonary vascular resistance ratio which is modulated in accordance with the ventilatory state. Important in

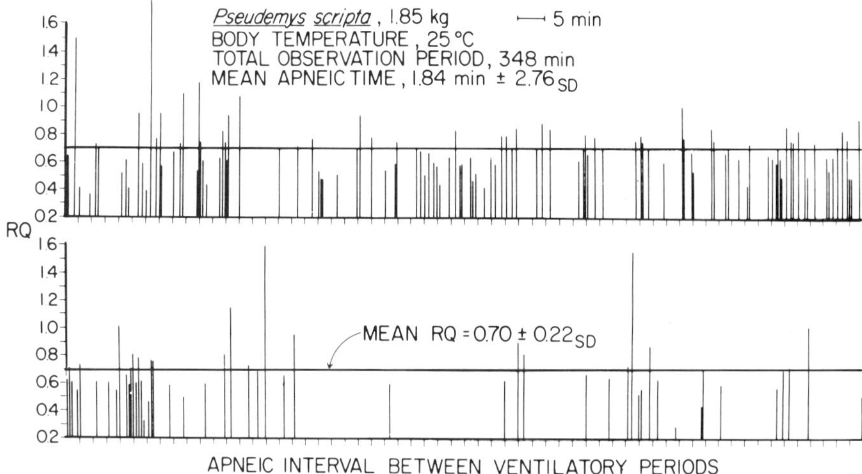

Figure 11 Great variations in RQ are associated with successive ventilatory cycles in a fasting turtle. The horizontal axis provides a time scale from which apneic times between ventilatory bouts are indicated. Total observational period was 348 min. The time scale is useful only for determining apneic times because time associated with ventilation is omitted. The mean RQ of 0.7 is indicated by the horizontal line. Observations commence at the left of the top panel and terminate at the right of the bottom panel. (Reprinted from White and Ackerman, 1979, with permission of the University of Chicago Press.)

this respect is the parasympathetic (vagal) pulmonary arterial vasoconstrictor system that is present in lungfishes, lunged amphibians, and reptiles (White and Hicks, 1987). This system appears to be absent in mammals and birds. Such alterations in pulmonary perfusion and ventilation may be expected to profoundly alter cardiopulmonary and peripheral gas transport. During the breath-holding phase of the ventilatory cycle of turtles the efflux of O_2 from the lung is at a steady rate, reflecting the O_2 consumption of the animal. However, CO_2 entry to the lung is at a rate far below its metabolic production. Yet, during the brief ventilatory bouts of fasting turtles, an RQ of 0.7 to 0.75 is recovered in the expired gas (Ackerman and White, 1979). This does not characterize each breathing bout and long-term collections demonstrate great variability in RQ with over- and undershoots around the long-term mean value (Fig. 11).

The low Re of lung gas during breath holding, calculated by the method of Otis (1964), shows a progressive decline from the termination of ventilation, reaching values of around 0.05 (Fig. 12). A study by White (1985) demonstrated that at the close of a 21-min breath hold the P_{CO_2} of the lung gas had risen by

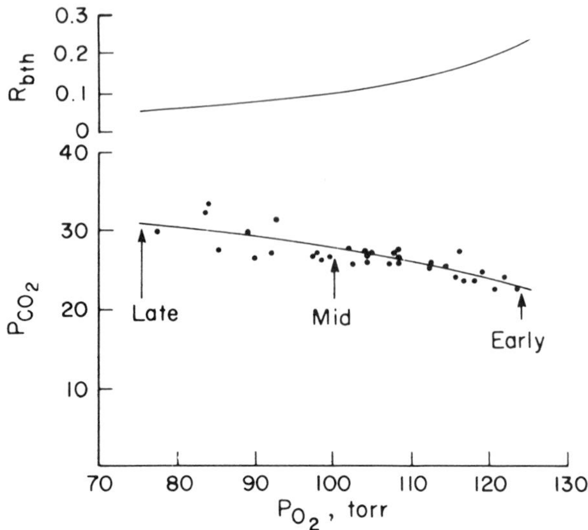

Figure 12 Partial pressures of O_2 and CO_2 of lung gas during normal breath holds of a turtle at 25°C. The upper frame displays respiratory exchange ratios calculated by the method of Otis (1964). The calculations take into account the effects of lung shrinkage and changing levels of the respiratory gases and N_2. (Reprinted from White, 1985, with permission of The Benzon Foundation, Copenhagen.)

8 torr, whereas PO_2 fell by 50 torr from the initial postventilatory levels. The continued uptake of O_2 at levels reflecting the metabolic rate is attributable to rising O_2 conductance in the presence of declining pulmonary blood flow. This can be accounted for by the progressively increasing blood β values for O_2 as the pulmonary arterial and venous points shift to steeper portions of the O_2 dissociation curve. In the example cited, pulmonary blood flow fell by 58%, whereas β increased 3.7-fold, resulting in a 2.2-fold increase in G_{perf} for O_2. A progressive increase in the pulmonary venous to pulmonary arterial O_2 content difference also characterizes breath holding. A right Bohr shift was minimal because the equilibrium conditions for O_2 loading were CO_2-sparse owing to low Re in the lung gas.

The behavior of the CO_2 transport characteristics of blood stand in contrast to those of O_2. The declining blood flow associated with breath holding is associated with a progressive decrease in βCO_2 and thus G_{perf} CO_2 declines. The usually expected positive pulmonary artery to pulmonary venous PCO_2 gradient becomes increasingly negative following the initial phase of breath holding. This counterclockwise rotation of the pulmonary arterial point around an axis connected to the pulmonary venous point is a consequence of an increased Haldane effect and the demonstrably declining blood–lung CO_2 flux (declining R values). It has been shown on theoretical grounds that should the Haldane factor (h) exceed the respiratory exchange ratio (R), blood β should become negative and will progressively decline to lower negative values as R/h diminishes (Kim et al., 1966; Meyer et al., 1976). The observations in the turtle suggest that this effect may be a routine event during breath holding in lower vertebrates. It has recently been verified in resting, intact alligators by Hicks and White (personal observations).

While negative pulmonary arterial–pulmonary venous P_{CO_2} gradients characterize most of the breath-hold period, a small positive CO_2 flux from blood to lung persists. It seems probable that CO_2 is transported from lungs to blood (reverse flux) in the afferent segment of the pulmonary capillaries; and, as oxygenation of blood occurs primarily in the efferent limb, the CO_2-combining capacity is reduced (Haldane effect) with release of CO_2 and net positive transport to the lungs.

The different behaviors in O_2 and CO_2 transport across the lungs is importantly influenced by right-to-left intracardiac shunting in the turtle. First, the reduction in pulmonary blood flow is a factor in influencing G_{perf} for both gases, whereas right-to-left shunt favors increased Pv – Pa O_2 content difference as breath holding progresses (increase Haldane effect). This effect promotes negative β for CO_2 and contributes to a decline in the magnitude of βCO_2 and, thus, CO_2 flux from blood to lung gas. A right-to-left (R:L) shunt thus minimizes CO_2 transport to the lungs and represents, in effect, a CO_2 shunt away from the lungs and to tissues, including the blood. At the end of a 21-min breath hold it is estimated that only 17.8% of the CO_2 produced found its way into the lungs, whereas 26.4% was buffered in blood and 55.8% in other tissues (White, 1985). The venous admixture with arterialized blood and the progressive acidification at the tissue level are factors favoring a right Bohr shift and, thus, offloading of O_2 to tissues. The maintenance of a CO_2-sparse lung, on the other hand, creates conditions minimizing a right Bohr shift at the level of the lungs and is a factor favoring extraction of the lung O_2 stores to low P_{O_2} levels during protracted breath holding, such as during driving.

Although it is clear that rapid offloading of CO_2 from blood to lungs occurs during brief breathing bouts, the precise mechanisms of cyclic release (Ackerman and White, 1979) have not been clearly defined. It is likely that left-to-right (L:R) intracardiac shunt, which reduces the transpulmonary Haldane effect, an increase in G_{perf} CO_2 (increase in $\dot{V}_b$ and βCO_2), and improved blood-lung gas gradients combine to produce the rapid release of CO_2 during the brief ventilatory bouts. Quantitation of these factors is difficult because of the rapidity of the events.

To the cardiologist, patterns of human intracardiac shunting that resemble those of lower vertebrates, are a serious and life-threatening finding. Unlike lower vertebrates, these patterns occur in a rhythmically breathing species and shunts cannot be periodically reversed in relationship to a particular phase of an intermittent ventilatory cycle. As far as the reptilian example is concerned, the presence of R:L shunt is largely confined to the variously protracted breath-holding periods—and it contributes to a CO_2-sparse environment at the level of the lung which minimizes the rate and magnitude of a right Bohr shift. The converse effect in tissues augments a right Bohr shift and tissue O_2 uptake. But, the imbalances in CO_2 distributions are reversed when breathing again commences, R:L shunt diminishes while L:R shunt increases and the CO_2 of metabolism is emitted to the atmosphere while O_2 stores are replenished. A major difference, then, between a human with an intracardiac defect and the turtle is the rhythmic breathing pattern and high rate of metabolism of the former and the ability of the latter to modulate both the intensity and direction of shunting in relationship to the phase of the intermittent respiratory cycle.

B. Rhythms in Carbon Dioxide Homeostasis

Repetitive behavioral states, such as rest–activity cycles, are accompanied by physiological and biochemical alterations that are poorly appreciated. This is, in part, due to the behavioral patterns of investigators who tend toward pursuing their work in accordance to their personal intrinsic rest–activity patterns. Yet, the often neglected nighttime hours constitute a time sector in which fundamental alterations in physiological control mechanisms occur that are as "normal" to the lives of animals as during daylight hours. Sleep research in humans, although far in advance of comparative studies of "behavioral sleep" in lower vertebrates, has suffered a historical latency of blooming, for as Dement comments in his *Forward* to *Physiology in Sleep* (1980): "Far too prematurely, there was a conceptual closure about these issues and a feeling there was no need to carry out redundant observations on sleeping organisms." One aspect of "alteration in state" involves CO_2 homeostasis and its possible implications as a determinant of metabolic intensity and alterations in level and direction of biochemical processes.

Slow-wave sleep in humans is characterized by a reduction in minute ventilation and in O_2 consumption of 10 to 20% (Sullivan, 1980). A change in ventilatory control of CO_2 is evident because alveolar ventilation falls more than expected in response to the metabolic change. There is a decrease in respiratory sensitivity to CO_2 and an accompanying rise in arterial P_{CO_2}. Thus, a respiratory acidosis characterizes slow-wave sleep. It also seems that the slow-wave/rapid eye movement (REM) sleep ratio may be linked to the level of metabolism preceding sleep. This is implied in a study of sleep stages in athletes before and after exercise (Shapiro et al., 1981). Before undertaking a 92-km marathon, the

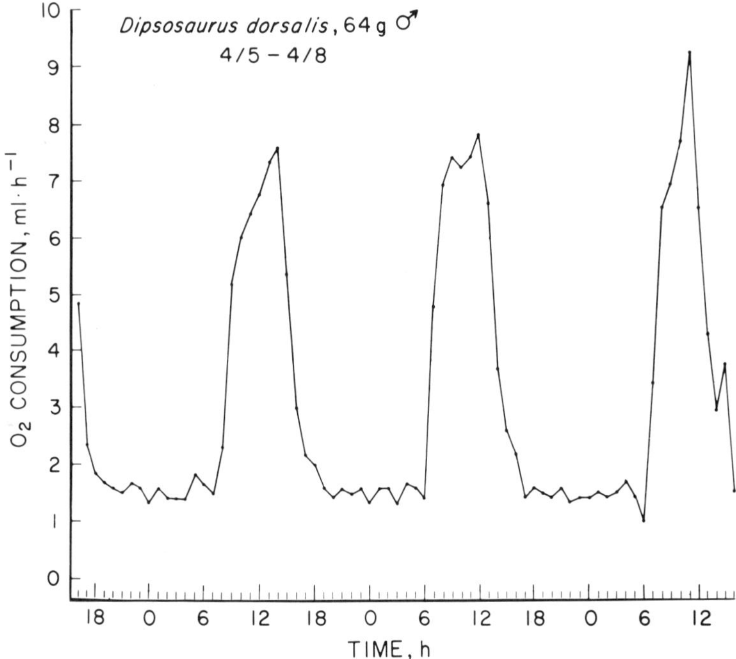

Figure 13 Diurnal cycles in oxygen consumption of a Desert iguana, *Dipsosaurus dorsalis*, at constant temperature and darkness. (Personal observations.)

total sleep time of the five athletes involved in the study averaged 420 min, of which 20% was spent in slow-wave sleep. After the marathon, total sleep time was extended on nights 1 and 2 to around 500 min, whereas slow-wave sleep accounted for approximately 40% of sleep time. The authors concluded that these results support the sleep-restoration hypothesis. The results also suggest that the time spent in slow-wave sleep, and thus in respiratory acidosis relative to REM or wakefulness, may be responsive to the metabolic events of the activity portion of the diurnal cycle.

Rest–activity cycles in metabolism are of common occurrence in lower vertebrates. Figure 13 illustrates such cycles in the lizard *Dipsosaurus dorsalis* at a constant temperature of 25°C and in total darkness in which a relatively constant minimum metabolism recurs on a regular nocturnal basis. These periods are referred to as *behavioral sleep* without reference to sleep stages, there being no equivalent criteria for mammalian sleep stages. Bickler (1986) has shown that such nocturnal periods in *Dipsosaurus* are associated with a significant elevation in blood P_{CO_2} of 4 to 7 torr and a decline in pH of slightly greater than 0.1 pH units relative to the waking state. Using the dimethyl oxazolidine dione (DMO)

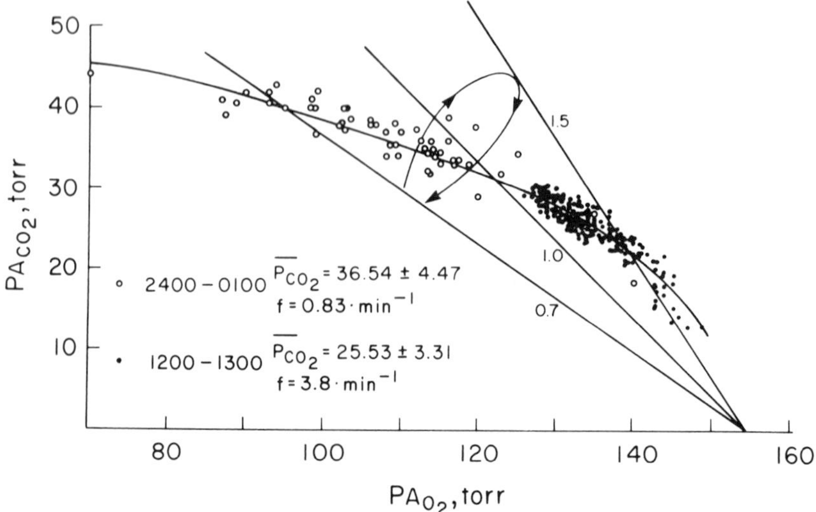

Figure 14 End-expired O_2 and CO_2 for individual breaths during 1200–1300 and 2400–0100 hrs on a single day in a turtle at a constant body temperature of 25°C. Reference RQ lines (0.7–1.5) are shown. Variations between these extremes are encountered at intervening times of the 24-hr cycle. (Personal observations.)

technique to estimate intracellular pH, he found that the pHs of skeletal muscle, esophagus, and liver were about 0.2 units lower at night than during the day. Heart pH was not demonstrably altered. Ventilatory frequency fell at night, indicating that the observed extra- and intracellular acidosis was of respiratory origin. Hicks and Riedesel (1983) demonstrated recurrent nocturnal hypoventilation in the garter snake that was suggestive of a diurnal rhythm in acid-base state.

White, Weinstein, and Palacios (personal observations), by following end-expired P_{CO_2} levels in turtles over several days at constant temperature, observed diurnal variations in O_2 consumption in which high levels of CO_2 correlated with nocturnal periods of behavioral sleep when metabolism was low relative to waking hours. They contrasted the end-expired values of CO_2 of four animals over 20 days during nocturnal maxima and daytime minima (2400-0100 h vs. 1200-1300 h), finding a significant elevation in the mean end expired P_{CO_2} of 8.6 torr during the nocturnal phase. The data base represented a total of 1666 breaths during midday and 1015 during the nocturnal period of measurements. Nocturnal respiratory frequency fell to 60% of the midday period. Comparisons of breaths collected during 1800 to 1900 h and 0600 to 0700 h showed no significant differences in end-expired P_{CO_2}. The P_{O_2} – P_{CO_2} diagram, based on end-expired gases of a single turtle, is shown in Figure 14. The data indicate that a wide range of R values may be encountered between the extreme of night and daytime oscillations.

These collective observations indicate that rest–activity cycles of humans, turtles, and lizards share a common pattern in which the sensitivity of the respiratory system to CO_2 declines during rest (behavioral sleep in reptiles; slow-wave sleep in humans). In both instances, respiratory acidosis characterizes the resting state relative to that of the waking state. This is reflected, in *Dipsosaurus*, in a reduction in intracellular pH in muscle and liver. The mechanisms governing the oscillations of CO_2 balance are obscure. It is as if the neural mechanisms of respiration shift from a lower CO_2 (or, proton)-stimulated threshold to a higher threshold. The association of the transient acidosis with minimal metabolism needs investigation directed at cause and effect. Does the relative acidosis of behavioral sleep in reptiles, or slow-wave sleep in humans, play a role of modulating the metabolism of the organism? Are there indications that the CO_2 retention phase of the cycle is restorative in some manner, i.e., are certain anabolic pathways stimulated during CO_2 retention, whereas catabolic ones are depressed relative to the activity and waking states?

That alterations in the P_{CO_2} of blood may be related to varying levels of aerobic metabolism is implied by studies of mammalian preparations. Among the earliest demonstrations of an "antimetabolic" effect of CO_2 is the 1927 study of Cordier (cited in Stupfel, 1974) in which it was shown that the O_2 consumption of the curarized rabbit with the medulla oblongata sectioned, was reduced by 14% when ventilated with 4.2% CO_2 in 21% O_2. Subsequently, it was shown that aerobic metabolism of isolated canine hindlimb (Harken, 1976), artificially ventilated dogs (Cain, 1970), and hyperventilating humans (Karetsky and Cain, 1970) varies inversely with Pa_{CO_2} (directly with arterial pH). In addition to the impact of CO_2, or $[H^+]$, on metabolism, it seems clear that CO_2 may act as an anesthetic agent. This has been long known to entomologists who routinely use CO_2 as an immobilizing agent. Less widely appreciated is that an increase in inspired CO_2 of 10 torr lowers the anesthesia endpoint for N_2O by 50 torr (McAleavy et al., 1961). Thus, CO_2 has five times the anesthetic potency of N_2O, and the two agents are additive when used together (Severinghaus, 1974).

Malan (1985) makes the case that the respiratory acidosis of hibernating mammals provids a means of reversible inhibition of various nervous and metabolic processes, which contributes to the sparing of energy reserves. Similar arguments may be made for sleep, a state that may functionally resemble hibernation, at least in stages 3 and 4 (slow-wave sleep). Among the metabolic processes inhibited by CO_2 retention (and associated acidosis) are glycolysis in red cells (Tomoda et al., 1977) and skeletal muscle (Fidelman et al., 1982) where the main pH effect is directed at a rate-limiting enzyme, phosphofructokinase (PFK). Here, PFK is sensitive to relatively small alterations in pH (about 0.1–0.2

pH units) such that the active tetramer reversably dissociates into inactive dimers under the acid condition (White and Somero, 1981). It may be argued that the converse effect, i.e., stimulation of key control sites in gluconeogenesis may characterize the CO_2 retention phases of sleep-wake or normothermia-hibernation cycles. Here one may cite fructose bisphosphatase (FBPase), which may be activated by pH changes of 0.1 to 0.3 units (Horecker et al., 1975). Additionally, falling pH activates another regulatory enzyme of gluconeogenesis, phosphoenolpyruvate carboxykinase (PEPCK) (Hochachka and Somero, 1984). The effects of CO_2 retention and its associated decline in pH on these two critical regulatory sites of gluconeogenesis may be adequate to favor glycogen synthesis during periods of falling pH (sleep, hibernation). It must be emphasized that such linkages with CO_2 retention (acid) states can only be inferred at this stage of our knowledge. From the preceding biochemical examples, the overall inhibition of oxidative metabolism through the agency of CO_2 retention (respiratory acidosis) should be viewed as a net resultant of both stimulated and inhibited processes.

Among other systems in which the elimination of an acidotic state has been correlated with a sharp rise in the activity level of the system are: respiration in developing echinoderm embryos, protein synthesis rates in embryos, activation of bacterial metabolism following spore germination, and metabolic rate in brine shrimp embryos after cyst hydration (Nuccitelli and Heiple, 1982).

All of these observations and inferences suggest an important role for endogenously produced CO_2 (and protons) in the control of metabolic processes. Alterations in CO_2 homeostasis in such states as sleep, estivation, torpor, and hibernation, are likely to be of regulatory importance for both overall metabolic intensity and stimulation or inhibition of specific biochemical pathways. Future work should be directed at acquiring a deeper appreciation of the role of the smoke of the metabolic fire in modulating the intensity of the very flame from which it is produced.

References

Ackerman, R. A., and White, F. N. (1979). Cyclic carbon dioxide exchange in the turtle, *Pseudemys scripta*. *Physiol. Zool.* *52*:378-389.

Albery, W. J., and Lloyd, B. B. (1967). Variation of chemical potential with temperature. In *Development of the Lung*. Edited by A. V. S. de Reuck, R. Porter. London, J. and A. Churchill, Ltd., pp. 30-33.

Aoyagi, K., Piiper, J., and May, F. (1965). Alveolarev Gasaustausch und Kreislauf am narkotisierten Hund bei Spontanatmung und bei kuntslicher Beatmung. *Pflügers Arch. Gesamte Physiol.* *286*:311-316.

Bickler, P. E. (1986). Day-night variations in blood and intracellular pH in a lizard, *Dipsosaurus dorsalis*. *J. Comp. Physiol.* *156*:853-857.

Brattstrom, B. H. (1965). Body temperatures of reptiles. *Am. Midl. Nat. 73*: 376-422.

Burton, R. F. (1986). The role of imidazole in the control of breathing. *Comp. Biochem. Physiol. 83A*:333-336.

Cain, S. M. (1970). Increased oxygen uptake with passive hyperventilation of dogs. *J. Appl. Physiol. 28*:4-7.

Davies, D. G., Thomas, J. L., and Smith, E. N. (1982). Effect of body temperature on ventilatory control in the alligator. *J. Appl. Physiol. 52*:114-118.

Dejours, P. (1972). Comparison of gas transport by convection among animals. *Respir. Phsysiol. 14*:96-104.

Dejours, P., Garey, W. F., and Rahn, H. (1970). Comparison of ventilatory and circulatory flow rates between animals in various physiological conditions. *Respir. Physiol. 9*:108-117.

Dement, W. C. (1980). Forward. In *Physiology in Sleep*. Edited by J. Orem and C. D. Barnes. New York, Academic Press, pp. xi-xii.

Ekeland, L. G., and Holmgren, A. (1964). Circulatory and respiratory adaptation during long-term, non-steady state exercise, in the sitting position. *Acta Physiol. Scand. 62*:240-255.

Fidelman, M. L., Seekolzer, K. B., Walsh, K. B., and Moore, R. D. (1982). Intracellular pH mediates action of insulin on glycolysis in frog skeletal muscle. *Am. J. Physiol. 242*:C87-C93.

Fishman, A. P., Delaney, R. G., Laurent, P., and Szidon, J. P. (1984). Blood shunting in lungfish and humans. In *Cardiovascular Shunts*. Edited by K. Johansen and W. Burggren. Copenhagen, Munksgaard, pp. 88-95.

Fishman, A. P., DeLaney, R. G., Laurent, P., and Szidon, J. P. (1985). Blood shunting in lungfish and humans. In *Cardiovascular Shunts*. Edited by K. Johansen and W. Burggren. Copenhagen, Munksgaard, pp. 88-99.

Harken, A. H. (1976). Hydrogen ion concentration and oxygen uptake in an isolated canine hindlimb. *J. Appl. Physiol. 40*:1-5.

Hicks, J. W., and Riedesel, M. L. (1983). Diurnal ventilatory patterns in the garter snake, *Thamnophis elegans. J. Comp. Physiol. 149*:503-510.

Hitzig, B. M., and Jackson, D. C. (1978). Central chemical control of ventilation in the unanesthetized turtle. *Am. J. Physiol. 235*:R257-R264.

Hitzig, B. M. (1982). Temperature-induced changes in turtle CSF pH and central control of ventilation. *Respir. Physiol. 49*:205-222.

Hochachka, P. W., and Somero, G. N. (1984). *Biochemical Adaptation*. Princeton, Princeton University Press, pp. 178-179.

Horecker, B. L., Melloni, E., and Pontremoli, S. (1975). Fructose-1, 6-biphosphatase: Properties of the neutral enzyme and its modification by proteolytic enzymes. *Adv. Enzymol. Relat. Areas Mol. Biol. 42*:193-226.

Howell, B. J., Baumgardner, F. W., Bondi, K., and Rahn, H. (1970). Acid-base balance in cold-blooded vertebrates as a function of body temperature. *Am. J. Physiol. 218*:600-606.

Jackson, D. C. (1971). The effect of temperature on ventilation in the turtle, *Pseudemys scripta elegans. Respir. Physiol. 18*:178-187.

Jackson, D. C., Palmer, S. E., and Meadow, W. L. (1974). The effects of temperature and carbon dioxide breathing on ventilation and acid-base status of turtles. *Respir. Physiol. 20*:131-146.

Johansen, K. (1972). Heart and circulation in gill, skin and lung breathing. *Respir. Physiol. 14*:193-210.

Johansen, K. (1984). A phylogenetic overview of cardiovascular shunts. In *Cardiovascular Shunts*. Edited by K. Johansen and W. Burggren. Copenhagen, Munksgaard, pp. 17-32.

Karetsky, M. S., and Cain, S. M. (1970). Effects of carbon dioxide on oxygen uptake during hyperventilation in normal man. *J. Appl. Physiol. 28*:8-12.

Kim, T. S., Rahn, H., and Fahri, L. E. (1966). Estimation of true venous and arterial P_{CO_2} by gas analysis of a single breath. *J. Appl. Physiol. 21*:1338-1344.

Kinney, J. L., Matsuura, D. T., and White, F. N. (1977). Cardiorespiratory effects of temperature in the turtle. *Respir. Physiol. 31*:309-325.

Kroncke, G. M., Nichols, R. D., Mendenhall, J. T., Myerowitz, P. D., and Starling, J. R. (1986). Ectothermic philosophy of acid-base balance to prevent fibrillation during hypothermia. *Arch. Surg. 121*:303-304.

Lundblad, R. L., and Noyes, C. M. (1984). *Chemical Reagents for Protein Modification*, Vol. 1. Boca Raton, Fla., CRC Press, pp. 105-125.

Malan, A. (1985). Acid-base regulation during hibernation. In *Acid-Base Regulation and Body Temperature*. Edited by H. Rahn and O. Prakash. Dordrecht, Martinus Nijhoff, pp. 33-53.

McAleavy, J. C., Way, W. L., Alstatt, A. H., Guadagni, N. P., and Severinghaus, J. W. (1961). The effect of P_{CO_2} on the depth of anesthesia. *Anesthesiology 22*:260.

Meyer, M., Worth, H., and Scheid, P. (1976). Gas-blood CO_2 equilibrium in parabronchial lungs of birds. *J. Appl. Physiol. 41*:302-309.

Nattie, E. E. (1986a). Diethyl pyrocarbonate (an imidazole binding substance) inhibits rostral VLM CO_2 sensitivity. *J. Appl. Physiol. 61*:843-850.

Nattie, E. E. (1986b). Intracisternal diethyl pyrocarbonate inhibits rabbit central chemosensitivity. *Respir. Physiol. 64*:161-176.

Nuccitelli, R., and Heiple, J. M. (1982). Summary of the evidence and discussion concerning the involvement of pH_i in the control of cellular functions. In *Intracellular pH: Its Measurement, Regulation and Utilization in Cellular Function*. Edited by R. Nuccitelli and D. W. Deamer. New York, Allen R. Liss, pp. 567-586.

Otis, A. B. (1964). Quantitative relationships in steady-state gas exchange. In *Handbook of Physiology*, Vol. 1, Sect. 3, Respiration. Edited by W. O. Fenn and H. Rahn. Baltimore, Waverly Press, pp. 681-698.

Peters, J. P., and Van Slyke, D. D. (1931). *Hemoglobin and Oxygen, Carbonic Acid and Acid-Base Balance*. Baltimore, Waverly Press, p. 868.

Piiper, J., and Scheid, P. (1977). Comparative physiology of respiration: Functional analysis of gas exchange organs in vertebrates. In *International Review of Physiology*, Vol. 14, Respiration Physiology II. Edited by J. G. Widdicombe. Baltimore, University Park Press, pp. 219-253.

Rahn, H., and Howell, B. J. (1976). Bimodel gas exchange. In *Respiration in Amphibious Vertebrates*. Edited by G. M. Hughes. New York, Academic Press, pp. 271-285.

Randall, D. J. and Cameron, J. N. (1973). Respiratory control of arterial pH as temperatures changes in rainbow trout *Salmo gairdneri. Am. J. Physiol. 225*:997-1002.

Reeves, R. B. (1972). An imidazole alphastat hypothesis for vertebrate acid-base regulation. *Respir. Physiol. 14*:219-236.

Romer, A. S. (1972). Skin breathing-primary or secondary? *Respir. Physiol. 14*:183-192.

Rosenthal, T. B. (1948). The effect of temperature on the pH of blood and plasma in vitro. *J. Biol. Chem. 173*:25-30.

Severinghaus, J. W. (1974). Carbon dioxide transport. In *Carbon Dioxide and Metabolic Regulations*. Edited by G. Nahas and K. E. Schaefer. Heidelberg, Springer-Verlag, pp. 138-143.

Shapiro, C. M., Bortz, R., Mitchell, D., Bartel, P., and Jooste, P. (1981). Slow-wave sleep: A recovery period after exercise. *Science 214*:1253-1254.

Shelton, G., and Boutilier, R. G. (1982). Apnea in amphibians and reptiles. *J. Exp. Biol. 100*:245-273.

Shelton, G., and Boutilier, R. G. (1982). Apnea in amphibians and reptiles. In *Control and Coordination of Respiration and Circulation*. Edited by P. J. Butler. London, Cambridge University Press, pp. 245-273.

Somero, G. N., and White, F. N. (1985). Enzymatic consequences under alphastate regulation. In *Acid-Base Regulation and Body Temperature*. Edited by H. Rahn and O. Prakash. Dordrecht, Martinus Nijhoff, pp. 55-80.

Stupfel, M. (1974). Carbon dioxide and temperature regulation of homeothermic mammals. In *Carbon Dioxide and Metabolic Regulations*. Edited by G. Nahas and K. E. Schaefer. Heidelberg, Springer-Verlag, pp. 163-186.

Sullivan, C. E. (1980). Breathing in sleep. In *Physiology in Sleep*. Edited by J. Orem and C. D. Barnes. New York, Academic Press, pp. 213-272.

Swain, J. A., White, F. N., and Peters, R. M. (1984). The effect of pH on the hypothermic fibrillation threshold. *J. Thorac. Cardiovasc. Surg. 87*:445-451.

Tomoda, A., Tsuda-Hirota, S., and Minakami, S. (1977). Glycolysis of red cells suspended in solutions of impermeable solutes: Intracellular pH and glycolysis. *J. Biochem. (Tokyo) 81*:697-701.

Weinstein, Y., Ackerman, R., and White, F. N. (1986). Influence of temperature on the CO_2 dissociation curve of the turtle *Pseudemys scripta. Respir. Physiol. 63*:53-63.

White, F. N. (1969). Redistribution of cardiac output in the diving alligator. *Copeia 3*:567-570.

White, F. N. (1976). Circulation. In *Biology of the Reptilia*, Vol. 5. Edited by C. Gans and W. Dawson. New York, Academic Press, pp. 275-334.

White, F. N. (1985). Role of intracardiac shunts in pulmonary gas exchange in chelonian reptiles. In *Cardiovascular Shunts*. Edited by K. Johansen and W. Burggren. Copenhagen, Munksgaard, pp. 296-309.

White, F. N., and Bickler, P. E. (1987). Cardiopulmonary gas exchange in the turtle: A model analysis. *Am. Zool. 27*:31-39.

White, F. N., Bickler, P., and Yacoe, M. (1985). Gas exchange in intermittently breathing turtles. In *Circulation, Respiration and Metabolism, Current Comparative Approaches*. Edited by R. Gilles. Heidelberg, Springer-Verlag, pp. 139-148.

White, F. N., and Hicks, J. W. (1987). Cardiovascular implications of the transition from aquatic to aerial respiration. In *Comparative Physiology: Life in Water and on Land*. Edited by P. Dejours, L. Bolis, C.R. Taylor, and E. R. Weibel. Fidia Research Series. Padova, Liviana Press, pp. 93-106.

White, F. N., and Ross, G. (1966). Circulatory changes during experimental diving in the turtle. *Am. J. Physiol. 211*:15-18.

White, F. N., and Somero, G. N. (1982). Acid-base regulation and phospholipid adaptations to temperature: Time courses and physiological significance of modifying the milieu for protein function. *Physiol. Rev. 62*:40-90.

Part Four

Fluid Balance

16

Comparative Aspects of Interstitial Fluid Balance

ALAN R. HARGENS*

University of California
and Veterans Administration Medical Center
San Diego, California

I. Introduction

The foundations for our present understanding of fluid exchange between the blood and tissue spaces were firmly laid by two pioneering physiologists, Carl Ludwig and Ernest Starling. Ludwig (1861) hypothesized that interstitial fluid is formed by filtration of blood through the capillary wall during periods of elevated capillary blood pressure. Starling (1896) proposed that blood volume is maintained and edema is prevented by the colloid osmotic pressure of blood proteins. These basic theories provide the framework of our present knowledge of fluid exchange between blood and interstitial fluids.

Various ideas about the direction and magnitude of interstitial fluid pressure have been argued forcefully by many investigators during the past 20 years. Frequently, these controversies dominated many studies of transport dynamics between blood, interstitial fluid, and peripheral lymph. Sometimes arguments

---

**Present affiliation*: NASA –Ames Research Center, Moffett Field, California.

concerning whether interstitial fluid pressure was positive or negative (with reference to atmospheric or ambient pressure) led to colorful debates about the validity and utility of one pressure-measuring technique over another. Most workers in this field today, however, agree that some tissues (e.g., subcutaneous, peritoneal, synovial, and lung tissues) normally have negative interstitial fluid pressure, whereas other tissues (muscle enclosed by fascia and filtering organs such as the liver and kidney) normally contain positive pressures within their interstitial fluids. During the past 20 years, our understanding of interstitial fluid pressure dynamics has advanced markedly, partly because of these controversies but, also, as a result of the availability of new technology (macro- and microtechniques) for measuring pressures in blood, tissue, and peripheral lymph.

Several reviews have comprehensively treated interstitial pressures, interstitial volume regulation, and lymph formation (Guyton, 1976; Aukland and Nicolaysen, 1981; Brace, 1981; Taylor, 1981; Casley-Smith, 1982; Effros, 1984; Granger et al., 1984; Hargens, 1987), and it is beyond the scope of this chapter to treat these topics with equal depth. Also, an earlier volume *Lung Water and Solute Balance*, edited by Professor Norman Staub (1978) in this same series of monographs, systematically treats fluid and solute exchange in the lung. Therefore, my chapter will primarily focus upon comparative aspects of interstitial fluid balance, emphasizing our own laboratory techniques for measuring hydrostatic and colloid osmotic pressures and providing examples in which these techniques have illuminated basic mechanisms of interstitial fluid balance in a wide variety of animals.

II. Basic Research Tools for Measuring Fluid Pressures in Tissue and Blood

Twenty years ago we developed techniques for basic science studies of interstitial fluid pressure and colloid osmotic pressure during the 1967 R/V *Alpha Helix* Expedition to the Amazon River (Scholander et al., 1968). The wick catheter technique was used to examine pressure-volume relationships in animal tissues and a simple colloid osmometer was employed to assess blood samples from Amazon animals. These techniques were refined during subsequent expeditions from Scripps Institution of Oceanography (University of California, San Diego) to investigate physiological adaptations of Antarctic penguins, polar fishes, and Pacific salmon. Later studies using the same techniques focused upon normal transcapillary fluid balance in humans, fluid shifts related to simulated weightlessness in preparation for a Space Shuttle project, and orthostatic adaptations in the giraffe.

A. Wick Catheter

The wick catheter was developed at Scripps Institution of Oceanography, UCSD during 1966-1971. Previous needles and catheters used for measuring interstitial fluid pressure required saline infusion to maintain patency of the probe. This requirement precluded measurements of negative fluid pressure in tissue, a concept that Arthur Guyton pioneered in the early 1960s. Although Guyton's capsule (1963) provided very dynamic measurements of tissue fluid pressure, it was large and required implantation for 6 weeks before any determinations could be made. The wick catheter was developed to provide immediate, equilibrium measurements of tissue fluid pressure without saline infusion (Fig. 1). Microscopic channels of free fluid between the wick fibers maintained catheter patency and offered a relatively large pickup area for sensing changes in tissue pressure.

Scholander's dream of a floating laboratory to study physiological adaptations throughout the world became a reality in 1965 with the christening of

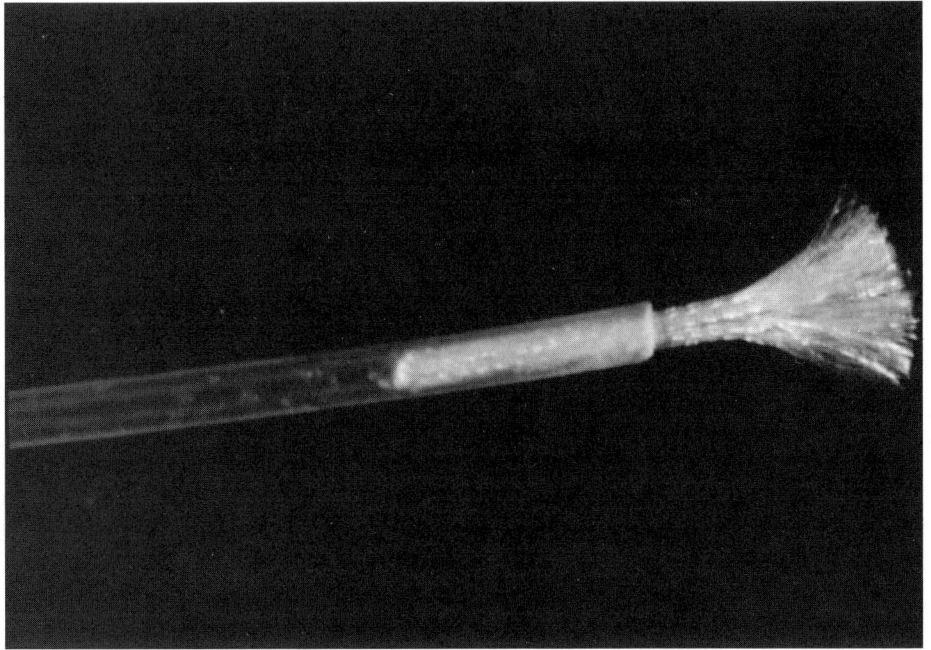

Figure 1 Close-up view of wick catheter tip showing microscopic wick fibers that provide contact with tissue fluids and maintain catheter patency without saline infusion. (From Adair et al., 1983.)

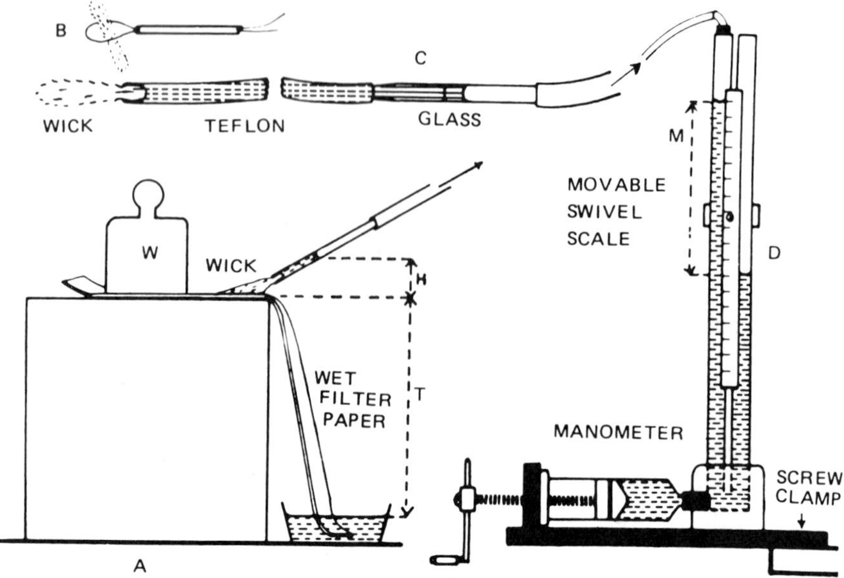

Figure 2 Principles of measuring negative water pressure. (A) Measuring negative pressure in wet filter paper using wick-containing capillary tube, connected to manometer (D) that balances the meniscus. Water tension T (in cm H_2O) = manometer reading M + capillarity C – hydrostatic height of meniscus H. (B) Pulling wick into tubing by means of thread. (C) Wick assembly with read-out meniscus in clean capillary tube. (D) Field-type manometer. W, weight to hold filter paper. (From Scholander et al., 1968.)

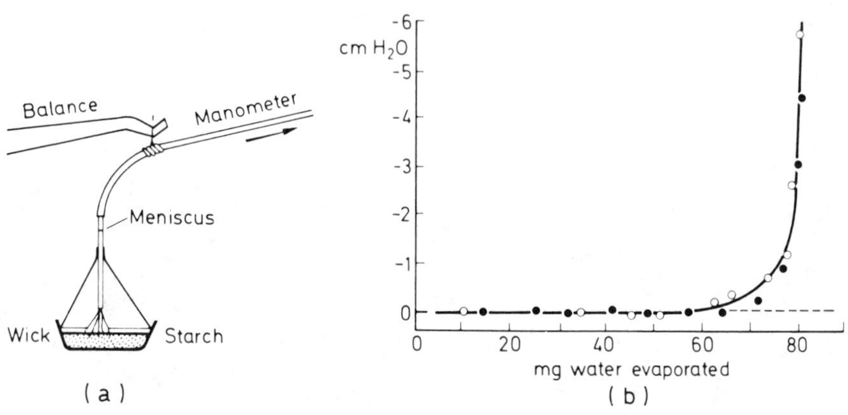

Figure 3 Wick technique in model system. (a) Simultaneous measurement of water loss and tension in sedimented starch. (b) Water tension (measured by wick catheter) versus water loss (measured by torsion balance in sedimented corn (o) and potato starch (●). The sharp increase in negative water pressure occurs when the water surface evaporates down to the sedimented grains. (From Hammel and Scholander, 1976.)

the R/V *Alpha Helix*. The maiden voyage of this NSF-supported research vessel was to the Great Barrier Reef of Australia where plants living in sea water and "air-breathing" fishes were studied. The *Alpha Helix*'s second major expedition was to the Amazon River Basin and it was here we developed the wick technique (Scholander et al., 1968). A simple catheter system made from Teflon tubing, a cotton wick, glass tube, and custom manometer were designed especially for field-type research "where electronic gadgetry was useless," according to Scholander (Fig. 2). The system was thoroughly tested to assure that it accurately measured only hydrostatic fluid pressures, especially under conditions of negative fluid pressures where other techniques were found inoperative. The wick technique was also tested in model systems of dehydration, for example, in monitoring development of negative pressure in starch suspensions during water evaporation (Fig. 3). These initial studies were extended to measurement of fluid pressure in subcutaneous, peritoneal, and muscle tissues (Fig. 4) during the Amazon Expedition.

The basic principles for measuring tissue fluid pressure in animals were applied and refined for intracompartmental studies in humans. For example, intramuscular fluid pressures in the forearm could be measured instanteously

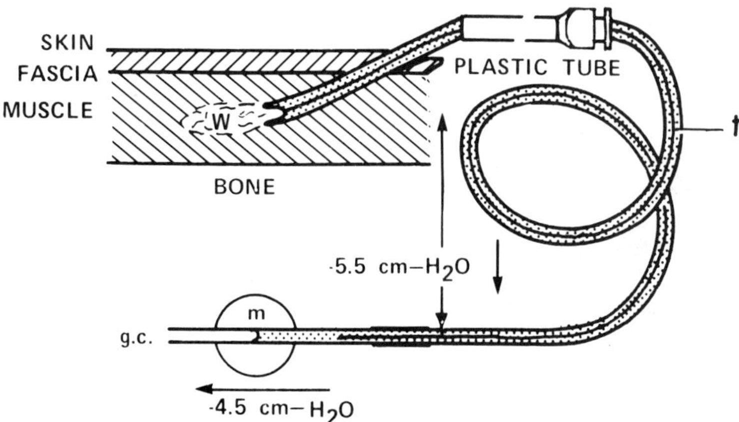

Figure 4 Principles of measuring tissue fluid pressure in muscle using the wick technique. Wick (w) is held within tubing by thread (t). Glass capillary (g.c.) is adjusted vertically until read-out meniscus (m) is stationary, indicating equilibrium is reached. Here, intramuscular fluid pressure equals hydrostatic height (-5.5 cm H_2O) plus capillary (-4.5 cm H_2O) to give -10 cm H_2O.

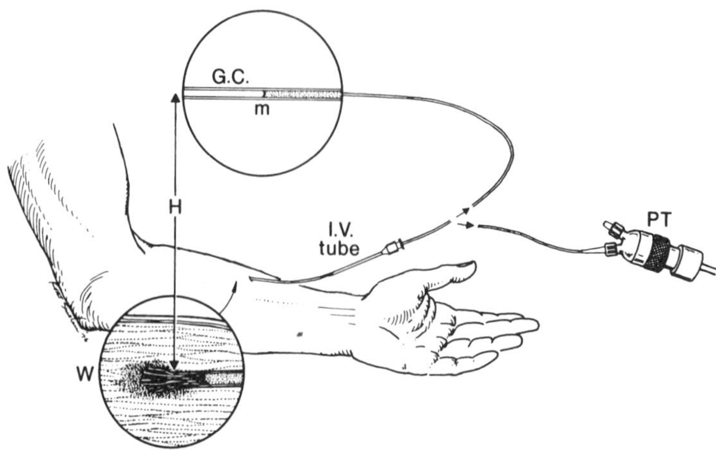

Figure 5 Wick catheter for measuring intracompartmental (volar forearm) fluid pressure. The sterile, heparinized catheter is connected to a read-out glass capillary tube (G.C.) where the meniscus (m) is held stationary by adjusting its hydrostatic height (H) above the wick (W). Meniscus movement is followed microscopically. Subtracting the capillarity of the glass tube (G.C.) from the equilibrium height (H) yields muscle fluid pressure in cm H_2O. Alternatively, the wick catheter can be connected to a pressure transducer (PT) zeroed to the wick's hydrostatic level (W). The IV tube shields the wick catheter during the latter's entry into muscle. (From Hargens et al., 1977.)

using the glass capillary technique or continuously using a pressure transducer (Fig. 5). Revisions of the original technique included use of braided suture for wick material, smaller catheter tubing, improved techniques to minimize trauma during insertion, heparinized saline to prevent coagulation, and sterilization of all system components to minimize risks of infection.

B. Colloid Osmometer

Colloid osmometers have been available for over a century but recent improvements in membrane and pressure-sensing technology make their use more general and reliable. Colloid osmometry is important for studying (1) the capacity of blood to absorb tissue fluid, specifically edema fluid; (2) the colloid osmotic pressure of interstitial fluid that counteracts the colloid osmotic pressure of blood; and (3) the ability of a tissue matrix (e.g., nucleus pulposus of the intervertebral disk) to swell. The importance of these phenomena in tissue fluid homeostasis will become evident later in this chapter.

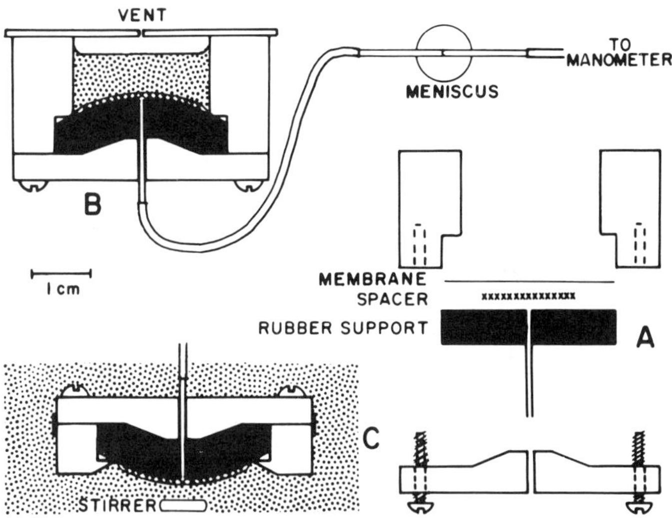

Figure 6 Colloid osmometer uses a stretch mounting for its membrane. (A) Exploded cross section showing assembly. (B) Osmometer for measuring colloid osmotic pressure. (C) Submerged osmometer. (From Hargens and Scholander, 1969.)

Our first colloid osmometer was again developed for field physiology research where electric power was not always available (Fig. 6). Principles for measuring osmotic pressures were similar to those outlined previously for the wick catheter technique. Basically, our new technique employed a stretch mounting for membranes to measure weak osmotic pressures accurately to within 1% (Hargens and Scholander, 1969).

All techniques for measuring negative tissue fluid or osmotic pressures use the "push" or "pull" technique to release trapped fluid (Fig. 7). Scholander and colleagues (1965) employed the push technique to verify experimentally Dixon's transpiration model (1914) for the ascent of fresh water sap in all vascular plants. Briefly, Scholander and coworkers placed a cut branch in a pressure bomb and compressed the plant tissue until the water meniscus returned to its initial position at the cut surface (Fig. 8). Recently, we employed a similar technique to measure the enormous swelling pressure of tissues with a high glycosaminoglycan content (e.g., nucleus pulposus). Previous osmometric techniques are unreliable because of cavitation (gas bubble formation) on the side of the membrane opposite the swelling tissue.

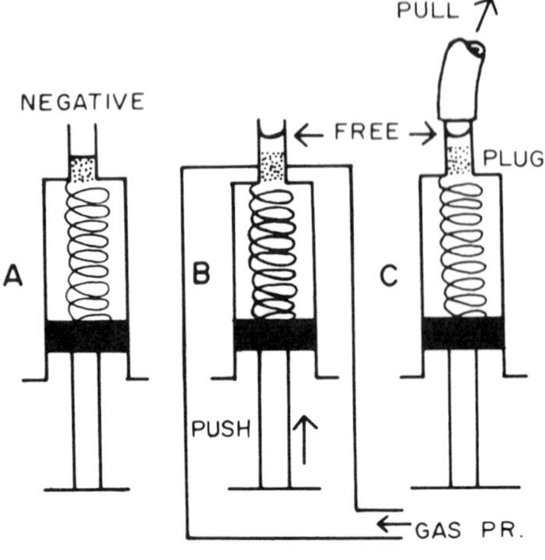

Figure 7 Two principles of measuring negative fluid pressure. (A) System with unknown fluid pressure in frictionless syringe with expansion spring in barrel and porous plug in nozzle. Negative fluid pressure can be measured by (B) "push" technique (compression of system by gas pressure) to free meniscus or (C) "pull" technique (suction) to free meniscus in nozzle. Both techniques measure the compression of the spring (swelling pressure) that produces negative fluid pressure. (From Hammel and Scholander, 1976.)

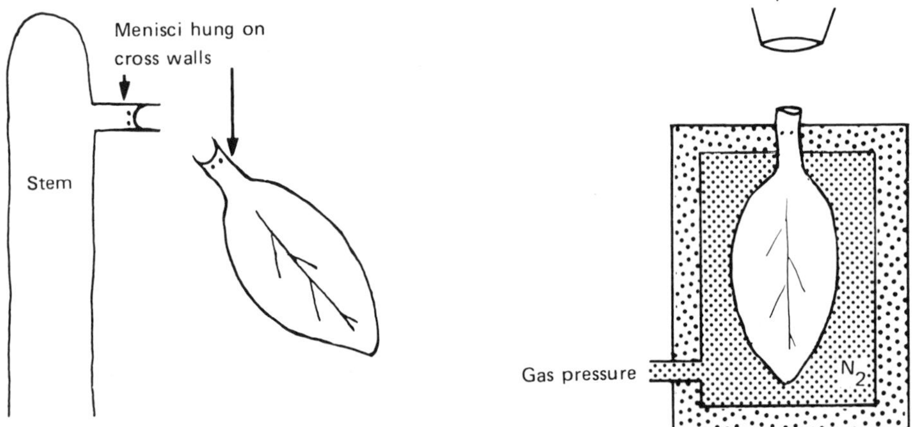

Figure 8 Scholander's technique for measuring sap pressure in vascular plants (Scholander et al., 1965). Left: After cutting off leaf, sap retracts back to first cross walls when xylem pressure is negative. Right: Applying the push method of Figure 7, the leaf is enclosed in a pressure chamber and compressed by N_2 at pressure (P) until sap appears at the cut surface. The sap pressure in then – P. (From Scholander, 1972.)

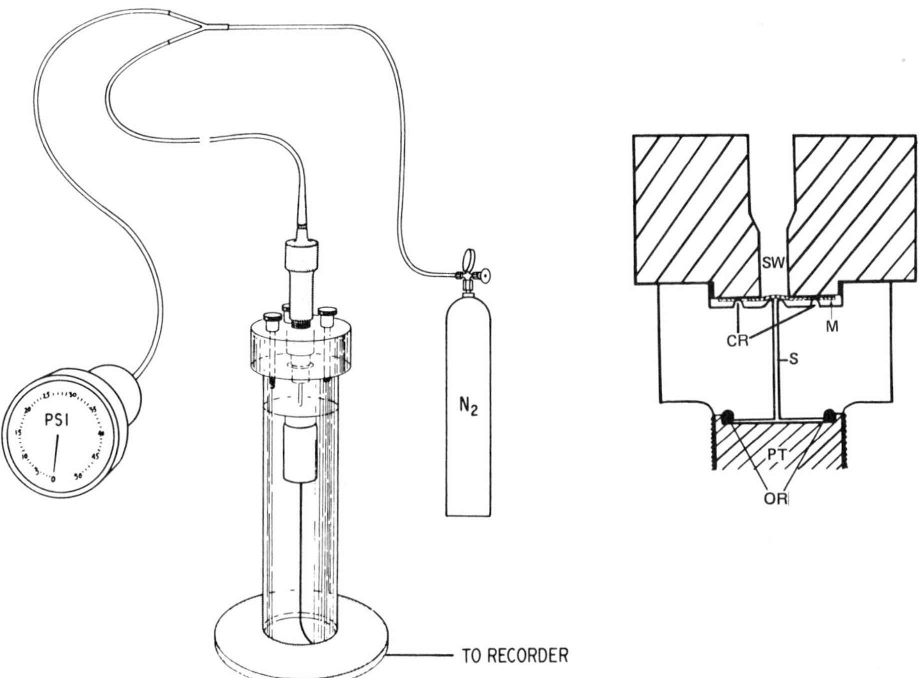

Figure 9 New compression-type osmometer for measuring swelling pressure of nucleus pulposus. Left: Plexiglas osmometer mounted on stand with N_2 gas inlet at top. The osmometer is connected to a N_2 gas source, precision pressure gauge, and pressure transducer. Transmembrane pressure gradients are continuously measured by a strip-chart recorder. Right: Cross section of osmometer with sealing of membrane by the crimp rings (CR) on the screw-down Plexiglas plate. Nucleus pulposus is placed in the sample well (SW) on top of the membrane (M). Pressure gradients across the membrane are transmitted by the fluid column (S) and monitored by the pressure transducer (PT) fitted tightly to bottom of osmometer by an O ring (OR).

Our new compression-type osmometer (Fig. 9) consists of a sample chamber over a rigid Millipore filter (0.5 μm pore diameter). Samples of nucleus pulposus are compressed over the membrane by nitrogen gas to prevent swelling of the tissue. Equilibrium swelling pressure is reached within 10 min and measured by a Heise precision gauge. Pressure gradients across the membrane are detected using a low-volume displacement, pressure transducer and nullified using the pressurized gas.

III. Basic Science Studies of Tissue Fluid Balance

A. Amazon Studies of Reptiles

The wick catheter and colloid osmometer were first used to investigate interstitial fluid pressure in Amazon animals (Scholander et al., 1968). These experiments were undertaken during the 1967 R/V *Alpha Helix* Expedition to the Amazon River. This and other NSF-sponsored, field-research expeditions by the *Alpha Helix* allowed cross-fertilization of ideas between colleagues from the United States, Europe, and the country where the expedition was located. These

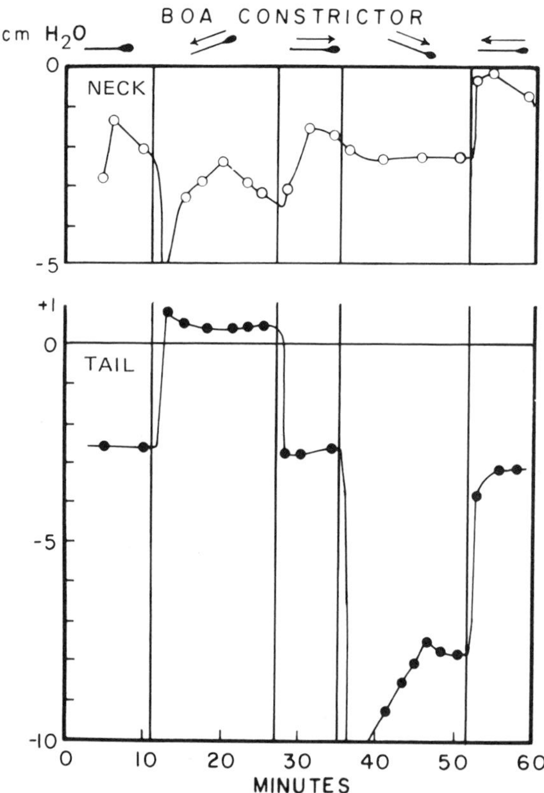

Figure 10 Hydrostatic compensation of tissue fluid pressure in neck (top) and tail (bottom) of a tilted boa constrictor. Wick catheters were placed subcutaneously and the snake's posture is indicated at top (arrows indicate direction of gravitational flow of fluids). (From Scholander et al., 1968.)

expeditions fortified the concept that interdisciplinary team efforts pay great dividends in terms of scientific progress and international cooperation. Researchers who participated in these expeditions worked and lived together around the clock for periods of 1 to 2 months.

One of our first wick studies addressed the question of how snakes, particularly tree-climbing species, such as the boa constrictor, prevented edema in their tail or head as they climbed up or down a tree. To study tissue pressures in 3 to 4 m long boas and anacondas, we built wooden troughs to hold the snakes and inserted wick catheters in the neck and tail during head-up and head-down tilting. Briefly, we found that interstitial fluid and blood ultrafiltration flowed very slowly to dependent tissues and that snakes have good, short-term mechanisms for edema prevention, considering that the pressure gradients in our snakes were at least 200–300 cm H_2O during tilt (Fig. 10). Development and relief of edema were studied in toads and crocodiles during our Amazon project. Subcutaneous and peritoneal pressures were slightly negative, but tourniquet application raised pressure to about + 5 cm H_2O. This positive pressure decreased with tourniquet removal (Fig. 11).

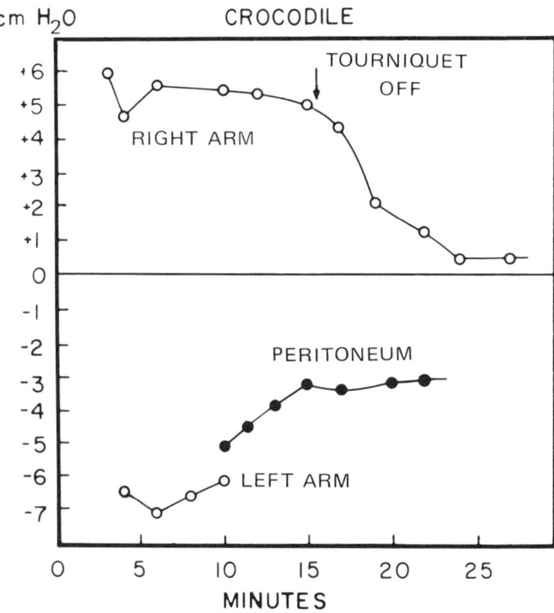

Figure 11 Relief of subcutaneous edema in forelimb of crocodile upon removal of tourniquet. (From Scholander et al., 1968.)

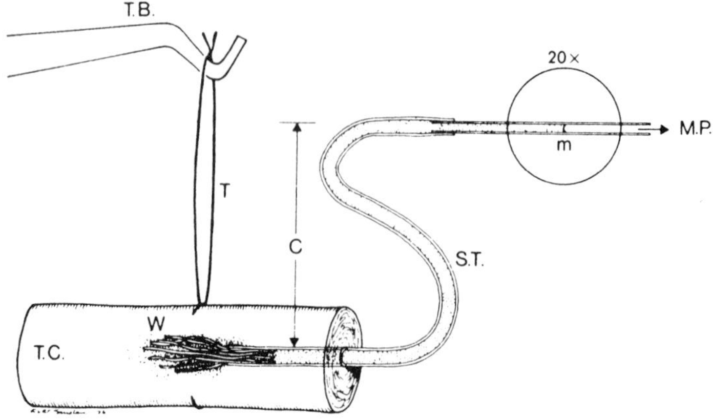

Figure 12 Pressure–water loss relations in tissue cylinder (T.C.) are followed by saline-filled tubing (S.T.) fitted with wick (W). Fluid pressure equals the applied manometric pressure (M.P.) when the meniscus (m) is held stationary at a height equal to the capillarity (C). Meniscus movement is monitored microscopically (20x). Tissue specimen is connected by a thread (T) and weighed by torsion balance (T.B.) to quantitate water loss during dehydration. (From Hargens, 1977.)

B. Pressure–Volume Relations in Animals and Plants

Our Amazon, and later, studies included analysis of pressure–volume relationships in dehydrating tissues, using the wick technique to measure fluid pressure and a torsion balance to follow water loss (Fig. 12; Hargens, 1977; Hargens et al., 1978a). These experiments documented striking differences between animals and plants in terms of their tissue compliance during water loss (Fig. 13).

C. Antarctic Studies of Penguins and Fishes

During a subsequent expedition to the Antarctic, we investigated tissue pressures with increased body temperature in birds and freezing resistance in fishes (Hargens, 1972; Hargens et al., 1978b). Briefly, we found that warming the feet of adelie penguins produced a significant rise in subcutaneous pressure (Fig. 14), probably caused by increased blood flow and ultrafiltration across the capillaries in the penguins' relatively noncompliant foot tissues. Separate studies of fishes living just beneath the polar sea ice at -1.8°C (Hargens, 1972) indicated

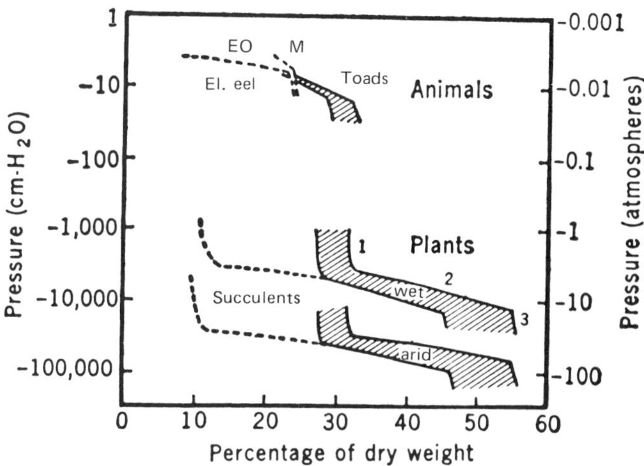

Figure 13 Tension buildup in tissue fluids of animals and plants during dehydration. Dry weight is given as a percentage of total weight. Symbols are electric organ in eel (EO) and toad muscle (M). Plants are separated into "wet" species of Amazon and arid species of California desert. Plant dehydration includes (1) turgor, (2) no turgor, and (3) negative turgor (cellular packing). Pressures in plants are four orders of magnitude more negative than those in animals because plants have salt-rejecting membranes in their "vascular system," whereas animals do not. (From Scholander et al., 1968.)

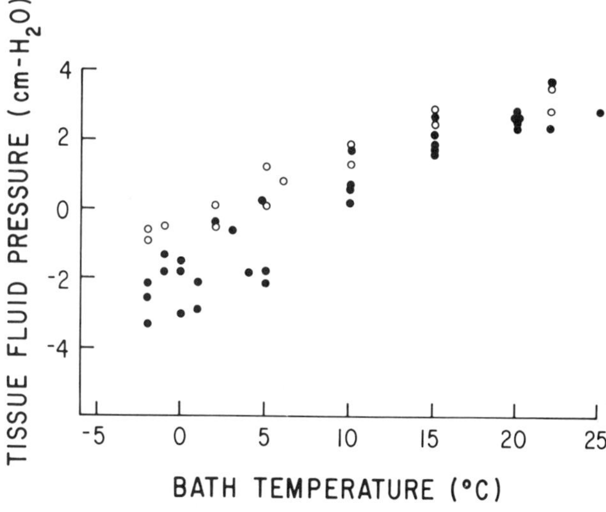

Figure 14 Development of subcutaneous edema in web feet of five adelie penguins upon warming in brine bath (solid points). Relief of web foot edema by cooling in brine bath (open circles). (From Hargens et al., 1978b).

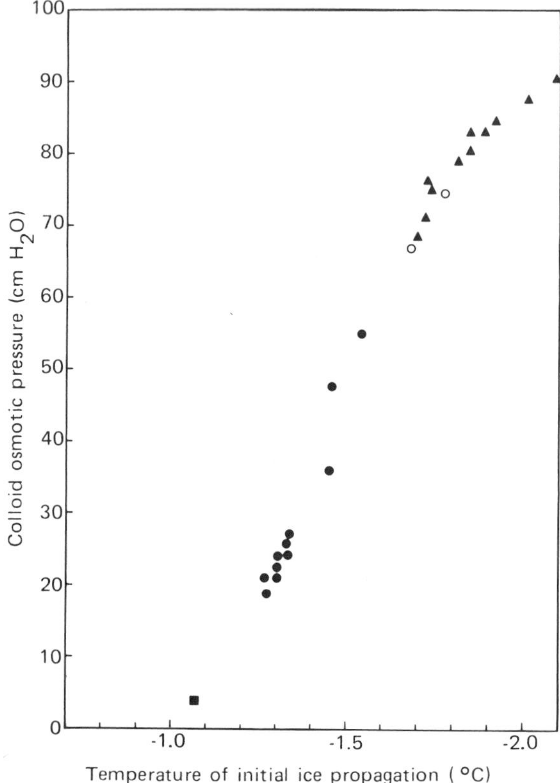

Figure 15 Temperature of initial ice propagation correlates with serum colloid osmotic pressures of Antarctic fishes. (From Hargens, 1972.)

that their high plasma colloid osmotic pressure provided these species with a natural "antifreeze" (Fig. 15).

D. Edema in Spawning Salmon

During the last leg of the 1968 *Alpha Helix* Expedition to the Bering Sea, we investigated tissue fluid balance in spawning Pacific salmon. By comparing freshly caught ocean specimens with those caught just upstream in rivers, the wick technique demonstrated that salmon become edematous during their spawning run (Fig. 16). The increase of tissue fluid pressure in all four species

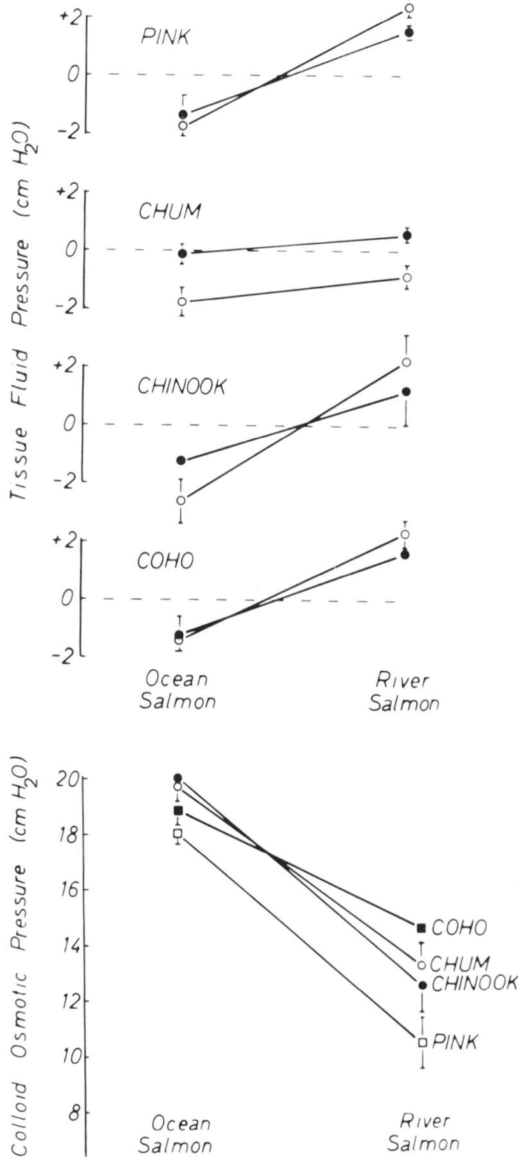

Figure 16 Top: Development of edema in four species of Pacific salmon upon migration from ocean to river water. Solid points are peritoneal fluid pressures and open circles are subcutaneous fluid pressures. Bottom: Loss of blood colloid osmotic pressure of Pacific salmon upon migration to spawning grounds. (From Hargens and Perez, 1975.)

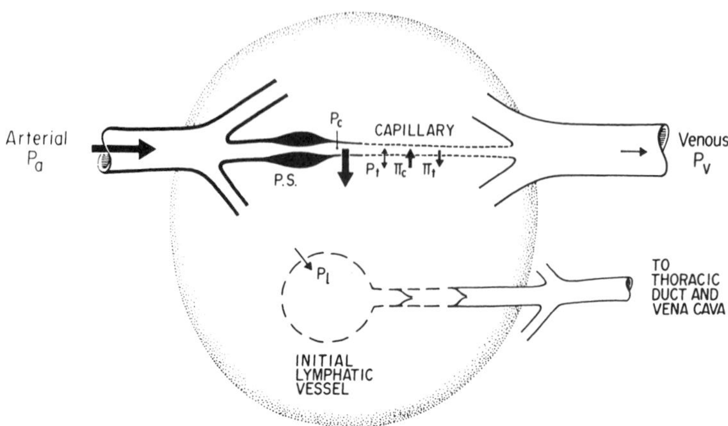

Figure 17 Fluid transport across capillary wall is determined by blood pressure (P_c), tissue fluid pressure (P_t) (positive or negative), blood colloid osmotic pressure (Π_c) and tissue fluid colloid osmotic pressure (Π_t). Capillary surface area and blood flow are regulated by precapillary sphincters (P.S.). Usually there is net fluid filtration out of the capillary, and this ultrafiltrate is returned through the lymphatic system. (From Hargens, *Handbook of Bioengineering*, Chap. 19, 1987.)

was probably caused by a reduction of blood colloid osmotic pressure, as measured by our simple field-type osmometer (Hargens and Perez, 1975). These results for Pacific salmon shed light on mechanisms by which transcapillary fluid balance is maintained. Basically, both blood and interstitial fluid have hydrostatic pressures as well as colloid osmotic pressures (Fig. 17). Although these pressures are greater in blood than in the interstitium, all four pressures are important for fluid homeostasis across the capillary membrane (Hargens, 1981). Interestingly, we found that animals with low blood pressure have relatively high capillary permeability to proteins (Fig. 18), thus reducing the gradient of colloid osmotic pressure $\sigma_p (\Pi_c - \Pi_t)$ across the capillary wall, according to the Starling equilibrium for transcapillary fluid transport J_{TC} (Hargens, 1981):

$$J_{TC} = L_p A[(P_c - P_t) - \sigma_p (\Pi_c - \Pi_t)],$$

where L_p = hydraulic conductivity
A = capillary surface area
P_c = capillary blood pressure
P_t = tissue fluid pressure

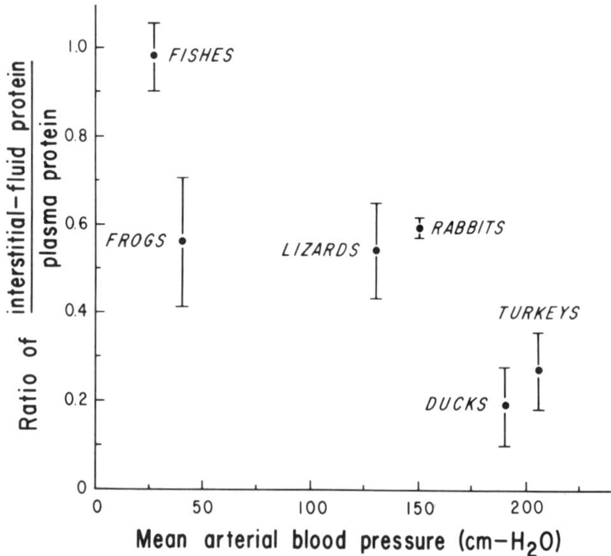

Figure 18 Reduction of tissue fluid/plasma protein ratio with higher arterial blood pressures in vertebrates. (From Hargens et al., 1974.)

σ_p = reflection coefficient of plasma proteins
Π_c = capillary colloid osmotic pressure
Π_t = tissue fluid colloid osmotic pressure

E. Normal Transcapillary Fluid Balance in Humans

Our initial comparative studies of Starling pressures in various animals were later extended to humans (Tables 1 and 2). In these studies, empty wick catheters were employed to collect 5-10 μl samples of interstitial fluid for measurement of colloid osmotic pressure. This technique was validated against other methods in subcutaneous tissues of normal human thorax (Fig. 19). We found that little or no suction in empty wick catheters provides the most reliable samples of interstitial fluid (Fig. 20).

F. Tissue Fluid Shifts Associated with Simulated Weightlessness in Humans

In 1979, NASA funded our Definition Phase Study for a Space Shuttle project to examine fluid shifts resulting from weightlessness. It is known that astronauts

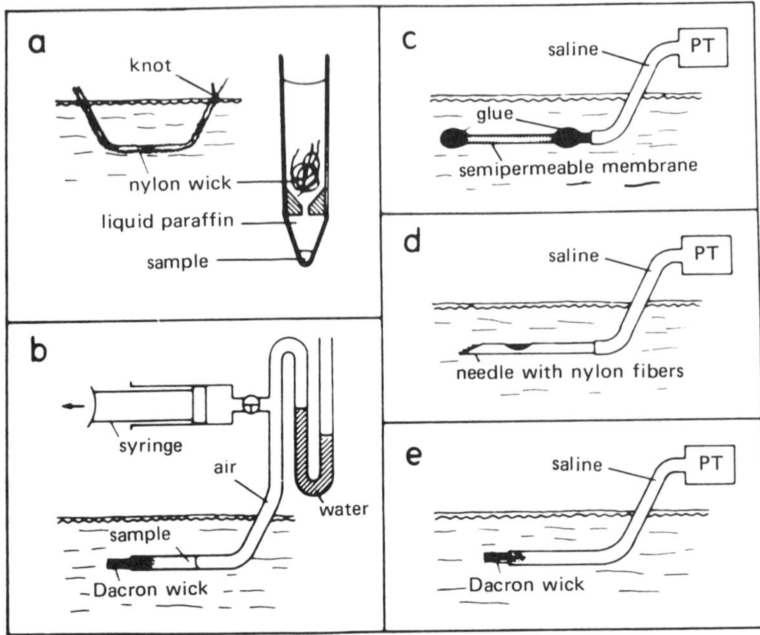

Figure 19 Methods of tissue fluid collection (a and b) and for direct measurements of tissue fluid colloid osmotic (c) and hydrostatic (d and e) pressures in human subcutaneous tissue. (a) Implanted wick, (b) empty wick catheter, (c) implantable colloid osmometer, (d) wick-in-needle, and (e) wick catheter. PT represents pressure transducer. (From Noddeland et al., 1982.)

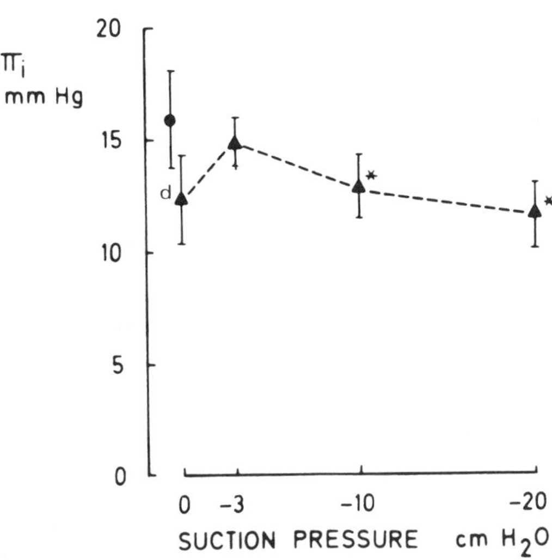

Figure 20 Effect of suction pressure on colloid osmotic pressure of tissue fluid (Π_t) sampled by empty wick catheters. Data identified by "d" were affected by dilution error. (From Noddeland et al., 1982.)

Table 1 Normal Transcapillary Pressures in Human Subcutaneous and Skeletal Muscle Tissues [Mean ± *SD*; (*n* = Number of Subjects)]

	Measured π_c (mm Hg)	Calculated π_t (mm Hg)	Measured P_t (mm Hg)	Measured P_c (mm Hg)
Subcutaneous tissue	27 ± 1.8 (19)	8.6 ± 1.0 (15)	-0.7 ± 0.4 (19)	29 ± 9.4 (6)[a]
Skeletal muscle tissue	27 ± 1.8 (19)	7.9 ± 1.2 (12)	2.2 ± 2.4 (19)	–

[a]Limited to measurements in fingernail-fold capillaries of six male subjects.
[b]Measurements of P_c were not attempted in skeletal muscle.
Source: Hargens et al., 1981.

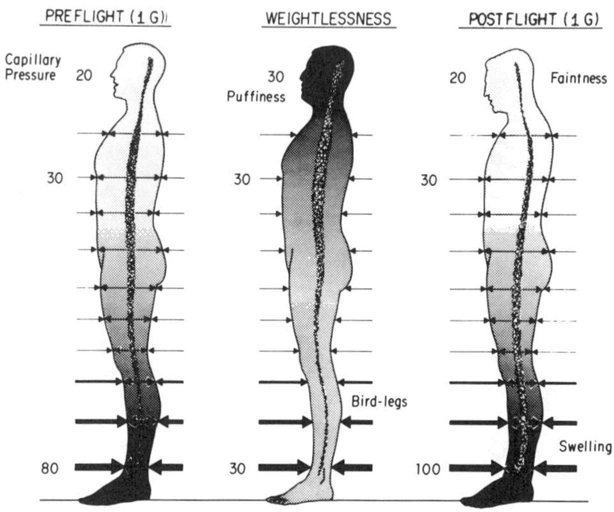

Figure 21 Hypothetical shifts in capillary blood pressure and tissue fluid during space flight and readjustment to Earth's gravity. Because weightlessness eliminates all hydrostatic gradients, blood pools in the central and upper veins and capillary blood pressure in the feet drops from 80 to 30 mm Hg. Facial edema and lower leg dehydration follow within hours. Upon return to Earth's gravity, precapillary smooth-muscle tone may be insufficient to prevent swelling and pain in the lower extremities by myogenic mechanisms. Thus, mean capillary blood pressure could rise to levels of 100 mm Hg or higher. Mean capillary blood pressure at heart level probably remains constant before, during, and after weightlessness. Each number represents a hypothetical capillary blood pressure at a given tissue level while standing during preflight, space flight, and postflight conditions. (From Hargens, 1981.)

Table 2 Normal Transcapillary Pressures in Subcutaneous and Skeletal Muscle Tissues of a Single Human Subject [Mean ± *SD*; (n = 6 Measurements)]

	Measured π_c (mm Hg)	Measured π_t[a] (mm Hg)	Measured P_t (mm Hg)	Measured P_c (mm Hg)	Calculated filtration equilibrium P_c (mm Hg)
Subcutaneous tissue	28 ± 0.6	9.1 ± 1.0	-1.3 ± 0.5	31 ± 11[b]	16
Skeletal muscle tissue	28 ± 0.6	8.3 ± 1.6	0.5 ± 1.5	—[a]	18

[a]Measured directly in 5-μl samples.
[b]Limited to fingernail-fold capillaries.
[c]Measurements of P_c were not attempted in skeletal muscle.
Source: Hargens et al., 1981.

experience headaches and facial edema during zero G exposure (Fig. 21), so we investigated fluid shifts and tissue fluid pressures in eight normal volunteers who were tilted head-down at 5° for 8 h (Fig. 22). Most of the initial loss of leg volume during head-down tilt represented a passive shift of venous blood toward the head. Facial edema, headache, and a pronounced diruesis were associated with this redistribution of blood volume (Fig. 23). As measured by the wick catheter, tissue fluid pressures of subcutis and muscle of the leg documented a significant dehydration of these tissues during simulated weightlessness. Thus, head-down tilt for several hours does change tissue fluid pressure but not to the degree expected from the induced gravitational pressure gradient. These results support and extend our original Amazon work concerning tilted snakes which were short-term studies of about 0.5 h in each position. Our recent human experiments provided evidence that head-down tilt represents a procedure that simulates many features of actual weightlessness in humans. Also, our techniques should prove useful to quantitate fluid shifts associated with weightlessness and subsequent readjustment to Earth's gravity.

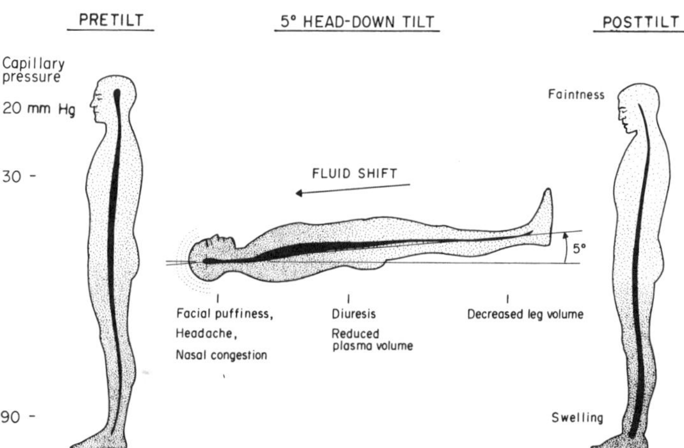

Figure 22 Summary of physiological responses to weightlessness simulation by 5° head-down tilt. Most of the responses depicted were documented in our 8-h study. The steep gradient of capillary blood pressure from head to foot during standing is probably lost during head-down tilt. Venous blood is immediately shifted cephaled upon exposure to head-down tilt. (From Hargens, 1983.)

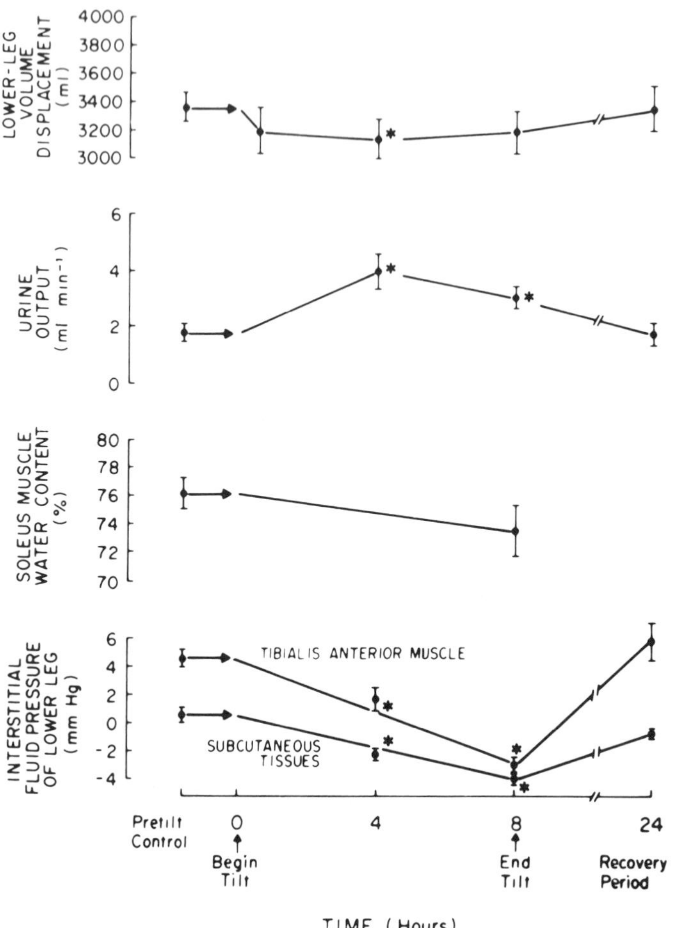

Figure 23 Significant fluid shifts during 5° head-down tilt are indicated by reduced volume (–190 ml) of lower leg, elevated urine output, decreased water content of soleus muscle, and decreased tissue fluid pressures in muscle and subcutis. *Denotes significant change ($p < 0.05$) from pretilt control. (From Hargens, 1983.)

G. Orthostatic Adaptation in the Giraffe

Recently we organized a physiological expedition to study orthostatic adaptation in the giraffe. The giraffe is unique in terms of extreme hydrostatic pressure gradients in its cardiovascular system. After capture in the field, transcapillary fluid pressures were studied in feet and neck tissues of four standing giraffes (3.1-3.5 m tall) sedated with 150 to 200 mg azaperone and 10 to 25 mg detomidine. Near the forelimb fetlock joint, mean digital arterial and venous blood pressures were 260 and 150 mm Hg, respectively, during upright position (Fig. 24). Carotid and jugular pressures were 110 and 16 mm Hg, respectively. Mean interstitial fluid pressures in the foot, as measured by subcutaneous wick catheters, were + 5.9 mm Hg at the fetlock joint and + 44 mm Hg under tight skin and fascia above this joint. Subcutaneous fluid pressure in the neck was + 0.7 mm Hg. Mean colloid osmotic pressures of blood, foot subcutaneous fluid, and neck subcutaneous fluid were 27, 15, and 1 mm Hg, respectively. However, interstitial fluid samples from feet were often contaminated by blood. As monitored by radiotelemetry, these pressures were highly variable with exercise and altered posture.

Calculating the transcapillary pressure gradients for a standing giraffe based upon our static results: $J_{Tc} = L_pA[(P_c - P_t) - \sigma_p (\Pi_c - \Pi_t)]$, where σ_p is very close to unity because giraffes have extraordinarily low protein concentrations and correspondingly low colloid osmotic pressures in their tissue fluids (see Fig. 24). Therefore, plugging pressure values into the Starling equation for the giraffe neck gives:

$$J_{TC} = L_pA[(20 - 1) - 1.0\,(27 - 1)\text{ mm Hg}] = L_pA\,(-7\text{ mm Hg})$$

and, thus, there is a net *reabsorption* pressure gradient in neck capillaries to prevent edema. However, performing the same analysis to our Starling pressure data for giraffe feet gives net *filtration* pressures of + 88 to + 152 mm Hg, depending on the capillary pressure and site examined in the leg. Thus, during upright posture, giraffes are prone to severe dependent edema because they maintain this position most of the day and night (we never observed them sleeping in a totally recumbent position).

However, our radiotelemetry results indicate that blood pressures and tissue fluid pressures vary greatly during normal ambulation. We even recorded some negative values for venous and tissue pressures in giraffe legs that deserve future, more detailed analyses. Therefore, another conclusion we made from this project was that fluid balance and other types of physiological studies in a stationary or an anesthetized animal may give a false or incomplete picture of underlying mechanisms that operate during normal exercise. In summary, our results suggest that edema is prevented in dependent giraffe tissues by: (1) rela-

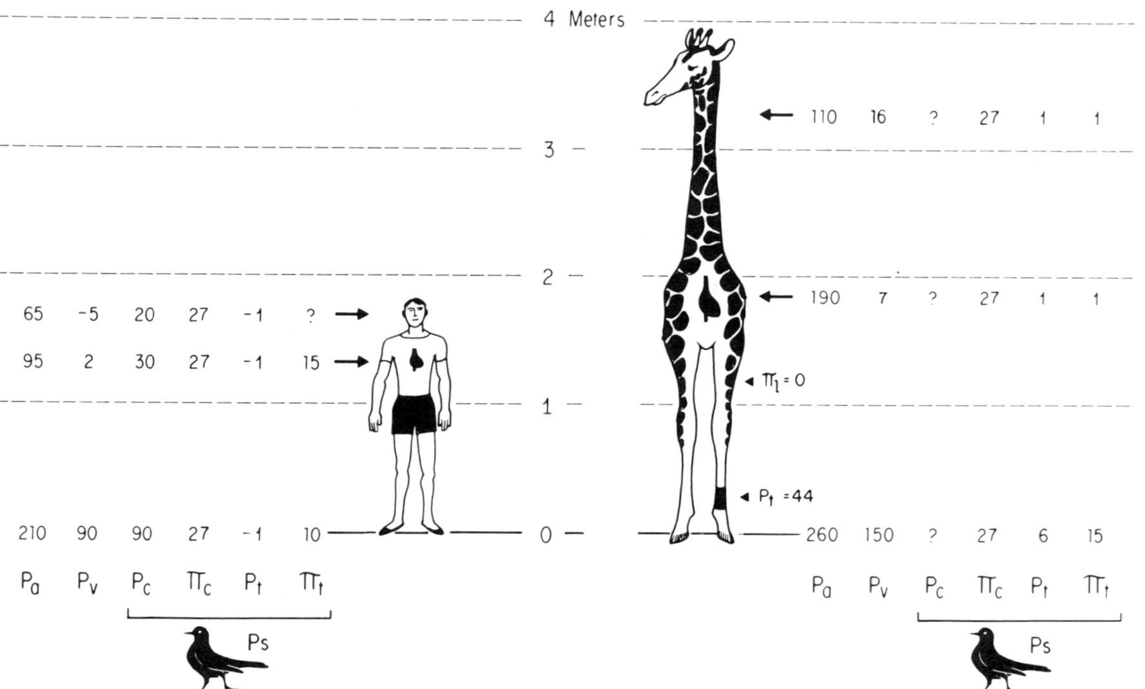

Figure 24 Meaned values for the four Starling pressures (signified by Starling birds) in humans and giraffes in the standing posture. Note that subcutaneous fluid pressure just above the giraffe foot averaged + 44 mm Hg, which is considered pathological in human tissues. This provides evidence that parts of the giraffe leg are wrapped by tight skin and fascia that act as a *g*-suit. (From Hargens et al., 1987.)

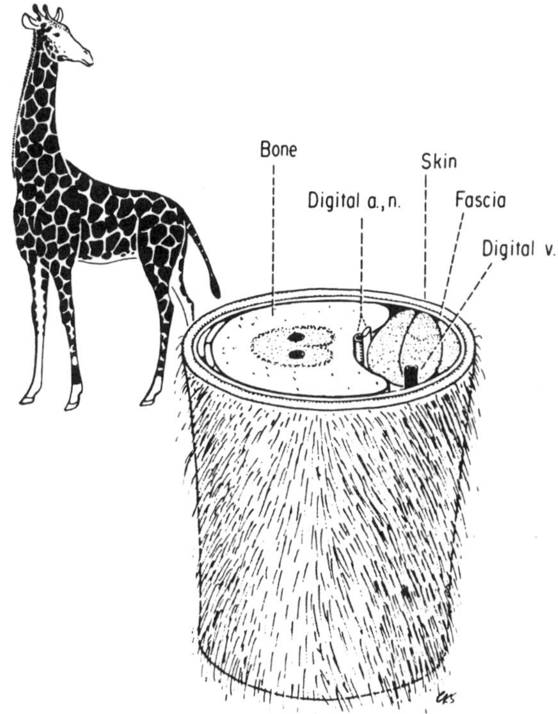

Figure 25 Tight skin and fascia that surround all major blood vessels and tissues of the leg probably act as a *g*-suit to prevent dependent swelling in the giraffe. (From Hargens et al., 1987.)

tively impermeable capillaries, (2) a *g*-suit effect by the tight skin and fascia of the leg (Fig. 25), and (3) altered transcapillary pressures with exercise.

IV. Colloid and Tissue Osmometry

A. Reduced Osmotic Pressure of Deoxygenated Sickle Cell Hemoglobin

In these studies our long-term objective was to improve treatment of patients with sickle cell disease by understanding volume control and oxygen transport of erythrocytes containing sickle cell hemoglobin (Hb S). Sickling of deoxygenated erythrocytes containing Hb S results from an aggregation of Hb S tetramers into a gel of long, multistranded polymers (Ross et al., 1975). The Hb S molecule differs from normal hemoglobin by a single amino acid substitution in each β-globin polypeptide chain (Ingram, 1956). This turns the erythrocytes into long, stiff convolutes. The major factors that promote high Hb S gelation are low oxygen tension and low pH (Briehl and Ewert, 1973). Distortion and stiffening of the cells, even though the erythrocytes are generally smaller than normal, give rise to many of the clinical manifestations of the sickle cell anemia.

Perutz and Mitchison (1950) proposed that Hb S cell volume is lost during sickling. Because the loss of water by cells containing Hb S would lead by itself to higher intracellular hemoglobin concentrations, both speed and extent of aggregation would increase as these cells are exposed to hypoxia. A unified reevaluation of the osmotic mechanism implied to us that the osmotic behavior of Hb S may substantially change during sickling.

The osmotic effect on Hb S was measured after oxygenation and deoxygenation in a wide range of concentrations obtained by a simple dilution procedure, going from 35 to 2.5 g of hemoglobin per 100 ml (Hargens et al., 1980). similarly, the osmotic behavior of normal hemoglobin (Hb A) was studied in its oxygenated and deoxygenated states in the same range of concentration.

Venous blood was drawn from subjects homozygous for Hb S or Hb A. The anticoagulant-treated samples were centrifuged at 1300 × *g* and washed three times with 0.9% NaCl. The packed cells were lysed in an equal volume of distilled water, followed by extraction of membrane lipids with an equal volume of chloroform. Cell debris was removed by centrifugation at 1300 × *g* for 15 min, and the hemolysate was carefully removed by aspiration. The resulting hemoglobin solution was dialyzed and concentrated, using a membrane with a molecular mass exclusion limit of 25,000. These purified hemoglobin solutions were concentrated to slightly above 33 g/100 ml and subsequently diluted to produce a series of hemoglobin concentrations from 35–2.5 g/100 ml. Each hemoglobin sample was placed in a glass tonometer and equilibrated at 22°C with humidified gas [PO_2 was 100 mm Hg and 0 mm Hg for oxy- and deoxy-forms, respectively; the remaining gas was N_2 (1 mm Hg = 133 Pa)]. During each measurement of osmotic pressure, the respective gases were continuously passed over the sample. Osmotic pressure in the purified Hb solution was measured in a simple, flowthrough gas colloid osmometer that combined membrane rigidity with accuracy to within 1 %(Fig. 26). A dialysis membrane with a molecular mass retention of 10,000 was stretched over a lens paper spacer and rubber support to maintain membrane rigidity so that osmotic pressures up to 500 mm Hg were measurable.

The osmotic pressure of normal hemoglobin, Hb A, was the same for oxygenated and deoxygenated Hb at all concentrations (Fig. 27). Furthermore, it

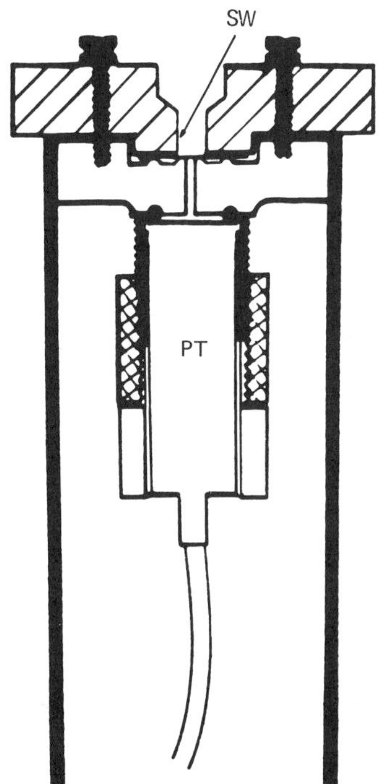

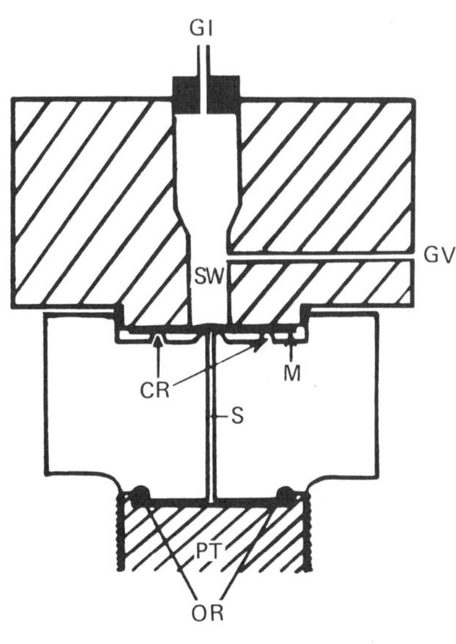

Figure 26 Osmometer for measuring Hb osmotic pressure. Left: Axial section of osmometer consisting of base attached to insulated and screw-down top with sample well (SW). Right: Close-up axial section showing O ring (OR) seal with pressure transducer (PT), saline-filled reference solution (S), compression ring (CR) to maintain membrane seal, and stretch mounted membrane (M), sample well (SW), gas vent (GV), and gas inlet (GI).

is clear that the osmotic pressures of normal oxy- and deoxyhemoglobin molecules increase more rapidly than an increase in their molar concentrations, the line labeled "van't Hoff contribution" in Figure 27. This deviation of osmotic pressure from the van't Hoff line is characteristic of large molecules.

The osmotic pressure of all oxy-Hb S samples (Fig. 28) was not distinguishable from the osmotic pressure of either oxy-Hb A or deoxy-Hb A at the same concentration. In other words, the curve for oxy-Hb S in Figure 28 will superimpose on the curve for oxy-Hb A and deoxy-Hb A in Figure 27. On the other hand, the osmotic pressure of all deoxy-Hb S samples was markedly less than for the oxy-Hb S samples (see Fig. 28). At 35 g/100 ml, a concentration

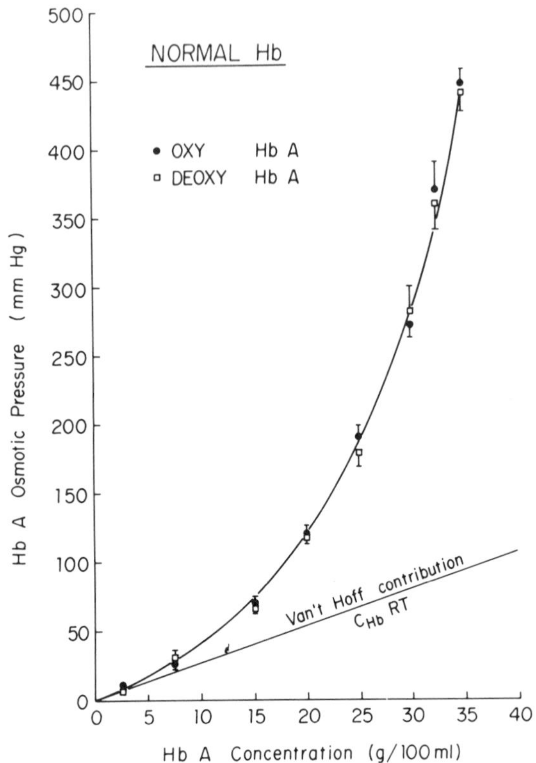

Figure 27 Osmotic pressure of oxy-Hb A (closed circles) and deoxy-Hb A (open squares) solutions as a function of concentration. Samples contained 0.05 M Tris-HCl buffer (pH 7.2), 0.1 M KCl, and 0.02 M NaCl, and were adjusted to an osmolality of 295 Osm/kg with distilled water at the beginning of each experiment. There is no significant difference between the two curves represented here and, in addition, there is no statistically significant difference between these curves and that shown for oxy-Hb S in Figure 28. Each point represents the mean of four determinations and the bars represent ± 1 SD of the mean. The magnitude of the kinetic, van't Hoff contribution to osmotic pressure is indicated by the solid line near the bottom of the figure, assuming hemoglobin has a molecular weight of 68,000. C_{Hb}, molar concentration of hemoglobin; R, gas constant; T, absolute temperature. (From Hargens et al., 1980.)

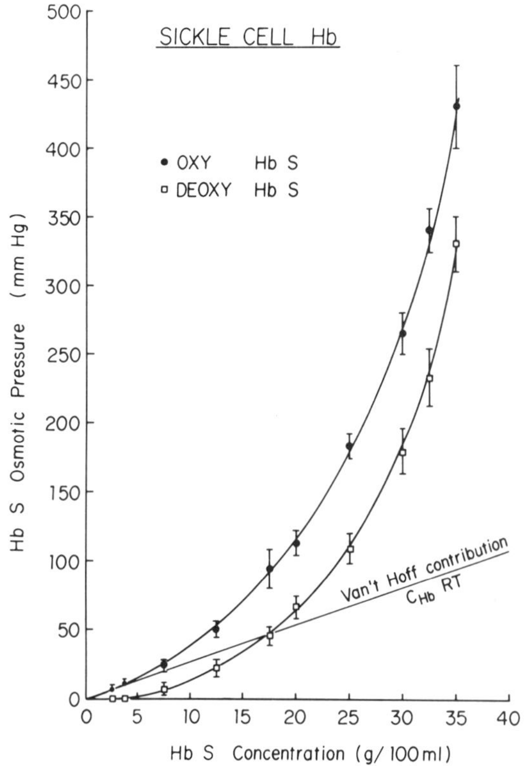

Figure 28 Osmotic pressure measurement on solutions of Hb S in oxy- (closed circles) and deoxy- (open squares) forms. Experimental conditions are the same as for Figure 27. Each point represents the mean of four determinations and the bars represent ± 1 SD of the mean. The broken line represents a regression plot of the difference in mean osmotic pressure between oxy- and deoxy-Hb S. (From Hargens et al., 1980.)

within physiological limits, osmotic pressure of deoxy-Hb S was approximately 100 mm Hg less than that for oxy-Hb S. At the lowest concentrations, the osmotic pressure of deoxy-Hb S was not measurably above zero.

With deoxygenation, the increased density and rigidity of cells homozygous for Hb S (SS cells) are probably caused by polymerization, lost random-translational (thermal) motion, and reduced osmotic pressure of Hb S tetramers. Under these conditions, the ability of hemoglobin tetramers to facilitate oxygen diffusion may be reduced or eliminated. Loss of Hb S osmotic pressure caused by polymerization of deoxy-Hb S probably decreases both intracellular water and facilitated diffusion of oxygen, initiating a vicious cycle of more polymerization, less osmotic pressure, less intracellular water, less Hb S translational motion, and less facilitated diffusion of oxygen until the deoxy-SS cell is transformed into a vaso-occlusive, irreversibly sickled cell. Thus, the pathophysiology of sickle cell disease may be primarily attributed to loss of translational motion and osmotic pressure of Hb S with deoxygenation.

B. Reduced Swelling Pressure with Hydration or Enzyme Treatment of Human Nucleus Pulposus

On the basis of studies of imbibition pressure in isolated samples of umbilical tissue (Hargens, 1981), elastic recoil or electrostatic expansion forces primarily cause a tissue matrix to swell when excess fluid is available. With elimination of electrostatic and associated Donnan effects between anionic charges in the matrix (by placing the tissue in a solution with high salt concentration), only a small shift of the volume-pressure relationship occurs. This suggests that electrostatic expansion (swelling) of glycosaminoglycan (GAG) macromolecules within the tissue matrix provides the primary mechanism for tissue swelling (Fig. 29). In an unstressed tissue matrix (Fig. 29B), the imbibition pressure of these macromolecules is balanced by the external loading pressure such that there is no fluid pressure gradient across the tissue boundary. Normally, therefore, GAG tends to swell and imbibe fluid, whereas this tendency is prevented by constraining properties of collagen and external loading pressures. If external loading pressure increases or imbibition pressure decreases by GAG loss (Fig. 29A), the matrix is compressed and fluid is lost. On the other hand, if external pressure decreases or imbibition pressure increases, fluid is absorbed (Fig. 29C). The intervertebral disk may be a tissue in which these fluid pressure-volume relationships apply. For example, Figure 29A could explain water loss from the nucleus pulposus during weight lifting (increased load) and Figure 29C could explain the swelling of the nucleus pulposus during sleep (decreased load). During abnormal conditions of severe dehydration or edema, any tissue can assume a compacted or expanded state, respectively.

The swelling pressure of nucleus pulposus depends mainly on fixed-charge density with lesser contributions from osmotic and excluded volume factors (Maroudas et al., 1985). Chemonucleotyic enzymes may reduce fixed-charge density by releasing sulfate groups of the glycosaminoglycans from the nucleus-annulus-vertebral endplate complex. Addition of water will also reduced fixed-charge density by dilution of sulfate groups.

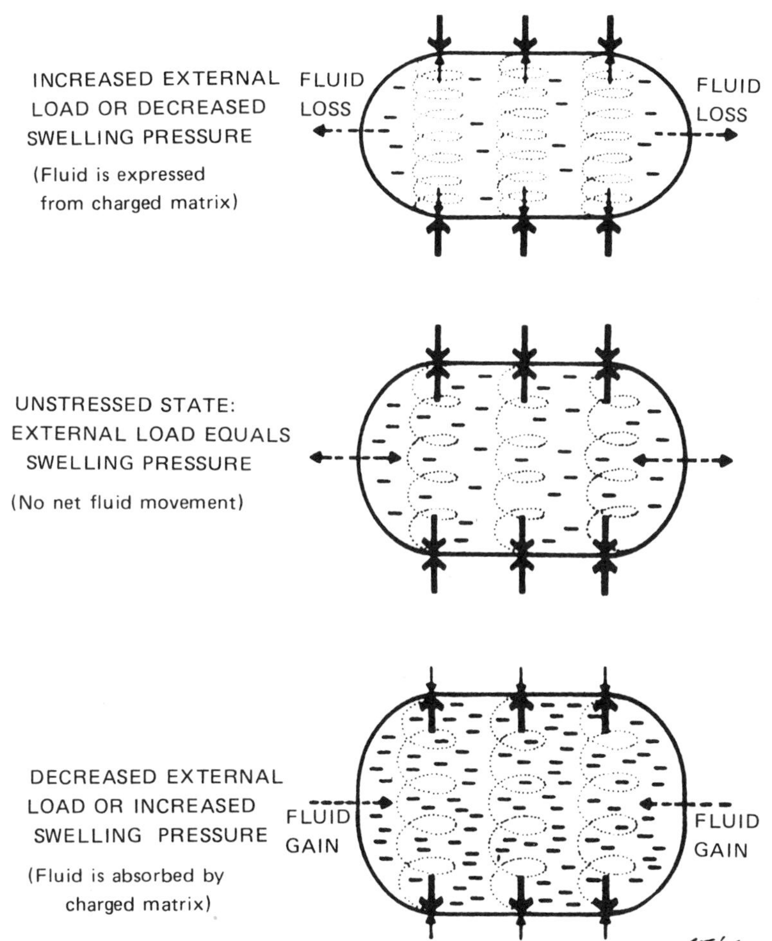

Figure 29 Relationship between external loading pressure, expansion pressure (swelling due to imbibition or osmosis), and tissue fluid pressure during compression (A), unstressed state (B), and expansion (C) of tissue matrix. (From Hargens, 1986.)

V. Summary

The two basic research tools developed to measure tissue fluid pressure (wick catheter) and osmotic pressure (colloid osmometer) have undergone extensive validation and refinement over the past 22 years. Using these techniques, we have undertaken basic science investigations of edema in Amazon reptiles, pressure-volume relations in animals and plants, adaptive physiology of Antarctic penguins and fishes, edema in spawning salmon, tissue fluid balance in humans under normal conditions and during simulated weightlessness, and orthostatic adaptation in a mammal with high and variable blood pressures—the giraffe. Following and sometimes paralleling this basic research have been several clinical applications related to use of our colloid osmometer and wick technique. Applications of the osmometer have included (1) reduced osmotic pressure of sickle cell hemoglobin with deoxygenation and (2) reduced swelling pressure of human pulposus with hydration or certain enzymes.

References

Adair, T. H., Hogan, R. D., Hargens, A. R., and Guyton, A. C. (1983). Techniques in the measurement of tissue fluid pressures and lymph flow. In *Techniques in the Life Sciences*, Vol. P3/1. Edited by R. J. Linden. County Clare, Ireland, Elsevier Scientific Publishers Ireland Ltd., 1-27.

Aukland, K., and Nicolaysen, G. (1981). Interstitial fluid volume: Local regulatory mechanisms. *Physiol. Rev. 61*:556-643.

Brace, R. A. (1981). Progress toward resolving the controversy of positive vs. negative interstitial fluid pressure. *Circ. Res. 49*:281-297.

Briehl, R. W., and Ewert, S. (1973). Effects of pH, 2,3-diphosphoglycerate and salts on gelation of sickle cell deoxyhemoglobin. *J. Mol. Biol. 80*:445-458.

Casley-Smith, J. R. (1982). Mechanisms in the formation of lymph. In *International Review of Physiology IV*, Vol. 26. Edited by A. C. Guyton and J. E. Hall. Baltimore, University Park Press, pp. 147-187.

Dixon, H. H. (1914). *Transpiration and the Ascent of Sap in Plants*. London, Macmillan, 216 pp.

Effros, R. M. (1984). Pulmonary microcirculation and exchange. In *Handbook of Physiology*, Section 2: The Cardiovascular System, Vol. IV Microcirculation, Part 2, Baltimore, American Physiological Society, pp. 865-915.

Granger, H. J., Laine, G. A., Barnes, G. E., and Lewis, R. E. (1984). Dynamics and control of transmicrovascular fluid exchange. In *Edema*. Edited by N. C. Staub and A. E. Taylor. New York, Raven Press, pp. 189-228.

Guyton, A. C. (1963). A concept of negative interstitial pressure based on pressures in implanted perforated capsules. *Circ. Res. 12*:399-414.

Guyton, A. C. (1976). Interstitial fluid pressure and dynamics of lymph formation. *Fed. Proc. 35*:1861-1862.

Hammel, H. T., and Scholander, P. F. (1976). *Osmosis and Tensile Solvent*. Berlin, Springer-Verlag, 133 pp.

Hargens, A. R. (1972). Freezing resistance in polar fishes. *Science 176*:184-186.

Hargens, A. R. (1977). Pressure-volume relationships in dehydrating animal tissues. *Comp. Biochem. Physiol. 56A*:363-367.

Hargens, A. R. (1981). *Tissue Fluid Pressure and Composition*. Baltimore, Williams & Wilkins, 275 pp.

Hargens, A. R. (1983). Fluid shifts in vascular and extravascular spaces during and after simulated weightlessness. *Med. Sci. Sports Exercise 15*:421-427.

Hargens, A. R. (1986). *Tissue Nutrition and Viability*. New York, Springer-Verlag, 312 pp.

Hargens, A. R. (1987). Interstitial fluid pressure and lymph flow. In *Handbook of Bioengineering*. Edited by R. Skalak and S. Chien. New York, McGraw-Hill, pp. 19.1-19.25.

Hargens, A. R., and Perez, M. (1975). Edema in spawning salmon. *J. Fish. Res. Board Can. 32*:2538-2541.

Hargens, A. R., and Scholander, P. F. (1969). Stretch mounting for osmotic membranes. *Microvasc. Res. 1*:417-419.

Hargens, A. R., Millard, R. W., and Johansen, K. (1974). High capillary permeability in fishes. *Comp. Biochem. Physiol. 48A*:675-680.

Hargens, A. R., Akeson, W. H., Mubarak, J., Owen, C. A., and Garetto, L. P. (1977). Tissue fluid states in compartment syndromes. *Recent Adv. Basic Microculatory Res. 15*:108-111.

Hargens, A. R., Akeson, W. H., Mubarak, S. J., Owen, C. A., Evans, K. L., Garetto, L. P., Gonsalves, M. R., and Schmidt, D. A. (1978a). Fluid balance within canine anterolateral compartments and its relationship to compartment syndromes. *J. Bone Joint Surg. 60A*:499-505.

Hargens, A. R., Scholander, P. F., and Orris, W. L. (1978b). Positive tissue fluid pressure in the feet of antarctic birds. *Microvasc. Res. 15*:239-244.

Hargens, A. R., Bowie, L. J., Lent, D., Carreathers, S., Peters, R. M., Hammel, H. T., and Scholander, P. F. (1980). Sickle-cell hemoglobin: Fall in osmotic pressure upon deoxygenation. *Proc. Natl. Acad. Sci. USA 77*:4310-4312.

Hargens, A. R., Cologne, J. B., Menninger, F. J., Hogan, J. S., Tucker, B. J., and Peters, R. M. (1981). Normal transcapillary pressures in human skeletal muscle and subcutaneous tissues. *Microvasc. Res. 22*:177-189.

Hargens, A. R., Millard, R. W., Pettersson, K., van Hoven, W., Gershuni, D. H., and Johansen, K. (1987). Transcapillary fluid balance in giraffe. In *Interstitial-Lymphatic Liquid and Solute Movement*. Edited by N. C. Staub, J. C. Hogg, and A. R. Hargens. Basel, S. Karger, pp. 195-202.

Ingram, V. M. (1956). A specific chemical difference between the globins of normal human and sickle-cell anaemia haemoglobin. *Nature 178*:792-794.

Ludwig, C. F. (1861). *Lehrbuch der Physiologie des Menschen*, Vol. I and II. Leipzig, C. F. Winter.

Maroudas, A., Ziv, I., Weisman, N., and Venn, M. (1985). Studies of hydration and swelling pressure in normal and osteoarthritic cartilage. *Biorheology 22*:159-169.

Noddeland, H., Hargens, A. R., Reed, R. K., and Aukland, K. (1982). Interstitial colloid osmotic and hydrostatic pressures in subcutaneous tissue of human thorax. *Microvasc. Res. 24*:104-113.

Perutz, M. F., and Mitchison, J. M. (1950). State of hemoglobin in sickle-cell anaemia. *Nature 166*:677-679.

Ross, P. D., Hofrichter, J., and Eaton, W. A. (1975). Calorimetric and optical characterization of sickle cell hemoglobin gelation. *J. Mol. Biol. 96*:239-256.

Scholander, P. F. (1972). Tensile water. *Amer. Sci. 60*:584-590.

Scholander, P. F., Hammel, H. T., Bradstreet, E. D., and Hemmingsen, E. A. (1965). Sap pressure in vascular plants. *Science 148*:339-346.

Scholander, P. F., Hargens, A. R., and Miller, S. L. (1968). Negative pressure in the interstitial fluid of animals. *Science 161*:321-328.

Starling, E. H. (1896). On the absorption of fluids from the connective tissue spaces. *J. Physiol. (Lond.) 19*:312-326.

Staub, N. C. (1978). *Lung Water and Solute Exchange*. Vol. 7 of Lung Biology in Health and Disease. Edited by C. Lenfant. New York, Marcel Dekker, 568 pp.

Taylor, A. E. (1981). Capillary fluid filtration. Starling forces and lymph flow. *Circ. Res. 49*:557-575.

17

Fluid Balance in Vertebrate Lungs

ALLAN W. SMITS*

University of Massachusetts
Amherst, Massachusetts

I. Introduction

The movement of fluid across capillary membranes has long been of interest to physiologists. Since the early interpretations of fluid filtration by Bartholin (1653), the relationship between plasma and lymph as demonstrated by Hewson (Gulliver, 1846), the significance of transcapillary pressures (Starling, 1896), to the modern day estimation of tissue water by positron emission tomography (Schuster et al., 1986), substantial efforts have been made to explain the transcapillary balance of fluid in tissues.

No other organ has kindled such interest in this regard as the lung. The lung possesses two extravascular compartments (interstitium and alveolus) in which fluid may accumulate (Fig. 1). Fluid build up in either of these spaces (called edema), particularly in the alveolus, may cause a substantial limitation to the diffusion of gases, resulting in severe respiratory insufficiency. Clinical interest in understanding the causes of pulmonary edema and, thus, the appropri-

---

**Present affiliation*: University of Texas, Arlington, Texas.

Research and writing of this contribution were financially supported by a Parker B. Francis Fellowship in Pulmonary Physiology.

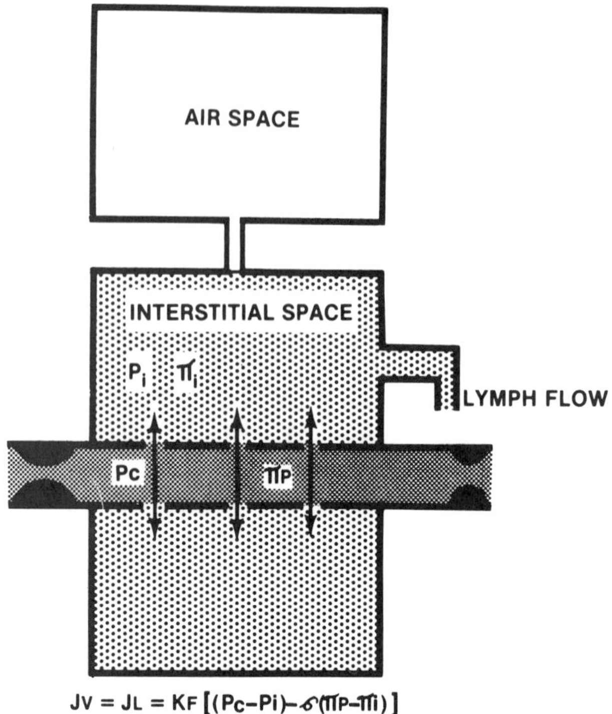

Figure 1 A schematic illustration of the mammalian pulmonary capillary-tissue-lymphatic system. The net transvascular fluid filtration rate (J_V) or lymph flow (J_L) is determined by the hydraulic conductivity (K_F) and protein reflection coefficient (σ) of the capillary endothelium, and by the four transcapillary Starling forces (see text). The alveolar epithelial membrane is highly impermeable to solute flux (compared with the capillary endothelium) and represents a high resistance to fluid movement into the air spaces. Regulation of P_c (and thus J_V) is determined by the precapillary/postcapillary resistance ratio as adjusted by local smooth-muscle tone of the arteries and veins. (From Malik, 1985.)

ate measures to reverse the tissue fluid imbalance has, by necessity, directed pulmonary research in recent times. The result is a substantial and rapidly growing knowledge of tissue fluid balance in the mammalian lung.

Unfortunately, in the apparent sparsity of data for nonmammalian vertebrates, the concepts of tissue fluid balance in mammalian lungs have been assumed to be applicable to all vertebrate lungs. Given the incredible diversity in pulmonary vascular architecture and physiology across the vertebrate classes, there is little basis for this assumption. Ironically, the basis for transcapillary fluid balance was initiated using nonmammalian models (Starling, 1896; Landis,

1926, 1927; Drinker, 1927). Research on nonmammalian vertebrates since those early studies, however, has largely been phenomenological.

Recent studies on the structure and function of pulmonary microcirculations in nonmammalian vertebrates have revealed fundamental differences in the way these organisms regulate fluid partitioning in their lungs. Although these differences represent exciting examples of vertebrate adaptation in their own context, they may also provide useful insights into the mechanisms operating in the balance (or imbalance) of tissue fluid in mammalian lungs.

This chapter presents the first comparative review of fluid balance in vertebrate lungs. Given that thorough and excellent reviews already exist for mammalian vertebrates (Staub, 1974, 1978; Taylor et al., 1985; Taylor and Rippe, 1986), I will discuss the similarities and differences in morphology and physiology of vertebrate microcirculation as a basis for explaining phenomenological differences in lung fluid balance between mammalian and nonmammalian vertebrates.

II. Determinants of Transcapillary Exchange

The rate and direction of fluid movement across capillaries is determined by two major factors; the algebraic sum of the fluid pressures on both sides of the capillary wall and the permeability of the capillary membrane to solutes. Integration of these factors by Kedem and Katchalsky (1958) into the well-known expression $J_v = J_L = K_f[(P_c - P_i) - \sigma(\pi_p - \pi_i)]$, represents the most currently accepted model of transcapillary fluid exchange, and is schematically shown in Figure 1. Dissecting this equation, we see the four Starling forces (in parentheses) which represent the hydrostatic fluid pressures inside (P_c) and outside (P_i) the capillary, and the colloid osmotic (oncotic) pressure in the capillary plasma (π_p) and in the interstitial fluid (π_i). The extent to which these forces are realized further depends upon the permeability of the capillary to proteins (σ; the osmotic reflection coefficient) and the hydraulic conductivity (K_f) of the capillary membrane to bulk fluid flow.

Three essential aspects of this relationship are that (1) the factors on the right-hand side of this equation rarely equal zero (causing lymph flow, J_L), (2) the Starling pressures are neither fixed nor independent of one another, and (3) the permeability of the membrane varies between tissues and may be modulated. Clearly, these considerations suggest that this equation be used as but a model of the complex forces governing microvascular fluid flux, for as we shall see, the diversity of lung architecture among the vertebrates is substantial (see Chapters 6, 7, and 8). The following discussion compares and contrasts the vertebrate groups with respect to the available information on the transcapillary fluid forces and capillary permeability. The significance of such comparisons will become evident in the later sections in which data on pulmonary filtration rates in conscious, resting vertebrates are presented and comparative role of the lymphatic system is reviewed.

III. Transcapillary Fluid Forces

A. Capillary Hydrostatic Pressure

The first reliable measurements of capillary hydrostatic pressure (P_c) in any tissue were made in the frog mesenteric capillary by Landis (1926). His ingenious yet simple experiments established the minimum pressure necessary to cause zero transcapillary flow (no filtration or absorption). Landis (1927) extended these measurements (using a micropipet and manometer) to demonstrate the now-familiar relationship between P_c and the rate of fluid movement across the capillary wall (Fig. 2). These studies provided the experimental basis for a wide variety of techniques that are now currently used to measure this basic relationship and its permutations in mammalian lungs. Isogravimetric perfusion of whole lungs (e.g., Guyton and Lindsey, 1959; Drake et al., 1978), vascular occlusion measurements (e.g., Parker et al., 1983; Townsley et al., 1986), and direct measurement via servo-null micropipets (Lai-Fook, 1981, 1982; Lai-Fook and Kaplowitz (1984) all indicate that P_c in lungs of mammals average between 8 and 10 mm Hg.

Unfortunately, direct measurement of P_c within lungs of nonmammalian vertebrates have not, to my knowledge, been made. Available evidence from anesthetized animals indicate that P_cs in lower vertebrate lungs may be similar to those in mammals. Maloney and Castle (1970) measured intravascular pres-

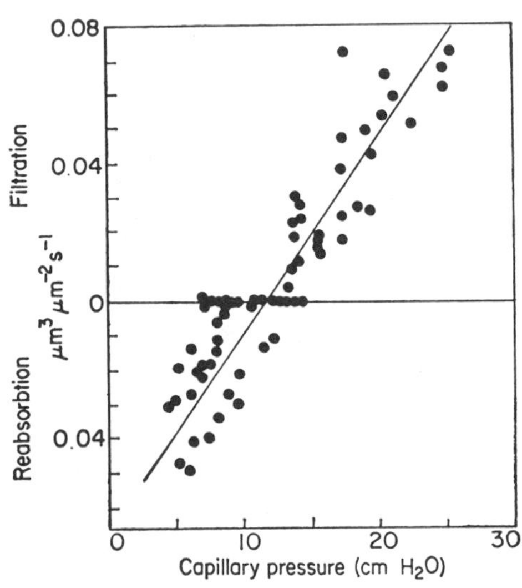

Figure 2 Net transcapillary fluid movement as a function of capillary pressure (P_c) determined by Landis (1927) in single capillaries of the frog mesentery. (From Michel, 1972).

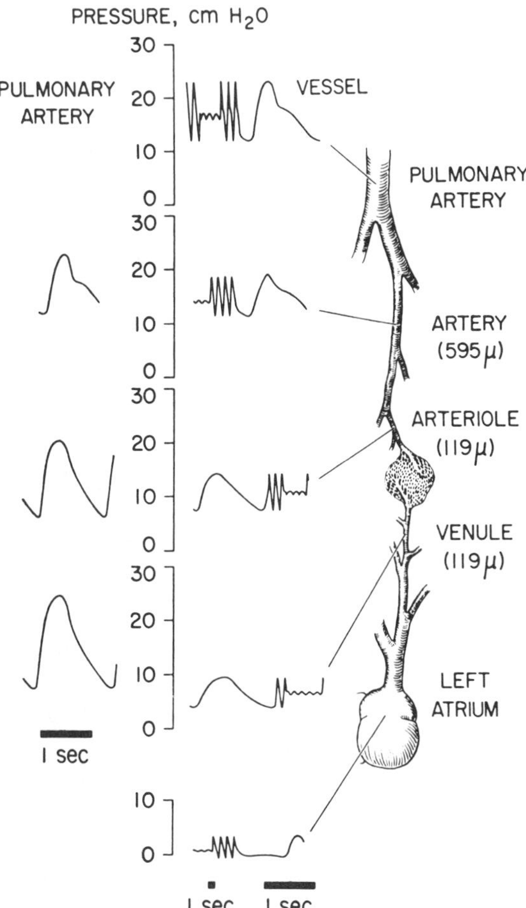

Figure 3 Dynamic intravascular pressures measured across the pulmonary vascular hierarchy of the bullfrog (*R. catesbeiana*), using servo-null micropipets. Simultaneously measured pressures in the pulmonary artery are shown on the left hand side of the figure. (From Maloney and Castle, 1970.)

sure on both sides of the pulmonary capillary bed in the frog (*Rana catesbeiana*) at a variety of arterial perfusion pressures (Fig. 3). At 20 to 25 mm Hg–the mean pulmonary arterial pressures known to exist in resting, conscious frogs (Shelton and Jones, 1968)–the mean arteriolar (ca. 10 mm Hg) and venular (ca. 8 mm Hg) pressures approximate the P_c measured in mammalian lungs. These estimates agree well with estimates of P_c made by Smits and West (unpublished data) on pulmonary arterial wedge pressure in *Bufo marinus* (7-8 mm Hg), and direct micropipet measurement of pressures in pulmonary arterioles (about 100 μm in diameter) of 8 to 10 mm Hg in *R. pipiens* (Smits, unpublished).

It must be emphasized that measurements of P_c in lungs of anesthetized vertebrates may not be representative of their normal P_c, and this may be particularly true for lower vertebrates. The undivided ventricle of amphibians and most reptile hearts is the single force generator that pumps blood to both systemic and pulmonary circuits in parallel (versus in series in birds and mammals). Hemodynamically, this means that blood pressures and flows in the common pulmonary artery may be similar to those in the aortas, and commonly exceed pulmonary arterial pressure measured in mammals by 10 to 20 mm Hg (Shelton and Jones, 1965, 1968; Johansen and Burggren, 1980). As but one example of this, pond turtles (*Chrysemys*) show a pulmonary arterial pressure at rest of 22/10 mm Hg (systolic/diastolic) and an incredible 60/22 mm Hg after activity (Shelton and Burggren, 1976). The degree to which these pressures are realized in the lung is under exquisite neural control by a vascular sphincter located in the extrinsic pulmonary artery proximal to the lung (see Chaps. 22, 23; Luckhardt and Carlson, 1921b; March, 1961; Milsom et al., 1977; Burggren, 1977; deSaint-Aubain and Wingstrad, 1979). This sphincter, now identified in numerous species of amphibians and reptiles, can produce variations in pulmonary blood flow, ranging from near zero to over 90% of the cardiac output.

However, because vasomotion of this arterial segment is cholinergically mediated through the vagus nerve, the neurally controlled tone appears abolished or heavily dampened in anesthetized animals. In *Bufo marinus*, anesthesia typically results in a complete dilatation of the sphincter and elevated pulmonary blood pressures downstream (West and Smits, unpublished). Clearly, this variable resistance upstream from the lung of lower vertebrates is a major determinant of the hydrostatic pressure realized at the capillary, and its influence must be seriously considered by comparative physiologists interested in the pulmonary transcapillary pressures in these lower vertebrates.

In contrast, the anatomical separation of the pulmonary and systemic circuits in birds and mammals permits the generation of lower pulmonary arterial pressures (10–15 mm Hg; e.g., Powell et al., 1985; Guyton, 1981). Thus, the distribution of vascular resistances *within* the lung might be comparatively more important in regulating P_c in mammals than in other vertebrates. Mammals exquisitely control P_c by adjusting both pre- and postcapillary resistance (see review by Dawson, 1984). Dramatic changes in P_c in the mammalian lung are also buffered passively (without neural control) by a relatively compliant and recruitable microcirculation, resulting in a decrease in pulmonary vascular resistance (PVR) when blood pressure and flow to the lung are elevated (Fishman, 1963; West, 1974).

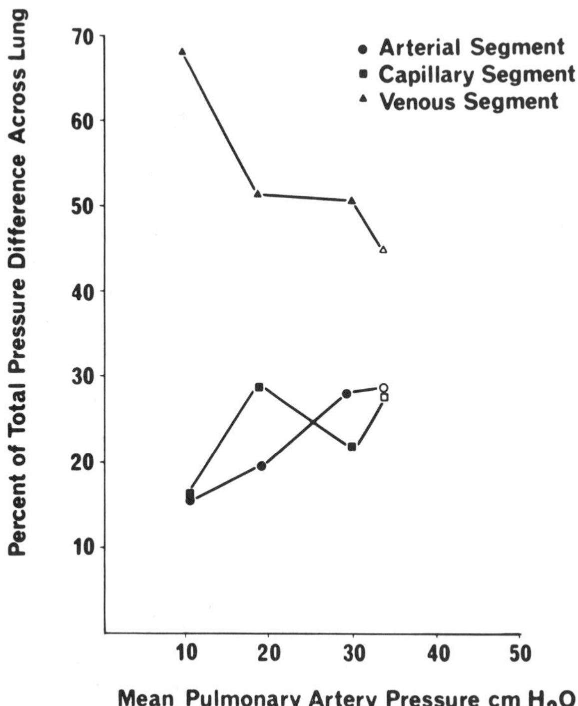

Figure 4 Contribution of the arterial (> 100 μm diameter), capillary, and venous (> 100 μm diameter) sites to the pulmonary vascular resistance (PVR) in the bullfrog (*R. catesbeiana*) lung, expressed as a percentage of the total PVR at various pulmonary arterial pressures. Note the dramatic decrease in venous resistance with increasing arterial pressure. Closed symbols: $P_{alv} > P_V$; open symbols $P_{alv} < P_V$. (From Maloney and Castle, 1970.)

Similar reductions in PVR in response to increased pulmonary blood flow (and associated pressure increase) have also been observed in amphibian lungs (Smits et al., 1986). In lungs of the frog, *R. catesbeiana*, the major pressure drop is apparently in the venous segment (Fig. 4; Maloney and Castle, 1970), rather than evenly distributed across the microcirculation as in mammals (Lineham et al., 1982; Michel et al., 1984). When pulmonary hydrostatic pressure is increased, the contribution of venous resistance to the total PVR decreases dramatically (see Fig. 4).

Indeed, the changes in PVR caused by the passive changes (distention and recruitment of capillaries) in the microcirculation may be representative of all alveolar-type lungs, given that the sheetlike architecture of microcirculation and

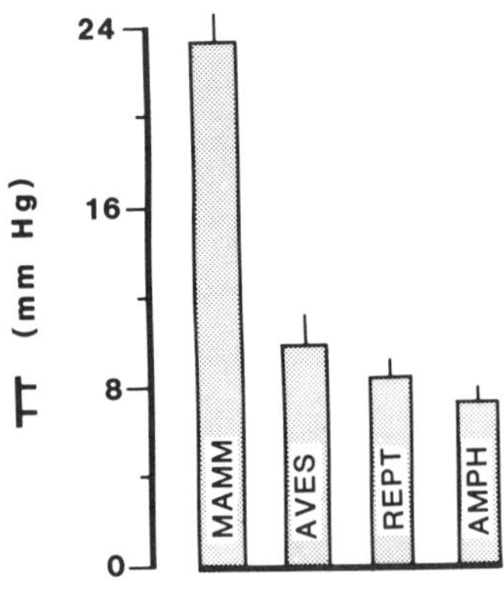

Figure 5 Mean colloid pressures (π_p) of blood plasma measured in four vertebrate classes. Vertical lines above bars represent the standard error for each group. Number of species (N) and samples (n) included in the analysis for each group are: Mammalia 56,58; Aves 3,3; Reptilia 8,8; and Amphibia 5,12, respectively. (From White, 1924; Krough and Nakazawa, 1927; Landis, 1927; Keyes and Hill, 1934; Campbell and Turner, 1937; Prather et al., 1968; Scholander et al., 1968; Zweifach and Intaglietta, 1968, 1971; Sturkie, 1954; Horowitz and Borut, 1973; Hattingh et al., 1980; Hillman et al., 1987.)

the vascular compliance are very similar across the vertebrate taxa (Maloney and Castle, 1969; Farrell, 1981; Farrell and Sobin, 1985).

Little is known about either active or passive circulatory resistance in the parabronchial bird lung. In distinct contrast to alveolar lungs, PVR is relatively insensitive to changes in pulmonary blood flow (Powell et al., 1985). Such an invariant PVR in bird lungs could result from a dominant and fixed resistance located proximal to the capillaries, or from a noncompliant microvasculature; however, neither of these possibilities has yet been demonstrated.

B. Capillary Oncotic Pressure

The presence of proteins (primarily albumin, globulin, fibrinogen) in blood and lymph imparts a colloid osmotic (or oncotic) pressure (π_p) to these fluids that opposes transcapillary hydrostatic pressure. The original and still useful relationship between the number and types of solutes and π_p was described by Landis and Pappenheimer (1963). In mammals the oncotic pressure of "normal" plasma (25-30 mm Hg subatmospheric) is typically sufficient to oppose P_c.

Despite the relatively meager amount of data on π_p in nonmammalian vertebrates, the available information clearly indicates that π_ps are not the same in all vertebrate groups (Fig. 5). All nonmammalian species (including birds) appear to have lower π_ps than mammals. Early observers (Landis, 1927; Michel, 1972) of this difference in π_p between mammals and lower vertebrates suggested that this correlated well with the differences in central blood pressure between the vertebrate groups, but birds appear to be the obvious exception that invalidates this argument. This difference in plasma oncotic pressure between mammalian and nonmammalian vertebrates also appears unrelated to the proportions of proteins in the different vertebrate groups. For example, Hillman et al. (1987) have recently shown that the measured π_p of plasma from toads (*B. marinus*) was not significantly different from a calculated π_p based on the equation derived by Landis and Pappenheimer (1963) for mammals.

Given the assumptions of the equation in Figure 1, the consequences of these differences in π_p between the vertebrate groups are very important and suggest three possibilities. First, the other three transcapillary pressures are sufficiently different (e.g., lower P_c and π_i, higher P_i) in nonmammalian vertebrates to compensate for their lower π_p. Second, lung microvascular permeability is substantially different among the vertebrate groups. Third, there is a substantially larger net filtration in the lungs (and other tissues) of nonmammalian vertebrates. The likelihood of each of these possibilities will be discussed.

C. Interstitial Hydrostatic Pressure

Measurement of the Starling forces on the interstitial side of the capillary have proved to be one of the most challenging goals in microvascular physiology (see Hargens, 1987). This is particularly true for the lung because (1) exposing the lung for such measurements disturbs the pressure-sensitive environment of the pleural cavity, and (2) the pericapillary interstitium that separates the vascular and alveolar spaces is too thin to permit accurate pressure measurements (Lai-Fook, 1981). Although measured values for interstitial or tissue fluid pressure (P_i) in mammals are variable and highly dependent on the technique, the animal, and the tissue location, it appears that P_i in nonedematous mammal lungs is typically 0 to 5 mm Hg below atmospheric pressure (Meyer et al., 1968; Lai-Fook, 1981; Taylor and Rippe, 1986). This is clearly the range of P_i over which interstitial fluid volume is maintained within normal limits in mammalian lungs (Fig. 6). Positive P_is appear coincident with large increases in extravascular water volume in these mammalian lung preparations (Parker et al., 1978; Taylor et al., 1981). Subatmospheric P_is are not unique to the lung, because subatmospheric pressures have been recorded in most other tissues, with the exception of skeletal muscle that is bound tightly by fascia (see Chap. 18 for review).

No measurements of P_i have been made in the lungs of nonmammalian vertebrates. Subatmospheric P_is have been reported for subcutaneous locations in toads (*Pipa americana*, Scholander et al., 1968; *B. marinus*, Hillman et al., 1987), frogs (*R. catesbeiana*, Stromme et al., 1969; Hillman et al., 1987), a lizard (*Iguana iguana*, Stromme et al., 1969), and snakes (*Boa constrictor*, Scholander et al., 1968; *Pituophis melanoleucus*, Stromme et al., 1969), and crocodiles (*Caiman niger*, Scholander et al., 1968). Whether or not a similar magnitude of negative pressure (favoring transcapillary filtration) exists in pulmonary inter-

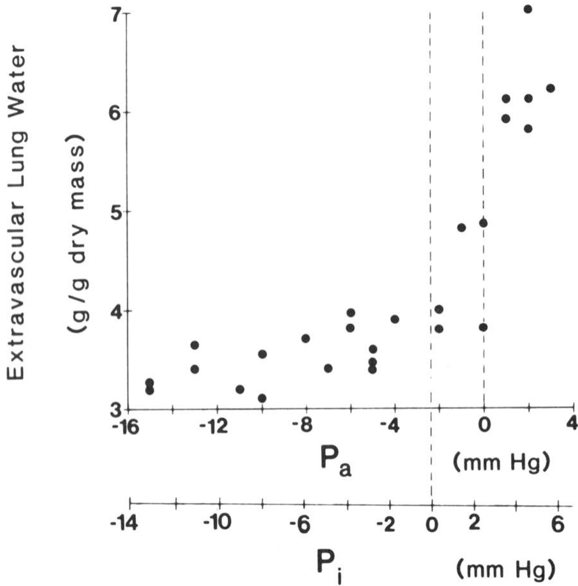

Figure 6 Changes in extravascular (interstitial) lung water in relation to the interstitial fluid pressure (P_i) and alveolar fluid pressure (P_a) measured by Parker et al., 1978. Note the large increase in lung water when P_i approaches zero.

stitia of birds and lower vertebrates remains in question. Alveolar-type lungs that are ventilated by aspiration (mammals, reptiles) would most likely follow this pattern because of the similar pressure gradient necessary to expand the lungs. However, because transpulmonary pressure has such a profound effect on P_i (Lai-Fook, 1979, 1981; Jasper and Goldberg, 1984), the interstitial pressures developed in the noncompliant bird lungs or the positive-pressure-inflated lungs of amphibians may be quite different.

The latter, involving amphibian lungs, represents a novel analogy to the controversial method of human respiratory therapy called positive end-expiratory pressure (PEEP). The PEEP therapy has been used to increase blood oxygenation in patients with severe pulmonary edema by maintaining a positive intrapulmonary air pressure throughout the ventilatory cycle (Ashbaugh and Petty, 1973; Cross and Hyde, 1978). Although PEEP does not appear to reduce the degree of extravascular edema (Staub, 1974; Van Der Zee et al., 1986), prevention of further edema and improved oxygenation may result from a reversal of the transcapillary pressures favoring filtration by an elevation of P_i (Cross and Hyde, 1978). Many amphibians demonstrate "natural" PEEP as they inflate and maintain lung volume using a positive pressure buccal pump. The changes in P_i, produced by intrapulmonary pressures of 0 to 5 cm H_2O, that are normally developed in lungs of frogs and toads (West and Jones, 1975; MacIntyre and Toews, 1976) are not known. However, experimental inflation of lungs of intact toads (*B. marinus*), resulting in an increase in intrapulmonary pressure from 0.5 up to 5 cm H_2O can reverse the net direction of transcapillary fluid flux from filtration to absorption (Smits, unpublished). Whether this results from elevation in P_i alone or from a general reduction in perfusion pressure through the Starling resistor effect has yet to be determined.

D. Interstitial Oncotic Pressure

Lung interstitial oncotic pressure (π_i) has perhaps been the most difficult of transcapillary forces to measure accurately because of the inaccessibility of true pericapillary or interstitial fluid. In fact, π_i at the site of filtration has not been directly measured (Taylor and Rippe, 1986). Rather, estimates of π_i in mammals are based on samples of lymph collected from lung lymphatics (Staub, 1974; Vreim et al., 1976; Staub et al., 1981), preferably from prenodal lymphatics (Staub et al., 1981; Adair et al., 1982; Taylor and Rippe, 1986). Given that π_i is highly influenced by (1) capillary permeability, (2) capillary filtration and lymph flow, and (3) π_p, it is inappropriate to assign a single value to π_i. The ratio of protein concentration in lung lymph to that of plasma (C_L/C_P) averages 0.75 in nonedematous, noninjured mammalian lungs. Thus, the π_i (based on the Landis-Pappenheimer equation and 7.5 g protein per 100 ml plasma) is approximately 18 mm Hg (Taylor et al., 1985; Taylor and Rippe, 1986).

To my knowledge, samples of interstitial fluid (or even lymph) from lungs of nonmammalian vertebrates have yet to be collected and assayed. Nonpulmonary lymphatic or interstitial fluid collected from a variety of nonmammalian vertebrates contains, on the average, comparatively less protein ($C_L/C_P = 0.2$ to 0.6; Hargens et al., 1974; Smits, 1986; Hillman et al., 1987) than measured in the interstitial fluid of mammalian lungs.

Regardless of the actual values for pulmonary π_i in nonmammalian vertebrates, the important consideration in lung fluid balance is the transcapillary oncotic pressure gradient. Because π_p averages only 8 to 10 mm Hg (effectively half that observed in mammals), any oncotic pressure gradient established across the capillary would amount to precious little. Thus, the $[\sigma(\pi_p - \pi_i)]$ term of the equation describing transcapillary fluid flux (Fig. 1) in nonmammalian vertebrates is comparatively small in contrast to mammals.

IV. Capillary Permeability

Although the previous discussion has shown how embarrasingly little we know about the magnitude of transcapillary forces operating in the nonmammalian lung, the literature is more enlightening in the area of microvascular permeability. In fact, recent studies on solute fluxes in frog lungs have been very instructive in describing the general characteristics of vertebrate alveolar epithelium (Gatzy, 1967, 1975; Kim and Crandall, 1982, 1983).

Important factors in capillary permeability include the characteristics of the capillary endothelium and alveolar epithelium, the ultrastructural basis for net water and macromolecular movement, and the net hydrostatic and osmotic forces involved. A full discussion of this complex subject is inappropriate to this chapter (for reviews see Michel, 1972; Granger and Perry, 1983; Taylor et al., 1985; and Effros et al., 1986).

In brief, the permeability of capillary endothelium in mammals has been largely defined by the hydraulic conductance (K_f, commonly called the filtration coefficient) and the osmotic reflection coefficient (σ). The K_f (in ml · min^{-1} · (mm Hg)$^{-1}$ · 100 g^{-1}), a weight-specific measure of fluid flow across the capillary as a function of the hydrostatic driving pressure, is comparatively high in lungs compared with other tissues in the body (Mortillaro and Taylor, 1983; Taylor and Rippe, 1986). However, if corrections are made for the higher capillary area in the lung, the hydraulic conductivity of lung capillaries is, in fact, as low or lower than skeletal muscle or intestine (Taylor and Rippe, 1986). The osmotic reflection coefficient (σ) is a unitless measure of the resistance of capillaries to the passage of proteins, and ranges from zero in highly permeable capillaries (e.g., liver) to a value of 1.0 in capillaries that are effectively impermeable to proteins (e.g., brain). The lung reflection coefficient for all protein (0.75) is typically low in comparison with other tissues (heart = 0.9, skeletal muscle = 0.95, intestine = 0.92; see table and references in Taylor and Rippe, 1986). Similar to other tissues with continuous-type capillaries, transcapillary movement of proteins appears to occur across two or more size-dependent pathways or "pores" with small (50–80 Å) and large (200–300 Å) radii (Blake and Staub, 1978; McNamee and Staub, 1979; Granger and Perry, 1983; Taylor et al., 1985; Parker et al., 1986).

There have been numerous studies on capillary permeability in amphibians (e.g., Danielli, 1940; Curry et al., 1976; Mason et al., 1977; Crone, 1979; Michel, 1979; Olesen et al., 1984). Unfortunately, they do not allow a direct comparison with mammalian literature because, first, the experiments concern permeabilities in nonpulmonary vasculature and, second, the techniques used (single capillary permeability) may provide substantially different results than "whole-organ" preparations. Given that capillary permeabilities may vary significantly between tissues of the same species (as noted earlier), it would be inappropriate and misleading to use these studies to make even the most general comparisons. Direct comparisons of endothelial permeability in vertebrate lungs await whole-organ estimates of K_f and σ in nonmammalian species.

Two indirect lines of research suggest structural similarities in both the endothelial and epithelial layers of the vertebrate capillary. Drinker (1927) and

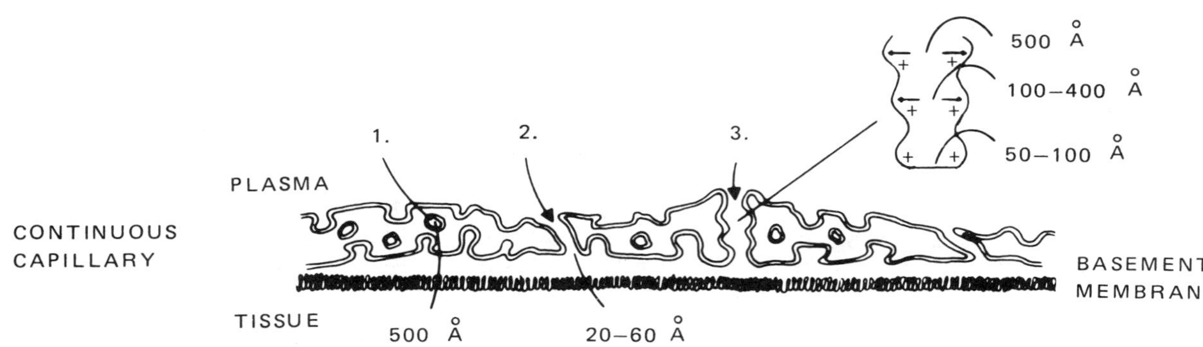

Figure 7 Schematic illustration of the mammalian pulmonary "continuous" capillary wall, indicating three routes by which solutes of various sizes (in Ångstrom units) might move across this barrier: (1) Plasmalemmal vesicles; (2) junctions between adjacent endothelial cells; (3) transendothelial junctions of variable width. (From Taylor and Granger, 1984, modified by Taylor et al., 1985.)

Danielli (1940) were the first to observe that certain protein or formed elements in the plasma were necessary to maintain normal permeability in the frog mesenteric capillary, independently of the colloid osmotic forces. These observations, confirmed by Landis and Pappenheimer (1963) and Renkin (1968), led to early hypotheses concerning a permeability-regulating interaction between blood-borne substances and the endothelium. The importance of such permeability modulation was seemingly "rediscovered" in frog mesenteric capillaries (Levick and Michel, 1973; Mason et al., 1977; Michel, 1979) and, more recently, in mammalian skeletal muscle and lung capillaries (Diana et al., 1980; Watson, 1983, 1984; Haraldsson and Rippe, 1984; Rippe et al., 1985). Because only small amounts of albumin (0.1 g/100 ml plasma) are necessary to maintain or restore normal hydraulic conductivity of the endothelium (Mason et al., 1977; Rippe et al., 1985), it is thought that albumin proteins (and possibly other types of protein) exert their effects by adhering to the walls of the endothelium or by interacting with the glycocalyx coating the endothelium (Curry and Michel, 1980; Turner et al., 1983; Curry, 1985; Huxley and Curry, 1985).

Although limitations in ultrastructural microscopy still prevent us from visualizing differences in exchange pathways in vertebrate pulmonary endothelium, the similar effect of albumin on both amphibian and mammalian endothelial permeability suggests a uniform pattern of capillary architecture among the vertebrates.

If the structure of the endothelium is comparatively uniform across vertebrate taxa, it raises some interesting questions about the effect of temperature on K_f and permeoselectivity of the microcirculation in lower vertebrates. Ectothermic vertebrates commonly undergo 10 to 20°C changes in body temperature on a hourly or a daily basis. These temperature variations can drastically change blood viscosity by as much as 2 to 3 centipoise (cp) (Langille and Crisp, 1980)! Such changes in viscosity not only alter the apparent peripheral resistance of the organ being perfused, but may have direct effects on the geometry of trancapillary membrane "pores." In the only study known to address this issue, Wolf and Watson (1985) found that the capillary filtration coefficient (a measure that represents the product of permeability and perfused surface area) in the perfused cat hindlimb decreased more in the cold (5-10°C) than could be predicted by the temperature-induced viscosity changes. Their analyses indicated that these effects most likely were due to changes in capillary permeability, specifically in the geometry of the protein-independent pathways for water movement. Considering the exponential effect of temperature on physiological processes, the effect of temperature on capillary permeability deserves more attention in the future.

More concrete evidence for structural uniformity is provided by studies of the alveolar epithelium, the boundary ultimately responsible for preventing interstitial fluid in the lung from entering the alveoli. As one might predict, the epithelium has been shown to be more resistant (less permeable) to solute diffusion than the endothelium, and this is true for lungs of both mammals (Taylor et al., 1965; Wangensteen et al., 1969; Taylor and Garr, 1970; Effros et al., 1986) and amphibians (Gatzy, 1967,1975; Crandall and Kim, 1981; Kim and Crandall, 1983). The pore radii (estimated by the diffusion rates of different-sized solutes) for mammalian and frog alveolar epithelia (0.6–1.0 nm and 0.8–0.9 nm, respectively) are in good agreement with and much smaller than the pore radius estimated for the pulmonary endothelium (7.5–15 nm; Wangensteen et al., 1969; Taylor and Garr, 1970). Multiple sizes of pores (heteropore populations) have been identified in both mammalian and amphibian alveolar epithelia (Theodore et al., 1975; Kim and Crandall, 1983); however, the population of large-sized pores (5–8 nm) appears to be minute in both groups.

The common features of capillary structure suggest that in both mammals and amphibians (and presumably other vertebrates) the alveolar epithelium is the major structural barrier preventing alveolar edema. Interestingly, these structural similarities have led some physiologists to promote the use of the anatomically simpler frog lung as a model for studying pulmonary edema (Kim and Crandall, 1982; Schaeffer et al., 1984).

V. Rates of Pulmonary Filtration

In light of the previous considerations of the hydrostatic and osmotic forces encouraging transcapillary fluid exchange and the structural basis for capillary resistance to this exchange, we shall now view the net result in terms of the fluid flux actually measured in vertebrate lungs.

For a long time, there has been indirect evidence that fluid movement between systemic intravascular and extravascular compartments is quite labile in lower vertebrates. Both Isayama (1924) and Conklin (1930) measured enormous rates of lymph production and recirculation in the frog. On the basis of lymph flows through the posterior lymph hearts in frogs, Isayama (1924) estimated that the entire plasma volume was recirculated 50 times daily! The high ratios of interstitial-plasma protein concentrations discovered in lower vertebrates by Hargens et al. (1974) have also been interpreted to reflect either high capillary permeability or greater filtration in these animals. More recently, hemorrhage experiments in the turtle *Pseudemys scripta* (Smits and Kozubowski, 1985) and the snake *Elaphe obsoleta* (Lillywhite and Smith, 1981; Lillywhite et al., 1983; Smits and Lillywhite, 1985) have shown amazing capacities for systemic transcapillary mobilization of interstitial fluid. Further, snakes have been shown to transiently filter up to 20% of their blood volume following brief locomotory activity (Lillywhite and Smits, 1984). Collectively, these studies indicate that, in comparison to mammals, amphibians and reptiles either have a great mis-

Table 1 Pulmonary Filtration Rates of Vertebrate Species[a]

Species	$ml \cdot min^{-1}$	$ml \cdot h^{-1} \cdot kg^{-1}$	Ref.
Toad (*Bufo marinus*) conscious, at rest temp = 20-22°C	0.21	43.8	Smits et al. (1986)
Toad (*B. marinus*) $n = 7$, BM = 0.29 kg, conscious, bilateral denerv. of pulmocut. baroreceptors	2.24	466.2	Smits et al. (1986)
Iguanid lizard (*Sauromalus hispidus*) BM = 0.55 kg, temp = 22-25°C; conscious at rest	0.87	94.9	Smits and Burggren (unpublished)
Varanid lizard (*Varanus exanthematicus*) BM = 1.75 kg, temp = 22°C; conscious, at rest	0.22	7.5	Smits and Burggren (unpublished)
Pond turtle (*Chrysemys scripta*) BM = 1.0 kg, temp = 22-23°C; conscious, volun. diving	0-2.0	0-120.0	Burggren (1981)
Dog BM = 22 kg, temp = 37°C; anesth., closed chest; spontan. breathing, RLD	0.043	0.12	Courtice (1951, 1963)
Cat BM = 4 kg, temp = 37°C; anesth., closed chest; spontan. breathing, RLD	0.009	0.13	Courtice (1963)
Rat BM = 0.3 kg, temp = 37°C; anesth., closed chest; spontan. breathing, RLD	0.002	0.33	Schooley (1958)

Table 1 (continued)

Species	$ml \cdot min^{-1}$	$ml \cdot h^{-1} \cdot kg^{-1}$	Ref.
Rabbit BM = 2.5 kg, temp = 37°C; anesth., closed chest; spontan. breathing, RLD	0.005	0.12	Hughes et al. (1956)
Sheep BM = 50 kg, temp = 37°C; anesth., closed chest; spontan. breathing, RLD	0.093	0.11	Boston et al. (1965) Humphreys et al. (1967)
Sheep BM = 35 kg, temp = 37°C; conscious, CMN	0.13	0.18	Brigham et al. (1974) Staub (1971)
Human BM = 70 kg	0.09-0.18	0.07-0.14	Blake (1978)

[a]Values for mammalian species were calculated from Staub (1974).
[b]Minimum and maximum values during apnea (diving) and breathing.

match between the transcapillary Starling forces, such that filtration is favored, or the capillary resistance to fluid movement is comparatively low, or both.

Does this lability of fluid exchange demonstrated in systemic tissues also hold true within the lungs of lower vertebrates? The available measurements of net pulmonary filtration in vertebrate lungs clearly indicate that it does (Table 1). Mass-specific comparisons of the net pulmonary transcapillary exchange demonstrate that these amphibians and reptiles filter fluid into the lung at rates that exceed those of mammals by two orders of magnitude!

The first evidence of this "wet lung" syndrome was demonstrated by Burggren (1982) in the aquatic pond turtle, *Chrysemys scripta*. Using the concentration of erythrocytes in blood samples drawn simultaneously from pulmonary arterial and venous sites as indicators of net transcapillary exchange, Burggren (1982) correlated changes in the degree and direction of pulmonary fluid exchange with the intermittent-breathing pattern (and associated hemodynamics) of these diving reptiles (Fig. 8). Large increases in pulmonary blood flow during breathing (common in many lower vertebrates) in conscious, voluntarily diving turtles resulted in as much as 20 to 30% of the fluid entering the lung being filtered and left behind in the pulmonary extravascular spaces. Sharp reductions in pulmonary perfusion during diving (apnea) reduced the rate of filtration to minimum levels and, occasionally, actually initiated net absorption. Pul-

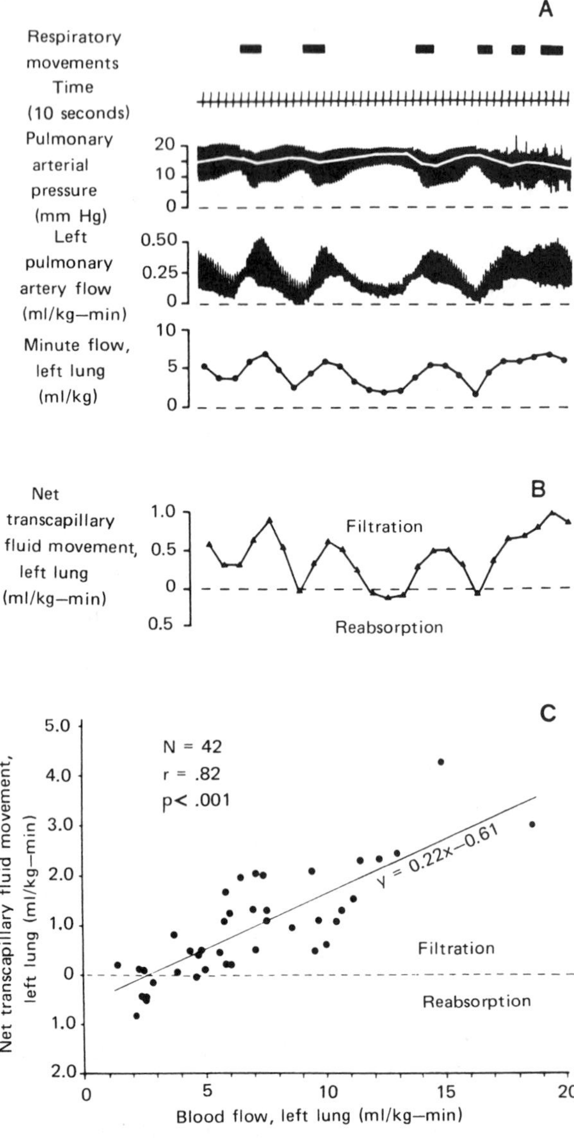

Figure 8 Pulmonary hemodynamics and respiratory movements (A) in a 1-kg aquatic turtle (*Chrysemys scripta*) during normal intermittent breathing, and the concurrent changes in net transcapillary fluid flux in the lungs (B). Note (1) the close correlation between the periods of ventilation, pulmonary blood flow, and lung filtration, and (2) the prevalent filtration bias. (C) Correlation plot of net transcapillary fluid flux and pulmonary blood flow in *Chrysemys*. (From Burggren, 1982.)

monary arterial pressure, measured close to the heart, was not significantly related to the degree of pulmonary filtration in this study. However, because of the variable impedance established by vasomotion proximal to the lung parenchyma (discussed earlier with regard to P_c), pressures measured proximal to the lungs may bear little relation to the pressures actually exerted at the capillary.

Recent support for this wet lung syndrome and the influence of pulmonary blood flow in filtration in turtles has come from similar studies on amphibians. Smits et al. (1986) found comparatively high rates of pulmonary filtration in resting, conscious toads (0.21 ml · min^{-1} in *B. marinus*; see Table 1). Further, they showed that the 10-fold increase in pulmonary filtration observed after baroreceptor denervation was most closely related to the increase in pulmonary blood flow that accompanied this experimental treatment. In light of Smith's (1979) study on *B. marinus*, indicating a vagally mediated control over the distribution of blood flow within the lung, Smits et al. (1986) have proposed that flow-related changes in net pulmonary filtration (induced by denervation of baroreceptor afferents carried in the vagus nerve) might best be explained by an increase in capillary recruitment. This recruitment would result in an increased P_c being applied over a larger surface area, ultimately increasing pulmonary filtration.

Considering the magnitude of these pulmonary filtration rates, one must question whether these animals tolerate incredible accumulations of fluid in the lung interstitium, or whether their pulmonary lymphatics are exceptionally effective. Evidence for the latter scenario is supplied by several studies. Turtles in Burggren's (1982) study alternated between states of pulmonary filtration and absorption in phase with periods of breathing and apnea, respectively (see Fig. 8). However, the very large net filtration that prevailed, if calculated on the basis of mammalian lymph flow, would reduce the turtle's blood volume by 70% in 1 h. Similar deficits in plasma volume resulting from net pulmonary filtration can be calculated for the toad, *B. marinus*. Denervation of the pulmocutaneous baroreceptors in the toad (Smits et al., 1986) caused pulmonary filtration to increase sufficiently (average = 2.24 ml · min^{-1}) to reduce the toad's plasma volume by 5 to 10%/min! Systemic hematocrit increased transiently during the initial stages of this filtration condition (indicating a net plasma loss), but returned to control values within 0.5 h. Clearly, neither the turtle nor toad could be expected to maintain any sort of circulatory or respiratory homeostasis if even a small proportion of the pulmonary filtrate remained in the lung.

Direct tests for pulmonary edema in toad lungs have recently been conducted in which fluid partitioning in lungs from control and pulmocutaneous barodenervate toads were made (Smits, unpublished). Extremely high pulmonary blood pressure and flow induced by barodenervation (three to four times greater than control levels) persisted for 1 h. Although lungs from barodenervate

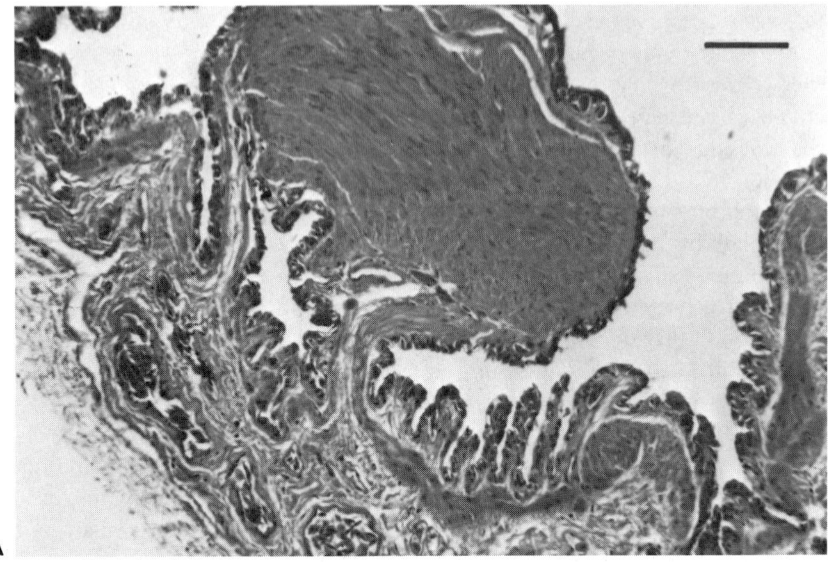

Figure 9 Photomicrographs showing lung structure in the sea snake, *Aipysurus laevis*, from a normal lung (A) and from the lung of a snake tilted 45° head-up for 20 min in air (B and C). Lung sections from the tilted snake exhibit numerous ruptured capillaries and an accumulation of erythrocytes within the foveolae. Sections were taken approximately 42 cm posterior to the lung apex. Size bars = 100 μm. (From Lillywhite, unpublished.)

toads had significantly higher total water and blood volumes than lungs of control toads, the interstitial volumes were similar. This is perhaps the strongest direct evidence yet that pulmonary lymphatics in these animals are very effective in preventing the accumulation of extravascular fluid. Recent studies by Van Rossum and Parsons (1985) on perfusion of the frog lung in situ also support this phenomenon of exceptional lymphatic return. Saline-perfused lungs of *R. pipiens* in their study did not become edematous, even in experiments in which the volume of pulmonary venous recovery was only 90% of the pulmonary arterial inflow. At their experimental perfusion rates and durations, nearly 4 ml of perfusate might have accumulated in these frog lungs that normally weigh less than 1 g! Such an accumulation, as tested by Van Rossum and Parsons (1985) by weighing lungs after the experiment, did not occur.

The only known case of pulmonary edema in lower vertebrates is that demonstrated in aquatic sea snakes by Lillywhite (unpublished). Histological examinations of the single lung of *Aipysurus laevis* following head-up tilting (out of water) indicate substantial accumulation of lung fluid and rupturing of

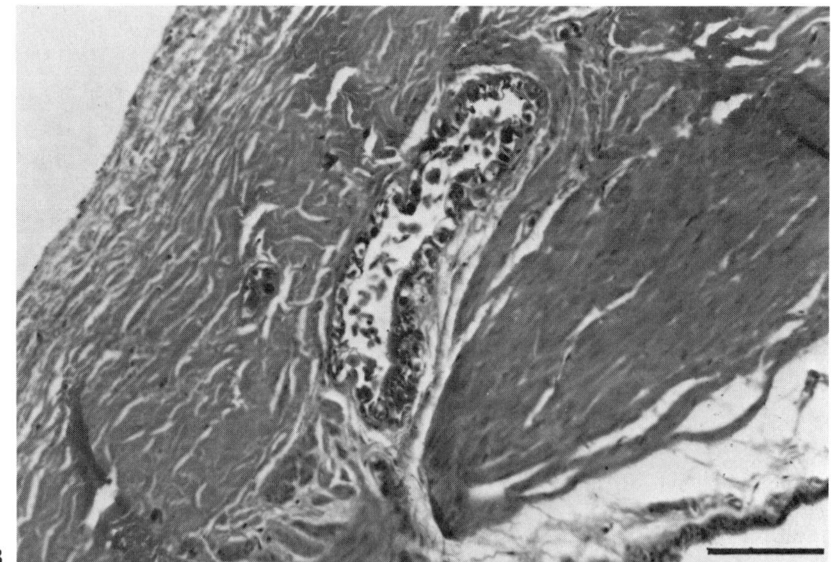

B

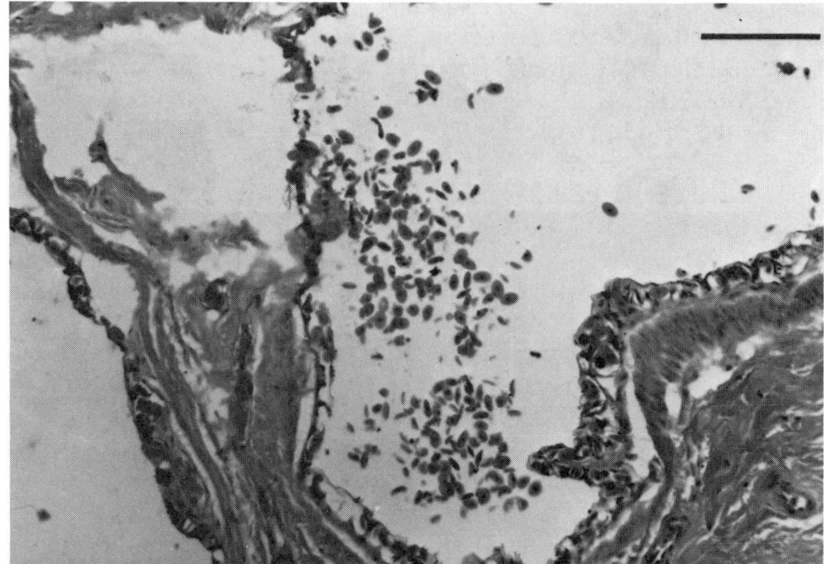

C

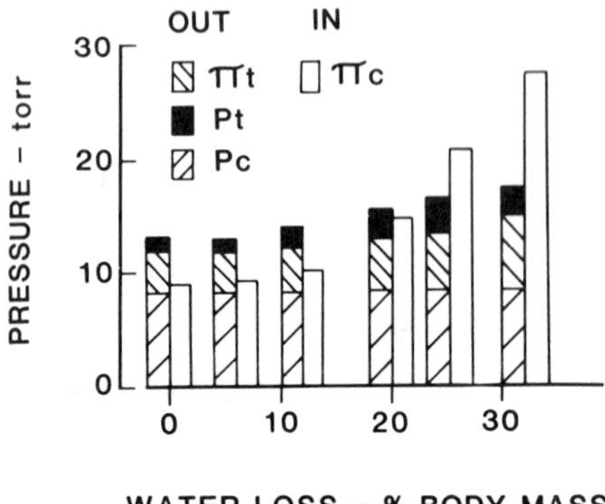

Figure 10 Summary of transcapillary forces in the integument of the toad (*B. marinus*) at various stages of dehydration. Note that the outward forces (favoring filtration) are not balanced by inward forces (favoring absorption) until body water loss exceeds 20% of the body mass. (From Hillman et al., 1987.)

capillaries, as evidenced by abundant erythrocyte accumulation in the lung foveolae (Fig. 9). Although this represents an experimentally induced and therefore unnatural edema, these findings illustrate how cardiorespiratory adaptations to an aquatic niche have influenced the physiology of lung function in these reptiles. In contrast to terrestrial snakes, these aquatic snakes have very low circulatory pressures, a less developed barostatic response, and possess a much longer lung that extends from the head to the cloaca (Lillywhite and Pough, 1983). The apparent net result of these characteristics when these animals are tilted head-up in the air is (1) P_c in the dependent lung vasculature increases because of the hydrostatic column of pressure in the lung pulmonary blood vessels, (2) there is a less effective cardiogenic capacity to maintain blood pressure and venous return, and (3) a hydrostatic gradient resists the flow of lymph away from the lung. These gravity-induced increases in transmural forces apparently do not develop when these snakes are at home in their aquatic environment (Lillywhite and Pough, 1983).

At present, this "filtration bias" in the lungs of these lower vertebrates is a newly described phenomenon, presumably based on a "mismatch" of the transcapillary Starling forces or comparatively high capillary permeability. The only study that has tested this hypothesis is that by Hillman et al. (1987), who measured transcapillary forces in nonpulmonary tissues of the marine toad (*B. marinus*) and the bullfrog (*R. catesbeiana*). Their estimations of the four transcapillary pressures (the first complete set ever for a lower vertebrate) show a clear filtration bias of 4 to 5 mm Hg (Fig. 10). Because their value for P_c was based on central venous pressure, the net transcapillary pressure gradient is probably underestimated by several millimeters of mercury. Interestingly, this net filtration in *Rana* and *Bufo* was not curtailed until these amphibians had lost over 20% of their body mass by dehydration. Clearly, the filtration bias demonstrated in the lungs of *Bufo* (Smits et al., 1986; see Table 1) might be largely related to the findings of Hillman et al. (1987) if a similar disequilibrium of Starling forces occurs in the pulmonary microcirculation.

VI. Lymphatic Return

The comparative study of lymphatics has its origins in excellent descriptive work on the morphology and physiology of lymphatic vessels and lymph hearts (Priestly, 1878; Gaupp, 1896; Isayama, 1924; Winterstein, 1925; Conklin, 1930; Kampmeier, 1969). These and more recent studies have stressed the importance of the lymphatics to circulatory homeostasis in response to a variety of circumstances ranging from the edema safety factor in mammalian lungs (see Taylor and Rippe, 1986) to the maintenance of blood volume during hemorrhage and dehydration in amphibians and reptiles (Middler et al., 1968; Smits, 1986; Hillman et al., 1987).

Unfortunately, little investigation of lymphatic function in the vertebrate comparative context has developed beyond these few observations, a situation apparently rooted in the difficulty of working on (or even visualizing) these translucent vessels. This paucity of data is particularly evident for the comparative structure and function of lung lymphatics and, thus, disappointing in the context of this chapter. All lunged vertebrates apparently exhibit pulmonary lymphatics as discrete vessels or perivascular spaces that largely parallel the pulmonary vasculature. In amphibians, at least, lymph may also flow directly into the peritoneal-pleural spaces into adjoining lymph sinuses (Ecker, 1889).

Based on the comparatively high filtration bias observed in amphibians and reptiles, differences obviously must exist in the capacitance of the lymphatic systems of these animals. Two differences in lymphatic design in lower vertebrates, which may explain lymphatic effectiveness, are large and extensive lymph sinuses and contractile lymph "hearts." Both amphibians and reptiles have capacious intra- and extracoelomic sinuses that serve as collecting sites or reservoirs for filtered plasma (Kampmeier, 1969). Two distinct examples of this are the subcutaneous lymph sacs of anuran amphibians (Carter, 1979) and the lateral abdominal lymph sacs of iguanid lizards (*Sauromalus*; Smits, 1986). By default, these compliant lymph sinuses bestow a comparatively high extracellular fluid volume (Smits, 1986). Historically, this has been interpreted as an adaptation to dehydration stress. However, this deserves reexamination in light of the comparatively high rates of transcapillary filtration.

Also unique within the lymphatic systems of lower vertebrates are lymph hearts; not simply enlarged, contractile vessels but discrete, pulsatile chambers under neural control that propel substantial amounts of lymph from the lymph sinuses back into the blood vessels (Isayama, 1924; Conklin, 1930; Baustian, 1986). The rapid onset of tissue edema and decreases in blood volume when

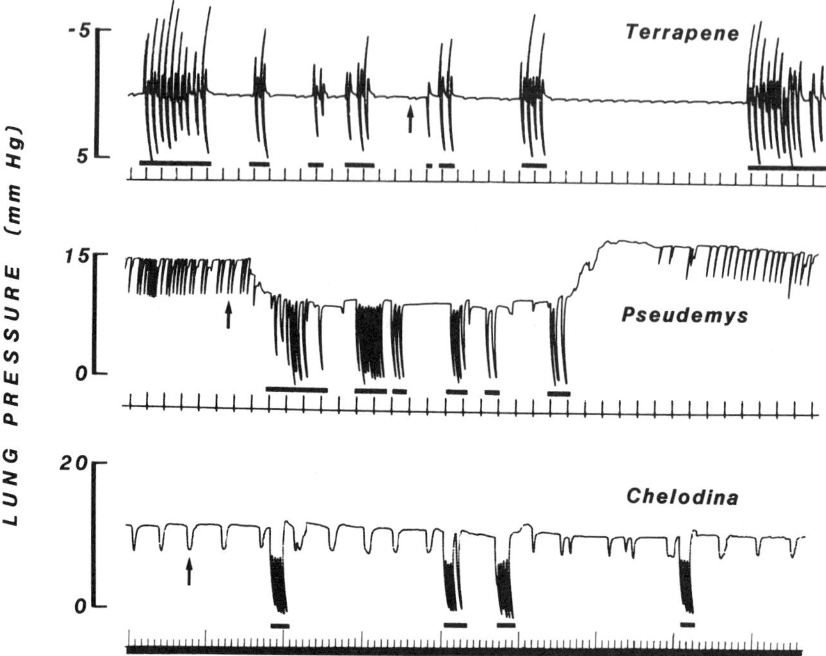

Figure 11 Changes in intrapulmonary pressure in three species of turtles (*Terrapene carolina*, terrestrial; *Pseudemys scripta*, aquatic; *Chelodina longicollis*, aquatic) resulting from ventilation (marked by solid lines) and from lung automatism during periods of apnea (marked by arrows). Time marks for the two upper panels and the lower panel are 10 s and 1 min, respectively. (From Burggren, Smits, and Evans, unpublished.)

these lymph hearts are chemically or neurally inhibited is well documented (Conklin, 1930; Zwemer and Foglia, 1943; Baustian, 1986). Lymph hearts are typically paired structures exhibited in both thoracic and sacral locations in amphibians and in only sacral locations in most reptiles. The size of these lymph propulsors also varies enormously from a few millimeter in most lower vertebrates to 11 mm (over one-fourth the body length!) in the frog *Breviceps* (Kampmeier, 1969). Clearly, these lymph hearts are essential in maintaining the recirculation of plasma back into the intravascular space; the direct importance of these lymph propulsors to pulmonary fluid balance has yet to be determined.

The mechanical events associated with ventilation of the lungs is also known to play an important role in pulmonary lymphatic return, at least in mammals (Staub, 1974; Aldelda et al., 1986). Many nonmammalian species of vertebrate do not breathe in regular cycles but ventilate their lungs intermittently. This is particularly evident in aquatic amphibians and reptiles that may remain under water for minutes to hours (see Shelton and Boutilier, 1982). Without the regular mechanical "massage" of the lung during periods of apnea, lymphatic return by mechanical assistance might be of minor importance. However, lungs of these lower vertebrates do not remain stationary during periods of apnea, but instead exhibit "lung automatism." Rhythmic contraction and relaxation (independent of the ventilatory cycle) occur in both excised lungs (Carlson and Luckhardt, 1920; Luckhardt and Carlson, 1921a; Tsuchiya, 1959) and lungs in conscious animals (Smits, Burggren, and Evans, unpublished). The frequency and magnitude of these lung movements appear to vary considerably (Fig. 11), and may induce changes in intrapulmonary pressure that exceed 5 mm Hg. The prevelence of smooth-muscle bands in the lungs of lower vertebrates (Jackson and Pelz, 1918; Berger, 1973; Smith and Campbell, 1976; Smith and Satchell, 1987; Chap. 6) and the apparent sympathetic and parasympathetic innervation of these bands (Burnstock, 1969; Berger, 1973; Nilsson, 1985) suggest that lower vertebrates have autonomic control over the contractile state of the lung. Whether or not the primary role of lung automatism is to facilitate pulmonary lymphatic return has yet to be demonstrated.

VII. Summary

This chapter has provided information from a rather diverse literature concerning factors that influence transcapillary fluid exchange in vertebrate lungs. Admittedly, many direct comparisons across the vertebrate taxa of the ultrastructure of the capillary membrane and the fluid forces operating across the pulmonary microcirculation are not yet possible. Particularly lacking is information about tissue fluid balance in the parabronchial bird lung.

From a phenomenological viewpoint, rates of transcapillary filtration suggest fundamental differences between mammals and lower vertebrates in the degree of transvascular fluid exchange. In the hemodynamically low-pressure lung of mammals, where capillary hemodynamics are largely regulated in the microcirculation, net filtration is normally comparatively low. In contrast, high pulmonary arterial pressures in lower vertebrates, attenuated primarily by vascular resistance proximal to the lung, may result in an extremely variable capillary pressure sufficient to induce pulmonary filtration rates substantially higher than those measured in mammals. The apparent lack of edema in lower vertebrate lungs suggests that very effective mechanisms of pulmonary lymph removal are present.

These exciting phenomenological differences now invite comparative pulmonary physiologists to work "inductively" to discover the specific differences in capillary permeability, transcapillary fluid forces, and lymphatic design among the vertebrates. Both in vivo and in vitro methodologies, similar to those already applied to the study of mammalian lungs, will provide the most efficient means to determine the taxonomic differences in pulmonary transvascular exchange. Future discoveries in the comparative physiology of pulmonary tissue fluid balance will be greatly facilitated by collaborative efforts between basic and applied pulmonary physiologists, with promises of numerous dividends to each.

Acknowledgments

I extend my sincere appreciation to H. Lee, L. Smith, and K. Smits for technical assistance, and to P. Kimmel and W. Burggren for critical reviews of earlier drafts of this chapter.

References

Adair, T., Moffat, D. S., and Guyton, A. C. (1982). Lymph flow and composition is modified by the lymph node. *Am. J. Physiol. 243*:H351-H359.

Albelda, S. M., Hansen-Flaschen, J. H., Lankin, P. N., and Fishman, A. P. (1986). Effects of increased ventilation on lung lymph flow in unanesthetized sheep. *J. Appl. Physiol. 60*:2063-2070.

Ashbaugh, D. G., and Petty, T. L. (1973). Positive end-expiratory pressure: Physiology, indications and contraindications. *J. Thorac. Cardiovasc. Surg., 65*:165-170.

Bartholin, T. (1653). Dubia anatomica de lacteis thoracis. Publice proposita. Martzan, Copenhagen.

Baustian, M. (1986). The contribution of the lymph hearts in compensation for acute hypovolemic stress in the toad *Bufo marinus*. Unpublished MS Thesis. Portland State University. June, 1986.

Berger, P. J. (1973). Autonomic innervation of the visceral and vascular smooth muscle of the lizard lung. *Comp. Gen. Pharmacol. 4*:1-10.

Bieter, R. N., and Scott, F. H. (1928). Blood pressure and blood protein determinations in the frog. *Proc. Soc. Exp. Biol. Med. 25*:832-834.

Blake, L. H. (1978). Mathematical modeling of steady state fluid and protein exchange in the lung. In *Lung Water and Solute Exchange*, Vol. 7. Edited by N. C. Staub. *Lung Biology in Health and Disease*. Exec. editor, C. Lenfant. New York, Marcel Dekker, pp. 99-128.

Blake, L. H., and Staub, N. C. (1978). Pulmonary vascular transport in sheep: A mathematical model. *Microvasc. Res. 12*:197-220.

Boston, R. W., Humphreys, P. W., Reynolds, E. O. R., and Strang, L. B. (1965). Lymph flow and clearance of fluid from the lungs of the foetal lamb. *Lancet 2*:473-474.

Brigham, K. L., Woolverton, W. C., and Staub, N. C. (1974). Reversible increase in pulmonary vascular permeability after *Pseudomonas aeruginosa* bacteremia in unanesthetized sheep. *Chest 65* (Suppl.):515-535.

Burggren, W. W. (1977). The pulmonary circulation of the chelonian reptile: Morphology, haemodynamics and pharmacology. *J. Comp. Physiol. B 116*:303-323.

Burggren, W. W. (1982). Pulmonary blood plasma filtration in reptiles: A "wet" vertebrate lung. *Science 215*:77-78.

Burnstock, G. (1969). Evolution of the autonomic innervation of visceral and cardiovascular systems in vertebrates. *Pharmacol. Rev. 21*:247-324.

Campbell, M. L., and Turner, A. H. (1937). Serum protein measurements in the lower vertebrates. I. The colloid osmotic pressure, nitrogen content, and refractive index of turtle serum and body fluid. *Biol. Bull. 73*:504-510.

Carlson, A. J., and Luckhardt, A. B. (1920). Studies on the visceral sensory nervous system. III. Lung automatism and lung reflexes in Reptilia (turtles: *Chrysemys elegans* and *Malacoclemys lesueurii*; snake: *Eutenia elegans*). *Am. J. Physiol. 54*:261-306.

Carter, D. B. (1979). Structure and function of the subcutaneous lymph sacs in the Anura (Amphibia). *J. Herpetol. 13*:321-327.

Conklin, R. E. (1930). The formation and circulation of lymph in the frog. II. Blood volume and pressure. *Am. J. Phsyiol. 95*:91-97.

Courtice, F. C. (1951). Extravascular protein and the lymphatics. *Aust. N.Z. Assoc. Adv. Sci. 28*:115-119.

Coutice, F. C. (1963). Lymph flow in the lungs. *Br. Med. Bull. 19*:76-79.

Crandall, E. D., and Kim, K. J. (1981). Transport of water and solutes across bullfrog alveolar epithelium. *J. Appl. Physiol. 50*:1263-1271.

Crone, C. (1979). Permeability of single capillaries compared with results from whole-organ studies. *Acta Physiol. Scand. 463*:75-80.

Cross, C. E., and Hyde, R. W. (1978). Treatment of pulmonary edema. In *Lung Water and Solute Exchange*, Vol. 7. Edited by N. C. Staub. *Lung Biology in Health and Disease*. Exec. editor, C. Lenfant. New York, Marcel Dekker, pp. 471-525.

Curry, F. E. (1985). Effect of albumin on the structure of the molecular filter at the capillary wall. *Fed. Proc. 44*:2610-2613.

Curry, F. E., Mason, J. C., and Michel, C. C. (1976). Osmotic reflection coefficients of capillary walls to low molecular weight hydrophilic solutes measured in single capillaries of the frog mesentary. *J. Physiol. (Lond.) 261*:319-336.

Curry, F. E. and Michel, C. C. (1980). A fiber matrix model of capillary permeability. *Microvasc. Res. 20*:96-99.

Danielli, J. F. (1940). Capillary permeability and oedema in the perfused frog. *J. Physiol. (Lond.) 98*:109-129.

Dawson, C. A. (1984). Role of pulmonary vasomotion in physiology of the lung. *Physiol. Rev. 64*:544–616.

Diana, J. N., Keith, B. J., and Fleming, B. P. (1980). Influence of macromolecules on capillary filtration coefficients in isolated dog hindlimbs. *Microvasc. Res. 20*:106–107 (abstr.).

Drake, R. E., Gaar, K. A., and Taylor, A. E. (1978). Estimation of the filtration coefficient of pulmonary exchange vessels. *Am. J. Physiol. 234*:H266–H274.

Drinker, C. K. (1927). The permeability and diameter of the capillaries in the web of the brown frog (*Rana temporaria*) when perfused with solutions containing pituitary extract and horse serum. *J. Physiol. (Lond.) 63*:249–269.

Ecker, A. (1889). *The Anatomy of the Frog*. (Translation by G. Haslan). Oxford, Clarendon Press. 449 pp.

Effros, R. M., Mason, G. R., Silverman, P., Reid, E., and Hukkanen, J. (1986). Movement of ions and small solutes across endothelium and epithelium of perfused rabbit lungs. *J. Appl. Physiol. 60*:100–107.

Farrell, A. P. (1981). Relations between capillary dimensions and transmural pressure in the turtle lung. *Respir. Physiol. 45*:13–24.

Farrell, A. P., and Sobin, S. S. (1985). Sheet blood flow: Its application in predicting shunts in respiratory systems. In: *Cardiovasculat Shunts: Phylogenetic, Ontogenetic and Clinical Aspects*. Edited by K. Johansen and W. Burggren. Munksgaard, Copenhagen. pp. 269–278.

Fishman, A. P. (1963). Dynamics of the pulmonary circulation. In *Handbook of Physiology*. Vol. 2, Sec. 2. Circulation. Washington, American Physiological Society, pp. 1667–1743.

Gatzy, J. T. (1967). Bioelectric properties of the isolated amphibian lung. *Am. J. Physiol. 213*:425–431.

Gatzy, J. T. (1975). Ion transport across the excised bullfrog lung. *Am. J. Physiol. 228*:1162–1171.

Gaupp, E. (1896). In *Anatomie des Frosches*. Edited by A. Eckers and R. Wiedersheim. Braunschweig, F. Vieweg und Sohn.

Granger, D. N., and Perry, M. A. (1983). Permeability characteristics of the microcirculation. In *The Physiology and Pharmacology of the Microcirculation*, Vol. 1. Edited by N. A. Mortillaro. New York, Academic Press, pp. 157–208.

Gulliver, G. (1846). The works of William Hewson, FRS, edited with an introduction and notes. London, Sydenham Society.

Guyton, A. C., and Lindsey, A. E. (1959). Effect of elevated left atrial pressure and decreased plasma protein concentration on the development of pulmonary edema. *Circ. Res. 7*:649–657.

Guyton, A. C. (1981). *Textbook of Medical Physiology*, 6th ed. Philadelphia, W. B. Saunders, 1704 pp.

Haraldsson, B., and Rippe, B. (1984). Higher albumin clearance in rat hind-quarters perfused with pure albumin solution than with serum as perfusate. *Acta Physiol. Scand. 122*:93-95.

Hargens, A. R., Millard, R. W., and Johansen, K. (1974). High capillary permeability in fishes. *Comp. Biochem. Physiol. A 48*:675-680.

Hattingh, J., DeVos, V., Bomzon, L., Marcus, E., Jooste, C., and Chertkow, S. (1980). Comparative physiology of colloid osmotic pressure. *Comp. Biochem. Physiol. A 67*:203-206.

Hillman, S. S., Zygmunt, A., and Baustian, M. (1987). Transcapillary fluid forces during dehydration in two amphibians. *Physiol. Zool. 60*:339-345.

Horowitz, M., and Borut, A. (1973). Blood volume regulation in dehydrated rodents: Plasma colloid osmotic pressure, total osmotic pressure and electrolytes. *Comp. Biochem. Physiol. A 44*:1261-1265.

Hughes, R. A., May, A. J., and Widdecombe, J. C. (1956). The output of lymphocytes from the lymphatic system of the rabbit. *J. Physiol. (Lond.) 132*:384-389.

Humphreys, P. W., Normand, I. C. S., Reynolds, E. O. R., and Strang, L. B. (1967). Pulmonary lymph flow and the uptake of liquid from the lungs of the lamb at the start of breathing. *J. Physiol. (Lond.) 193*:1-29.

Huxley, V. H., and Curry, F. E. (1985). Albumin modulation of capillary permeability: Test of an adsorption mechanism. *Am. J. Physiol. 248*:H264-H273.

Isayama, S. (1924). Uber die Geschwindigkeit des Flussigkeitsanstauches zwischen Blut und Gewebe. *Z. Biol. 82*:101-106.

Jackson, D. E., and Pelz, M. D. (1918). A contribution to the physiology and pharmacology of chelonian lungs. *J. Lab. Clin. Med. 3*:344-347.

Jasper, A. C., and Goldberg, H. S. (1984). Change in extra-alveolar perimicrovascular pressure with lung inflation. *J. Appl. Physiol. 57*:772-776.

Johansen, K., and Burggren, W. W. (1980). Cardiovascular function in lower vertebrates. In *Hearts and Heart-Like Organs*, Vol. 1. Edited by G. H. Bourne. New York, Academic Press, pp. 61-117.

Kampmeier, O. F. (1969). *Evolution and Comparative Morphology of the Lymphatic System*. Springfield, Charles C. Thomas, 375 pp.

Kedem, O., and Katchalsky, A. (1958).Thermodynamic analysis of the permeability of biological membranes to nonelectrolytes. *Biochim. Biophys. Acta 27*: 229-246.

Keyes, A., and Hill, R. M. (1934). The osmotic pressure of the colloids in fish sera. *J. Exp. Biol. 11*:28-34.

Kim, K. J., and Crandall, E. D. (1982). Alveolar water and solute permabilities at different lung volumes. *J. Appl. Physiol. 52*:1498-1505.

Kim, K. J., and Crandall, E. D. (1983). Heteropore populations of bullfrog alveolar epithelium. *J. Appl. Physiol. 54*:140-146.

Krough, A., and Nakazawa, F. (1927). Beitrage zur Messung des kolloidosmotischen Druckes in biologischen Flussigkeiten. *Biochem. Z. 188*:241-258.

Lai-Fook, S. J. (1979). Perivascular interstitial fluid pressure measured by 2-5 μ micropipets in isolated dog lung. *Physiologist 22*:74 (abstr.).

Lai-Fook, S. J. (1981). Interstitial pressure in the lung. In *Tissue Fluid Pressure and Composition*. Edited by A. R. Hargens. Baltimore, Williams and Wilkins, pp. 125-134.

Lai-Fook, S. J. (1982). Perivascular interstitial fluid pressure measured by micropipettes in isolated dog lung. *J. Appl. Physiol. 53*:737-743.

Lai-Fook, S. J., and Kaplowitz, M. R. (1984). Alveolar liquid pressure measured using micropipets in isolated rabbit lungs. *Respir. Physiol. 57*:61-72.

Landis, E. M. (1926). The capillary pressure in frog mesentery as determined by microinjection. *Am. J. Physiol. 75*:548-570.

Landis, E. M. (1927). Microinjection studies of capillary permeability. II. The relationship between capillary pressure and the rate at which fluid passes through the walls of single capillaries. *Am. J. Physiol. 82*:217-238.

Landis, E. M., and Pappenheimer, J. R. (1963). Exchange of substances through the capillary walls. In *Handbook of Physiology*. Edited by W. F. Hamilton and P. Dow. Vol. II, Circulation. Washington, American Physiological Society, pp. 961-1033.

Langille, B. L., and Crisp, B. (1980). Temperature dependence of blood viscosity in frogs and turtles: Effect on heat exchange wih environment. *Am. J. Physiol. 239*:R248-R253.

Levick, J. R., and Michel, C. C. (1973). The effect of bovine albumin on the permeability of frog mesenteric capillaries. *Q. J. Exp. Physiol. 58*:67-85.

Lillywhite, H. B., Ackerman, R. A., and Palacios, L. (1983). Cardiorespiratory responses of snakes to experimental hemorrhage. *J. Comp. Physiol. 152*: 59-65.

Lillywhite, H. B., and Pough, F. H. (1983). Control of arterial pressure in aquatic sea snakes. *Am. J. Physiol. 244*:R66-R73.

Lillywhite, H. B., and Smith, L. H. (1981). Hemodynamic responses to hemorrhage in the snake. *Elaphe obsoleta obsoleta. J. Exp. Biol. 94*:275-283.

Lillywhite, H. B., and Smits, A. W. (1984). Lability of blood volume in snakes and its relation to activity and hypertension. *J. Exp. Biol. 110*:267-274.

Linehan, J. H., Dawson, C. A., and Rickaby, D. A. (1982). Distribution of vascular resistance and compliance in a dog lung lobe. *J. Appl. Physiol. 53*:158-168.

Luckhardt, A. B., and Carlson, A. J. (1921a). Studies on the visceral sensory nervous system. VI. Lung automatism and lung reflexes in *Cryptobranchus* with further notes on the physiology of the lung of *Necturus. Am. J. Physiol. 55*:212-222.

Luckhardt, A. B., and Carlson, A. J. (1921b). Studies on the visceral sensory nervous system. VIII. On the presence of vasomotor fibers in the vagus nerve to the pulmonary vessels of the amphibian and reptilian lung. *Am. J. Physiol. 56*:72-112.

MacIntyre, D. H., and Toews, D. P. (1976). The mechanism of lung ventilation and the effects of hypercapnia on respiration in *Bufo marinus. Can. J. Zool. 54*:1364-1374.

McNamee, J. E., and Staub, N. C. (1979). Pore models of sheep lung microvascular barrier using new data on protein tracers. *Microvasc. Res. 18*:229-244.

Malik, A. B. (1985). Mechanisms of neurogenic pulmonary edema. *Circ. Res. 57*: 1-18.

Maloney, J. E., and Castle, B. L. (1969). Pressure-diameter relations of capillaries and small blood vessels in frog lung. *Respir. Physiol. 7*:150-162.

Maloney, J. E., and Castle, B. L. (1970). Dynamic intravascular pressures in the microvessels of the frog lung. *Respir. Physiol. 10*:51-63.

March, H. W. (1961). Persistence of a functioning bulbous cordis homologue in the turtle heart. *Am. J. Physiol. 201*:1109-1112.

Mason, J. C., Curry, F. E., and Michel, C. C. (1977). The effect of proteins upon the filtration coefficient of individually perfused frog mesenteric capillaries. *Microvasc. Res. 13*:185-202.

Meyer, B. J., Meyer, A., and Guyton, A. C. (1968). Interstitial fluid pressure. V. Negative pressure in the lungs. *Circ. Res. 22*:263-271.

Michel, C. C. (1972). Flows across the capillary wall. In *Cardiovascular Fluid Dynamics*, Vol. 2. Edited by D. H. Bergel. New York, Academic Press.

Michel, C. C. (1979). The investigation of capillary permeability in single vessels. *Acta Physiol. Scand. 463*:67-74.

Michel, C. C., and Turner, M. R. (1981). The effect of molecular charge on the permeabilities of frog mesenteric capillaries to myoglobin. *J. Physiol. (Lond.) 316*:51P-52P.

Michel, R. P., Hakim, T. S., and Chang, H. K. (1984). Pulmonary arterial and venous pressures measured with small catheters in dogs. *J. Appl. Physiol. 57*:309-314.

Middler, S. A., Kleeman, C. R., and Edwards, E. (1968). Lymph mobilization following acute blood loss in the toad, *Bufo marinus. Comp. Biochem. Physiol. A 24*:343-353.

Milsom, W. K., Langille, B. L., and Jones, D. R. (1977). Vagal control of pulmonary vascular resistance in the turtle. *Can. J. Zool. 55*:359-367.

Mortillaro, N. A., and Taylor, A. E. (1983). Fluid exchange in the microcirculation. In *The Physiology and Pharmacology of the Microcirculation*, Vol. 1. Edited by N. A. Mortillaro. New York, Academic Press, pp. 143-158.

Nilsson, S. (1985). *Autonomic Nerve Function in the Vertebrates*. Berlin, Spinger-Verlag.

Olesen, S.-P., De Saint-Aubain, M. L., and Bundgaard, M. (1984). Permeabilities of single arterioles and venules in the frog skin: A functional and morphological study. *Microvasc. Res. 28*:1-22.

Parker, J. C., Guyton, A. C., and Taylor, A. E. (1978). Pulmonary interstitial and capillary pressures estimated from intra-alveolar fluid pressures. *J. Appl. Physiol. 44*:267-276.

Parker, J. C., Kvietys, P. R., Ryan, K. P., and Taylor, A. E. (1983). Comparison of isogravimetric and venous occlusion capillary pressures in isolated dog lungs. *J. Appl. Physiol. 55*:964-968.

Parker, J. C., Rippe, B., and Taylor, A. E. (1986). Fluid filtration and protein clearances through large and small pore populations in dog lung capillaries. *Microvasc. Res. 31*:1-17.

Perry, M. A., Colebatch, J. G., Glover, W. E., and Roddie, I. C. (1986). Measurement of capillary pressure in humans using a venous occlusion method. *J. Appl. Physiol. 60*:2114-2117.

Powell, F. L., Hastings, R. H., and Mazzone, R. W. (1985). Pulmonary vascular resistance during unilateral pulmonary arterial occlusion in ducks. *Am. J. Physiol. 249*:R39-R43.

Prather, T. W., Gaar, K. A., and Guyton, A. C. (1968). Direct continuous recording of plasma colloid osmotic pressure of whole blood. *J. Appl. Physiol. 24*:602-605.

Priestly, J. (1878). An account of the anatomy and physiology of Batrachian lymph hearts. *J. Physiol. (Lond.) 1*:1-19.

Renkin, E. M. (1968). Exchange of substances through capillary walls. In *Circulatory and Respiratory Mass Transport*. Edited by G. E. W. Wolstenholme and J. Knight. Ciba Foundation Symposium, London, Churchill.

Rippe, B., Townsley, M. I., and Taylor, A. E. (1985). Effects of plasma- and cell-free perfusates on filtration coefficient of perfused canine lungs. *J. Appl. Physiol. 58*:1521-1527.

de Saint-Aubain, M. L., and Wingstrand, K. G. (1979). A sphincter in the pulmonary artery of the frog *Rana temporaria* and its influence on blood flow in skin and lungs. *Acta Zool. (Stockholm) 60*:163-172.

Schaeffer, J. D., Kim, K. J., and Crandall, E. D. (1984). Effects of cell swelling on flow across alveolar epithelium. *J. Appl. Physiol. 56*:72-77.

Scholander, P. F., Hargens, A. R., and Miller, S. L. (1968). Negative pressures in the interstitial fluids of animals. *Science 161*:321-328.

Schooley, J. (1958). Lymphocyte output and lymph flow of thoracic and right lymphatic duct in anesthetized rats. *Proc. Soc. Exp. Biol. Med. 99*:511-513.

Shelton, G., and Boutilier, R. G. (1982). Apnoea in amphibians and reptiles. *J. Exp. Biol. 100*:245-273.

Shelton, G., and Burggren, W. (1976). Cardiovascular dynamics of the chelonia during apnoea and lung ventilation. *J. Exp. Biol. 64*:323-343.

Shelton, G., and Jones, D. R. (1965). Pressure and volume relationships in the ventricle, conus and arterial arches of the frog heart. *J. Exp. Biol. 43*:479-488.

Shelton, G., and Jones, D. R. (1968). A comparative study of central blood pressures in five amphibians. *J. Exp. Biol. 49*:631-643.

Shuster, D. P., Marklin, G. F., and Mintun, M. A. (1986). Regional changes in extravascular lung water detected by position emission tomography. *J. Appl. Physiol. 60*:1170-1178.

Smith, D. G. (1979). Factors affecting oxygen exchange in isolated, saline-perfused lungs of *Bufo marinus. Comp. Biochem. Physiol. A 62*:655-659.

Smith, D. G., and G. Campbell. (1976). The anatomy of the pulmonary vascular bed in the toad *Bufo marinus. Cell Tissue Res. 165*:199-213.

Smith, R. V., and Satchell, D. G. (1987). Innervation of the lung of the Australian snake-necked tortoise, *Chelodina longicollis. Comp. Biochem. Physiol. C 87*:439-444.

Smits, A. W. (1986). Accessory lymph sacs and body fluid partitioning in the lizard, *Sauromalus hispidus. J. Exp. Biol. 121*:165-177.

Smits, A. W., and Kozubowski, M. M. (1985). Partitioning of body fluids and cardiovascular responses to circulatory hypovolaemia in the turtle, *Pseudemys scripta elegans. J. Exp. Biol. 116*:237-250.

Smits, A. W., and Lillywhite, H. B. (1985). Maintenance of blood volume in snakes: Transcapillary shifts of extravascular fluids during acute hemorrhage. *J. Comp. Physiol. B 155*:305-310.

Smits, A. W., West, N. H., and Burggren, W. W. (1986). Pulmonary fluid balance following pulmocutaneous baroreceptor denervation in the toad. *J. Appl. Physiol. 61*:331-337.

Starling, E. H. (1896). On the absorption of fluid from the connective tissue spaces. *J. Physiol. (Lond.) 19*:312-326.

Staub, N. C. (1971). Steady state pulmonary transvascular water filtration in unanesthetized sheep. *Circ. Res. 28/29* (Suppl. 1):135-139.

Staub, N. C. (1974). Pulmonary edema. *Physiol. Rev. 54*:678-811.

Staub, N. C. (1978). Lung fluid and solute exchange. In *Lung Water and Solute Exchange*. Edited by N. C. Staub. Vol. 7. *Lung Biology in Health and Disease*. Exec. editor, C. Lenfant. New York, Marcel Dekker, pp. 3-16.

Staub, N. C., Flick, M., Perel, A., Landolt, C., and Vaughan, T. R. (1981). Lymph as reflection of interstitial fluid. In *Tissue Fluid Pressure and Composition*. Edited by A. R. Hargens. Baltimore, Williams & Wilkens, pp. 113-123.

Stromme, S. B., Maggert, J. E., and Scholander, P. F. (1969). Interstitial fluid pressure in terrestrial and semiterrestrial animals. *J. Appl. Physiol. 27*:123-126.

Sturkie, P. D. (1954). *Avian Physiology*. Ithaca, N. Y., Comstock Publishers, 423 pp.

Taylor, A. E., and Garr, K. A. (1970). Estimation of equivalent pore radii of pulmonary capillary and alveolar membranes. *Am. J. Physiol. 218*:1133-1140.

Taylor, A. E., and Granger, D. N. (1984). Exchange of macromolecules across the microcirculation. In *Handbook of Physiology*. Edited by E. M. Renkin and C. C. Michel. The Cardiovascular System. Vol. IV, Part 1. Microcirculation. Bethesda, American Physiological Society, pp. 867-920.

Taylor, A. E., Grimbert, F., Rutili, G., Kvietys, P. R., and Parker, J. C. (1981). Pulmonary edema: Changes in Starling forces and lymph flow. In *Tissue Fluid Pressure and Composition*. Edited by A. R. Hargens. Baltimore, Williams & Wilkens, pp. 135-143.

Taylor, A. E., Guyton, A. C., and Bishop, V. S. (1965). Permeability of the alveolar membrane to solutes. *Circ. Res. 16*:353-362.

Taylor, A. E., and Rippe, B. (1986). Pulmonary edema. In *Physiology of Membrane Disorders*. Edited by T. E. Andreoli, J. F. Hoffman, D. D. Fanestil, and S. G. Schultz. New York, Plenum, pp. 1025-1039.

Taylor, A. E., Townsley, M. I., and Korthuis, R. J. (1985). Macromolecule transport across the pulmonary microvessel wall. *Exp. Lung Res. 8*:97-123.

Theodore, J., Robin, E. D., Gaudio, R., and Acevedo, J. (1975). Transalveolar transport of large polar solutes (sucrose, inulin, and dextran). *Am. J. Physiol. 229*:989-996.

Townsley, M. I., Korthuis, R. J., Rippe, B., Parker, J. C., and Taylor, A. E. (1986). Validation of double occlusion method for $P_{c,i}$ in lung and skeletal muscle. *J. Appl. Physiol. 61*:127-132.

Tsuchiya, S. (1959). Lung automatism in the Japanese toad. *J. Physiol. Soc. Jpn. 21*:272-279.

Turner, M. R., Clough, G., and Michel, C. C. (1983). The effect of cationised ferritin and native ferritin upon the filtration coefficient of single frog capillaries: Evidence that proteins in the endothelial cell coat influence permeability. *Microvasc. Res. 25*:205-222.

Van Der Zee, H., Cooper, J. A., Hakim, T. S., and Malik, A. B. (1986). Alterations in pulmonary fluid balance induced by positive end-expiratory pressure. *Respir. Physiol. 64*:125-133.

Van Rossum, G. D. V., and Parsons, D. S. (1985). Vascularly perfused frog lung: Effects of metabolic conditions on adenine nucleotides and inorganic ions. *Q. J. Exp. Physiol. 70*:1-14.

Vreim, C. E., Snashall, P., and Staub, N. C. (1976). Protein composition of lung fluids in anesthetized dogs with acute cardiogenic edema. *Am. J. Physiol. 231*:1466-1469.

Wangensteen, O. D., Wittmers, L. E., Jr., and Johnson, J. A. (1969). Permeability of the mammalian blood gas barrier and its components. *Am. J. Physiol. 216*:719-727.

Watson, P. D. (1983). Effects of blood-free and protein-free perfusion on CFC in the isolated cat hindlimb. *Am. J. Physiol. 245*:H911-H919.

Watson, P. D. (1984). Effect of plasma and red blood cells on water permeability in cat hindlimb. *Am. J. Physiol. 246*:H818-H823.

West, J. B. (1974). *Respiratory Physiology*. Baltimore, Williams & Wilkens, 185 pp.

West, N. H., and Jones, D. R. (1975). Breathing movements in the frog *Rana pipiens*. I. The mechanical events associated with lung and buccal ventilation. *Can. J. Zool. 53*:332-344.

White, H. (1924). On glomerular filtration. *Am. J. Physiol. 68*:523-529.

Winterstein, H. (1925). *Handbuch der vergleichende Physiologie*. Vol. 1. Jena.

Wolf, M. B., and Watson, P. D. (1985). Effect of temperature on transcapillary water movement in isolated cat hindlimb. *Am. J. Physiol. 249*:H792-H798.

Zweifach, B. W., and Intaglietta, M. (1968). Mechanics of fluid movement across single capillaries in the rabbit. *Microvasc. Res. 1*:83-101.

Zweifach, B. W., and Intaglietta, M. (1971). Measurement of blood plasma colloid osmotic pressure. II. Comparative study of different species. *Microvasc. Res. 3*:83-88.

Zwemer, R. L., and Foglia, V. G. (1943). Fatal loss of plasma volume after lymph heart destruction in toads. *Proc. Soc. Exp. Biol. Med. 53*:14-17.

18

Ion Transfer Processes as Mechanisms for Acid-Base Regulation

NORBERT HEISLER

Max Planck Institute for Experimental Medicine
Göttingen, Federal Republic of Germany

I. Introduction

Acid-base regulation in living organisms is characterized by the balance between the release of acid-base relevant ions (e.g., H^+, OH^-, and HCO_3^-) to the body fluids, either by endogenous metabolic production or by introduction from the environment, and the elimination of those ions from the biological fluid system (Fig. 1). Release of acid-base relevant ions to the body fluids is counteracted by various mechanisms, such as changes in CO_2 gas exchange, transient buffering, and transmembrane and transepithelial ion transfer. Release and elimination usually take place at different sites, which are interconnected by the circulating blood as the main convective transport medium in vertebrates. The complexity of such biological systems, with numerous fluid compartments, and the relative inaccessibility of body compartments other than readily available extracellular fluids, such as central venous and arterial blood, have often prohibited closer understanding of systemic acid-base regulation. Acid-base analysis in fluid compartments representing a minor fraction of the total body mass (> 8% for blood) must necessarily result in incomplete and misleading conclusions about the overall organismic pattern. The transport of acid-base relevant ions by the

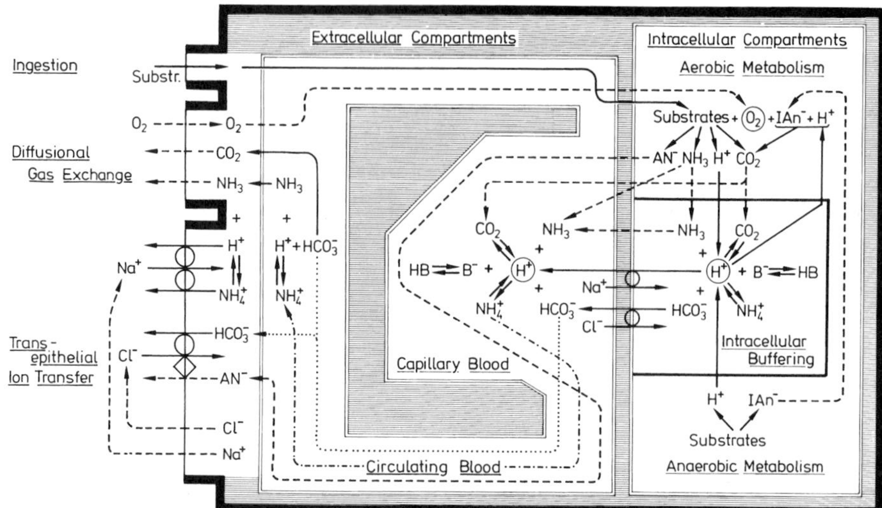

Figure 1 Schematic general representation of the acid-base regulation as the interaction between production and buffering of surplus acid-base relevant ions, convective transport by the circulating blood, the diffusional gas exchange, and transmembrane and transepithelial ion transfer mechanisms. Nonvolatile metabolic end products are eliminated by ionic exchange processes; CO_2 and NH_3 are present in the organisms, mainly in ionic form (HCO_3^- and NH_4^+) but are eliminated by nonionic diffusion.

blood from the site of production in intracellular tissue compartments to the site of elimination by metabolic processes or permanent excretion, certainly an important factor for the evaluation of the acid-base regulation, is completely discounted by exclusive blood analysis. Interestingly, the transepithelial elimination of acid-base relevant ions has rarely been taken into consideration, in spite of the fact that the analogous exchange of respiratory gases is commonly studied by respiratory physiologists.

Recent developments in technology and experimental approaches have facilitated a more comprehensive description of systemic acid-base regulation, taking the status of the intracellular space, transmembrane and transepithelial ion fluxes, and the distribution and buffering of surplus acid-base relevant ions in various body fluid compartments into account. Analyses of fast, dynamic processes related to the involved mechanisms and their limiting factors, however, are still scarce.

This chapter is intended to delineate current approaches to systemic acid-base analysis with some representative (sometimes the only available) examples for analysis of certain regulatory processes. No attempt is made (and also prohibited by space limitations) to present a general review of acid-base regulation. The reader is thus referred to other relevant recent publications (e.g., Heisler, 1986, ed.).

II. Basic Concepts

A conventional acid-base analysis includes measurements of pH, P_{CO_2}, and determination of $[HCO_3^-]$ by either direct measurement (e.g., Van Slyke, Capnicon L, reviewed in Heisler, 1988c) or, more often, calculation based on the Henderson-Hasselbach equation (for constants see Heisler, 1986a). The amount of surplus acid-base relevant ions can be determined from the buffering properties of the respective fluid compartment (see Heisler, 1986a). This concept, with its fundamentals laid by the work of Arrhenius (1887), Henderson (1909), Sϕrensen (1912), Hasselbalch (1916), Van Slyke (1917, 1922), Brϕnsted (1923), and other pioneers in this field, is widely distributed and technical improvements have led to the high reliability and accuracy of this approach.

Another system, the strong ion difference concept (SID; Stewart, 1978), is generally compatible and describes the acid-base interrelations on the basis of the strong ions, which maintain osmolarity in the body fluids and balance the charges of the weak acid and base buffer systems. The strong ion difference is accordingly equivalent to the *buffer bases* (a term coined by Singer and Hastings, 1948). Any changes in the difference between the activity of positively and negatively charged strong ions are stoichiometrically equivalent to the changes in buffer ions (buffer bases) and, thus, represent the amount of acid-base relevant ions bound by the buffer system (*base excess*, Siggaard-Andersen and Engel, 1960; Siggaard-Andersen, 1962, 1974).

Evidently, there is no principal difference between these two concepts, and their respective descriptions of the acid-base status are equivalent. Practical limitations, however, disqualify the SID concept for most physiological studies, except for some marginal applications. This is due to its inherent relatively low accuracy. The SID can only be determined by measurement of the activity of all individual strong ions. The high background of the major ions (e.g., Na^+, K^+, Cl^-) in body fluids (100-300 mM, up to 600 mM in osmoconforming marine species) leads to errors in the mM range (even assuming an optimistic sD of ± 2% for electrolyte determinations), whereas changes in the amount of H^+ ions bound in blood of < 0.3 mM can be detected on a background of 24 mM plasma $[HCO_3^-]$ (mammals) with conventional acid-base analytical techniques. This does not even take into account that the activity, rather than the ion concentrations, is seldom measured for determination of the SID, which can be misleading when nominally strong ions combine with formation of weak complex ions (or vice versa). Reactions of this type, for instance, are the formation of magnesium-phosphate compounds, such as Mg ATP^-, or of inorganic phosphate during ATP cleavage. With the typically high intracellular concentrations of organic phosphate compounds (ATP, IPP, etc.) misestimates in the range of several mM must be expected (see Heisler, 1986a). The uncertainty provided by the fact that the variety of strong ions in biological (especially intracellular) compartments are often not completely known and, thus, can seldom be completely determined, is difficult to estimate, and such an estimate may exceed the error of a conventional status determination by orders of magnitude.

Because physiological studies rely heavily on the acquisition of appropriate data, the SID concept is apparently unsuitable for even the most conventional single-compartment analyses. Accordingly, more advanced studies, taking into account dynamic processes, such as transmembrane and transepithelial acid-base relevant ion transfer, have almost exclusively utilized extensions of the more conventional system based on determination of pH, P_{CO_2}, $[HCO_3^-]$, and buffering properties, a type of analysis also applied in this chapter.

III. Experimental Approaches and Parameters

Biological systems are open for the exchange of gases and ions. Accordingly, any complete description of acid-base regulatory processes must include the transmembrane (between intra- and extracellular space) and transepithelial (between extracellular space and environment) ion transfer processes, in addition to the status description by pH, P_{CO_2}, and $[HCO_3^-]$ in one or several extracellular and intracellular body fluid compartments. However, the transfer of acid-base relevant ions, such as H^+, OH^-, and HCO_3^-, cannot yet be monitored directly. This is because these ions are in equilibrium with numerous other substances, such that any labels are readily exchanged according to the continuous cycling reactions resulting from thermodynamic activity. Ionic transfer must, therefore, be deduced from its effect on the acid-base status in one or more of the involved fluid compartments.

Although the species of acid-base relevant ions that is actually transferred across membranes and epithelia is uncertain, the addition of H^+ ions will result in the same effect as the removal of either OH^- or HCO_3^-, as long as the whole system is in equilibrium. This can generally be assumed when the hydration-dehydration reaction of CO_2 is catalyzed by carbonic anhydrase. Disequilibrium may occur for limited periods when carbonic anhydrase is not available. Although this is an important factor for the diffusive elimination of CO_2 in aquatic organisms (see Heisler, 1988a) and can be utilized as a tool for the evaluation of acidification mechanisms (e.g., "disequilibrium pH" in the kidney tubule, see Sullivan, 1986), it usually has little effect for acid-base analyses because of the delays involved in the measurement of relevant parameters (for uncatalyzed reaction times, see Kern, 1960).

The considerations and models to be outlined are based on the buffering capabilities and the changes in pH and $[HCO_3^-]$ of various body and extracorporeal fluid compartments. Acid-base relevant ions are expressed as *bicarbonate equivalents* because of the role of bicarbonate as an indicator substance in the determination of the nonbicarbonate buffer value by CO_2 titration (see Heisler, 1986a, 1988a). The approaches can just as well be viewed in terms of *H^+ ion equivalents* with the appropriate adjustment of signs and direction of ion transfers.

A. Approach 1

Acid-base relevant ion transfer processes between the intracellular and extracellular compartments of tissues were first quantitatively determined in isolated Ringer suspended tissues (Heisler and Piiper, 1972). The amount of bicarbonate-equivalent ions transferred to the Ringer solution as the extension of the extracellular space is:

$$\Delta HCO^-_{3\,i\rightarrow e} = \Delta[HCO_3^-]_r \cdot (V_r + M_t \cdot F_{H_2O} \cdot Q_e) - \Delta HCO^-_{3\,NBr} \tag{1}$$

where: M_t = tissue mass, F_{H_2O} = fractional water content of the tissue, Q_e = fractional extracellular space. Indices r and NB refer to parameters in Ringer solution and to nonbicarbonate buffering, index i → e to the direction (intracellular, i, to extracellular, e) of bicarbonate equivalent transfer, respectively. V = volume.

The kinetics of intracellular pH adjustment can be followed by inserting $\Delta HCO^-_{3\,i\rightarrow e}$ values (determined by frequent application of Equation 1 into Equation 6 (Approach 3), expressing $[HCO_3^-]$ by P_{CO_2} and pH_i, and solving the resulting equation by computer iteration (see Heisler and Neumann, 1980; Heisler, 1984a).

Simultaneous measurement of the transmembrane ion transfer and the change in intracellular pH allows determination of the total intracellular nonbicarbonate buffer value in the intact tissue, as long as no nonsteady-state acid-base relevant metabolic processes (e.g., production of lactic acid) are involved:

$$\beta_{NBi} = \frac{\Delta[HCO_3^-]_i}{-\Delta pH_i} + \frac{\Delta HCO^-_{3\,i\rightarrow e}}{-\Delta pH\{M_t \cdot F_{H_2O} \cdot (1 - Q_e)\}} \tag{2}$$

where: index i refers to the intracellular tissue compartment.

B. Approach 2

A similar two-compartment model as in Approach 1 can be applied to describe the bicarbonate-equivalent transfer in an isolated, blood-perfused, tissue preparation.

$$\Delta[HCO_3^-]_{i \to e} = \Delta[HCO_3^-]_{pl} \cdot (\dot{Q}_{pl} + M_t \cdot FH_2O \cdot Q_e) - \Delta pH_{pl} \cdot \beta_{NBpl} \cdot$$

$$\dot{Q}_{pl} + (\Delta[HCO_3^-]_{ery} - \Delta pH_{ery} \cdot \beta_{NBery}) \cdot \dot{Q}_{ery} \qquad (3)$$

where: indices pl and ery designated plasma and erythrocyte values, respectively. $\dot{Q}$ is plasma or erythrocyte flow (in terms of water volume). The effect of oxygenation/deoxygenation of hemoglobin (Bohr/Haldane effect) has to be taken into account during determination of the second line term of Equation 2.

A disadvantage of this approach is that the total amount of bicarbonate-equivalent ions usually has to be extrapolated from discontinuous measurements in the inflowing and outflowing perfusate and from average flow values, whereas in Approach 1 integration is automatically and more accurately provided by accumulation of transferred ions in the extended extracellular space, the Ringer solution.

The nonbicarbonate buffer value is determined according to Equation 2, and intracellular pH kinetics are modeled, as outlined for Approach 1.

C. Approach 3

The following two approaches are applicable to intact animals. Approach 3 is suitable to determine the amount of bicarbonate-equivalent ions transferred across the cell membrane of an intracellular fluid compartment, based on the changes in intracellular pH, $[HCO_3^-]$, and the intracellular buffering capabilities.

Changes in intracellular pH elicit production of bicarbonate on the basis of nonbicarbonate buffering of CO_2:

$$\Delta[HCO_3^-]_{NBi} = -\Delta pH_i \cdot \beta_{NBi} \qquad (4)$$

where: β_{NB} = the nonbicarbonate buffer value.

Shifts in buffer pK′ values induced by changes in temperature or other mechanisms (see Heisler, 1986a) must be subtracted from the changes in pH:

$$\Delta[HCO_3^-]_{NBi} = \beta_I(\Delta pK_I - \Delta pH_i) + \beta_{II}(\Delta pK_{II} - \Delta pH_i) \qquad (5)$$

$$\ldots + \beta_N(\Delta pK_N - \Delta pH_i)$$

where: indices I, II, to N refer to buffer systems with different changes in pK′ values.

The difference between the changes in $[HCO_3^-]$ and the amount per unit intracellular water volume produced or decomposed by buffering, or by effectors of nonsteady-state conditions (index NST, e.g., lactic acid production), multiplied by the intracellular volume yields the amount of bicarbonate equivalents transferred from an individual intracellular compartment to the extracellular space:

$$\Delta HCO^-_{3\,i\rightarrow e} = (\Delta[HCO^-_3]_{NBi} - \Delta[HCO^-_3]_i - \Delta[HCO^-_3]_{NST}) \cdot V_i \tag{6}$$

For steady-state conditions the term $\Delta[HCO^-_3]_{NST}$ can be neglected, and the effect of transmembrane transfer of bicarbonate equivalents for intracellular pH adjustment can be evaluated by simulating the intracellular fluid compartment as a semiclosed buffer system (open for only molecular CO_2). Then, the changes in pH expected without transmembrane transfer processes can be modeled by setting $\Delta HCO^-_{3\,i\rightarrow e}$ to zero, expressing $\Delta[HCO^-_3]_i$ by pH and P_{CO_2} values according to the Henderson-Hasselbalch equation, and solving the resulting equation by computer iteration (see Heisler and Neumann, 1980; Heisler, 1984a).

The overall intracellular to extracellular bicarbonate-equivalent transfer as the sum of $\Delta HCO^-_{3\,i\rightarrow e}$ of all tissues leads to an estimate of the transepithelial bicarbonate-equivalent transfer ($\Delta HCO^-_{3\,e\rightarrow env}$):

$$\Delta HCO^-_{3\,e\rightarrow env} = \sum_1^n (\Delta HCO^-_{3\,i\rightarrow e} - \Delta HCO^-_3 e + \Delta HCO^-_{3\,NBe}) \tag{7}$$

Because information on transmembrane bicarbonate transfer is usually limited, $\Delta HCO^-_{3\,e\rightarrow env}$ is more appropriately determined directly from release and uptake of bicarbonate equivalents at epithelial sites (see Approach 4).

D. Approach 4

This whole-animal approach takes the direction opposite that of Approach 3 and is based on the bicarbonate-equivalent transfer at various epithelial sites of the organism. The transepithelial bicarbonate-equivalent transfer is:

$$\begin{aligned}\Delta HCO^-_{3\,e\rightarrow env} &= (\Delta[HCO^-_3]_{env} - \Delta[NH^+_4]_{env} - \Delta pH_{env} \cdot \beta_{NBenv}) \cdot V_{env} \\ &\quad + ([HCO^-_3]_u - [NH^+_4]_u - TA_u) \cdot V_u \ldots . \\ &\quad \ldots + [HCO^-_3]_n - [NH^+_4]_n - TA_n) \cdot V_n\end{aligned}$$

where: indices e, env, and u designate extracellular space, environmental (water), or urine values, respectively. n represents all other excretion sites such as rectal, sweat and salt glands, intestine, etc. TA = titratable acidity.

For aquatic species, this equation can be applied for both open flow-through systems (Δ then refers to the difference between inflowing and outflowing water, and V to a volume of water per unit of time), as well as for closed water recirculation systems (see Heisler et al., 1976; Heisler, 1978) for which Δ refers to differences for a certain period, and V represents the volume of the recirculated water. In aquatic animals, such as fishes and amphibians, the first-line term, measured in the environmental water, is quantitatively more important, whereas the second-line term (urine values) is quantitatively predominant in terrestrial species.

The overall transfer of bicarbonate equivalents between extracellular space and intracellular fluid compartments can be determined from the transepithelial transfer, the amount of bicarbonate produced by nonbicarbonate buffering, and the change in bicarbonate concentration in the extracellular space:

$$\Delta HCO^-_{3\,i\rightarrow e} = \Delta HCO^-_{3\,e\rightarrow env} + \Delta[HCO^-_3]_e \cdot V_e - \Delta HCO^-_{3\,NBe} \tag{9}$$

The amount of bicarbonate-equivalent ions produced by nonbicarbonate buffering in the extracellular compartment (including blood) is:

$$\Delta HCO^-_{3\,NBe} = \Delta pH_e \cdot \beta_{NBe} \cdot (V_e - V_{pl}) + \Delta pH_e \cdot \beta_{NBpl} \cdot V_{pl} + \Delta pH_{ery} \cdot \beta_{NBery} \cdot V_{ery} \tag{10}$$

The overall transmembrane bicarbonate-equivalent transfer determined by this approach can be introduced into Equation 6 (Approach 3) and allows an estimate of the intracellular pH adjustment kinetics, taking for granted that the transfer kinetics are similar in most tissues (a prerequisite valid for only few species, mainly fishes).

If the changes in the amount of intracellular bicarbonate of all intracellular compartments are known, or an average value can be determined from mean whole-body intracellular pH measurements, the overall amount of bicarbonate produced (or decomposed) by intracellular nonbicarbonate buffering can be calculated as:

$$\Delta HCO^-_{3\,NBi} = \Delta HCO^-_{3\,i\rightarrow e} + \sum_{1}^{n} (\Delta[HCO^-_3]_i \cdot V_i) \tag{11}$$

Extrapolations for the pH_i adjustment kinetics and for the overall buffering capability, however, should be viewed with a certain amount of discretion. They can be considered to yield reliable (and certainly valuable) estimates only if a large fraction of the intracellular compartments has been investigated (such as for fish with their large proportion of white musculature; see Heisler, 1978, 1982, 1984a).

IV. Acid-Base Relevant Ion Transfer Processes

A. Temperature Changes

The first studies of the acid-base status in heterothermal animals indicated a considerable variability of pH between mammalian values and values higher than 7.8, suggesting that pH in lower vertebrates was regulated loosely, or not at all (e.g., Austin et al., 1927; Dill and Edwards, 1935; Edwards and Dill, 1935; Dill et al., 1935). Winterstein (1954) was the first to state that the acid-base status in heterothermal animals should not be evaluated on the basis of a constant pH, and suggested the neutrality of water expressed by the $[OH^-]/[H^+]$ ratio as a reference system (a concept also independently developed by Rahn, 1966, 1967). Systematic studies by Robin (1962) suggested a regulated correlation between temperature and pH in turtles, a proposition confirmed later by numerous other studies (for review see Heisler, 1986c). To explain the observed regulatory pattern, Reeves (1972; Reeves and Malan, 1976) propounded that pH in all body compartments was regulated by appropriate changes in P_{CO_2} induced by adjustment of ventilation, such that pH changed with temperature in parallel with the pK′ of biological histidine-imidazole moieties. It was claimed that this was achieved without any transmembrane and transepithelial ion transfer processes and at constant bicarbonate concentration (see Heisler, 1986c).

The large number of relevant studies conducted in the meantime has not confirmed the general concept of this hypothesis (see Heisler, 1986c; Boutilier and Heisler, 1988). The pH of plasma changes with temperature–in most of studied species–much less (average $\Delta pH/\Delta t$: - 0.011 U/°C; see Heisler, 1986c) than expected from the $\Delta pK'/\Delta t$ of imidazole compounds (-0.018 to 0.024 U/°C, Edsall and Wyman, 1958; Heisler, 1986c). Also, the pH in intracellular compartments (for review: Heisler, 1986c) and the magnitude of temperature-induced changes in ventilation are generally do not conform with Reeves' hypothesis (Glass et al., 1985).

A central feature of the imidazole alphastat hypothesis is the adjustment of pH without any transmembrane and transepithelial ion transfers (Reeves, 1972; Reeves and Malan, 1976). To date, there is only limited information on this point, collected exclusively in fishes. This may be related to the fact that transepithelial ion transfer processes can be determined more directly and accurately in a closed water recirculation system (see Heisler, 1984b, 1986a) than by collection of urine and other excreted fluids of terrestrial animals. The results vary among species: the elasmobranch, *Scyliorhinus stellaris*, and the freshwater channel catfish, *Ictalurus punctatus*, both reversibly exchange bicarbonate-equivalent ions with the environmental water [Table 1, column (5); Heisler, 1978; Cameron and Kormanik, 1982] upon changes in temperature, whereas the tropical freshwater teleost, *Synbranchus marmoratus*, behaves as a whole animal more like a semiclosed buffer system with little, and insignificant, ion exchange with the environmental water [Table 1 (5); Heisler, 1984a].

The overall transmembrane bicarbonate-equivalent ion transfer (determined by Approach 4), however, is much larger in *S. marmoratus*, and takes place in a direction opposite that in the other two fish species [see Table 1, (4)]. The data available for *Scyliorhinus* and *Synbranchus* also allow approximate determination of the transmembrane transfer by Approach 3. Because the characteristics of the intracellular body compartments are known to only a certain (although large) extent (54 and 75%, respectively), the remainder of the body mass is considered to behave like white musculature. The results of these

Table 1 Production of Bicarbonate in Intracellular Body Compartments, Changes in the Amount of Intracellular and Extracellular Bicarbonate, and Transfer of Bicarbonate-Equivalent Ions Among Intracellular and Extracellular Fluid Compartments and the Environmental Water upon an Increase in Body Temperature by 10°C in Three Fish Species[a]

			Approach 3			Approach 4		
Species	Tissue	ICS[c] volume	ΔHCO^-_{3NBi} (1)	ΔHCO^-_{3i} (2)	$\Delta HCO^-_{3i \to e}$ (3)	$\Delta HCO^-_{3i \to e}$ (4)	$\Delta HCO^-_{3e \to w}$ (5)	Ref.
Scyliorinus stellaris	White muscle	357	0.19	0.07	0.12			Heisler and Neumann, 1980
	Red muscle	35	0.26	-0.01	0.27			Heisler et al., 1980
	Other tissues	340	0.18[d]	0.06[d]	0.12[d]			
	Total	732			0.51			
						0.77	0.41	Heisler, 1978
Ictalurus punctatus						0.36	0.55	Cameron and Kormanik, 1982
Synbranchus marmoratus	White muscle	600	-0.21	-0.38	-1.83			Heisler, 1984a
	Other tissues	201	-0.74[d]	-0.13[d]	-0.61[d]			
	Total	801			-2.44	-2.01	(-0.08)[e]	Heisler, 1984a

[a]Data have been analyzed for comparison (where possible) by application of two different approaches (3 a:d 4, see text).
[b]Values expressed as mmol/kg body water.
[c]ICS, intracellular space, ml water/kg body water.
[d]Other tissues treated as white muscle.
[e]Transfer statistically insignificant.

Table 2 Changes of pH with Temperature In Vivo (*iv*), and in the Respective Compartments Modeled as Semiclosed Buffer Systems (cl′; Approach 4 and 3, see text) in Some Selected Fish Species[a]

Species	Body compartment	$\Delta pH_{iv}/\Delta t$ (in vivo)	$\Delta pH_{cl}/\Delta t$ (semiclosed buffer system)	$\frac{\Delta pH_{cl}}{\Delta pH_{iv}}$	Ref.
Scyliorhinus stellaris	White muscle ICS	-0.018	-0.017	0.95	Heisler et al., 1980
	Red muscle ICS	-0.031	-0.013	0.41	
	Heart muscle ICS	-0.007	-0.016	2.28	
	ECS	-0.011	-0.021	1.90	
Synbranchus marmoratus	White muscle ICS	-0.009	-0.017	1.89	Heisler, 1984a
	Heart muscle ICS	-0.003	-0.021	7.00	
	ECS	-0.017	-0.003	0.17	
Salmo gairdneri	ECS	-0.013	-0.001	0.07	Randall and Cameron, 1973
Cynoscion arenarius	ECS	-0.013	-0.002	0.15	Cameron, 1978
Ictalurus punctatus	ECS	-0.013	-0.007	0.53	Cameron and Kormanik, 1982a

[a]Values for the ratio $\Delta pH_{cl}/\Delta pH_{iv}$ higher or lower than 1 indicate that the in vivo PCO_2 attained after the change in temperature is too high or too low, respectively, to conform with the semiclosed buffer system (see text). ICS = intracellular space, ECS = extracellular space.

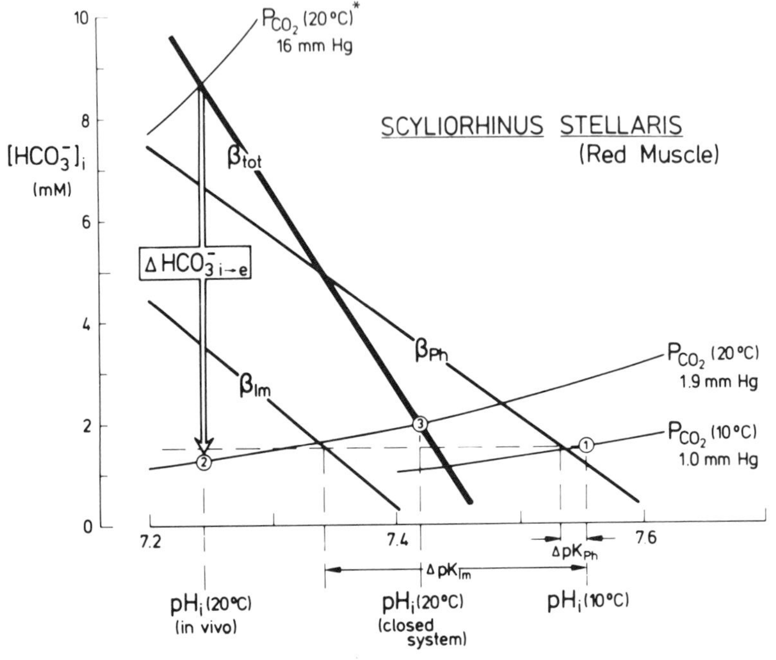
SCYLIORHINUS STELLARIS
(Red Muscle)
[HCO3-]i
(mM)
PCO2 (20°C)*
16 mm Hg
βtot
βPh
βIm
Δ HCO3- i→e
PCO2 (20°C)
1.9 mm Hg
PCO2 (10°C)
1.0 mm Hg
ΔpKPh
ΔpKIm
pHi (20°C)
(in vivo)
pHi (20°C)
(closed
system)
pHi (10°C)

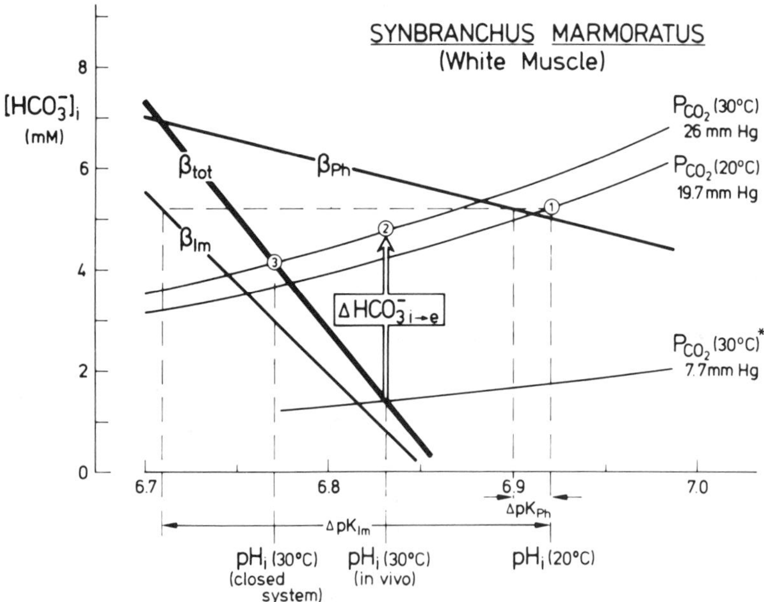
SYNBRANCHUS MARMORATUS
(White Muscle)
[HCO3-]i
(mM)
PCO2 (30°C)
26 mm Hg
PCO2 (20°C)
19.7 mm Hg
PCO2 (30°C)*
7.7 mm Hg
βtot
βPh
βIm
Δ HCO3- i→e
ΔpKPh
ΔpKIm
pHi (30°C)
(closed
system)
pHi (30°C)
(in vivo)
pHi (20°C)

extrapolations [see Table 1, (3)] conform rather well with those of Approach 4 [Table 1, (4)], being different by only 33 or 21% for *S. stellaris* and *S. marmoratus*, respectively.

The effect of bicarbonate-equivalent transmembrane ion transfer processes, and the contribution of buffering and changes in P_{CO_2} for the pH adjustment in individual tissues is well illustrated by modeling the respective fluid compartment as semiclosed buffer systems (open for CO_2) on the basis of experimental data on intracellular pH and temperature-dependent buffer values. This is performed by setting $\Delta HCO^-_{3\,i\rightarrow e}$ in Equation 6 (for the intracellular compartments), and $\Delta HCO^-_{3\,i\rightarrow e}$ and $\Delta HCO^-_{3\,e\rightarrow env}$ in Equation 9 (for the extracellular space) to zero (no transfer) and by solving the resulting equations (see preceding discussion). The pH-temperature coefficients expected for such semiclosed buffer systems (at the same P_{CO_2} as in vivo) are, with few exceptions, largely different from the values observed in vivo (Fig. 2; Table 2), underlining the importance of acid-base relevant ion transfer processes. The negative temperature coefficients of phosphatelike ($\Delta pK/\Delta t < -0.002$ U/°C) and imidazolelike buffers ($\Delta pK/\Delta t < -0.02$ U/°C; Edsall and Wyman, 1958, see Heisler, 1986c) certainly support a decrease in pH with rising temperatures. Changes of P_{CO_2} in the range of physiological values, however, has little influence on the finally adjusted $\Delta pH/\Delta t$ value because of the steep nonbicarbonate buffer line, especially in the intracellular compartments (see Fig. 2, β_{tot}). Changing the temperature by 10°C, required adjustement of P_{CO_2} from about 1 mm Hg to 16 mm Hg in red muscle of *Scyliorinus* (10-20°C), and from about 20 to less than 8 mm Hg in white muscle of *Synbranchus* (20-30°C) for pH adjustment exclusively on the basis of semiclosed system buffering, values that cannot be attained at all during normal conditions in these animals (Heisler et al., 1980; Heisler, 1980; Heisler, 1982; see Heisler, 1984, 1986b). Accordingly, the final adjust-

---

Figure 2 Intracellular pH regulation during changes in temperature by 10°C. pH is changed in vivo from points (1) to (2). A large fraction of bicarbonate produced (*Scyliorhinus stellaris*) or decomposed (*Synbranchus marmoratus*) intracellularly according to nonbicarbonate buffering of imidazolelike ($\Delta pK/\Delta t$ about -0.021 U/°C) and phosphatelike ($\Delta pK/\Delta t$ about -0.002 U/°C) buffers is transferred in vivo across the cell membrane ($\Delta HCO^-_{3\,i\rightarrow e}$). (Note: ascending arrow indicates transfer into, descending arrow indicates transfer out of the intracellular compartment.) Regulation on the basis of semiclosed system buffering (i.e., in vivo PCO_2 values, but no ionic transfer) would result in a shift of pH to point (3) as the intersection of the total nonbicarbonate buffer line ($\beta_{tot} = \beta_{Im} + \beta_{Ph}$) with the PCO_2 isopleth for the new temperature. The in vivo $\Delta pH/\Delta t$ could be achieved in vitro only with changes in PCO_2 (PCO_2*) that cannot be attained in vivo (based on Approach 3, see text). (Data from Heisler et al., 1980; Heisler and Neumann, 1980.)

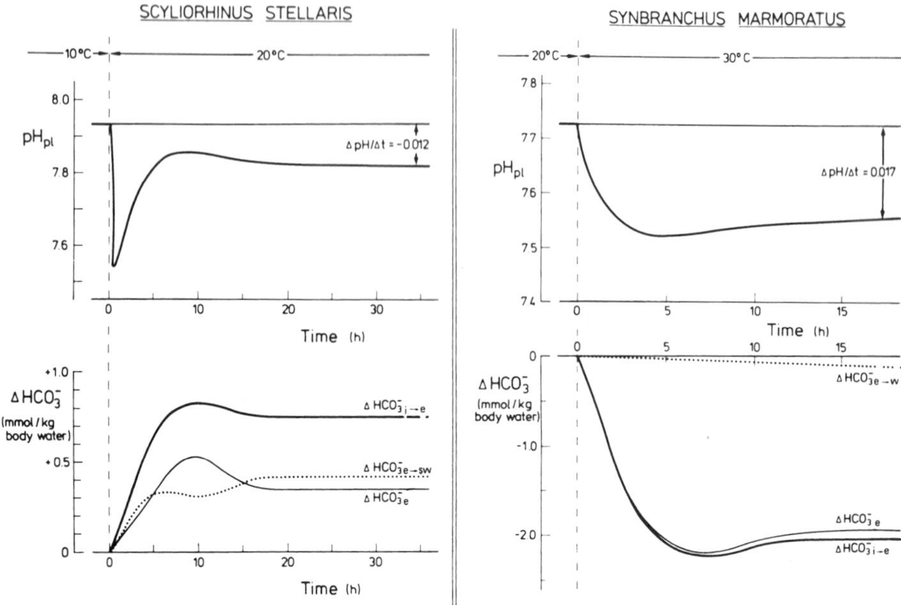

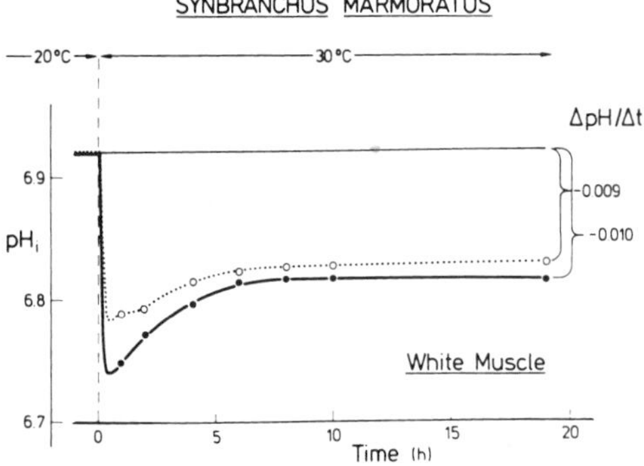

Figure 3 Time course of the changes in extracellular pH, the amount of extracellular bicarbonate ($\Delta HCO_{3\,e}^-$), the bicarbonate-equivalent ion transfer processes among intracellular and extracellular body compartments ($\Delta HCO_{3\,i\rightarrow e}^-$), and the environmental water ($\Delta HCO_{3\,e\rightarrow sw}^-$ or $\Delta HCO_{3\,e\rightarrow w}^-$) in the marine elasmobranch *Scyliorhinus stellaris* and the freshwater teleost *Synbranchus marmoratus* upon a 10°C step-change in temperature (Approach 4, see text). Adjustment of intracellular pH in white muscle of *Synbranchus* is delayed similarly to extracellular pH (C) (based on Approaches 3 and 4, see text). (Data from Heisler, 1978, 1984a.)

ment of pH is mainly the result of considerable bicarbonate-equivalent transfer (see Fig. 2, $\Delta HCO^-_{3\,i \to e}$), which may occasionally exceed the actual intracellular bicarbonate concentration by severalfold.

The kinetics of these transfer processes are relatively slow (Fig. 3), especially when compared with the transfer rates observed during more extensive acid-base disturbances, e.g., during environmental hypercapnia and during lactacidosis following exhaustive muscular activity (see later). In both of the two studied species, they are not complete before 15 to 20 h after the change in temperature. These ion transfer processes will not only affect pH regulation in terms of absolute values, but they also evidently dominate the adjustment kinetics. Extracellular pH is affected by both the transmembrane and transepithelial ion transfers and stabilizes only after about 15 to 20 h (see Fig. 3). As estimated, based on the intracellular buffering properties of *Synbranchus* white muscle (which represents 75% of the body mass), and the overall transmembrane bicarbonate-equivalent transfer (Approaches 4 and 3), adjustment of intracellular pH in this tissue will be delayed to 7 to 10 h after the change in temperature (see Fig. 3; Heisler, 1984a).

This exemplary evaluation emphasizes the predominant role of acid-base relevant ion transfer processes during changes in temperature. Although the negative temperature coefficients of the nonbicarbonate buffers (discussed earlier) support the decrease in pH with rising temperature toward the in vivo values, this is often counteracted by the in vivo changes in P_{CO_2}, rather than being supported (e.g., white muscle of *Synbranchus*, Fig. 2; and heart muscle of *Synbranchus* and *Scyliorhinus*; see Heisler et al., 1980, Heisler, 1984a). At least in those few species that have been studied relative to ion transfer processes and pH adjustment kinetics, in addition to intracellular and extracellular acid-base status descriptions, it has become evident that simple semiclosed system buffering, the basis of the alphastat hypothesis, is not a major factor in pH regulation after changes in temperature.

B. Hypercapnia

In erythrocytes, the transfer of acid-base relevant ions across the cell membrane during changes in P_{CO_2} is a well-known mechanism (Hamburger shift), supporting the convective transport of metabolically produced CO_2 (buffered as HCO_3^-) from the tissues to the gas exchange site. Although transmembrane ion transfer in the tissues is a mechanism undoubtedly required to deal with the normal production of nonvolatile acid-base relevant metabolic endproducts, such processes only recently have received adequate attention.

Transmembrane Transfer In Vitro

Experiments in isolated, Ringer-suspended rat diaphragm indicated for the first time that during changes in P_{CO_2}, bicarbonate-equivalent ions were transferred

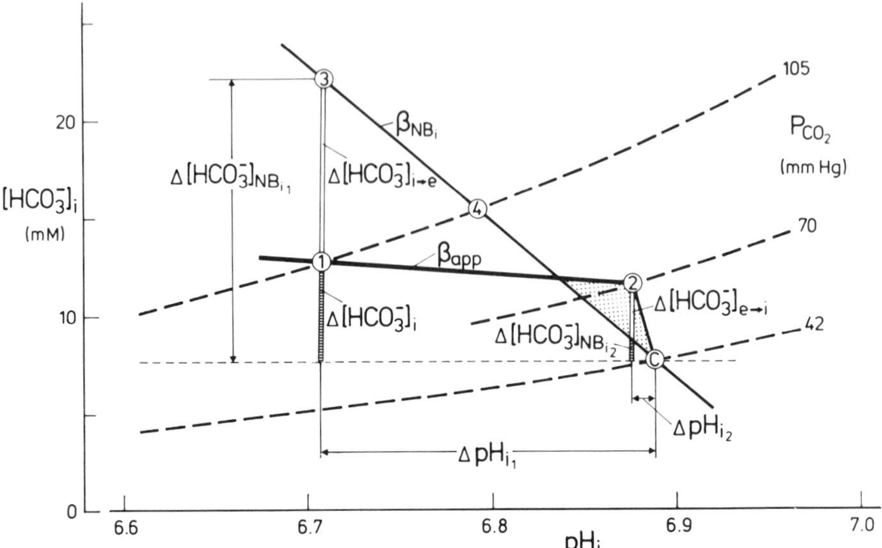

Figure 4 Changes in intracellular pH and bicarbonate concentration in rat diaphragm muscles during hypercapnia. The line labeled β_{app} represents the apparent buffer line with pH and $[HCO_3^-]$ values determined during various levels of hypercapnia, whereas β_{NBi} is the total nonbicarbonate buffer line of the intracellular space. During higher levels of hypercapnia, the intracellular $[HCO_3^-]$ is elevated for compensation a little higher than at lower levels of hypercapnia. A large fraction of bicarbonate produced by intracellular nonbicarbonate buffering ($\beta_{NBi} \cdot \Delta pH_{i1}$) is transferred to the extracellular space ($\Delta HCO_{3\,i\to e}^-$), (1) to (3), Approach 1 and 3). With a semiclosed system buffering pH would have been deflected by only (C) to (4) rather than by (C) to (1) (Approach 3, see text). At lower levels of hypercapnia, bicarbonate is gained from the extracellular space ($\Delta HCO_{3\,e\to i}^-$, shaded area), supporting compensation of the elevated PCO_2 and leading to an extremely high apparent buffer value [(C) to (2)], and concurrent extreme pH_i protection. (Based on data from Heisler and Piiper, 1971, 1972; Heisler, 1975.)

across tissue cell membranes (Fig. 4, $\Delta HCO_{3\,i\to e}^-$; Heisler and Piiper, 1972; see Approach 1). A considerable fraction of the bicarbonate produced intracellularly by nonbicarbonate buffering was released to, and could be measured in, the Ringer solution suspending the diaphragms. It was demonstrated that this resulted in a considerable underestimate in the total nonbicarbonate buffer value, if this was determined as the ratio of the changes in intracellular $[HCO_3^-]$ and pH (see Fig. 4, $\Delta[HCO_3^-]_i$, ΔpH_{i1}). In fact, evaluation of the data on the basis of this "open buffer system" concept (Heisler and Piiper, 1971; see Heisler,

1986a) resulted in an apparent buffer value, which was in good agreement with previous in vivo determinations (e.g., Irving et al., 1932; Waddell and Butler, 1959; Brown and Goott, 1963; Clancy and Brown, 1966; Schloerb et al., 1967; Burnell, 1968; Saborowski et al., 1970). When, however, the amount of bicarbonate-equivalents transferred to the extended extracellular space of the diaphragms was referred back to the intracellular space (see Fig. 4, $\Delta[HCO_3^-]_{NBi1}$, Approach 1), the resulting total nonbicarbonate buffer value complied very well with measurements in homogenates of the same tissue (Heisler and Piiper, 1971). This comparison also suggests that in the studies just cited, bicarbonate-equivalent ionic transfer contributed significantly to intracellular pH regulation.

Closer analysis in rat diaphragms of the process by application of the opposite approach (Approach 3, Eq. 6), on the basis of the intracellular nonbicarbonate buffer value and changes in pH, indicated that the extent and direction of bicarbonate-equivalent ion transfer between intra- and extracellular compartments depended very much upon the extent of the respiratory acid–base disturbance (see Fig. 4; Heisler, 1975). A moderate rise in P_{CO_2} and reduction in extracellular pH resulted in a net transfer of bicarbonate to the intracellular space, rather than in a release, as originally found during severe respiratory acid–base disturbances in the same preparation. The accumulation of additional bicarbonate originating from the extracellular space yielded an extremely high apparent intracellular buffer value (Heisler, 1975) [see Fig. 4, line (C)-(2)]. Although such extreme protection of pH_i appears to be limited to a range of extracellular pH values between 7.15 and 7.4 (or by a bicarbonate concentration limit in the range of about 12 to 14 mmol; see Fig. 4), the apparent buffer value of rat heart muscle (Clancy and Brown, 1966; Lai et al., 1973) is generally much higher than the chemical nonbicarbonate buffer value (Gonzalez et al., 1979), at least in the range of physiological pH values. This pH protection is the result of similar bicarbonate equivalent ion transfer mechanisms (Strome et al., 1977) as in the rat diaphragm, which is evidently even further stimulated during cardiac hypertrophy (Saborowski et al., 1973; Gonzalez et al., 1979).

Hypercapnia In Vivo

In living animals, hypercapnia can be induced by various processes. Elevated levels of CO_2 in the environment are rare in terrestrial animals, but are frequently encountered by aquatic species and readily transferred to their body fluids by the large gas exchange surface areas of gills and skin. Hypercapnia may also develop at normal environmental P_{CO_2} as a result of gas exchange limitations (e.g., in aquatic animals burrowed and estivating in dried out soil, and during pathological conditions such as emphysema and asthma in higher vertebrates) and because of changes in the O_2 content of the breathing medium (e.g., transition water to air breathing, environmental water hyperoxia). Hypercapnia of regulatory origin is rare in higher vertebrates and occurs only when the setpoint values of the ventilatory system are offset during physiological transitions (e.g., during hibernation) and because of pathological events (e.g., Pickwick syndrome).

The initial response to hypercapnia is a general fall in plasma and intracellular pH values. The magnitude of this fall depends on the relative increase in P_{CO_2} according to the exponential relationship between P_{CO_2} and pH of the Henderson-Hasselbalch equation. With some remarkable exceptions, however, pH recovers toward control values soon after initiation of hypercapnia by elevation of the bicarbonate concentration, partially or even completely compensating the elevation in P_{CO_2}.

Role of Buffering

Two main mechanisms are involved in the compensatory elevation of bicarbonate concentration. Production of bicarbonate by nonbicarbonate buffering of CO_2, especially in the well-buffered intracellular compartments may contribute significantly. The fraction of compensation supplied by this mechanism, however, is proportional to the deflection of pH in the respective compartment. Accordingly, the contribution of nonbicarbonate buffering is largest in those animals that are barely compensating, but comparatively small or negligible in those with close to complete compensation (see Fig. 6). The fractional contribution also changes during the time course of compensation, being reduced with the degree of pH recovery brought about by other mechanisms (see Fig. 5).

Another kind of buffering is the mobilization of carbonate from the osteal structures of the animal. This mechanism is certainly involved in bicarbonate elevation during long-term hypercapnia (e.g., Biebisch et al., 1955; Burnell, 1971; Schaefer, 1980) and during long-term metabolic acidosis (e.g., Leman et al., 1966; Jackson and Heisler, 1982), but its role in short-term disturbances has not yet been resolved. It apparently does not play any significant role in the teleost fish, *Ictalurus punctatus*, (Cameron, 1985), and, as judged from changes in plasma [Ca^{2+}] and [Mg^{2+}], it does not contribute significantly to compensation of hypercapnia in the freshwater turtle, *Pseudemys scripta elegans* (Silver and Jackson, 1985).

Bicarbonate-Equivalent Ion Transfer

The largest contribution to the compensation of hypercapnia is clearly supplied by acid–base relevant ion transfer mechanisms. The rate of bicarbonate gain is severalfold larger in fishes and in amphibia than in man (Table 3), although the uptake rate is, at least in freshwater fishes, apparently linked to the bicarbonate and counterion concentrations in the environmental water, and may well be reduced considerably under adverse conditions (see Heisler, 1984b, 1986b). This sensitivity of fishes resides in the direct contact with the environmental water of

Table 3 Maximal Transepithelial Acid-Base Relevant Ion Transfer Rates

Species	Conditions		Transfer rate (μmol/kg body water)	Transfer rate/ SMR	Ref.
	Exercise-induced lactacidosis $[Lact^-]_{pl}$ (mM)	Hypercapnia P_{CO_2} (mm Hg)			
Scyliorhinus stellaris	<15		14.3	0.41[a]	Holeton and Heisler, 1983
	>15		15.7	0.45[a]	Heisler et al., 1976
		8.2	15.3	0.43[a]	
		10.3	14.7	0.42[a]	Heisler and Nuemann, 1977
Conger conger	<10		9.3		Holeton et al., 1986
	10–20		10.4		
	>20		9.8		
		10.1	15.3		Toews et al., 1983
Salmo gairdneri	<15		24.1	0.43[b]	Holeton et al., 1983
	>15		26.3	0.47[b]	
Cyprinus carpio		37.2	5.3	0.13[c]	Claiborne and Heisler, 1986
Bufo marinus		40.6	5.1	0.11[d]	Toews and Heisler, 1982
		40.0	23.5	0.43[d]	

Table 3 (continued)

Species	Conditions: Exercise-induced lactacidosis $[Lact^-]_{pl}$ (mM)	Conditions: Hypercapnia P_{CO_2} (mm Hg)	Transfer rate (μmol/kg body water)	Transfer rate/ SMR	Ref.
Dog	Acute NH_4Cl acidosis		<3	0.02[c]	Pitts, 1945a,b
	Chronic NH_4Cl acidosis		<7	0.03[c]	
Man	Severe diabetic acidosis		<7.5	0.03[c]	Pitts, 1948

Data for standard metabolic rate (SMR):
[a] 34.8 μmol/min · kg^{-1} body water: Randall et al., 1976.
[b] 55.3 μmol/min · kg^{-1} body water: Ultsch et al., 1980.
[c] 39.1 μmol/min · kg^{-1} body water: Ultsch et al., 1980.
[d] 55 μmol/min · kg^{-1} body water: Jackson and Braun, 1979. (data for bullfrog, *Rana catesbeiana*)
[e] 298 μmol/min · kg^{-1} body water: Scotto et al., 1984.
SMR = standard metabolic rate.

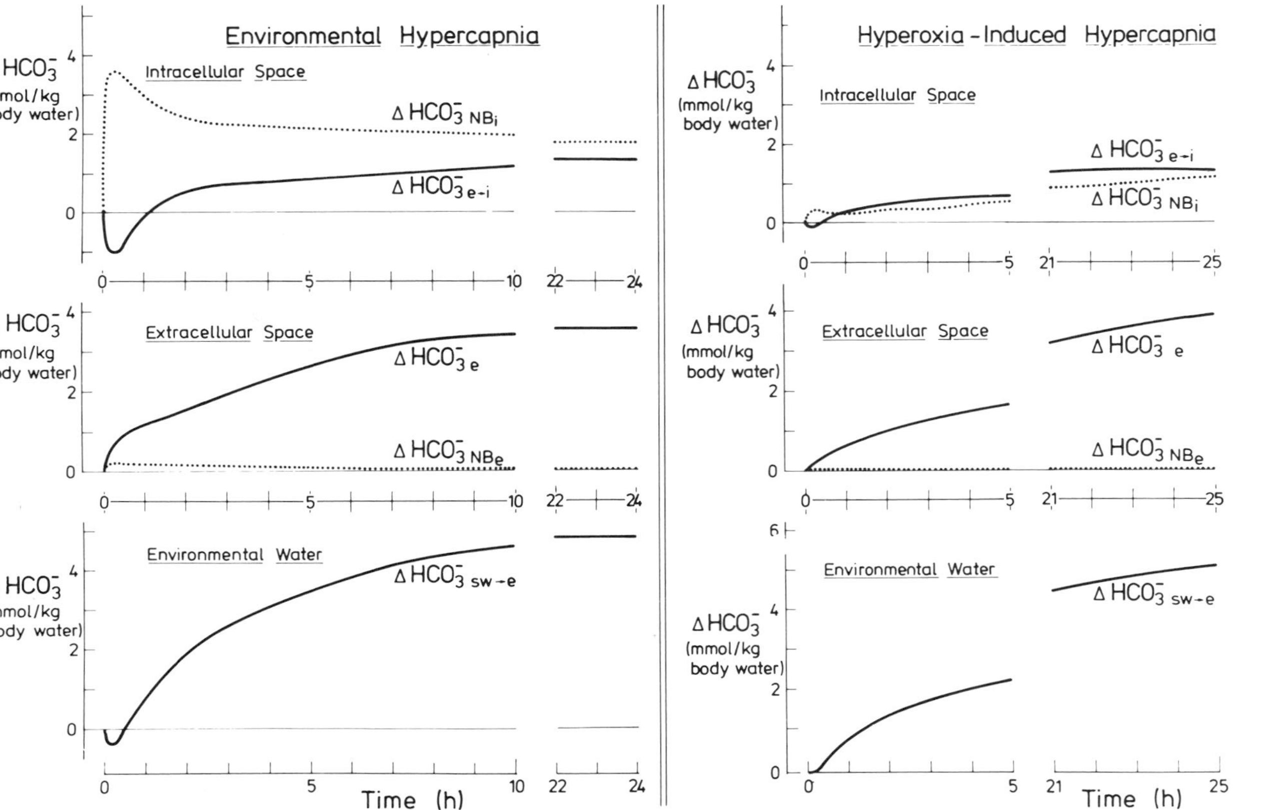

Figure 5 Contribution of nonbicarbonate buffering (index NB) and the transfer of bicarbonate-equivalent ions (indices e→i and sw→e) to the compensatory bicarbonate accumulation in the body fluids of *S. stellaris* during environmental and hyperoxia-induced hypercapnia. e = extracellular, i = intracellular, sw = seawater.

the branchial epithelium, which is responsible for usually more than 95% of the ion transfer (for review see Heisler, 1984b, 1986b). Semiterrestrial animals, relying more on renal mechanisms, are little affected by such factors.

As a typical pattern, at least in some lower vertebrates, it has emerged that during the initial phase of rapidly imposed environmental hypercapnia the well-buffered intracellular space supports compensation of the extracellular space by a transmembrane bicarbonate-equivalent shift (e.g., Heisler et al., 1976; Toews et al., 1983; Boutilier and Heisler, 1988; Fig. 5, left panel) before the transepithelial bicarbonate-equivalent uptake is sufficiently activated. As a maladaptive response, a loss of bicarbonate-equivalents to the environment often occurs during the initial stage of hypercapnia (see Fig. 5, left panel). This phenomenon may be viewed as an expression that the bicarbonate threshold of the ion retaining and resorbing structures is not yet adjusted to the different conditions with plasma bicarbonate levels already elevated by blood nonbicarbonate buffering and by transfer from the intracellular space. The initial release of bicarbonate-equivalents may then, in turn, represent a similar lack of adjustment at the cell membrane level. After full activation of the transepithelial transfer, the amount of bicarbonate originally supplied by the intracellular space is returned, and bicarbonate gained from the environment is accumulated in both the extracellular and intracellular compartments (see Fig. 5). With rising bicarbonate concentration and restoration of pH toward control values, the contribution of nonbicarbonate buffering to the overall compensation is reduced to insignificant levels in the extracellular space and to about half in the intracellular compartments (see Fig. 5).

About the same elevation in plasma P_{CO_2}, induced by an increase of the O_2 content of the breathing medium (see Dejours, 1975, 1981), results in a slightly different regulatory pattern from that observed during environmentally imposed hypercapnia. The reduction in ventilation leading to hypercapnia in the body fluids is finely adjusted and matched to the uptake rate of bicarbonate-equivalent ions, resulting in only small changes of pH in the body fluids (Heisler et al., 1981, 1988; see Heisler, 1988b). Under these conditions, the role of buffering during the initial stages of hyperoxia-hypercapnia is very small (see Fig. 5, right panel) and, only after several days, rises to values similar to those found during environmental hypercapnia (cf. Heisler et al., 1987). Also, the bicarbonate-equivalent uptake rate is generally lower than during environmental hypercapnia, and the "overflow" effects of bicarbonate from intracellular to extracellular space and to the environment are very much reduced or completely avoided (see Fig. 5, right panel).

Limits of Compensation

The extent of hypercapnic compensation by accumulation of bicarbonate in the body fluids is quite variable among animal classes, even among individual species of classes. Fishes generally manage to compensate for the shift in extracellular pH (at constant bicarbonate concentration; see Heisler, 1986c) by more than 80%, with some notable exceptions (*Cyprinus carpio*, about 50%, Claiborne and Heisler, 1984, 1986; *Synbranchus marmoratus*, 0%, Heisler, 1982). In amphibians, which may be subjects of extreme environmental hypercapnia (see Heisler et al., 1982), the compensation of plasma pH is comparatively poor (0-35%), with the Amazonian apodan *Typhlonectes compressicauda* representing another remarkable exception (80% compensation; Toews and Macintyre, 1978). The degree of compensation in Reptilia, at least in the only two studied species, is similar to that in many Amphibia (*Tupinambis nigropunctatus*, 28 or 36%, at 4 or 7% inspired F_{CO_2} for 72 h, respectively, Glass and Heisler, 1986; *Chrysemys picta bellii*, 35%, Silver and Jackson, 1986). In higher vertebrates, moderate hypercapnia is usually rather well compensated (increase of P_{CO_2} in plasma < 1.4-fold), whereas more extensive elevations of P_{CO_2} (which is usually the case in experiments with lower vertebrates) drastically reduce the extent of compensation to values similar to those in reptiles and amphibians (for references see Woodbury, 1965).

Although environmental factors, such as the water composition (see Heisler and Neumann, 1977; Heisler, 1984b, 1986b, 1988b)—especially the bicarbonate and the exchange counterion concentrations—and behavioral factors, such as air breathing (see Heisler, 1982), may also be involved, the extent of compensation appears to be closely linked to the maximal bicarbonate concentration that can be attained in the animal plasma. A critical review of relevant literature suggests that certain plasma bicarbonate concentrations are never surpassed. These values are apparently absolute limits for individual species, whereas some variability exists among species. For most lower vertebrates (fishes, amphibians, and reptiles, with few exceptions) the plasma bicarbonate threshold appears to fall into a range of 23 to 33 mmol (Fig. 6), with the fishes at the lower end, and the reptiles (27-45 mmol) and the higher vertebrates (40-50 mmol) tending toward the higher end of this range, or exceeding it (27-45 mmol).

Complete compensation of elevated plasma P_{CO_2} implies elevation of the bicarbonate concentration by the same factor as that for the rise in P_{CO_2} (see Heisler, 1986c). According to the maximal bicarbonate concentration, the extent of compensation is closely related to the initial (control) bicarbonate concentration. It is evident that fishes with their primarily low $[HCO_3^-]$ can raise bicarbonate to a much larger extent than reptiles and most amphibia. The only fishes that achieve less than almost complete compensation are actually those with high control values (*Cyprinus*, about 50%, $[HCO_3^-]_c = 14$ mmol; *Synbranchus*, 0%, $[HCO_3^-]_c = 24$ mmol), and the exception from the general pattern of poor compensation in amphibians, *Typhlonectes*, has a control $[HCO_3^-]$ of only about 12 mmol.

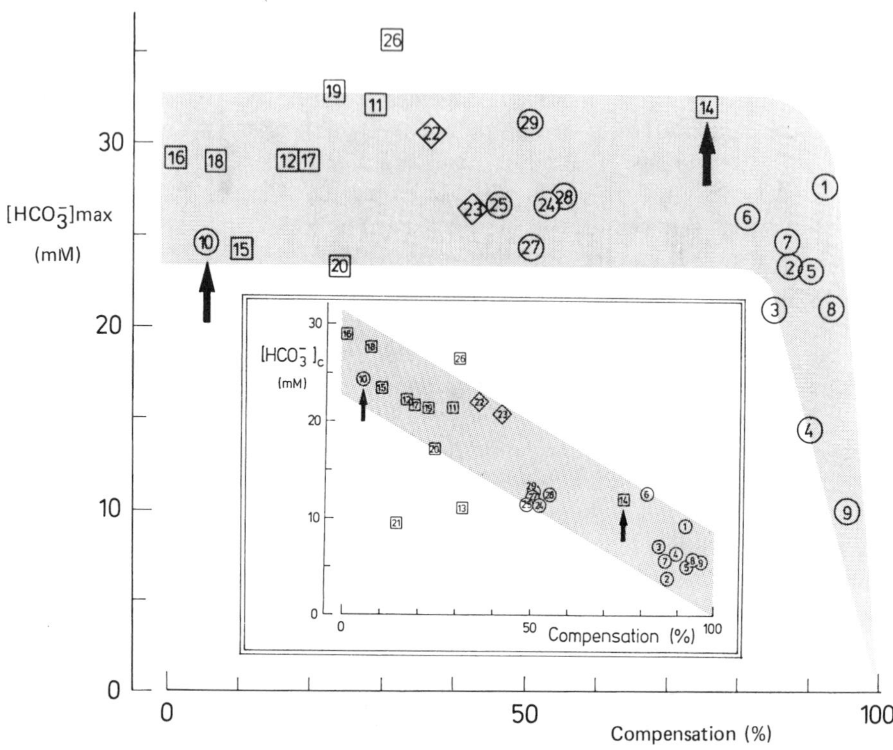

Figure 6 Maximal bicarbonate concentration and degree of pH compensation attained during hypercapnia in fishes (circles), amphibia (squares) and reptiles (rhombs). Insert: Relationship between control bicarbonate concentration ([HCO_3^-]$_c$) and degree of compensation during hypercapnia. Arrows indicate remarkable exceptions from the general pattern of animal classes (see text). [Species and data sources: (1) *Salmo gairdneri*: Janssen and Randall, 1975; (2) *S. gairdneri*: Eddy et al., 1977; (3) *Scyliorinus stellaris*: Heisler et al., 1976a; (4) *Ictalurus punctatus*: Cameron, 1980; (5) *Conger conger*: Toews et al., 1983; (6) *Cyprinus carpio*: Claiborne and Heisler, 1986; (7) *Scyliorinus stellaris*: Heisler et al., 1981; (8) *S. stellaris*: Heisler et al., 1981; (9) *S. stellaris*: Heisler et al., 1980; (1) *Synbranchus marmoratus*: Heisler, 1982; (11) *Bufo marinus*: Toews and Heisler, 1982. (12) *B. marinus*: Boutlier et al., 1979; (13) *Cryptobranchus aleganiensis*: Boutilier and Toews, 1981; (14) *Typhlonectes compressicauda*: Toews and Macintyre, 1978; (15) *Siren lacertina*: Heisler et al., 1982; (16) *Amphiuma means*: Heisler et al., 1982; (17) *Ambystoma tigrinum* (larvae): Hicks and Stiffler, 1980; (18) *Xenopus laevis*: Boutilier, 1981; (19) *B. marinus*: Toews and Kirby, 1985; (20) *A. tigrinum*: Stiffler et al., 1983; (21) *Necturus maculosus*: Stiffler et al., 1983; (22) *Tupinambis nigropunctatus*: M. L. Glass and N. Heisler, 1986; (23) *T. nigropunctatus*: M. L. Glass and N. Heisler, 1986; (24) *Cyprinus carpio*: J. B. Claiborne and N. Heisler, 1986; (25) *C. carpio*: Claiborne and Heisler, 1984; (26) *B. marinus*, Boutilier and Heisler, 1988; (27–29) *C. carpio*: N. A. Andersen and N. Heisler, unpublished.]

This pattern, indirectly indicating the existence of a species-specific plasma bicarbonate threshold, is confirmed by some more direct experimental evidence. Specimens of incompletely compensating species were exposed to environmental hypercapnia until a new steady state had been attained. When bicarbonate was then directly infused into the blood stream, the extent of compensation was improved only transiently before the infused bicarbonate was quantitatively released to the environment (*Siren lacertina*, Heisler et al., 1982; *Cyprinus carpio*, Claiborne and Heisler, 1986; *Tupinambis nigropunctatus*, Glass and Heisler, 1986; *Bufo marinus*, Boutilier and Heisler, 1988).

Regulation of Intracellular pH

The largest fraction of the bicarbonate gained by transepithelial transfer is usually accumulated in the extracellular body compartments (see Fig. 5). Nevertheless, the intracellular pH is generally very well compensated, typically to a larger extent than the extracellular pH. This is especially evident when little or no extracellular compensation takes place, such as in the air-breathing teleost fish, *S. marmoratus* (Heisler, 1982), the amphibians, *Siren lacertina* (Heisler et al., 1982) and *B. marinus* (Toews and Heisler, 1982). But also in fishes with pronounced extracellular pH compensation ($\Delta pH < -0.15$; for review, see Heisler, 1984b, 1986b; Heisler et al., 1988) the intracellular pH usually exceeds the extracellular pH compensation ($\Delta pH < -0.07$) (Fig. 7). This phenomenon of preferential intracellular versus extracellular pH regulation is supported by the primarily lower bicarbonate concentrations in the intracellular body compartments. Almost complete compensation is achieved by transmembrane transfer of bicarbonate-equivalent ions, which quantitatively would hardly effect the extent of extracellular compensation (see Fig. 7; Heisler, 1982; Heisler et al., 1982). This pattern of pH protection, even at the expense of the extracellular space, suggests a view of the membranes of the intracellular body compartments as the "second defense line" for body fluid homiostasis. The intracellular body compartments may accordingly represent an analogue to Claude Bernards "milieu interieur."

C. Lactacidosis

The main end product of anaerobic glycolysis in vertebrates is lactic acid, which is produced in large quantities during periods of environmental hypoxia or anoxia. It is also produced when the oxygen demand to tissues exceeds the oxygen supply by gas exchange with the environment and the convective transport by the blood to the site of consumption. This may be related to failure of ventilatory and circulatory mechanisms, or to anemia, but it is most frequently encountered during transient periods of an excessively high energy demand during escape and predatory activities, which is then supplied by anaerobic metabolism.

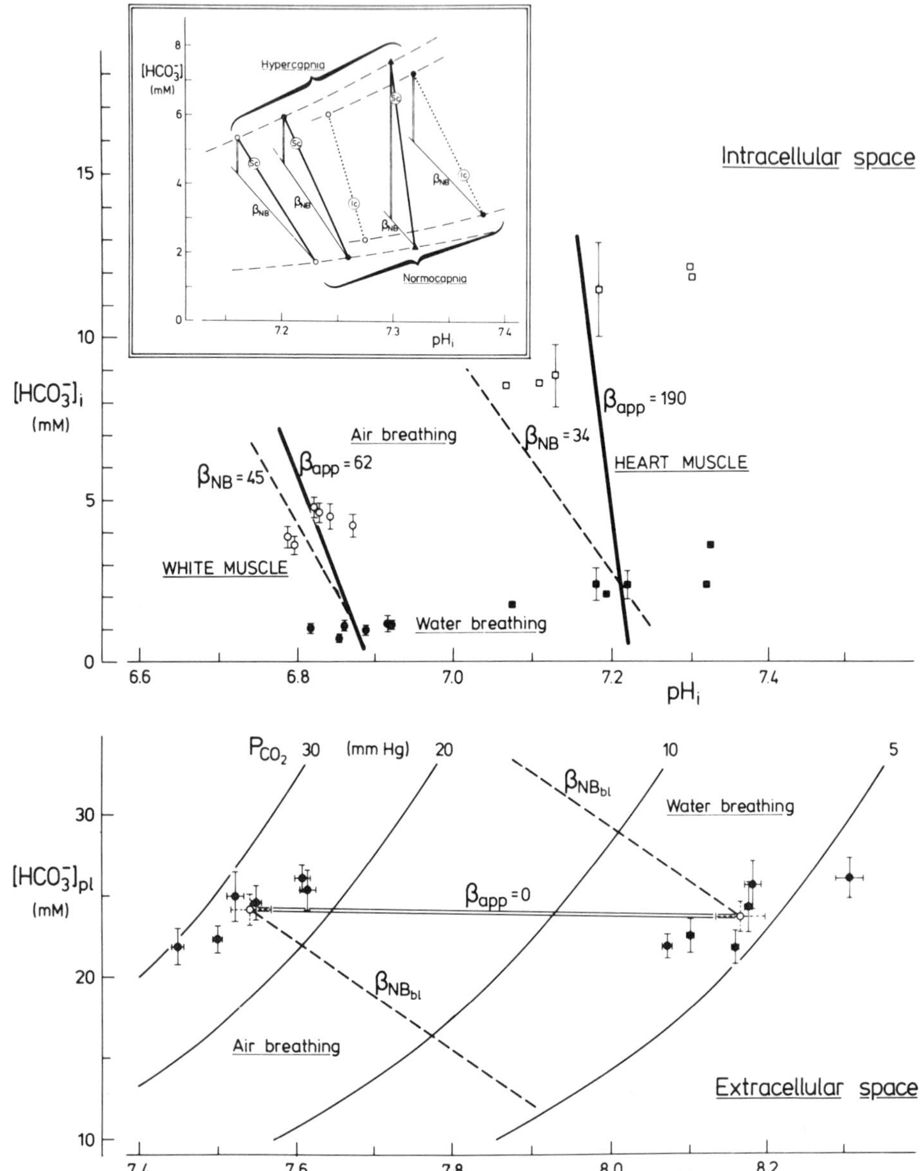
Intracellular space
[HCO3-]i (mM)
pHi
Air breathing
Water breathing
WHITE MUSCLE
HEART MUSCLE
βNB = 45
βapp = 62
βNB = 34
βapp = 190
Hypercapnia
Normocapnia
Extracellular space
[HCO3-]pl (mM)
pHpl
PCO2 (mm Hg)
βNBbl
βapp = 0

While cleavage of creatine phosphate and ATP as the other components of the "oxygen debt" is repaid by resynthesis within short periods (see Piiper and Spiller, 1970) at the site of energy production (e.g., white musculature), lactic acid is removed from the body fluids mainly by futher aerobic metabolism to CO_2 (or resynthesis to glycogen) in only a few tissues (e.g., liver, heart, and red muscle), with a comparatively delayed time course. According to its low pK value (about 3.9) lactic acid is dissociated into H^+ and lactate (La^-) ions immediately upon production and, therefore, represents a considerable stress factor for the acid-base regulation.

Characteristics of Acid-Base Regulation During Lactacidosis in Vivo

A complete evaluation of the acid-base regulation, including transmembrane and transepithelial ion fluxes, requires a considerable amount of experimental data, which are scarce for animal species other than the elasmobranch fish, *Scyliorhinus stellaris*. The following analysis based on those data certainly cannot be transferred directly to other species, especially terrestrial animals (which lack the important capability of aquatic animals for transient translocation of surplus H^+ ions to the environment), but may provide an overview of the facilities and limitations of acid-base regulation during lactacidosis (Approaches 4 and 3).

In *S. stellaris*, an average of about 16 mmol/kg body water of lactic acid was accumulated in the intracellular muscle fluid compartments during exhausting anaerobic activity, equivalent to an average muscle cell water concentration of about 36 mM (Holeton and Heisler, 1983). The dissociation products, H^+ and La^- ions are gradually released to the extracellular space. The H^+ ions are eliminated initially from the muscle cells to the extracellular space, at an ex-

---

Figure 7 Intracellular pH compensation during hypercapnia. In spite of completely uncompensated air-breathing-induced hypercapnia and associated acidosis in the extracellular space (lower panel), the intracellular pH of *Synbranchus marmoratus* is almost completely restored by elevation of the bicarbonate concentration (upper panel), similar to the extent of intracellular compensation observed during environmental hypercapnia in water-breathing fishes [Insert: intracellular pH and [HCO_3^-] of *Scyliorinus stellaris* (Sc) and *Ictalurus punctatus* (Ic) during normocapnia and hypercapnia. Filled circles: white muscle; open circles: red muscle; triangles: heart muscle.] The bicarbonate elevation is brought about by intracellular nonbicarbonate buffering (β_{NB}), and by bicarbonate-equivalent ion transfer to the intracellular space (difference between β_{NB} and β_{app}, in the insert indicated by vertical double lines (Approach 3, see text). (Data from Heisler et al., 1976; Heisler, 1980, 1982; Cameron, 1985.)

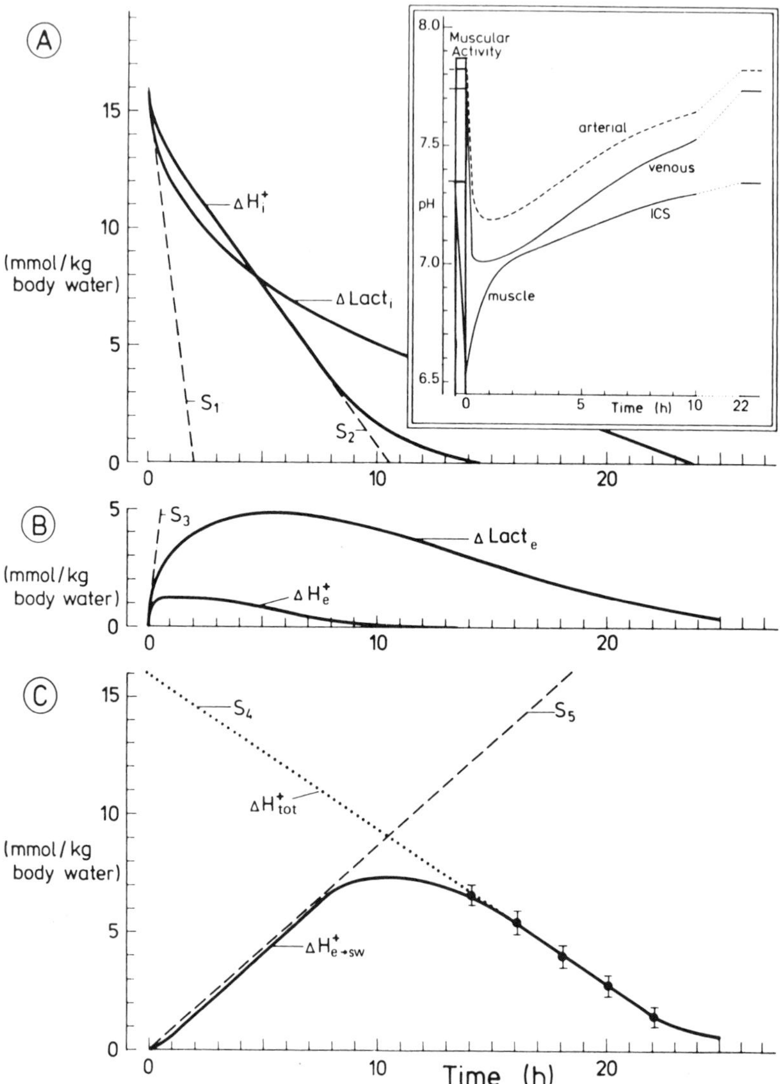

Figure 8 Kinetics of elimination of surplus H^+ and La^- ions from the intracellular muscle compartments [(A), indices i] to the extracellular space [(B), indices e], and to the environmental water [(C), index e→sw] after exhausting muscular activity in the elasmobranch *S. stellaris*. Transfer and lactic acid metabolization rates are indicated by S_1–S_5 (Approach 4). Insert: changes of extracellular and intracellular muscle pH (Approaches 3 and 4, see text). (Data from Holeton and Heisler, 1983; Heisler and Neumann, 1980; Heisler, 1978.)

tremely high rate (> 150 μmol/min · kg body water; S_1, Fig. 8). This elevates the amount of H^+ ions bound extracellularly at a rate (S_3, Fig. 8) smaller than that of the intracellular-extracellular transfer (S_1) by only the rate of lactic acid metabolism (see S_4, Fig. 8). This tremendous rate of initial H^+ efflux from the muscle cells, compared with the maximal transepithelial transfer rate, certainly represents an underestimate of the real transmembrane transfer rate; any dislocation of H^+ equivalents into nonmuscular intracellular compartments, facilitated by the concurrent reduction of extracellular pH, cannot be taken into account given the available data. Furthermore, the process must be considered to be perfusion limited (Neumann et al., 1983).

This initial high rate of H^+ transfer is reduced to about 25 μmol/min · kg (see Fig. 8, S_2), mainly as a result of an *equilibrium limitation* (Holeton and Heisler, 1983). Extracellular pH in the small volume of poorly buffered extracellular fluid (see Fig. 8, insert) is reduced to such an extent by transfer of only about 8% of the amount of originally produced H^+ ions that equilibrium (although at a reduced level) between intracellular and extracellular pH is achieved. This eliminates the driving force for any further H^+ equivalent transfer in excess of the rate of H^+ removal from the extracellular space (ECS) by other mechanisms (observe the plateau in ΔH^+_e curve, S_5, S_4, Fig. 8). After having attained pH equilibrium, the time course of pH normalization therefore depends only on the rate of lactic acid metabolism (about 11 μmol/min · kg, S_4) and the transfer rate of H^+ equivalents to the environmental water ($\Delta H^+_{e \rightarrow env}$, about 14 μmol/min · kg, S_5). When all surplus H^+ ions are removed from the organism with normalization of intracellular and extracellular pH, metabolism of lactic acid continues with H^+ ions being taken up from the environment at the metabolic rate (S_4, about 11 μmol/min · kg), which is slightly lower than the maximal branchial transfer rate (S_5, about 14 μmol/min · kg; see Table 3).

This evaluation emphasizes the important role of transepithelial acid-base relevant ion transfer processes for the acid-base regulation of this and other aquatic animal species (see Heisler, 1986, ed.). Transient transfer of H^+ equivalents to the environment facilitates early normalization of pH in the body fluids long before the original stress factor, lactic acid, has been completely removed from the system. A typical feature of the described regulatory pattern is the preferential restoration of intracellular pH (see Fig. 8, insert), suggesting a priority of intracellular over extracellular pH regulation, similar to the conditions observed during hypercapnia (see Heisler, 1986c).

Efflux Kinetics of Lactate and Hydrogen Ions

Although the elimination kinetics of La^- and H^+ ions from muscle cells in *S. stellaris* can be distinguished clearly (see Fig. 8A), the amount of lactate actually released from the cellular compartment is not much different from that of

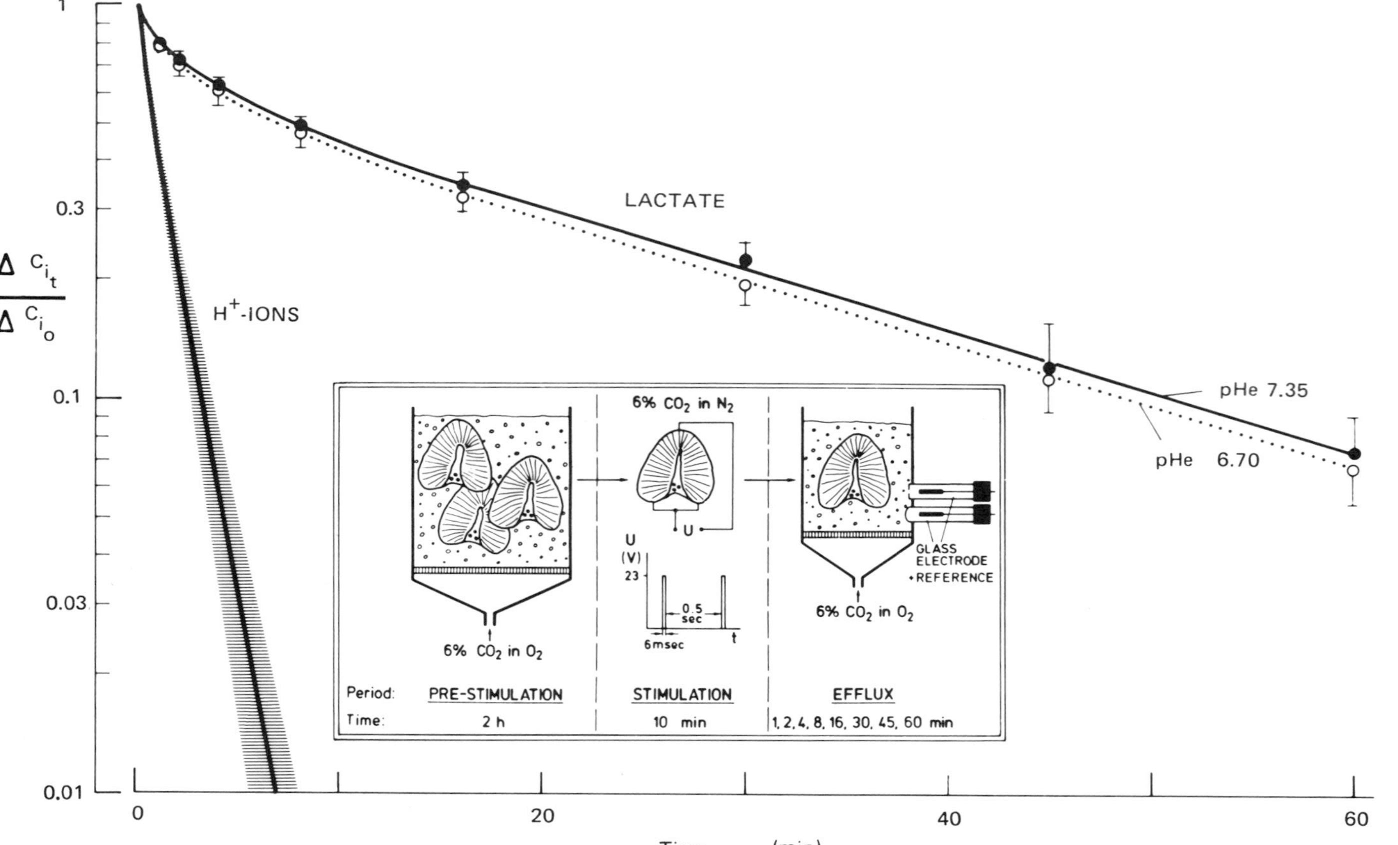

LACTATE
H+-IONS
pHe 7.35
pHe 6.70
Δ C_it / Δ C_io
1
0.3
0.1
0.03
0.01
0
20
40
60
Time (min)
6% CO2 in O2
6% CO2 in N2
U (V)
23
0.5 sec
6 msec
t
U
GLASS ELECTRODE +REFERENCE
6% CO2 in O2
Period: PRE-STIMULATION STIMULATION EFFLUX
Time: 2 h 10 min 1, 2, 4, 8, 16, 30, 45, 60 min

Figure 9

H^+, at least during the first 8 h of the experiment. This feature conforms well with data obtained in experiments on the isolated perfused dog gastrocnemius muscle (Hirche et al., 1975), on superfused (Mainwood and Worsley-Brown, 1975) and perfused frog muscle (Boutilier et al., 1985), and in various whole-animal experiments (for references seen Benade' and Heisler, 1978). In those experiments the ratio of H^+/La^- transferred to the extracellular space was usually approximately unity and seldom exceeded a factor of 2.

The similarity in the amounts of La^- and H^+ eliminated from muscle cells, however, cannot be taken as an indication that the efflux (or elimination) time constants of these two dissociation products are the same, or similar, because the steady-state distribution patterns of La^- and H^+ are rather different. Lactate is distributed across the cell membrane either according to the membrane potential (main transfer form: La^-) or according to the intracellular-extracellular pH differences (main transfer form: lactic acid). In both, equilibrium is achieved when most of the La^- has been transferred to the extracellular space (ECS). In contrast, the distribution of H^+ is mainly determined by the distribution of the nonbicarbonate buffer capacity, which in fishes is much higher in intracellular tissue compartments than in the ECS (Heisler, 1986a, 1986d).

Accordingly, the absolute transfer rate for H^+ will be reduced and will have already approached zero when a much smaller fraction of the total amount of H^+ than La^- has been transferred. When taking into account the different asymptotes of La^- and H^+ elimination (the extracellular plateau ranges, Fig. 8B), the efflux rate constants actually differ by a factor of about 12 (Holeton and Heisler, 1983).

This rough estimate conforms rather well with results of experiments in isolated Ringer-suspended rat diaphragms (Fig. 9, insert) and frog sartorius muscles (Approach 1; Benade' and Heisler, 1978). Those experiments indicated that H^+ ions were eliminated 12 (diaphragm) to 40 times (sartorius) faster (half time of the efflux) than La^- ions (see Fig. 9). This remarkable difference in efflux rate constants suggests that H^+ and La^- rather than the nondissociated lactic acid are actually transferred across the cell membrane. This proposition is supported by the independence of the efflux time constant of La^- from intra-

---

Figure 9 Efflux kinetics of La^- and H^+ ions from isolated Ringer-suspended rat diaphragm muscles. Insert: experimental procedure and apparatus. The efflux of H^+ ions was monitored continuously, the occurrence of La^- in the Ringer solution was measured at the indicated times after stimulation. ΔC_{it} and ΔC_{i0} are the changes in intracellular amounts of La^- and H^+ ions at time t and time zero. (For details see Benadé and Heisler, 1978.)

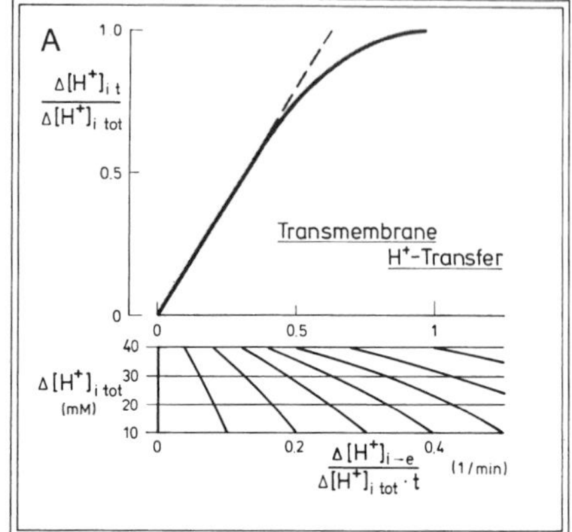
A
Transmembrane H⁺-Transfer
Δ[H⁺]i t / Δ[H⁺]i tot
Δ[H⁺]i tot (mM)
Δ[H⁺]i→e / Δ[H⁺]i tot · t (1/min)

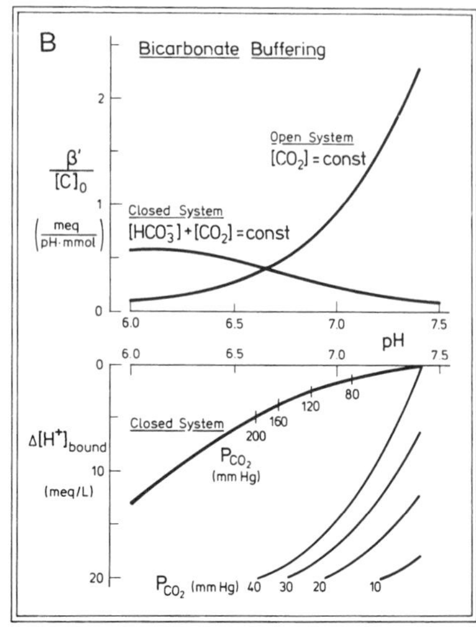
B
Bicarbonate Buffering
β′ / [C]0 (meq / pH·mmol)
Open System
[CO2] = const
Closed System
[HCO3⁻] + [CO2] = const
pH
Δ[H⁺]bound (meq/L)
Closed System
PCO2 (mm Hg)
PCO2 (mm Hg) 40 30 20 10

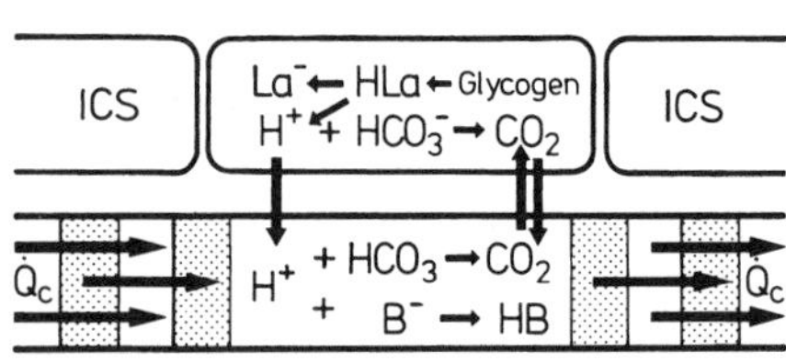
ICS
La⁻ ← HLa ← Glycogen
H⁺ + HCO3⁻ → CO2
ICS
Q̇c
H⁺ + HCO3 → CO2
+ B⁻ → HB
Q̇c

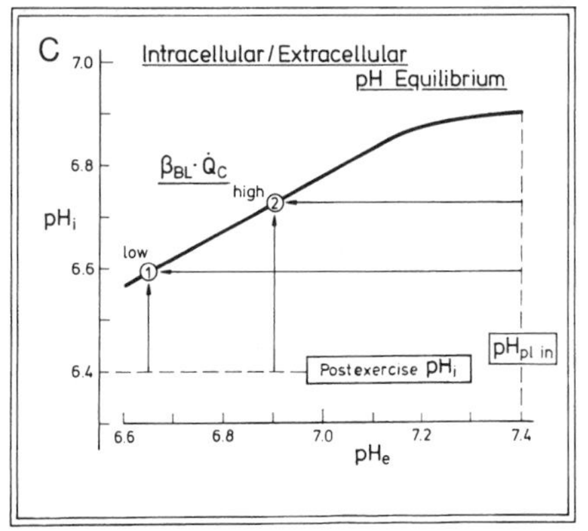
C
Intracellular / Extracellular pH Equilibrium
βBL · Q̇C
high
low
pHi
pHpl in
Postexercise pHi
pHe

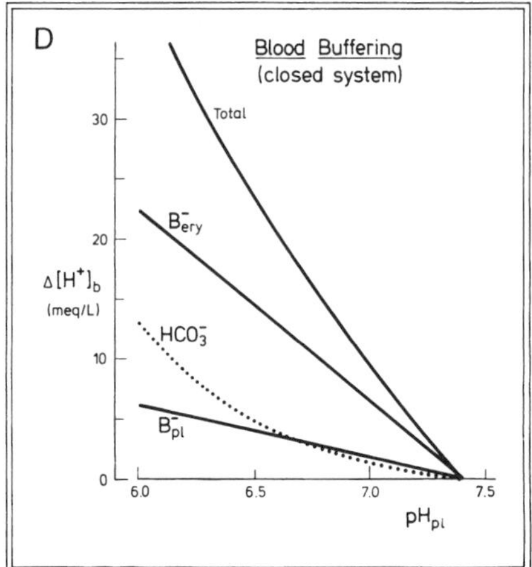
D
Blood Buffering (closed system)
Total
B⁻ery
Δ[H⁺]b (meq/L)
HCO3⁻
B⁻pl
pHpl

cellular and extracellular pH in isolated suspended muscles and by comparison with the efflux time constants of partially charged (DMO) and uncharged substances (tritiated water and antipyrine) (Heisler et al., 1977, 1978; Heisler, 1988d).

Limiting Factors for Hydrogen Ion Elimination from Perfused Muscle Tissues

The *equilibrium limitation* of transmembrane H^+-equivalent ion transfer during lactacidosis in *S. stellaris* (Holeton and Heisler, 1983; see Fig. 8), induced by the low extracellular, in comparison with the intracellular, buffer capacity (buffer value × volume) results in a similar delay in the efflux of H^+ ions from muscle cells as observed in the preceding experiments with perfused and superfused muscle preparations. The experimental conditions, however, are hardly comparable. In heavily exercised fishes more than 40% of the body weight (equivalent to the entire muscle mass) is loaded with H^+ ions to be eliminated to the comparatively small and poorly buffered extracellular space (15-20% of the body weight), whereas superfused and perfused isolated muscle preparations are continuously supplied with fresh super-/perfusate of normal pH and P_{CO_2}. Similar conditions apply for most in vivo experiments, during which exercise usually is performed in only selected muscle groups.

The original pH and P_{CO_2} composition of the perfusate, however, will be not maintained when H^+ ions are released from the cells past the interstitial space into the capillary fluid. Similarly, as with reduction of pH in the bulk extracellular fluid of *Scyliorhinus*, the local reduction in capillary pH may lead to an equilibrium between intracellular and capillary-interstitial pH. The amount

---

Figure 10 Parameters for a model simulation of the H^+ elimination kinetics from perfused rat diaphragm muscles on the basis of data from isolated Ringer-suspended diaphragm muscles (Approaches 2 and 3, see text). (A) Specific transmembrane H^+ transfer rate (x-axis) as a function of the amount of surplus intracellular H^+ ions ($\Delta H^+]_{itot}$) and the remaining intracellular H^+ ions at time, t, (y-axis). (Data of Benadé and Heisler, 1978; N. Heisler, A. J. S. Benadé, and H. Weitz, unpublished.) (B) Bicarbonate buffering in fluid systems closed or open for molecular CO_2. (C) Correlation between intracellular (pH_i) and extracellular pH (pH_e) at equilibrium (rat diaphragm, Heisler, 1975). Post exercise pH_i restoration toward control values is reduced at lower (1) as compared with higher (2) pH_e values, which are a function of the buffer capacity of the perfusate ($\beta_{BL} \cdot \dot{Q}_c$). pH_{pl} is the plasma pH of blood entering muscle capillaries. (D) Buffering of H^+ ions in blood of normal hematocrit by erythrocyte and plasma nonbicarbonate buffers (B^-_{ery} and B^-_{pl}) and blood bicarbonate, after reduction of pH from 7.4 to lower values in a system closed for molecular CO_2. See text.

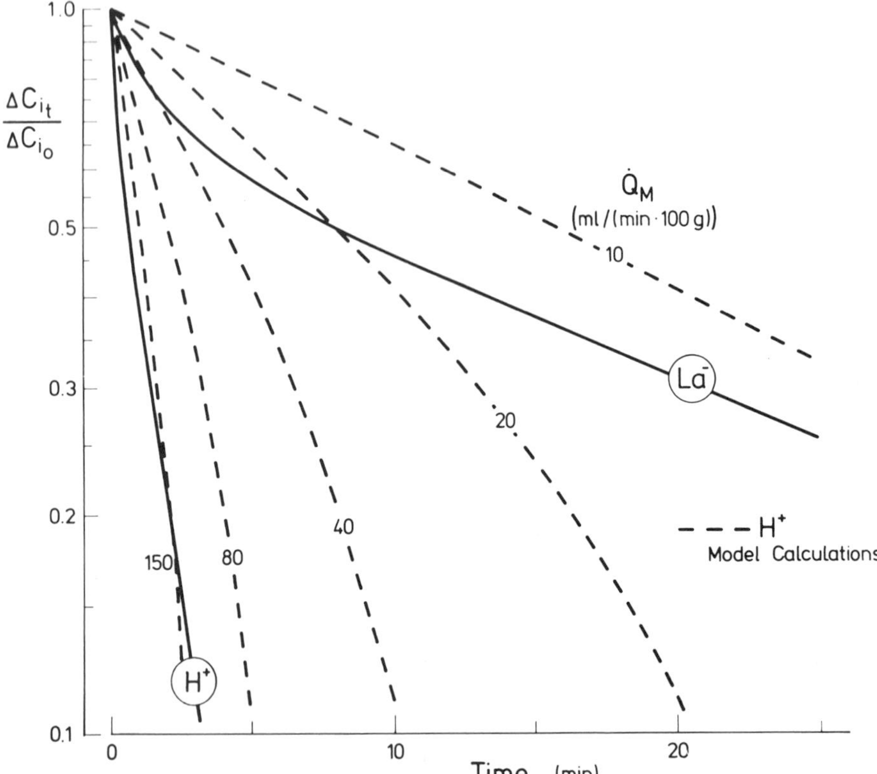

Figure 11 Model simulation of the expected H^+ ion efflux rate from isolated perfused rat diaphragm muscles (dashed lines) compared with the measured efflux of H^+ and La^- in Ringer-suspended diaphragms (solid lines) (Data of Benadé and Heisler, 1978; see Fig. 9). ΔC_{io} is the fraction of surplus H^+ ions still in the intracellular space at time t, $\dot{Q}_M$ = muscle perfusion. H^+ and La^- elimination kinetics are similar at low perfusion rates. The extremely fast elimination kinetics of H^+ ions from isolated Ringer-suspended diaphragms can be expected in blood-perfused preparations only at extremely high perfusion rates. See text.

of H^+ ions taken up by the capillary fluid per unit of time before pH_i/pH_e equilibrium is attained is a function of the buffering capabilities and the volume supplied to the interface of H^+ transfer.

The buffering capabilities of extracellular fluids with respect to the addition of nonvolatile H^+ ions are largely determined (especially in air breathers) by the bicarbonate buffer system. However, because of its low pK_1' value the bicarbonate system is an effective buffer only when the CO_2 resulting from buffering H^+ ions is removed by the gas exchange structures (open-buffer system; Fig. 10B). Blood passing the muscle tissue must be considered as a closed-buffer system (see Heisler, 1986a,c) and the effective buffering capability is, accordingly, rather limited (see Fig. 10B). Surplus CO_2 is not eliminated from the buffer system and cannot even diffuse into the muscle tissue because a large proportion of the intracellular HCO_3^- has been transferred to molecular CO_2 by the H^+ ions produced during muscular activity. The tissue P_{CO_2} value attained after buffering of transferred H^+ ions is, accordingly, higher than that of the blood.

Because bicarbonate buffering is rather limited, resulting from the closed-system conditions, H^+ ions transferred from muscle tissue to blood must be bound primarily by nonbicarbonate buffers (Fig. 10D). The lower (closed-system) buffer value can be compensated for only by increased flow through the muscle tissue. Conditions are worse with perfusate that does not contain red blood cells and, more so, when nonbicarbonate buffers are completely lacking. With such conditions, equilibrium limitation of H^+ efflux by the largely reduced perfusate pH (blood or electrolyte solution) during capillary passage is a most likely mechanism.

The extent to which this mechanism contributes to the comparatively delayed efflux of H^+ ions from muscles in vivo can be quantified by model calculations (combination of Approaches 2 and 3) based on the numerous data available for isolated Ringer-suspended rat diaphragms, such as the H^+ ion transfer kinetics (Fig. 10A; Benadé and Heisler, 1978), the mammalian blood buffer value (Fig. 10B and D; Nissen and Heisler, 1973), the buffer value of the intracellular space of rat diaphragm (Heisler and Piiper, 1971, 1972), and the steady-state correlation between intracellular and extracellular pH (Fig. 10C; Heisler, 1975). The amount of H^+ that is transferred across the cell membrane during a short time interval until pH equilibrium has been established between the amount of blood available and the intracellular space is calculated according to the specified perfusion rate. Integration then yields the predicted efflux curve for a specified perfusion rate.

The model indicates that the H^+ elimination rates for "perfused" rat diaphragm muscles are largely dependent on the rate of perfusion (Fig. 11). At normal hematocrit, low perfusion rates in the range of 10–20 ml/(min · 100 g) will result in about the same efflux kinetics for H^+ and La^-, whereas an ex-

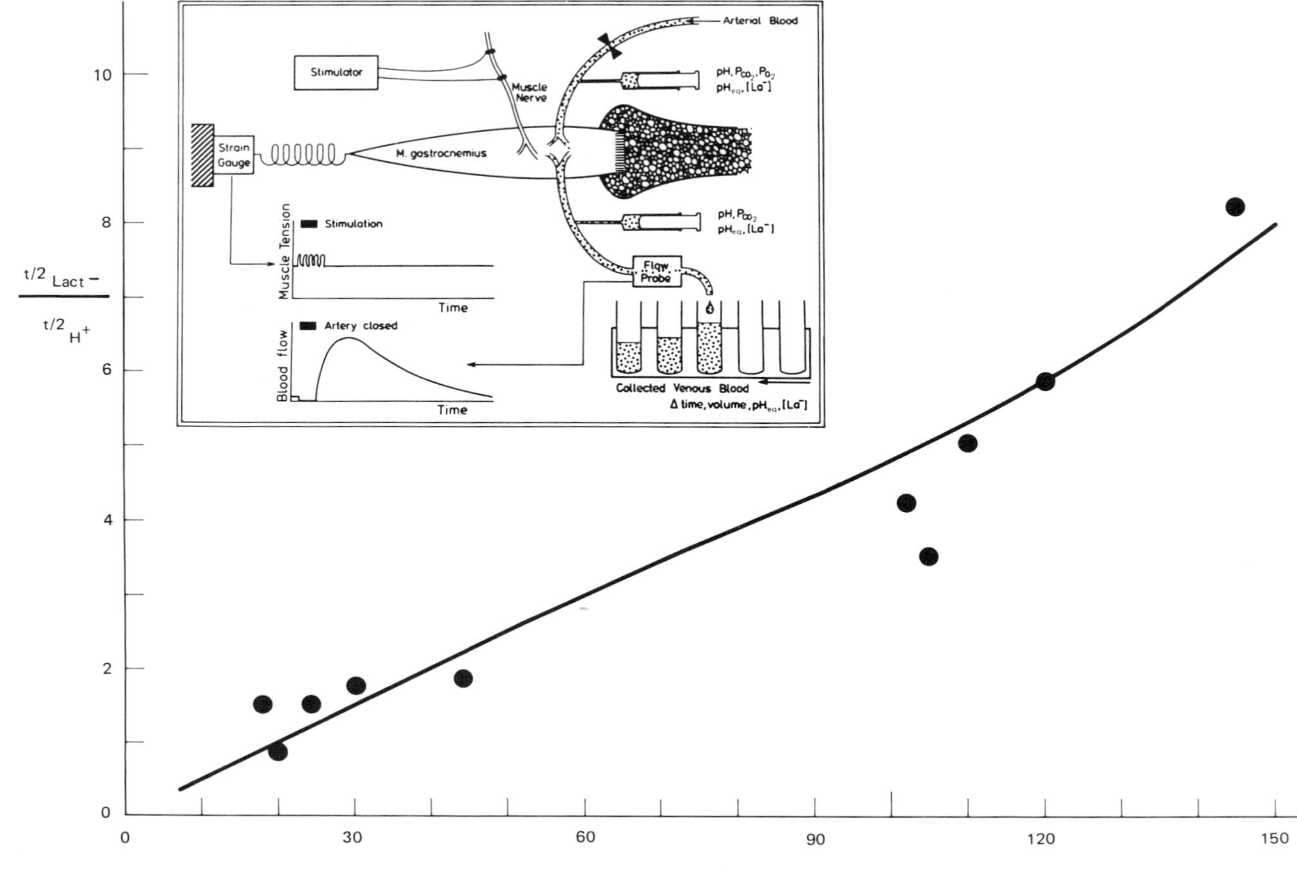

Stimulator
Muscle Nerve
Arterial Blood
pH, P_{CO_2}, P_{O_2}
pH_{eq}, $[La^-]$
Strain Gauge
M. gastrocnemius
pH, P_{CO_2}
pH_{eq}, $[La^-]$
Stimulation
Muscle Tension
Time
Flow Probe
Artery closed
Blood flow
Time
Collected Venous Blood
Δ time, volume, pH_{eq}, $[La^-]$
$\frac{t/2\ Lact^-}{t/2\ H^+}$
0
2
4
6
8
10
0
30
60
90
120
150
Peak Muscle Blood Flow (ml/(min·100 g))

Figure 12

tremely high blood perfusion would be required (150-200 ml/(min · 100 g)) to achieve similar efflux kinetics for H^+ as obtained in the isolated Ringer-suspended rat diaphragm and frog sartorius muscles (Benadé and Heisler, 1978). Such high muscle perfusion rates are seldom attained in vivo. The model suggests, accordingly, that limited perfusion rates are responsible for the observed discrepancy between the perfused muscle preparations and the Ringer-suspended preparations.

Actually, the efflux rate ratios expected from the rat diaphragm model calculations closely resemble those of recent experiments in isolated blood-perfused dog gastrocnemius muscles (Fig. 12, insert; N. Heisler, A. J. S. Benadé and H. Weitz, unpublished). After stimulation during circulatory arrest, the efflux rate ratio of La^-/H^+ ions was widely variable, in the range of 1 to 8.5, but was highly correlated with the peak blood flow through the muscle (range: 18-145 ml/(min · 100 g) (see Fig. 12, solid circles). When the data from the dog gastrocnemius study are compared with those obtained from the diaphragm model calculations (see Fig. 12, solid line), it becomes evident that the muscle perfusion rate is one of the most limiting factors for H^+ elimination from muscle cells.

V. Concluding Remarks

A large number of directly determined parameters, such as transepithelial acid-base relevant ion fluxes; intracellular and extracellular pH and buffer values; bicarbonate concentrations; PCO_2 and body fluid compartment volumes, have been utilized in this chapter together with model calculations and indirect approaches for an analysis of inaccessible in vivo transmembrane ion transfer processes and kinetic values. With all of their limitations, these approaches and models have provided valuable information that is not available by any other method. They have indicated that acid-base relevant ion transfer processes are generally involved during homeostatic regulation in various kinds of acid-base disturbances, have evidenced that these transfer mechanisms are an essential part of the acid-base regulation, and have indicated some of the limiting factors. The description of the processes necessarily had to be incomplete and limited to very

---

Figure 12 Ratio of elimination half-times of La^- and H^+ ions as a function of muscle blood flow in isolated perfused dog gastrocnemius muscle (solid points; N. Heisler, A. J. S. Benadé, and H. Weitz, unpublished data) compared with predictions of model calculations (solid line) on the basis of blood buffering, intracellular–extracellular pH equilibria, and the transmembrane H^+-equivalent transfer rate determined in rat diaphragm muscles. (Benadé and Heisler, 1978.) See text.

few species because of the general lack of relevant data. The large diversity of habitats and the adaptational variety of animals accordingly requires extensive future studies to arrive at a more comprehensive delineation of acid-base regulation.

References

Arrhenius, S. (1887). Über die Dissoziation der im Wasser gelösten Stoffe. *Z. Physikal. Chem. 1*:631-648.

Austin, J. H., Sunderman, F. W., and Camack, J. G. (1927). Studies in serum electrolytes. II. The electrolyte composition and the pH of a poikilothermous animal at different temperatures. *J. Biol. Chem. 72*:677-685.

Benadé, A. J. S., and Heisler, N. (1978). Comparison of efflux rates of hydrogen and lactate ions from isolated muscles in vitro. *Respir. Physiol. 32*: 369-380.

Brønsted, J. N. (1923). Einige Bemerkungen über den Begriff der Säuren und Basen. *Rec. Trav. Chim. Pays-Bas 42*:718-728.

Brown, E. B., and Goott, B. (1963). Intracellular hydrogen ion changes and potassium movement. *Am. J. Physiol. 204*:765-770.

Boutilier, R. G. (1981). Gas exchange and transport during intermittent breathing in the aquatic amphibian, *Xenopus laevis*. Ph.D. Thesis, Univ. East Anglia, Norwich, England.

Boutilier, R. G., and Toews, D. P. (1981). Respiratory, circulatory and acid-base adjustments to hypercapnia in a strictly aquatic and predominantly skin breathing urodele, *Cryptobranchus alleganiensis*. *Respir. Physiol. 46*: 177-192.

Boutilier, R. G., and Heisler, N. (1988). Regulation of the acid-base status of the anuran amphibian *Bufo marinus* during environmental hypercapnia. *J. Exp. Biol. 134*:79-98.

Boutilier, R. G., Randall, D. J., Shelton, G., and Toews, D. P. (1979a). Acid-base relationships in the blood of the toad *Bufo marinus*. I. The effects of environmental CO_2. *J. Exp. Biol. 82*:331-344.

Boutilier, R. G., Emilio, M. G., and Shelton, G. (1985). The effects of mechanical work on water and electrolyte distribution in amphibian skeletal muscle. *J. Exp. Biol. 120*:333-350.

Burnell, J. M. (1968). In vivo response of muscle to changes in CO_2 tension or extracellular bicarbonate. *Am. J. Physiol. 215*:1376-1312.

Burnell, J. M. (1971). Changes in bone sodium and carbonate in metabolic acidosis and alkalosis. *J. Clin. Invest. 50*:327-331.

Cameron, J. N. (1978). Regulation of blood pH in teleost fish. *Respir. Physiol. 33*:129-144.

Cameron, J. N. (1980). Body fluid pools, kidney function, and acid-base regulation in the freshwater catfish *Ictalurus punctatus. J. Exp. Biol. 86*:171-185.

Cameron, J. N. (1985). The bone compartment in a teleost fish, *Ictalurus punctatus*: Size, composition and acid-base response to hypercapnia. *J. Exp. Biol. 117*:307-318.

Cameron, J. N., and Kormanik, G. A. (1982). Intracellular and extracellular acid-base status as a function of temperature in the freshwater channel catfish, *Ictalurus punctatus. J. Exp. Biol. 99*:127-142.

Claiborne, J. B., and Heisler, N. (1984). Acid-base regulation in the carp (*Cyprinus carpio*) during and after exposure to environmental hypercapnia. *J. Exp. Biol. 108*:25-43.

Claiborne, J. B., and Heisler, N. (1986). Acid-base regulation and ion transfers in the carp (*Cyprinus carpio*): pH compensation during graded long- and short-term environmental hypercapnia and the effect of bicarbonate infusion. *J. Exp. Biol. 126*:41-61.

Clancy, R. L., and Brown, E. B., Jr. (1966). In vivo CO_2 buffer curves of skeletal and cardiac muscle. *Am. J. Physiol. 211*:1309-1312.

Dejours, P. (1975, 1981). *Principles of Comparative Respiratory Physiology*. 1st and 2nd ed. Amsterdam, Elsevier/North-Holland.

Dill, D. B., and Edwards, H. T. (1935). Properties of reptilian blood. IV. The alligator (*Alligator mississippiensis* Daudin). *J. Cell. Comp. Physiol. 6*:243-254.

Dill, D. B., Edwards, H. T., Bock, A. V., and Talbott, J. H. (1935). Properties of reptilian blood. III. The chuckwalla (*Sauromalus obesus* Baird). *J. Cell. Comp. Physiol. 6*:37-42.

Eddy, F. B., Lomholt, J. P., Weber, R. E., and Johansen, K. (1977). Blood respiratory properties of rainbow trout (*Salmo gairdneri*) kept in water of high CO_2 tension. *J. Exp. Biol. 67*:37-47.

Edsall, J. T., and Wyman, J. (1958). *Biophysical Chemistry*. New York, Academic Press.

Edwards, H. T., and Dill, D. B. (1935). Properties of reptilian blood. II. The gila monster (*Heloderma suspectum* Cope). *J. Cell. Comp. Physiol. 6*:21-35.

Giebisch, G., Bergern, N., and Pitts, R. F. (1955). The extrarenal response to acute acid-base disturbances of respiratory origin. *J. Clin. Invest. 34*:231-245.

Glass, M. L., and Heisler, N. (1986). The effect of hypercapnia on the arterial acid-base status in the tegu lizard, *Tupinambis nigropunctatus. J. Exp. Biol. 122*:13-24.

Glass, M. L., Boutilier, R. G., and Heisler, N. (1985). Effects of body temperature on respiration, blood gases and acid-base status in the turtle *Chrysemys picta bellii. J. Exp. Biol. 114*:37-51.

Gonzalez, N. C. (1986). Acid-base regulation of mammals. In *Acid-Base Regulation in Animals*. Edited by N. Heisler. Amsterdam, Elsevier Biomedical Press, pp. 175-202.

Gonzalez, N. C., Wemken, H. G., and Heisler, N. (1979). Intracellular pH regulation of normal and hypertrophic rat myocardium. *J. Appl. Physiol. Respir. Environ. Exercise Physiol. 47*:651-656.

Hasselbach, K. A. (1916). Die reduzierte und regulierte Wasserstoffzahl des Blutes. *Biochem. Z. 74*:56-62.

Heisler, N. (1975). Intracellular pH of isolated rat diaphragm muscle with metabolic and respiratory changes of extracellular pH. *Respir. Physiol. 23*: 243-255.

Heisler, N. (1978). Bicarbonate exchange between body compartments after changes of temperature in the larger spotted dogfish (*Scyliorhinus stellaris*). *Respir. Physiol. 33*:145-160.

Heisler, N. (1980). Regulation of the acid-base status in fishes. In *Environmental Physiology of Fishes*. Edited by M. A. Ali. New York, Plenum, pp. 123-162.

Heisler, N. (1982). Intracellular and extracellular acid-base regulation in the tropical freshwater teleost fish *Synbranchus marmoratus* in response to the transition from water breathing to air breathing. *J. Exp. Biol. 99*: 9-28.

Heisler, N. (1984a). Role of ion transfer processes in acid-base regulation with temperature changes in fish. *Am. J. Physiol. 246*:R441-R451.

Heisler, N. (1984b). Acid-base regulation in fishes. In *Fish Physiology*, Vol. XA, Edited by W. S. Hoar and D. J. Randall. Academic Press, New York and London, pp. 315-340.

Heisler, N. (1986 ed.). *Acid-Base Regulation in Animals*. Edited by N. Heisler. Amsterdam, Elsevier Biomedical Press, 492 pp.

Heisler, N. (1986a). Buffering and transmembrane ion transfer processes. In *Acid-Base Regulation in Animals*.Edited by N. Heisler. Amsterdam, Elsevier Biomedical Press, pp. 3-47.

Heisler, N. (1986b). Acid-base regulation in fishes. In *Acid-Base Regulation in Animals*. Edited by N. Heisler. Amsterdam, Elsevier Biomedical Press, pp. 309-356.

Heisler, N. (1986c). Comparative aspects of acid-base regulation. In *Acid-Base Regulation in Animals*. Edited by N. Heisler. Amsterdam, Elsevier Biomedical Press, pp. 397-450.

Heisler, N. (1986d). Mechanisms and limitations of fish acid-base regulation. In *Fish Physiology: Recent Advances*. Edited by S. Nilsson and S. Holmgren. London, Croom-Helm, pp. 24-49.

Heisler, N. (1988a). Acid-base regulation in fishes: I. Mechanisms. In *Acid Toxicity and Aquatic Animals*. Edited by R. Morris. Society of Experimental Biology Seminar Series. London, Cambridge University Press.

Heisler, N. (1988b). Acid-base regulation in elasmobranch fishes. In *Physiology of Elasmobranch Fishes*. Edited by T. J. Shuttleworth. Heidelberg, Springer-Verlag.

Heisler, N. (1988c). Parameters and methods in acid-base physiology. In *Techniques in Comparative Respiratory Physiology: An Experimental Approach*. Edited by C. R. Bridges and P. J. Butler. Society of Experimental Biology Seminar Series, London, Cambridge University Press.

Heisler, N. (1988d). Lactin acid elimination from muscle cells. Edited by J. Grote. Akademie der Wissenschaften und der Literatur, Mainz, Wiesbaden, Franz Steiner Verlag.

Heisler, N., and Neuman, P. (1977). Influence of sea water pH upon bicarbonate uptake induced by hypercapnia in an elasmobranch (*Scyliorhinus stellaris*). *Pflügers Arch. 368* (Suppl.):R19.

Heisler, N., and Neumann, P. (1980). The role of physico-chemical buffering and of bicarbonate transfer processes in intracellular pH regulation in response to changes of temperature in the larger spotted dogfish (*Scyliorhinus stellaris*). *J. Exp. Biol. 85*:99-100.

Heisler, N., and Piiper, J. (1971). The buffer value of rat diaphragm muscle tissue determined by PCO_2 equilibration of homogenates. *Respir. Physiol. 12*:169-178.

Heisler, N., and Piiper, J. (1972). Determination of intracellular buffering properties in rat diaphragm muscle. *Am. J. Physiol. 222*:747-753.

Heisler, N., Weitz, H., and Weitz, A. M. (1976). Hypercapnia and resultant bicarbonate transfer processes in an elasmobranch fish. *Bull. Eur. Physiopathol. Respir. 12*:77-85.

Heisler, N., Weitz, H., and Rothe, K. F. (1977). Efflux kinetics of hydrogen and lactate ions from isolated rat diaphragm. *Proc. Int. Union Physiol. Sci. 13*:315.

Heisler, N., Weitz, H., Rothe, K. F., and Wiese, G. (1978). Analysis of lactate elimination from isolated rat diaphragms. *Pflügers Arch. 373*:R41.

Heisler, N., Neumann, P., and Holeton, G. F. (1980). Mechanisms of acid-base adjustment in dogfish (*Scyliorhinus stellaris*) subjected to long-term temperature acclimation. *J. Exp. Biol. 85*:89-98.

Heisler, N., Holeton, G. F., and Toews, D. P. (1981). Regulation of gill ventilation and acid-base status in hyperoxia-induced hypercapnia in the larger spotted dogfish (*Scyliorhinus stellaris*). *Physiologist 24*:305.

Heisler, N., Forcht, G., Ultsch, G. F., and Anderson, J. F. (1982). Acid-base regulation in response to environmental hypercapnia in two aquatic salamanders, *Siren lacertina* and *Amphiuma means*. *Respir. Physiol. 49*:141-158.

Heisler, N., Toews, D. P., and Holeton, G. F. (1988). Regulation of ventilation and acid-base status in the elasmobranch of *Scyliorhinus stellaris* during hyperoxia-induced hypercapnia. *Respir. Physiol. 71*:227-247.

Henderson, L. J. (1909). Das Gleichgewicht zwischen Basen und Säuren im tierischen Organismus. *Ergeb. Physiol. Biol. Chem. Exp. Med. 427*:255-325.

Hicks, G. H., and Stiffler, D. F. (1980). The effects of temperature and hypercapnia on acid-base status of larval *Ambystoma tigrinum*. *Fed. Proc. 39*: 1060.

Hirche, H., Hombach, V., Langohr, H. D., Wacker, U., and Busse, J. (1975). Lactic acid permeation rate in working gastrocnemius of dogs during metabolic alkalosis and acidosis. *Pflügers Arch. 356*:209-222.

Holeton, G. F., and Heisler, N. (1983). Contribution of net ion transfer mechanisms to the acid-base regulation after exhausting activity in the larger spotted dogfish (*Scyliorhinus stellaris*). *J. Exp. Biol. 103*:31-46.

Irving, L., Forster, H. C., and Ferguson, J. K. W. (1932). The carbon dioxide dissociation curve of living mammalian muscle. *J. Biol. Chem. 95*:95-113.

Leman, J., Jr., Litzow, J. R., and Lennon, E. J. (1966). The effects of chronic acid loads in normal man: Further evidence for the participation of bone mineral in the defense against chronic metabolic acidosis. *J. Clin. Invest. 45*:1608-1614.

Mainwood, G. W., and Worsley-Brown, P. (1975). The effects of extracellular pH and buffer concentration on the efflux of lactate from frog sartorius muscle. *J. Physiol. 250*:1-22.

Neumann, P., Holeton, G. F., and Heisler, N. (1983). Cardiac output and regional blood flow in gills and muscles after exhaustive exercise in rainbow trout (*Salmo gairdneri*). *J. Exp. Biol. 105*:1-14.

Nissen, P., and Heisler, N. (1973). Pufferung und Verteilung von Bikarbonat in Erythrocytensuspensionen mit verschiedenen Zellkonzentrationen. *Pflügers Arch. 343*:221-234.

Kern, D. M. (1960). The hydration of carbon dioxide. *J. Chem. Educ. 37*:14-23.

Lai, Y. L., Attebery, B. A., and Brown, E. B., Jr. (1973a). Mechanisms of cardiac muscle adjustment to hypercapnia. *Respir. Physiol. 19*:123-129.

Lai, Y. L., Atteberry, B. A., and Brown, E. B., Jr. (1973b). Intracellular adjustments of skeletal muscle, heart, and brain to prolonged hypercapnia. *Respir. Physiol. 19*:115-122.

Jackson, D. C., and Braun, B. A. (1979). Respiratory control in bullfrogs: Cutaneous versus pulmonary response to selective CO_2 exposure. *J. Comp. Physiol. 129B*:339-342.

Jackson, D. C., and Heisler, N. (1982). Plasma ion balance of submerged anoxic turtles at 3°: The role of calcium lactate formation. *Respir. Physiol. 49*: 159-174.

Janssen, R. G., and Randall, D. J. (1975). The effect of changes in pH and P_{CO_2} in blood and water on breathing in rainbow trout, *Salmo gairdneri*. *Respir. Physiol. 25*:235-245.

Piiper, J., and Spiller, P. (1970). Repayment of O_2 debt and resynthesis of high-energy phosphates in gastrocnemius muscle of the dog. *J. Appl. Physiol. 28*:657-662.

Pitts, R. F. (1945). The renal regulation of acid-base balance with special reference to the mechanism for acidifying the urine. *Science 102*:49-54, 81-85.

Pitts, R. F. (1948). Renal excretion of acid. *Fed. Proc. 7*:418-426.

Rahn, H. (1966). Development of gas exchange. Evolution of the gas transport system in vertebrates. *Proc. R. Soc. Med. 59*:493-494.

Rahn, H. (1967). Gas transport from the environment to the cell. In *Development of the Lung*. Edited by A. V. S. de Reuck and R. Porter. London, Churchill, pp. 3-23.

Randall, D. J., and Cameron, J. N. (1973). Respiratory control of arterial pH as temperature changes in rainbow trout. *Am. J. Physiol. 225*:997-1002.

Randall, D. J., Heisler, N., and Drees, F. (1976). Ventilatory response to hypercapnia in the larger spotted dogfish *Scyliorhinus stellaris. Am. J. Physiol. 230*:590-594.

Robin, E. D. (1962). Relationship between temperature and plasma pH and carbon dioxide tension in the turtle. *Nature 135*:249-251.

Reeves, R. B. (1972). An imidazole alphastat hypothesis for vertebrate acid-base regulation: Tissue carbon dioxide content and body temperature in bullfrogs. *Respir. Physiol. 14*:219-236.

Reeves, R. B., and Malan, A. (1976). Model studies of intracellular acid-base temperature responses in ectotherms. *Respir. Physiol. 28*:49-63.

Saborowski, F., Scholand, C., Lang, D., and Albers, C. (1973). Intracellular pH and CO_2 combining curve of hypertrophic cardiac muscle in rats. *Respir. Physiol. 18*:171-177.

Saborowski, F., Usinger, W., and Albers, C. (1970). Das intracelluläre pH des Muskels in Abhängigkeit vom CO_2-Druck. *Pflügers Arch. 319*:R4.

Schaefer, K. E., Pasquale, S., Messier, A. A., and Shea, M. (1980). Phasic changes in bone CO_2 fractions, calcium, and phosphorus during chronic hypercapnia. *J. Appl. Physiol. 48*:802-811.

Schloerb, P. R., Blackburn, G. L., and Grantham, J. J. (1967). Carbon dioxide dissociation curve in potassium depletion. *Am. J. Physiol. 212*:953-956.

Scotto, P., Rieke, H., Schmitt, H. J., Meyer, M., and Piiper, J. (1984). Blood-gas equilibration of CO_2 and O_2 in lungs of awake dogs during prolonged rebreathing. *J. Appl. Physiol. Respir. Envir. Exercise Physiol. 57*:1354-1359.

Siggaard-Andersen, O. (1974). *The Acid-Base Status of Blood*. Copenhagen, Munksgaard.

Siggaard-Andersen, O., and Engel, K. (1960). A new acid-base nomogram. An improved method for calculation of the relevant blood acid-base data. *Scand. J. Clin. Lab. Invest. 12*:311-314.

Siggaard-Andersen, O. (1962). The pH, log P_{CO_2} blood acid-base nomogran revised. *Scand. J. Clin. Lab. Invest. 14*:598-604.

Silver, R. B., and Jackson, D. C. (1985). Ventilatory and acid-base responses to long term hypercapnia in the freshwater turtle, *Chrysemys picta bellii. J. Exp. Biol. 114*:661-672.

Singer, R. B., and Hastings, A. B. (1948). An improved clinical method for the estimation of disturbances of the acid-base balance of human blood. *Medicine (Baltimore) 27*:223-242.

Sørensen, S. P. L. (1912). Über die Messung und Bedeutung der Wasserstoffionenkonzentration bei biologischen Prozessen. *Ergeb. Physiol. Biol. Chem. Exp. Med. 12*:394-532.

Stiffler, D. F., Tufts, B. L., and Toews, D. P. (1983). Acid-base and ionic balance in *Ambystoma tigrinum* and *Necturus maculosus* during hypercapnia. *Am. J. Physiol. 245*:R689-R694.

Strome, D. R., Clancy, R. L., and Gonzalez, N. C. (1976). Myocardial CO_2 buffering: Role of transmembrane transport of H^+ or HCO_3^- ions. *Am. J. Physiol. 230*:1037-1041.

Stewart, P. A. (1978). Independent and dependent variables of acid-base control. *Respir. Physiol. 33*:9-26.

Sullivan, L. P. (1986). Renal mechanisms involved in acid-base regulation. In *Acid-Base Regulation in Animals.* Edited by N. Heisler. Amsterdam, Elsevier Biomedical Press, pp. 83-137.

Toews, D. P., and Heisler, N. (1982). The effects of hypercapnia on intracellular and extracellular acid-base status in the toad *Bufo marinus. J. Exp. Biol. 97*:79-86.

Toews, D. P., and Macintyre, D. (1978). Respiration and circulation in an apodan amphibian. *Can. J. Physiol. 56*:998-1004.

Toews, D. P., and S. Kirby (1985). The ventilation and acid-base physiology of the toad, *Bufo marinus*, during exposure to environmental hyperoxia. *Respir. Physiol. 59*:225-229.

Toews, D. P., Holeton, G. F., and Heisler, N. (1983). Regulation of the acid-base status during environmental hypercapnia in the marine teleost fish *Conger. J. Exp. Biol. 107*:9-20.

Ultsch, G. R., Ott, M. E., and Heisler, N. (1980). Standard metabolic rate, critical oxygen tension, and aerobic scope for spontaneous activity of trout (*Salmo gairdneri*) and carp (*Cyprinus carpio*) in acidified water. *Comp. Biochem. Physiol. 67A*:329-335.

Van Slyke, D. D. (1917). Studies of acidosis. II. A method for the determination of carbon dioxide and carbonates in solution. *J. Biol. Chem. 30*:347-368.

Van Slyke, D. D. (1922). On the measurement of buffer values and on the relationship of buffer value to the dissociation constant of the buffer and the concentration and the reaction of the buffer system. *J. Biol. Chem. 52*: 525-570.

Waddell, W. J., and Butler, T. C. (1959). Calculation of intracellular pH from the distribution of 5,5-dimethyl-2,4-oxazolidinedione (DMO). Application to skeletal muscle of the dog. *J. Clin. Invest. 38*:720-729.

Winterstein, H. (1954). Der Einfluss der Körpertemperatur auf das Säure-Basen-Gleichgewicht im Blut. *Arch. Exp. Pathol. Pharmakol. 223*:1-18.

Woodbury, J. W. (1965). Regulation of pH. In *Physiology and Biophysics*. Edited by T. C. Ruch and H. D. Patton. Philadelphia: W. B. Saunders, pp. 899-934.

Part Five

Mechanics and Control of Breathing

19

Comparative Aspects of Vertebrate Pulmonary Mechanics

WILLIAM K. MILSOM

University of British Columbia
Vancouver, British Columbia, Canada

I. Introduction

From a mechanical viewpoint, the design of vertebrate respiratory systems has been subject to two major sets of constraints. The first is the need to satisfy the primary function of the lung as an organ of gas exchange. These constraints include the need to reduce the diffusion gradient between air and blood while providing adequate ventilation and perfusion of the exchange surface. The second set of constraints arises from the need to satisfy other physiological, environmental, and behavioral demands. A quick consideration of the consequences of the long, thin body of a snake or the rigid shell of a turtle on the design of the respiratory pump; the hydrostatic pressures encountered by diving animals on the structure of the lungs and chest wall; and the modifications associated with vocalization on the development of the lungs and respiratory passages in many species, indicate the magnitude of these constraints. The literature is rich with the details of comparative studies of respiratory structure and function in air-breathing vertebrates, which outline the diversity of existing solutions to the different sets of constraints imposed on different species. This chapter will survey some of the consequences of these solutions on respiratory mechanics.

Table 1 Respiratory Variables in Mammals Expressed as Allometric Equations

Variable	Units	Allometric equation: Body mass (kg)	Allometric equation: Metabolic rate (ml O_2/min)
		Function-related variables	
Oxygen consumption	ml/min	$11.6\ M_b^{0.76}$	—
Minute volume	ml/min	$379\ M_b^{0.80}$	$6.4\ MR^{1.06}$
Pulmonary surface area[a]	m^2	$131\ M_b^{0.76}$	$2.22\ MR^{1.00}$
Power of breathing	g · cm/min	$962\ M_b^{0.78}$	$16.4\ MR^{1.03}$
Cardiac output	ml/min	$187\ M_b^{0.81}$	$3.2\ MR^{1.07}$
Total airway resistance	cm H_2O/(L/sec)	$24.4\ M_b^{-0.70}$	$0.41\ MR^{-0.92}$
Mean expiratory flow rate	ml/min	$101\ M_b^{0.77}$	$1.72\ MR^{1.02}$
		Size-related variables	
Total lung weight	g	$11.3\ M_b^{0.99}$	
Vital capacity	ml	$56.7\ M_b^{1.03}$	
Functional residual capacity (V_{LR})	ml	$24.1\ M_b^{1.13}$	
Tidal volume	ml	$7.69\ M_b^{1.04}$	
Dead space	ml	$2.76\ M_b^{0.96}$	
Total compliance	ml/cm H_2O	$1.56\ M_b^{1.04}$	
Work/breath	g · cm	$17.1\ M_b^{1.08}$	
		Function X size-related variables	
Respiratory rate	/min	$53.5\ M_b^{-0.26}$	
Time constant	s	$0.04\ M_b^{0.30}$	
		Size-independent variables	
C_T/V_{LR}	ml/cm H_2O/ml	0.065	(RME = 0.01)
$V_T/C_T = \Delta P$	cm H_2O	4.93	(RME = 0.09)
W/V_T	g · cm/ml	2.22	(RME = 0.04)

Source: [a]Tenney and Remmers, 1963. All other values from Stahl, 1967.

Several excellent papers and reviews already address certain aspects of this topic in great detail (Agostini et al., 1959; Crossfill and Widdicombe, 1961; Tenney and Remmers, 1963; Stahl, 1967; Spells, 1969; Tenney and Tenney, 1970; Leith, 1976). The treatment presented here, however, attempts to be more comprehensive, focusing on basic trends and principles that are common to all vertebrate respiratory systems and highlighting those areas that look most fruitful for future study.

A. Lung Structure

To meet the constraints placed on the respiratory system for gas exchange, lungs must be designed to match their diffusing capacity to metabolic demands. Metabolic demands, on the other hand, vary greatly between vertebrate groups, particularly between the ectotherms and endotherms as well as within any given group, as a function of both life-style and body size. The structure and function of vertebrate gas exchangers are reviewed earlier in this volume but several points relevant to our discussion of pulmonary mechanics will be presented again, briefly.

Effects of Body Size

Kleiber (1961), and many others, have demonstrated that for all vertebrates, oxygen consumption varies roughly with the three quarters power of body weight (mass; $M_b{}^{0.75}$). As a consequence, one would expect that respiratory variables related to gas exchange should also scale $M_b{}^{0.75}$. Extensive literature reviews by several authors indicate that this is so (Zeuthen, 1953; Hemmingsen, 1960; Stahl, 1967; Hutchison et al., 1968). Thus, we see in Table 1 that for mammals, the total amount of gas ventilated each minute, the alveolar surface area available for gas exchange, the perfusion of the lungs, and the minute work or power required to move the gas, all vary in direct proportion to metabolic rate. Interestingly, size (rather than function)-related variables of the respiratory system scale as the first power of body weight ($M_b{}^1$). As a consequence, variables such as lung weight, total lung volume, dead space volume, and tidal volume, remain the same relative to body weight in mammals of all sizes. The physiological consequences of these trends have been reviewed elsewhere (Piiper and Scheid, 1972; Piiper, 1982). Pertinent to our discussion, and as pointed out by Tenney and Remmers (1963), as mammals decrease in size, their lung volume will decrease in direct proportion to their body weight, whereas the internal surface area of the lung decreases in direct proportion to metabolic rate (or $M_b{}^{0.75}$). One consequence of these two trends is that there must be an increase in the internal partitioning of the lung and, thus, a decrease in alveolar dimensions (Table 2). Similar trends have now been described for several of these vari-

Table 2 Values for Various Respiratory Measurements in Eight Species of Mammal

Species	Units	Mouse	Rat	Guinea pig	Rabbit	Monkey	Cat	Dog	Man
Body weight	kg	0.03	0.25	0.69	2.4	2.5	3.7	12.6	70
Tidal volume	ml	0.18	1.55	3.7	16	20	34	144	400
Tidal pressure swing	cm H_2O	3.6	4.3	3.2	2.9	1.7	2.6	3.8	4.5
Respiratory frequency	/min	109	97	42	39	33	30	21	16
Minute volume	ml/min	0.02	0.16	0.13	0.6	0.7	0.96	3.1	6.4
Lung compliance	ml/cm H_2O	0.05	0.39	1.26	6.0	12.3	13.4	40	200
	ml/cm H_2O/ml	0.11	0.12	0.15	0.3	0.12	0.16	0.12	0.07
Mean alveolar diameter	μ	39	59	83	94	89	133	74	166
Lung resistance	cm H_2 O/L/sec	480	90	59	25	8.6	11.5	1.3	0.9
Time constant	sec	0.03	0.04	0.08	0.15	0.1	0.14	0.06	0.18

Source: Adapted from Crosfill and Widdicombe, 1961.

variables in birds, reptiles, and amphibia (Hutchison et al., 1968; Tenney and Tenney, 1970; Perry, 1983).

Pulmonary mechanics will reflect pulmonary structure and, thus, will also be influenced by these allometric relationships. As one example, because all mammalian lungs have similar elastic properties, the total compliance of the respiratory system is primarily a function of the volume of the system and scales to M_b^1. Total airway resistance, however, is primarily a function of airway diameter and, given the relative increase in airway dimensions with increasing body size that has just been described, it is not surprising that this variable scales with $M_b^{0.75}$ (see Table 1). Thus, as animals decrease in size, the total compliance of the respiratory system will remain relatively unchanged, whereas the total airway resistance will increase. Consequently, the time constant for passive lung emptying will not decrease that much, restricting the extent to which breathing frequency can increase to meet increasing weight-specific metabolic demands, while expiration still remains a passive process (see Table 2). We will return to a consideration of the mechanical consequences of such changes shortly.

It should be noted that there is tremendous variability in the literature values used to construct these allometric relationships. As a consequence, animals of any body weight may deviate from predicted values for any variable by over ± 50% (Stahl, 1967). As pointed out by Leith (1976), some of this variation may simply be "noise" caused by variations in methods of measurement, but some is undoubtedly "signal" resulting from real differences attributable to adaptation or specialization among species. The net result is that although these equations or relationships are extremely useful for revealing general trends common to vertebrates as a whole, they are not particularly useful as predictive tools applied to any one given species. Deviations from these general trends, however, can be a useful means of revealing physiological specializations resulting from other constraints. (Taylor et al. in Chapter 3 discuss more details and principles of scaling.)

Effects of Phylogeny and Life-Style

The basic structure of the respiratory system differs markedly among different vertebrate groups. According to the type classification system proposed by Duncker (1978), all mammals possess a bronchoalveolar lung, whereas all birds possess a parabronchial-type lung. Reptiles, on the other hand, possess a continuum of lung structures that have been categorized as unicameral, paucicameral, and multicameral. The unicameral lung consists of an undivided single chamber in which the respiratory surfaces are elaborations of the lung wall. In paucicameral lungs, the central lumen of the lung is subdivided by a small number of large septa, and in the multicameral lung, a cartilage-reinforced, intrapulmonary bronchus connects a number of separate chambers (Duncker, 1978).

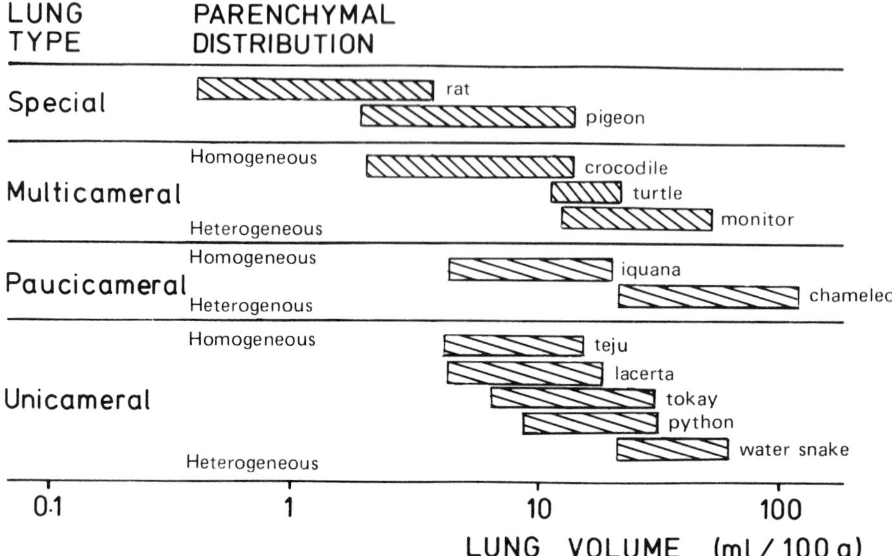

Figure 1 Lung volumes in various reptiles, rat, and pigeon (lung and air sacs), grouped according to lung structure. The lower limit of each bar indicates V_{LR}, the upper limit, VC. (Modified from Perry, 1983.)

Perry (1983) has reviewed the trends that exist in lung structure among the reptiles, birds, and mammals. Lung volumes vary extensively in size among the vertebrates, from less than 1.0 to over 100 ml/100 g (Fig. 1). Although there is much variation within each group, in general, the lungs of reptiles tend to be larger than those of birds which, in turn, are larger than those of mammals. Within each structural type of lung, larger lungs usually exhibit a more heterogeneous distribution of parenchyma than do smaller lungs. These trends, both within and between groups, to some extent reflect constraints placed upon the lungs that are not associated with an increasing gas exchange surface, per se. Large, flexible, saclike regions of the lungs of various vertebrates play putative roles in gas storage, buoyancy control, locomotion, communication, and behavioral displays (Perry, 1983).

The constraints imposed by the need for gas exchange will be most clearly reflected in the anatomical diffusion factor (ADF) of the lung. This variable represents the anatomically measurable component of the diffusing capacity of lung tissue (Dto_2) for oxygen and is equal to the respiratory surface area to harmonic mean thickness ratio of the air-blood tissue barrier. The graphic representation of ADF shown in Figure 2 (from Perry, 1983) clearly depicts the trend of increasing respiratory surface area (per gram of bodyweight), decreasing air-

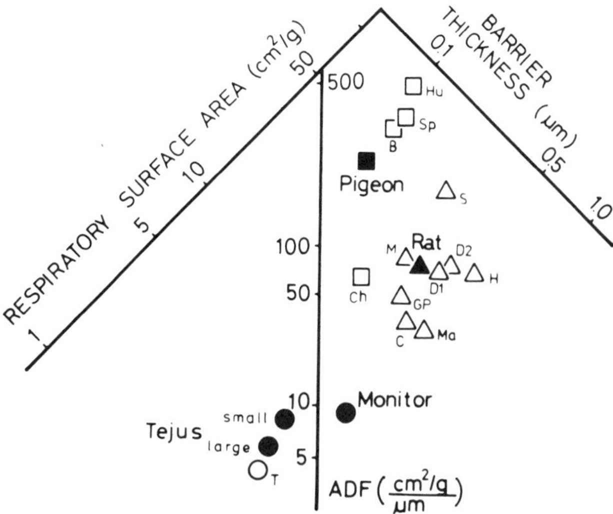

Figure 2 Respiratory surface area plotted against the harmonic mean thickness of the air–blood tissue barrier. The quotient of these two parameters, the air diffusion (ADF), can be read off against the vertical axis. ($DLO_2 = KLO_2 \cdot ADF$.) Open circles = reptiles, open triangles = mammals, open squares = birds. Darkened symbols represent animals in a similar body weight range (approximately 55 g). Abbreviations: reptiles: T, turtle; mammals: C, cow; D, dog; GP, guinea pig; H, horse; M, mouse; Ma, man; R, rat; S, shrew; birds: B, budgerigar; Ch, chicken; Hu, hummingbird; Sp, sparrow. (From Perry, 1983.)

blood tissue barrier thickness, and increasing anatomical diffusion factor, as one progresses from reptiles, through mammals, to birds. It is noteworthy that in many instances, different strategies of increasing surface area or decreasing barrier thickness are employed to attain similar levels of ADF (compare chicken, rat, and horse, for instance). Although the significance of these differences is not at all clear, there is a definite trend for both increasing surface area and decreasing barrier thickness with increasing metabolic rate. In Figure 3, the morphometrically determined diffusing capacity of the air–blood tissue barrier (DtO_2) is plotted against metabolic rate for many of the same species. This figure, also taken from the work of Perry (1983), clearly illustrates the correlation that exists between increasing metabolic demand (both resting and maximal) and the diffusing capacity of the lungs. Although the diffusing capacities plotted here are morphometric and not physiological, and are all calculated using the Krogh diffusion constant for oxygen of the rat lung (this constant has not been measured for most of the species depicted here), the trends that such calcula-

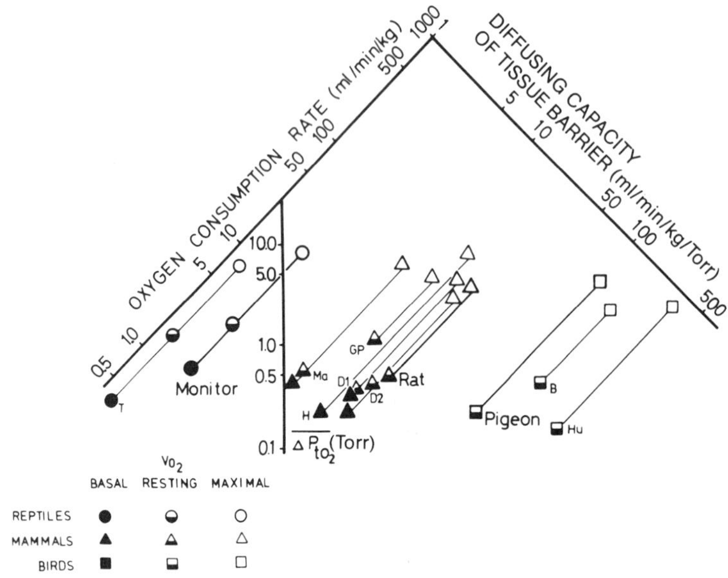

Figure 3 Oxygen consumption rate plotted against diffusing capacity of the tissue barrier. The quotient of these two parameters (ΔPto_2) represents the partial pressure difference between air and blood in the lung and is read off against the vertical axis. Values for reptiles, mammals, and birds are given under basal and/or resting and maximal conditions. Abbreviations as in Fig. 2. (From Perry, 1983.)

tions reveal are probably quite valid. The slope of the relationship shown here (ΔPto_2) has torr as the unit. Although this measure is not identical with the physiologically determined alveolar-arterial partial pressure difference, it is probably, nontheless, a good indicator of alveolar-arterial Po_2 differences (see Perry, 1983 for discussion). This index shows a clear increase in the degree of equilibration between arterial blood and alveolar gas, under resting conditions, again progressing from reptiles, through mammals, to birds, which is reduced, but still present, even under conditions of maximal oxygen uptake.

What these trends again demonstrate, are a decrease in lung volume per unit body weight, but an increase in lung partitioning and complexity associated with increased metabolic demands. As with changes in body size, these changes will have a large influence on the mechanics of the respiratory system.

B. Ventilatory Pumps

To also meet the constraints placed on the respiratory system for gas exchange, respiratory pumps must be designed to provide sufficient ventilation to match metabolic demands. The design of these pumps is heavily influenced by the constraints of nonrespiratory functions. As such, they represent the results of multiple experiments in design, each with its own unique features. This is the topic of several earlier chapters in this volume and I only wish to point out here that the mechanics of the entire respiratory system will also be heavily influenced by the constraints on, as well as the design of, these pumps.

II. Static Mechanics

The resting position of the respiratory system with the glottis open and the lungs equilibrated to atmospheric pressure is generally referred to in mammals as the functional residual capacity (FRC) or resting lung volume (V_{LR}). This volume is determined by a static balance of forces that varies tremendously from species to species. In mammals, which possess a diaphragm and in which the lungs are contained in a true pleural cavity, relaxation volume is a static balance of forces between lungs and chest wall. In most laboratory mammals, at V_{LR}, the lungs tend to collapse and the chest wall to spring out with the balance of these two forces establishing V_{LR} (Agostoni et al., 1959; Agostoni and Hyatt, 1986). This is not true for all mammals, however, for in many other mammals such as the seal, mouse, and hamster, the chest wall is extremely compliant and recoils inward over almost the entire range of vital capacity (Leith, 1976; Koo et al., 1976). As a consequence, in these species at resting volume, the chest wall rests on the lungs, which resist further collapse only because the airways are closed, preventing any more gas from leaving the lung. In these latter species, V_{LR} is equal to residual volume (RV), which is equal to the trapped gas volume (V_{tr}) of the lungs. Although this represents an extreme example, as a general rule, the more compliant the chest wall, the smaller V_{LR}. This same situation occurs in the amphibia (Gans, 1970; Hughes and Vergara, 1978).

In reptiles, in which the lungs do not reside in a separate pleural cavity and that lack a true diaphragm, the forces that determine V_{LR} arise not only from the lungs and chest wall but also from the viscera. The lungs in these species lie attached to the dorsal surface of the pleuroperitoneal cavity, and in many instances ventral mesopneumonia anchor the ventromedial surfaces of the lungs to underlying viscera (Gans and Hughes, 1967; Perry and Duncker, 1978). In those few species that have been studied with the airways open to the atmosphere, even though the lungs tend to collapse and the chest wall to spring out, the weight of suspended viscera also acts to expand the lungs (Gans and Hughes, 1967; Perry and Duncker, 1978). The situation is not dissimilar in birds (King,

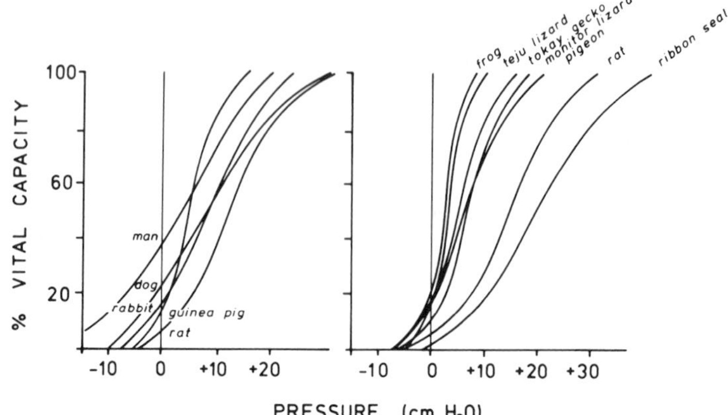

Figure 4 Mean pressure–volume curves for the respiratory systems of several species. (Mammalian data from Agostoni et al., 1959; Leith, 1976. Bird and reptile data from Perry and Duncker, 1980. Frog data from Hughes and Vergara, 1978.)

1966). Here, however, the lungs interdigitate strongly with the ribs in the dorsal body wall and are attached ventrally to the pulmonary aponeurosis, a thin membrane that stretches tightly across the ventromedial surfaces of the lungs from the midline to attach to the ribs at the junction of the vertebral and sternal parts. Although many authors feel that this arrangement precludes any expansion or contraction of the lungs (Fedde et al., 1963), there is strong evidence that some volume changes associated with ventilation do occur (see King, 1966 for review). Most of the ventilatory gas flow, however, is due to expansion and compression of the air sac system whose resting volume is determined very much like the resting lung volume in reptiles (King, 1966).

Figure 4 depicts the static relationship between the transpulmonary pressure and volume of the respiratory system for a number of different vertebrate species. When the lungs are open to atmospheric pressure, the static balance of forces in the different species produce resting lung volumes that range from almost zero (the ribbon seal) to almost 40% (man) of vital capacity. In determining the V_{LR}, the static balance of forces acting on the respiratory system at rest also determine the inspiratory and expiratory reserve volumes of the lungs. In terrestrial mammals, the expiratory reserve volume (ERV), that volume of air which can be actively expelled beyond a normal, passive expiration, decreases with decreasing body size (see Fig. 4; Agostoni et al., 1959), whereas the inspiratory reserve volume (IRV) increases proportionately. For animals such as the ribbon seal, there is no ERV; thus, all increases in tidal volume must come from increases in inspiratory effort (Leith, 1976). It then follows that the development and strategy of recruitment of the various inspiratory and expiratory muscle groups in different species will also reflect this static balance of forces, and vice versa. Consequently, nonrespiratory constraints on the design of the body wall will greatly affect the partitioning of TLC.

Note, that V_{LR} is not necessarily the volume at which the lungs normally reside. Although most terrestrial mammals relax between breaths with the glottis open, many marine mammals and all reptiles and amphibians relax at end inspiration against a closed glottis (breath holding or glottal trapping) and, hence, at a much larger lung volume then that determined by static forces alone (Gans, 1970; Gans and Clark, 1978). One consequence of this is to increase lung gas stores and reduce the swings in arterial gas tensions that would occur between breaths.

The abscissa in Figure 4 represents the pressure required to inflate (positive) or deflate (negative) each respiratory system over its entire vital capacity. The shapes of the curves indicate that respiratory systems behave stiffly (small change in volume for a large change in deforming pressure) as they approach maximum and minimum volumes. Over much of the total volume range, however, they behave in a relatively linear fashion. The slope of the relationship between volume and pressure over this linear portion of the range, an indication of the stiffness of the system, is the static compliance of the system (C). Figure 4b demonstrates the greater compliance of the respiratory systems of reptiles and birds relative to those of mammals.

Figure 5 illustrates the relative contributions of the compliance of the lungs alone and the body wall alone to the total compliance of the respiratory system in different vertebrate species. This is a double logarithmic plot and both compliance and respiratory tract volume are normalized to body weight. When expressed this way, the lungs, body wall, and total respiratory system of birds and reptiles appear to be from one to three orders of magnitude more compliant than those of mammals. The quotient of these variables (the slope of the relationship between weight-specific compliance and lung volume) is the specific compliance (C/V_L) of the respiratory system and can be read off against the vertical axis in the figure. Because it is the function of the respiratory system that is under consideration, it seems more logical to normalize mechanical and functional variables to the size of the respiratory system, rather than to the size of the animal. When expressed in this fashion, it can be seen that the body wall compliance of most vertebrates is remarkably similar. The turtle, with its rigid shell, depends on movements of the flank cavities and pectoral girdle for volume change (McCutcheon, 1943; Gans and Hughes, 1967) and, not surprisingly, has a specific body wall compliance an order of magnitude stiffer than that of most other vertebrates. There is a large degree of variation in the specific compliance of the lungs of different species, which to some extent reflects variations in lung

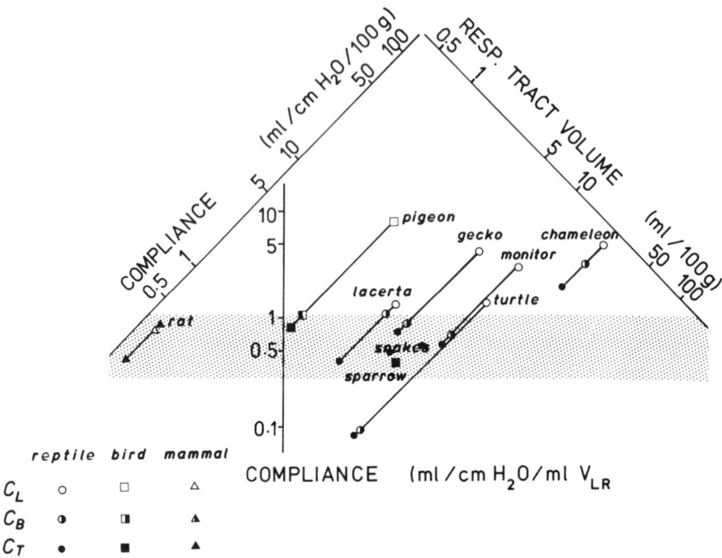

Figure 5 Relationship between specific compliance and respiratory tract volume in seven reptilian, two avian, and one mammalian species. The quotient of these two parameters is the volume-standardized compliance (C/V_{LR}), which is read off against the vertical axis. C_L, C_B, and C_T are the compliances of the lungs (and air sacs in birds), body wall, and total system, respectively. The stippled area indicates the range of C_T/V_{LR} values found in most species. (Modified from Perry and Duncker, 1980.)

architecture and lung volume (Perry and Duncker, 1980). The large, heterogeneous lungs of reptiles and lung-air sac systems of birds are much more compliant than are those of the relatively small homogeneous lungs of mammals. The scaling equations of Stahl (1967) indicate that the specific compliance for mammals should be independent of body weight ($C_T/V_{LR} = 1.56\ M_b{}^{1.04}/56.7\ M_b{}^{1.03} = 0.065$ ml/cm H_2O/ml; see Table 1). Although the logarithmic scales used in Figure 5 mask a 25-fold range of values from that of the turtle (and most mammals, not shown here) to that of the chameleon, specific compliance is also consistent among the vertebrate classes, despite the tremendous diversity in body structure and lung architecture found among these groups. It should be noted, however, that despite this relatively narrow range of values, there is one fundamental difference. In mammals, C_T is primarily determined by the specific compliance of the lungs, whereas in the birds and reptiles, C_T is primarily determined by the specific compliance of the body wall. As a consequence, the source of the recoil pressure responsible for passive deflation of the system following inspiration can vary tremendously from species to species.

One consequence of this difference is that with increasing inflation, it is the lungs in mammals that increase dramatically in stiffness and appear to set the TLC, whereas in the birds and reptiles, this is due to a sudden increase in the stiffness of the body wall. Apparently, with the larger, more heterogeneous lungs of birds and reptiles, expansion of the body wall restricts the TLC of the respiratory system as a whole.

On the other hand, the cause of the increase in stiffness or decrease in compliance as gas is withdrawn from the lungs at volumes approaching RV, is due to an increase in the stiffness of the body wall in almost all vertebrates (Leith, 1976; Agostoni and Hyatt, 1986). However, there are examples in which the body wall is exceptionally compliant, as in the ribbon seal or the mouse (Leith, 1976), and here, it is the decrease in compliance of the lungs resulting from airway closure and air trapping that causes the respiratory system to behave in this fashion.

Finally, it should be noted from Figure 4 that all lungs, regardless of species (from amphibians to mammals) or body size (only three of seven orders of magnitude are shown here) are powered by similar changes in transpulmonary pressure (Agostoni et al., 1959; also see Table 2). This suggests that there are real limits to the extent of transpulmonary pressure swings that can be used to power ventilation, but the exact nature of the limiting factors remains unknown. That aside, the same change in transpulmonary pressure of 2 to 5 cm H_2O will expand the lungs by 1 tidal volume in each species, by over 50 L in a whale but under 0.1 ml in a shrew (Stahl, 1967; Leith, 1976).

The lung anatomy of reptiles, more so than that of mammals, reflects the influence of many nonrespiratory constraints. Many aquatic species of reptile rely on lung volume changes for buoyancy control (Jackson, 1969; Milsom, 1975). Large excursions of lung volume are utilized to alter body shape in behavioral displays associated with reproduction, territoriality, and defense (Perry and Duncker, 1978; Perry, 1983). Many species of reptiles, as well as birds, rely on large excursions in lung volume for vocalization (King, 1966; Gans and Maderson, 1973; Perry, 1983). Given the preceding discussion, it is noteworthy that the development of large, heterogeneous lungs in these species for these various functions also increase their relative compliance and, consequently, reduces the distending pressures required for their inflation. Changes in lung volume of over 4 V_{LR} can often be achieved with a transpulmonary pressure of only 2 to 3 cm H_2O (Perry, 1983). However, because the total respiratory system compliance in birds and reptiles is more a function of the specific compliance of the body wall than that of the lungs, this depends upon the presence of a flexible body wall. Interestingly, the large changes in lung volume associated with buoyancy control in the chelonia—animals with rigid shells and relatively stiff body walls—are compensated with decreases in the volume of the urinary bladder to hold total body volume relatively constant (Jackson, 1971). As a consequence, these animals achieve a much larger lung volume for the same distending pressure, completely circumventing the limitations of the rigid body wall.

III. Dynamic Mechanics

Given the importance of ventilation for proper pulmonary function, it is somewhat surprising how little work has been done on the dynamic mechanics of nonmammalian respiratory systems. Despite this, the work that has been done provides some interesting insights and raises a number of provocative hypotheses.

During ventilation, dynamic forces are applied to the system that are met by equal and opposing forces developed by the system (Newton's third law of motion). For the respiratory system, the applied pressure is opposed by pressures related to the volume, flow, and volume acceleration of the respiratory system. The mechanical properties related to these pressures are dynamic compliance, flow resistance, and inertance. The following discussion will deal only with very selected aspects of the first two properties.

The compliance of the lung and respiratory system are affected by the rate of inflation or the frequency of ventilation; the higher the ventilation frequency, the stiffer the behavior of the system. Thus, the dynamic compliance during ventilation is less than the corresponding static compliance obtained by step inflation of the lungs to similar volumes. In most mammals, this reduction in compliance is small (10% reduction over a 10-fold increase in ventilation frequency) (Sullivan and Mortola, 1987). It is generally believed to be due to airflow resistance or regional differences in peripheral flow resistance (Otis et al., 1956), although in young rats, the viscoelastic properties of the lungs also cause them to stiffen during ventilation in proportion to the rate of stress relaxation of the tissue (Sullivan and Mortola, 1987). This is also true in the turtle (Vitalis and Milsom, 1968a) although, here, the effect is somewhat large (67% reduction over a sixfold increase in ventilation frequency). In the gecko, the decrease in compliance with increasing frequency is also large (50-70% reduction over a 10-fold increase in ventilation frequency), but this apparently is solely due to viscoelastic properties of the body wall (Milsom and Vitalis, 1984). This data suggests that stress relaxation in reptilian respiratory systems greatly exceeds that found in mammalian systems, although the reasons for this are not clear. Some of the consequences of this, however, will be discussed shortly.

The magnitude of the flow resistive forces that must be overcome during ventilation are a function of the flow resistance and the rate of movement of gas and tissues. These, in turn, are a function of the dimensions of the respiratory system. The flow resistance of the airways will decrease as lung volume increases because the airway dimensions increase, as discussed earlier (Crosfill and Widdicombe, 1961; Tenney and Remmers, 1963; Rodarte and Rehder, 1986). The flow resistance of lung tissue and the chest wall should decrease with increasing lung volume because the pressure associated with tissue viscous resistance is proportional to the linear velocity of tissue, and, for a given volume change, the linear movement of tissue decreases as the volume increases (Grimsby et al., 1968). One would also expect that flow resistance would be less in heterogeneous lungs compared with homogeneous lungs of equal size as a result of the large expansible chambers. Given the trend of increasing homogeneity and decreasing alveolar dimensions with an increasing weight-specific metabolic rate, described earlier, one would also expect to see a good correlation between total resistance and metabolic rate. In mammals, at least, this is exactly what occurs, total airway resistance = 24.4 $M_b^{-0.7}$ or, therefore, = 0.41 metabolic rate$^{-0.92}$ (see Tables 1,2).

Because the total compliance of the respiratory system of mammals scales to M_b^{1}, whereas the total airway resistance roughly scales to $M_b^{-0.75}$, the time constant for the respiratory system ($T = R \times C$) will roughly scale to $M_b^{0.25}$ (see Tables 1,2). This time constant is the time required for the lungs to empty 63% during a passive expiration and can be used to give us an indication of the time required for a passive expiration following glottal opening. If the expiratory interval (T_E) of a breath is assumed to be a fixed proportion of the total breath length (T_{TOT}) and respiratory frequency scales to $M_b^{-0.26}$ (see Tables 1,2) and $f = 60/T_{TOT}$, then T_E will scale to $M_b^{0.26}$. Thus, we see that the time required for passive expiration changes in parallel with the time available under resting conditions. Because tidal volume scales to M_b^{1}, however, the airflow velocity associated with expiration (V_T/T_E) will scale to $M_b^{0.75}$ and, thus, we will see an increase in expiratory flow rates with increasing size (see Table 1).

Similar considerations allow us to make some predictions about resting breathing patterns. For most mammals, tidal volume (and lung volume) scales to M_b^{1}. As a consequence, weight-specific tidal volume will be relatively constant for most mammals. Without getting too far ahead of ourselves, Otis et al. (1950) have predicted based on energetic considerations, that the optimal tidal volume for most mammals is twice the dead space volume of the respiratory system. The allometric relationships developed by Stahl (1967) indicate that V_T = 7.69 $M_b^{1.04}$, whereas V_D = 2.76 $M_b^{0.96}$. From these relationships we see that $V_T \simeq 2.8\ V_D$, which is not such a bad fit considering that the predictions of Otis et al. (1950) were based on considerations of anatomical rather than physiological dead space, which is bound to be much larger. Be that as it may, given

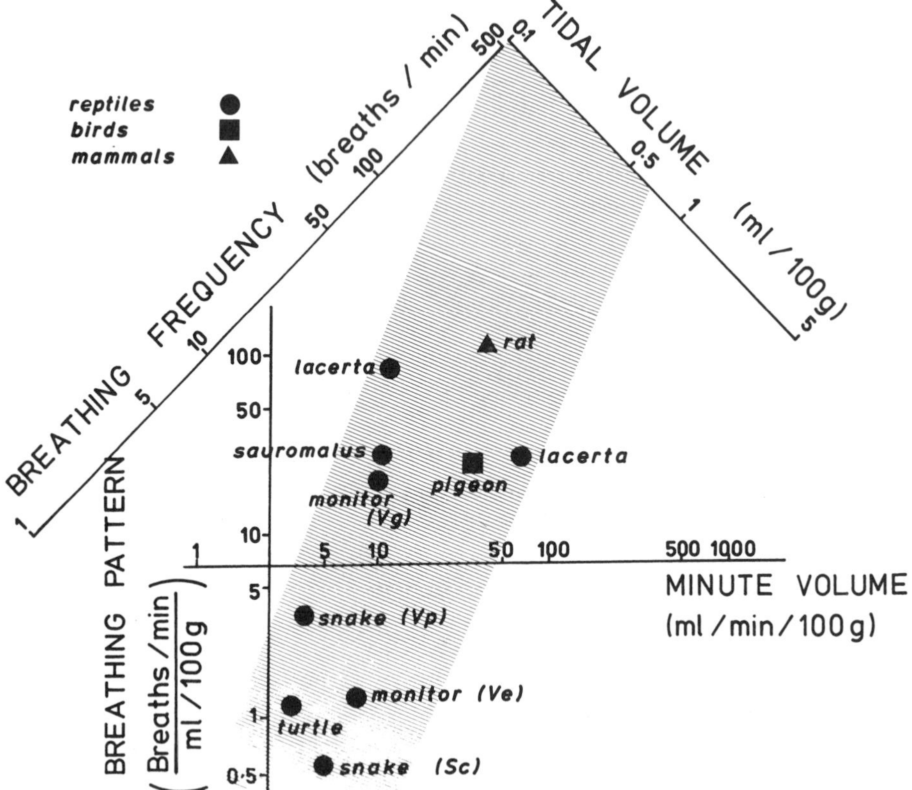

Figure 6 Relationship between breathing frequency and tidal volume in seven reptilian, one avian, and one mammalian species under resting conditions. The breathing pattern index (f/V_T) is indicated on the vertical axis and minute volume ($\dot{V}_E = f \times V_T$) on the horizontal axis. Abbreviations: Sc, *Spalerosophis cliffordi*; Ve, *Varanus exantematicus*; Vg, *V. gouldii*; Vp, *Vipera palestinae*. (Modified from Perry and Duncker, 1980.)

these relationships, because minute ventilation ($\dot{V}_E$) is proportional to the metabolic demands of the animal and, thus, scales to $M_b^{0.75}$, breathing frequency should scale to $M_b^{-0.25}$. The data presented by Stahl (1967) and Crosfill and Widdicombe (1961) indicate that this is indeed so; $f = 53.5\ M_b^{-0.26}$ (see Tables 1,2). What these numbers tell us is that small animals with relatively high weight-specific metabolic rates, will breath with a relatively high-frequency, low tidal volume breathing pattern, whereas larger animals, with relatively low weight-specific metabolic rates, will breath with relatively low frequencies but higher tidal volumes. The same general trend also applies across the vertebrate classes.

Figure 6 is a graphic representation of this phenomenon adapted from the work of Perry and Duncker (1980). This is a double logarithmic plot of weight-specific tidal volume plotted against breathing frequency for seven reptilian, one avian, and one mammalian species. All data shown are for animals under resting conditions at normal or preferred body temperatures. The vertical axis in this diagram represents the quotient of breathing frequency/tidal volume which the authors term a breathing pattern index. Increasing values represent a transition to a relatively high-frequency, low tidal volume breathing pattern. The horizontal axis in this diagram is minute ventilation. The cross-hatched area indicates the trend toward a high breathing pattern index with increasing levels of resting minute ventilation (i.e., increasing resting metabolic rate) progressing from reptiles to birds and mammals.

There is also a decrease in V_{LR} (or FRC) and ERV associated with decreasing body weight or increasing weight-specific metabolic rate. Agostoni et al. (1959) suggested that (large) mammals, breathing at a lower frequency, require a relatively large FRC (or V_{LR}) to contain, within small limits, changes in composition of the alveolar air resulting from the breathing cycle. It could also be argued that animals with relatively large FRC (V_{LR}) and, therefore, relatively large gas stores, need to replenish those stores less often but require a larger V_T to do so.

Given the diversity of structure and function found in vertebrate respiratory systems, numerous exceptions to these general trends are common and invariably provide further insights into the design of respiratory systems. In this regard, Crosfill and Widdicombe (1961), in a study of eight mammalian species (see Table 2), noted that the time constant for the respiratory system of the dog was exceptionally short relative to predictions based on the body weight of these animals. They also noted, however, that of all the species they studied, the dog most commonly breathed rapidly and shallowly to dissipate body heat and, for this function, a short time constant would be a distinct advantage. This reduced time constant in the dog was primarily because of a relative reduction in flow resistance.

Unlike most mammals, the respiratory pause occurs at end-inspiration in many marine mammals, as well as the reptiles and amphibians (Gans, 1970; Kooyman, 1973; Kooyman and Sinnett, 1979; Kooyman and Cornell, 1981). Each breath commences with expiration followed immediately by inspiration. Although much, if not all, of the energy required for expiration could theoretically be derived from the static recoil of the system, as in most mammals, expiration is an active process in all of these species (Gans, 1970; Kooyman and Sinnett, 1979; Kooyman and Cornell, 1981). In fact, in amphibians and reptiles, the tidal volume of each breath quite often cycles below V_{LR} (Gans and Hughes, 1967; Gans, 1970). Thus, intrapulmonary pressure often rises before the onset of airflow, and pressure–volume and volume–flow relationships exceed

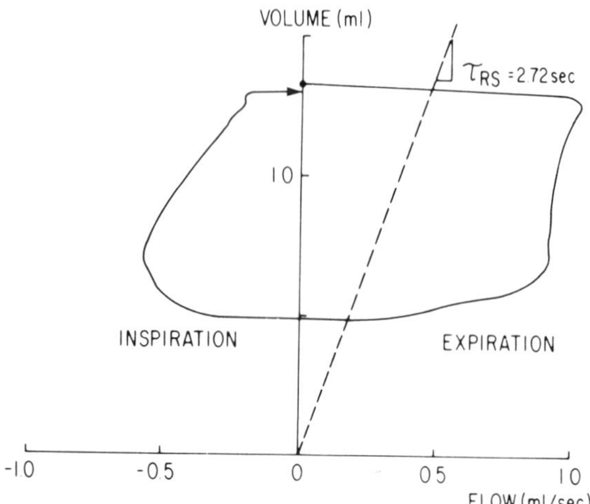

Figure 7 Volume–flow diagram of a single breath in a garter snake. The interrupted line shows the passive volume–flow course predicted from independent measurements of resistance and C_T. (From Bartlett et al., 1986.)

the passive characteristics of the system (Fig. 7). In Figure 7, the volume–flow relationship during a single breath in a snake is shown. The passive flow relations of the respiratory system of the snake are represented by the line drawn through the origin of the volume–flow diagram, the slope of which is equal to the time constant of the system (Bartlett et al., 1986). Combinations of volume and flow lying to the right of this line must include active expiratory effort. Thus, expiratory flow is greater than can be attributed to the passive mechanical properties of the system throughout almost the entire expiration. Expiratory muscle activity increases throughout deflation, providing the respiratory system with dynamic stiffening (Rosenberg, 1973) that, when added to the frequency-dependent increase in dynamic compliance discussed earlier, acts to maintain relatively high and constant flow rates throughout much of the expiration, despite the shrinking of lung volume and the attendant decrease in passive recoil pressure (Bartlett et al., 1986).

The use of active expiration in marine mammals has been suggested to reduce the time required for these animals to renew lung gases at the waters surface (Kooyman and Sinnett, 1979; Kooyman and Cornell, 1981). Because V_T may almost equal VC in these animals, lung stores can be renewed rapidly, in a single breath. In the reptiles and amphibians, the passive time constant for the respiratory systems is relatively long (2–14.6 s; Bartlett et al., 1986; Morgan and Milsom, unpublished) and passive expiration is more than 10 times slower than in most mammals (0.03 s, mouse; 0.18 s, human; Crosfill and Widdicombe,

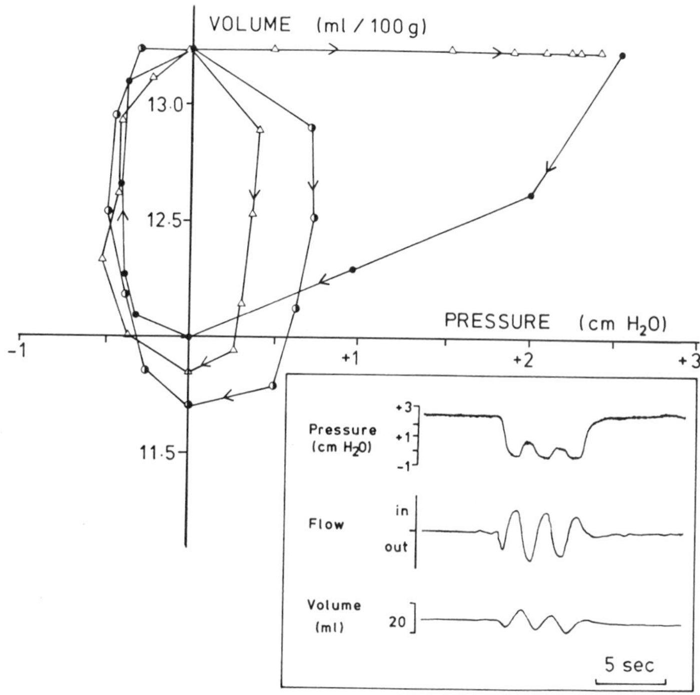

Figure 8 Pressure–volume diagram of a breathing episode in an awake, spontaneously breathing turtle (*Chrysemys picta*). Arrows indicate the direction of change during the first (filled circles), second (half-filled circles), and third (open triangles) breath of the episode. The inset shows the pressure, flow, and volume changes associated with the three breaths. (From Morgan and Milsom, unpublished.)

1961). Although the use of passive expiration could restrict breathing frequency (4–30/min) and be a great disadvantage in aquatic species, the presence of active expiration in terrestrial species of reptiles with extremely low respiratory frequencies suggests such teleological arguments should be used with caution.

There are situations in which reptiles do appear to utilize the passive mechanical properties of the respiratory system to power expiration. One well-documented example occurs during quiet respiration in the caiman (*Caiman crocodilus*) while resting submerged at the water's surface (Gans and Clark, 1976). Gans and Clark have shown that as the trunk of the caiman is immersed, the pattern of muscular activity shifts; expiration becomes passive, and inspiration requires increased muscular effort. This transition implies some form of feedback control, the mechanism of which remains unexplored. Although corresponding myographic data is not available for the turtle, the pressure–volume relationships of spontaneously breathing animals resting at the water's surface suggest a somewhat more complex picture (Fig. 8). The insert in Figure 8 shows the volume, airflow, and intrapulmonary pressure changes associated with an episode of three breaths in a turtle floating in an aquarium. The intrapulmonary pressure is almost 3 cm H_2O during the breath-holding period, a consequence of both elastic recoil and the hydrostatic head of the water. The first expiration closely follows the passive pressure–volume relationship for this animal (not shown) but the pressure changes associated with the subsequent two expirations are much smaller, suggesting that the hydrostatic pressure of the water column is not transmitted through to the lungs. In other words, expiratory braking occurs that could be due to either active (muscular tone in the flank cavities arising from either inspiratory or slowly contracting expiratory muscles) or passive processes (high flow resistance of the tissues of the body wall). The rapid increase in pressure following the last breath of the sequence, once the glottis closes and the respiratory muscles relax, suggests that it is the former. Unfortunately, there is insufficient data to pursue such considerations further, but the relationship between breathing pattern, expiratory muscle activity, and respiratory time constants in reptiles certainly deserves further investigation. The sum of the data suggests that expiratory flow rates in these animals are quite closely and actively controlled.

IV. Energetics

A. Mechanical Cost of Breathing

In generating pressure and, hence, flow in the respiratory system, the respiratory muscles perform work to overcome the forces associated with the dynamic properties we have just discussed. At low respiratory frequencies, most of this work is required to overcome the elastic forces resisting lung inflation, which will be a function of the tidal volume and the compliance of the system (Agostoni et al., 1970; Roussos and Campbell, 1986). Given that both of these latter two variables scale with M_b^{1} in most mammals, the cost of taking a breath also scales to M_b^{1}. As a consequence, the relative cost of taking a breath (i.e., the cost per milliliter) should be the same for mammals of all sizes ($\simeq$ 2.2–2.5 g · cm/ml) (see Table 1). The minute work or power of breathing will simply be a function of the work per breath times the respiratory frequency, which will scale to $M_b^{0.75}$ ($W = 962\ M_b^{0.78}$, Stahl, 1967). Thus, weight-specific metabolic rate, minute ventilation, and minute work of breathing all increase in parallel with decreasing body size (see Table 1).

Comparative data for nonmammalian vertebrates are scarce. Perry and Duncker (1980) have calculated the elastic work of resting breathing based on static compliance measurements for a number of species of reptiles as well as the pigeon. When these values are expressed per unit of minute ventilation, they also yield a value for the relative cost of breathing (0.01-0.06 g · cm/ml). Although the data are insufficient to yield any trends that may exist as a function of body size or lung type within the reptiles, they do indicate that because of both higher compliances and a lower breathing pattern index, the relative cost of ventilation in reptiles and birds is one to three orders of magnitude lower than in mammals. Although recent measurements of the total cost of breathing in the turtle and gecko (Milsom and Vitalis, 1984; Vitalis and Milsom, 1986a,b) yield values that are predictably higher than the elastic work calculated by Perry and Duncker (0.02-0.2 g · cm/ml), they are nonetheless one to two orders of magnitude lower than those recorded in mammals. Perry and Duncker (1980) suggest that the dramatic increase in the work of breathing seen in mammals may account for the presence of the muscular diaphragm in this class, which is lacking in all other vertebrates.

B. Optimal Frequency of Breathing

It has been well established on theoretical grounds that in all vertebrates, at any given level of total ventilation, mechanical work decreases as respiratory frequency increases, with a concomitant decrease in tidal volume (Roussos and Campbell, 1986). This is because the work required to overcome elastic forces is inversely proportional to frequency, whereas that required to overcome nonelastic forces is independent of frequency (Otis, 1954). The same, however, is not true for alveolar ventilation. For any given level of alveolar ventilation, there is an optimal frequency at which the cost of ventilation is minimal (Otis et al., 1950). As pointed out by Otis (1954), to maintain a constant level of alveolar ventilation with increasing respiratory frequency and decreasing tidal volume, actually requires an increase in total ventilation. This is required to offset the proportionate increase in dead space ventilation. As a consequence, increasing frequency tends to increase elastic work because of the increase in total ventilation, while at the same time it tends to decrease elastic work because of the decrease in tidal volume. It is because of these opposite effects of frequency on elastic work that an optimum frequency occurs although nonelastic work also determines the exact nature of the relationship between minute work and breathing frequency (Otis, 1954; Roussos and Campbell, 1986).

Figure 9 illustrates such relationships for three species of vertebrate; a lizard, a turtle, and a mammal. The curves labeled *total* represent the relationship between the total cost of ventilating the entire respiratory system and the respiratory frequency at a constant level of alveolar ventilation in each animal. Clearly, there is an optimal frequency at which minute work is a minimum in each. Despite this, the site and nature of the forces responsible for the generation of this work are significantly different. The work required to inflate the

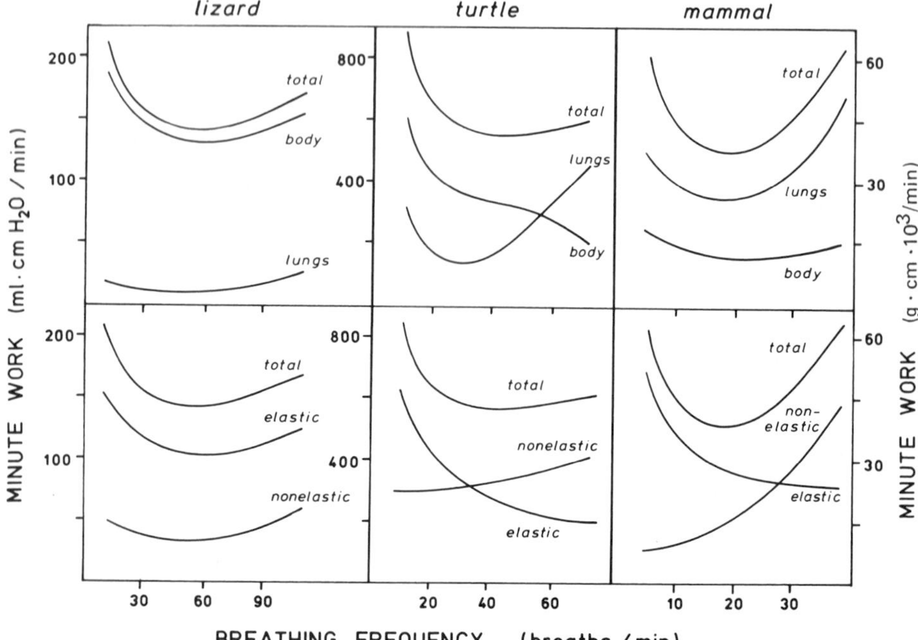

Figure 9 Upper panels: The minute work required to ventilate the lungs, body compartment, and total respiratory system in a lizard, turtle, and mammal, at a constant level of alveolar ventilation, as a function of ventilation frequency. Lower panels: The amount of minute work required to overcome elastic and nonelastic forces in the total respiratory system, at a constant level of alveolar ventilation, as a function of ventilation frequency in the same three species. Values for minute work for the lizard and turtle are in ml · cm H_2O/min (left hand axis); those for the mammal are in g · cm/min (right hand axis). [Data from Milsom and Vitalis, 1984 (lizard); Vitalis and Milsom, 1986a (turtle); and Otis et al., 1950 (mammal).]

lungs as a percentage of the total work of breathing increases in the sequence: gecko < turtle < mammal. This hierarchy also reflects the increasing complexity of lung architecture (Perry, 1983). Given the simple structure of their lungs, the total work of breathing in the Tokay gecko is almost entirely required to overcome elastic forces arising from the body wall at all frequencies and tidal volumes (Milsom and Vitalis, 1984). In turtles, the mechanical work required to inflate the respiratory system is required to overcome both elastic and nonelastic forces over the entire range of frequencies studied. At low frequencies, elastic forces predominate, with these forces residing primarily in the body wall and cavity. The work required to overcome nonelastic forces, however, predominates at high frequencies, with the lungs contributing an increasing portion of this work (Vitalis and Milsom, 1986a). In mammals, the work required to inflate the respiratory system is primarily required to overcome elastic forces at low pump frequencies and nonelastic forces at high pump frequencies, but in both instances, these forces reside primarily in the lungs (Otis et al., 1950; Agostoni et al., 1959). Despite these vast differences in the pulmonary mechanics of each group, the interaction between pulmonary mechanics and the relative costs of dead space ventilation invariably produce an optimal frequency.

The correspondence between these calculated and predicted optimal breathing frequencies and observed breathing frequencies, in all species that have been studied, is striking (Agostoni et al., 1959; Crosfill and Widdicombe, 1961; Milsom and Vitalis, 1984; Vitalis and Milsom, 1986b). It strongly suggests that alveolar ventilation is regulated according to the principle of minimum effort as postulated by Rohrer (1925). It has been suggested that this correlation may be somewhat coincidental and that the frequency of spontaneous ventilation corresponds more closely with that associated with the minimum force required by the respiratory muscles (Mead, 1960). The difference in these predicted frequencies is not large, and given the shape of the relationships between minute work or minimum force and respiratory frequency, there is very little difference in energy cost between breathing patterns utilizing either one (Otis, 1954). At present, the physiological mechanisms that underlie this phenomenon remain unclear, although the data attests to their universality.

The calculations of optimal tidal volume and respiratory frequency, discussed earlier, all assume a continuous breathing pattern with passive expiration (Otis, 1954; Roussos and Campbell, 1986). For several mammals (diving species in particular), as well as the reptiles and amphibians, breathing is periodic and, as we have seen, expiration is active (Milsom, 1988). The consequences of active expiration for predictions of optimal breathing pattern are small. Recent measurements of the mechanical cost of ventilation in spontaneously breathing lizards and turtles produced values that were not significantly different from those calculated from mechanical studies on pump-ventilated animals with passive expiration (Milsom, 1984, Morgan and Milsom, unpublished). Presumably the increased cost of active expiration was small and offset by stored energy resulting from the active expiration that was available to help power inspiration. The consequences of periodic breathing for predictions of optimal breathing frequency, however, are another matter. There are two general patterns of periodic breathing commonly seen in these animals. One consists of single breaths separated by relatively short periods of breath holding; the other consists of episodes of, more or less, continuous breathing separated by much longer periods of breath holding (see inset, Fig. 8). On theoretical grounds, continuous breathing in the episodic breathers should correspond closely to predicted patterns based on the mechani-

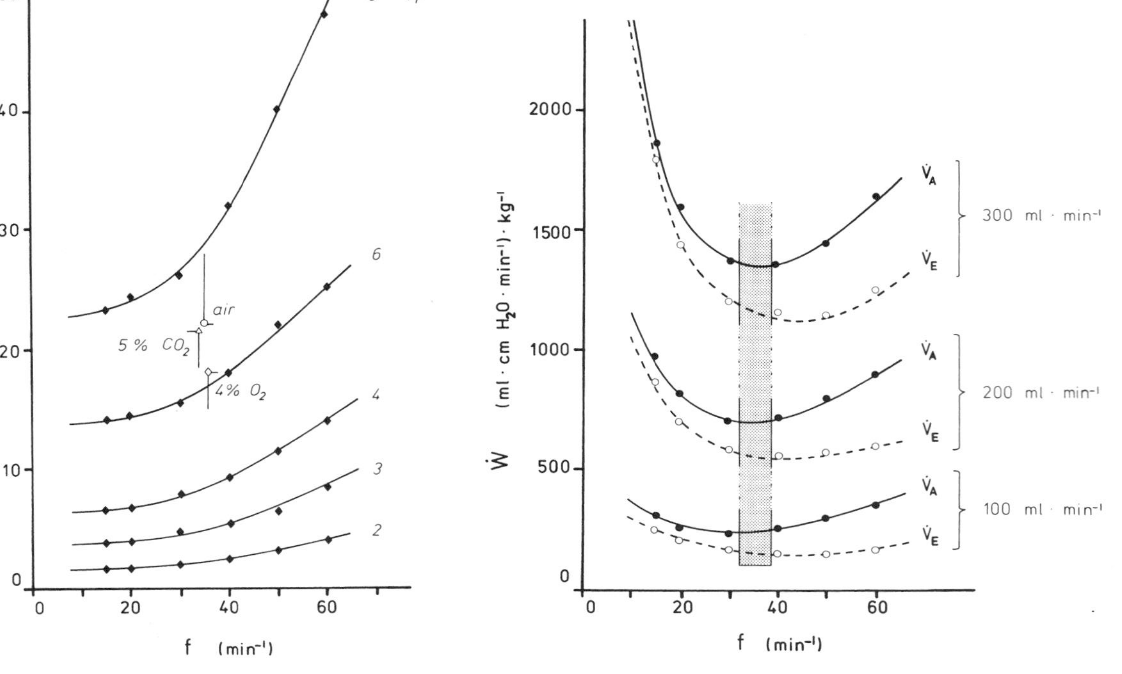

Figure 10 Left-hand panel: The relationship between the work/breath and ventilation frequency for various levels of tidal volume (V_T) in the turtle (*Pseudemys scripta*). The open symbols represent the mean values ± SEM of V_T and intantaneous breathing frequency ($f' = 60/T_{TOT}$) measured from six animals spontaneously breathing air (circle), 5% CO_2 in air (triangle), or 4% O_2 in N_2 (diamond). Right-hand panel: The minute work or power required to produce various constant levels of alveolar ($\dot{V}_A$) and total ($\dot{V}_I$) ventilation as a function of breathing frequency. The stippled area represents the range of instantaneous breathing frequencies (f') measured in spontaneously breathing animals. (From Vitalis and Milsom, 1986a,b).

cal considerations discussed earlier. This is certainly true for the turtle, *Pseudemys scripta* (Vitalis and Milsom, 1986a,b). In the right-hand panel of Figure 10, the power required to maintain a constant level of alveolar ventilation is plotted, along with that required to maintain a constant level of total ventilation as a function of ventilation frequency. Note that, because of dead space ventilation, minute work is always greater for any given level of alveolar ventilation when compared with a similar level of total ventilation and that the difference increases as frequency increases because of the proportionate increase in dead space ventilation along with rising nonelastic forces. The shaded area in this panel indicates the range of instantaneous-breathing frequencies measured in spontaneously breathing animals and corresponds quite closely with the pump frequencies that require the minimum rate of work to maintain a constant level of alveolar ventilation. They correspond less well to those frequencies at which the minimum work is required to maintain a constant level of total ventilation (Vitalis and Milsom, 1986a,b).

The optimal breathing frequency for animals that take only single breaths followed by a variable pause, however, should be determined from an analysis of the work per breath, rather than the minute work of breathing. Marine turtles and tortoises exhibit such patterns (Shelton, et al., 1985; Milsom, 1988) and, if the pulmonary mechanics and respiratory variables of these species are similar to those of *P. scripta*, the work of breathing associated with such a pattern can be analyzed using the left-hand panel in Figure 10. This panel displays the mechanical cost required to produce single breaths at various tidal volumes as a function of the instantaneous ventilation frequency ($60/T_{TOT} = f'$). The values of V_T and f' for spontaneously breathing *P. scripta* when breathing various gas mixtures are placed on the graph for comparison. These work/breath curves illustrate that for any given frequency, the smaller V_T, the lower the cost of each breath. A low V_T, however, will compromise alveolar ventilation and gas exchange. Presumably, the need to keep V_T sufficiently large to maintain alveolar ventilation, and the increased mechanical work associated with increases in V_T, interact to produce the resting level of V_T. At any given V_T, the work/breath decreases as breathing frequency decreases. There are physiological and behavioral factors, however, that should restrict breath duration from becoming too long. A very long breath in a spontaneously breathing animal would require a slow, controlled expiration and inspiration that would require expiratory braking as well as dissipate the stored elastic energy that partially powers both expiration and inspiration. It would also tie up accessory respiratory muscles that frequently subserve other roles in reptiles (Gans, 1970) as well as reduce the breath-holding period, which would serve to restrict dive lengths in aquatic and semiaquatic species. Given the shape of the relationship between work/breath and ventilation frequency shown in Figure 10, the decrease in mechanical work associated with a fall in ventilation frequency below the f' measured in spontaneously breathing animals is minute compared with the large increase in the work/breath associated with an increase in breathing frequency above that value. The value of f′ measured in spontaneously breathing animals may, thus, represent a compromise between mechanical and biological constraints.

With increasing metabolic demands, animals that exhibit periodic breathing can increase the tidal volume of each breath, increase the speed of the breath, or simply reduce the total period of breath holding by taking more breaths per minute. The data presented here would suggest that it is less costly to restrict changes in V_T and f′ and take more breaths of a similar length and depth (in an episode or individually) and, thus, shorten the nonventilatory period, than it is to increase V_T or shorten T_{TOT}. This is in fact what is seen in most reptiles (see Shelton et al., 1985; Milsom, 1988 for reviews). The hypothesis would predict that a reduction in T_{TOT} would occur only when ventilation was sufficiently elevated that all periods of breath holding had disappeared.

C. Oxidative Cost of Breathing and Breathing Efficiency

Because it is not possible to measure the oxygen consumption of the respiratory muscles directly, the general method for determining the oxidative cost of ventilation is to measure the total oxygen consumption of the animal at several different levels of ventilation, assuming that the increments in oxygen uptake represent the metabolic cost of the increase in ventilation (Otis, 1954; Agostoni et al., 1970; Roussos and Campbell, 1986). The oxygen cost of resting ventilation can be estimated by extrapolation. Although many investigators have made such measurements on humans, few data are available for other species. Table 3 lists the oxidative cost of resting ventilation for human, dog, turtle, and frog. These values are presented as absolute values normalized to body weight, as milliliters of O_2 consumed per liter of gas moved and as a percentage of the resting metabolic rate. Whereas the oxidative cost per liter of gas ventilated is roughly an order of magnitude greater in the turtle than in mammals, the cost of ventilation in the frog is surprisingly low. Despite this, when differences in metabolic rate and minute ventilation are taken into account, the relative cost of ventilation as a fraction of the total oxygen consumption of the animal is an order of magnitude greater for both species of lower vertebrate compared with mammals.

Knowing the oxidative cost of ventilation as well as the mechanical cost, the efficiency of the respiratory pump can be calculated. Table 3 lists the calculated efficiencies for the same four species. Given the difficulties of measuring both the total mechanical work of breathing as well as the oxidative cost of breathing, these calculations are only rough indications of efficiency. They do indicate, however, that with the exception of the turtle, the mechanical efficiency of breathing is approximately 1 to 15%. The reasons for the low efficiency in the turtle are not clear but probably stem from the indirect coupling of the

Table 3 Cost and Efficiency of Breathing in Different Vertebrates

	Oxidative cost			Mechanical cost	Efficiency	
Species	kcal/min/kg	%$\dot{V}O_2$	ml/L	kcal/kg/min	%	Ref.
Human	1.64×10^{-1}	1-2	0.5-1	3.74×10^{-4}	3-10	1
Dog	1.44×10^{-4}	0.6	0.2	2.13×10^{-5}	15	2
Turtle	$5\text{-}20 \times 10^{-4}$	10-30	5-15	1.25×10^{-6}	0.1-0.25	3-5
Frog	4.06×10^{-4}	5	0.5-0.7	3.25×10^{-6}	8	6-8
Trout	2.49×10^{-4}	1-7	0.1-0.3	2.49×10^{-6}	0.6-1.2	9,10

Sources: 1. Otis et al., 1950; 2. Robertson et al., 1977; 3. Kinney and White, 1976; 4. Vitalis and Milsom, 1986a; 5. Morgan and Milsom, unpublished; 6. West and Jones, 1974; 7. Boutilier, 1984; 8. Emilio, 1974; 9. Jones and Schwarzfeld, 1974; 10. Davis and Randall, 1973.

respiratory pump to lung ventilation in these animals. In turtles, ventilation is powered by muscles associated with the pectoral girdle and flank cavities. To effect lung ventilation, these muscles must expand and contract the entire body cavity. Several of the muscles involved in this process are principally involved in locomotion, with only an accessory role in ventilation (Gans and Hughes, 1967). Data from the trout are included in this table for comparison. It can be seen that the oxidative cost of pumping water over the gills in this species is consistent with the cost of aerial ventilation in higher vertebrates but that the efficiency of the branchial pump is also quite low (Jones and Schwarzfeld, 1974).

In mammals, the work of breathing is a small fraction of the total energy turnover of resting animals. As a consequence, it is usually considered of minor physiological importance (Otis, 1954). The cost at higher levels of ventilation does become significant because the oxygen cost of breathing is known to increase dramatically with breathing frequency, at least in humans (Roussos and Campbell, 1986). This, however, has not been sufficient to stimulate much research in this area. The data for the lower vertebrates presented here indicate that even at rest, the oxygen cost of breathing is a major fraction of their total metabolic rate. The oxidative cost during periods of strenuous activity could become prohibitive. This indicates the importance of strategies that optimize the work of breathing in these species and suggests that such considerations are of more than academic interest.

V. Conclusions

The work presented in this chapter deals mainly with considerations of pulmonary mechanics associated with resting ventilation.

In general, relative to body volume, the total lung capacity of reptiles exceeds that of birds, which exceeds that of mammals. The larger lungs of reptiles tend to be more heterogeneous in parenchymal distribution reflecting increasing effects of nonrespiratory constraints on the design of the respiratory system.

Weight-specific metabolic rate increases from reptiles, through mammals, to birds and, furthermore, increases with decreasing body size in any one group. Associated with increasing weight-specific metabolic rate is a decrease in total lung volume but an increase in lung partitioning such that alveolar dimensions decrease and surface area increases. There is also a trend toward decreasing tissue barrier thickness, increasing diffusion capacity, and a reduction in the alveolar–arterial oxygen partial pressure difference.

The static forces that operate to establish the resting lung volume of each species also establish both the inspiratory and expiratory reserve capacities. It follows, therefore, that the development and strategy of recruitment of inspiratory and expiratory muscles will vary from species to species reflecting this static balance of forces and vice versa. Nonrespiratory constraints on the design of the respiratory system greatly affect the partitioning of TLC.

Although the compliance of the respiratory system of reptiles and birds is one to three orders of magnitude greater than that of mammals, the specific compliance of these respiratory systems (C_T/V_{LR}) is remarkably similar. In mammals, however, total compliance is primarily a function of the compliance of the lungs, whereas in birds and reptiles, it is primarily a function of the compliance of the body wall. This suggests that despite the similarities in specific compliance, the primary source of the recoil pressure is very different.

All respiratory systems, from amphibians to mammals, and spanning seven orders of magnitude in size, are powered by similar changes in transpulmonary pressure.

Although the dynamic compliance of the respiratory system of mammals is relatively frequency-independent, that of reptiles decreases dramatically with increasing ventilation frequency (50–70% over a 10-fold increase in f) because of viscoelastic properties of the lungs and body wall. Despite this, the time constant of the respiratory system, an indication of the time required for passive expiration, is still an order of magnitude greater in reptiles than in mammals. This long time constant may necessitate the active expiration that is routinely found in this group. In mammals, the respiratory time constant is relatively short and changes in parallel with T_E, the time available for passive expiration.

As predicted from allometric equations, animals with high, weight-specific metabolic rates tend to breath with high frequency, and low tidal volume-breathing patterns are associated with species with low, weight-specific metabolic rates. Resting-breathing patterns, thus, reflect the changes in pulmonary mechanics resulting from differences in lung architecture associated with difference in metabolic demand.

The mechanical work of breathing is size-independent within any group but one to two orders of magnitude greater in mammals than in birds and reptiles. It has been suggested that this may account for the presence of a muscular diaphragm in mammals.

There are vast differences in the relative contributions of elastic and nonelastic forces arising from the lungs and body wall in establishing the minute work or power required for ventilation in different vertebrates. Despite this, the interaction of the relative cost of dead space ventilation invariably produces an optimum combination of tidal volume and breathing frequency which minimizes the power required for ventilation. These optimal combinations of V_T and f correspond closely with observed resting-breathing patterns in all species that have been studied.

In animals that exhibit periodic breathing, such as the lower vertebrates, the most economical way to increase ventilation is to reduce the periods of breath holding and take more breaths at this optimal combination of V_T and f. The changes in spontaneous breathing observed in these species are consistent with these predictions.

The relative oxidative cost of ventilation (ml $\dot{V}O_2$/L $\dot{V}E$) is roughly the same in those few vertebrates that have been studied, as is the efficiency of breathing (1-15%). (The turtle is a rather inefficient exception.) Relative to resting metabolic rate, however, the cost of ventilation is much greater in the lower vertebrates (5-30% resting $\dot{V}O_2$) and could become prohibitive with increasing ventilation, emphasizing the importance of strategies that optimize breathing patterns in these species.

References

Agostoni, E., Campbell, E. J. M., and Freedman, S. (1970). Energetics. In *The Respiratory Muscles*. Edited by E. J. M. Campbell, E. Agostoni, and J. Newsom Davis. London, Lloyd-Luke, pp. 115-137.

Agostoni, E., and Hyatt, R. E. (1986). Static behaviour of the respiratory system. In *Handbook of Physiology*. Sect. 3. The Respiratory System. Vol. III. Mechanics of Breathing, Part 1. Edited by A. P. Fishman, P. T. Macklem, J. Mead, and S. R. Geiger. Washington, American Physiological Society, pp. 113-130.

Agostoni, E., Thimm, F. F., and Fenn, W. O. (1959). Comparative features of the mechanics of breathing. *J. Appl. Physiol. 14*:679-683.

Bartlett, D., Jr., Mortola, J. P., and Doll, E. J. (1986). Respiratory mechanics and control of the ventilatory cycle in the garter snake. *Respir. Physiol. 64*:13-27.

Boutilier, R. G. (1984). Characterization of the intermittent breathing pattern in *Xenopus laevis. J. Exp. Biol. 110*:291-309.

Crosfill, M. L., and Widdicombe, J. G. (1961). Physical characteristics of the chest and lungs and the work of breathing in different mammalian species. *J. Physiol. 158*:1-14.

Davis, J. C., and Randall, D. J. (1973). Gill irrigation and pressure relationships in rainbow trout (*Salmo gairdneri*). *J. Fish. Res. Board Can. 30*:99-104.

Duncker, H. R. (1978). Funktionsmorphologie des Atemapparates und Coelom-Gliederung bei Reptilien, Vogeln und Saugern. *Verh. Dtsch. Zool. Ges. 1978*:99-132.

Emilio, M. G. (1974). Gas exchanges and blood gas concentrations in the frog *Rana ridibunda. J. Exp. Biol. 60*:901-908.

Fedde, M. R., Burger, R. F., and Kitchell, R. L. (1963). Localization of vagal afferents involved in the maintenance of normal avian respiration. *Poult. Sci. 42*:1224-1236.

Gans, C. (1970). Strategy and sequence in the evolution of the external gas exchangers of ectothermal vertebrates. *Forma Functio 3*:61-104.

Gans, C., and Clark, B. (1976). Studies on ventilation of *Caiman crocodilus* (Crocodilia:Reptilia). *Respir. Physiol. 26*:285-301.

Gans, C., and Clark, B. D. (1978). Air flow in reptilian ventilation. *Comp. Biochem. Physiol. 60a*:453-457.

Gans, C., and Hughes, G. M. (1967). The mechanism of lung ventilation in the tortoise *Testudo graeca* Linne. *J. Exp. Biol. 47*:1-20.

Gans, C., and Maderson, P. F. A. (1973). Sound production mechanisms in recent reptiles: Review and comment. *Am. Zool. 13*:1195-1203.

Grimsby, G., Takishima, T., Graham, W., Macklem, P., and Mead, J. (1968). Frequency dependence of flow resistance in patients with obstructive lung disease. *J. Clin. Invest. 47*:1455-1465.

Hemmingsen, A. M. (1960). Energy metabolism as related to body size and respiratory surfaces and its evolution. *Rep. Steno Mem. Hosp. Nord. Insulinlab. 9*:1-110.

Hughes, G. M., and Vergara, G. A. (1978). Static pressure-volume curves for the lung of the frog (*Rana pipiens*). *J. Exp. Biol. 76*:149-165.

Hutchison, V. H., Whitford, W. G., and Kohl, M. (1968). Relation of body size and surface area to gas exchange in anurans. *Physiol. Zool. 41*:65-85.

Jackson, D. C. (1969). Buoyancy control in the freshwater turtle, *Pseudemys scripta elegans. Science 166*:1649-1651.

Jackson, D. C. (1971). Mechanical basis for lung volume variability in the turtle *Pseudemys scripta elegans. Am. J. Physiol. 220*:754-758.

Jones, D. R., and Schwarzfeld, T. (1974). The oxygen cost to the metabolism and efficiency of breathing in the trout (*Salmo gairdneri*). *Respir. Physiol. 21*:241-254.

King, A. S. (1966). Structural and functional aspects of the avian lungs and air sacs. *Int. Rev. Gen. Exp. Zool. 2*:171-267.

Kinney, J. L., and White, F. N. (1977). Oxidative cost of ventilation in a turtle, *Pseudemys floridana. Respir. Physiol. 31*:327-332.

Kleiber, M. (1961). *The Fire of Life*. New York, John Wiley & Sons.

Koo, K. W., Leith, D. E., Scherter, C. B., and Snider, G. L. (1976). Respiratory mechanics in normal hamsters. *J. Appl. Physiol. 40*:936-942.

Kooyman, G. L. (1973). Respiratory adaptations in marine mammals. *Am. Zool. 13*:457-468.

Kooyman, G. L., and Cornell, L. H. (1981). Flow properties of expiration and inspiration in a trained bottle-nosed porpoise. *Physiol. Zool. 54*:55-61.

Kooyman, G. L., and Sinnett, E. E. (1979). Mechanical properties of the harbour porpoise lung. *Respir. Physiol. 36*:287-300.

Leith, D. E. (1976). Comparative mammalian respiratory mechanics. *Physiologist 19*:485-510.

McCutcheon, F. H. (1943). The respiratory mechanism in turtles. *Physiol. Zool. 16*:255-269.

Mead, J. (1960). Control of respiratory frequency. *J. Appl. Physiol. 15*:325-327.

Milsom, W. K. (1975). Development of buoyancy control in juvenile Atlantic loggerhead turtles, *Caretta caretta. Copeia 1975*:758-762.

Milsom, W. K. (1984). The interrelationship between pulmonary mechanics and the spontaneous breathing pattern in the Tokay lizard, *Gekko gecko. J. Exp. Biol. 113*:203-214.

Milsom, W. K. (1988). Control of arrhythmic breathing in aerial breathers. *Can. J. Zool. 66*:99-108.

Milsom, W. K., and Vitalis, T. Z. (1984). Pulmonary mechanics and the work of breathing in the lizard, *Gekko gecko. J. Exp. Biol. 113*:187-202.

Otis, A. B. (1954). The work of breathing. *Physiol. Rev. 34*:449-458.

Otis, A. B., Fenn, W. O., and Rahn, H. (1950). Mechanics of breathing in man. *J. Appl. Physiol. 2*:592-607.

Otis, A. B., McKerrow, C. B., Bartlett, R. A., Mead, J., McIlroy, M. B., Selverstone, N. J., and Radford, E. P. (1956). Mechanical factors in the distribution of pulmonary ventilation. *J. Appl. Physiol. 8*:427-443.

Perry, S. F. (1978). Quantitative anatomy of the lungs of the red-eared turtle, *Pseudemys scripta elegans. Respir. Physiol. 35*:245-262.

Perry, S. F. (1983). Reptilian lungs. *Adv. Anat. Embryol. Cell. Biol. 79*:1-81.

Perry, S. F., and Duncker, H. R. (1978). Lung architecture, volume and static mechanics in five species of lizards. *Respir. Physiol. 34*:61-81.

Perry, S. F., and Duncker, H. R. (1980). Interrelationship of static mechanical factors and anatomical structure in lung evolution. *J. Comp. Physiol. 138*: 321-334.

Piiper, J. (1982). Respiratory gas exchange at lungs, gills and tissues: Mechanisms and adjustments. *J. Exp. Biol. 100*:5-22.

Piiper, J., and Scheid, P. (1972). Maximum gas transfer efficacy of models of fish gills, avian lungs and mammalian lungs. *Respir. Physiol. 14*:115-124.

Robertson, C. H., Jr., Pagel, M. A., and Johnson, R. L., Jr. (1977). The distribution of blood flow, oxygen consumption, and work output among the respiratory muscles during unobstructed hyperventilation. *J. Clin. Invest. 59*:43-50.

Rodarte, J. R., and Rehder, K. (1986). Dynamics of respiration. In *Handbook of Physiology*. Sect. 3. The Respiratory System. Vol. III. Mechanics of Breathing. Part I. Edited by A. P. Fishman, P. T. Macklem, J. Mead, and S. R. Geiger. Washington, American Physiological Society, pp. 131-144.

Rohrer, F. (1925). Physiologie der Atembewegung. In *Handbuch der normalen und pathologisch Physiologie*, Vol. 2. Edited by A. T. J. Bethe, G. von Bergman, G. Embden, and A. Ellinger. Berlin, Springer-Verlag, pp. 70-127.

Rosenberg, H. I. (1973). Functional anatomy of pulmonary ventilation in the garter snake, *Thamnophis elegans. J. Morphol. 140*:171-184.

Roussos, C., and Campbell, E. J. M. (1986). Respiratory muscle energetics. In *Handbook of Physiology*. Sect. 3. The Respiratory System. Vol. III. Mechanics of Breathing. Part 2. Edited by A. P. Fishman, P. T. Macklem, J. Mead, and S. R. Geiger. Washington, American Physiological Society, pp. 481-509.

Shelton, G., Jones, D. R., amd Milsom, W. K. (1985). Control of breathing in ectothermic vertebrates. In *Handbook of Physiology*. Sect. 3. The Respiratory System. Vol. II. Control of Breathing. Part 2. Edited by A. P. Fishman, N. S. Cherniack, J. G. Widdicombe, and S. R. Geiger. Washington, American Physiological Society, pp. 857-909.

Spells, K. E. (1969). Comparative studies in lung mechanics based on a survey of literature data. *Respir. Physiol. 8*:37-57.

Stahl, W. R. (1967). Scaling of respiratory variables in mammals. *J. Appl. Physiol. 22*:453-460.

Sullivan, K. J., and Mortola, J. P. (1987). Age related changes in the rate of stress relaxation within the rat respiratory system. *Respir. Physiol. 67*: 295-309.

Tenney, S. M., and Remmers, J. E. (1963). Comparative quantitative morphology of the mammalian lung: Diffusing area. *Nature 197*:54-56.

Tenney, S. M., and Tenney, J. B. (1970). Quantitative morphology of cold-blooded lungs: Amphibia and Reptilia. *Respir. Physiol. 9*:197-215.

Vitalis, T. Z., and Milsom, W. K. (1986a). Pulmonary mechanics and the work of breathing in the semi-aquatic turtle, *Pseudemys scripta*. *J. Exp. Biol.* *125*:137–155.

Vitalis, T. Z., and Milsom, W. K. (1986b). Mechanical analysis of spontaneous breathing in the semi-aquatic turtle, *Pseudemys scripta*. *J. Exp. Biol.* *125*: 157–171.

West, N. H., and Jones, D. R. (1975). Breathing movements in the frog, *Rana pipiens*. II. The power output and efficiency of breathing. *Can. J. Zool.* *53*:345–353.

Zeuthen, E. (1953). Oxygen uptake as related to body size in organisms. *Q. Rev. Biol.* *28*:1–12.

20

Control of Breathing
Effects of Temperature

DONALD C. JACKSON

Brown University
Providence, Rhode Island

I. Introduction

A major theme in comparative respiratory physiology in recent years has concerned the effects of changes in body temperature. Because of its pervasive influences on relevant chemical constants and interactions, temperature has particularly pronounced effects on respiratory control. Ectotherms are the animals of primary interest because of their variable body temperatures, but endotherms under the special circumstances of hibernation and hypothermia are also important subjects for consideration.

Ectotherms that experience substantial fluctuations in body temperature exhibit changes in physiological variables that suggest temperature-dependent adjustments in homeostatic state. The conventional regulated variables of the respiratory system (blood P_{CO_2}, pH, and P_{O_2}) are all influenced significantly by temperature in most animals that have been studied. Such variations represent a challenge to physiologists to understand their basis and significance, as well as an opportunity to uncover fundamental principles of respiratory control not apparent in the isothermal state.

This chapter will address some of the recent directions and controversies in the comparative physiology of respiratory control that relate to temperature variation. Obviously, many aspects of comparative respiratory control, such as the diversity of control mechanisms, the identity and characterization of receptor mechanisms, and phylogenetic analysis, are not considered here, but interested readers can consult an excellent recent review by Shelton et al. (1986) for a comprehensive treatment of the subject.

II. Physical Effects of Temperature

A consideration of the manifold effects of temperature on the physical properties of the respiratory system must lead one to expect an impact on the control of breathing. These various effects, which will only be summarized here, are so complex, however, that no firm prediction would be possible given only these considerations. Furthermore, the integrative physiological responses to temperature are unpredictable a priori, and these may dominate the overall response of the control system.

The exchange and transport of respiratory gases, O_2 and CO_2, are markedly affected by temperature. The solubilities of both gases change inversely with temperature; CO_2 solubility increases more than threefold between 40 and 0°C and O_2 solubility more than doubles over the same range (Dejours, 1975). Gas diffusion increases with temperature, but in proportion to absolute temperature, so that changes within the physiological temperature range are comparatively small; indeed, in the liquid phase, when gas solubility is taken into account as it is in the Krogh diffusion constant, rate of diffusion down a constant partial pressue differential only increases by about 1% per degree Celsius. Temperature has complex effects on the exchange and transport of O_2 because of the direct thermal effect on reaction rates between O_2 and hemoglobin and the inverse effect on the affinity of hemoglobin for O_2.

Temperature effects on solution chemistry are of particular importance. The ionization constant of water and the dissociation constants of weak acids and bases are all temperature-dependent. However, the magnitude of the dependencies, dpK/dT, which are determined by the respective enthalpies of ionization (ΔH^o) are quite different for the various equilibria. Consequently, not all dissociable groups will remain unchanged when temperature is varied and a new homeostatic state is achieved. In addition, the direct effect of temperature on the acid-base state of solution will depend on the solution's composition. This is important because of the different buffer components of the extracellular and intercellular fluids and of the intracellular compartments of different tissues.

Finally, temperature affects cellular metabolism through effects on reaction rates and on enzyme properties. This is apparent at the organism level as the metabolic Q_{10} effect, which is typically a two- to threefold increase in metabolic rate per 10°C increase in body temperature. Exceptions to the general rule, however, are common. Metabolic adaptations can preserve constant metabolism over a range of temperatures ($Q_{10} = 1$) or Q_{10} can be much larger than 2 to 3, as in many ectotherms at the low end of their temperature range.

III. Effect of Temperature on Regulated Variables

A. Respiration in Air Versus Water

It is now well established that the conventional variables of the respiratory system vary with temperature in most ectothermic vertebrates. In air breathers, blood PCO_2 rises and pH falls with body temperature (Reeves, 1977). Blood PO_2 change has been measured less frequently but, like PCO_2, also usually increases with temperature. In water breathers, blood pH varies inversely with temperature in a fashion similar to the aerial species, but the blood gases do not change in any consistent manner (Cameron, 1984).

B. PCO_2

In the air-breathing vertebrates, but not in the water breathers, these blood changes can be related to apparent temperature-dependent changes in respiratory control. The rise in PCO_2 as a function of body temperature is associated with a fall in the ratio between ventilation and metabolic rate, the so-called air convection requirement. For example, at 10°C the turtle, *Pseudemys scripta*, has an air convection requirement (in milliliters air per milliliters O_2) of 60 to 65 and a blood PCO_2 of 14 torr; at 30°C, the values are 22 ml/ml and 32 torr, respectively (Jackson et al., 1974). In each case, the values represent "normal" values for that temperature. In the terminology of isothermal respiratory physiology, a progressive hypoventilatory shift occurs as temperature rises, but current understanding of ectothermic physiology would lead to the conclusion that at each temperature, normal respiratory homeostasis prevails. Similar temperature-related changes have been reported for a variety of air-breathing ectotherms.

C. Blood pH: The Alphastat Hypothesis

Definition

Fundamental to an understanding of these temperature effects is the identity of the regulated variable or variables of the control system. The prevailing view, developed by Reeves (1972), is that the net charge state of proteins, specifically the imidazole group of histidine, is the key variable defended. The fractional dissociation of imidazole is denoted αIm and the maintenance of this dissociation is termed alphastat regulation. The alphastat hypothesis, and the concept of con-

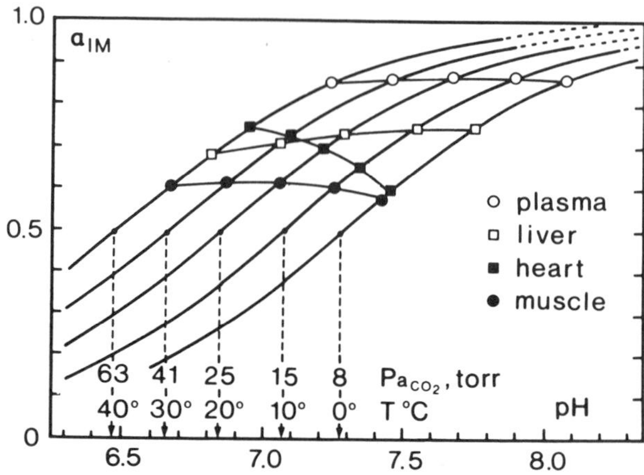

Figure 1 α-Imidazole (αIm) for tissues of the turtle, *Pseudemys scripta*, as a function of body temperature: plasma, skeletal muscle, cardiac muscle, and liver. (From Malan et al., 1976.)

stant relative alkalinity (Rahn, 1967) that preceded it, have proved to be important organizing principles for comparative acid-base physiology and have provided a framework for subsequent work in this field. The alphastat hypothesis is attractive because of the fundamental importance of charge state to protein structure-function relations and, thereby, its clear homeostatic relevance. Titration away from the optimal state may cause structural changes in proteins, leading to disturbances in binding or catalytic functions. By defending α_{Im}, these and other critical protein functions may be maintained throughout an ectotherm's normal temperature range. The regulation of α_{Im} in plasma and several tissues is illustrated in Fig. 1 (Malan et al., 1976).

Pros and Cons

The alphastat hypothesis has become a standard against which results in this field are measured, but when data have not matched theory, it has also been an object for critical challenges. In a broad sense, the extracellular, or blood, data have conformed to the hypothesis, although the slopes of the relationship, dpH/dT, have usually failed to reach the values predicted for complete alphastat regulation (Heisler, 1986). Striking exceptions to the hypothesis have also been reported, particularly among the mammallike varanid lizards, that exhibit only a slight pH change with temperature, significantly removed from the alphastat standard (Wood et al., 1981). The major discrepancy and disagreement concerning the efficacy of the alphastat hypothesis have concerned intracellular pH. Clearly, this is the site of prime importance because multiple functions are performed by temperature- and pH-sensitive macromolecules within the cellular environment. Two recent reviews, one supporting the application of alphastat theory to the intracellular milieu (Somero, 1986) and one challenging its validity (Heisler, 1986) epitomize the current state of affairs. The major points of these important contributions to the topic will be summarized.

In his review, Somero (1986) makes two important assumptions based on cited data: first, that intracellular pH of various tissues falls by about -0.015-0.020 U/°C rise in body temperature; and second, that the pK of imidazole groups that are exposed to cell water has temperature-dependence similar to the cell pH-dependence, and the fractional dissociation of these groups is near 0.5 at physiological pH. Together, these properties ensure that the key imidazole groups are poised at maximal sensitivity to acid-base change, a state that should confer maximal responsiveness to pH-sensitive functions of proteins when cell pH deviates from its optimal value. For example, midrange activity of the glycolytic regulatory enzyme, phosphofructokinase (PFK), shifts to lower pH as temperature rises, in parallel to alphastat control. A fall in pH at any temperature inhibits glycolysis by an inactivation of PFK. Inactivation is, at least in part, due to a dissociation of the enzyme from a tetrameric to a dimeric form. The pK of lactate dehydrogenase (LDH) is also close to pHi, and the LDH pK changes in response to temperature in parallel to pHi, therefore, the regulatory function of this enzyme in directing the reaction either toward lactate or toward the tricarboxylic acid cycle is maximally sensitive (Wilson, 1977). Other enzymes also have been reported to have activity optima that are matched to alphastat regulation (Park and Hong, 1976).

Somero discusses additional pH-sensitive cellular phenomena that may retain optimal function under conditions of alphastat regulation. The binding of PFK to intracellular sites, either on band 3 protein in erythrocytes or on actin in skeletal muscle, is in its midrange-sensitive state only under alphastat pH conditions. Finally, the binding of calcium to calmodulin is pH sensitive and appears to be due to a single imidazole group. Calmodulin's affinity for calcium may be stabilized by alphastat-based pH regulation.

Heisler (1986) challenges the validity of the two key assumptions of the Somero review, as well as other critical prerequisites of the alphastat hypothesis. The first is that dpH/dT of blood and tissue fluids of ectothermic vertebrates approximates the -0.015-0.020 U/°C required by alphastat theory. Most recorded blood values are below this range and 59 published slopes cited by Heisler, including data from reptiles, amphibians, and fishes, average -0.0124 ± 0.0035 U/°C. This compilation includes the varanid lizards, well-known nonconformers to alphastat control, and overall slopes from studies that included temperatures outside the usual range for the species. Nonetheless, the slopes are low, as they also are for many intracellular compartments, although the variability of the intracellular values is much greater, and certain tissues appear to have slopes consistently removed from the alphastat norm. For example, red muscle dpH/dT is usually high, 0.025 or more, and heart muscle is often low, 0.010 or less. The grand mean for 39 measurements on tissues from ectotherms is 0.0132 ± 0.0080 U/°C. Heisler also questions the choice of the imidazole pK and of its temperature-dependence. For blood values, the hemoglobin and plasma protein dpK/dT can be obtained using isoelectric technique, or by measuring the pH–temperature relationship of purified protein solutions (Reeves, 1976), although not without some question about the in vivo applicability (Cameron, 1984). Intracellular values are more difficult to obtain because of the diversity of proteins and the heterogeneity of microscopic imidazole pK values. Various proteins doubtless have different values, but whether or not key enzymes have properties matched to normal pH control is still an open question. Heisler contends, based on cited data, and in contrast to Somero (1986), that the dpH/dT slopes for optimal activity for most studied enzymes exceed both the measured pH slopes and the ideal alphastat slope.

Heisler concludes that pH regulation in response to temperature change is the same as that which occurs isothermally, involving compartmental buffering, ventilatory control of P_{CO_2}, and transmembrane and transepithelial ion transfers. Alphastat theory holds that no ion transfers are required but that the thermal effect on buffer equilibria and the appropriate regulation of P_{CO_2} will bring all compartments to their proper pH (Reeves, 1977).

The resolution of this controversy is clearly not at hand. The alphastat concept in its most extreme form, in which all body fluid compartments smoothly move on the pH–temperature slope to their respective ideal values with no ionic transfers required, is probably not tenable. Other key molecular considerations may share importance with protein charge state, such as membrane phosphate groups, as Heisler (1986) suggests. The answer must come from new approaches directed at the cellular milieu. The unarguable fact remains, however, that pH of various body fluid compartments changes in a consistent manner with body temperature. The alphastat hypothesis is still our best working model until a better one is brought forward to replace it.

Alphastat Model for Respiratory Control

An important contribution of the alphastat hypothesis has been to provide a unifying model for respiratory control that applies to endotherms and ectotherms alike. According to this model (Reeves, 1977), strategically positioned imidazole groups within the respiratory center, perhaps at a key site in a chemoreceptor channel protein, are poised to respond to deviations in pH. Normal pH is of course temperature-dependent, but normal acid–base homeostasis at each temperature would require temperature-independent imidazole-α. It is the regulation of α-imidazole, not of pH or P_{CO_2}, that would be the basis for respiratory control at any temperature, according to this view. A difficulty with testing this hypothesis is that α-imidazole is one of a number of dependent variables of the acid–base system (Stewart, 1981), each of which is affected by a change in acid–base state. An ingenious experimental approach to circumvent this problem has recently been devised by Nattie (1986a,b). The acylating agent, diethyl pyrocarbonate (DEPC), reacts with histidine imidazole to form a relatively stable product with a half-life of 55 h. Nattie (1986a) introduced this substance into the cerebrospinal fluid (CSF) of conscious rabbits and observed the effect on ventilation and on ventilatory control. Although DEPC is not without complicating properties, its presence in the CSF bathing the central chemoreceptors significantly attenuated the ventilatory response of the animals to acid infused into the CSF and to hypercapnic gas mixtures without affecting the integrative response of the central controller to peripheral hypoxic drive. These data provide supporting evidence for the alphastat model of respiratory control, but further evidence will be necessary to prove it. Additional support for the model has come from experiments showing a temperature-independent relationship between air convection requirement and blood α_{Im} in the alligator (Davies et al., 1982) and between ACR and cerebrospinal fluid α_{Im} in the turtle, *Pseudemys scripta* (Hitzig, 1982). These studies will be discussed further when respiratory sensitivity is considered.

D. Oxygen

An alphastat chemoreceptor presupposes that normal respiratory control is acid–base linked. There is evidence in certain animals that oxygen plays an important, if not a dominant, role in normal control. This is clearly true in fishes in which respiratory control and acid–base control are largely uncoupled processes. Blood pH of fish falls regularly with temperature, as in other ectotherms, but the control is accomplished primarily by ion transport processes and not by ventilatory control of P_{CO_2} (Cameron, 1984; Heisler, 1984). Changes in ambient and internal O_2 levels drive gill ventilation, and the control state is positioned to respond to either a rise in P_{O_2} (with hypoventilation) or to a fall in P_{O_2} (with hyperventilation). The role of O_2 in normal ventilatory control is less obvious in air-breathing ectotherms because, as in mammals, consistent steady-state responses to changes in inspired or arterial P_{O_2} are not apparent until well below ambient levels. Recently, however, Wood (1984) pointed out that the arterial O_2 saturation of a variety of reptiles, including lizards and turtles, is nearly constant across a range of body temperatures, although because of changes in affinity, arterial P_{O_2} varies directly with temperature. It is not clear how this apparent regulation relates to normal control of breathing, but the apneic threshold in various intermittent breathers has also been associated with a response to O_2 level (to be discussed shortly).

IV. Effect of Temperature on Ventilatory Responsiveness

A. Variability of Respiratory Homeostasis

For an ectotherm to function over a range of temperatures, it is necessary for respiratory homeostasis to be maintained. That this occurs has been amply documented in many animals by the similar variance in blood PCO_2 values at temperatures throughout their usual range (e.g., Cameron, 1984; Jackson, 1978). Consequently, the coupling between ventilation and metabolic rate is not disturbed by temperature change, although as already discussed, the ratio between these variables falls with temperature in air breathers.

B. Responses to Changes in Respiratory Gases

A further measure of respiratory responsiveness as a function of temperature has been obtained by exposing animals to inspired gas mixtures with elevated PCO_2 or reduced PO_2. Of particular interest are the air breathers in which blood gas values vary with temperature. Do such variations reflect a change in respiratory sensitivity or a shift in the control state with no change in sensitivity? Available data, at least for CO_2 responsiveness, appear to favor the latter alternative, i.e., temperature-independent sensitivity. The response to O_2, on the other hand, changes as a function of temperature.

Carbon Dioxide

Three studies have explicitly addressed the problem of CO_2 response at different temperatures, two on freshwater turtles (Jackson et al., 1974; Funk and Milsom, 1986) and one on the alligator (Davies et al., 1982). In the first of these (Jackson et al., 1974), control V_E of *P. scripta* was independent of temperature, an observation not observed in the other studies nor in most studies of other species in which $\dot{V}_E$ increases with temperature. Nonetheless, these three studies obtained essentially the same result. By the various criteria selected, ventilatory control was not affected by temperature. In the study by Jackson et al. (1974), the relationship between air convection requirement ($\dot{V}_E/\dot{V}_{O_2}$) and either inspired CO_2 (between 0 and 6%) or $PaCO_2$ was parallel at 10, 20, and 30°C, although shifted to the left at each lower temperature. In the study by Funk and Milsom (1986) on *Chrysemys picta*, the percentage changes in a variety of ventilatory variables (including $\dot{V}_E$, V_T, f, and $\dot{V}_E/\dot{V}_{O_2}$) were not significantly different at 10, 20, and 30°C in response to gases containing between 0 and 8%

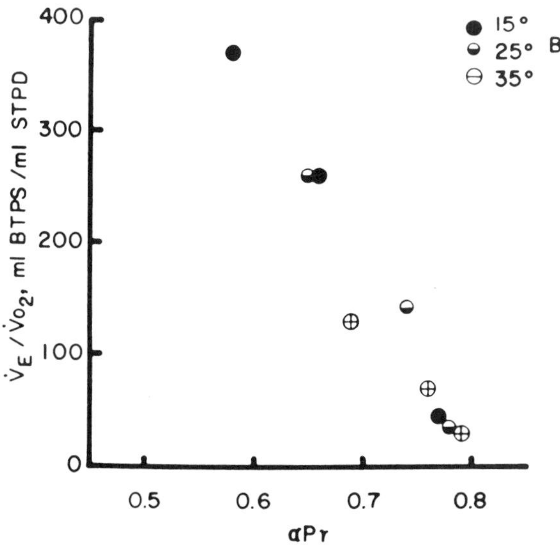

Figure 2 Ventilation of the American alligator, normalized to $\dot{V}_{O_2}$, plotted as a function of plasma α-imidazole. (From Davies et al., 1982.)

CO_2. These authors use their results to argue against alphastat regulation, citing the low dpH/dT in this and other studies. They propose that their results (and those of Jackson et al.) can be explained by an equal temperature effect (Q_{10}) on metabolic rate and on CO_2 sensitivity. In other words, CO_2 sensitivity per se is not temperature invariant, but CO_2 sensitivity normalized to $\dot{V}_{O_2}$ is. They further propose that normal resting ventilation, as well as the response to CO_2, can be explained by this putative Q_{10} coupling. In contrast, the study by Davies et al. (1982) on the American alligator uses a different criterion, and one that supports the alphastat concept. Their blood pH values are transformed to α_{Im}, assuming a value for dpK_{Im}/dT, and the normalized ventilation ($\dot{V}_E/\dot{V}_{O_2}$) for 15, 25, and 35°C, and for 0, 5, and 10% CO_2 at each temperature, is plotted as a function of α_{Im} (Fig. 2). The CO_2 response plotted in this fashion appears to be independent of temperature. The common feature of each of these analyses is the normalization of the ventilation to $\dot{V}_{O_2}$; without normalization, the response expressed simply as the change in $\dot{V}_E$ per torr P_{CO_2} is temperature-dependent.

Further support for both the temperature independence of respiratory control linked to acid-base balance and for the alphastat hypothesis was provided by Hitzig (1982). In this study of central mechanisms in the turtle, *P.*

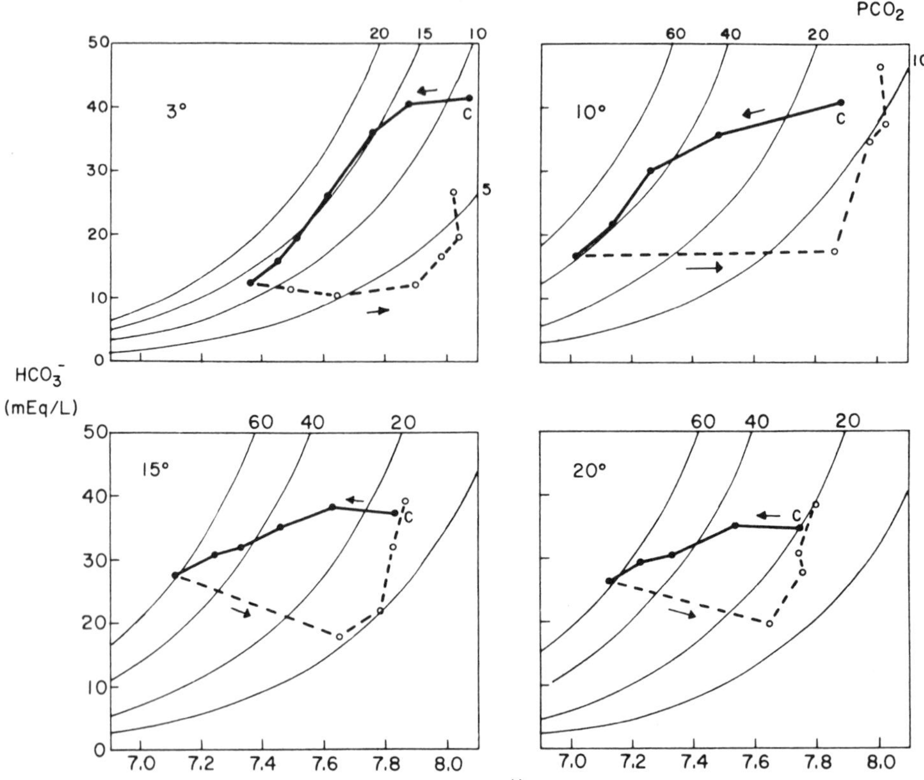

Figure 3 pH-HCO_3 diagrams showing blood acid–base changes of the turtle, *Chrysemys picta bellii*, under control conditions (C), during anoxic submergence (solid lines and circles), and during recovery from anoxia (dashed lines and open circles). Total anoxic periods were 12 h at 30°C, 3 days at 15°C, 10 days at 10°C, and 12 weeks at 3°C. Note the compensatory respiratory alkalosis that occurs during the early phases of recovery at each temperature. (From Herbert and Jackson, 1985.)

scripta, the pH of CSF samples, obtained from unanesthetized animals at 10, 20, and 30°C, was found to vary by -0.015 U/°C, in line with alphastat control. In addition, $\dot{V}_E$ normalized to $\dot{V}_{O_2}$ varied as a single function of CSF α_{Im} at 20 and 30°C for experiments in which CSF pH was altered by ventricular perfusion. Furthermore, the data obtained earlier on the goat by Pappenheimer et al. (1965), using a similar protoctol, fell nearly on the same line.

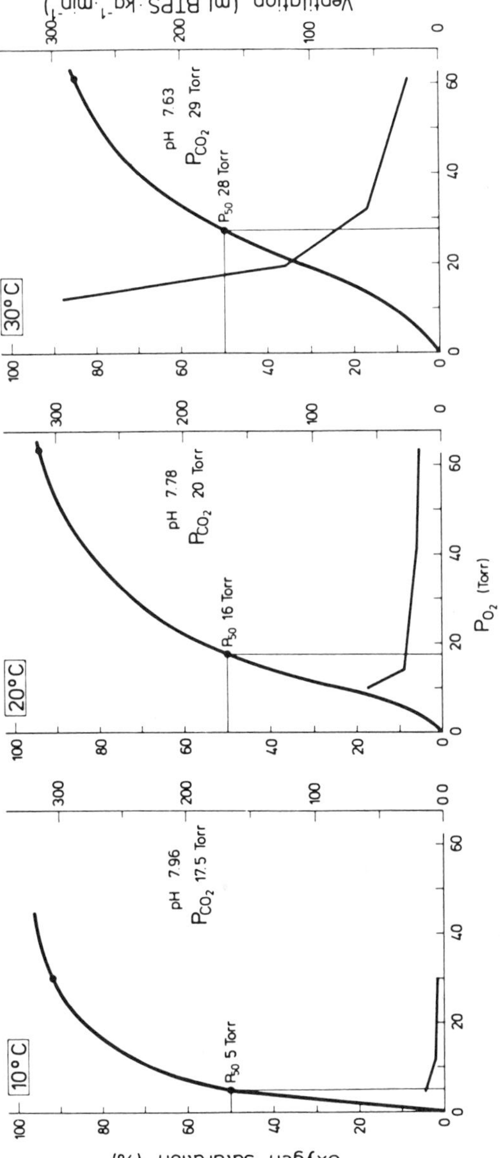

Figure 4 Ventilation and blood O_2 saturation of the turtle, *Chrysemys picta*, plotted as functions of blood PO_2 at various temperatures. Values for P_{50} and in vivo arterial PO_2 points are indicated on the dissociation curves. Note that ventilation increases above the normoxic level as PO_2 nears the P_{50} of blood (Glass et al., 1983).

A final experimental observation that reveals vigorous respiratory sensitivity across a range of temperatures is the hyperventilation that occurs in freshwater turtles following prolonged anoxic submergence (Herbert and Jackson, 1985). At 3, 10, 15, and 20°C, $PaCO_2$ fell substantially below control levels during the early stages of the recovery process, permitting a rapid return of blood pH to its normal value at each temperature, although the animals still experienced a severe metabolic acidosis (Fig. 3).

Oxygen

Hypoxic sensitivity, in contrast to CO_2 sensitivity, is distinctly temperature-dependent. Measurements of the ventilatory response to hypoxic gas mixtures at various temperatures have been made on two species of turtles, *P. scripta* by Jackson (1973) and *Chrysemys picta* by Glass et al. (1983), and in a preliminary report on a lizard, the Mexican black iguana (Dupré et al., 1984). In each study the threshold PO_2 for eliciting increased ventilation decreased when temperature fell. The principal explanation advanced by Jackson (1973) relates to the inverse relationship between air convection requirement and temperature, a pattern that is required for normal temperature-dependent, acid-base balance. Low temperature ventilation, although appropriate for PCO_2 control, is excessive for O_2 uptake, and therefore a reduction in ambient O_2 will not elicit a ventilatory response as readily as at higher temperature. Glass et al. (1985), on the other hand, emphasize the importance of blood affinity for O_2, which increases as temperature falls. Saturation can occur at lower PO_2 as temperature falls; thus, lower O_2 levels can be tolerated before ventilation must increase (Fig. 4). At each temperature, increased ventilation occurred when arterial O_2 saturation fell to about 50%. These results, and a nearly temperature-independent O_2 saturation in this and in other studies, have led to the suggestion by Wood (1984) that O_2 content is a regulated variable in air-breathing ectotherms. Similarly, White and Somero (1982) point out that the critical PO_2, the level below which excess lactate appears in the blood, is a direct function of temperature in the turtle, *P. scripta*.

V. Intermittent Breathing

A. Nonventilatory Period and Apneic Threshold

In aquatic or semiaquatic air-breathing ectotherms, lung ventilation is typically periodic, occurring as bouts of breathing separated by apneic intervals of variable duration (Shelton and Boutilier, 1982). An important variable of an intermittent-breathing pattern is the apneic interval or nonventilatory period (NVP). During the NVP, lung and blood gases change in the direction of lower PO_2 and higher PCO_2, the rate of change determined by the rate of metabolism and by the size of the lung and tissue gas stores and capacities. The PO_2 falls faster than the rise in PCO_2 because of greater tissue capacity for CO_2 and, additionally in some cases, because of extrapulmonary loss of CO_2. The assumption is that at some point the fall in PO_2 and the developing hypercapnia, coupled possibly to feedback from any accompanying changes in lung volume, combine to activate the next bout of breathing. This point is referred to as the apneic threshold and could occur at a variety of combinations of chemoreceptor and mechanoreceptor input. The formula by which these various inputs sum to drive breathing is not understood nor is it certain that these factors all contribute. There are also undoubtedly substantial species differences (Shelton and Boutilier, 1982). Experimental results have revealed lack of consistency in apneic and end points (e.g., Burggren and Shelton, 1979; Lenfant et al., 1970; Shelton and Boutilier, 1982; Toews et al., 1971). The signals for turning off the bout of breathing and commencing the next NVP are also poorly understood, although an important role of PCO_2 has been suggested (Shelton, 1986).

B. Are Intermittent Breathers Facultative Air Breathers?

The intermittency and apneic threshold concept suggest a somewhat different basis for respiratory pattern generation than in continuously breathing animals, such as most fishes, birds, and mammals (Shelton et al., 1986). In the latter groups, an intrinsic breathing rhythm is thought to reside in the medullary respiratory center that is modulated by peripheral and higher center input. In the periodic breathers, ventilation may be driven entirely by receptor input, or alternatively, a central rhythm generator is intermittently turned on and off by receptor input. These animals can be considered facultative breathers in which apnea persists as long as no activating input from chemoreceptors or mechanoreceptors arouses the respiratory center. For many air-breathing fishes, this is the normal circumstance; lung ventilation is initiated only if the aquatic environment becomes hypoxic, otherwise they rely on branchial respiration. In other air-breathing fish (Johansen, 1970) and in bimodal amphibians (Lenfant and Johansen, 1967) and reptiles (Wood and Lenfant, 1976), aerial gas exchange is usually a regular and necessary (albeit intermittent) occurrence and these animals are thus denoted obligate air breathers.

Many of these "obligate" air breathers, however, stop ventilating their lungs when body temperature is very low. The otherwise inadequate branchial or cutaneous exchange surfaces can satisfy the greatly depressed metabolic requirements in certain air-breathing fish (Rahn et al., 1971), amphibians (Whitford and Hutchison, 1965), and reptiles (Ultsch et al., 1984). Presumably, the apneic threshold may never be reached under very cold, hypometabolic conditions. But if the activity level rises, or if temperature goes up promoting higher metabolic rate, then ventilation may again be initiated. Multiple factors participate in eliciting the drive to breathe: metabolic rate is obvious because of its effect on the rate of change of controlled variables; the exchange capacity of nonpulmonary surfaces; and the changing requirements for control, because of temperature-dependent, acid-base regulation and temperature-dependent hemoglobin affinity for O_2. A careful investigation is needed to define how these various factors interrelate near the transition temperature below which breathing may not occur.

VI. Cutaneous Gas Exchange

A. Is It a Passive Process?

The complete reliance on nonpulmonary or, in gill-less species, cutaneous gas exchange at low temperature introduces the question of how control of gas exchange occurs in this state. The problem is even broader because a large group of amphibians, the plethodontid salamanders, rely exclusively on their skin and buccopharygeal surfaces for exchange at all temperatures, and most amphibians and many reptiles and fish utilize their skin for a substantial fraction of total gas exchange. For many years, the skin has been regarded as a passive, poorly controlled avenue of exchange, based on experimental data from both exclusively skin-breathing (Boutilier et al., 1980; Gatz et al., 1975; Moalli et al., 1981) and bimodal (Gottlieb and Jackson, 1976; Jackson and Braun, 1979; Mackenzie and Jackson, 1978) amphibians, and on a theoretical analysis indicating that exchange is diffusion-limited and, therefore, not subject to effective control (Gatz et al., 1975).

B. Evidence for the Existence of Control Mechanisms

The passive nature of cutaneous exchange has recently been challenged by Feder and Burggren (1985) who argue that potentially effective control can occur both by altering ambient convection (Burggren and Feder, 1986) and by cutaneous capillary recruitment (Burggren and Moalli, 1984). In addition, recent studies by Malvin and Hlastala (1986a,b), using inert gas flux into a ventilated capsule placed on the ventral surface of the frog (*Rana pipiens*), report significant local adaptive changes in gas exchange, presumably resulting from blood flow responses. An argument against control has been that increased gas flux, such as occurs when metabolic rate rises, is attributable primarily to increased partial pressure gradient for O_2 or CO_2 across the skin surface (Boutilier et al., 1980; Mackenzie and Jackson, 1978). Recently, however, Full (1986) has recorded O_2 uptake by lungless plethodontid salamanders up to 10 times the resting level, a result difficult to imagine without some adaptive increase in cutaneous exchange capacity.

Despite the impressive case that is being made in support of control of cutaneous exchange, I know of no convincing examples of effective homeostatic control arising solely from skin gas exchange. It is now evident, however, that adaptive augmentation of gas flux is possible, so the likelihood for homeostatically relevant control is high. The experimental search for control should focus on species, such as the plethodonts, that are exclusive skin breathers, or on larger (and more easily studied) bimodal species at the low temperatures at which the lungs are not ventilated. For example, Pinder (1985) recently observed that bullfrogs (*R. catesbeiana*) submerged at 5°C could maintain normoxic $\dot{V}_{O_2}$ from ambient P_{O_2} down to about 80 torr, strongly suggesting an adaptive control mechanism. Occasionally, an observation that appears to be active control is actually a passive process. For example, the large predominantly skin-breathing salamander, *Cryptobranchus alleganiensis*, exhibits alphastat-type blood pH control between 10 and 30°C, even when denied access to air, but this was explained by the rise in metabolic rate with temperature producing an elevated blood P_{CO_2} that was appropriate for alphastat pH control (Moalli et al., 1981).

VII. Variable Temperature in Mammals

Although mammalian body temperatures are normally confined within narrow limits, large changes do occur in those species that hibernate or become torpid, and during experimental or clinical hypothermia. These animals, or those that are managing them, confront the same thermal challenges to physiological homeostasis as do the ectotherms. The best solution, however, may not be the same in the different circumstance because the priorities may differ. Many ectotherms carry out normal life functions over a wide range of body temperatures, and regulatory stability appropriate for these functions must be preserved. Hibernators, on the other hand, have as a prime consideration the conservation of energy resources with the important requirement that the profound reduction of temperature and function be reversible. The management of hypothermic animals or patients must be based on the control of respiratory gases and other homeostatic variables that is best suited to the situation. The question is what criteria should be used?

A. Hibernation

It is well documented in a variety of hibernating mammals that a rather profound respiratory acidosis develops during entry and persists until arousal (Malan, 1982). The blood P_{CO_2} measured at the hibernating temperature may actually be lower than the euthermic level, but when the value is temperature corrected based on solubility effect, the considerable hypercapnia is revealed. The blood pH is also close to the euthermic pH when each is measured at the corresponding body temperature, but on the basis of alphastat control, the pH during hibernation is quite acidotic, some 0.45 below the pH appropriate for alphastat control. Likewise, it is considerably less than the blood pH observed in ectotherms at the same temperature. For example, the blood pH of the ground squirrel, *Citellus tridecemlineatus*, at 5°C was 7.39 and its blood P_{CO_2} was 35 torr (Kent and Peirce, 1967); in contrast, values of the bullfrog *R. catesbeiana*, at the same temperature were 8.08 and 5.5 torr, respectively (Howell et al., 1970). Although acid-base control of hibernators differs from ectotherms, their breathing pattern like many ectotherms is intermittent, and prolonged apneic periods of an hour or more may occur (Malan, 1982). The apparent respiratory acidosis of hibernating mammals is not considered a failure of the control system but, instead, like the fall in body temperature (Heller, 1979), represents a shift of the regulatory state. Hibernating animals respond to changes in inspired gas (high CO_2 or low O_2) by increased respiratory activity, and they show similar variance in the blood values of the regulated variables (Malan, 1982).

An important current question in this field concerns the adaptive significance of respiratory acidosis during hibernation. Malan (1986) argues that the acidosis may act to depress metabolism, perhaps through inhibition of key regulatory enzymes such as PFK. The acidosis occurs during entry into hibernation, and is rapidly reversed by increased ventilation during arousal. If this is true, the low metabolism during hibernation is due to two factors: (1) the direct effect temperature on cellular metabolism (Q_{10} effect) and (2) the further depressant effect of acidosis.

B. Hypothermia

The question of respiratory and acid-base control during hypothermia is of enormous importance because of the large number of patients undergoing surgical procedures that employ hypothermia. Should the management of these patients be based on the ectotherm model in which blood pH rises as temperature falls, or on the hibernators model in which blood pH remains nearly unchanged; The hibernation model is attractive because metabolic depression is surely a goal in the surgical setting. The acid-base response of a hibernator is complex, however, and goes beyond the regulation of blood pH. Cell pH regulation in the European hamster at 6°C ranged from alphastat-type control in the heart and liver, to blood-type regulation in skeletal muscle and brain (Malan et al., 1985). Ectotherm-type control is attractive because of the functional significance of protein charge state regulation. Again, however, the question of intracellular acid-base state is a difficult one. A functional study comparing the two strategies indicated improved cardiac performance in dogs using the ectotherm model (McConnell et al., 1975). On the question of metabolic depression, a recent study by Willford et al. (1986) on hypothermic (29°C) domestic pigs found that metabolic rate was significantly lower in the alphastat group (compared with the pH-stat group), in contrast to the hypothesis regarding the hibernators. A sympathetic discharge in response to the relative acidosis of the pH-stat animals was suggested as the basis for the difference. Clearly, multiple factors are at play in adjusting to a new thermal state. Lessons from comparative physiology, from ectotherms and hibernating mammals, can contribute insights into a rational approach to this important problem (White, 1981).

References

Boutilier, R. G., McDonald, D. G., and Toews, D. P. (1980). The effects of enforced activity on ventilation, circulation and blood acid-base balance in the aquatic gill-less urodele *Cryptobranchus alleganiensis*; a comparison with the semi-terrestrial anuran, *Bufo marinus. J. Exp. Biol. 84*:289-302.

Burggren, W. W., and Feder, M. E. (1986). Effect of experimental ventilation of the skin on cutaneous gas exchange in the bullfrog. *J. Exp. Biol. 121*:445-450.

Burggren, W., and Moalli, R. (1984). "Active" regulation of cutaneous gas exchange by capillary recruitment in amphibians: Experimental evidence and a revised model for skin respiration. *Respir. Physiol. 55*:379-392.

Burggren, W. W., and Shelton, G. (1979). Gas exchange and transport during intermittent breathing in chelonian reptiles. *J. Exp. Biol. 82*:75-92.

Cameron, J. N. (1984). Acid-base status of fish at different temperatures. *Am. J. Physiol. 246*:R452-R459.

Davies, D. G., Thomas, J. L., and Smith, E. N. (1982). Effect of body temperature on ventilatory control in the alligator. *J. Appl. Physiol. Respirat. Environ. Exercise Physiol. 52*:114-118.

Dejours, P. (1975). *Principles of Comparative Respiratory Physiology*. Amsterdam, North-Holland, p. 22.

Dupré, R. K., Hicks, J. W., and Wood, S. C. (1984). Ventilatory responses of the Mexican black iguana to hypercapnia and hypoxia at different temperatures. *Physiologist 27*:285.

Feder, M. E., and Burggren, W. W. (1985). Cutaneous gas exchange in vertebrates: Design, patterns, control and implications. *Biol. Rev. 60*:1-45.

Full, R. J. (1986). Locomotion without lungs: Energetics and performance of a lungless salamander. *Am. J. Physiol. 251*:R775-R780.

Funk, G. D., and Milsom, W. K. (1986). Effects of changes in temperature and inspired CO_2 on the breathing pattern of turtles (*Chrysemys picta*). *Proc. Int. Union Physiol. Sci. 16*:534.

Gatz, R. N., Crawford, E. C., Jr., and Piiper, J. (1975). Kinetics of inert gas equilibration in an exclusively skin-breathing salamander, *Desmognathus fuscus. Respir. Physiol. 24*:15-29.

Glass, M. L., Boutilier, R. G., and Heisler, N. (1983). Ventilatory control of arterial PO_2 in the turtle *Chrysemys picta bellii*: Effects of temperature and hypoxia. *J. Comp. Physiol. 151*:145-153.

Gottlieb, G., and Jackson, D. C. (1976). The importance of pulmonary ventilation in respiratory control in the bullfrog. *Am. J. Physiol. 230*:608-613.

Heisler, N. (1984). Role of ion transfer processes in acid-base regulation with temperature changes in fish. *Am. J. Physiol. 246*:R441-R451.

Heisler, N. (1986). Comparative aspects of acid-base regulation. In *Acid-Base Regulation in Animals*. Edited by N. Heisler. Amsterdam, Elsevier, pp. 397-450.

Heller, H. C. (1979). Hibernation: Neural aspects. *Ann. Rev. Physiol. 41*:305-321.

Herbert, C. V., and Jackson, D. C. (1985). Temperature effects on the responses to prolonged submergence in the turtle *Chrysemys picta bellii*. I. Blood acid-base and ionic changes during and following anoxic submergence. *Physiol. Zool. 58*:655-669.

Hitzig, B. M. (1982). Temperature-induced changes in turtle CSF pH and central control of ventilation. *Respir. Physiol. 49*:205-222.

Howell, B. J., Baumgardner, F. W., Bondi, K., and Rahn, H. (1970). Acid-base balance in cold-blooded vertebrates as a function of body temperature. *Am. J. Physiol. 218*:600-606.

Jackson, D. C. (1973). Ventilatory response to hypoxia in turtles at various temperatures. *Respir. Physiol. 18*:178-187.

Jackson, D. C. (1978). Respiratory and CO_2 conductance: Temperature effects in a turtle and a frog. *Respir. Physiol. 33*:103-114.

Jackson, D. C., and Braun, B. A. (1979). Respiratory control in bullfrogs: Cutaneous versus pulmonary response to selective CO_2 exposure. *J. Comp. Physiol. 129*:339-342.

Jackson, D. C., Palmer, S. E., and Meadow, W. L. (1974). The effects of temperature and carbon dioxide breathing on ventilation and acid-base status of turtles. *Respir. Physiol. 20*:131-146.

Johansen, K. (1970). Air breathing in fishes. In *Fish Physiology* IV. Edited by W. S. Hoar and D. J. Randall. London, Academic Press, pp. 361-411.

Kent, L. M., and Peirce, E. C. II (1967). Acid-base characteristics of hibernating animals. *J. Appl. Physiol. 23*:336-340.

Lenfant, C., and Johansen, K. (1967). Respiratory adaptations in selected amphibians. *Respir. Physiol. 2*:247-260.

Lenfant, C. K., Johansen, K., Peterson, J. A., and Schmidt-Nielsen, K. (1970). Respiration in the fresh water turtle *Chelys fimbriata*. *Respir. Physiol. 8*:261-275.

Mackenzie, J. A., and Jackson, D. C. (1978). The effect of temperature on cutaneous CO_2 loss and conductance in the bullfrog. *Respir. Physiol. 32*:313-323.

Malan, A. (1982). Respiration and acid-base state in hibernation. In *Hibernation and Torpor in Mammals and Birds*. Edited by C. P. Lyman, J. S. Willis, A. Malan, and L. C. H. Wang. New York, Academic Press, pp. 237-282.

Malan, A. (1986). pH as a control factor in hibernation. In *Living in the Cold: Physiological and Biochemical Adaptations*. Edited by H. C. Heller, X. J. Musacchia, and L. C. H. Wang. New York, Elsevier, pp. 61-70.

Malan, A., Rodeau, J. L., and Daull, F. (1985). Intracellular pH in hibernation and respiratory acidosis in the European hamster. *J. Comp. Physiol. B 156*:251-258.

Malan, A., Wilson, T. L., and Reeves, R. B. (1976). Intracellular pH in cold-blooded vertebrates as a function of body temperature. *Respir. Physiol. 28*:29-47.

Malvin, G. M., and Hlastala, M. P. (1986a). Regulation of cutaneous gas exchange by environmental O_2 and CO_2 in the frog. *Respir. Physiol. 65*: 99-111.

Malvin, G. M., and Hlastala, M. P. (1986b). Effects of lung volume and O_2 and CO_2 content on cutaneous gas exchange in frogs. *Am. J. Physiol. 251*: R941-R946.

McConnell, D. H., White, F. N., Nelson, R. L., Goldstein, S. M., Maloney, J. V., DeLand, E. C., and Buckbe, G. D. (1975). Importance of "alkalosis" in maintenance of ideal blood pH during hypothermia. *Surg. Forum 26*:263-265.

Moalli, R., Meyers, R. S., Ultsch, G. R., and Jackson, D. C. (1981). Acid-base balance and temperature in a predominantly skin-breathing salamander, *Cryptobranchus alleganiensis. Respir. Physiol. 43*:1-11.

Nattie, E. E. (1986a). Intracisternal diethylpyrocarbonate inhibits central chemosensitivity in conscious rabbits. *Respir. Physiol. 64*:161-176.

Nattie, E. E. (1986b). Imidazole binding by diethylpyrocarbonate inhibits rostral ventrolateral medulla chemosensitivity. *Fed. Proc. 45*:872.

Pappenheimer, J. R., Fenci, V., Heisey, S. R., and Held, D. (1965). Role of cerebral fluids in control of respiration as studied in unanesthetized goats. *Am. J. Physiol. 208*:436-450.

Park, S. P., and Hong, S. K. (1976). Properties of toad skin Na-K-ATPase with special reference to effect of temperature. *Am. J. Physiol. 231*:1356-1363.

Pinder, A. W. (1985). Respiratory physiology of the frogs *Rana catesbeiana* and *Rana pipiens*: Influences of hypoxia and temperature. Ph.D. Dissertation, Univ. of Massachusetts, Amherst.

Rahn, H. (1967). Gas transport from the external environment to the cell. In *Development of the Lung*. Edited by A. V. S. de Rerck and R. Porter. *London, Churchill, pp. 3-23.*

Rahn, H., Rahn, K. B., Howell, B. J., Gans, C., and Tenney, S. M. (1971). Air breathing of the garfish (*Lepisosteus osseus*). *Respir. Physiol. 11*:285-307.

Reeves, R. B. (1972). An imidazole alphastat hypothesis for vertebrate acid-base regulation: Tissue carbon dioxide content and body temperature in bullfrogs. *Respir. Physiol. 14*:219-236.

Reeves, R. B. (1977). The interaction of body temperature and acid-base balance in ectothermic vertebrates. *Ann. Rev. Physiol. 39*:559-586.

Shelton, G. (1986). The evolution of breathing control systems and their influence on steady and unsteady states in lower vertebrates. *Proc. Int. Union Physiol. Sci. 16*:532.

Shelton, G., and Boutilier, R. G. (1982). Apnoea in amphibians and reptiles. *J. Exp. Biol. 100*:245-273.

Shelton, G., Jones, D. R., and Milsom, W. K. (1986). Control of breathing in ectothermic vertebrates. In *Handbook of Physiology*. Section 3. The Respiratory System. Control of Breathing. Vol. II. Edited by N. S. Cherniack and J. G. Widdicombe. Washington, American Physiological Society, pp. 857-909.

Somero, G. N. (1986). Protons, osmolytes, and fitness of internal milieu for protein function. *Am. J. Physiol. 251*:R197-R213.

Stewart, P. A. (1981). *How to Understand Acid-Base*. New York, Elsevier.

Toews, D. P., Shelton, G., and Randall, D. J. (1971). Gas tensions in the lungs and major blood vessels of the urodele amphibian *Amphiuma tridactylum*. *J. Exp. Biol. 55*:47-61.

Ultsch, G. R., Herbert, C. V., and Jackson, D. C. (1984). The comparative physiology of diving in North American freshwater turtles. I. Submergence tolerance, gas exchange, and acid-base balance. *Physiol. Zool. 57*:620-631.

White, F. N. (1981). A comparative physiological approach to hypothermia. *J. Thorac. Cardiovasc. Surg. 82*:821-831.

White, F. N., and Somero, G. (1982). Acid-base regulation and phospholipid adaptations to temperature: Time courses and physiological significance of modifying the milieu for proton function. *Physiol. Rev. 62*:40-90.

Whitford, W. G., and Hutchison, V. H. (1965). Gas exchange in salamanders. *Physiol. Zool. 38*:228-242.

Willford, D. C., Hill, E. P., and White, F. C. (1986). Oxygen consumption rates, cardiac output, and ventricular dP/dt during hypothermia with different pH strategies. *Physiologist 29*:178.

Wilson, T. L. (1977). Interrelations between pH and temperature for the catalytic rate of the M4 isozyme of lactate dehydrogenase from goldfish (*Carassium auratus* L.). *Arch. Biochem. Biophys. 179*:378-390.

Wood, S. C. (1984). Cardiovascular shunts and oxygen transport in lower vertebrates. *Am. J. Physiol. 247*:R3-R14.

Wood, S. C., and Lenfant, C. J. M. (1976). Respiration: Mechanics, control and gas exchange. In *Biology of the Reptilia*. Edited by C. Gans and W. R. Dawson. Vol. 5. Physiology A. New York, Academic Press, pp. 225-274.

Wood, S. C., Johansen, K., Glass, M. L., and Hoyt, R. W. (1981). Acid-base regulation during heating and cooling the lizard, *Varanus exanthematicus*. *J. Appl. Physiol.* *50*:779-783.

Part Six

Diving Physiology

21

Diving Physiology
Lungfish

ALFRED P. FISHMAN, R. J. GALANTE, and A. I. PACK

University of Pennsylvania
and Hospital of the University of Pennsylvania
Philadelphia, Pennsylvania

I. Introduction

The dipnoan lungfish possess both gills and lungs that are used in gas exchange. These two complementary systems for gas exchange require not only individual control mechanisms but also synchronizing mechanisms to match ventilation, blood flow, and metabolism while the lungfish is submerged, gulping a breath of air, or air breathing uninterruptedly during estivation. Therefore, study of this species affords an unusual opportunity for insight into the evolution of lungs or lunglike organs and into the organization of fundamental neural control mechanisms related to the respiration and circulation.

The present chapter describes current understanding of the ventilatory and circulatory control mechanisms in this species.

The original studies reported here have been generously supported by the National Heart, Lung, and Blood Institute (HL08805).

II. Genus

There are three living genera of dipnoan lungfish. They are found in Australia (*Neoceratodus fosteri*), South America (*Lepidosiren*), and in various areas of Africa (*Protopterus*). There are different species of *Protopterus–P. aethiopicus, P. annectens, P. amphibius*, and *P. dolloi*–although most studies have been performed on *P. aethiopicus*. Although all of these fish have many common features, there are important differences. In particular, *Neoceratodus* is the only facultative air-breathing form that usually inhabitats well-aerated waters (Grigg, 1965b). In contrast, in both *Lepidosiren* (Johansen and Lenfant, 1967) and *Protopterus* (Johansen and Lenfant, 1968; McMahon, 1970), the gills are so rudimentary that the fish cannot survive without air breathing, i.e., they are obligate air breathers. Because most of the investigative studies have been done in either *Protopterus* or *Lepidosiren*, the material in the rest of this chapter is relevant to these genera.

III. Anatomy of the Gas Exchange Systems

A. Lungs

The structure of the lungs has been described for *P. aethipicus* (Parker, 1892) and *Neoceratodus* (Grigg, 1965a). In both fish the lungs extend as long, hollow sacs along the dorsal portion of the abdominal cavity (Fig. 1). The dorsal surface of each lung is attached to the body wall beneath the ribs such that when the lung expands it does so primarily in the ventral direction. Toward the mouth

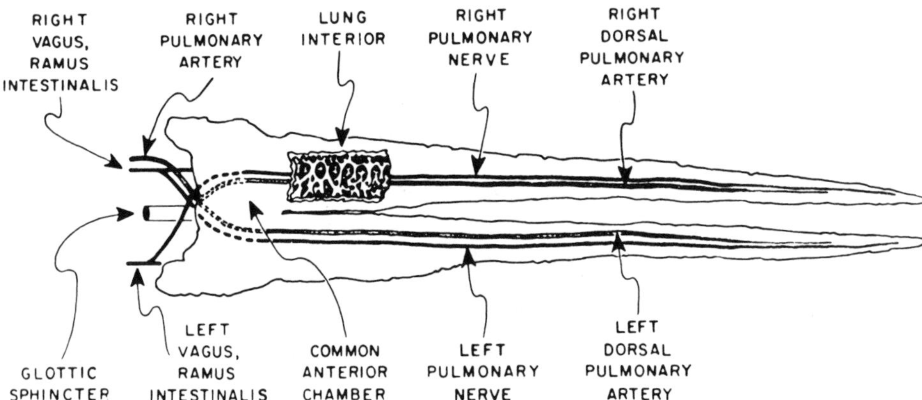

Figure 1 Schematic diagram of structure of lungs in *P. aethiopicus*. For further details see text. (Redrawn from DeLaney et al., 1983.)

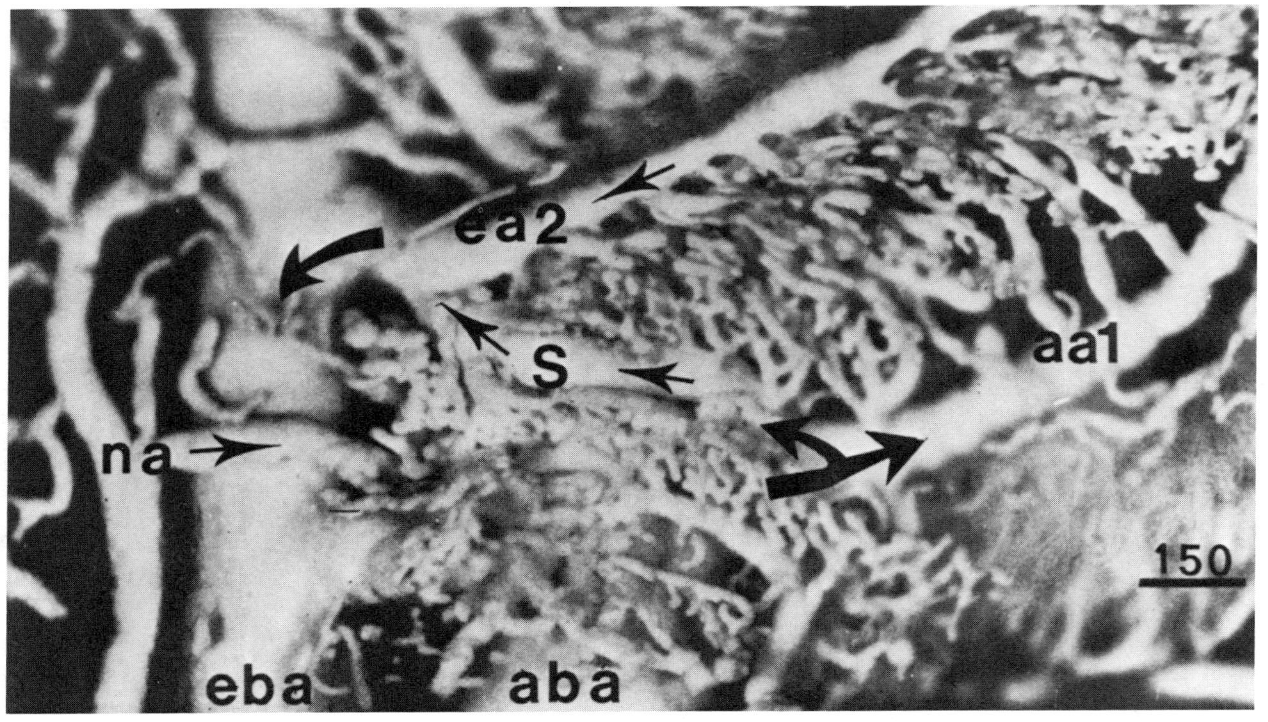

Figure 2 Photograph of microfil cast showing vascular supply of an arch IV primary lamella in *P. aethiopicus*. The arrows indicate direction of flow. The abbreviations are explained in text. (From Laurent et al., 1978.)

the two lungs merge to form a common anterior chamber. This is connected to a muscular glottic sphincter by a short pneumatic duct (see Fig. 1). Within the lung there are trabeculae that extend into the central cavity. These trabeculae increase the surface area for gas exchange and are, in consequence, more pronounced in the cephalad part of the lung. Within these trabeculae and surrounding the lung, there is smooth muscle. The muscular nature of the organ probably reflects the fact that because the lung is filled with gas while the fish is submerged it acts not only as an organ for gas exchange but also for control of buoyancy. Thus, active control of lung volume is likely to be essential. Not unexpectedly, therefore, the lung is richly innervated. Each sac is supplied by a separate branch from the ramus intestinalis of the vagus nerve that runs on the dorsal surface of the lung to its distal end (see Fig. 1).

B. Gills

The structure of the gills in lungfish has been most extensively described for *P. aethiopicus* (Laurent et al., 1978). This lungfish, like others, has six branchial arches (Parker, 1892; Chardon, 1961). Arch I has, however, only a single row of gill primary lamellae, whereas arches II and III are almost totally devoid of lamellae. Thus, these arches are unimportant in gas exchange. Arches IV and V do, however, play a role in gas exchange because they support two rows of primary lamellae. Arch VI, like arch I, has again only a single row of lamellae. This relative lack of lamellae on many of the gill arches is found in both *Protopterus* and *Lepidosiren*. However, in *Neoceratodus*, which can survive solely with gill breathing, lamellae are found on all gill arches (Sewertzoff, 1924).

On the arches each lamella is provided with a blood supply by a series of parallel afferent arteries (aal) that arise from an afferent branchial artery (aba) (Fig. 2). The afferent arteries progressively bifurcate to supply the lamellae and then reconnect to form the corresponding efferent artery (ea2). At the base of each primary lamella there is a large "shunt" vessel(s) that connects directly the afferent to efferent branchial artery (see Fig. 2). This gill shunt is under active vasomotor control and plays an important role in circulatory control. This is discussed in Section VIII on Key Elements in Circulatory Control. In addition there is a nutrient artery (na) that is a collateral branch of the efferent branchial artery (see Fig. 2).

IV. Mechanisms of Ventilation

A. Lung

The mechanism of pulmonary ventilation in the lungfish has been studied by a variety of techniques–cineradiography (Jesse et al., 1967; Bishop and Foxon, 1968; McMahon, 1969); simultaneous recording of pressures in lung, opercular

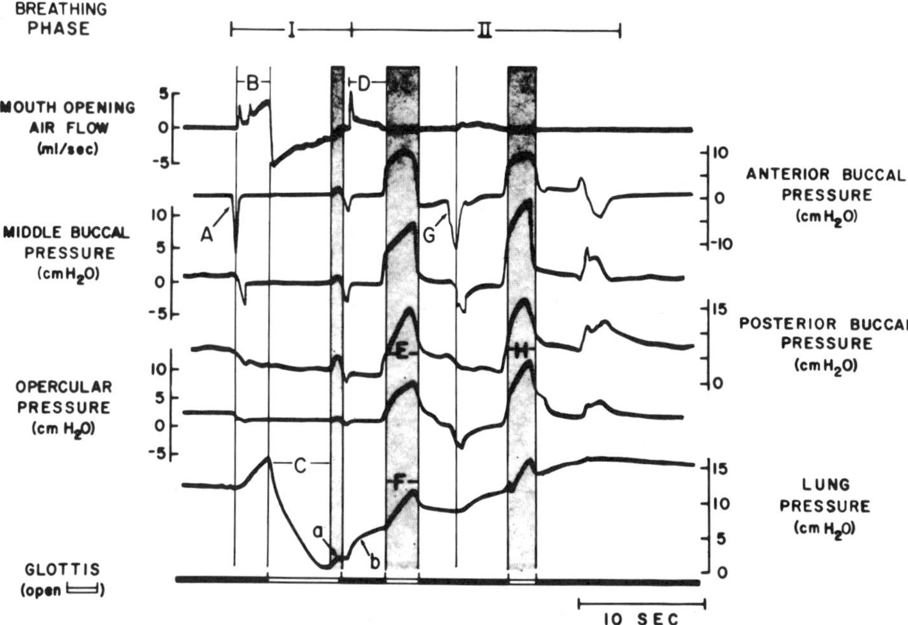

Figure 3 Simultaneous recording of pressure at various points in buccal cavity, in opercular cavity, and lung together with a measure of airflow through the mouth during a lung breath in an estivating lungfish. The opening and closing of the glottis are illustrated diagrammatically at the foot of the figure. During the first phase of the breathing act (see phase I), air is aspirated into the mouth where it mixes with gas expelled from the lung. During the second phase (II) the lung is inflated by the action of the buccal force pump (shaded areas). Further details are described in text. (From DeLaney and Fishman, 1977.)

and buccal cavities (McMahon, 1969; DeLaney and Fishman, 1977); and simultaneous recording of electromyographic activity from a number of muscles (McMahon, 1969). These various studies lead to the same conclusion, i.e., that to ventilate its lungs, the lungfish employs a buccal force pump mechanism that is similar in many respects to that found in amphibians (Jongh and Gans, 1969; West and Jones, 1975; MacIntyre and Toews, 1976).

The mechanism is complex, but the essential features are shown in Figure 3. This figure is from a lungfish in estivation, i.e., where it is surviving completely out of water. There are differences in the ventilatory pattern compared with that in aquatic life, but the major features are identical. At the onset of a lung breath (left side of figure), the muscles in the floor of the mouth relax, creating a negative pressure in the anterior buccal cavity (A in Fig. 3). In consequence air enters the mouth (B in Fig. 3). During this phase of the cycle the glottis is closed and a positive intrapulmonary pressure is maintained. At this time the axial muscles may contract and intrapulmonary pressure may become increasingly positive. Thereafter, when the glottis opens (C in Fig. 3) there is airflow from the lung into the buccal cavity. Thus, gas just sucked into the mouth mixes with gas expelled from the lung into the buccal cavity. Thereafter, there is a rhythmic series of contractions of the buccal musculature that are coordinated with opening and closing of the glottis to refill the lung (E and H in Fig. 3). The gas entering the lung is, therefore, at least partially rebreathed. Finally, excess gas in the buccal cavities is expelled through the opercula with the glottis closed.

B. Gill

Just as the mechanism for pulmonary ventilation is similar to that in amphibia, the mechanism for gill ventilation (McMahon, 1969) is similar to that described for fish (Hughes and Ballintijn, 1965; Ballintijn and Hughes, 1965). The muscles closing the jaw act in concert with the muscles of the buccal flow and the constrictor hyoideus muscle, action of which closes the opercular flap, to create a rhythmic pumping of water over the gills. This pumping action involves active aspiration of water through the mouth into the buccal cavity and active exhalation of water over the gills and out of the operculum (McMahon, 1969).

V. Relative Role of Gills and Lung in Gas Exchange

In lungfish, gills play a more important role in CO_2 exchange than in O_2 exchange. This reflects their rudimentary structure and the higher solubility of CO_2 in water. The relative role of the two gas exchange systems has been studied quantitatively by analysis of expired gas from the lung and exhaled water from the opercula (McMahon, 1970). In these studies, the lung contributed an average of 91.7% of the O_2 exchange (range 86.5-94.0%) but an average of only 32.5% of CO_2 is excreted by the lung. The remainder is excreted through the gills, with the skin also playing possibly some role (Cunningham, 1934).

VI. Ventilatory Control Mechanisms

A. Two Pattern Generators

As outlined earlier, the muscular basis for pulmonary ventilation is similar to the buccal force mechanism that is found in amphibia. Likewise, the muscular basis for gill ventilation is similar to the mechanism for ventilation in fish. Thus,

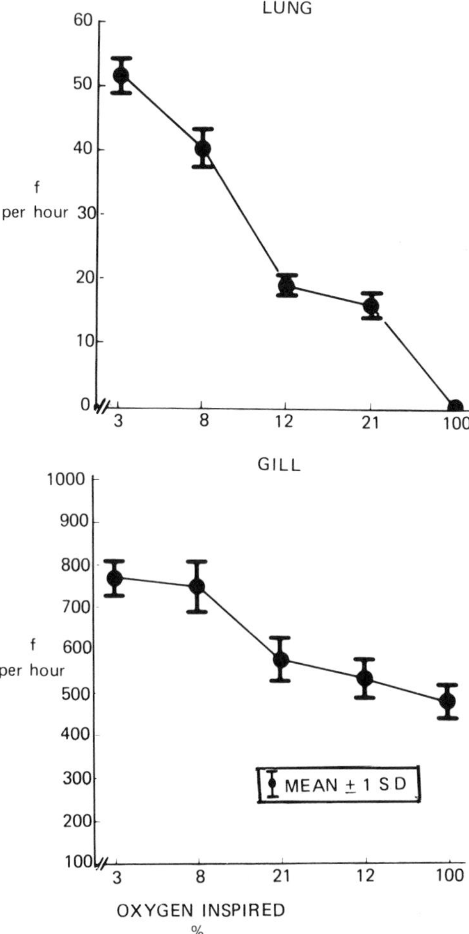

Figure 4 Effect of hypoxia in both water and air on frequency of lung (left side of figure) and gill (right side of figure) respiration in *Protopterus*. Hypoxia increases the frequency of both aerial and aquatic respiration, but the effect on lung ventilation is more marked. Hyperoxia depresses both modes of respiration and causes complete cessation of aerial respiration. (From Jesse et al., 1967.)

the lungfish brain must contain neural networks that generate both patterns of activity. These "patterns" may engage the same muscles, but in different ways, as part of highly programmed behaviors. In viewing ventilatory control, therefore, it is convenient to consider these two separate networks for gill and pulmonary ventilation. Each network may receive different afferent inputs. Alternatively, if each network receives the same afferent stimulus, its relative effect on the two networks may be different. Finally, because each of the pattern generators provide input to at least certain common muscles, there must be mechanisms to coordinate their action. In what follows we review the effect of different afferent inputs on each of the networks and then synthesize the overall properties of the networks and their interaction. The networks are believed to be situated in the medulla because both pulmonary and gill ventilation continue essentially unaltered when the brain is transected through the diencephalon and at the caudal end of the medulla (unpublished observations).

B. Effect of Hypoxia

The most fundamental of respiratory stimuli is hypoxia. Hypoxia in the lungfish is known to stimulate both lung and gill ventilation (Jesse et al., 1967). In initial experiments, both the Po_2 of water and that of the gas inspired were changed simultaneously (Jesse et al., 1967). Hypoxia in this setting increased the frequency of both pulmonary and gill ventilation (Fig. 4). The relative effect of hypoxia on the frequency of lung breaths is, however, much more marked. In later experiments the separate effects of alteration of Po_2 in the water and that in the gas inspired were examined (Johansen and Lenfant, 1968). In *Protopterus*, variations of Po_2 in the water are without effect on the frequency of either gill or pulmonary ventilation. In contrast, alterations of the Po_2 of the gas being inspired into the lungs produces marked changes in the frequency of lung breaths. This lack of effect of hypoxic water indicates that the dipnoan lungfish do not possess the chemoreceptors monitoring environmental Po_2 that have been thought to exist in some fish (Eclancher, 1975; Eclancher and Dejours, 1975; Smatresk et al., 1986). Dipnoan lungfish are different in this regard from holostean air-breathing fish in whom aquatic hypoxia increases the frequency of air breaths (Johansen et al., 1970; Randall et al., 1981; Smatresk et al., 1986). In these fish, aquatic hypoxia may depress gill ventilation (Johansen et al., 1970; Smatresk et al., 1986). Aquatic hypoxia also increases the frequency of air breathing in larval anurans (tadpoles) (West and Burggren, 1982; Feder, 1983). The lack of effect of aquatic hypoxia in dipnoi presumably reflects the relative lack of importance of gills for O_2 exchange described previously. Because gills contribute so little to O_2 exchange, hypoxia in the water will have negligible effects on systemic Po_2. Support for this argument comes from the observations that hypoxia in water does stimulate breathing in *Neoceratodus* in which gills are more efficient (Johansen et al., 1967).

In the lungfish, not only is breathing stimulated by hypoxia, but hyperoxia inhibits respiration. Indeed, hyperoxia causes a complete cessation of pulmonary ventilation (Jesse et al., 1967). Thus, the pattern generator for pulmonary ventilation is inoperative unless it receives an afferent stimulus related to hypoxia. This necessary role of hypoxia is not unique to the lungfish; it is also found in some other species (Heisler, 1982; Hughes and Singh, 1971; Smatresk et al., 1986).

Although the important role of hypoxia in ventilatory control in the lungfish is evident, the mechanism by which this is sensed remains elusive. Sectioning

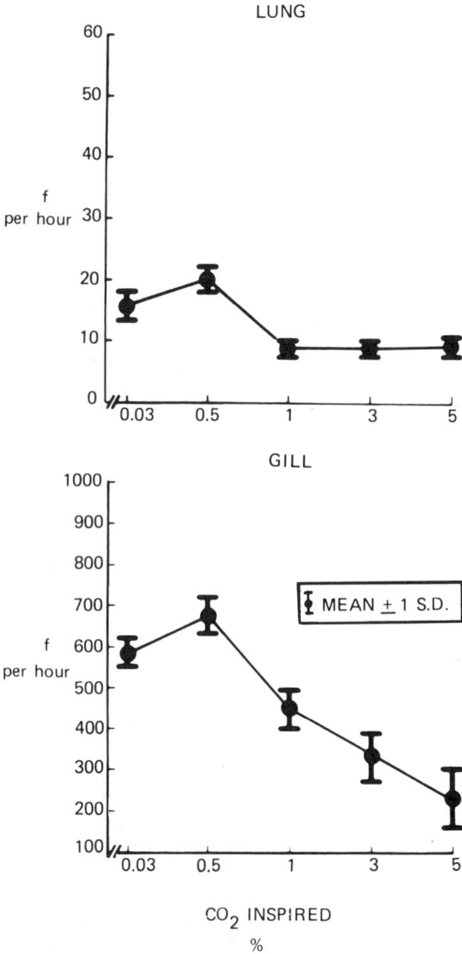

Figure 5 Effect of hypercarbia in both water and air on frequency of pulmonary and gill ventilation in *Protopterus*. Low levels of CO_2 increased the frequency of both, whereas higher levels inhibited ventilation. This inhibitory effect of hypercapnia is more marked on the gills. The data shown are the mean ± SD from eight experiments in two fish. (From Jesse et al., 1967.)

of the nerves supplying the branchial arches reduces the ventilatory response to hypoxia (Lahiri et al., 1970). However, careful histological study of the vasculature of the branchial arches does not reveal an organized collection of glomus-like cells (unpublished observations). It seems unlikely, therefore, that the lungfish possess an organized chemoreceptor.

C. Effect of Hypercapnia

Hypercapnia also affects gill and pulmonary ventilation in lungfish (Jesse et al., 1967; Johansen et al., 1967; Johansen and Lenfant, 1968). When both P_{CO_2}

in water and in inspired gas are altered simultaneously, low levels of hypercapnia ($< 0.5\%$) stimulate both pulmonary and gill ventilation (Fig. 5), but higher levels reduce the frequency of oscillation of both generators. This inhibitory effect is more marked for the gills; progressive increases in P_{CO_2} cause a progressive reduction in the rate of gill ventilation but not in pulmonary ventilation (see Fig. 5). Hypercapnia in water also has different effects on gill and lung ventilation (Johansen and Lenfant, 1968). When 5% CO_2 in air is bubbled through water, there is a reduction in the gill ventilation rate and an increase in the frequency of air breathing. Because these changes occur without significant change in the P_{CO_2} of arterial blood, they may be mediated by alteration in some afferent stimulus from the gills themselves. However, as with hypoxia, the sensory mechanisms mediating these hypercapnic responses are unknown, and it is currently uncertain whether or not there is a structure equivalent to the central chemoreceptor in mammals.

D. Afferent Input from the Lung

Although chemical-sensing mechanisms are poorly understood, much more is known about mechanoreceptors in the lung. In the lungfish lung there are both slowly adapting and rapidly adapting receptors (DeLaney et al., 1983). The former increase their firing with progressive inflation of the lung. Stretch receptors are found that are active even when the lungs are at atmospheric pressure, whereas others are recruited as the lung is expanded. The firing of these receptors seems to be most closely related to transpulmonary pressure. The slowly adapting receptors also have, however, a dynamic component to their response such that their firing during ramp inflations is greater than while the lung is static. Not unexpectedly, this dynamic response is a function of inflation rate.

Stretch receptor discharge is, however, not solely dependent on mechanical stimuli. Their firing is affected by variations in intrapulmonary CO_2 concentration. Specifically, hypercapnia inhibits receptor discharge (DeLaney et al., 1983). This effect is not small because 6% CO_2 causes a 40 to 60% reduction in firing. The effect of hypercapnia is not instantaneous because there are distinct dynamics, the transient response in firing following reductions in P_{CO_2} being faster than that associated with increases. Although CO_2 affects the firing of stretch receptors, the lungfish lacks the specialized CO_2 receptors that are found in the lungs of birds (Fedde and Peterson, 1970) and reptiles (Fedde et al., 1977).

The lung also contains rapidly adapting receptors that fire briefly during lung inflation and deflation. As in mammals (Pack and DeLaney, 1983), the response of these receptors is particularly dependent on the rate of inflation, but the inflation rate is not the only determinant of the firing of this receptor type.

The response characteristics of pulmonary mechanoreceptors in dipnoi are similar to those described in related species, although some differences have

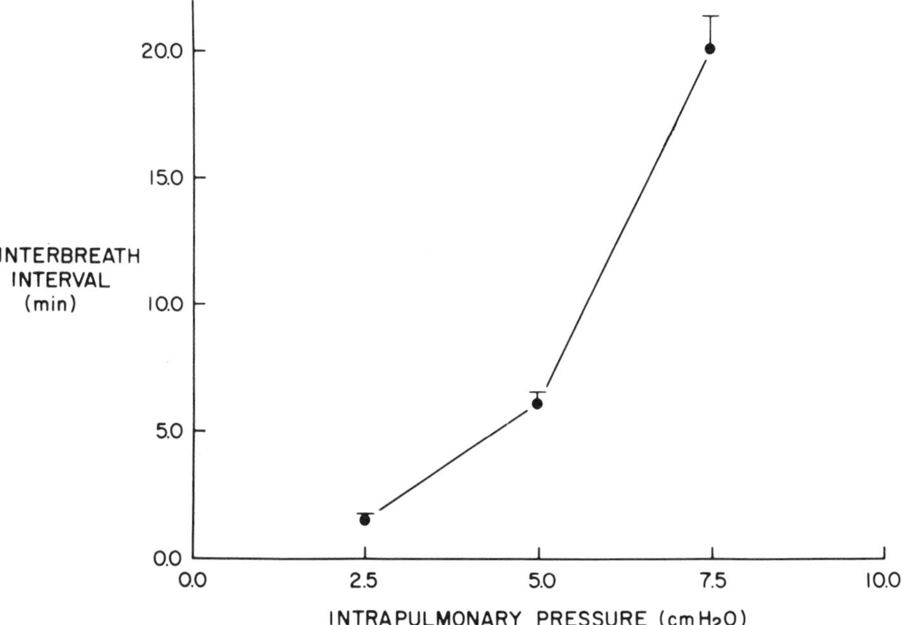

Figure 6 Relationship between interval between lung breaths and intrapulmonary pressure in a single lungfish. Each point represents the mean of six measurements at each of the three levels of pressure.

been reported. In frogs both slowly adapting and rapidly adapting receptors are found (Taglietti and Casella, 1966; McKean, 1969; Milsom and Jones, 1977), with the response of frog slowly adapting receptors being inhibited by increases in CO_2 concentration (Milsom and Jones, 1977). Likewise, in the holostean air-breathing fish, *Lepisosteus oculatus* (spotted gar), both types of receptor have been reported, with CO_2 exerting an inhibitory effect on the firing of slowly adapting receptors (Smatresk and Azizi, 1987). In another holostean air-breathing fish, *Amia calva*, all receptors found were of the slowly adapting type and were insensitive to changes in CO_2 concentration (Milsom and Jones, 1985). The number of receptors studied was, however, small ($n = 10$). Thus, the absence of rapidly adapting receptors in *Amia calva* may be only apparent and reflect just the small sample of receptors studied.

The receptor studies in dipnoi indicate that the brain stem receives afferent information both about the overall degree of lung inflation and the rate of inflation. It seems likely that this information plays a role in ventilatory control. Certainly, lung deflation can precipitate a lung breath (DeLaney et al., 1974; unpublished observations) suggesting that Hering-Breuer reflexes are operative in the lungfish. Indeed, we have recently demonstrated that the interval between lung breaths, called by some the nonventilatory period (NVP) (Glass and Johansen, 1976; Milsom and Jones, 1980), is influenced by the degree of lung inflation (Fig. 6). But in lungfish, alterations in lung inflation not only affect the afferent input from stretch receptors but also the magnitude of the pulmonary O_2 store. Thus, at high lung volumes arterial PO_2 should fall slower during the interval between lung breaths. Hence, at least part of the effect of lung inflation on the duration of the nonventilatory period may be mediated by differences in arterial PO_2. Such differences, however, do not explain the results we have obtained. We have observed, in another preparation we have employed, in which gas was continuously blowing through both lungs before exiting, thereby maintaining intrapulmonary and arterial PO_2 constant, that variations in intrapulmonary pressure have profound effects on the duration of the interbreath interval. Thus, the lungfish has an extremely active Hering-Breuer reflex of the expiratory-promoting type. The processing characteristics of this reflex are unknown but may share some characteristics of that for control of expiratory duration in mammals (Knox, 1973) because lung inflations early in the interbreath interval produce less prolongation of the interval than inflations later in the interval (unpublished observations).

Afferent information from stretch receptors also plays a role in the duration of the lung breath itself. Hence, in preliminary studies, we have observed that inflation of the lung just after the onset of an air breath prematurely terminates action of the buccal force pump. In contrast, occlusion of the glottis produces a marked prolongation of the action of this muscular system (unpublished observations). Such features are similar to that of the Hering-Breuer inspiratory-terminating reflex in mammals (Clark and von Euler, 1972).

In dipnoi lungfish, pulmonary afferent information may play other important roles. For example, DeLaney et al. (1983) have suggested that afferent information from pulmonary stretch receptors may be used to regulate lung volume by a vasovagal reflex loop because pulmonary smooth muscle is under vagal efferent control. Control of lung volume is particularly important in the lungfish because the lung serves as a hydrostatic organ to control buoyancy, as well as for gas exchange. Support for this hypothesis comes from recent studies in the holostean air-breathing fish, gar, which showed the expected changes in vagal efferent outflow to the lung in response to alterations in pulmonary pressure (Azizi and Smatresk, 1986).

Afferent information from stretch receptors may also be involved in the regulation of pulmonary blood flow. This is discussed more fully later in Sections VIII and IX.

Afferent information from the lung, however, plays little, if any, role in control of gill ventilation. We have observed that inflation of the lung between

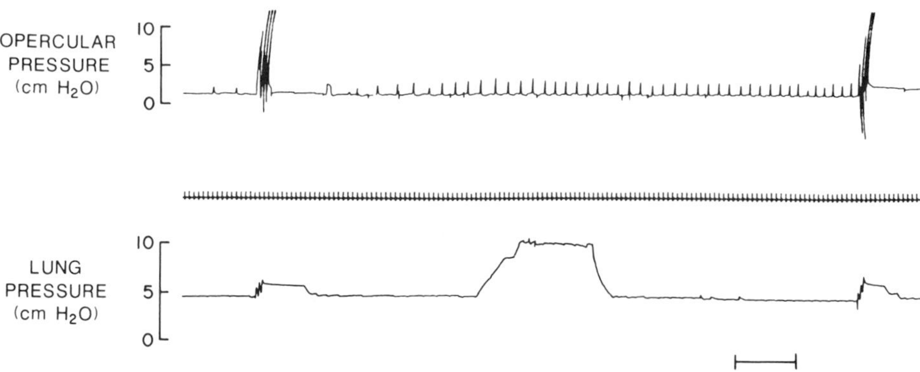

Figure 7 Effect of lung inflation between lung breaths on frequency of gill ventilation. As is seen in the figure, lung inflation is without effect on the frequency of gill ventilation in *Protopterus.*

lung breaths produces no alteration in the frequency of gill ventilation (Fig. 7). This observation is in contrast to that in bullfrog tadpoles in whom lung inflation produces a slowing of gill frequency (West and Burggren, 1983).

E. Afferent Input from Mechanoreceptors in Branchial Arches

It seems more likely that frequency of the gill ventilation will be altered by afferent information from mechanoreceptors in the region of the gills. Certainly, it is known that stimulation of branchial mechanoreceptors in elasmobranches reflexly slows gill frequency (Satchell and Way, 1962). Moreover, electrical stimulation of the epibranchial vagus ganglia in carp during the inspiratory (opening) phase of the cycle causes a premature termination of that phase (Ballintijn et al., 1983). But whether or not such receptors exist in lungfish is currently unknown. Somewhat crude, albeit provocative, observations do suggest, however, that mechanical stimuli to the branchial arches reflexly alter gill frequency. Thus, Johansen and Lenfant (1968) observed that mechanical agitation of the water increased the frequency of gill ventilation.

F. Temperature

Temperature might also be anticipated to affect the activity of both pattern generators. In fish, increased temperature increases the frequency of gill ventilation (for review see Shelton et al., 1986), whereas in frogs, increased temperature also stimulates the action of the buccal force pump (Smyth, 1939). In other air-

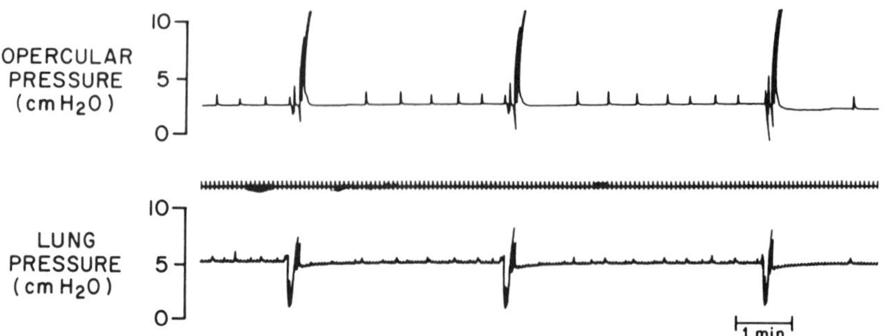

Figure 8 Recordings of opercular and intrapulmonary pressure in a preparation in which intrapulmonary pressure was maintained, more or less constant, as was arterial PO_2. With the lung breath there was a brief period during which intrapulmonary pressure fell. This presumably is due to loss of the seal at the glottis as the glottis was dilated with the air breath. After a lung breath, there is a period of inhibition of gill ventilation. It is proposed that this inhibition is generated by the pattern generator for pulmonary ventilation.

breathing fish, increased temperature increases the frequency of aerial respiration (Johansen et al., 1970; Horn and Riggs, 1973; Smatresk and Cameron, 1982; Yu and Woo, 1985). In lungfish we have observed that raising core temperature does increase both the frequency of gill and lung ventilation. However, neither we nor others have quantified this relationship and, in particular, examined the relative effect of temperature on the two oscillatory systems.

G. Interaction Between Two Pattern Generators: A Hierarchical System

These observations indicate that the two generators receive certain common information related to the chemical status of the fish. The relative effect, however, of a given stimulus, e.g., hypoxia, on the two systems is different. Each pattern generator may receive, moreover, "private" information. Thus, we have demonstrated that pulmonary stretch receptor information has no effect on the gill system and, likewise, it may be that afferent information from branchial mechanoreceptors has no effect on pulmonary ventilation.

What remains to be determined, however, is how crucial afferent systems are in operation of these networks and how much is intrinsic to the network itself. Certainly, for the pattern generator for pulmonary ventilation some degree of hypoxic stimulation is crucial because hyperoxia causes it to stop. For this network the two important afferents are those related to hypoxia and pulmonary stretch receptor information. It seems likely that these afferents play a major

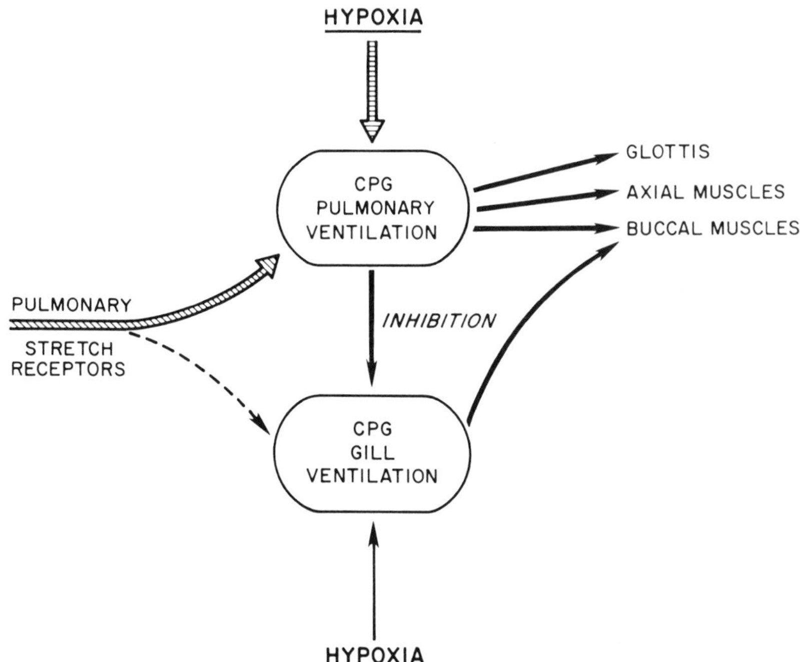

Figure 9 Model of separate pattern generators for pulmonary and gill ventilation. The two neural circuits receive similar afferent inputs, but the strength of their action in the two networks is different. Hypoxia has a pronounced effect on pulmonary ventilation but little effect on gill ventilation. The afferent activity from pulmonary stretch receptors likewise has pronounced effects on pulmonary ventilation but no effect on gill ventilation. The pattern generators are organized in a hierarchical way such that operation of the pulmonary generator inhibits the gill generator. There is currently no evidence of the reverse link whereby action of the pattern generator for gill ventilation alters that for pulmonary ventilation.

role in determining the duration of the nonventilatory period. During this period, arterial PO_2 progressively falls (Johansen and Lenfant, 1968; McMahon, 1970), albeit at a rate slower than that of the PO_2 of pulmonary gas. Simultaneously, lung volume declines because the O_2 uptake from the lung is greater than the CO_2 exchange into the lungs. Both of these changes are in direction to provide stimuli—lower PO_2, lower lung volume—that act to shorten the interbreath interval. The system is not, however, totally dependent on the time variation of those afferent inputs. We have observed that in the preparation just described the pulmonary system cycles when arterial PO_2 and lung volume are maintained constant. Hence, this generator has inherent rhythmicity, provided sufficient tonic afferent stimulation is present.

These pattern generators must also interact, because they compete for some of the same muscles. It has long been known that following a lung breath, there is a slowing of gill ventilation (Jesse et al., 1967; McMahon, 1969) and an acceleration before a lung breath (Johansen and Lenfant, 1968; McMahon, 1969). This phenomenon has been described in other species—the air-breathing teleost fish *Anabas* (Singh and Hughes, 1973), the holostean air-breathing fish, *Amia calva* (Johansen et al., 1970), and in the bullfrog tadpole (West and Burggren, 1983). In the latter species, it was proposed that the inhibition of gill ventilation following a lung breath was reflexly produced by the increased activity of pulmonary stretch receptors. However, this cannot be so in lungfish because we have not demonstrated a reflex of this type. Moreover, in lungfish in which we have used our previously described flow-through preparation to maintain constancy of PO_2 and intrapulmonary pressure, we have also observed a period of inhibition of gill ventilation after a lung breath (Fig. 8). Immediately after such a breath there is a period with no gill movement and thereafter, gill frequency increases exponentially to the steady-state value it assumes in the nonventilatory period. Because in our preparation, afferent inputs are maintained more or less constant, this implies that this inhibition of gill ventilation is not reflexly mediated, as proposed by West and Burggren (1983), but is rather a feature that is intrinsic to the networks. We envisage, therefore, a hierarchical system of two pattern generators (Fig. 9). Action of the lung generator may provide an inhibitory influence on the pattern generator for gill ventilation. This inhibitory influence seems to decline exponentially after a lung breath, thereby releasing the generator for gill ventilation from inhibition and allowing it to resume its normal activity. This period after a lung breath may correspond to what has become known in mammals as the postinspiratory phase of the respiratory cycle (Richter, 1982; Ballantyne and Richter, 1984; Richter et al., 1986). During this phase of the mammalian respiratory cycle, there is widespread inhibition of respiratory neurons, both inspiratory and expiratory.

VII. Overview of the Circulation

Just as for ventilation, there needs to be complex circulatory control to coordinate gas exchange from the gills and lungs. Before considering this, it is essential to review the basic features of the circulation of the lungfish. The heart of the lungfish has been studied by a number of investigators using anatomical (Spencer, 1893; Robertson, 1913; Bugge, 1960; Johansen et al., 1968; Szidon et al., 1969; Arbel et al., 1977), electrophysiological (Szidon et al., 1969; Arbel et al., 1977) and hemodynamic (Johansen et al., 1968; Szidon et al., 1969) techniques.

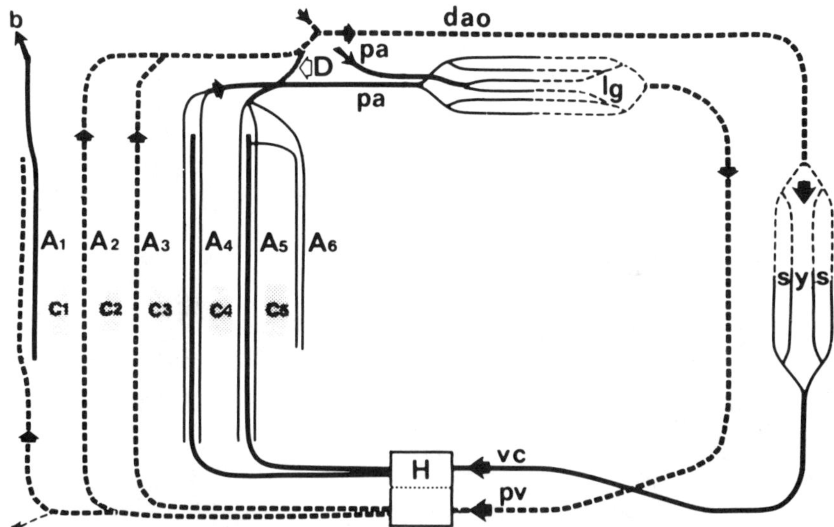

Figure 10 Schematic diagram showing the arrangement of the circulation in *Protopterus*. The following abbreviations are used: A1 to A6, arches I–VI; b, brain; D, ductus; dao, dorsal aorta; H, heart; lg, lung; pa, pulmonary artery; pv, pulmonary vein; sys, systemic circulation. For further details see text. (From Laurent et al., 1978.)

The heart is surrounded by a thick, relatively rigid pericardium (Johansen et al., 1968; Szidon et al., 1969). This rigidity results in intrapericardial pressure falling during ventricular systole, thereby aiding venous return by an aspiration mechanism. The systemic venous return empties into a single, thin-walled sinus venosus which acts as a reservoir to store the venous return during ventricular ejection. In contrast, pulmonary veins from both lungs unite to form a single pulmonary vein that empties directly into the left atrium. The atria have a septum that divides the atria into two separate chambers. The degree of septation is different in the different genera of lungfish. It is most marked in *Lepidosiren* and least in *Neoceratodus*, which retains more piscine characteristics, including the ability to support gas exchange requirements by gill ventilation. The ventricles also have a muscular septum, but this is incomplete at its cranial end such that there is a communication between the two ventricles. As with the atria, the degree of septation varies in the different genera. The ventricles empty into what is known as the bulbus, which is subdivided into two channels–ventral and dorsal. The ventral and dorsal channels of the bulbus supply different gill arches (Fig. 10). The ventral channel supplies the first three gill arches. Only the first of these three anterior arches retains well-developed lamellae; it is known as the

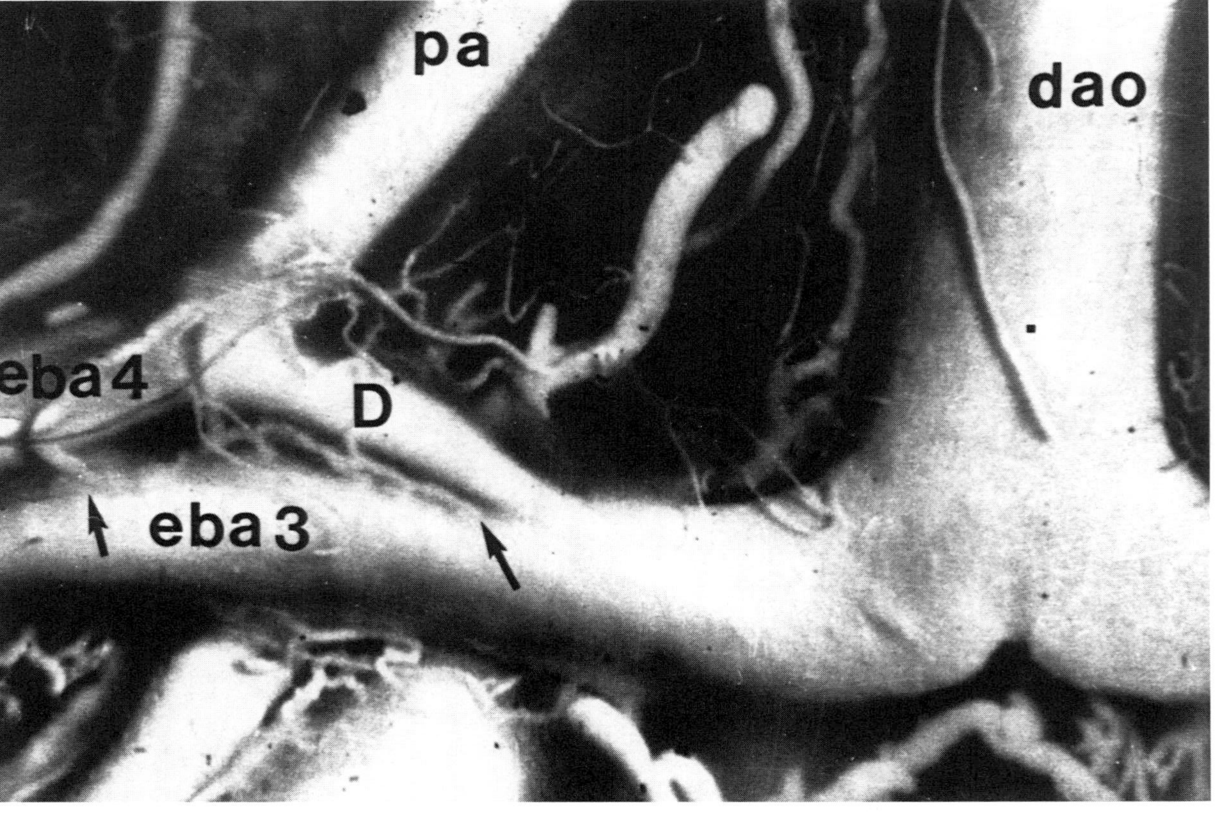

Figure 11 Microfil cast preparation from *Lepidosiren* showing arrangement of ductus arteriosus (D), pulmonary artery (pa), and dorsal aorta (dao). eba4 is the effect vessel from the posterior branchial arches, eba3 from the anterior arches (see Fig. 10). Arrows show the vasovasorum as tributaries of eba3. (Modified from Fishman et al., 1985.)

hyoidean hemibranch. The efferent arteries from arch I deliver blood to the internal carotid arteries, which are the major blood supply to the brain. The other two arches (arches II and III) can be considered as true aortic arches. As discussed earlier in *Protopterus* and *Lepidosiren*, they are virtually devoid of lamellae and do not contribute to gas exchange. Blood vessels from these arches unite to form the dorsal aorta (see Fig. 10). The blood they contain comes largely from the left side of the heart, i.e., it is oxygenated blood from the lung.

In contrast, the dorsal part of the bulbus supplies afferent arteries to arches IV through VI. This blood comes largely from the right side of the heart and is deoxygenated. Efferent arteries from arch IV and V join to form the pulmonary artery (see Fig. 10). There is a ductus vessel connecting the dorsal aorta and pulmonary artery (Fig. 11).

Although the ventricles are not completely separated, there is little mixing between the circulation in the right and left side of the heart. This has been shown by angiography and injection of india ink (Szidon et al., 1969). Contrast material injected into the single pulmonary vein preferentially opacified the ventral channel of the bulbus and first three gill arches, although the aorta was opacified faintly. Conversely, after injection into the vena cava, the dorsal channel of the bulbus and gill arches IV through VI were opacified. There was, however, some faint opacification of the first three gill arches. The degree of mixing between the right and left circulations within the heart has been measured by Johansen et al. (1968) using simultaneous blood gas analysis at various points within the circulation. As expected, the degree of mixing varies in the different genera with mixing being greatest in *Neoceratodus*. The most complete data were obtained for *Protopterus*, in whom the degree of mixing varied during the interval between lung breaths. After a lung breath the proportion of pulmonary venous blood present in the anterior arches (systemic circulation) was 95%, reducing to 65% before the next breath. This in part reflects changes in pulmonary blood flow during the interval.

VIII. Key Elements in Circulatory Control

The circulation in the lungfish supports both gill and pulmonary gas exchange. However, the relative amount of gas exchange by each route varies with time. After a lung breath pulmonary gas exchange is maximal but subsequently declines during the interbreath interval. Thus, the circulation has to adjust such that there are temporal variations in the relative perfusion of gills and lungs. The lungfish possess a number of important controlling elements that permit this adjustment.

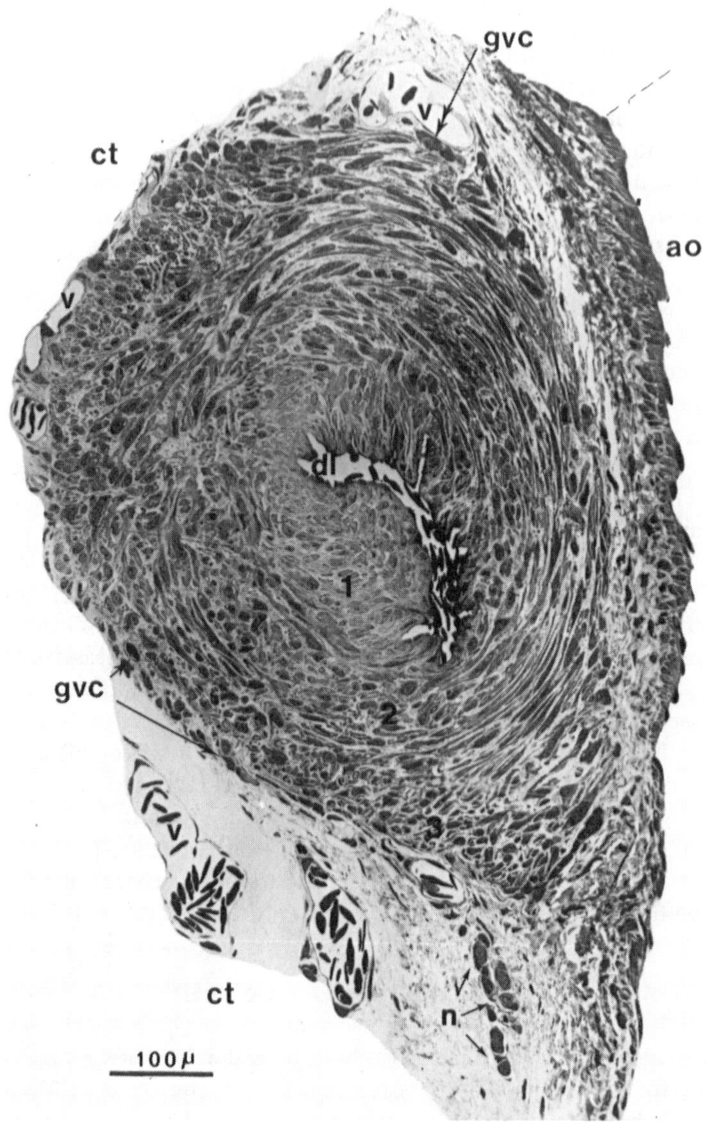

Figure 12 A cross section of the ductus arteriosus of *Protopterus*. There are many layers of smooth muscle in the media. The innermost (1) and outermost layers are arranged longitudinally, whereas the middle layer is circular. In this specimen the lumen (dl) is very narrow. Small vessels (v) and neurons (n) lie outside the media. Granular vesicle cells (gvc) are indicated. (From Fishman et al., 1985.)

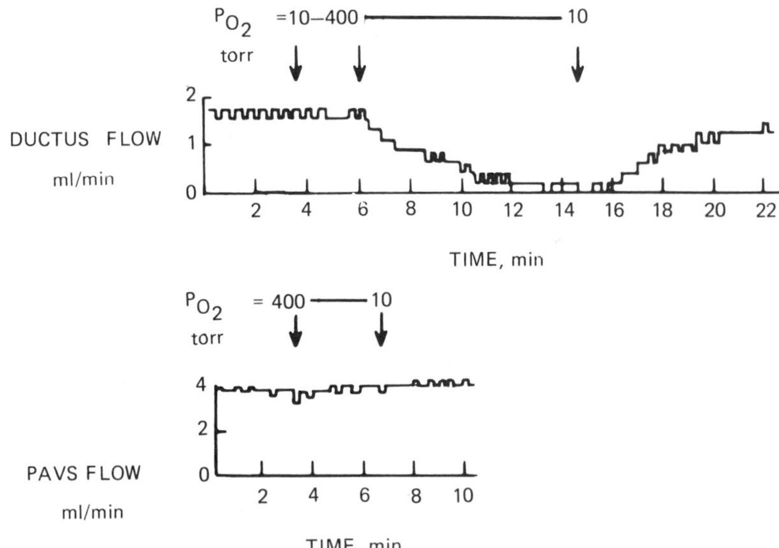

Figure 13 Recordings of flow through the ductus and pulmonary artery vasomotor segment (PAVS) during constant-pressure perfusion of eba4 (see Fig. 11). Switching from hypoxic perfusate (PO_2 = 10 torr) to well-oxygenated perfusate (PO_2 = 400 torr) markedly reduced flow through the ductus, whereas flow through the PAVS was unaltered. (From Fishman et al., 1985.)

A. Ductus Arteriosus

One of these important elements is the ductus arteriosus which joins the pulmonary artery and dorsal aorta (see Fig. 11). The ductus is extremely muscular and its media contains many layers of smooth-muscle cells (Fig. 12). In the figure there are about 30 layers of cells, which contrasts with five to seven layers in the dorsal aorta. The smooth-muscle cells in the inner and outer part of the media are organized longitudinally such that their contraction shortens the ductus. The cells in the middle are more circular so that their contraction tends to shut the lumen.

Nerve bundles, neurons, and granular vesicle cells often are found within the ductus structure. Myelinated and nonmyelinated fibers penetrate the media from the adventitia. Cholinergic-type endings are found in close contact with the smooth muscle, and there is an extremely large number of cholinergic nerve endings, one nerve profile for every four to six muscle profiles (Fishman et al., 1985). This suggests an extremely important neural control of the ductus arteriosus in the lungfish, although this has not yet been directly assessed.

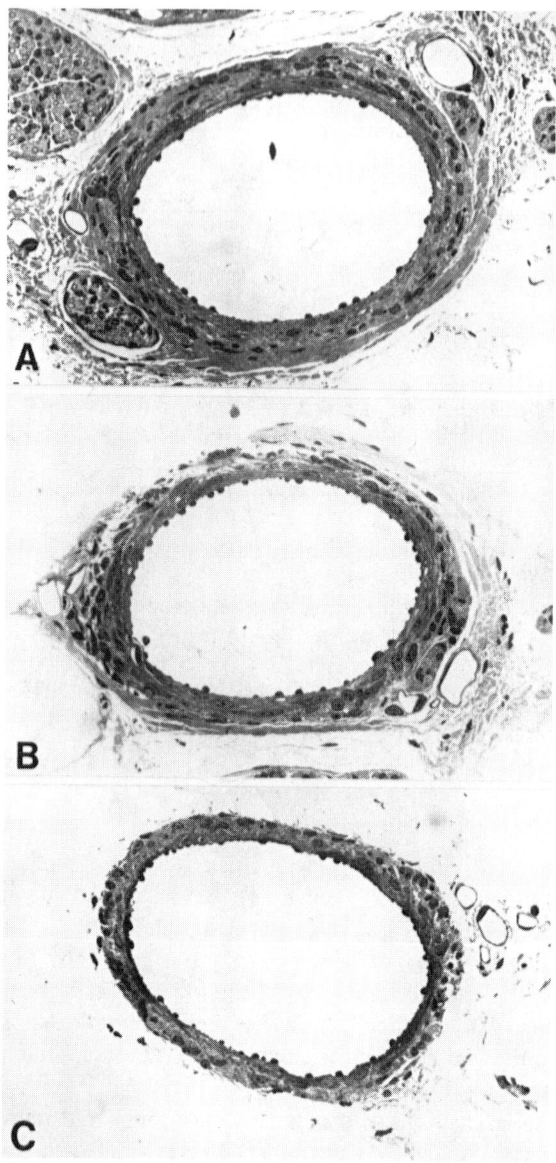

Figure 14 A cross section of three different levels of the extrinsic pulmonary artery in *Lepidosiren*. The levels are as follows: A, close to ductus; B, at middle distance between ductus and lung; C, close to lung. The vessel is relatively thick at its origin and decreases as the lung is approached. (Original magnification × 30). (From Fishman et al., 1985.)

Given the large number of cholinergic nerve endings, it is somewhat surprising that acetylcholine has relatively weak effects on the ductus that causes vasodilatation in the lungfish. In contrast, the ductus is very sensitive to norepinephrine which causes vasoconstriction. It seems unlikely, however, that norepinephrine is released by neural mechanisms because in the lungfish, the adrenergic nervous system is not prominent (Abrahamsson et al., 1979). It has been proposed that the granular vesicle cells may store and release norepinephrine (as well as dopamine, which dilates the ductus) (Fishman et al., 1985), although there is no proof of this.

The ductus is not only sensitive to these neurotransmitters but also to hypoxia. Hypoxia causes, as in mammals, dilatation of the ductus, whereas hyperoxia constricts the ductus (Fig. 13, top panel). Thus the direct effects of variations in O_2 tension are added to neural influences on the ductus.

B. Pulmonary Artery Vasomotor Segment

A second key controlling element is the pulmonary artery vasomotor segment (PAVS) that controls the resistance of the pulmonary circulation. This structure has been identified histologically. At the origin of the pulmonary artery there is a thickened segment of the vascular wall that extends distally from the ductus to affect approximately one-third of the extrapulmonary part of the pulmonary artery (Fishman et al., 1985) (Fig. 14). At maximum thickness, the media of the PAVS consists of eight to ten smooth-muscle fibers oriented obliquely. The innervation of the PAVS seems less than that for the ductus. Neurons are scattered throughout the adventitia. Postganglionic axons are found in the media and amyelinated bundles are seen close to smooth-muscle cells. As in the ductus, granular vesicle cells are present.

The responses of the PAVS are different from those of the ductus. Local PO_2 has no effect on the pulmonary artery vasomotor segment (see Fig. 13, bottom panel). Acetylcholine constricts the PAVS, although, as discussed before, it dilates the ductus, whereas dopamine and norepinephrine are without effect (Fishman et al., 1985).

Pulmonary artery vasomotor segments have also been described in other species–frog (De Saint-Aubain et al., 1979) and turtles (Milsom et al., 1977; Burggren, 1977). As in the lungfish, acetylcholine constricts the PAVS, whereas epinephrine is without effect. In turtles, a definite neural influence on the PAVS has been demonstrated (Milsom et al., 1977). Stimulation of the vagus nerve constricts the extrinsic pulmonary artery. Physiological studies reveal that the increase in pulmonary artery pressure when the vagus nerve is stimulated is almost entirely caused by constriction in the proximal pulmonary artery. The effect can be demonstrated at relatively low stimulation thresholds, e.g., lower than that necessary to induce bradycardia. Although neural vagal control of the PAVS has not been demonstrated in the lungfish, it seems likely that it exists.

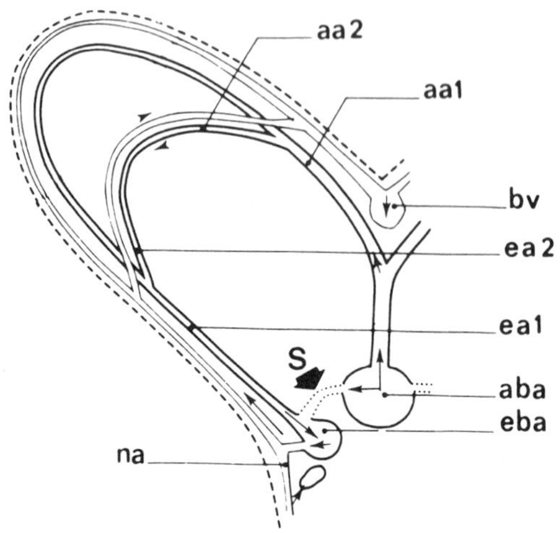

Figure 15 Schematic of the vasculature of the primary lamellae on branchial arches IV–VI. Small arrows indicate direction of blood flow. Large arrow (S) indicates the afferent–efferent shunt. Other abbreviations are: aa1 and aa2, primary and secondary afferent arteries; aba, afferent branchial artery; bv, branchial vein; ea1 and ea2, primary and secondary efferent arteries; eba, efferent branchial artery; na, nutrient artery. (Modified from Laurent et al., 1978.)

C. Gill Shunts

The third major controlling element are gill shunts. These were discussed briefly in Section III (see Fig. 1). The shunts are short vessels that connect directly the afferent to efferent branchial arteries at the base of primary lamellae on branchial arches IV through VI (Fig. 15). In histological sections they have a thick muscular layer suggesting, thereby, that they have a role in vasomotor control (Laurent et al., 1978). Certainly, changes in caliber of this vessel will alter both the passage followed by blood through the primary lamellar structure and the resistance of the branchial vessels. Although these shunt vessels seem capable of exerting an important controlling influence, there is little data for this. It is reported that innervation of the gill is sparse (Laurent et al., 1978), hence, direct neural control may be limited. Pharmacological studies show that acetylcholine increases branchial resistance, whereas epinephrine and norepinephrine produce vasodilation of the branchial circulation (Johansen et al., 1968; Johansen and Reite, 1967). Such shunts are also described in amphibians, and here, too, appear to be under neurohumoral control (Fige, 1936).

IX. Circulatory Adjustments for Gill and Lung Ventilation

Alterations in the setting of these three key conduits presumably underlie the changes that take place in the lungfish circulation when it switches from aerial to gill ventilation. The largest change in the circulation is the increase in pulmonary blood flow that occurs with an air breath (Johansen et al., 1968; Szidon et al., 1969). This change is large; with a breath the pulmonary blood flow increases to about four times the prebreath value (Johansen et al., 1968). Between breaths pulmonary blood flow declines toward zero (Szidon et al., 1969). Other circulatory adjustments also accompany air breaths. If intervals between air breaths are long, i.e., more than 4 min, cardiac output tends to increase with each air breath. Moreover, branchial vascular resistance often decreases in association with each spontaneous air breath (Johansen et al., 1968).

These changes are probably partly mediated by central neural mechanisms, i.e., as part of the programmed behavior, and partly by reflex circulatory adjustments secondary to lung inflation. Evidence of the former is the observation that the increase in pulmonary blood flow can precede the breathing act (Johansen et al., 1968). Relative to the latter, artificial lung inflation in lungfish has been shown to produce tachycardia and an increase in pressure in both systemic and pulmonary arteries (Johansen et al., 1968).

Similar circulatory adjustments occur in other intermittently breathing animals with both gill and aerial ventilation. In amphibia (Shelton, 1970; Emilio and Shelton, 1972) and air-breathing teleost fish (Singh and Hughes, 1973; Farrell, 1978), there is a tachycardia and an increase in blood flow to the gas exchange organ synchronous with the air breath. Likewise in aquatic reptiles that breathe intermittently, there is an increase in heart rate (ventilation tachycardia) (Burggren, 1975) and blood flow to the lungs (Shelton and Burggren, 1976) in association with the resumption of ventilation.

Although these circulatory adaptations with air breathing in the lungfish are known, the precise mechanisms mediating them are not understood. The large change in pulmonary blood flow with air breathing suggests a critical role for the PAVS. Reductions in the tone of this may be partly centrally mediated because pulmonary blood flow can change in anticipation of an air breath (Johansen et al., 1968). A vagovagal reflex related to lung inflation is also likely to be operative. Certainly in turtles, who also have a PAVS (Milsom et al., 1977), lung inflation produces marked alterations in pulmonary blood flow (Johansen et al., 1977). Inflation of the lung leads to an increase in pulmonary blood flow, whereas deflation of the lung causes heart rate and pulmonary blood flow to decrease sharply (Johansen et al., 1977). Added to these effects could be reduction in resistance of the pulmonary circulation produced by the higher intrapulmonary O_2 concentration that follows an air breath. It seems likely, moreover, that with air breathing there are changes in the other key controlling elements of the circulation. The drop in branchial resistance suggests that gill shunts are opened with air breathing, although whether this occurs or how it is mediated is unknown. The higher arterial PO_2 with the air breath should also lead to constriction of the ductus arteriosus.

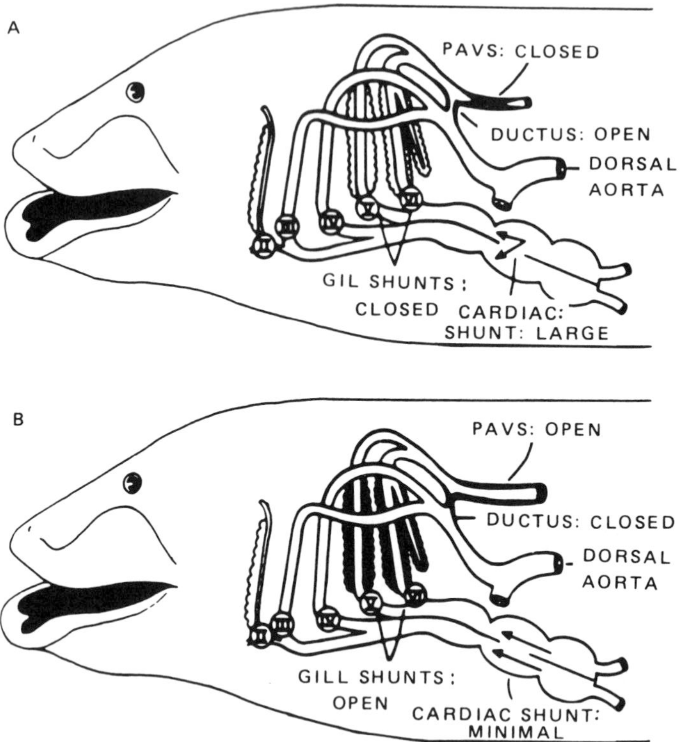

Figure 16 Schematic representations of the proposed circulatory adjustments for gill ventilation during submersion (A) and pulmonary ventilation during aerial respiration (B). The concepts are discussed in the text. (From Fishman et al., 1985.)

Given these considerations, conceptual models of how the lungfish's circulation is organized for aerial and gill ventilation have been proposed (Fishman et al., 1985). During submersion the fish is apneic; the lung O_2 store is low and the lung receives little blood flow. The gills continue to function for CO_2 exchange and osmotic equilibration. In this mode (Fig. 16A, upper panel) the gill shunts are closed so that gill lamellae are perfused, PAVS is closed to prevent perfusion of the lung, and the ductus arteriosus is open. In contrast, during air breathing (see Fig. 16B, lower panel) gill shunts are envisaged to be open such that flow bypasses the gill lamellae. The PAVS is open, but the ductus is closed. In this mode there is separation of the two circulations. Oxygenated blood from the lungs perfuses the anterior arches and dorsal aorta, whereas deoxygenated blood from the systemic circulation perfuses the posterior arches and then the lung.

X. Ventilatory and Circulatory Control During Bimodal Respiration: Conclusions

In this chapter we have reviewed how gill and pulmonary ventilation in the dipnoan lungfish are controlled and the circulatory adaptations to accommodate both. The picture that emerges is of an intricate control system. Although many of the features of control of pulmonary ventilation are similar to those in mammals, complexities are added because of the presence of gill ventilation. It seems likely that there are two respiratory pattern generators, one to produce gill ventilatory movements and the other pulmonary ventilation, the circuits being organized in a hierarchical fashion. The pattern generators may also contain elements related to cardiovascular control because air breathing requires a marked readjustment of the pattern of the circulation. To these centrally generated patterns are added important modifying effects produced by reflexes secondary to lung inflation and hypoxia. Such reflexes affect ventilatory movements and the performance of the key controlling elements in the circulation. These considerations lead us to believe that a future challenge in this species is to unravel the neural circuits that produce pulmonary and gill ventilation and how they interact. Many of the features of the mammalian respiratory pattern generator must be present in the lungfish. It is obvious, however, that with evolution there is loss of the intricate neural controls required for bimodal respiration. What use, if any, such mechanisms were put to is likely to be a fascinating area of study.

References

Abrahamsson, T., Holmgren, S., Nilsson, S., and Pettersson, K. (1979). Adrenergic and cholinergic effects on the heart, the lung, and the spleen of the African lungfish, *Protopterus aethiopicus. Acta Physiol. Scand. 107A*: 141-147.

Arbel, E. R., Liberthson, R., Langendorf, R., Pick, A., Lev, M., and Fishman, A. P. (1977). Electrophysiological and anatomical observations on the heart of the African lungfish. *Am. J. Physiol. 232*:H24-34.

Azizi, S. Q., and Smatresk, N. J. (1986). Relationships between vagal efferent activity and pressure in the air-breathing organ of gar. *Physiologist 29*:177 (abstr.).

Ballantyne, D., and Richter, D. W. (1984). Post-synaptic inhibition of bulbar inspiratory neurones in the cat. *J. Physiol. (Lond.) 348*:67-87.

Ballintijn, C. M., and Hughes, G. M. (1965). The muscular basis of the respiratory pumps in the trout. *J. Exp. Biol. 43*:349-362.

Ballintijn, C. M., Roberts, B. L., and Luiten, P. G. M. (1983). Respiratory responses to stimulation of branchial vagus nerve ganglia of a teleost fish. *Respir. Physiol. 51*:241-257.

Bishop, I. R., and Foxon, G. E. H. (1968). The mechanism of breathing in the South American lungfish *Lepidosiren paradoxa*; a radiological study. *J. Zool. (Lond.) 154*:263-272.

Bugge, J. (1960). The heart of the African lungfish, *Protopterus. Vidersk. Medd. Dan. Naturhist. Foren. 123*:193-210.

Burggren, W. W. (1975). A quantitative analysis of ventilation tachycardia and its control in two chelonians, *Pseudemys scripta* and *Testudo graeca. J. Exp. Biol. 63*:367-380.

Burggren, W. (1977). The pulmonary circulation of the chelonian reptile, morphology, hemodynamics and pharmacology. *J. Comp. Physiol. 136*:303-323.

Chardon, M. (1961). Contribution a l'etude du systeme circulatoire a la respiration des Protopteridae. *Ann. Tervuum Mus. R. Afr. Centr. Sci. Zool. 103*: 53-97.

Clark, F. J., and von Euler, C. (1972). On the regulation of depth and rate of breathing. *J. Physiol. (Lond.) 222*:267-295.

Cunningham, J. T. (1934). Experiments in the interchange of oxygen and carbon dioxide between the skin of *Lepidosiren* and the surrounding water and the probable emission of oxygen by the male *Synbranchus. Proc. Zool. Soc. Lond. 102*:875-887.

DeLaney, R. G., and Fishman, A. P. (1977). Analysis of lung ventilation in the aestivating lungfish *Protopterus aethiopicus. Am. J. Physiol. 233*:R181-R187.

DeLaney, R. G., Lahiri, S., and Fishman, A. P. (1974). Aestivation of the African lungfish *Protopterus aethiopicus*: Cardiovascular and respiratory function. *J. Exp. Biol. 61*:111-128.

DeLaney, R. G., Laurent, P., Galante, R., Pack, A. I., and Fishman, A. P. (1983). Pulmonary mechanoreceptors in the dipnoi lungfish *Protopterus* and *Lepidosiren. Am. J. Physiol. 244*:R418-R428.

DeSaint-Aubain, M. L., and Wingstrand, K. G. (1979). A sphincter in the pulmonary artery of the frog *Rana temporaria* and its influence on blood flow in skin and lungs. *Acta Zool. (Stockholm) 60*:163-172.

Eclancher, B., and Fontaine, M. (1975). Controle de la respiration chez les poissons teleosteens: Reactions respiratoires a des changements rectangulaires de l'oxygenation du milieu. *C. R. Acad. Sci. Ser. D. 280*:307-310.

Eclancher, B., and Dejours, P. (1975). Controle de la respiration chez les poissons teleosteens: Existence de chemorecepteurs physiologiquement analogues aux chemorecepteurs des vertebres superieurs. *C. R. Acad. Sci. Ser. D 280*:451-453.

Emilio, M. G., and Shelton, G. (1972). Factors affecting blood flow to the lungs in the amphibian, *Xenopus laevis. J. Exp. Biol. 56*:67-77.

Farrell, A. P. (1978). Cardiovascular events associated with air breathing in two teleosts, *Hoplerythrinus unitaeniatus* and *Arapaima gigos. Can. J. Zool. 56*:953-958.

Fedde, M. R., Kuhlmann, W. D., and Scheid, P. (1977). Intrapulmonary receptors in the Tegu lizard. I. Sensitivity to CO_2. *Respir. Physiol. 29*:35-48.

Fedde, M. R., and Peterson, D. F. (1970). Intrapulmonary receptor responses to changes in airway gas composition in *Gallus domesticus. J. Physiol. 209*: 609-625.

Feder, M. E. (1983). Responses to acute aquatic hypoxia in larvae of the frog *Rana berlandieri. J. Exp. Biol. 104*:79-95.

Fige, F. H. J. (1936). The differential reaction of the blood vessels of a branchial arch of *Amblystoma tigrinum* (Colorado axoloth). I. The reaction to adrenaline, oxygen and carbon dioxide. *Physiol. Zool. 9*:79-101.

Fishman, A. P., DeLaney, R. G., and Laurent, P. (1985). Circulatory adaptation to bimodal respiration in the dipnoan lungfish. *J. Appl. Physiol. 59*:285-294.

Glass, M. L., and Johansen, K. (1976). Control of breathing in *Acrochordus javanicus*, an aquatic snake. *Physiol. Zool. 49*:328-340.

Grigg, C. (1965a). Studies on the Queensland lungfish *Neoceratodus fosteri* (Krefft). I. Anatomy, histology and functioning of the lung. *Aust. J. Zool. 13*:243-253.

Grigg, C. (1965b). Studies of the Queensland lungfish *Neoceratodus fosteri* (Krefft). III. Aerial respiration in relation to habits. *Aust. J. Zool. 13*:413-421.

Heisler, N. (1982). Intracellular and extracellular acid-base regulation in the tropical fresh-water teleost fish *Synbranchus marmoratus* in response to the transition from water breathing to air breathing. *J. Exp. Biol. 99*:9-28.

Horn, M. H., and Riggs, C. D. (1973). Effects of temperature and light on the rate of air breathing of the bowfin, *Amia calva. Copeia 4*:653-657.

Hughes, G. M., and Ballintijn, C. M. (1965). The muscular basis of the respiratory pumps in the dogfish (*Scyliorhinus canicula*). *J. Exp. Biol. 43*:363-383.

Hughes, G. M., and Singh, B. N. (1971). Gas exchange with air and water in an air-breathing catfish, *Saccobranchus (Heteropneustes) fossilis. J. Exp. Biol. 55*:667-682.

Jesse, M. J., Shub, C., and Fishman, A. P. (1967). Lung and gill ventilation of the African lungfish. *Respir. Physiol. 3*:267-287.

Johansen, K., Burggren, W., and Glass, M. (1977). Pulmonary stretch receptors regulate heart rate and pulmonary blood flow in the turtle, *Pseudemys scripta. Comp. Biochem. Physiol. 58A*:185-191.

Johansen, K., Hanson, D., and Lenfant. C. (1970). Respiration in a primitive air breather, *Amia calva. Respir. Physiol. 9*:162-174.

Johansen, K., and Lenfant, C. (1967). Respiratory function in the South American lungfish *Lepidosiren paradoxa. J. Exp. Biol. 46*:205-218.

Johansen, K., and Lenfant, C. (1968). Respiration in the African lungfish *Protopterus aethiopicus*. II. Control of breathing. *J. Exp. Biol. 49*:453-468.

Johansen, K., Lenfant, C., and Grigg, G. C. (1967). Respiratory control in the lungfish, *Neoceratodus fosteri* (Krefft). *Comp. Biochem. Physiol. 20*:835-854.

Johansen, K., Lenfant, C., and Hanson, D. (1968). Cardiovascular dynamics in the lungfishes. *Z. Vgl. Physiol. 59*:157-186.

Johansen, K., and Reite, O. B. (1967). Effects of acetylcholine and biogenic amines on pulmonary smooth muscle in the African lungfish, *Protopterus aethiopicus. Acta Physiol. Scand. 71*:248-252.

Jongh, H. J. De, and Gans, C. (1969). On the mechanism of respiration in the bullfrog *Rana catesbeiana*: A reassessment. *J. Morphol. 127*:259-290.

Knox, C. K. (1973). Characteristics of inflation and deflation reflexes during expiration in the cat. *J. Neurophysiol. 36*:284-295.

Lahiri, S., Szidon, J. P., and Fishman, A. P. (1970). Potential respiratory and circulatory adjustments to hypoxia in the African lungfish. *Fed. Proc. 29*: 1141-1148.

Laurent, P., DeLaney, R. G., and Fishman, A. P. (1978). The vasculature of the gills in the aquatic and aestivating lungfish (*Protopterus aethiopicus*). *J. Morphol. 156*:173-208.

MacIntyre, D. H., and Toews, D. P. (1976). The mechanics of lung ventilation and the effects of hypercapnia on respiration in *Bufo marinus. Can. J. Zool. 54*:1364-1374.

McKean, T. A. (1969). Linear approximation of the transfer function of pulmonary mechanoreceptors of the frog. *J. Appl. Physiol. 27*:775-781.

McMahon, B. R. (1969). A functional analysis of the aquatic and aerial respiratory physiology of an African lungfish *Protopterus aethiopicus* with reference to the evolution of vertebrate lung ventilation mechanisms. *J. Exp. Biol. 51*:407-430.

McMahon, B. R. (1970). The relative efficiency of gaseous exchange across the lungs and gills of an African lungfish *Protopterus aethiopicus. J. Exp. Biol. 52*:1-15.

Milsom, W. K., and Jones, D. R. (1977). Carbon dioxide sensitivity of pulmonary receptors in the frog. *Experientia 33*:1167-1168.

Milsom, W. K., and Jones, D. R. (1980). The role of vagal afferent information and hypercapnia in control of the breathing pattern in chelonia. *J. Exp. Biol. 87*:53-63.

Milsom, W. K., and Jones, D. R. (1985). Characteristics of mechanoreceptors in the air-breathing organ of the holostean fish, *Amia calva. J. Exp. Biol. 117*:389-399.

Milsom, W. K., Langille, B. L., and Jones, D. R. (1977). Vagal control of pulmonary vascular resistance in the turtle *Chrysemys scripta. Can. J. Zool. 55*:359-367.

Pack, A. I., and DeLaney, R. G. (1983). Response of pulmonary rapidly adapting receptors during lung inflation. *J. Appl. Physiol. 55*:955-963.

Parker, W. N. (1892). On the anatomy and physiology of *Protopterus aethiopicus. Trans. R. Irish Acad. 30*:111-230.

Randall, D. J., Cameron, J. N., Daxboeck, C., and Smatresk, N. (1981). Aspects of bimodal gas exchange in the bowfin, *Amia calva L* (Actinopterygii: Amiiformes). *Respir. Physiol. 43*:339-348.

Richter, D. W. (1982). Generation and maintenance of the respiratory rhythm. *J. Exp. Biol. 100*:93-107, 1982.

Richter, D. W., Ballantyne, D., and Remmers, J. E. (1986). How is the respiratory rhythm generated? A model. *News Physiol. Sci. 1*:109-112.

Robertson, J. (1913/14). The development of the heart and vascular system of *Lepidosiren paradoxa. Q. J. Microsc. Sci. 59*:53-152.

Satchell, G. H., and Way, H. K. (1962). Pharyngeal proprioceptors in the dogfish *Squalus acanthias. J. Exp. Biol. 39*:243-250.

Sewertzoff, A. N. (1924). Die Entwicklung der Kiemen und Kiemenbogengefässe der Fische. *Z. Wiss. Zool. 121*:494-556.

Shelton, G. (1970). The effect of lung ventilation on blood flow to the lungs and body of the amphibian, *Xenopus laevis. Respir. Physiol. 9*:183-196.

Shelton, G., and Burggren, W. W. (1976). Cardiovascular dynamics of the chelonia during apnoea and lung ventilation. *J. Exp. Biol. 64*:323-343.

Shelton, G., Jones, D. R., and Milsom, W.K. (1986). Control of breathing in ectothermic vertebrates. In *Handbook of Physiology.* Sect. 3: The Respiratory System (A. P. Fishman, ed.). Vol. II: Control of Breathing, Part 1 (N. S. Cherniack, J. G. Widdicombe, eds.) Bethesda, American Physiological Society, pp. 857-909.

Singh, B. N., and Hughes, G. M. (1973). Cardiac and respiratory responses in the climbing perch *Anabas testudineus. J. Comp. Physiol. 84*:205-226.

Smatresk, N., and Cameron, J. (1982). Respiration and acid-base physiology of the spotted gar, a bimodal breather. I. Normal values and the responses to serum hypoxia. *J. Exp. Biol. 96*:263-280, 1982.

Smatresk, N. J., Burleson, M. L., and Azizi, S. Q. (1986). Chemoreflexive responses to hypoxia and NaCN in longnose gar: Evidence for two chemoreceptor loci. *Am. J. Physiol. 251*:R116-R125.

Smatresk, N. J., and Azizi, S. Q. (1987). Characteristics of lung mechanoreceptors in spotted gar, *Lepisosteus oculatus. Am. J. Physiol. 252*:R1066-R1072.

Smyth, D. H. (1939). The central and reflex control of respiration in the frog. *J. Physiol. (Lond.) 95*:305-327.

Spencer, W. B. (1893). Contributions to our knowledge of Ceratodus. I. The blood vessels. *Proc. Linnean Soc. N.S. Wales, Macleay Memorial Volume* pp. 1-34.

Szidon, J. P., Lahiri, S., Lev, M., and Fishman, A. P. (1969). Heart and circulation of the African lungfish. *Circ. Res. 25*:23-38.

Taglietti, V., and Casella, C. (1966). Stretch receptor stimulation in frog lungs. *Pflügers Arch. 292*:297-308.

West, N. H., and Burggren, W. W. (1982). Gill and lung ventilatory responses to steady-state aquatic hypoxia and hyperoxia in the bullfrog tadpole. *Respir. Physiol. 47*:165-176.

West, N. H., and Burggren, W. W. (1983). Reflex interactions between aerial and aquatic gas exchange organs in larval bullfrogs. *Am. J. Physiol. 244*:R770-R777.

West, N. H., and Jones, D. R. (1975). Breathing movements in the frog *Rana pipiens*. I. The mechanical events associated with lung and buccal ventilation. *Can. J. Zool. 53*:332-344.

Yu, K. L., and Woo, Y. S. (1985). Effects of ambient oxygen tension and temperature on the bimodal respiration of an air-breathing teleost, *Channa maculata. Physiol. Zool. 58*:181-189.

22

Diving Physiology
Amphibians

ROBERT G. BOUTILIER

Dalhousie University
Halifax, Nova Scotia, Canada

I. Introduction

Amphibians represent a diverse group, ranging from animals that spend most of their time underwater to those that rarely, if ever, engage in diving. Although all of these animals ventilate their lungs in a periodic fashion, the relative breath-holding capabilities can vary enormously. Presumably, such differences in the diving strategies are related to the wide diversity in the form and function of the aerial and aquatic exchangers, their relative efficacy for gas exchange, and the degree of aquatic or terrestrial adaptation of the animals themselves. Much of the earlier work on amphibians examined the limits of tolerance to enforced submersion by which the investigator controlled the frequency and duration of diving. Under such circumstances, even the most well-adapted divers, such as *Xenopus*, develop a lactacidosis. This apparent reliance on anaerobiosis has long been considered an important part of these animals' energy metabolism during a

The author's research is supported by operating grants from the Natural Sciences and Engineering Research Council of Canada.

dive. However, more recent investigations of animals allowed to dive and surface freely have shown that most voluntary dives are aerobic, requiring little, if any, recruitment of anaerobic pathways. It appears, instead, that these animals are able to manage their O_2 stores quite effectively, replenishing the stores during periods of lung ventilations at the surface and monitoring the stores such that an anaerobic component is avoided in the dive.

II. Utilization of Diving Oxygen Stores

The primary concern for a diving animal is being able to supply the tissues with adequate O_2 for the duration and activities of the dive as well as being able to tolerate or eliminate any undesirable end products of metabolism. The highly permeable skin of most diving amphibians is beneficial for both functions be-

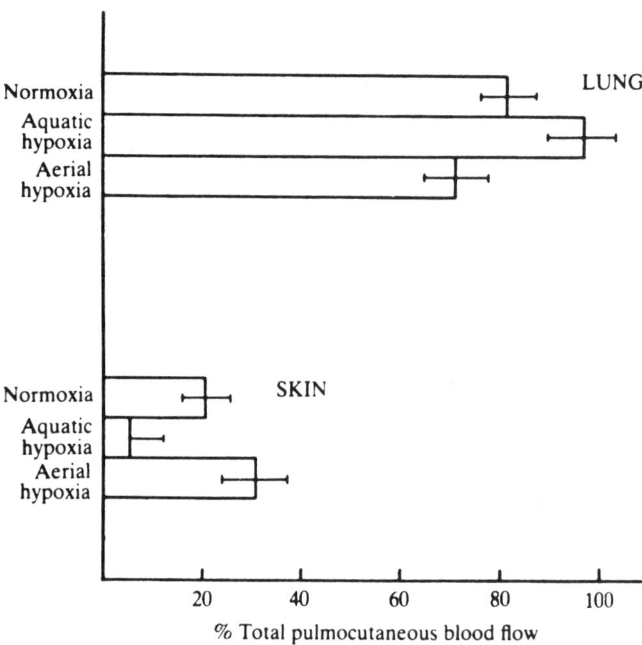

Figure 1 Histogram showing the relative flow of pulmocutaneous blood in voluntarily diving bullfrogs (*Rana catesbeiana*), subjected to normoxic ($PO_2 \sim 155$ torr), aquatic hypoxia ($PO_2 \sim 40$ torr) delivered only at the skin, and aerial hypoxia ($PO_2 \sim 40$ torr) delivered only at the lungs. Radioactive microspheres were injected via a cannula, 10 min into a dive. Data are means from seven experiments at 20°C. (From Boutilier et al., 1986a.)

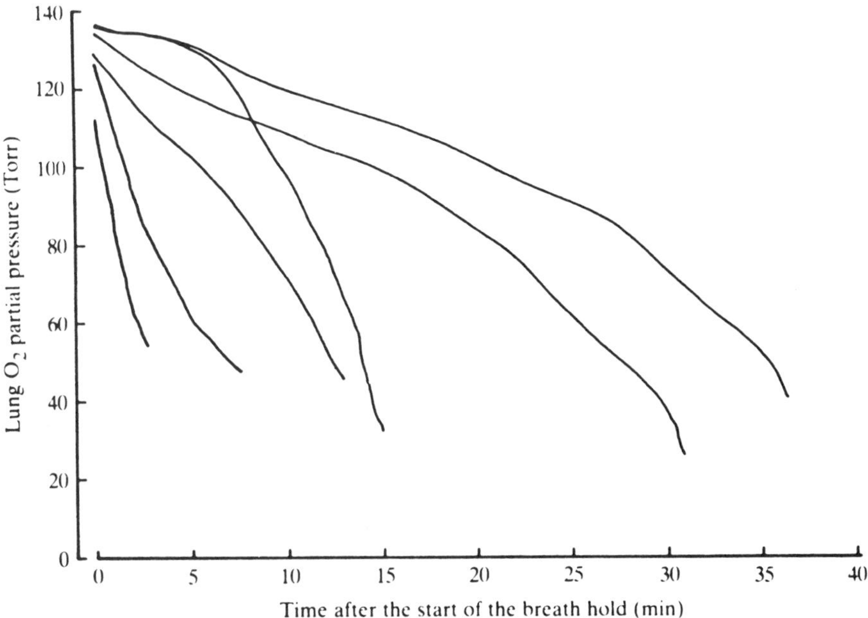

Figure 2 Continuous records of lung gas PO_2 during periods of voluntary diving in six *X. laevis*. Breathing stopped and a voluntary dive began at time zero in all animals. The data were obtained from an O_2 electrode in an extracorporeal lung gas circuit. Temperature = 25°C. (From Boutilier and Shelton, 1986c.)

cause it can be used to tap environmental sources of O_2 during a dive as well as acting as an avenue for the elimination of CO_2. Oxygen in the aquatic environment can, through exchanges with the skin, act as a substantial O_2 store from which supplies can be taken throughout the dive. However, it can also be a potential liability to the body O_2 store during periods of aquatic hypoxia, when the possibility exists for the O_2 gained by air breathing to be lost transcutaneously after the animal dives (Boutilier et al., 1986a).

Body O_2 stores in amphibians are found, as in other vertebrates, in the blood, lungs, and muscle tissue. Blood O_2 capacities and blood volumes of amphibians have not often been assessed using comparable methods, and thus, it is difficult to make any firm statements at this stage about whether or not the blood of diving amphibians is especially well suited as an O_2 store, as is true for some diving mammals (reviewed by Butler and Jones, 1982). Little more is known about the volumes of gas carried in the lungs or of the way in which the lung might act as an O_2 store during a dive. Certainly, the lung can be used as a source of O_2 during a dive as evidenced by measurements of alveolar O_2 depletion in voluntarily diving *Amphiuma* (Toews, 1971; Toews et al., 1971), *Xenopus* (Boutilier and Shelton, 1986c), and *Rana pipiens* (T. Vitalis and G. Shelton, personal communication).

The incompletely divided circulation of amphibians permits variable perfusion and selective distribution of blood to various sites of gas exchange (Shelton and Boutilier, 1982; Malvin and Boutilier, 1985) and appears to offer a good deal of control over the way in which the lung O_2 stores are utilized during a voluntary dive (Boutilier et al., 1986a; Boutilier and Shelton, 1986c). For example, the relative lung perfusion of voluntarily diving *Rana* is increased during water hypoxia and reduced with lowered inspired P_{O_2} (Fig. 1). This mechanism can be interpreted in two ways; first, it may be seen as a readjustment of blood flow to the gas exchange site with the greatest potential for O_2 uptake or, alternatively, as a mechanism to prevent O_2 loss from body O_2 stores at exchange sites of low O_2 tension. Sudden changes in the rates of O_2 extraction from the lungs of voluntarily diving, but otherwise quiescent, *Xenopus* (Fig. 2) also suggest that factors in additional to the metabolic rate of the cells are important in determining the rates at which the O_2 stores are used in the various storage compartments. Further studies on *Xenopus*, in which the lungs were rendered progressively hypoxic during the course of a voluntary dive (Boutilier, Butler and Evans, in Boutilier, 1988), indicated that the animals were able to shut down pulmonary perfusion to conserve their remaining O_2 stores.

III. Model of Oxygen Exchange, Storage, and Transport

A. Oxygen Stores

Over the past 20 years, there have been numerous studies carried out on the African clawed toad, *X. laevis*, one of the best adapted anuran divers. These studies have made it possible to develop an idealized model of the O_2 exchange, storage, and transport system of a 100-g *Xenopus* at 25°C during a dive (Fig. 3; Boutilier and Shelton, 1986c). The model operates on a pulmonary O_2 uptake of 55 μl/min, and a cutaneous O_2 uptake of 15 μl/min, to give a total O_2 consumption of the cells at 70 μl/min (all values derived from experimental measurements of Emilio and Shelton, 1980). The main O_2 stores are found in the lungs and blood; tissue stores were considered to be negligible. The total blood volume of 13 ml (Emilio and Shelton, 1980) has been subdivided into arterial and venous compartments as shown in Figure 3, whereas the diving lung gas volume has been estimated at 8 ml (Boutilier and Shelton, 1986b).

The extent of the O_2 stores in the lungs and various blood compartments are shown on the model (Fig. 3 A) by plotting P_{O_2} against the O_2 capacitances ($B_{O_2} = \Delta V_{O_2}/\Delta P_{O_2}$; Piiper, 1982). Oxygen capacitance is proportional to the

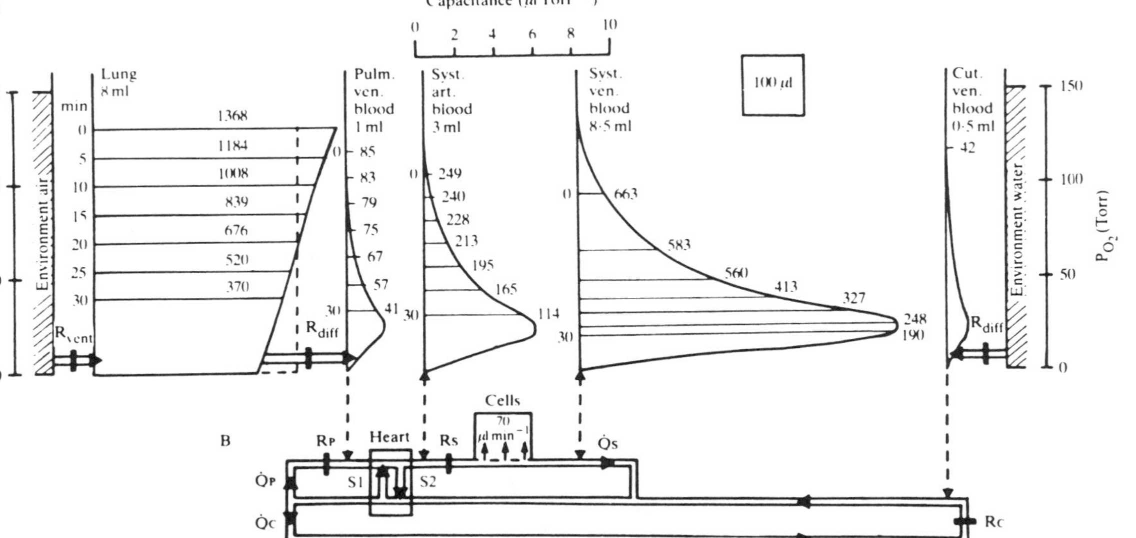

Figure 3 Model of (A) O_2 exchange, O_2 storage, and (B) O_2 transport in *X. laevis* (100 g at 20–25 °C). In A, arrows indicate the direction of O_2 movement in the system, PO_2 gradient per unit of O_2 transfer being determined by ventilation (R_{vent}), diffusive (R_{diff}), and perfusion (not shown) resistances. During dive, R_{vent} is infinite and no environmental O_2 is transferred to the lung; skin O_2 transfer is constant at 15 μl/min. Oxygen stores in lung, pulmonary venous, systemic arterial, systemic venous, and cutaneous venous blood are shown as areas (note 100 μl calibration square) by plotting store capacitances against PO_2. The volumes of air and blood making up each store are also given. The reduction in O_2 content of each store (in μl; figures shown at the right of each store) during a 30-min dive is shown for 5-min intervals. The capacitance relationships for the lung are derived from calculations of $\Delta VO_2/\Delta PO_2$ based on the assumptions that PCO_2 changed by only 3 torr, water vapor pressure remained constant, and the volume of N_2 in the lung was unchanged throughout the dive. If N_2 is also absorbed, there will be even more pronounced decreases in lung O_2 capacitance values as PO_2 falls. In B, large arrows indicate pulmonary ($\dot{Q}_p$), cutaneous ($\dot{Q}_c$) and systemic (Q_s) blood flows, whose rates are determined, in a large part, by respective peripheral resistances (R_p, R_c, R_s). In the heart, arrows show right-to-left (S_1) and left-to-right (S_2) shunts. (From Boutilier and Shelton, 1986c.)

volume (V) of the storage medium (V_{gas} or V_{blood}) and its capacitance coefficient (β_{gas} or β_{blood}) for oxygen:

$$BO_2 = V_{gas} \times \beta O_{2,gas} \text{ or } V_{blood} \times \beta O_{2,blood} \quad (1)$$

The volume of O_2 released by lowering the oxygen partial pressure from P_1 to P_2 is (for example, in the lung):

$$\Delta VO_2 = V\beta O_{2,gas} (P_1 - P_2) = BO_{2,gas} (P_1 - P_2) \quad (2)$$

According to this analysis, the O_2 liberated or absorbed by each of the stores constitutes a change in area in Fig. 3 A (note 100 μl O_2 calibration square). Neither blood nor lung O_2 stores are of constant capacitance as PO_2 levels change. Variations in the shapes of the areas representing blood stores are attributable to changes in the blood O_2 capacitance coefficients as a function of PO_2 (Boutilier and Shelton, 1986a), the volume of blood being constant. In the lung store, there are apparent increases in capacitance at high PO_2 levels because the lung volume declines during a dive, $\beta O_{2,gas}$ being constant. The dashed line in the lung store illustrates the line of constant capacitance that would occur if lung volume was also constant (at 8 ml) throughout the dive.

In the model (Fig. 3 A), changes in the O_2 store of each compartment (except for cutaneous venous blood), are plotted at 5-min intervals on the basis of data where the lung gas PO_2 falls linearly from a predive level of 130 torr to 40 torr (see Fig. 2). Thereafter, the stores were estimated using blood-gas O_2 equilibration data (Boutilier and Shelton, 1986c) and blood O_2 dissociation curves (Boutilier and Shelton, 1986a). The O_2 content of systemic venous blood (C_{sv}) at the beginning of the dive (time zero) was calculated from the cell O_2 consumption ($\dot{V}O_2$), systemic arterial O_2 content (C_{sa}), and a systemic blood flow rate of ($\dot{Q}_s$) of 14 ml/min (Shelton, 1970):

$$C_{sv} = C_{sa} - \dot{V}O_2/\dot{Q}_s \quad (3)$$

The total amount of O_2 in the systemic venous store ($VO_{2,svs}$) is the product of the blood O_2 content (Boutilier and Shelton, 1986a) and the systemic venous blood volume:

$$VO_{2,svs} = C \times V_{sv} \quad (4)$$

The decline in the systemic venous O_2 store was, thereafter, calculated at 5-min intervals as the difference between the O_2 consumption of the cells ($VO_{2,cells}$) and that taken up cutaneously ($VO_{2,cut}$), as well as that coming from stores in lung gas ($VO_{2,gas}$), pulmonary venous blood ($VO_{2,pv}$), and systemic arterial blood ($VO_{2,sa}$), namely:

$$\Delta VO_{2,svs} = VO_{2,cells} - VO_{2,cut} - \Delta VO_{2,gas+pv+sa} \quad (5)$$

B. Regulation of Oxygen Supplies

It is clear from the model that the lung constitutes an important O_2 store from which supplies can be "metered out" during a dive. In addition to a substantial diving lung volume, the alveolar PO_2 following a breathing episode can reach levels as high as 140 to 150 torr (Boutilier and Shelton, 1986c), owing to the comparatively low dead space of these anatomically simple lungs (Smith and Rapson, 1977). It follows, too, that the blood leaving the lungs is also highly saturated with oxygen, despite there being less than complete blood-gas equilibrium (Boutilier and Shelton, 1986c) across the comparatively thick gas to blood barrier (Weibel, 1972).

Certainly, the systemic venous blood is also an important O_2 store, and one that is called upon extensively in the early stages of the modeled dive. The advantage of an early use of this store is one of reducing the PO_2 of the venous return and of the pulmocutaneous blood supply, as long as shunt 2 (S_2) is relatively small. Such conditions would facilitate continued O_2 uptake from the lung and skin even if the flow to these areas ($\dot{Q}_p$, $\dot{Q}_c$) were to become reduced. It is also easy to see how cutaneous O_2 uptake could be increased under these conditions, especially so if there were simultaneous recruitment of skin capillaries (see Burggren and Moalli, 1984). The early use of the venous store occurs as a result of a reduction in systemic blood flow (calculated from a rearranged Equation 3) from 14 ml/min at time zero to 6 ml/min at 5 min, 4 ml/min at 10 min, and 3 ml/min thereafter. Reductions such as these can be produced by increasing systemic resistance (R_s) or decreasing cardiac output, both of which occur as part of the "diving response" in this animal (Shelton, 1970; Emilio and Shelton, 1972).

The model can also be used to predict how other O_2 storage locations could be utilized throughout the course of a dive, their rate of use being determined in large part by the gas concentration differences and the rates of perfusion. For example, selective pulmonary vasoconstriction would lead to an increase in the resistance of the pulmonary circuit (R_p increase, Fig. 3 B), thereby causing $\dot{Q}_p$ to fall more than $\dot{Q}_s$, increasing shunt 1 and, thereby, conserving the stores in the lung and pulmonary vein. Under these conditions, the systemic and venous blood O_2 stores would be used more rapidly than is shown (see Fig. 3 A), facilitating even greater possibilities for cutaneous gas exchange. During the course of such a dive, the ever-diminishing blood PO_2 would presumably lead to a progressively increasing extraction of O_2 from the lung O_2 store. Marked changes in the O_2 depletion rates of the lung during prolonged voluntary dives have indeed been observed in these animals (see Fig. 2). In more active animals, lung O_2 extraction rates are high in the early stages of the dive (Boutilier and Shelton, 1986c), during which time blood flow to the lungs continues to be elevated at predive levels (Emilio and Shelton, 1972). Under such circumstances (maintained R_p decrease) there would be less likelihood of selective store useage because the arterial-venous PO_2 differences would not be increased and PO_2 levels in all parts of the storage system would move closer together than is detailed in the model.

It is important to remember that, despite such attempts to model gas exchange in lower vertebrates, these animals are more than capable of changing metabolic rates, blood flow distribution patterns, and their behavior throughout the course of a breathing-diving cycle. The present model examines only one of doubtless several and varied forms of O_2 store utilization during a dive.

IV. Gas Exchange and Respiratory Control

A. Acid-Base Balance

The skin of amphibians is extremely effective in CO_2 removal, usually excreting about 75% of that which is metabolically produced in gill-less forms (Hutchison et al., 1968). This facility for ridding the body cutaneously of an end product that is potentially disruptive to blood pH is particularly important during a dive, when the skin becomes the sole gas exchanger with the environment. Other diving vertebrates, with less permeable skin, must have comparatively greater abilities to either buffer the CO_2 produced or to tolerate wider excursions in blood and tissue pH.

Voluntary "Aerobic" Dives

In voluntarily diving *Amphiuma* (Toews et al., 1971) and *Xenopus* (Boutilier and Shelton, 1986b), blood PCO_2 levels increase during the initial few minutes of a dive, after which they appear to reach a near equilibrium state. In *Amphiuma*, the skin was found to be extremely effective in ameliorating any significant build up of CO_2, either during voluntary dives (Toews et al., 1971) or after injections of CO_2 into the lungs (Fig. 4). Measurements of blood pH accompanying such PCO_2 changes in voluntarily diving *Xenopus* have shown that a small respiratory acidosis develops over the first 10 min of a dive, with the acid-base state eventually reaching a new homeostasis that, thereafter, lasts as long as the dive. Presumably, the development of these new steady states for blood and lung gas PCO_2 (i.e., Fig. 5), are the result of the skin being able to eliminate all of the CO_2 being produced by the resting metabolism. It is important to add, however, that because the CO_2 capacitances of the tissues and blood are also quite large, CO_2 storage also has a role to play in the acid-base homeostasis of diving. Such stores are subsequently mobilized and released to the atmosphere during episodes of lung ventilation; this cyclic CO_2 exchange is bound to be more pronounced in animals with less permeable cutaneous surfaces.

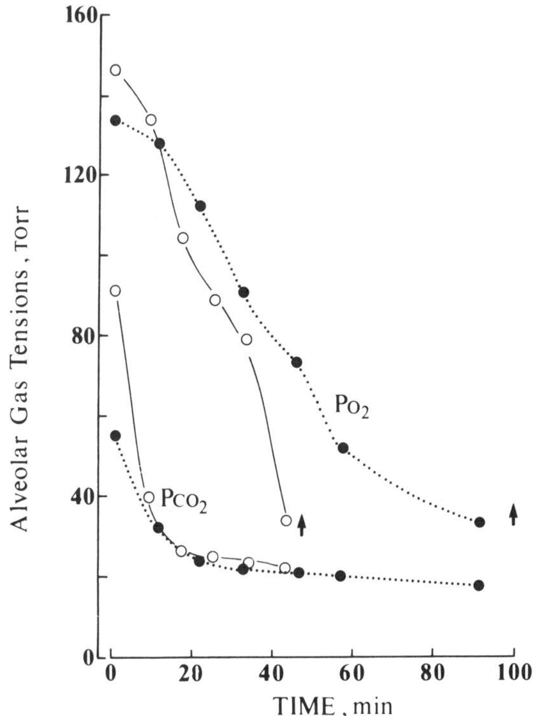

Figure 4 The removal of high levels of CO_2 and normal levels of O_2 from the lungs of two voluntarily diving *Amphiuma tridactylum* at 15°C. Carbon dioxide–air mixtures were injected into the lungs shortly after each animal voluntarily dived. Note that the extremely high levels of PCO_2 (normal $PACO_2$ of this animal is ~ 14 torr) did not stimulate breathing. Breathing times are marked by vertical arrows. (Adapted from Toews, 1971, with permission.)

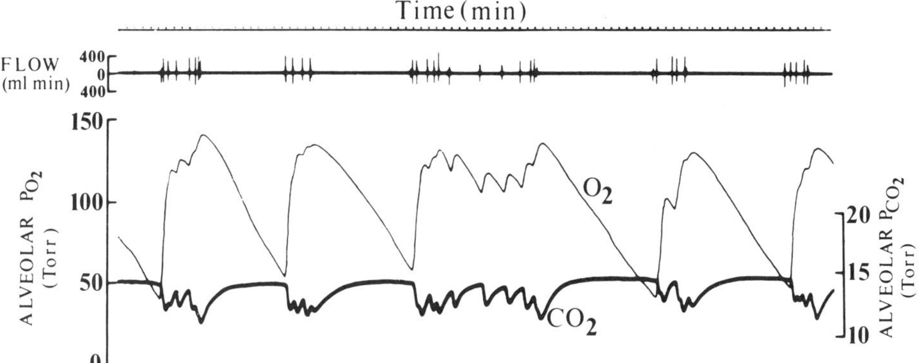

Figure 5 Continuous recordings of lung ventilation (shown as vertical deflections produced by gas flowing through a blowhole fitted with a pneumotachograph) and corresponding lung gas tensions in voluntarily diving and surfacing *Xenopus* at 25°C. The traces of lung ventilation are adjusted in time to take account of the delay in the extracorporeal loop used for lung gas partial pressure measurement. Animal in air-equilibrated water and breathing air at a blowhole. (From Boutilier and Shelton, 1986c.)

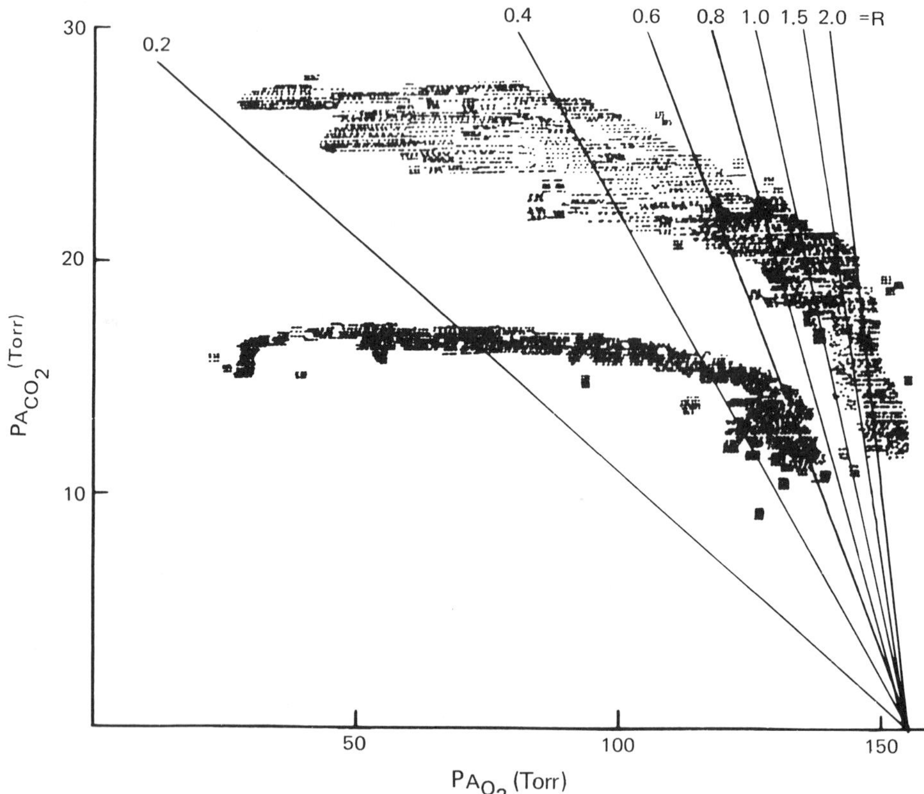

Figure 6 The relationships between alveolar PO_2 (PAO_2) and PCO_2 ($PACO_2$) in *X. laevis* during voluntary diving and surfacing in air-equilibrated conditions (lower plot) and subjected on the next day to aquatic hypercapnia (upper plot). Hypercapnia was administered by equilibrating the tank water with a 1% CO_2/ 99% air mixture; however, the animal was breathing air when ventilating its lungs at a surface blowhole. Lung R lines are shown from 0.2 to 2.0. Temperature = 25°C. (From Boutilier and Shelton, 1986c.)

"Anaerobic" Dives

Clearly, the acid-base state of a diving animal can be markedly affected if for any reason the animal must resort to anaerobic metabolism. In a variety of amphibians, such circumstances lead to a combined respiratory and metabolic lact-acidosis (Lenfant and Johansen, 1967; Jones, 1972; Emilio, 1974; Emilio and Shelton, 1980), recovery from which is usually several times longer than the dive itself (Boutilier and Shelton, 1986a,b; Toews and Boutilier, 1986). The large respiratory component of the acidosis occurs as a result of dehydration of plasma bicarbonate with protons of anaerobic origin. Whereas the animal can immediately begin to offset the increased PCO_2 levels by hyperventilation upon sufacing, readjustment of the HCO_3^-/CO_2 equilibrium is more complex and time-consuming, requiring renal and/or transcutaneous net uptake of bicarbonate equivalent ions (Boutilier and Heisler, 1988). Such dives are obviously quite energetically costly in comparison with the purely respiratory nature of aerobic dives and are probably avoided whenever possible.

B. Ventilatory Readjustment of Oxygen and Carbon Dioxide Stores Following a Dive

During a dive, the changes in blood and lung gas PCO_2 are much smaller than those of PO_2 as a consequence of greater capacity for tissue CO_2 storage and transepithelial elimination. Indeed, in the latter stages of a dive, the instantaneous gas exchange ratio of the lung often reaches zero (Fig. 6) and lung volume declines as more O_2 is taken up than is replaced by CO_2. Upon surfacing to breathe, therefore, there is a need to recharge not only the O_2 stores (primarily in blood and lungs) but also to discharge the body of builtup stores of CO_2 (primarily in blood and tissues). When blood and tissue PCO_2 levels increase even higher, as they do during anaerobic dives or periods of aquatic hypercapnia (Boutilier and Shelton, 1986b,c), the considerable hyperventilation upon surfacing results in lung R values that are much higher than the metabolic RQ of the animal (see Fig. 6). These elevated R values are attributable to the different rates at which the O_2 and CO_2 stores are adjusted during ventilation. Because most of the diving O_2 store is located in the blood and lungs, it can be readjusted much faster than can CO_2, which must be mobilized from stores in the blood, tissues, and cells. Certainly, the capacity for increasing pulmonary blood flow during periods of lung ventilation (Shelton, 1970; Johansen et al., 1970; West and Burggren, 1984) must aid in reducing the amount of time required for complete readjustment of the gas stores (see also Wood, 1984).

Upon surfacing from a dive, the efficacy with which O_2 and CO_2 stores are readjusted may depend, in a large part, upon the gas-carrying properties of blood (Lenfant and Johansen, 1967; Jokumsen and Weber, 1980; Boutilier and Shelton, 1986a). In *Xenopus* blood, for example, a high Bohr and Haldane effect, (Boutilier and Shelton, 1986a) in comparison with more semiterrestrial anurans (Tazawa et al., 1979; Boutilier and Toews, 1981), seems particularly well matched to the animal's predominantly aquatic existence and periodic nature of air breathing. Thus, whereas deoxygenated blood may be used as an effective storage site for the delivery of CO_2 to the lungs during breathing (or skin during a dive), the comparatively high Bohr effect represents an adaptation to facilitate delivery of the O_2 store to the tissues during a dive. It has also been suggested that such biochemical adaptations may be evolutionarily linked to the changes in respiratory blood flow that occur during intermittent ventilation in these animals. Such changes are made possible by the undivided ventricle (Shelton, 1976; West and Burggren, 1984) and in *Xenopus* appear to match the Haldane effect, with high blood flow to the lungs during breathing, and the Bohr effect, to an increasing movement of blood into the systemic circuit as a dive progresses (Shelton and Boutilier, 1982).

Adaptations for effective gas turnover are also seen at the level of the ventilatory apparatus itself. In *Amphiuma tridactylum* and *Siren lacertina*, for example, the entire lung receives fresh air with each inspiratory cycle as a result of a complete collapse of the lung during the exhalation that precedes the lung-filling phase (Martin and Hutchison, 1979). Such lung ventilations occur periodically between dives, lasting up to an hour or more (Toews et al., 1971), and the entire ventilatory cycle is over within 4 to 5 s, leaving little time for equilibration of blood and tissue compartments with lung gases. Interestingly, *Amphiuma* and *Siren* are particularly tolerant of high levels of CO_2 in their blood and tissues (Toews, 1971; Heisler et al., 1982). Combined with their ventilatory insensitivity to CO_2 (see Fig. 4) and a marked capacity for nonpulmonary CO_2 removal (Toews, 1971), this suggests that the lung ventilation cycle in *Amphiuma* (Martin and Hutchison, 1979) is primarily directed at recharging the O_2 stores in the lungs and blood. On the other hand, pulmonary ventilation in anuran divers is not only CO_2-sensitive, but it is also thought to play an important role in controlling CO_2 losses to the environment (Gottlieb and Jackson, 1976; Jackson and Braun, 1979; Boutilier, 1984). Upon surfacing, air breathing in these animals usually occurs as a series of lung ventilations (see Fig. 5; Boutilier, 1984, 1988) during which there is time for gas storage compartments in the blood and tissues to come into equilibrium with the lung gas pool.

C. Factors Affecting the Onset and Termination of Diving

Respiratory control of the onset and termination of a dive is thought to occur as a result of signals arising from chemo- and mechanosensitive receptors responding to changing conditions during breathing and diving. In amphibians, in which the gills or the skin are important avenues for CO_2 loss, it appears that falling levels of O_2 are the primary stimulus involved in the termination of a dive (Toews, 1971; Toews et al., 1971; Emilio and Shelton, 1974; Boutilier and Shelton, 1986b,c). Throughout the course of a dive, more O_2 is taken up from the lung than is replaced by CO_2 owing to the unevenly balanced exchange of O_2 and CO_2 that occurs across the skin of these animals (see Shelton et al., 1986). As a result, the volume of the lung will change more rapidly when the depletion rate of O_2 is high, and this in itself could furnish mechanosensitive information about the rate of use of the lung gas store. Certainly, pulmonary stretch receptors exist in the lungs of amphibians (reviewed by Jones and Milsom, 1982) and are thought to be important in the coordination of breathing and diving in these animals (Shelton and Boutilier, 1982; Boutilier, 1988). In *Xenopus*, for example, lung denervation leads to an overinflation of the lungs that is so great that the animals are unable to dive (Evans and Shelton, 1984). On the other hand, distension of the lungs of voluntarily diving *Amphiuma* with pure N_2 can be used to delay the onset of breathing (Toews, 1971). The delay can be further enhanced by injections of air or, even more so, with O_2, indicating that both mechano- and chemosensitive mechanisms are involved in bringing a dive to an end.

The rate of use of the lung O_2 store is thought to be a factor of some significance in *Xenopus* because dives end at higher values of alveolar PO_2 (PAO_2) when the decline is rapid than when it is slow (see Fig. 2). Dives also come to an end at relatively high PAO_2 values when $PACO_2$ levels become elevated during aquatic hypercapnia (see Fig. 6) or exercise (Boutilier and Shelton, 1986c). These conditions also lead to a marked increase in ventilation brought about by increasing the amount of time spent breathing at the surface (i.e., decreasing the duration of subsequent dives; Boutilier, 1984, 1988). Aquatic hypoxia elicits very similar ventilatory responses in *Xenopus* (Brett, 1980), *Rana catesbeiana* (Boutilier, unpublished observations), and *Amphiuma* (Toews, 1971). Whereas experiments on *Xenopus* suggest that elevated CO_2 levels modulate the sensitivity of a predominantly O_2-mediated emergence response (Boutilier and Shelton, 1986c), there appears to be no such interaction between the two respiratory gases in *Amphiuma* (Toews, 1971).

The information that brings ventilation to an end also appears to originate with mechano- and chemosensitive receptors. In *Amphiuma*, for example, less than full lung distension during a breathing cycle is enough to delay the onset of a dive and prolong the period of lung ventilation (Toews, 1971). Measurements of blood and lung gases in undisturbed *Xenopus* have shown that, after a voluntary dive, the readjustment of gas stores probably occurs within the first few breaths of a breathing episode (Boutilier and Shelton, 1986b; see Fig. 5). If, on the other hand, the animal has been highly active or exposed to hypercapnic water (see Fig. 6), the hyperventilation following a dive continues well beyond the point at which PAO_2 and PaO_2 are fully returned to normal. This suggests that breathing may continue until all of the builtup CO_2 stores have been removed from the body and that pH or PCO_2 may be more important than body oxygenation in determining the end of a breathing episode in *Xenopus*. In *Amphiuma*, however, the comparatively brief 4- to 5-s period for lung gas renewal (Martin and Hutchison, 1979), leaves hardly enough time for readjustment of blood and tissue stores of O_2, let alone CO_2 (Toews et al., 1971; Shelton, 1985). This, together with its large capacity for extrapulmonary CO_2 release (see Fig. 4) probably means that O_2, rather than CO_2, plays a more important role in effecting both the onset and termination of a dive in *Amphiuma*.

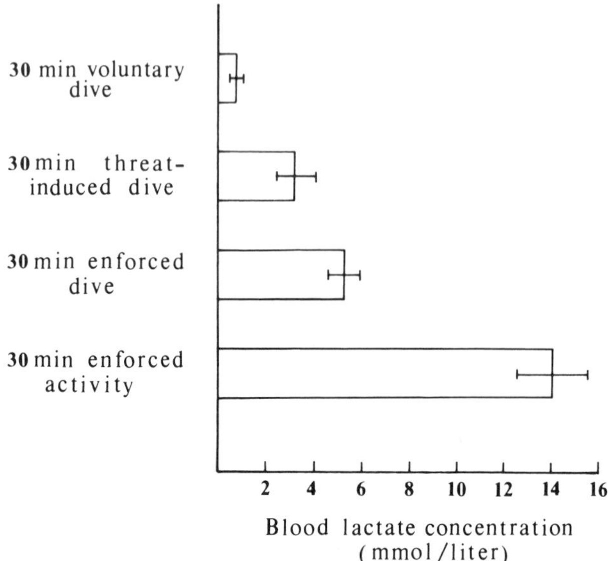

Figure 7 Lactate concentrations measured in blood taken from indwelling catheters in *X. laevis* subjected to various conditions at 20–25°C. Data for voluntary and enforced dives from Boutilier and Shelton (1986b), and for exercise from Boutilier et al. (1986b). Threat-induced dives are taken from unpublished material of the author.

V. Adaptations to Limited Oxygen Supplies

A. Diving Metabolism

As a way to extend diving time, many animals have the possibility of reducing their metabolic rate and, thus, the energetic demands of the dive. Indeed, O_2 uptake during enforced breath holding or submergence of anurans, decreases to between 45 and 80% of the predive value (Jones, 1967; Emilio and Shelton, 1980). Certainly, the pronounced asphyxial defense mechanisms of bradycardia, selective peripheral vasoconstriction, and anaerobiosis, which form the so-called diving reflex in higher animals (see Butler and Jones, 1982), would not seem very advantageous to an animal that respires cutaneously. Bradycardia occurs during both forced and voluntary dives, although to a much greater extent in the former (Jones and Shelton, 1964; Toews et al., 1971; Lillo, 1979). Although the bradycardia of voluntary diving is probably indicative of more widespread energetic savings, little work has been carried out in this area. The cardiorespiratory correlates associated with surfacing to breathe probably represent an "emergence reflex" as much, or even more so, than does the bradycardia of submergence represent a "diving reflex."

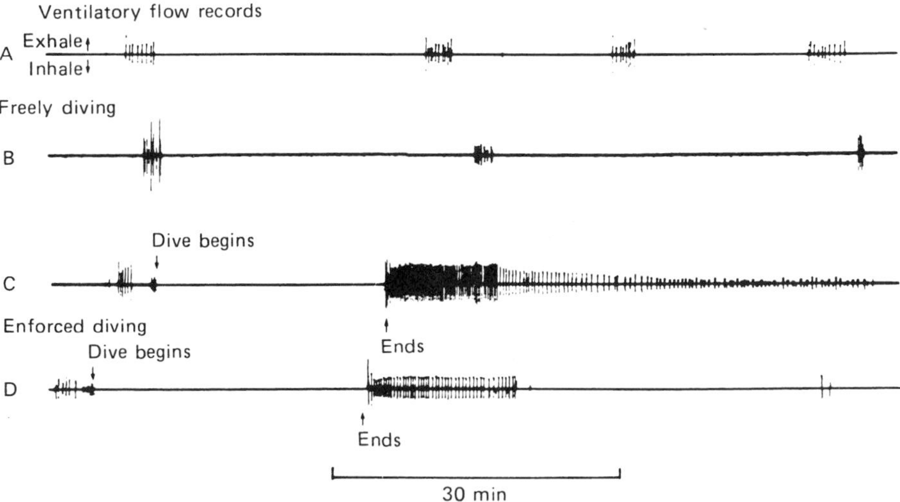

Figure 8 Lung ventilations and periods of breath holding showing intermittent ventilation pattern of voluntarily diving *Xenopus* (A,B) and the ventilation before and after two enforced dives of approximately 30-min duration (C,D). Breathing movements were detected when animals surfaced to breathe at a blowhole fitted with a pneumotachograph. The large increase in ventilation in the first breathing episode following an enforced dive is entirely due to the extra amount of time spent at the surface because breathing frequency and depth are not significantly different between pre- and postdive analyses. (From Boutilier and Shelton, 1986b.)

B. Anaerobiosis and Diving

Amphibians utilize anaerobic pathways during periods of functional tissue hypoxia brought on by environmental or organismal challenge (Rose and Drotman, 1967; Christiansen and Penny, 1973; Bennett, 1978; Toews and Boutilier, 1986; Fig. 7). Thus, during any extension of underwater activity (e.g., flight from predators or pursuit of prey), anaerobiosis can be used to extend the underwater activity range of the animal. It can also be argued that during relatively inactive dives, when O_2 stores are being slowly exploited, sudden bursts of mechanical power might require the activation of anaerobic pathways long before the O_2 stores are fully depleted, just as for animals on land. In addition, the O_2 content of the water and, thus, the relative capacity for extrapulmonary O_2 uptake (Boutilier et al., 1986a) might also influence the degree to which the anaerobic arsenal needs to be recruited during a prolonged or highly active dive. Unlike other diving vertebrates, this facility for extrapulmonary gas exchange affords a stopgap against total dependence on anaerobiosis when body O_2 stores run down.

In *Xenopus*, anaerobiosis is called upon during strenuous exercise, enforced diving, or when a voluntary dive is prolonged as the result of a threat being imposed at the surface (see Fig. 7). In the undisturbed *Xenopus*, however, even the longest dives are normally terminated long before the O_2 stores run out (see Figs. 2, 3, and 5), thereby eliminating the need to recruit anaerobic energy sources (Boutilier and Shelton, 1986a,b). It has been suggested that during threat-induced dives, brain centers higher than the medulla must be involved in overriding stimuli from chemical or mechanical receptors involved in the initiation of breathing (Boutilier and Shelton, 1986c; Boutilier, 1988). Diving times also appear to be extended, presumably beyond the aerobic capacity of the submerged animal, as a result of courtship (Halliday and Sweatman, 1976), one of doubtless several competitive interactions where underwater behavior patterns become incompatible with aerial gas exchange.

The O_2 debt and acid–base disturbance associated with enforced dives have a major impact on the frequency and duration of subsequent voluntary dives. In studies on *Xenopus*, restoration of acid–base balance and repayment of the O_2 debt after a 30-min "anaerobic" dive (see Fig. 7) can take upward of 4 h, whereas the effects of voluntary dives of similar duration are usually over with after the first few breaths upon surfacing (Emilio and Shelton, 1980; Boutilier and Shelton, 1986b,c). Marked differences in postdive activities are clearly seen when comparing the breathing behavior after forced and voluntary dives of similar duration (Fig. 8). The enforced anaerobic dive has a major impact on the subsequent aerobic diving schedule of the animal, effectively decreasing the time that can be devoted to underwater pursuits. Thus, although sudden bursts of activity associated with feeding or survival may well be traded off against the development of an oxygen debt, most routine dives are probably aerobic.

References

Bennett, A. F. (1978). Activity metabolism in the lower vertebrates. *Annu. Rev. Physiol. 400*:447–469.

Boutilier, R. G. (1984). Characterization of the intermittent breathing pattern in *Xenopus laevis*. *J. Exp. Biol. 110*:291–309.

Boutilier, R. G. (1988). Control of arrhythmic breathing in bimodal breathers: Amphibia. *Can. J. Zool. 66*:6–19.

Boutilier, R. G., Glass, M. L., and Heisler, N. (1986a). The relative distribution of pulmocutaneous blood flow in *Rana catesbeiana*: Effects of pulmonary or cutaneous hypoxia. *J. Exp. Biol. 126*:33–39.

Boutilier, R. G., Emilio, M. G., and Shelton, G. (1986b). The effects of mechanical work on electrolyte and water distribution in amphibian skeletal muscle. *J. Exp. Biol. 120*:333–350.

Boutilier, R. G., and Heisler, N. (1988). Acid-base regulation and blood gases in the anuran amphibian, *Bufo marinus*, during environmental hypercapnia. *J. Exp. Biol. 134*:79-98.

Boutilier, R. G., and Shelton, G. (1986a). Respiratory properties of blood from voluntarily and forcibly submerged *Xenopus laevis. J. Exp. Biol. 121*:285-300.

Boutilier, R. G., and Shelton, G. (1986b). The effects of voluntary and forced diving on ventilation, blood gases and pH in *Xenopus laevis. J. Exp. Biol. 122*:209-222.

Boutilier, R. G., and Shelton, G. (1986c). Gas exchange, storage and transport in voluntarily diving *Xenopus laevis. J. Exp. Biol. 126*:133-155.

Boutilier, R. G., and Toews, D. P. (1981). Respiratory properties of blood in a strictly aquatic and predominantly skin breathing urodele, *Cryptobranchus alleganiensis. Respir. Physiol. 46*:161-176.

Brett, S. S. (1980). Breathing and gas exchange in an aquatic amphibian, *Xenopus laevis*. Ph.D. dissertation, University of East Anglia, England.

Burggren, W., and Moalli, R. (1984). "Active" regulation of cutaneous gas exchange by capillary recruitment in amphibians: Experimental evidence and a revised model for skin respiration. *Respir. Physiol. 55*:379-392.

Butler, P. J., and Jones, D. R. (1982). The comparative physiology of diving in vertebrates. In *Advances in Comparative Physiology and Biochemistry*, Vol. 8, New York, Academic Press, pp. 179-364.

Christiansen, J., and Penny, D. (1973). Anaerobic glycolysis and lactic acid accumulation in cold submerged *Rana pipiens. J. Comp. Physiol. 87*:237-245.

Emilio, M. G. (1974). Gas exchanges and blood gas concentrations in the frog, *Rana ridibunda. J. Exp. Biol. 60*:901-908.

Emilio, M. G., and Shelton, G. (1972). Factors affecting blood flow to the lungs in the amphibian, *Xenopus laevis. J. Exp. Biol. 56*:67-77.

Emilio, M. G., and Shelton, G. (1974). Gas exchange and its effect on blood gas concentrations in the amphibian, *Xenopus laevis. J. Exp. Biol. 60*:567-579.

Emilio, M. G., and Shelton, G. (1980). Carbon dioxide exchange and its effects on pH and bicarbonate equilibria in the blood of the amphibian *Xenopus laevis. J. Exp. Biol. 83*:253-262.

Evans, B. K., and Shelton, G. (1984). Ventilation in *Xenopus laevis* after lung or carotid labyrinth denervation. In *Proceedings of the First Congress of Comparative Physiology and Biochemistry*. Liege, Belgium, A 75.

Gottlieb, G., and Jackson, D. C. (1976). Importance of pulmonary ventilation in respiratory control in the bullfrog. *Am. J. Physiol. 230*:608-613.

Halliday, T. R., and Sweatman, H. P. A. (1976). To breathe or not to breathe: The newt's problem. *Anim. Behav. 24*:551-561.

Heisler, N., Forcht, G., Ultsch, G., and Anderson, J. F. (1982). Acid-base regulation in response to environmental hypercapnia in two aquatic salamanders, *Siren lacertina* and *Amphiuma means. Respir. Physiol. 49*:141-158.

Hutchison, V. H., Whitford, W. G., and Kohl, M. (1968). Relation of body size and surface area to gas exchange in anurans. *Physiol. Zool. 41*:65-85.

Jackson, D. C., and Braun, B. A. (1979). Respiratory control in bullfrogs: Cutaneous versus pulmonary response to selective CO_2 exposure. *J. Comp. Physiol. 129*:339-342.

Johansen, K., Lenfant, C., and Hanson, D. (1970). Phylogenetic development of pulmonary circulation. *Fed. Proc. 29*:1135-1140.

Jokumsen, A., and Weber, R. E. (1980). Haemoglobin-oxygen binding properties in the blood of *Xenopus laevis*, with special reference to the influences of aestivation and of temperature and salinity acclimation. *J. Exp. Biol. 86*:19-37.

Jones, D. R. (1967). Oxygen consumption and heart rate of several species of anuran Amphibia during submergence. *Comp. Biochem. Physiol. 20*:691-707.

Jones, D. R. (1972). Anaerobiosis and the oxygen debt in an anuran amphibian, *Rana esculenta (L.). J. Comp. Physiol. 77*:356-382.

Jones, D. R., and Milsom, W. K. (1982). Peripheral receptors affecting breathing and cardiovascular function in non-mammalian vertebrates. *J. Exp. Biol. 100*:59-91.

Jones, D. R., and Shelton, G. (1964). Factors influencing submergence and heart rate in the frog. *J. Exp. Biol. 41*:417-431.

Lenfant, C., and Johansen, K. (1967). Respiratory adaptations in selected amphibians. *Respir. Physiol. 2*:247-260.

Lillo, R. S. (1979). Autonomic cardiovascular control during submergence and emergence in bullfrogs. *Am. J. Physiol. 237*:R210-R216.

Martin, K. M., and Hutchison, V. H. (1979). Ventilatory activity in *Amphiuma tridactylum* and *Siren lacertina* (Amphibia, Caudata). *J. Herpitol. 13*:427-434.

Malvin, G. M., and Boutilier, R. G. (1985). Ventilation-perfusion relationships in Amphibia. In *Circulation, Respiration, and Metabolism*. Edited by R. Gilles. Berlin, Springer-Verlag, pp. 114-124.

Piiper, J. (1982). Respiratory gas exchange at lungs, gills and tissues: Mechanisms and adjustments. *J. Exp. Biol. 100*:5-22.

Rose, F. L., and Drotman, R. B. (1967). Anaerobiosis in a frog, *Rana pipiens. J. Exp. Zool. 166*:427-432.

Shelton, G. (1970). The effect of lung ventilation on blood flow to the lungs and body of the amphibian, *Xenopus laevis. Respir. Physiol. 9*:183-196.

Shelton, G. (1976). Gas exchange, pulmonary blood supply, and the partially divided amphibian heart. In *Perspectives in Experimental Biology*. Edited by P. Spencer Davies. Oxford, Pergamon Press, pp. 247-259.

Shelton, G. (1985). Functional and evolutionary significance of cardiovascular shunts in the Amphibia. In *Cardiovascular Shunts*. Edited by K. Johansen and W. W. Burggren. Alfred Benzon Symposium 21, Copenhagen, Munksgaard, pp. 100-120.

Shelton, G., Jones, D. R., and Milsom, W. K. (1986). Control of breathing in ectothermic vertebrates. In *Handbook of Physiology*, Section 3, Vol. 2. Edited by N. S. Cherniack and J. G. Widdicombe. Washington, American Physiological Society, Bethesda, MD., pp. 857-909.

Shelton, G., and Boutilier, R. G. (1982). Apnoea in amphibians and reptiles. *J. Exp. Biol. 100*:245-273.

Smith, D. G., and Rapson, L. (1977). Differences in microvascular anatomy between *Bufo marinus* and *Xenopus laevis. Cell Tissue Res. 178*:1-15.

Tazawa, H., Mochizuki, M., and Piiper, J. (1979). Blood oxygen dissociation curve of the frogs *Rana catesbeiana* and *Rana brevipoda. J. Comp. Physiol. 129*:111-114.

Toews, D. P. (1971). Factors affecting the onset and termination of ventilation in the salamander, *Amphiuma tridactylum. Can. J. Zool. 49*:1231-1237.

Toews, D. P., and Boutilier, R. G. (1986). Acid-base regulation in the Amphibia. In *Acid-Base Regulation in Animals*. Edited by N. Heisler. Amsterdam, Elsevier, pp. 265-308.

Toews, D. P., Shelton, G., and Randall, D. J. (1971). Gas tensions in the lungs and major blood vessels of the urodele amphibian, *Amphiuma tridactylum. J. Exp. Biol. 55*:47-61.

Weibel, E. R. (1972). Morphometric estimation of pulmonary diffusion capacity. V. Comparative morphometry of alveolar lungs. *Respir. Physiol. 14*:26-43.

West, N. H., and Burggren, W. W. (1984). Control of pulmonary and cutaneous blood flow in the toad, *Bufo marinus. Am. J. Physiol. 247*:R884-R894.

Wood, S. C. (1984). Cardiovascular shunts and oxygen transport in lower vertebrates. *Am. J. Physiol. 16*:3-14.

23

Diving Physiology
Reptiles

ROGER S. SEYMOUR

University of Adelaide
Adelaide, South Australia, Australia

I. Introduction

Despite the importance placed by early workers on the role of the "diving response" in forced submergences in animals, it is now evident that natural, voluntary diving usually occurs aerobically in vertebrates. The classic picture of severe circulatory changes accompanying muscle ischemia and anaerobic metabolism, leading to pronounced acid-base disturbances, appears to be reserved for crucial situations involving offensive or defensive behavior underwater. Although the diving response may be of vital importance for survival of the animal, it is uncommon in routine dives. The major role of aerobic diving has been confirmed in reptiles by observing the temporal patterns of diving (e.g., Eckert et al., 1986; Rubinoff et al., 1986) and by measuring blood and body lactate in snakes (Seymour, 1979), lizards, (Gleeson, 1980a), turtles (Gatten, 1981), and crocodiles (Seymour et al., 1985).

The lung is the principal store of O_2 used during aerobic dives in most reptiles, although the blood may be important in a few species, and uptake of O_2 can occur through nonpulmonary gas exchange organs. This chapter deals with six aspects of pulmonary function: (1) the role of the lung as an O_2 source and

CO_2 sink, (2) the characteristics of gas transfer across the lung during intermittent ventilation, (3) the balance between nonpulmonary and pulmonary gas exchange, (4) the effect of deep diving and hydrostatic pressure on gas exchange, (5) the lung in buoyancy control, and (6) the effect of gravity on pulmonary circulation.

The coverage of this chapter is necessarily selective because the limited space will not accommodate the bulk of available information on aquatic reptiles. Indeed, most of what we know about pulmonary function in reptiles comes from aquatic species. Because only 8% of all reptiles are aquatic, the literature is, therefore, strongly biased.

More complete treatments of respiratory physiology of aquatic reptiles and extensive bibliographies can be found in Wood and Lenfant (1976), White (1976), Seymour (1982), Butler and Jones (1982), Glass and Wood (1983), Jackson (1985), and Lutz and Bentley (1985). Other aspects of the subject also appear in the present volume, principally within Chapters 7, 15, 19, and 20.

II. Oxygen Storage

Diving reptiles might be expected to have special adaptations for O_2 storage such as those that occur in endothermic divers (Butler and Jones, 1982), but no distinct trends appear (Seymour, 1982). Aquatic reptiles generally do not contain more O_2 than their terrestrial relatives, and sometimes considerably less. Lung volumes in voluntarily breathing reptiles are highly variable and probably relate to buoyancy in aquatic species (see Sect. VII), and maximum lung volumes are not correlated with diving behavior (Tenney and Tenney, 1970). Blood volumes, blood O_2 capacity, and muscle myoglobin concentration also do not correlate well with diving (Seymour, 1982). The conclusion is that the major differences between terrestrial and aquatic reptiles center around their ventilatory behavior. Breath holding has pronounced consequences for gas exchange.

III. Pulmonary Gas Exchange

A. Pattern of Breathing

Respiration in reptiles can be generally described as apneic. Periods of ventilation alternate with periods of breath holding in terrestrial as well as aquatic reptiles (Fig. 1). In aquatic species, however, the duration of apneic episodes is characteristically prolonged, and several breaths may be taken when the animal surfaces. Wholly terrestrial reptiles typically breathe more quickly and regularly. The aquatic pattern may persist when the reptile is removed from water, or it may shift to the terrestrial pattern. Exceptions to the aquatic pattern

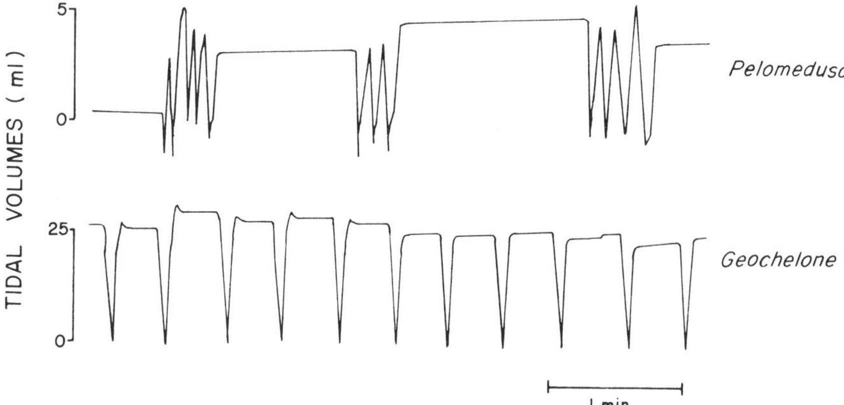

Figure 1 Patterns of ventilation in an aquatic (*Pelomedusa*) and a terrestrial (*Geochelone*) chelonian. (Adapted from Glass et al., 1978.)

appear in some marine turtles and snakes that often take only one breath between dives.

Intermittent ventilation results in unsteady gas exchange rates across the lung and large variation in blood gas tensions during the breathing cycle. This variability is greater in aquatic reptiles because of their typically longer apneic periods.

B. Gas Exchange During Apnea

Because of differences in CO_2 and O_2 capacitances of the lung gas and of body fluids, the kinetics of gas transfer across the lung depends on the duration of apnea. At the beginning of apnea, there is a rapid rate of CO_2 flux into the lung, but it quickly diminishes. Meanwhile, O_2 moves into the blood and the change in pulmonary P_{O_2} is greater than that of P_{CO_2}. The result is that the pulmonary respiratory exchange ratio ($R = \dot{V}_{CO_2}/\dot{V}_{O_2}$) decreases from values well above 1.0 during ventilation to values near zero (Fig. 2). A declining R value indicates storage of CO_2 in the carbonic buffer systems of the body or nonpulmonary CO_2 loss. In the semiaquatic turtle, *Pseudemys scripta*, storage of CO_2 is important because the overall value for R, integrated over several cycles of ventilation and apnea, approximates the estimated respiratory quotient of the fasting animal (Ackerman and White, 1979). It has been estimated that about 85% of the CO_2 produced by this turtle during apnea is stored in the body, only to be released during the brief ventilatory period (Burggren and Shelton, 1979). The slope of the P_{CO_2}-P_{O_2} diagram indicates the capacity of the body for holding

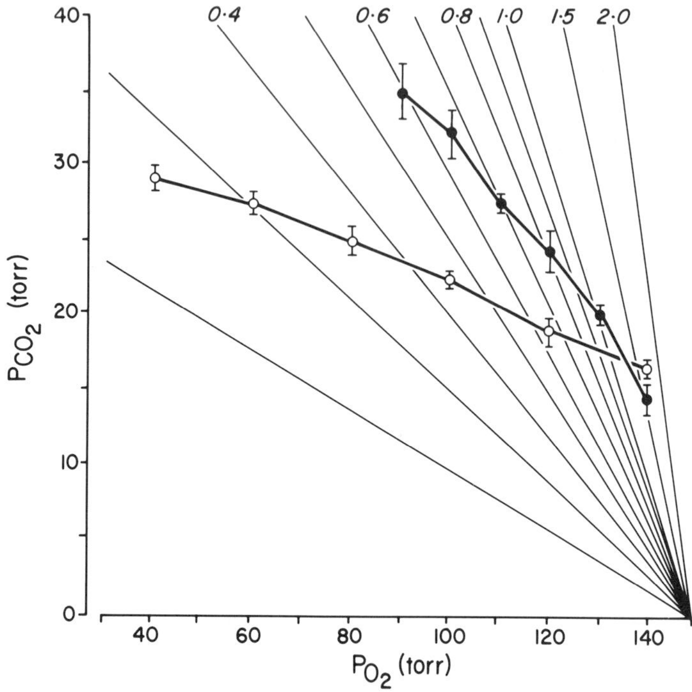

Figure 2 Relationship between PCO_2 and PO_2 in the pulmonary gas of an aquatic (*Pseudemys scripta*, open circles) and a terrestrial (*Testudo graeca*, filled circles) chelonian. The sloping lines indicate the pulmonary gas exchange ratio ($R = \dot{V}CO_2/\dot{V}O_2$). The data cross these lines, indicating that R decreases during breath holding. (Adapted from Burggren and Shelton, 1979.)

CO_2 as bicarbonate and carbamino compounds. The steeper slope for the terrestrial tortoise, *Testudo graeca* (see Fig. 2), suggests a lower CO_2 capacitance.

Considerable O_2 is removed from the lung during apnea. In *P. scripta*, for example, an estimated 88% of the O_2 requirement comes from the lung during a voluntary dive (Burggren and Shelton, 1979). In other species, however, O_2 storage in the blood is important, an extreme example being the aquatic file snakes, *Acrochordus* sp., with large blood volume and high O_2 saturation on both arterial and venous sides of the circulation (Feder, 1980; Seymour et al., 1981a).

The rate of O_2 uptake from the lung depends on the pulmonary blood flow and the venous–arterial O_2 content difference. There are several studies

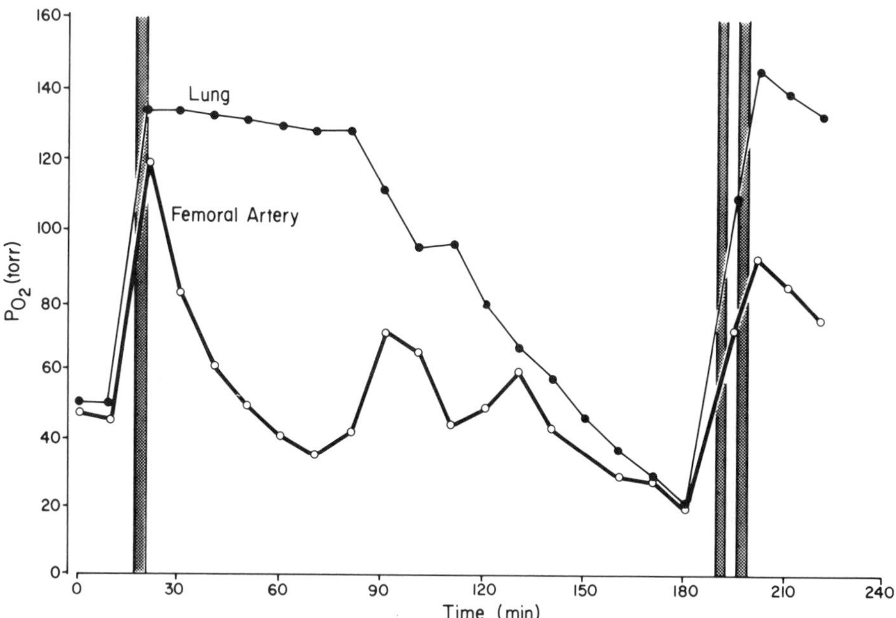

Figure 3 Relationship between PO_2 in the pulmonary gas and in systemic arterial blood of *Pseudemys scripta* between periods of ventilation (vertical bars). At the beginning of apnea, most O_2 is recruited from the blood, but later PO_2 decreases abruptly in the lung and increases in the blood, suggesting controlled shifts in pulmonary circulation. (Adapted from Burggren and Shelton, 1979).

that show cardiovascular control over the rate of O_2 recruitment during diving. In *P. scripta*, O_2 can be metered from the lung at more or less a constant rate during most short dives, but during longer dives, pulmonary PO_2 can dramatically change (Burggren and Shelton, 1979). An increased rate of O_2 recruitment is thought to result from an increase in pulmonary perfusion, and the arterialized blood PO_2 can actually rise during apnea (Fig. 3). In sea snakes, the fraction of venous blood bypassing the lung is high when pulmonary PO_2 is high, but it drops substantially when pulmonary PO_2 declines to levels at which the blood leaving the lung is no longer completely saturated (Fig. 4). Similarly, pulmonary blood flow and O_2 uptake from the lung of *Acrochordus arafurae* are low at the beginning of some dives, but can increase later (Fig. 5).

Continued O_2 uptake from the lung tends to concentrate the CO_2 there. In a short time, a seemingly paradoxical situation can arise in which the PCO_2

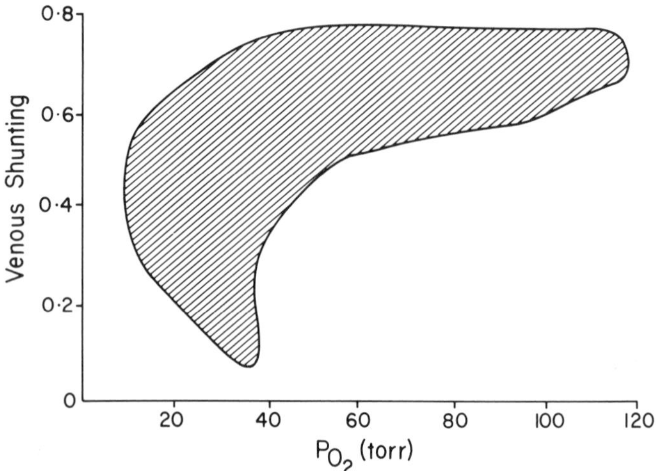

Figure 4 Fraction of venous blood shunted past the lung in relation to pulmonary PO_2 in sea snakes. The envelope includes all data from *Lapemis hardwickii* and *Acalyptophis peronii* (Seymour and Webster, 1975). Shunting is high when lung PO_2 is high, but declines at PO_2 corresponding to the steep portion of the Hb–O_2 equilibrium curves.

in the pulmonary vein becomes higher than that of the pulmonary artery (see Fig. 5), and the gradient for CO_2 flux appears reversed. However, it is not clear whether the lung actually becomes a source of CO_2 rather than a sink, because the oxygenation of the blood raises the PCO_2 without necessarily changing its CO_2 content (Haldane effect; White, 1985).

C. Gas Exchange During Ventilation

The CO_2 accumulated in the body during a breath hold is eliminated and the blood O_2 stores are replenished during the ventilatory period. To facilitate this exchange, there is often a substantial increase in pulmonary perfusion during the ventilatory period (Fig. 6). This may be accompanied by tachycardia, but also can result from increased stroke volume and from a shift in the pattern of central shunting. Cholinergic control of pulmonary flow exists in the pulmonary arteries, both proximally (in the pulmonary outflow tract of the heart) and distally (in the smaller arteries of the lung).

Despite an increase in pulmonary blood flow during ventilation, it is still low by mammalian standards, and considerable time may be required for equilibration between the body and the lung. Values of cardiac output taken from

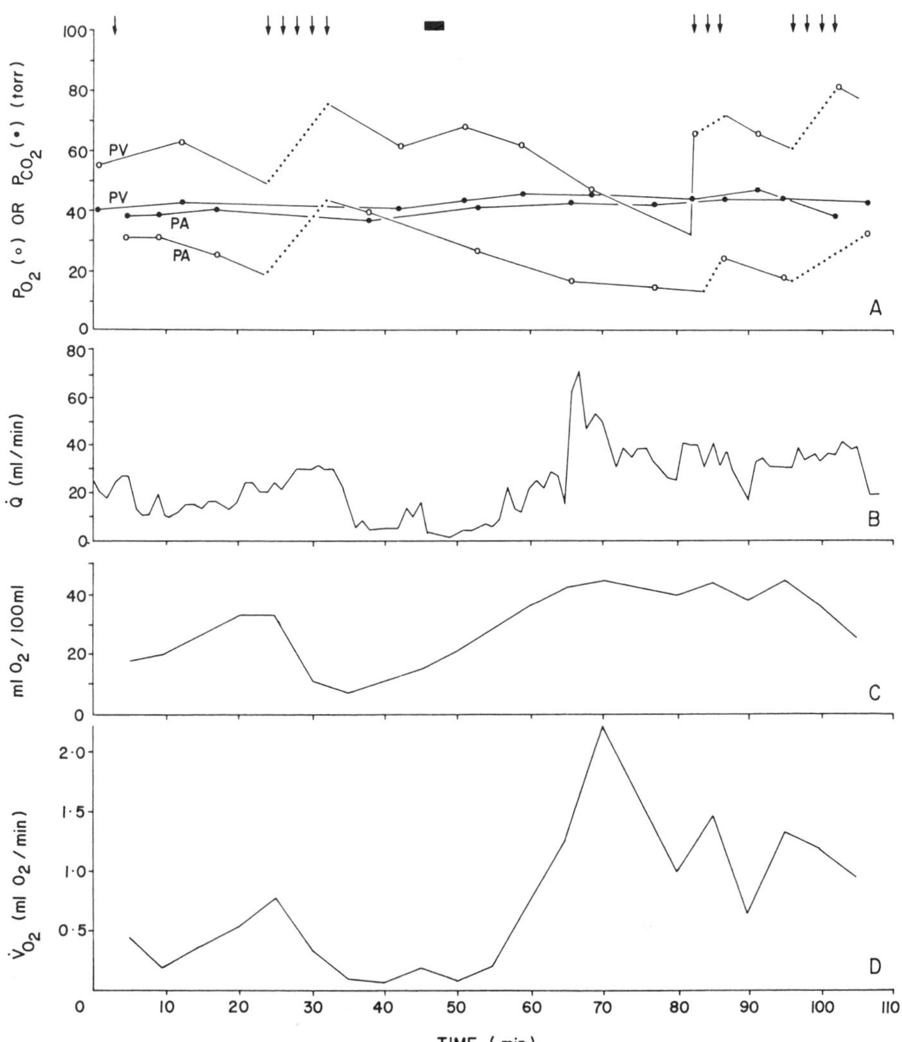

Figure 5 Gas tensions in the pulmonary artery and vein (A), total pulmonary blood flow (B), arterial–venous O_2 content difference (C) and rate of O_2 uptake from the lung (D) in diving snakes, *Acrochordus arafurae*. Arrows indicate individual breaths and the bar indicates a period of activity. Note that the PCO_2 is almost always higher in the pulmonary vein than in the artery and that the rate of O_2 uptake from the lung increases during apnea. (From Seymour et al., 1981a.)

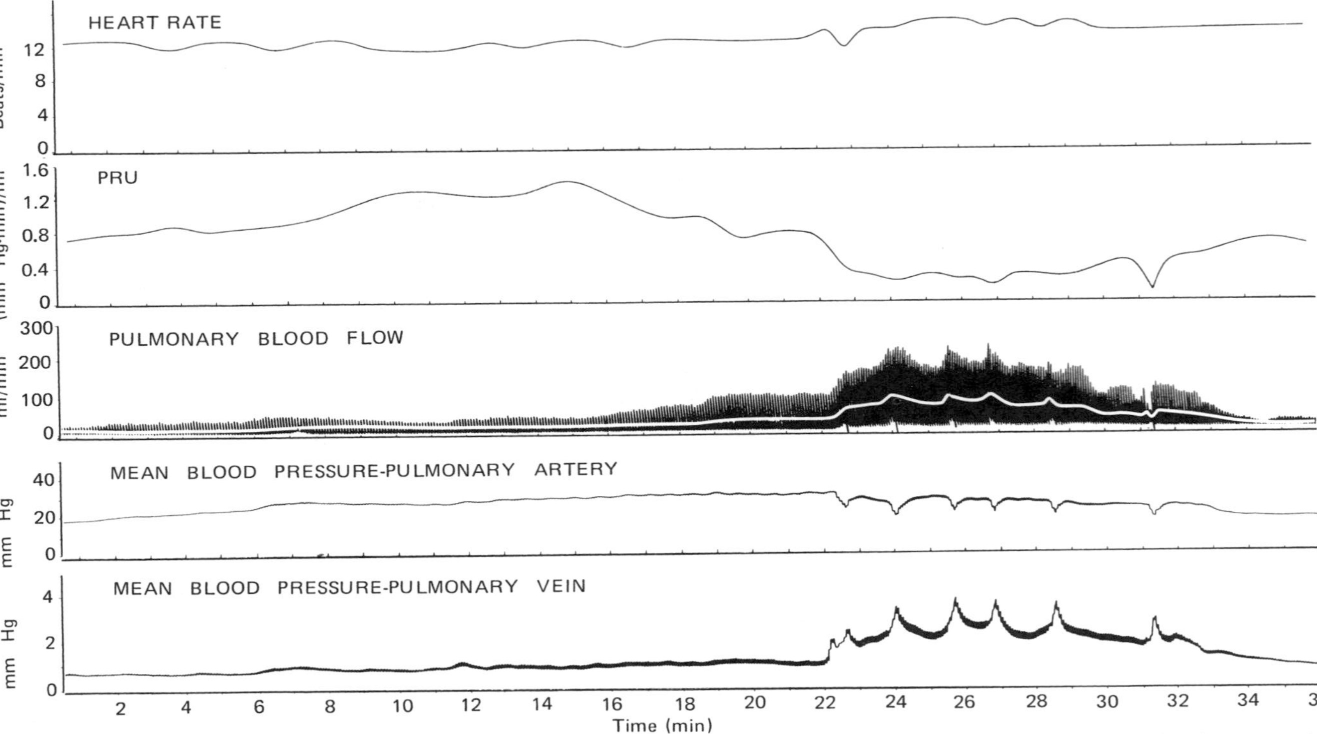

Figure 6 Heart rate, pulmonary peripheral resistance, instantaneous and mean pulmonary blood flow, and blood pressure in the aquatic snake, *A. arafurae*. The record shows a long period of apnea followed by a protracted ventilatory period during which six breaths are taken. The marked increase in blood flow results from decreased resistance, without much change in heart rate. (From Seymour, 1982.)

the literature indicate that it takes approximately 1 to 10 min to pass the entire blood volume through reptilian lungs. These periods probably determine the duration of the ventilatory period. An example comes from *A. arafurae* in which considerable O_2 is stored in the venous side of the circulation. To facilitate reoxygenation of this store, pulmonary flow increases from 6.8 ml/kg · min in apnea to 13.6 ml/kg · min during ventilation (Seymour et al., 1981a). With a blood volume of 133 ml/kg (Feder, 1980), it would require about 10 min to expose all of the blood to the lung, without any recirculation. The average duration of the ventilatory period (about 8 min) is close to the predicted requirement. During this period, the snake takes an average of 5.5 breaths, each separated by short breath holds of 0.5 to 2 min. It is calculated from metabolic rate, tidal volume, and pulmonary gas tensions that these multiple breaths are required to eliminate CO_2. Each breath can eliminate only 1.7 ml CO_2, but about 7.25 ml are produced during each diving cycle.

IV. Nonpulmonary Gas Exchange

The reptiles are generally characterized by a thick, cornified skin that reduces the rate of evaporative water loss. This feature, among others, allowed the radiation of reptiles into many terrestrial habitats where they did not have to rely on access to water. Fully terrestrial reptiles no longer needed cutaneous gas exchange that their amphibian ancestors presumably possessed, and a premium was placed on water conservation. However, multiple lines of reptiles successfully reinvaded the water where selection for nonpulmonary gas exchange was reestablished. Consequently, we now see redevelopment of cutaneous gas exchangers in aquatic snakes, and buccal, pharyngeal, and cloacal gas exchangers in aquatic turtles (Seymour, 1982; Feder and Burggren, 1985).

In sea snakes, cutaneous gas exchange is facilitated by a proliferation of cutaneous capillaries that are highly concentrated in the outermost zone of the dermis (Fig. 7; Rosenberg and Voris, 1980). It is remarkable that the redevelopment of cutaneous gas exchange was not necessarily accompanied by higher permeability of the skin to water (Dunson, 1986). However, water permeability of reptilian integument is related to the presence of cutaneous lipids (Roberts and Lillywhite, 1980), not scales (Bennett and Licht, 1975). Respiratory gases are lipid soluble and should not be greatly impeded by this barrier to water. Unfortunately, the relationship between cutaneous gas exchange capacity and permeability to water has not been well studied in reptiles.

Absolute rates of nonpulmonary gas exchange depend on body mass, but are generally higher in aquatic reptiles than in terrestrial species of the same mass (Seymour, 1982). There is indirect evidence that two groups of aquatic reptiles can satisfy all of their resting gas exchange requirements by nonpulmonary routes under certain conditions. Rates of nonpulmonary O_2 in small soft-shelled

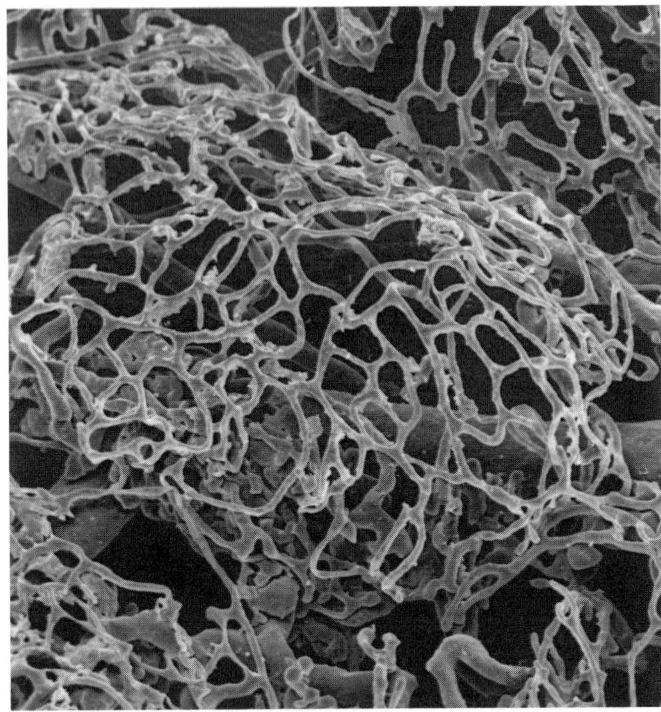

Figure 7 Vascular cast of the cutaneous capillaries of the sea snake, *Hydrophis fasciatus*. The subepidermal capillary network of an individual scale is shown above the underlying feeder vessels. (H. Rosenberg generously provided this unpublished scanning electron micrograph of a specimen supplied by H. Voris.)

turtles (*Trionyx*) (Dunson, 1960) and in some species of sea snakes (Seymour, 1982) are close to the minimum requirement of resting reptiles (Bennett and Dawson, 1976). Moreover, the early data from sea snakes may underestimate cutaneous exchange capacity because the measurements were made in chambers where (1) the PO_2 continually decreased, (2) the water was not well mixed, and (3) areas of the snake's skin pressed against the walls (Heatwole and Seymour, 1975a, 1978). These conditions would reduce O_2 diffusion into the animal. Additionally, some sea snakes can alter cutaneous perfusion under certain conditions, and they may voluntarily reduce arterial PO_2 below 10 torr (1.3 kPa) (Seymour and Webster, 1975). Such changes would increase both the effective surface area for diffusive exchange and the partial pressure gradient across the skin. Thus, it is likely that resting metabolic rates could be satisfied by O_2 uptake under favorable natural conditions in which well-oxygenated water moves over the skin by currents. If O_2 requirements are met cutaneously, CO_2 loss is not a problem because of its much higher coefficient of diffusion. Total reliance on the skin would account for the ability of certain sea snakes to rest quietly on the seabed throughout several hours of their daily cycle when they are not foraging (Dunson and Minton, 1978).

Gas exchange is fundamentally different in air and water. Because of the differences in O_2 and CO_2 capacitances of air and water, the blood P_{CO_2} of air breathers tends to be high and that of water breathers is very low (Rahn, 1966). The proposition that some reptiles can be essentially unimodal water breathers at rest might at first seem contrary to measured arterial P_{CO_2} in the region of 18 to 34 torr (2.4-4.5 kPa) (Seymour and Webster, 1975; Seymour, 1978). However, the parallel arrangement of the cutaneous and systemic circulation means that a considerable amount of blood is shunted away from the skin and CO_2 is retained in the body. The blood draining the skin probably has very low P_{CO_2} but, unfortunately, we have no confirming measurements because of difficulty in sampling the cutaneous veins. Cutaneous blood becomes mixed with systemic blood of higher P_{CO_2} because of right-to-left central shunting. The result is that most of the systemic tissues are exposed to a P_{CO_2} in the range normally experienced by air-breathing reptiles. A normal P_{CO_2} may be important to acid-base regulation in essentially water-breathing species that presumably recently evolved from totally air-breathing ancestors.

Although resting sea snakes might be able to remain submerged indefinitely under favorable conditions, foraging snakes apparently must return to the surface periodically to breathe. Submergence times of active snakes in the field are variable, lasting a few minutes to as much as 213 minutes (Heatwole, 1975; Rubinoff et al., 1986). Metabolic rates during swimming are presumably greater than can be supplied by cutaneous means, and the animals prefer to remain aerobic. However, *Pelamis platurus* may need to surface not only to gain O_2 but also to replenish lung volume for buoyancy control (see Sect. VII). Sometimes, the trips to the surface involve considerable energetic costs. For example, a snake feeding at 100 m depth requires about 10 min to make the trip to the surface and back (Heatwole and Seymour, 1975b; Heatwole et al., 1978). Cutaneous gas exchange is nevertheless valuable to deep divers by extending the time at depth. The long, deep dives of *P. platurus* are thought to be aerobic with most O_2 supplied cutaneously (Rubinoff et al., 1986). Among other species of sea snakes, there is a correlation between the extent of cutaneous gas exchange and diving depth. Deep-diving hydrophiines generally have higher rates of cutaneous O_2 uptake than do shallow-diving laticaudines (Heatwole and Seymour, 1975a, 1978).

Large diving reptiles rely less on nonpulmonary and more on pulmonary gas exchange than do small species (Seymour, 1982). This is explicable when one considers the allometry of cutaneous O_2 uptake and pulmonary O_2 storage. Because cutaneous O_2 uptake largely depends on the PO_2 gradient across the skin, the process appears to be strongly influenced by diffusion limitation. Therefore, the total rate of uptake depends on the surface area and thickness of the skin, although other factors, such as capillary recruitment, may affect this relationship (Feder and Burggren, 1985). Metabolic rate scales with body mass to the 0.80 power ($M_b^{0.80}$) in reptiles in general (Bennett and Dawson, 1976), but surface area scales only to the 0.67 power. Thus, larger species have relatively less surface area for exchange. Moreover, the skin of larger reptiles is thicker. In the few reptiles that have been examined, skin thickness is approximately proportional to $M_b^{0.4}$ (Smith, 1979). In a diffusion-limited system, the rate of transfer is proportional to the ratio of surface area divided by thickness. Therefore, the rate of cutaneous gas exchange should scale with $M_b^{0.27}$ (0.67-0.4). This exponent is in fact similar to those describing nonpulmonary O_2 uptake in soft-shelled turtles (0.23) (Dunson, 1960) and in selected terrestrial squamates (0.32) (Seymour, 1982).

The decrease in effectiveness of cutaneous gas exchange in large diving reptiles is compensated for by a greater capacity for O_2 storage in the lung, blood, and muscle. Scholander (1940) recognized that O_2 stores are directly proportional to body mass, and, because the mass-specific metabolic rates are smaller in larger animals, aerobic diving duration should increase in larger divers. This appears to be true in aerobically diving birds and mammals that doubtless lack significant nonpulmonary gas exchange capacity. Tolerance to forced dives involving anaerobic metabolism is even greater because of the reduced metabolic rate associated with the diving response (Butler and Jones, 1982). However, the exact correlations between body mass, nonpulmonary O_2 uptake, O_2 storage, and diving duration have yet to be fully analyzed in reptiles.

V. Balance Between Pulmonary and Cutaneous Gas Exchange

A. At Surface Pressure

Blood is supplied to the lung and skin in series. The skin receives systemic arterial blood derived exclusively from the intersegmental arteries in reptiles (Feder and Burggren, 1985). This is not the best arrangement for effective gas exchange because the cutaneous blood could be well saturated with O_2 and possess little capacity to obtain more.

However, the problem is ameliorated in reptiles because they possess a considerable degree of right-to-left venous shunting past the lungs. The total shunt derives from venous admixture, either in the hearts of noncrocodilian reptiles or through the foramen of Panizza in crocodilians (White, 1976) or within the lung itself (Seymour, 1978, 1983). The shunts dilute O_2-rich blood equilibrating with the pulmonary gas with O_2-poor venous blood. Central shunting is not constant, but tends to be high during ventilation and low during apnea (White, 1985; Burggren, 1985). On average, however, the degree of shunting appears to be correlated with the reliance on cutaneous gas exchange. For example, in voluntarily breathing crocodilians, cutaneous gas exchange is negligible (Wright, 1986), and there is little or no right-to-left shunt through the foramen of Panizza (White, 1969; Johansen, 1985). In noncrocodilians, intraventricular shunting is generally low when O_2 is plentiful in the lung and little nonpulmonary O_2 uptake occurs. Most measurements reveal venous shunts ranging up to about 30% of the systemic cardiac output (Seymour, 1982). Green turtles, *Chelonia mydas*, swimming aerobically at the surface, have almost no cutaneous exchange (Butler et al., 1984), a low venous shunt, and high saturation of arterial blood (Wood et al., 1984). However, in several species of aquatic snakes that are known to rely significantly on cutaneous gas exchange, the shunt normally represents about 50 to 70% of the systemic cardiac output, and the maximal saturation of systemic arterial blood is only 60 to 70%. This level of saturation corresponds to a PO_2 of about 40 torr (5.3 kPa) and ensures the maintenance of a favorable inward gradient for O_2 diffusion across the skin.

B. At Depth

Green turtles, *C. mydas*, have been observed at 290 m (Landis, 1965) and leatherback turtles, *Dermochelys coriacea*, have been tracked to 475 m (Eckert et al., 1986). The sea snake, *P. platurus*, dives deeper than 50 m (Rubinoff et al., 1986), and evidence suggests that other hydrophiine sea snakes feed at depths up to about 100 m (Heatwole and Seymour, 1975b). Because hydrostatic pressure increases about 1 atm/10 m depth, diving can have an enormous effect on pulmonary gas tensions.

Deep diving threatens cutaneous O_2 uptake because diving deeper than a few meters creates a net outward gradient between the lung and water. For example, if a sea snake begins a dive with a pulmonary PO_2 of about 120 torr (16 kPa) at the surface, compression increases it to equal to that of air-equilibrated seawater [about 150 torr (20 kPa)] at only 2.5 m depth. Because the ambient PO_2 in well-mixed water is independent of hydrostatic pressure, the outward PO_2 gradient increases with depth (Fig. 8).

Continued O_2 uptake from the seawater depends upon an ever-increasing isolation of pulmonary and cutaneous circuits. The pulmonary bypass shunts, which keep arterial saturation low at the surface, actually increase as the lung collapses during diving (Seymour, 1978). In the deep-diving hydrophiines, for example, arterial saturation remains low and practically independent of depth (see Fig. 8). Even at 41 m, the arterial PO_2 remains at about 40 torr (5.3 kPa) and the saturation at about 60%, despite a pulmonary PO_2 exceeding 500 torr (66 kPa).

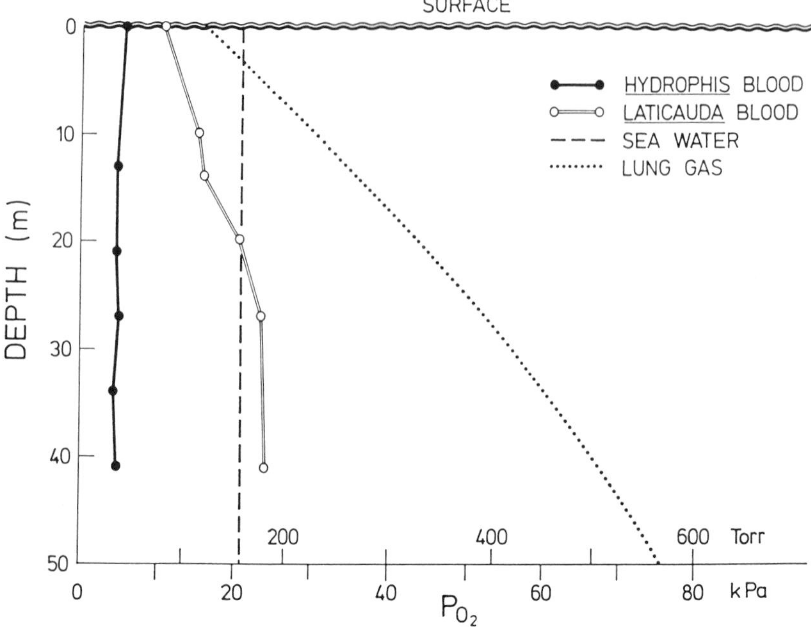

Figure 8 PO_2 in the blood of deep-diving (*Hydrophis* sp.) and shallow-diving (*Laticauda colubrina*) sea snakes during artificial compressions simulating dives to selected depth. Theoretical values of PO_2 in well-mixed seawater and in the lung of a snake during its swim from the surface are also indicated. (From Seymour, 1987b.)

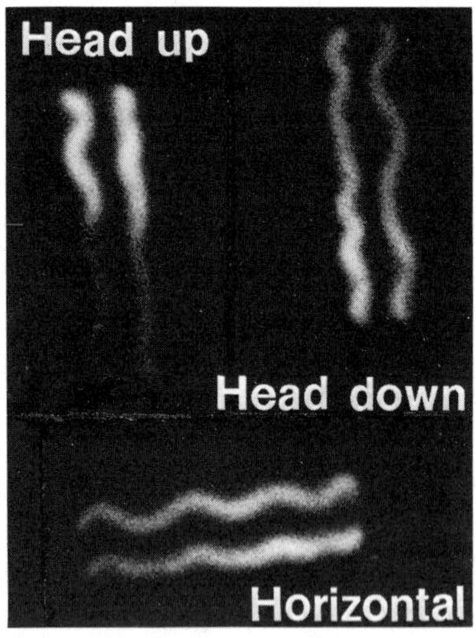

Figure 9 Gamma camera images of ^{133}Xe gas in the single lung of two sea snakes, *Pelamis platurus*, during tilting in water. (From Seymour et al., 1981b.)

Part of the increased shunt at depth apparently occurs by continued perfusion of collapsed portions of the lung. Another part stems from augmented intraventricular shunting, possibly resulting from increasing resistance in the pulmonary circuit. The distribution of lung gas, shown by x-rays and imaging of ^{133}Xe gas during compression, reveals a nonuniform collapse that depends on the orientation of the snake in the water (Seymour, 1978; Seymour et al., 1981b). During downward swimming, the anterior, well-vascularized tracheal and bronchial portions of the lung tend to collapse, but during upward swimming, the nonvascular saccular section collapses, forcing more gas into the vascular lung (Fig. 9). This is exactly the pattern of collapse that would provide greater effective shunting during the beginning of the dive when lung PO_2 is highest and reduced shunting during decompression when the PO_2 drops precipitously. More work is required, however, to establish detailed relationships between hydrostatic pressure, total pulmonary bypass, the pattern of lung perfusion, and cardiac output.

The overall level of shunting and its increase during compression seem to be related to reliance on cutaneous gas exchange and usual diving depths of a species. For example, the deep-diving hydrophiines have high cutaneous gas exchange capacity and a high prevailing shunt fraction, but shallow diving laticaudines have lower cutaneous gas exchange and a level of shunting similar to those in normal reptiles (Seymour, 1978, 1982). Figure 8 shows that the PO_2 in the blood of *Laticauda colubrina* begins to exceed that of seawater at hydrostatic pressures equivalent to 20 m depth. Fortunately, this snake does not normally dive deeper than 20 m, and it is in no danger of losing O_2 across the skin to the sea. Blood PO_2 in deep-diving *Hydrophis* sp. never exceeds that of the sea, even at 100 m.

VI. Decompression

Hydrostatic compression of the pulmonary gas during a dive increases its PN_2 and tends to drive N_2 into the body. If the N_2 content of the blood and other tissues exceeds a certain threshold, N_2 bubbles can form during decompression, leading to the syndrome called decompression sickness or "the bends" in humans. The threshold for bubble formation is about 4.7 ml N_2/100 ml blood in sea snakes (Seymour, 1978). Decompression sickness can occur after repeated breath-hold dives to a depth of only 25 m in humans (Paulev, 1965), and it has been shown theoretically that enough N_2 is present in the lungs of diving reptiles to saturate the body to bubble threshold (Seymour, 1978). Most freshwater reptiles do not appear to dive deep enough to experience decompression sickness, but marine turtles and snakes are in danger.

Sea snakes are protected from N_2 bubble formation by the same mechanism that keeps arterial PO_2 low (Seymour, 1974, 1978). The pulmonary bypass

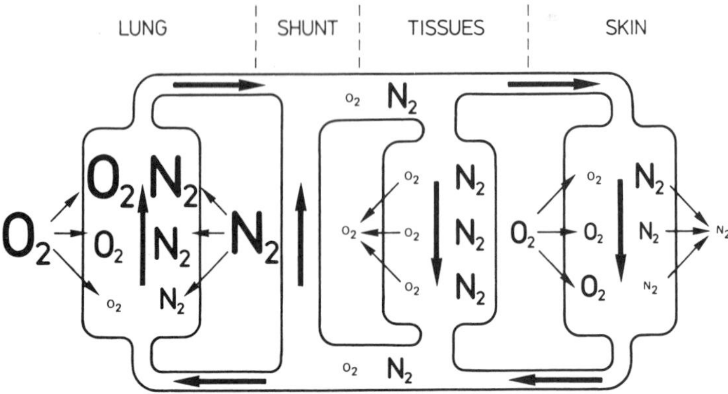

Figure 10 Diagrammatic representation of the circulatory system of a sea snake under hydrostatic pressure at depth. The size of the symbols indicates partial pressure, although the exact relationships are underemphasized for technical reasons. High pressures of O_2 and N_2 in the lung are diminished by powerful left-to-right shunts such that the tissue PO_2 and PN_2 are considerably lower. Arterial blood supplied to the skin can passively obtain O_2 and lose N_2. (From Seymour, 1987b.)

dilutes N_2-rich blood equilibrating in the lung with N_2-poor blood from the systemic veins (Fig. 10). Unlike O_2, however, N_2 is not consumed by the tissues and tends to build up in the body. Maintenance of low venous PN_2 would be impossible without a means of eliminating N_2 by nonpulmonary gas exchangers during a dive. Sea snakes can use their skin to lose N_2 and, as in O_2 uptake, the rate of flux depends on the PN_2 gradient between the arterial blood and the seawater. At the surface, the PN_2 in the blood is slightly higher than the atmospheric, because O_2 uptake from the lung and cutaneous CO_2 loss tend to concentrate the N_2 in the lung. The rate of N_2 loss through the skin is initially very small, but it increases when the snake dives as N_2 moves into the blood from the compressed lung. Although shunting tends to keep PN_2 lower in the arteries than in the lung, arterial PN_2 continues to increase until the gradient across the skin reaches a level at which the rate of cutaneous N_2 loss equals the rate of uptake from the lung. At this point, arterial PN_2 is maximal, and the value depends on several factors including cardiac output, pulmonary shunt fraction, cutaneous circuit fraction, N_2 capacitance of the blood, and the N_2 diffusion coefficient of the skin, none of which has been studied in detail. Nevertheless, it is clear that pulmonary shunt and cutaneous gas exchange protect sea snakes from bubble formation during decompression. Both factors are critical for protection.

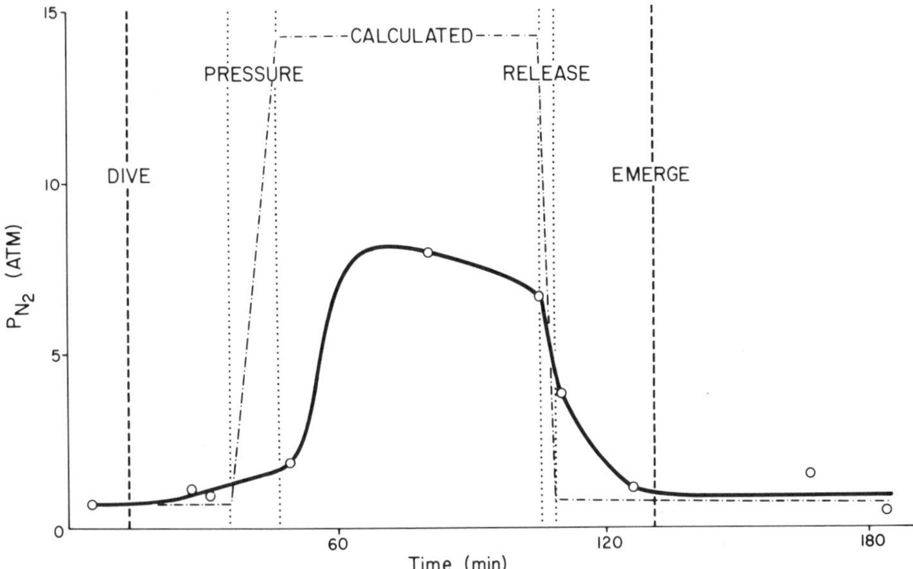

Figure 11 PN_2 in the arterial blood of the marine turtle, *Chelonia mydas*, before, during, and after artificial compression to 18.7 atm. Pulmonary PN_2 is calculated according to Boyle's law. (Adapted from Berkson, 1967.)

Bubbles form in the blood of artificially compressed sea snakes if either (1) the pulmonary shunt is reduced by lung inflation at ambient hydrostatic pressure, or (2) N_2 loss through the skin is reduced by high external PN_2 in the hyperbaric chamber (Seymour, 1978).

The submergence patterns of deep-diving leatherback turtles suggest that most dives occur aerobically (Eckert et al., 1986). The O_2 requirements must, therefore, be met either from the lung or through nonpulmonary routes. Turtles diving with air in the lungs experience a significant N_2 load, but Berkson (1967) showed that the arterial PN_2 remained about half that of the pulmonary PN_2 in green turtles artificially compressed to equivalent depths up to 180 m (Fig. 11). Nevertheless, he produced N_2 bubbles in the blood and fatal decompression sickness at depths to which the animals are known to dive in the field. Exactly how they avoid bubbles during deep, natural dives is not known, but it may be related to pulmonary isolation by central vascular shunts and a faculative ability to eliminate N_2 by nonpulmonary means. These mechanisms may have been unavailable or unused in Berkson's hyperbaric chamber.

VII. Buoyancy Control

Aquatic reptiles use the lung to control their specific gravity. Apparently achieving a body buoyancy appropriate for the depth leads to significant locomotory energy economy. Lung volumes are normally high, and the animal is positively buoyant, if it intends to remain at the surface, for example swimming marine iguanas *Amblyrhynchus cristatus* (Carpenter, 1966) or feeding *Pelamis platurus* (Graham et al., 1975). If the animal rests on the bottom, e.g., many turtles (Zug, 1971), lung volumes are lower. Of course lung volume affects diving duration, and bottom dwellers would seem to be disadvantaged, but the heavy shell of turtles (Jackson, 1969) and stomach stones of crocodilians (Cott, 1961) permit negative buoyancy with larger lung volumes.

The specific gravity of a diving animal depends on the absolute volume of pulmonary gas. This volume changes with hydrostatic compression, according to Boyle's law. Thus, neutral buoyancy occurs only at a single depth, above which the animal tends to rise to the surface and below which it tends to sink. During a dive, moreover, this point rises as gas is removed from the lung and the animal tends to become less buoyant.

Because reptiles appear incapable of resisting the hydrostatic compression of the lung (Berkson, 1967; Gaunt and Gans, 1969), the only way to achieve neutral buoyancy at a particular depth is to adjust lung volume at the beginning of a dive and then to find the depth resulting in neutral buoyancy and gradually move upward with it as the lung collapses. The only reptile known to do this is the pelagic sea snake, *P. platurus*, which apparently "plans" the depth of its dives and takes down the appropriate amount of gas (Graham et al., 1988). Snakes kept in tanks of depths up to 10 m eventually learn to dive with lung volumes consistently resulting in neutral buoyancy near the bottom. Naive snakes have variable lung volumes and are usually positively buoyant during dives in the same tanks. Furthermore, snakes tracked in the open ocean with pressure-sensitive ultrasonic transmitters show a recurring pattern of diving that suggests that they achieve neutral buoyancy at depths they choose before the dive (Rubinoff et al., 1986). The usual dive pattern consists of a rapid descent followed by a rapid ascent up to a depth that appears to result in neutral buoyancy (Fig. 12). During most of the time underwater (82%), however, the snakes gradually ascend until a point when they abruptly return to the surface. The period of gradual ascent is proposed to be a time during which the snake achieves a constant lung volume by matching the gradual loss of lung gas with expansion of the lung owing to a gradual reduction of hydrostatic pressure. Eventually, the snakes return to the surface to replenish lung gas.

If the gradual ascent phase of the dive represents maintenance of neutral buoyancy in the face of gas removal from the lung, the rate of ascent during this period is an indirect measure of the rate of gas removal from the lung. We have

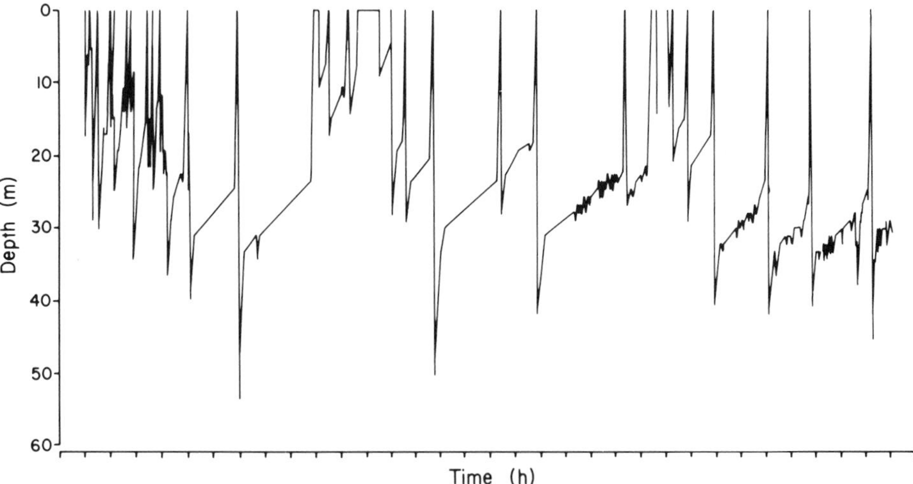

Figure 12 Pattern of diving in pelagic sea snakes, *P. platurus*, indicated by ultrasonic tracking. Dives are characterized by rapid descent, "bounce" ascent, gradual ascent, and finally, rapid ascent. The gradual ascent phase may represent maintenance of neutral buoyancy while lung volume declines as gas is removed from it. (Redrawn from Rubinoff et al., 1986.)

two reasons to expect that the rate of gradual ascent should increase the deeper the snake dives. First, greater hydrostatic compression increases pulmonary gas tensions and, therefore, increases the amount of gas dissolved in the pulmonary blood. Second, at higher pressure, a greater vertical distance is required to achieve the same change is lung volume (Boyle's law). However, Graham et al. (1988) report no significant correlation between gradual ascent rate and depth, indicating that the deeper the snake dives, the slower is the rate of recruitment of gas from the lung. These data are consistent with the idea that the level of effective pulmonary bypass increases with diving depth, tending to minimize the rates at which O_2 and N_2 are released from the lung.

VIII. Pulmonary Circulation and Gravity

The distribution of blood flow to the lungs of terrestrial animals is affected by gravity, which tends to make the blood flow to the dependent parts of the lung. This tendency causes inhomogeneity of ventilation/perfusion ratio in the lungs of animals (Farhi, 1985). The gravitational component of pulmonary blood pressure is higher in the capillaries at the bottom of the lung and, if pressure becomes high enough, pulmonary edema can result. Because of their body shape and length, snakes are the reptiles most affected by gravity. Indeed terrestrial and aquatic snakes show distinct differences in lung structure and blood pressure that are related to gravitational environment (Lillywhite, 1987; Seymour, 1988).

The lungs of snakes occupy most of the body cavity and are divided into vascular (tracheal and bronchial) and nonvascular (saccular) segments. The vascular lung of aquatic snakes is more extensive and, in some species, extends almost the entire length of the lung, up to about 90% of the body length. Tilting of sea snakes in air increases hydrostatic pressure in the pulmonary circulation and causes severe pulmonary edema and rupture of capillaries (Lillywhite, 1987). When tilted in water, however, the dependent part of the lung collapses completely (see Fig. 9), presumably preventing the development of high transmural pressure gradients in the pulmonary capillaries. Edema does not appear to be a problem in terrestrial and arboreal snakes because the vascular lung typically occupies less than 10% of the body length and hydrostatic pressure changes in the pulmonary circuit are small.

Terrestrial snakes generally have higher systemic blood pressures than do aquatic snakes (Seymour and Lillywhite, 1976; Seymour, 1987a), but pressures in the pulmonary arteries are similar in the two groups (Lillywhite, 1987). Thus, there appears to be a greater separation of pressure in the two circuits in terrestrial species, which may be related to prevention of pulmonary edema. Pressure separation is possible, despite the incompletely divided ventricle, because a powerful, cholinergically controlled, resistance occurs in the central or peripheral pulmonary arteries (Burggren, 1985; White, 1985).

IX. Summary

The characteristic apneic ventilation of reptiles is exaggerated in aquatic species. Shallow divers usually remain aerobic and satisfy their needs for O_2 by drawing on moderate stores in the lungs and blood. Most CO_2 is stored in the body during apnea and released during ventilation when pulmonary blood flow increases. The pattern of ventilation is related to metabolic rate, pulmonary blood flow, and gas capacitances of the body compartments.

Nonpulmonary gas exchange is important in several groups of aquatic species, and divers can take advantage of O_2 from the lung gas as well as the external water. The nonpulmonary gas exchanger is supplied with arterial blood of low O_2 content because of right-to-left venous shunts in the heart or the lungs. Because the shunts increase with depth in sea snakes, their cutaneous circulation is further protected from high pulmonary gas tensions during hydrostatic collapse of the lung. Deep-diving species have inherently higher shunts and greater capacity for cutaneous gas exchange than do shallow divers. Thus, there is a selective advantage for species with such a combination, for it not only facilitates O_2 uptake at greater depths, but it also prevents N_2 bubble formation during decompression. Some reptiles can satisfy all of their resting gas exchange requirements through skin, cloaca, or pharynx. These facultative unimodal water breathers maintain high circulating P_{CO_2} by perfusing the systemic tissues and gas exchangers in parallel.

Buoyancy control appears to be an important factor determining lung volumes. Some sea snakes appear to adjust lung volume to achieve neutral buoyancy at a desired depth. As gas is removed from the lung, they gradually ascend, presumably maintaining neutral buoyancy. Hydrostatic pressure collapses dependent parts of the elongate vascular lungs of sea snakes and prevents edema and capillary rupture resulting from high blood pressure.

References

Ackerman, R. A., and White, F. N. (1979). Cyclic carbon dioxide exchange in the turtle *Pseudemys scripta. Physiol. Zool. 52*:378-389.

Bennett, A. F., and Dawson, W. R. (1976). Metabolism. In *Biology of the Reptilia*, Vol. 5. Physiology A. Edited by C. Gans and W. R. Dawson. London, Academic Press, pp. 127-223.

Bennett, A. F., and Licht, P. (1975). Evaporative water loss in scaleless snakes. *Comp. Biochem. Physiol. 52A*:213-215.

Berkson, H. (1967). Physiological adjustments to deep diving in the Pacific green turtle (*Chelonia mydas agassizii*). *Comp. Biochem. Physiol. 21*:507-524.

Burggren, W. (1985). Hemodynamics and regulation of central cardiovascular shunts in reptiles. In *Cardiovascular Shunts*. Edited by K. Johansen and W. Burggren. Alfred Benzon Symposium 21, Copenhagen, Munksgaard, pp. 121-136.

Burggren, W. W., and Shelton, G. (1979). Gas exchange and transport during intermittent breathing in chelonian reptiles. *J. Exp. Biol. 82*:75-92.

Butler, P. J., and Jones, D. R. (1982). The comparative physiology of diving in vertebrates. *Adv. Comp. Physiol. Biochem. 8*:179-364.

Butler, P. J., Milsom, W. K., and Woakes, A. J. (1984). Respiratory, cardiovascular and metabolic adjustments during steady state swimming in the green turtle, *Chelonia mydas. J. Comp. Physiol. 154*:167-174.

Carpenter, C. C. (1966). The marine iguana of the Galapagos islands, its behavior and ecology. *Proc. Calif. Acad. Sci. 34*:329-376.

Cott, H. B. (1961). Scientific results of an inquiry into the ecology and economic status of the Nile crocodile (*Crocodilus niloticus*) in Uganda and Northern Rhodesia. *Trans. Zool. Soc. Lond. 29*:211-356.

Dunson, W. A. (1960). Aquatic respiration in *Trionyx spinifer asper. Herpetologica 16*:277-283.

Dunson, W. A. (1986). Estuarine populations of the snapping turtle (*Chelydra*) as a model for the evolution of marine adaptations in reptiles. *Copeia 1986*:741-756.

Dunson, W. A., and Minton, S. A. (1978). Diversity, distribution, and ecology of Philippine marine snakes (Reptilia, Serpentes). *J. Herpetol. 12*:281-286.

Eckert, S. A., Nellis, D. W., Eckert, K. L., and Kooyman, G. L. (1986). Diving patterns of two leatherback sea turtles (*Dermochelys coriacea*) during nesting intervals at Sandy Point, St. Croix, U.S. Virgin Islands. *Herpetologica 42*:381-388.

Farhi, L. E. (1985). Physiological shunts: Effects of posture and gravity. In *Cardiovascular Shunts*. Edited by K. Johansen and W. Burggren. Alfred Benzon Sympoisum 21. Copenhagen, Munksgaard, pp. 322-330.

Feder, M. E. (1980). Blood oxygen stores in the file snake, *Acrochordus granulatus*, and in other marine snakes. *Physiol. Zool. 53*:394-401.

Feder, M. E., and Burggren, W. W. (1985). Cutaneous gas exchange in vertebrates: Design, patterns, control and implications. *Biol. Rev.60*:1-45.

Gatten, R. E., Jr. (1981). Anaerobic metabolism in freely diving painted turtles (*Chrysemys picta*). *J. Exp. Zool. 216*:377-385.

Gaunt, A. S., and Gans, C. (1969). Mechanics of respiration in the snapping turtle, *Chelydra serpentina* (Linne). *J. Morphol. 128*:195-228.

Glass, M., Burggren, W. W., and Johansen, K. (1978). Ventilation in an aquatic and a terrestrial chelonian reptile. *J. Exp. Biol. 72*:165-179.

Glass, M. L., and Wood, S. C. (1983). Gas exchange and control of breathing in reptiles. *Physiol. Rev. 63*:232-260.

Gleeson, T. T. (1980). Lactic acid production during field activity in the Galapagos marine iguana *Amblyrhynchus cristatus. Physiol. Zool. 53*:157-162.

Graham, J. B., Gee, J. H., and Robison, F. S. (1975). Hydrostatic and gas exchange functions of the lung of the sea snake *Pelamis platurus. Comp. Biochem. Physiol. 50A*:477-482.

Graham, J. B., Gee, J. H., Motta, J., and Rubinoff, I. (1988). Subsurface buoyancy control by the sea snake *Pelamis platurus. Mar. Biol.* (in press).

Heatwole, H. (1975). Voluntary submergence times of marine snakes. *Mar. Biol. 32*:205-213.

Heatwole, H., and Seymour, R. (1975a). Pulmonary and cutaneous oxygen uptake in sea snakes and a file snake. *Comp. Biochem. Physiol. 51A*:399-405.

Heatwole, H., and Seymour, R. (1975b). Diving physiology. In *The Biology of Sea Snakes*. Edited by W. A. Dunson. Baltimore, London, University Park Press, pp. 289-327.

Heatwole, H., and Seymour, R. S. (1978). Cutaneous oxygen uptake in three groups of aquatic snakes. *Aust. J. Zool. 26*:481-486.

Heatwole, H., Minton, S. A., Jr., Taylor, R., and Taylor, V. (1978). Underwater observations on sea snake behaviour. *Rec. Aust. Mus. 31*:737-761.

Jackson, D. C. (1969). Buoyancy control in the freshwater turtle. *Science 166*: 1649-1651.

Jackson, D. C. (1985). Respiration and respiratory control in the green turtle, *Chelonia mydas. Copeia 1985*:664-671.

Johansen, K. (1985). A phylogenetic overview of cardiovascular shunts. In *Cardiovascular Shunts*. Edited by K. Johansen and W. Burggren. Alfred Benzon Symposium 21. Copenhagen, Munksgaard, pp. 17-32.

Landis, A. T., Jr. (1965). Research. *Undersea Tech. 6*:21.

Lillywhite, H. B. (1987). Circulatory adaptations of snakes to gravity. *Am. Zool. 27*:81-95.

Lutz, P. L., and Bentley, T. B. (1985). Respiratory physiology of diving in the sea turtle. *Copeia 1985*:671-679.

Paulev, P. (1965). Decompression sickness following repeated breath-hold dives. *J. Appl. Physiol. 20*:1028-1031.

Rahn, H. (1966). Aquatic gas exchange: Theory. *Respir. Physiol. 1*:1-12.

Roberts, J. B., and Lillywhite, H. B. (1980). Lipid barrier to water exchange in reptile epidermis. *Science 207*:1077-1079.

Rosenberg, H. I., and Voris, H. K. (1980). Cutaneous capillaries of sea snakes and their possible role in gas exchange. *Am. Zool. 20*:758.

Rubinoff, I., Graham, J. B., and Motta, J. (1986). Diving of the sea snake *Pelamis platurus* in the Gulf of Panama. I. Dive depth and duration. *Mar. Biol. 91*:181-191.

Scholander, P. F. (1940). Experimental investigations on the respiratory function in diving mammals and birds. *Hvalradets Skr. 22*:1-131.

Seymour, R. S. (1974). How sea snakes may avoid the bends. *Nature 250*:489-490.

Seymour, R. S. (1978). Gas tensions and blood distribution in sea snakes at surface pressure and at simulated depth. *Physiol. Zool. 51*:388-407.

Seymour, R. S. (1979). Blood lactate in free-diving sea snakes. *Copeia 1979*: 494-497.

Seymour, R. S. (1982). Physiological adaptations to aquatic life. In *Biology of the Reptilia*. Vol. 13, Physiology D. Edited by C. Gans and F. H. Pough. London, Academic Press, pp. 1-51.

Seymour, R. S. (1983). Functional venous admixture in the lungs of the turtle, *Chrysemys scripta. Respir. Physiol. 53*:99-107.

Seymour, R. S. (1987a). Scaling of cardiovascular physiology in snakes. *Am. Zool. 27*:97-109.

Seymour, R. S. (1987b). Physiological correlates of reinvasion of water by reptiles. In *Comparative Physiology: Life in Water and on Land.* Edited by P. Dejours, L. Bolis, C. R. Taylor, and E. R. Weibel. Padova, Liviana Press.

Seymour, R. S., and Lillywhite, H. B. (1976). Blood pressure in snakes from different habitats. *Nature 264*:664-666.

Seymour, R. S., and Webster, M. E. D. (1975). Gas transport and blood acid-base balance in diving sea snakes. *J. Exp. Zool. 191*:169-182.

Seymour, R. S., Bennett, A. F., and Bradford, D. F. (1985). Blood gas tensions and acid-base regulation in the salt-water crocodile, *Crocodylus porosus*, at rest and after exhaustive exercise. *J. Exp. Biol. 118*:143-159.

Seymour, R. S., Dobson, G. P., and Baldwin, J. (1981a). Respiratory and cardiovascular physiology of the aquatic snake, *Acrochordus arafurae. J. Comp. Physiol. 144*:215-227.

Seymour, R. S., Spragg, R. G., and Hartman, M. T. (1981b). Distribution of ventilation and perfusion in the sea snake, *Pelamis platurus. J. Comp. Physiol. 145*:109-115.

Smith, E. N. (1979). Behavioral and physiological thermoregulation of crocodiles. *Am. Zool. 19*:239-247.

Tenney, S. M., and Tenney, J. B. (1970). Quantitative morphology of cold-blooded lungs: Amphibia and Reptilia. *Respir. Physiol. 9*:197-215.

White, F. N. (1969). Redistribution of cardiac output in the diving alligator. *Copeia 1969*:567-570.

White, F. N. (1976). Circulation. In *Biology of the Reptilia*, Vol. 5, Physiology A. Edited by C. Gans and W. R. Dawson. London, Academic Press, pp. 275-334.

White, F. N. (1985). Role of intracardiac shunts in pulmonary gas exchange in chelonian reptiles. In *Cardiovascular Shunts*. Edited by K. Johansen and W. Burggren. Alfred Benzon Symposium 21. Copenhagen, Munksgaard, pp. 296-305.

Wood, S. C., and Lenfant, C. J. M. (1976). Respiration: Mechanics, control and gas exchange. In *Biology of the Reptilia*, Vol. 5, Physiology A. Edited by C. Gans and W. R. Dawson. London, Academic Press, pp. 225-274.

Wood, S. C., Gatz, R. N., and Glass, M. L. (1984). Oxygen transport in the green sea turtle. *J. Comp. Physiol. 154*:275-280.

Wright, J. C. (1986). Low to negligible cutaneous oxygen uptake in juvenile *Crocodylus porosus. Comp. Biochem. Physiol. 84A*:479-481.

Zug, G. R. (1971). Buoyancy, locomotion, morphology of the pelvic girdle and hindlimb and systematics of Cryptodiran turtles. *Misc. Publ. Mus. Zool. Univ. Mich. 142*:1-98.

24

Diving Physiology
Marine Mammals

GERALD L. KOOYMAN

Scripps Institution of Oceanography
University of California at San Diego
La Jolla, California

I. Introduction

Over the course of the last 15 years, major technical achievements have made possible detailed descriptions of the foraging behavior of marine tetrapods. As these studies are published and physiologists consider the patterns of dive behavior exhibited by various diving animals, it will no doubt modify previous interpretations of diving physiology and evoke questions that will lead to further research. My objective in this chapter is to briefly mention some of the most salient characteristics discovered and to point out the implications to diving physiology of marine mammals. The focus on marine mammals for this analysis is appropriate because the greatest amount of available information on diving behavior comes from this class, whereas such analysis on reptiles has occurred in just the last 2 or 3 years, and the work on birds is just beginning as of this writing.

This work was supported by USPHS HL-17731, NSF DCB84-07291, and UCSD RJ 148-5.

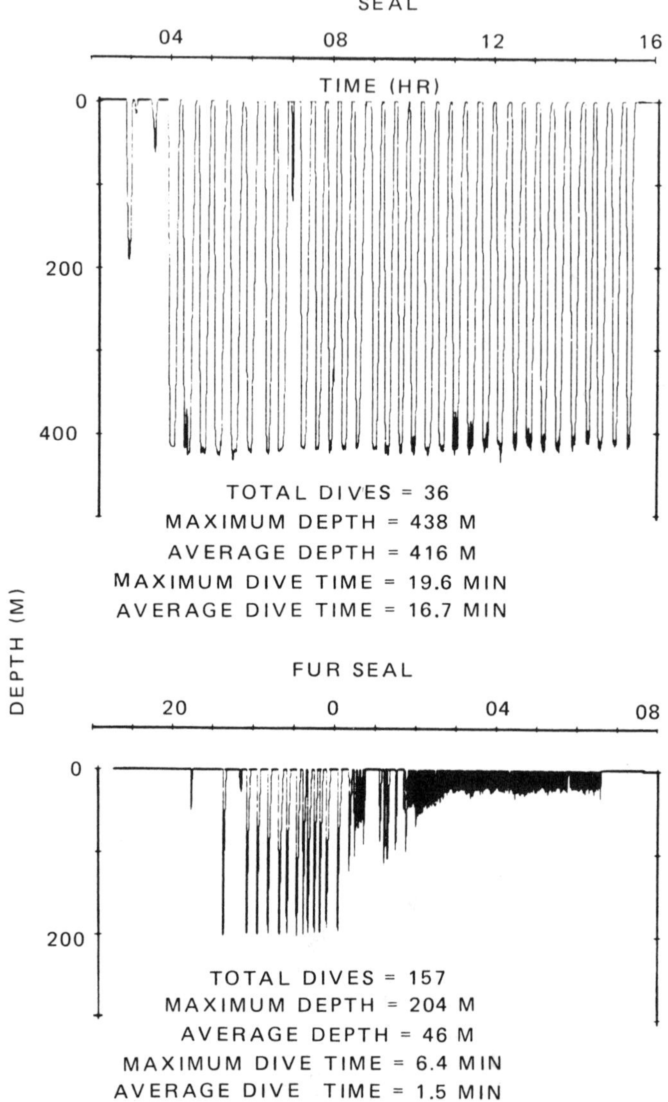

Figure 1 A single day of living activity (bout) for a Weddell seal, *Leptonychotes weddellii*, (upper) and South African fur seal, *Arctocephalus pusillus*, (lower). (From Kooyman, 1982.)

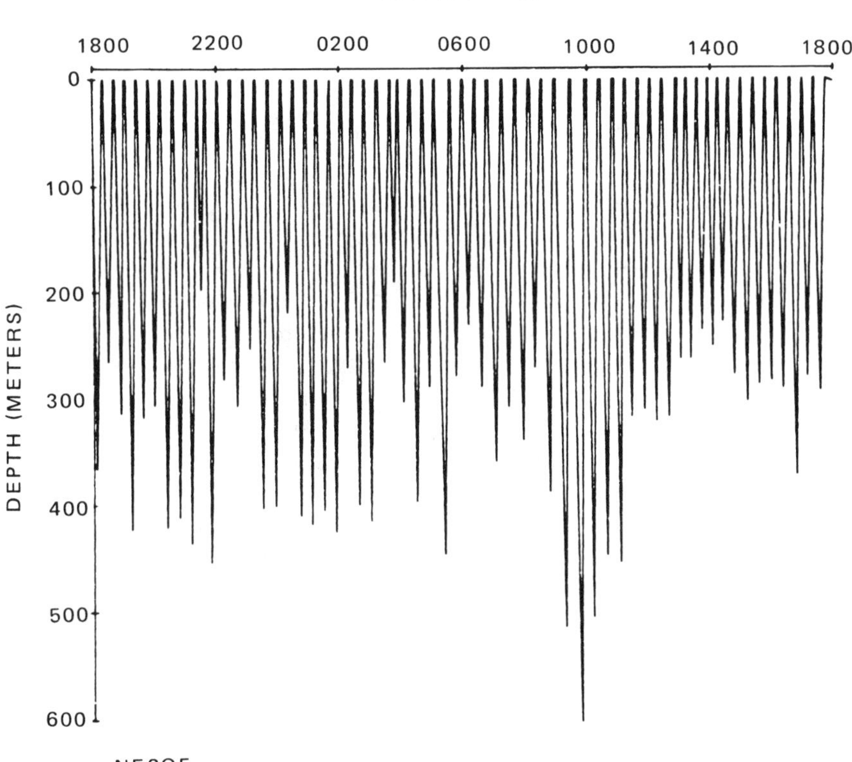

Figure 2 The fifth day of diving in an adult northern elephant seal female that followed this illustrated routine of continuous deep diving for the duration of the recorder's 11-day capacity. It should be noted that compression of a 24-h record has obscured time at depth and gives the dives the appearance of simple spikes.

The work on marine mammals has shown that this group might be divided behaviorally into two broad types: *divers* and *surfacers*. The differentiation was first expressed by Kramer (1988), a behavioral ecologist, and it has struck me as an appropriate and important classification. Divers are those animals that over a 24-h period at sea usually spend most of their time—more than 50%—on the surface. The dive periods are often circadian and usually occur in bouts that may last several hours as the animal hunts and captures prey. The bouts are best described as a series of dives, usually to a consistent depth, with a short surface interval between each dive for gas exchange. During the surface time, CO_2 is unloaded and O_2 stores are replenished. During a bout about 80 to 90% of the time is spent underwater. The duration of the dives most probably is dictated by O_2 stores and O_2 consumption rates; thus, the fur seal with its smaller O_2 store relative to its high metabolic rate makes comparatively short dives compared with the seal (Fig. 1). During the bout, the animals might be considered surfacers rather than divers, but this term seems more appropriate to another definition.

Surfacers are those animals that, based on present data, spend most of their time at sea underwater and surface only briefly for unloading and loading of CO_2 and O_2, respectively. Diving appears to be continuous, and as new data are accumulated it may reveal that breaks in this pattern may occur only seasonally for breeding or molting when the animals must be ashore. So far, there is only one example of this in mammals, the northern elephant seal, *Mirounga angustirostris* (Le Boeuf et al., 1985) (Fig. 2), but I suspect that as more species are studied others will be discovered. Indeed, the surfacer pattern has been described recently for the leatherback sea turtle, *Dermochelys coriacea*, (Eckert et al., 1986).

The objectives of the rest of this chapter are to discuss: (1) compression effects, (2) O_2 stores and aerobic limits, and (3) management of O_2 stores in light of these two patterns or categories. Much of the discussion will be necessarily hypothetical, but the examples may revise the perspective of many readers about how these animals work.

II. Compression Effects

In the past it has been generally accepted, I believe, that whatever adverse effects of compression may occur during a dive they are dissipated during recovery. A specific example is the elevated arterial N_2 tension, which may rise to as high as 2 to 6 atm absolute (ata) during a single dive, but soon falls to normal levels after the diver surfaces (Kooyman et al., 1973; Falke et al., 1985). However, the situation may be different in the more natural setting of a series of dives. During that time it is possible that a steady increment of N_2 may cause a rise of arterial and tissue N_2 to harmful levels after several dives.

The only measurements under these conditions have been on the bottlenose dolphin, *Tursiops truncatus*, trained to dive to 100 m. After 25 such dives of 1.5 min duration, with only brief surface intervals, the tissue P_{N_2} of the epaxial muscle at the end of the bout had risen to an apparent, but extrapolated, 2.1 ata (Ridgway and Howard, 1979). This suggests to me that arterial P_{aN_2} must have been, at times during the dive, much higher. Also, the recovery curve shows that clearance to normal atmospheric values took more than 20 min. Because no samples were taken during the course of the dive bout, the rate of N_2

Table 1 Dive Characteristics of a 280-kg Northern Elephant Seal Female During Her First 11 Days at Sea[a]

Day	No. of dives	Surface time (%)	Maximum depth (m)	Mean depth (m)	Maximum dive time (min)	Mean dive time (min)
1[b]	38	10	588	257 ± 140	30	22 ± 3.7
2	60	14	468	294 ± 78	30	21 ± 3.8
3	57	17	521	283 ± 106	32	21 ± 5.3
4	55	10	498	340 ± 67	28	24 ± 1.8
5	60	7	603	324 ± 109	28	21 ± 6.0
6	63	10	563	314 ± 127	28	20 ± 5.8
7	59	11	550	347 ± 112	26	21 ± 3.9
8	62	11	530	370 ± 88	25	21 ± 1.6
9	64	9	584	356 ± 95	23	20 ± 1.4
10	66	12	630	371 ± 114	24	19 ± 3.2
11[a]	69	12	581	387 ± 95	25	20 ± 1.6
Average[d]	61	11		333		21
Total	653					

[a]Mean ± 15D
[b]15.5 h
[c]26 h
[d]Neither day 1 nor 11 included in overall average.
Source: Le Boeuf et al. (1985).

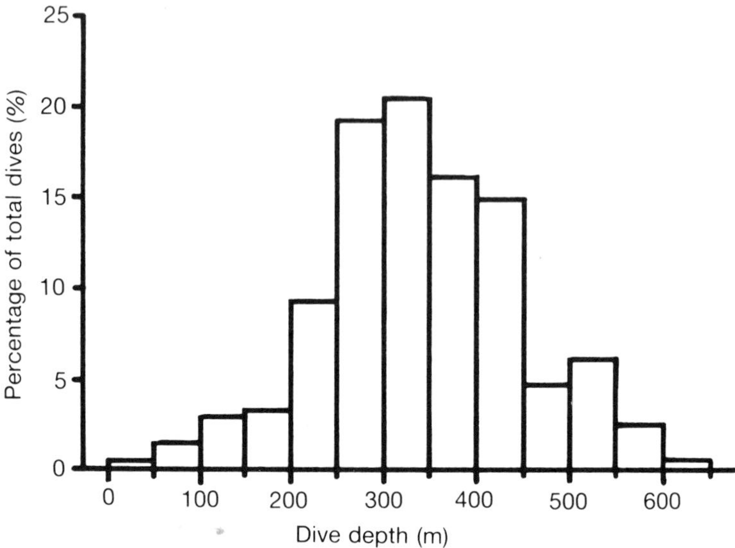

Figure 3 Frequency distribution of dive depths of the 11-day record of the same seal as in Figure 2. Total dives = 653. (From Le Boeuf et al., 1985.)

accumulation and whether or not it had reached some equilibrium are not known. It seems safe to conclude that during some of the dive bout, tissue PN_2 had more than doubled, and it might have climbed even further if the dive bout had been longer. Even with such a slow rate of PN_2 increase, it suggests that toward the end of a dive bout the N_2 tensions could be elevated to a level hazardous to the animal's health or that special tissue adaptations may be required to accommodate such tensions. However, the subsequent extended time at the surface would allow time for tissue and blood PN_2 to return to normal levels.

This concept of a steady rise in tissue PN_2 that is ameliorated by extended surface recovery after a bout may have to be revised for some species in light of the recent data on continuous diving. The nonstop deep diving of elephant seals allows no such recovery. The seals are seldom at the surface and rarely for extended periods (Table 1). Not only are they submerged for over 90% of the time, but when they dive it is always deep, seldom less than 200 m (Fig. 3). Even with the most conservative estimate of PN_2 occurring in elephant seals, which is based on single dives (Kooyman et al., 1973), the elephant seal may have tissue N_2 tensions of 2 to 3 ata or up to four times that of terrestrial mammals living at sea level. If the present observations of continuous diving over the first 2 to 3 weeks of a period at sea are found to reflect the general sea behavior of this beast, then this high tissue PN_2 would prevail for most of their life. At a PN_2 of 4 ata, the anesthetic effect is equivalent to about 15% of an anesthetizing dose of halothane (Winter and Miller, 1985). However, at depths of 200 m or greater the excitatory effect of compression of nervous tissue membranes would greatly override the low level anesthetic effect of N_2. Indeed the condition called high-pressure nervous syndrome (HPNS) is manifested as tremors in mammals at the equivalent 140 to 150 m and as convulsions at 500 m (Brauer, 1975). Such high pressure compresses and reduces the volume of the membrane of nervous tisse. This reduction in volume correlates with the excitatory properties of the nervous system (Winter and Miller, 1985). The site of action of soluble anesthetics may be by expanding the volume of the lipid membrane of nervous tissue and blocking its transmission. Indeed, the therapy of increasing the amount of N_2 in the membrane to 6.9 ata in saturation divers working at 690 m relieved them of HPNS. Could it be that some N_2 uptake in deep divers is beneficial for overcoming HPNS? And perhaps such persistent deep divers as elephant seals have a different membrane thickness and nervous conduction than terrestrial mammals, so that at depth they are in balance for alert and vigorous activity, whereas at the surface they are more soporific. There is no evidence for any of this speculation, but it is noteworthy that beached elephant seals are legendary for their sluggish behavior and sleeping apneuses, which may last 20 min in pups (Huntley and Costa, 1983) and probably longer in adults. Generally, the duration of the apneusis appears to be correlated with metabolic rate.

There is one final speculative point to be made relative to pressure that seems appropriate for this volume on the *Biology of the Lung in Health and Disease*. The primary function of the lung is gas exchange, and that is the task it does every minute of the day in most mammals. Yet, in the deep-diving animal involved in a bout of several hours duration (Weddell seal, *Leptonychotes weddellii*) or continuously (northern elephant seal) the lung must be atelectatic below 100 to 200 m, and that is where some of these animals spend most of their time. Therefore, during much of the life of the elephant seal, and perhaps other diving mammals, the lung must be gas free. How does this affect its inflation properties, the nature of ventilation/perfusion ratio distribution, and ultimately gas exchange characteristics during the brief encounters with the surface? Presumably, these dive schedules do not interfere with effective gas exchange because surface intervals remain consistently short. The fact suggests special surface tension and inflationary properties of the lung.

III. Aerobic Limits

When divers spend so much time at depth as illustrated in Figures 1 and 2, then the collapsed lung is almost functionless as an O_2 store. For seals this has little influence on the aerobic dive limit (ADL) because it represents only about 5%

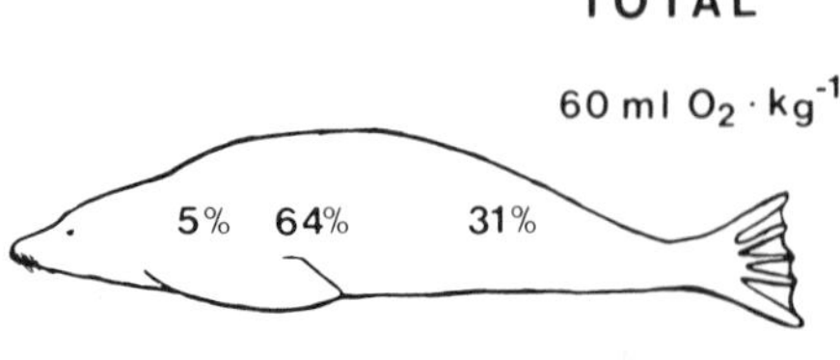

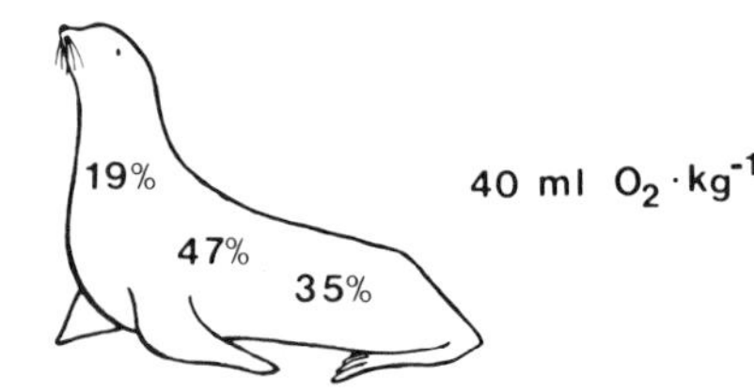

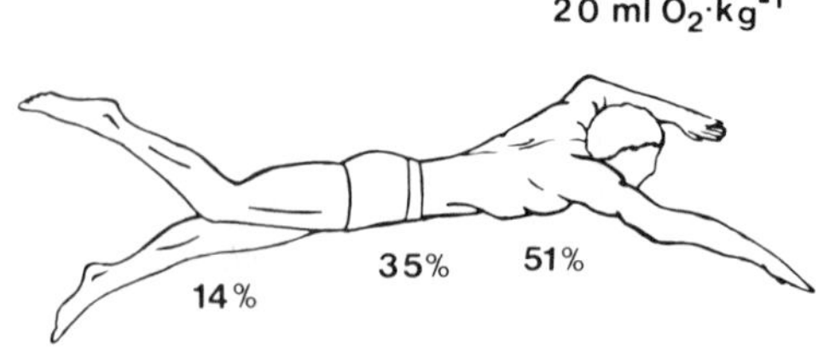

Figure 4 Approximate available lung, blood, and muscle O_2 stores in phocids, otariids (and dolphins), and man. (From Kooyman, 1985.)

of the total O_2 store (Fig. 4). For sea lions and dolphins, this may be a more serious loss because lung O_2 store is about 20% of the total O_2 stored based on calculations done for seals (Lenfant et al., 1970; Kooyman et al., 1980; Kooyman et al., 1983), fur seals, and sea lions (Lenfant et al., 1970; Gentry et al., 1986). These calculations take into account a reasonable estimate of the available blood and muscle O_2 store, as well as the lung store. The limit of their use in a so-called aerobic dive was defined by Kooyman (1985) as "the maximum breathhold that is possible without any increase in blood lactic acid [LA] concentration during or after the dive." This limit is dependent upon several variables in addition to O_2 stores. Some of these are the rate of O_2 consumption as well as LA production and consumption, and the nature of blood flow to O_2-consuming organs. The partitioning of the O_2 stores and their management is one of the exciting areas of present research on diving mammals.

We currently know little about this subject, but behavioral studies give us some concept of how closely it may be managed. Again, the elephant seal may be an exceptional example because they appear so mechanically precise in their dive habits. Over an 11-day period, the average dive duration of a 280-kg seal was 21 min with standard deviations for each 24 h or no greater than ± 6.0 min, and during four 24-h periods it was $< \pm$ 2.0 min. This dive duration is close to the calculated ADL of an elephant seal of about 450 kg in which the O_2 consumption rate is only slightly greater than the predicted resting rate. Because this seal had endured a long fast and lost most of its fat, the blood and muscle O_2 stores and metabolic rate may have been closer to those of a much larger seal than of its actual weight. It appears that the seal was striving to make maximum use of its O_2 store. Several assumptions were made to make the calculation, and much needs to be measured to understand clearly the management of internal resources. Although some of the pattern of management may be general for most marine mammals, others may be specific to groups. Seals tend to be slow swimmers, with apparently low metabolic rates, in which the lung store is of minor importance. Sea lions and dolphins may exhibit another pattern in which the lung store is of greater importance and, because of their high swim speeds, the metabolic rate may be higher. However, nothing is known about this group except the intriguing study of a trained bottlenose dolphin. This animal weighed 138 kg and, based on the end-tidal tensions which should reflect arterial O_2 tension, it returned to the surface with an end-tidal PO_2 of 18 torr after 4-min dives to 300 m depth (Ridgway et al., 1969). On the basis of the end-tidal O_2 tension, which should be slightly higher than arterial O_2 tension, it must have been near its breath hold limit. Again, the animal seemed to be utilizing fully its O_2 store.

IV. Recovery

In most instances, recovery from a dive is a time of rapid turnover of volatile metabolic products. Carbon dioxide is expired in such large quantities that the respiratory quotient initially exceeds 1.0 (Kooyman et al., 1973). The dissipation of CO_2 raises blood and tissue pH and enhances the rapid uptake of O_2 as it binds to hemoglobin and myoglobin. However, recovery from dives takes a new perspective when surfacers are considered. No longer can the course of recovery be regarded as an extended time to return acid–base conditions and metabolic imbalances to normal after a long dive (Fig. 5) or as a steady departure from normal during the dive bout. The recovery from dives is a process in which steady-state conditions prevail. There is no incremental increase in "O_2 debt," LA, and kidney and liver filtering. The exception would be the accumulation of food when an animal meets with good success during a series of lucky

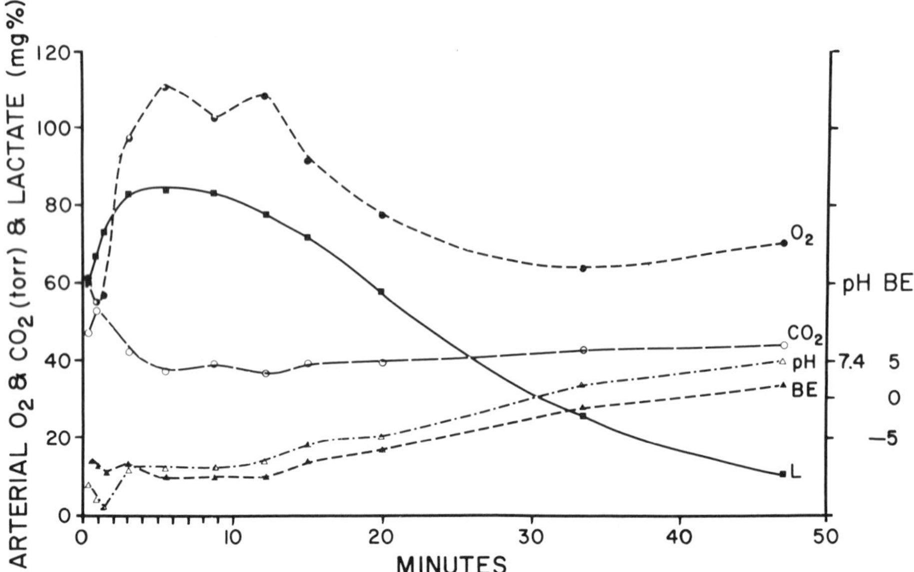

Figure 5 Arterial gas tensions, pH, base excess, and lactic acid levels of an adult Weddell seal during recovery from a 42.6-min dive. (From Kooyman et al., 1980.)

dives. During the unusual circumstances from which extra effort is required, such as an exceptionally long dive, the LA clearance may not take place during an extended recovery period, but, rather, over the course of the following dives.

A rare opportunity to sample blood and measure the LA concentration after an extended dive shows a steady decline of LA during the course of dives that followed a long dive (Fig. 6). In most instances, another extended dive is unlikely until the O_2 debt of the original dive is substantially reduced or eliminated. This does not mean that another extended dive is impossible, and a rare exception was probably observed recently.

After reviewing thousands of dives, from many records, of a variety of marine tetrapods, an example came to light. An adult, 400-kg female elephant seal, which a few days earlier had ended a 2-month fast during which she was nursing a pup, was engaged in continuous diving. In one series of dives, she accomplished a remarkable feat. She made a 48-min dive, followed by 40, 35, 36, 32, and 30-min dives before resuming the more normal 20- to 27-min dives. Given her size, at least all of these more than 30-min dives must have exceeded her aerobic dive limit if she was actively diving. No blood LA concentrations

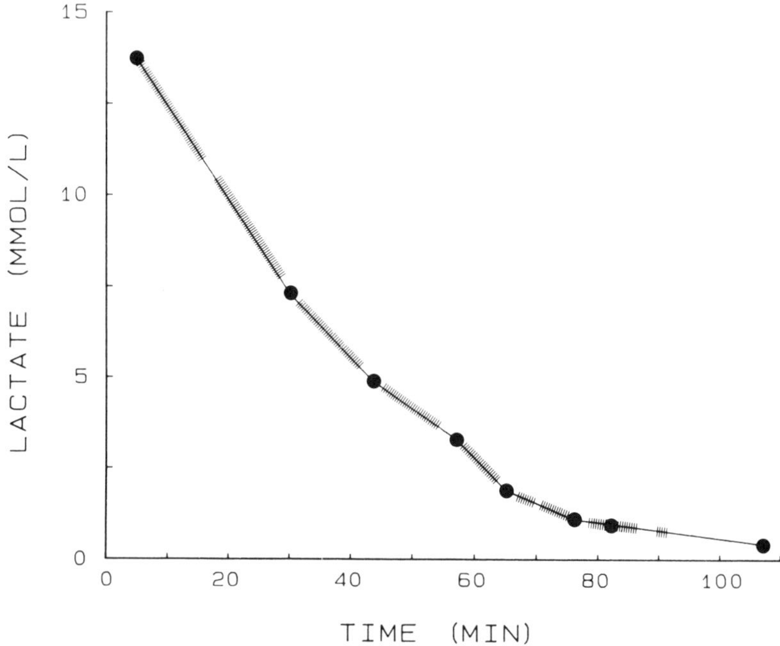

Figure 6 Decline in blood lactic acid concentration in a 205-kg immature Weddell seal in which a 33-min dive was followed by 10 shorter dives. The hatched marks on the curve indicate the dives and the closed circles the sample times.

were measured, but extrapolating similar data from a voluntarily diving Weddell seal of equal size, I have constructed a highly speculative blood LA profile through the course of this dive series (Fig. 7). It probably resembles a profile of a terrestrial animal involved in consecutive sprints. The final hypothetical peak [LA], assumes that:

1. Some aerobic consumption of LA continues throughout the dive by perfused organs. Consumption of LA occurs in nonperfused muscle also, as long as the internal O_2 store lasts. The rate of decline of blood LA is comparable with what has been measured in a Weddell seal (Kooyman et al., 1980).
2. Lactic acid is consumed at the surface during recovery by all organs capable of LA oxidation or resynthesis to glucose.
3. Lactic acid accumulation during the dive, and reflected in the post-dive peak, is similar to the amount and rate of increase in Weddell seals (Kooyman et al., 1980).

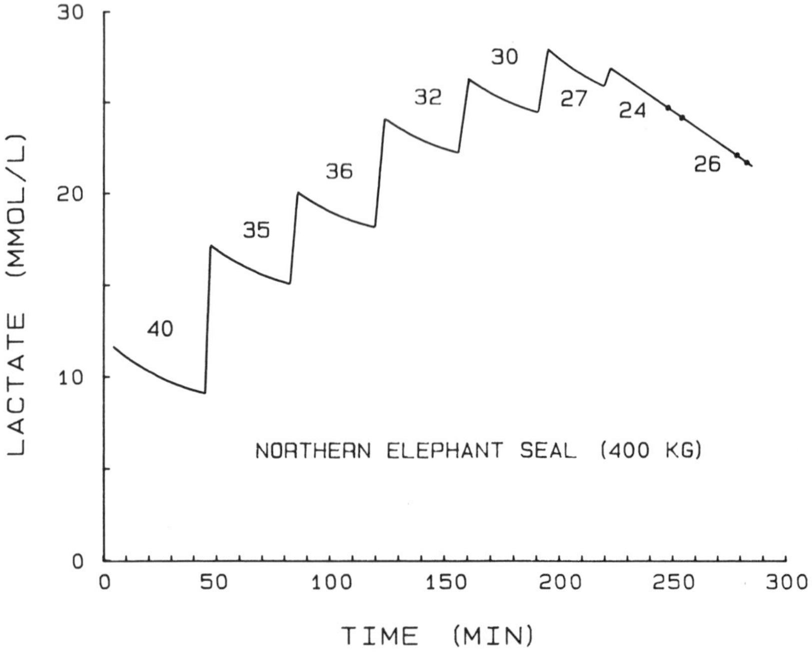

Figure 7 Hypothetical blood LA concentration during a series of dives that exceeded the aerobic dive limit of an adult, female northern elephant seal. The numbers near the slopes are the dive durations and the interval between the low and high point between slopes is the surface interval (about 2.2 min). See text for a detailed explanation.

Lactic acid accumulates to a final peak of about 27 mmol. This assumes a 25-min aerobic limit in which muscle and other organs are net consumers of LA during much of the dive. Also, when muscle O_2 is exhausted it becomes the major LA producer and is responsible for the incremental rise in peak blood [LA] after each dive. This description is a worst-possible-case condition. If the seal were resting and inactive during much of the submersion in some of the dives, then LA accrual would be less. The profiles of the last four dives (36–27 ft) suggest just that (Le Boeuf, personal communication).

Although this is a highly speculative account, it emphasizes the variance that continuous diving may have with our conventional views of metabolite management during diving. Serial diving is generally not addressed in studies or reviews of physiological responses to diving, but as we learn more about the behavior of these animals, the clarity of its importance to understanding the physiology of diving increases.

V. Summary and Conclusions

The emphasis of this chapter has been on recent observations on serial diving in discrete bouts and on continuous diving. Our understanding of the physiological processes involved in such diving activity is rudimentary. Specific examples reflect the impact on organs that are continuously exposed to high ambient pressure and to high N_2 tensions. Also, what is the size and availability of the O_2 store? Frequently, it appears to be nearly depleted in the course of a dive. The replenishment of the O_2 store and dissipation of LA may not be as conventional as previously reported from studies of single dives. Lactic acid accumulation resulting from an extended dive may be turned over in subsequent shorter dives. In short, a full understanding of diving physiology of natural divers will require more studies of serial diving.

Acknowledgment

I wish to thank M. Castellini, B. Le Boeuf, and P. Ponganis for the benefit of their discussions.

References

Brauer, R. W. (1975). The high pressure nervous syndrome: Animals. In *The Physiology and Medicine of Diving and Compressed Air Work*. Edited by P. B. Bennett and D. H. Elliott. Baltimore, Williams & Wilkins, pp. 231-247.

Eckert, S. A., Nellis, D. W., Eckert, K. L., and Kooyman, G. L. (1986). Diving patterns in two leatherback sea turtles (*Dermochelys coriacea*) during internesting intervals at Sandy Point, St. Croix, U.S. Virgin Islands. *Herpetologica 42*:381-388.

Falke, K. J., Hill, R. D., Qvist, J., Schneider, R. C., Guppy, M., Liggins, G. C., Hochachka, P. W., Elliott, R. E., and Zapol, W. M. (1985). Seal lungs collapse during free diving: Evidence from arterial nitrogen tensions. *Science 229*:556-558.

Gentry, R. L., Costa, D. P., Croxall, J. P., David, J. H. M., Davis, R. W., Kooyman, G. L., Majluf, P., McCann, T. S., and Trillmich, F. (1986). Synthesis and conclusions. In *Fur Seals: Maternal Strategies on Land and at Sea*. Princeton, Princeton University Press, pp. 220-264.

Huntley, A. C., and Costa, D. P. (1983). Sleep apnea: "Terrestrial diving" in the northern elephant seal. In *Breath-Hold Diving and Asphyxia*. I.U.P.S. Satellite Symposium, August 22-24, p. 9.

Kooyman, G. L. (1982). How marine mammals dive. In *A Comparison to Animal Physiology*. Edited by C. R. Taylor, K. Johansen, and L. Bolis. London, Cambridge University Press, pp. 151-160.

Kooyman, G. L. (1985). Physiology without restraint in diving mammals. *Mar. Mamm. Sci. 1*:166-178.

Kooyman, G. L., Castellini, M. A., Davis, R. W., and Maue, R. A. (1983). Anaerobic dive limits in immature Weddell seals. *J. Comp. Physiol. 151*:171-174.

Kooyman, G. L., Schroeder, J. P., Greene, D. G., and Smith, V. A. (1973). Gas exchange in penguins during simulated dives to 30 and 68 m. *Am. J. Physiol. 225*:1467-1471.

Kooyman, G. L., Wahrenbrock, E. A., Castellini, M. A., Davis, R. W., and Sinnett, E. E. (1980). Aerobic and anaerobic metabolism during voluntary diving in Weddell seals: Evidence of preferred pathways from blood chemistry and behavior. *J. Comp. Physiol. 138*:135-146.

Kramer, D. L. (1988). The behavioral ecology of air breathing by aquatic animals. *Can. J. Zool. 66*:89-94.

Le Boeuf, B. J., Costa, D. P., Huntley, A. C., Kooyman, G. L., and Davis, R. W. (1985). Pattern and depth of dives in two northern elephant seals. *J. Zool. (Lond.) 208*:1-7.

Lenfant, C., Johansen, K., and Torrance, J. D. (1970). Gas transport and oxygen storage capacity in some pinnipeds and the sea otter. *Resp. Physiol. 9*:277-286.

Ridgway, S. H., and Howard, R. (1979). Dolphin lung collapse and intramuscular circulation during free diving: Evidence from nitrogen washout. *Science 206*:1182-1183.

Ridgway, S. H., Scronce, B. L., and Kanwisher, J. (1969). Respiration and deep diving in the bottlenose porpoise. *Science 166*:1651-1654.

Winter, P. M., and Miller, J. N. (1985). Anesthesiology. *Sci. Am. 252*:124-131.

25

Diving Physiology
Birds

RICHARD STEPHENSON and DAVID R. JONES

University of British Columbia
Vancouver, British Columbia, Canada

I. Introduction

A major impediment to progress in the study of the physiology of diving has been, until relatively recently, a general reluctance of physiologists to consider all aspects of the diving habit (i.e., its evolution, its function in different species, and the behavioral characteristics of actual diving activities in naturally diving animals) when planning and interpreting experiments. Thus, for almost a century after the first laboratory experiments, it was almost universally accepted that all air-breathing vertebrates invoke the same stereotyped series of reflexes (the so-called diving response) upon submersion in water. The recent increase in interest in the responses to voluntary dives, made possible by the development of biotelemetry systems of small size and weight, has led to numerous demonstrations of the variability of responses to submersion in different situations. Documented observations of diving behavior in wild birds were available long before the advent of biotelemetry devices, yet these data were largely ignored, as were the few comments that were made to the effect that physiological responses observed in the laboratory may not represent those that occur in nature (e.g., Scholander, 1940; Eliassen, 1960).

Supported by grants from NSERCC and the B. C. and Yukon Heart Foundation.

Birds have evolved a range of methods by which they can obtain food from an aquatic habitat. There are numerous interspecific differences in such factors as body size, mode of propulsion, and duration and depth of dives, and it is to be expected, therefore, that with these differences in behavior there have evolved differences in the anatomical, physiological, and biochemical mechanisms that provide the means to optimize each behavior. Hence, although the emphasis in this chapter is on the nature and control of physiological adaptations and adjustments to submersion in various situations, a brief introductory account of the evolution of the diving habit in birds, the methods of propulsion used in various species (and the anatomical adaptations that enhance these), and the behavioral characteristics of observed diving activities in various species is presented to put the physiological observations into perspective.

II. Evolution of Diving Birds

The taxonomic and phylogenetic organization of the class Aves is based on evidence derived from palaeontological records of extant and extinct species and from comparative studies in the ecology, behavior, morphology, physiology, biochemistry, and genetics of living species. Theories relating to the origins and early evolution of birds are based, however, almost exclusively on the first of these: the fossil record, which has recently been reviewed by Olson (1985). However, the technique of DNA-DNA hybridization, in which phylogeny is reconstructed depending on the average difference between DNAs of living birds, often presents a challenge to the fossil record (Sibley and Ahlquist, 1986).

The first birds arose from reptilian ancestors, probably the pseudosuchian or the later coelorusaurian dinosaurs (Feduccia, 1980), during the Jurassic period (approximately 140 million years ago). Fossils from this period are scarce, but it is clear that the first aquatic birds arose relatively early in avian evolutionary history. There are fossils from the early Cretaceous period (approximately 135 to 65 million years ago) of two orders of toothed birds; Hesperornithiformes (e.g., *Enaliornis* spp. and *Hesperornis* spp.) which were flightless, foot-propelled diving birds, and Ichthyornithiformes (e.g., *Ichthyornis*) which were diving and flying birds. These primitive birds were initially believed to have given rise to the Gaviiformes (loons) and Podicipediformes (grebes), and to the Charadriiformes (shore birds), respectively (e.g., Brodkorb, 1963; Cracraft, 1982), although it is now generally accepted that these Cretaceous birds represented separate phyletic lines (Martin, 1983; Olson, 1985). In fact, Hou and Liu (1984) have proposed another order, the Gansuiformes, to represent the common ancestor of all the waterbirds. They claim that the Gansuiformes, which were present in the early Cretaceous period, were coeval with *Archaeopteryx* and gave rise to the Charadriiformes which, in turn, are widely believed to be the "primitive" lines from which most other aquatic birds are derived.

The Tertiary period (approximately 60 to 2 million years ago) was a time of rapid adaptive radiation in waterbirds (Brodkorb, 1971). The family Alcidae (auks, murres, puffins) are the most specialized divers of the present day Charadriiformes. These pelagic wing-propelled divers first appeared in the late Eocene (approximately 50 to 40 million years ago) as indicated by the fossils of *Hydrotherikornis oregonus* (Miller, 1931). The order Anseriformes (waterfowl) were derived from the early Charadriiformes of the late Cretaceous (approximately 100 million years ago) as indicated by fossils of the "intermediate" form, *Presbyornis*, "which had the head of a duck on the body of a shorebird" (Olson, 1985). Recent chemical analyses of protein electrophoretic data (e.g., Patton and Avise, 1986) and restriction endonuclease analysis of mitochondrial DNA (Kessler and Avise, 1984) confirm cladistic analysis of waterfowl phylogeny; that species of the genera *Aythya* (diving ducks) and *Anas* (dabbling ducks) are a monophyletic group and along with the ratites and gallinaceous birds are among the oldest groups of living birds (Ahlquist, personal communication).

The phylogenetic relationships of the Gaviiformes (loons), Podicipediformes (grebes), Pelecaniformes (including pelicans, gannets, cormorants, and snakebirds), Procellariformes (including the diving petrels), and the Sphenisciformes (penguins) are less certain. It is now generally accepted that the penguins descended from flying birds, rather than flightless ratites (Baker and Manwell, 1975; Simpson, 1975; Cracraft, 1982; Olson, 1985). It has been suggested on the basis of cladistic analysis (Cracraft, 1982), and at least partly supported by biochemical studies (Ho et al., 1976), that all of the mentioned orders are monophyletic, rather than convergent (Storer, 1956, 1960; Olson, 1985). This is confirmed by the technique of DNA-DNA hybridization, which suggests that these are among the most recently derived birds and are a sister group of the songbirds (Passeriformes).

Divergence of most waterbirds from a common ancestor would give a logical basis to the search for common physiological responses in diving birds, although there is no reason to suppose that divergence cannot occur at the physiological level, as well as at the morphological and biochemical levels. This is particularly true if a protracted period has elapsed since any two groups had a common ancestor. For instance, DNA-DNA hybridization indicates that it could be 100 million years since diving ducks and cormorants had a common ancestor, thus, similarities in diving physiology between these two groups may be convergent and probably have no real basis in phylogeny.

III. Adaptation in Diving Birds

The collective terms *aquatic birds* and *waterbirds* include species representing about half of the extant orders of birds. These birds exhibit various levels of specialization for an aquatic life-style ranging from those that feed at the air-water interface (e.g., gulls, skimmers, dabbling ducks, waders) to those that spend a considerable proportion of their time engaged in surface and subsurface swimming (e.g., diving ducks, grebes, loons, alcids, penguins). In keeping with this wide range of behaviors, aquatic species exhibit a spectrum of morphological and anatomical adaptations. An attempt is made here to define some general trends rather than provide a comprehensive comparative account.

Divers tend to have a dorsoventrally flattened (widened) body that promotes stability at the water surface, dense plumage that provides thermal insulation, and an enlarged uropygial gland to facilitate waterproofing the feathers (Raikow, 1985). In addition, the overall body shape tends to become more streamlined owing to narrowing of the pelvis and more posterior placement of the hind limbs (particularly in foot-propelled divers) such that the mass of the legs merges with the contours of the body (Storer, 1971). In foot-propelled divers, the hind limbs are often highly adapted for aquatic locomotion and the capacity for terrestrial locomotion is compromised. The surface area of the foot of divers is increased either by webbing (e.g., loons, ducks) or by lobation (e.g., grebes, rails) and the foot area/body weight ratio (the so-called paddle index) increases with increased diving abilities, at least in North American ducks (Raikow, 1973). Other hind-limb adaptations include reduction in femur length and increase in tibiotarsal length (Raikow, 1985). It is thought that the thigh muscles are used primarily to hold the short thigh relatively immobile during diving, whereas the power stroke is achieved by the extension of the foot, mainly as a result of contraction of the enlarged gastrocnemius muscle and its agonists (Wilcox, 1952; Owre, 1967; Raikow, 1970; Weinstein et al., 1984; Turner, 1986).

The use of the wings for underwater propulsion in addition to flight creates problems of adaptation because of the different physical requirements imposed by the two media, air and water. Birds originally evolved for flight, and the wings have a large surface area to produce lift, whereas the body density is low (containing a large gas volume in the respiratory apparatus and skeleton) to reduce wing loading per unit body volume. Thus, the wing surface area/body mass ratio is an important factor in determining wing size and maximum body size in flying birds. In water, however, the wings are not required to produce lift because the birds are supported by buoyant forces, and wing area is, therefore, not determined by total body mass. Instead, forward thrust must be produced in a relatively viscous medium, and this requires a fairly rigid wing, the size of which is dependent upon those factors that limit forward propulsion: cross-sectional area of the body (which determines body drag) and body density (which determines buoyancy). In those species that use the wings for both submerged swimming and aerial flight (e.g., alcids, diving petrels, dippers) a compromise in adaptation of body and wing structure must, therefore, take place and a bias toward one mode of locomotion will reduce the ability to utilize the other. Kinematics of wing-propelled swimming in penguins (Clark and Bemis, 1979), alcids (Spring, 1971), and the North American dipper, *Cinclus mexicanus* (Goodge, 1959) have been analyzed using motion photography and illustrate this point. Penguins, the most specialized divers produce thrust during both phases of the wing beat cycle (a powerful upstroke is aided by the highly developed supracoracoideus muscle; Raikow, 1985). The more flexible wings of the dipper and murres are held closer to the body during diving than during flight and forward thrust is produced mainly during the downstroke (Goodge, 1959; Spring, 1971).

Thus, diving birds are adapted to selective pressures that promote a relatively dense, large, and streamlined body (a larger mass in water may confer advantages in terms of reduced heat loss to the environment; increased oxygen storage capacity in lungs, blood, and muscle; and increased maximal swimming velocity) with relatively short, rigid wings, or enlarged foot area. The most extreme adaptations of this type are present in those species that are (or were) fully committed to an aquatic life-style (e.g., *Hesperornis*, great auk, penguins steamer ducks).

As mentioned previously, a low body density is advantageous to flying birds in that it reduces wing loading. It is also advantageous to surface-swimming birds, such as dabbling ducks and geese, in that it provides buoyancy. However, a high positive buoyancy represents a distinct disadvantage to diving birds because it increases the energetic cost of becoming, and remaining, submerged. Little information is available about buoyancy in birds; however, it appears that the buoyant force is lower in good divers (D. R. Jones, R. F. Berry, and R. Stephenson, unpublished observations). Positive buoyancy increases in the following order: double-crested cormorant (*Phalacrocorax auritus*), redhead duck (*Aythya americana*), mallard (*Anas platyrhynchos*), Pekin duck (*A. platyrhynchos*). Low buoyancy, as indicated by degree of skeletal pneumaticity and observations of the body position in the water when the birds are at the surface, is also correlated with good diving ability (e.g., Dehner, 1946; Bellairs and Jenkin, 1960; portman, 1950; Harrison, 1964; Owre, 1967; Casler, 1973; Butler and Woakes, 1984). There is some variability within this general trend, however, which is to be expected considering that body density is also important to flying abilities, particularly in larger birds, and that the lungs also function as an important site of oxygen storage in divers. Thus, several species of strong flyers that also dive (e.g., Pelecaniformes) have highly pneumatic skeletons (Richardson, 1939; Bellairs and Jenkin, 1960; Owre, 1967). The habit of plunging into the water from a height of several meters may be a behavioral strategy that has evolved to enable these relatively large birds to overcome the disadvantages of high buoyancy in diving while retaining the advantage of weight reduction for flight (Streseman, 1927–1934).

The volume of the respiratory system is also important in determining buoyancy, although few comparative studies have been made. It is difficult to distinguish any trends in lung–air sac volume related to diving activity from the data available, particularly because many of the earlier measurements were made by unreliable lung-cast techniques (see King, 1966, for references). If anything, divers appear to have slightly larger respiratory system volumes, which may be detrimental in terms of elevating buoyancy but confer greater advantages in oxygen storage capacity. Keijer and Butler (1982), using an inert gas washout technique, found the lung volume of a diving duck, the tufted duck (*Aythya fuligula*), to be greater than that of a dabbling duck, the mallard (*Anas platyrhynchos*), a difference that is likely to be even greater when allometric scaling factors are taken into account because in the larger *A. platyrhynchos*, the volume of the respiratory system is proportional to (body mass)$^{1.26}$ (Hudson and Jones, 1986). Furthermore, the data presented by Dehner (1946) also indicate a similar, but weak, trend in respiratory system volumes when comparing diving and dabbling ducks, although only if allometric factors are applied. It would appear, then, that the trend toward reduced buoyancy in divers may be achieved despite a contrary trend to increase buoyancy resulting from larger lung–air sac volumes.

Loss of air from beneath the feathers during submersion (Casler, 1973; Kooyman, 1975; Butler and Woakes, 1982b; Stephenson et al., 1986) and compression of the lungs at depth (Kooyman, 1975) may also play a role in buoyancy reduction during diving. Casler (1973) suggested that the approximately neutrally buoyant *Anhinga anhinga* may control buoyancy by regulating the amount of air held in the air sacs just before submergence, a mechanism that was first proposed by Streseman (1927–1934) for divers in general, and by Schorger (1947) specifically for the common loon, *Gavia immer*, and old-squaw, *Clanguia hyemalis*. Furthermore, the almost neutrally buoyant penguins often dive at end-inspiration (Kooyman et al., 1971) and may sometimes exhale while underwater (Kooyman, 1975), whereas the positively buoyant tufted duck, *Aythya fuligula*, dives after partial expiration (Butler and Woakes, 1979). The energetic significance of positive buoyancy in diving ducks has recently been determined for the lesser scaup, *Aythya affinis*. In this species, the subsurface buoyancy force (0.953N) is 3 times greater than the submerged drag force (0.35 N) at the measured diving velocity of 0.55 ms^{-1} (M. R. A. Heieis, D. R. Jones, and R. M. Blake, unpublished observations), and because approximately 85% of the active phase (descent and feeding period) of voluntary dives is spent spatially immobile while feeding on the bottom, work done to overcome buoyancy is many times greater than work done against body drag. In other species with reduced buoyancy and higher submerged swimming velocities (e.g., piscivorous species such as cormorants), this relationship is likely to be very different, and a comparative study would be most worthwhile.

Of all aquatic birds, the deepest and longest dives are performed by members of the order Sphenisciformes (penguins). Hydrostatic pressure increases by approximately 1 atm for every 10 m depth and this causes physiological problems to animals that submerge with air in their body. Compression of the lung-air sac gases will increase the partial pressure of oxygen, which will be beneficial in terms of lung oxygen store utilization, but it will also increase the partial pressure of nitrogen, which will enter the blood. This inevitably leads to the danger of succumbing to decompression sickness on ascent. If the rate of decompression exceeds the rate at which dissolved nitrogen can reenter lung gases then, when nitrogen tension exceeds the ambient pressure by 2.5 atm or more (Harvey et al., 1944a,b), bubbles may form in the blood leading to air embolisms. Kooyman et al. (1973) forcibly submerged Adelie and Gentoo penguins (*Pygoscelis adeliae* and *P. papua*, respectively) in a hyperbaric chamber and compressed them to simulated depths of 30 and 68 m. At 4 ata lung gases (O_2, CO_2, and N_2) equilibrated with the blood, but at 6.8 to 7.8 ata the arterial nitrogen was far below the equilibrium levels, indicating that at this pressure gas exchange was inhibited. Confirmation of inhibited gas exchange was obtained from measures of arterial P_{CO_2}, which was the same at 7.8 ata as it was at 4 ata. Thus, gas exchange is inhibited at depth, but given the lack of any evidence for a vascular shunt during submersion and difficulties associated with modeling complete lung collapse because of the physical structure of the lungs in birds, it is still unclear how birds avoid decompression sickness during rapid ascent from deep dives.

IV. Underwater Endurance Capacities and Natural Diving Behavior

The remarkable ability of aquatic birds to endure prolonged submersion, as compared with their terrestrial counterparts, has long been recognized. The search to discover the means and mechanisms by which this increased endurance capacity of aquatic birds is achieved has motivated most of the work in this field for over a century. Basically, as first proposed by Irving (1934, 1939), an enhanced endurance capacity is largely the result of an oxygen-conserving cardiorespiratory response that is evoked upon forced submersion into water (Fig. 3). The efficacy of the reflex adjustments that make up this response are enhanced in naturally aquatic species by means of the anatomical and biochemical adaptations that are discussed below.

Under normal circumstances, aquatic birds dive for only a small fraction of their maximum endurance capacities. It was pointed out by Kooyman et al. (1980) with reference to the Weddell seal, *Leptonychotes weddelli*, that by maintaining aerobic metabolism in all tissues during dives, a greater proportion of time could be spent submerged because on resorting to anaerobiosis, with its associated disturbance in acid-base balance, recovery time between dives will be

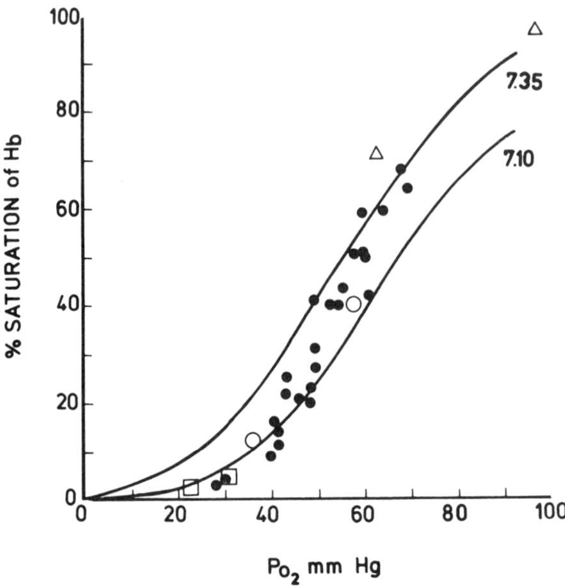

Figure 1 In vitro O_2 dissociation curves for duck blood illustrating the pronounced Bohr shift that occurs over a pH range representative of that which occurs during prolonged forced submergence. These curves, and the data illustrating arterial O_2 saturation and PO_2 during submersion (solid circles) are from Andersen and Lövö (1967). Data from Hudson and Jones (1986) (open symbols) illustrating arterial and venous O_2 saturation and PO_2 before submergence (triangles: pHa = 7.45, $pH\bar{v}$ = 7.38), at middive (circles: pHa = 7.27, $pH\bar{v}$ = 7.23), and at end-dive (squares; pHa = 7.11, $pH\bar{v}$ = 7.04) are also shown. It can be seen that at the low pH, which occurs at end-dive, venous and arterial blood are almost completely desaturated at the relatively high PO_2 of 20–30 mm Hg. This may explain why only approximately 75% of the O_2 stored in the lung–air sac system is available for use during submergence in the dabbling duck, *Anas platyrhynchos* (Hudson and Jones, 1986).

disproportionately increased. This probably applies to all diving birds and mammals. After short aerobic dives with little or no metabolic acidosis, a relatively short period of hyperventilation (associated with an increased cardiac output) will replenish oxygen stores and blow off accumulated carbon dioxide enabling dives to be performed in quick succession. This aerobic-diving strategy probably also serves an important antipredator function in that the period after a dive when escape from a predator would be impaired is reduced to a minimum. Thus, diving birds in their natural habitats are observed to perform dives of relatively short duration, which suggests that metabolism in these dives could be predominantly aerobic. Many dives (up to 40 or more) are usually performed with only a brief recovery period between each, and each series of dives is then followed by a longer period of rest at the water surface (Dewar, 1924; Kooyman et al., 1980; Jones and Furilla, 1987).

The aerobic dive limit and the maximum underwater endurance capacity are both dependent upon the magnitude of the usable oxygen stores in the body and upon the rate at which these stores are consumed. The major sites of oxygen storage are the lung-air sac system, the blood, and skeletal muscle. The relative importance of each probably varies according to body size and species (Hudson and Jones, 1986). Keijer and Butler (1982) concluded that the respiratory system represents a greater oxygen storage site in the tufted duck, *Aythya fuligula*, than in the mallard, *Anas platyrhynchos*. Unfortunately, because of the blood gas properties of ducks (see Fig. 1), only about 75% of this oxygen is usable during forced submergence (Hudson and Jones, 1986).

The size of the blood oxygen store is dependent upon the blood volume and the hemoglobin concentration. Strong flyers and divers tend to have blood volumes in the upper end of the range for all birds of approximately 45-175 $ml \cdot kg^{-1}$ (Bond and Gilbert, 1958; Lenfant et al., 1969; Huang et al., 1974; West, 1981; Keijer and Butler, 1982; Palacios et al., 1984; Hudson and Jones, 1986). Furthermore, an increased in overall levels of diving activity results in an increase in blood volume but no change in hemoglobin concentration in the tufted duck (R. Stephenson, D. L. Turner and P. J. Butler, unpublished observations). Avian hemoglobin concentrations, although affected by many factors, such as age, sex, and diet, usually fall within a range between 7 and 20 $mg \cdot 100\ ml^{-1}$. Good diving and flying ability tends to be correlated with values in the upper levels of this range (Lenfant et al., 1969; Murrish, 1970; Milsom et al., 1973; Balasch et al., 1974; Baumann and Baumann, 1977; Black and Tenney, 1980; West, 1981; Keijer and Butler, 1982; Freeman, 1984; Palacios et al., 1984; Maginniss, 1985).

The third significant site of oxygen storage is the myoglobin in skeletal muscle. Again, there appears to be a correlation between myoglobin concentrations and diving ability, with skeletal muscle concentrations ranging between approximately 0.3 and 10 $mg \cdot g^{-1}$ wet weight, with nondivers tending toward the lower end of this range (Pages and Planas, 1983; Palacios et al., 1984; Thomas, 1985) and aquatic birds such as ducks and geese toward the upper levels (Keijer and Butler, 1982; Snyder et al., 1984; R. Stephenson, D. L. Turner, and P. J. Butler, unpublished observations). Adult penguins, however, have exceptionally high myoglobin concentrations, approximately of the same order as that in marine mammals and an order of magnitude greater than that in some nondiving birds (Weber et al., 1974; Castellini and Somero, 1981; Baldwin et al., 1984). The primary role of myoglobin may be to facilitate the diffusion of oxygen from hemoglobin in the blood to cytochrome oxidase in the muscle

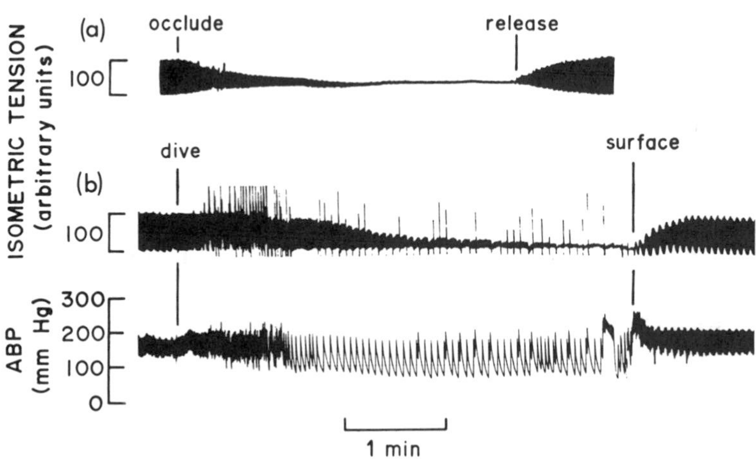

Figure 2 Traces of isometric tension (arbitrary units) developed by the tibialis anterior muscle of the Pekin duck, *Anas platyrhynchos*, during electrical stimulation at 3 H_Z. Traces illustrate: reduction in tension after occlusion of the ischiatic artery (a), and reduction in tension during forced submersion (b). Once a full "diving" bradycardia has developed [illustrated by arterial blood pressure (ABP) trace], the decline in tension during submersion followed a similar time course to that during complete occlusion of the arterial blood supply to the muscle. The contraction strength of perfused muscle did not decline after 45 min of stimulation in normally ventilating ducks. (From Jones and Furilla, 1987.)

mitochondria (Scholander, 1960; Wittenberg, 1970) and, in mammals, myoglobin is particularly important for the maintenance of normal cell function under conditions in which oxygen is in great demand (exercise) or in limited supply (hypoxia) (Cole, 1982, 1983). Not surprisingly, it has been found that aerobic endurance training (Pattengale and Holloszy, 1967; Hickson, 1981; Harms and Hickson, 1983) and exposure to high altitude (Reynafarje, 1962; Snyder et al., 1985) stimulated elevated myoglobin concentrations in mammals. Diving activity represents an energetic form of exercise in some birds (e.g., the tufted duck, *Aythya fuligula*; Woakes and Butler, 1983), and because this exercise is accompanied by apnea, there is likely to be a certain degree of hypoxia, particularly during long dives. Elevated myoglobin in avian divers may be an adaptation to improve oxygen delivery rather than storage, although in penguins, which dive deeply and may often have to use bursts of high-speed swimming to capture prey or avoid predators, myoglobin may serve as a store to fuel such burst activities. Duck leg muscles can maintain their strength of contraction for less than 30 s when the blood flow is occluded, and in forced submersion the strength of contraction decreases in a similar manner once bradycardia has been established (Fig. 2; Jones and Furilla, 1987). Furthermore, because myoglobin has a higher affinity for oxygen than hemoglobin has, myoglobin can act as a store only when muscle perfusion is reduced or Pa_{O_2} is very low. Because this is thought not to occur in most natural dives, it is, then, unlikely that myoglobin serves a storage function during most voluntary dives.

The oxygen transport properties of the blood are important in determining the efficacy of delivery of oxygen from stores to tissues. The oxygen affinity (described as oxygen tension at 50% saturation, P_{50}) of hemoglobin is an important determinant of the limiting partial pressures of oxygen under which oxygen can be loaded and unloaded at the lungs and tissues, respectively. A low P_{50} would favor uptake at the lung, whereas a high P_{50} would allow more efficient unloading at the tissues. Because of a high intra- and interspecific variability between P_{50} measurements in avian blood (Lutz, 1980), no clear trend for P_{50} and diving ability can be defined (Manwell, 1958; Lenfant et al., 1969; Milsom et al., 1973; Baumann and Baumann, 1977; Holle et al., 1977; Giardina et al., 1985; Maginniss, 1985).

The large Bohr factor ($= \Delta \log P_{50}/\Delta$ pH) in avian blood is close to the predicted optimum for oxygen delivery (Lapennas, 1983) and is not correlated with the diving habit (Manwell, 1958; Baumann and Baumann, 1977). Obviously, the change in pH and, therefore, the true impact of the Bohr effect during diving, will depend upon the buffering capacity of the blood. Indeed, the most consistent difference in the respiratory properties of the blood of aquatic versus terrestrial birds appears to be an increased buffering capacity in the former (Lenfant et al., 1969; Castellini and Somero, 1981; Murrish, 1982; Maginniss, 1985).

The Hill coefficient (n), which describes the degree of cooperativity of hemoglobin (and, therefore, the shape of the oxygen dissociation curve), is high in birds (Lenfant et al., 1969; Vandecasserie et al., 1973; Lutz et al., 1974; Scheipers et al., 1975; Wells, 1976; Maginniss, 1985). The reduction in cooperativity that occurs at low oxygen saturation is advantageous because it maximizes arteriovenous oxygen content differences when lung P_{O_2} is low (Lapennas and Lutz, 1982). The efficacy of stored oxygen utilization during voluntary dives is unknown. However, the white Pekin duck (*Anas platyrhynchos*) is not able to utilize all of its pulmonary oxygen store during forced submersion (Hudson and Jones, 1986). Only 4% of blood oxygen remains at the point of maximum underwater endurance (indicated by isoelectric EEG), whereas a full 25% of that in the air sacs is unused.

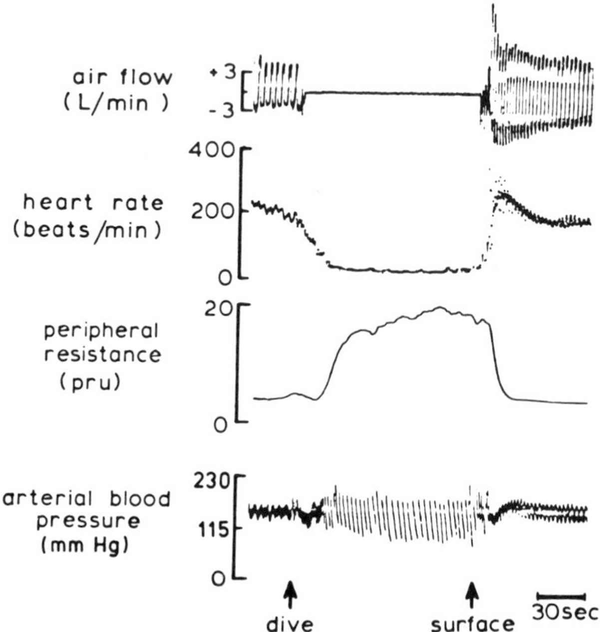

Figure 3 The O_2-conserving cardiorespiratory response evoked by a 1.9-min period of forced submergence in a domestic duck, *Anas platyrhynchos*. Apnea in the expiratory position, pronounced bradycardia, increased peripheral resistance (here measured as resistance to blood flow in one leg), and maintained arterial blood pressure during submergence are clearly illustrated. (From Butler and Jones, 1982.)

V. Metabolism and the Cardiorespiratory System in Aquatic Birds

A. The Responses During Forced and Voluntary Dives

There are two obvious differences between forced submergence and voluntary dives: (1) during forced submergence the bird is restrained and, therefore, inactive, whereas during natural dives the birds are physically active; and (2) during forced submergence the bird has no control over the duration of submergence, whereas voluntarily diving birds can usually control when they will return to the surface.

In view of these differences, it is not surprising that the metabolic (and associated cardiorespiratory) adjustments differ in the two situations. Birds become closed systems upon submersion in terms of gas exchange with the environment, and because the duration of forced submersion is out of the control of the animal, the logical response, as suggested by Irving (1934, 1939), is to reduce overall metabolic rate by reducing the level of aerobic metabolism or, in other words, to invoke an oxygen-conserving response. Such a response has been shown to occur during forced submergence in domestic ducks, *Anas platyrhynchos* (Scholander, 1940; Andersen, 1959; Pickwell, 1968). This overall reduction in metabolism to less than 20% of presubmersion levels in ducks (e.g., Pickwell, 1968) is the result of cardiorespiratory adjustments that basically consist of apnea accompanied by bradycardia, reduced cardiac output, and increased total peripheral resistance, with maintained arterial blood pressure (Fig. 3). Perfusion of hypoxia-tolerant tissues, notably skeletal muscle and viscera, is markedly reduced, whereas blood supply to the CNS, eyes, heart, and adrenal glands is maintained (Johansen, 1964; Jones et al., 1979). In the Pekin duck, *Anas platyrhynchos*, 75.2% of the total blood volume circulates within a central "heart-lung-brain" circulation after 2 to 5 min of forced submersion (M. R. A. Heieis and D. R. Jones, unpublished observations) in contrast to the suggestion that in seals, 85% of the blood volume is isolated in a slowly circulating peripheral pool that exchanges only slowly with blood in the central circulation (Murphy et al., 1980). Thus, in the Pekin duck, *A. platyrhynchos*, most of the blood oxygen store is accessible to the oxygen-dependent tissues (CNS and heart).

Unfortunately, relatively few studies have been performed on other species of birds. It is clear that the capacity to endure forced submersion is very variable between species. Redhead ducks, *Aythya americana*, of approximately 700 g body weight can withstand 6 to 8 min of forcible submersion (Furilla and Jones, unpublished observations), and by applying the allometric data of Hudson and Jones (1986), it can be calculated that the maximum endurance time of a Pekin duck of this size would be 5.3 min. The most probable explanation for increased endurance capacity in divers compared with dabblers is increased oxygen storage capacities and a more rapid onset of the oxygen-conserving response in divers. Having said that, many highly adapted divers, such as penguins, have rather low underwater endurance capacities compared with the domestic duck, a dabbling duck. It is probable that this variability in maximum submersion times results from a great variability in metabolic rate during submersion in different species. The domestic duck turns out to be rather exceptional in that it tolerates forced submergence well, struggling very little, whereas other species struggle violently and almost continuously during submersion (e.g., Scholander, 1940; Eliassen, 1960; Millard et al., 1973; Butler and Woakes, 1982a; Mangalam and Jones, 1984; Furilla and Jones, 1986). Indeed, the oxygen debt in penguins following forced submersion indicates that oxygen consumption was often greater than resting levels during submersion (Scholander, 1940). The very gradual development of bradycardia, the relatively rapid increase in blood lactate concentration, and the slow increase in muscle lactate concentration, all suggest that the oxygen-conserving response is relatively inefficient in penguins, at least during forced submersion.

The importance of the oxygen-conserving response to underwater endurance is indicated in several ways. If the cardiovascular response is abolished by administering an α-blocker to prevent peripheral vasoconstriction or if bradycardia is prevented by administering atropine (Butler and Jones, 1971), by pharmacological blockade of nasal receptors (Furilla and Jones, 1986), or by denervation of arterial chemoreceptors (Jones and Purves, 1970; Lillo and Jones, 1982), then the ability to tolerate prolonged forced submersion is compromised. Bryan and Jones (1980a,b) demonstrated the importance of the oxygen-conserving response by looking at the redox state of the cerebral hemispheres (monitoring changes in the quantity of NADH using a fluorometric technique) and the PO_2 of the hemispheric surface in domestic ducks and chickens. For a given decrease in tissue PO_2, ducks and chickens showed the same increase in NADH, indicating that both species are equally dependent on tissue PO_2 for maintenance of the redox state. In simulated dives, NADH increased much more slowly in the duck than the chicken, although NADH changes in the duck were accelerated after prevention of diving bradycardia with atropine.

It is probable that the endurance capacity of domestic ducks would be further increased if the rate of onset of the oxygen-conserving response was increased. In the frist 30 s of forced submergence, the fall in PaO_2 is identical between control and atropinized ducks (Butler and Jones, 1971), whereas in redhead ducks (*A. americana*), abolition of bradycardia by local anesthesia of the nasal passages caused a significant increase in the rate of reduction in PaO_2 compared with untreated ducks (Jones et al., 1987). The feedback mechanism initiating the oxygen-conserving response in dabbling ducks is inefficient because oxygen must initially be consumed before arterial chemoreceptors will be stimulated to evoke the response.

On the basis of observations of actual diving behavior as well as the results of laboratory experiments using several species of diving birds, Eliassen (1960) proposed that metabolic rate is at or above resting levels during voluntary dives. However, this was not generally accepted (e.g., Andersen, 1966) until over a decade later when actual measurements of cardiovascular variables were made in voluntarily diving birds. Telemetry of heart rate in Adelie and Gentoo penguins, *Pygoscelis adeliae* and *P. papua* (Millard et al., 1973) and tufted ducks, *A. fuligula* (Butler and Woakes, 1979) indicates that, if anything, metabolism is elevated above resting levels during voluntary dives, assuming a linear relationship between heart rate and oxygen consumption, which is the case in tufted ducks swimming on the surface (Fig. 4; Woakes and Butler, 1983, 1986). Millard et al. (1973) suggested that for penguins the response to voluntary diving represents a composite of responses to exercise and forced submersion, and Butler (1982) elaborated on this to suggest that in diving ducks the emphasis is on the exercise response.

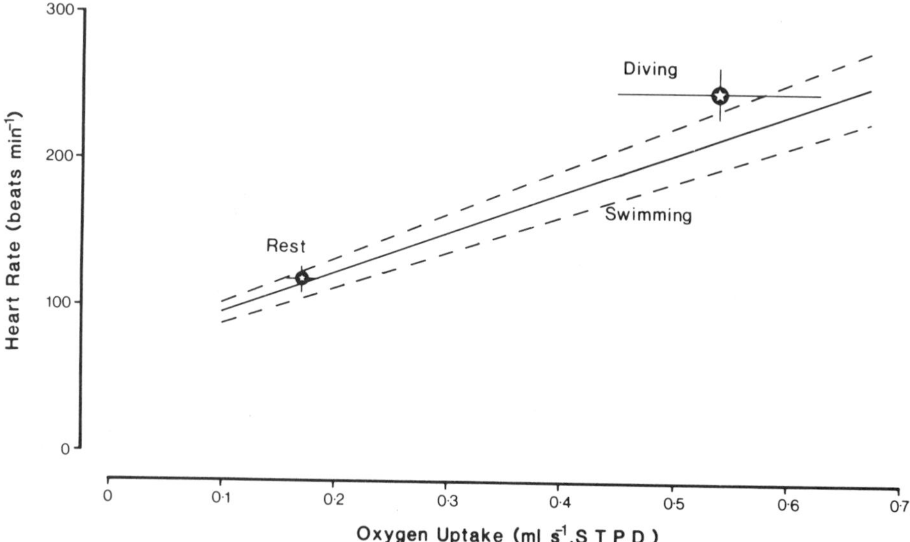

Figure 4 Relationship between heart rate (HR) and oxygen uptake ($\dot{V}O_2$) in resting, surface swimming, and diving tufted ducks, *A. fuligula.* The regression line represents the mean (± SE) relationship for five ducks swimming on a water flume at various speeds and is described by the following equation:

$$HR = 67.7 + 271.5\ (\pm 28.9) \cdot \dot{V}O_2$$

Points represent mean (± SE) heart rate at mean (± SE) levels of O_2 uptake for the same ducks at rest and during overall diving activities (i.e., measured over whole series of dives). (Data from Woakes and Butler, 1983, were reanalyzed, with permission, by Stephenson, 1987.)

By using a respirometry technique, Woakes and Butler (1983) estimated that oxygen uptake ($\dot{V}O_2$) during voluntary dives in the tufted duck, *A. fuligula,* increased to 3.5 times the resting level, a value similar to that measured during surface swimming at maximum sustainable speed ($0.78\ m \cdot s^{-1}$). Power output ($P_O = 0.59$ W) is correspondingly high in diving lesser scaup, *A. affinis,* most of the work being required to overcome the positive buoyancy of these diving ducks (M. R. A. Heieis, D. R. Jones, and R. A. Blake, unpublished observations) By using these data for P_O in *A. affinis* and the data of Woakes and Butler (1983) in *A. fuligula,* efficiency of underwater locomotion is calculated to be approximately 7%. In view of the low drag coefficients (Baudinette and Gill, 1985) and near neutral buoyancy of penguins, it is not surprising that oxygen consumption during voluntary diving behavior is close to resting values (Butler and Woakes, 1984). The average metabolic rate found during foraging (diving)

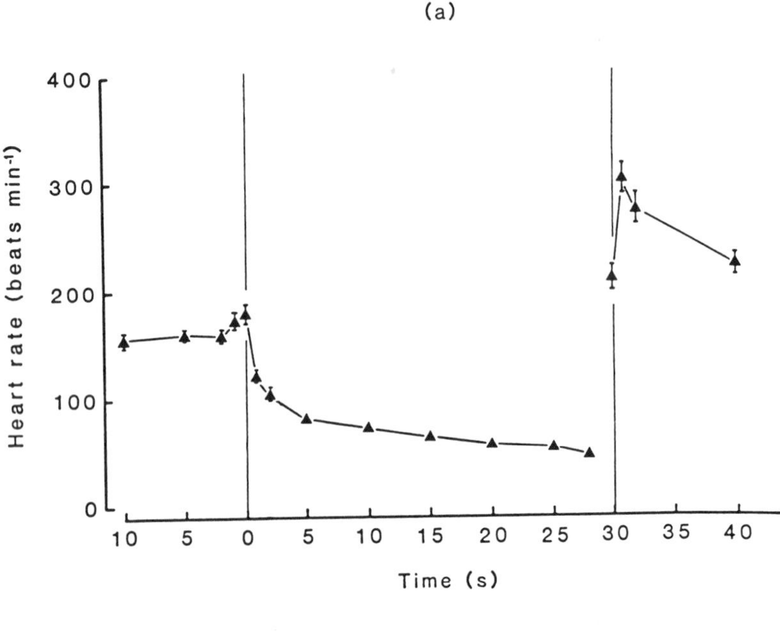

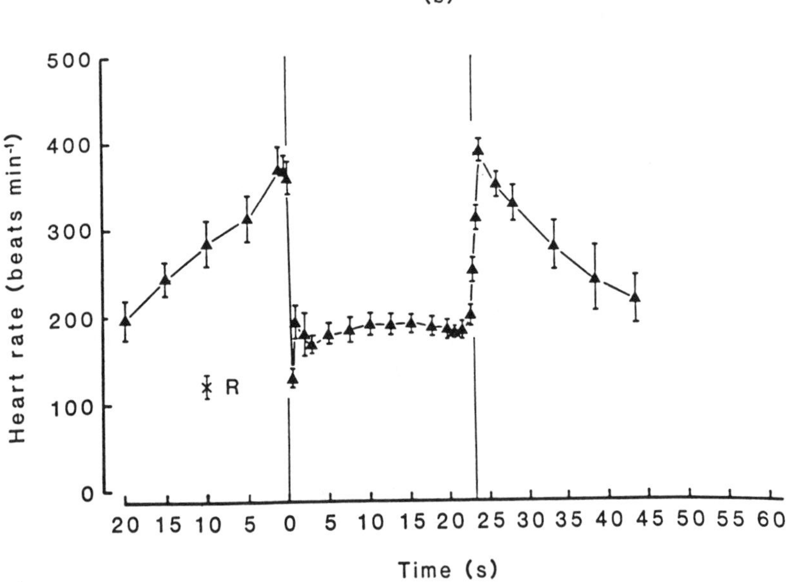

Figure 5 Mean heart rate (± SE) in tufted ducks, *A. fuligula*, during (a) forced submergence and (b) voluntary dives. Times of immersion (at time 0) and emersion are indicated by the vertical lines. R represents resting heart rate. (From Butler, 1988.)

activity as measured in penguins by utilizing the tritiated water techniques (Kooyman et al., 1982; Davis et al., 1983) revealed an average daily metabolic rate of 1.8 to 2.8 times the standard metabolic rate. These slightly higher values, compared with the respirometry studies of Butler and Woakes (1984), are probably a result of low environmental temperatures and increased proportion of time spent engaged in energetically more expensive surface swimming by free-ranging penguins (Baudinette and Gill, 1985). There is need for a comprehensive comparative study of power output requirements (drag and buoyancy) and metabolic responses (power input) under various circumstances encountered by various species in their natural habitats, as well as the laboratory, to test the generality of the preceding observations, which are presently restricted to diving ducks and penguins.

Diving cormorants and ducks exhibit markedly different heart rate responses to forced and voluntary submersion (Kanwisher et al., 1981; Butler and Stephenson, 1987; Fig. 5). A predive tachycardia (in excess of 300 beats · min^{-1}) in freely diving ducks is followed, upon immersion, by a rapid reduction in heart rate that then stabilizes at approximately 200 beats · min^{-1}, well above resting values (which are approximately 100 beats · min^{-1} in diving ducks), for the remainder of normal dives. Development of bradycardia is also rapid in onset during forced submergence, but in this situation, heart rates are lower than resting values until emersion (see Fig. 5). This is not true in all birds because the dipper shows similar responses in forced and voluntary dives (i.e., a profound bradycardia; Murrish, 1970), whereas in penguins and dabbling ducks there is very little change in heart rate from presubmergence levels during voluntary dives and only minute changes in the initial stages of forced submergence (Millard et al., 1973; Furilla and Jones, 1986). It is suggested that in diving ducks, when diving heart rate is higher than resting levels but lower than that during surface swimming at the same level of oxygen uptake (Woakes and Butler, 1983), perfusion of the active leg muscles is maintained and supply to inactive muscles may be reduced (Butler, 1982). That blood supply to the hind limbs is maintained during voluntary dives in the lesser scaup *A. affinis* has recently been confirmed (M. R. A. Heieis and D. R. Jones, unpublished observations). Voluntarily diving ducks, carrying an infusion pump attached as a backpack, were injected (in the base of the aorta) with macroaggregated albumin that was labeled with the gamma-emitter 99^{m} technetium. Organ trapping of the labeled protein, which was visualized uisng a gamma camera, produced a qualitative picture of blood flow distribution. Hind-limb perfusion was clearly maintained during voluntary dives but not during forced submersion (Fig. 6). Furthermore, Millard et al. (1973) found that femoral blood flow was reduced in voluntarily diving penguins, *Pygoscelis adeliae* and *P. papua*, as would be expected because the wings are used for propulsion in penguins.

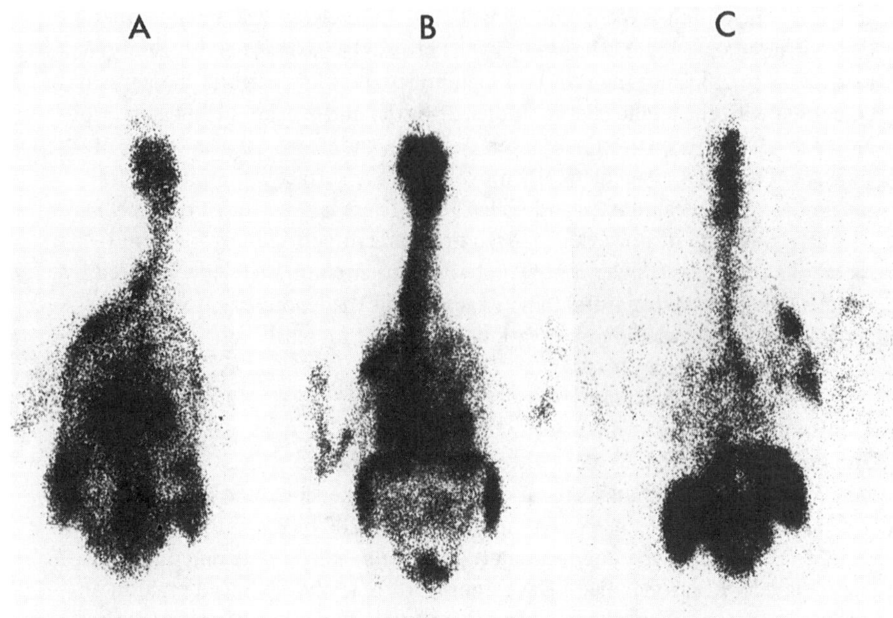

Figure 6 Blood flow distribution in a female lesser scaup, *A. affinis*, at rest (A), after 10 s of forced submergence (B), and after 5–10 s of voluntary diving (C). The images, obtained by the method of photographic visualization of organ-trapped, gamma-labeled macroaggregated albumin (MAA), are two-dimensional and, therefore, provide only a qualitative comparison of proportional blood flow to various body regions under different situations. Restriction of blood volume to a "central circulation" (thoracic and cranial areas) is apparent during forced submergence, whereas it is clear that during voluntary dives, perfusion of the legs is maintained.(Adapted from Jones, 1987.)

In addition to differences in cardiovascular and metabolic responses to forced and voluntary dives, it is now apparent that the response can vary depending upon the specific circumstances of individual dives. For example, as for several aquatic mammals, when unrestrained Humboldt penguins, *Spheniscus humboldti*, redhead ducks, *Aythya americana*, and tufted ducks, *A. fuligula*, are trapped underwater, they invoke a pronounced bradycardia that is similar to that seen during forced dives (Fig. 7) (Butler and Woakes, 1984; Furilla and Jones, 1986; Stephenson et al., 1986). In addition, tufted ducks that have to swim long distances underwater for food exhibit a more gradually developing bradycardia (Fig. 8; Stephenson et al., 1986). On the other hand, heart rate during escape dives in which the water surface is readily accessible in tufted ducks

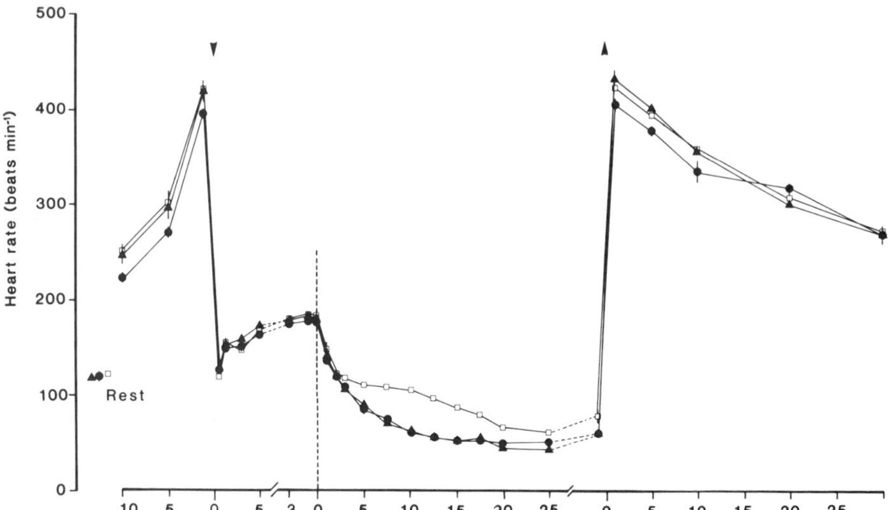

Figure 7 Mean (± SE) heart rate at rest and at specific times before during and after trapped dives in intact (closed circles), sham-operated (closed triangles), and carotid body denervated (open squares) tufted ducks, *A. fuligula*. Arrowheads represent the times of immersion and emersion, and the vertical dashed line represents the point at which the ducks apparently became aware that they were unable to reach the surface. (Data from Stephenson, 1987.)

(Stephenson, 1987) and redhead ducks (Furilla and Jones, 1986) is similar to that during normal-feeding dives. If heart rate is indicative of other circulatory adjustments and overall levels of metabolic rate, it is obvious that these are highly labile during diving activities under various conditions in conscious diving ducks (Butler and Stephenson, 1987).

B. Acid-Base Balance

Surprisingly, there are only two studies of acid-base balance during forced submersion (and none in voluntarily diving birds), both of which used the domestic duck, *Anas platyrhynchos*, (Andersen et al., 1965; Shimizu and Jones, 1987). Andersen et al. (1965) concluded that acidosis during the early period of submergence was largely respiratory and that a metabolic acidosis assumed increasing importance later in the dive. They concluded that the postdive acidosis was entirely metabolic, being due to release of lactate from tissues that had been hypoperfused in the dive. However, Andersen (1965) also reported an increase in the concentration of plasma potassium ions, $[K^+]$, during and after submersion, which would tend to offset any effects of increasing $[\text{lactate}^-]$ by reducing

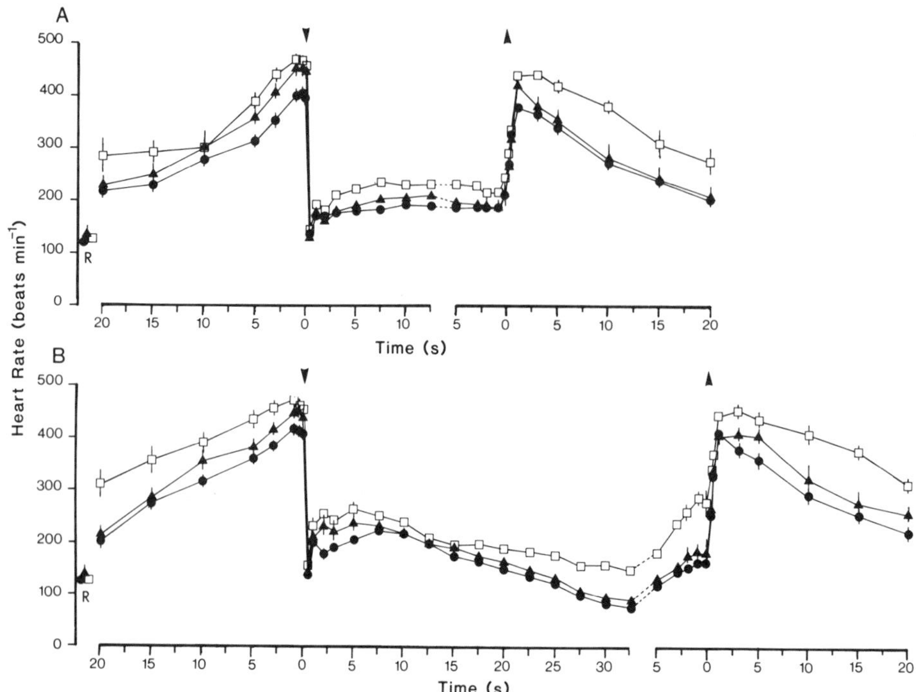

Figure 8 Mean (± SE) heart rate at rest (R) and at specific times before, during, and after (A) short (duration < 20 s, distance 2 m) and (B) extended (duration > 30 s, distance 11 m) dives in intact (closed circles), sham-operated (closed triangles, and carotid body denervated (open squares) tufted ducks, *A. fuligula*. Arrowheads represent the times of immersion and emersion (both at time = 0). (Adapted from Stephenson, 1987.)

strong ion difference (SID) (see Stewart, 1981, 1983). This prompted a more quantitative approach to acid-base balance during and after forced submersion by Shimizu and Jones (1987). Their conclusions were basically similar to those of Andersen et al. (1965), except that plasma sodium ions [Na^+], increased, more than plasma [K^+], along with plasma [$lactate^-$] during submersion, thereby countering any metabolic acidosis. Shimizu and Jones (1987), therefore, concluded that acidosis during submersion was entirely respiratory, a result of increased $PaCO_2$. During recovery $PaCO_2$ [Na^+], and [K^+] reached predive values by 3 min after emersion, and postdive acidosis largely resulted from a depression of SID caused by the much slower decline in plasma [$lactate^-$] in the recovery period (Fig. 9).

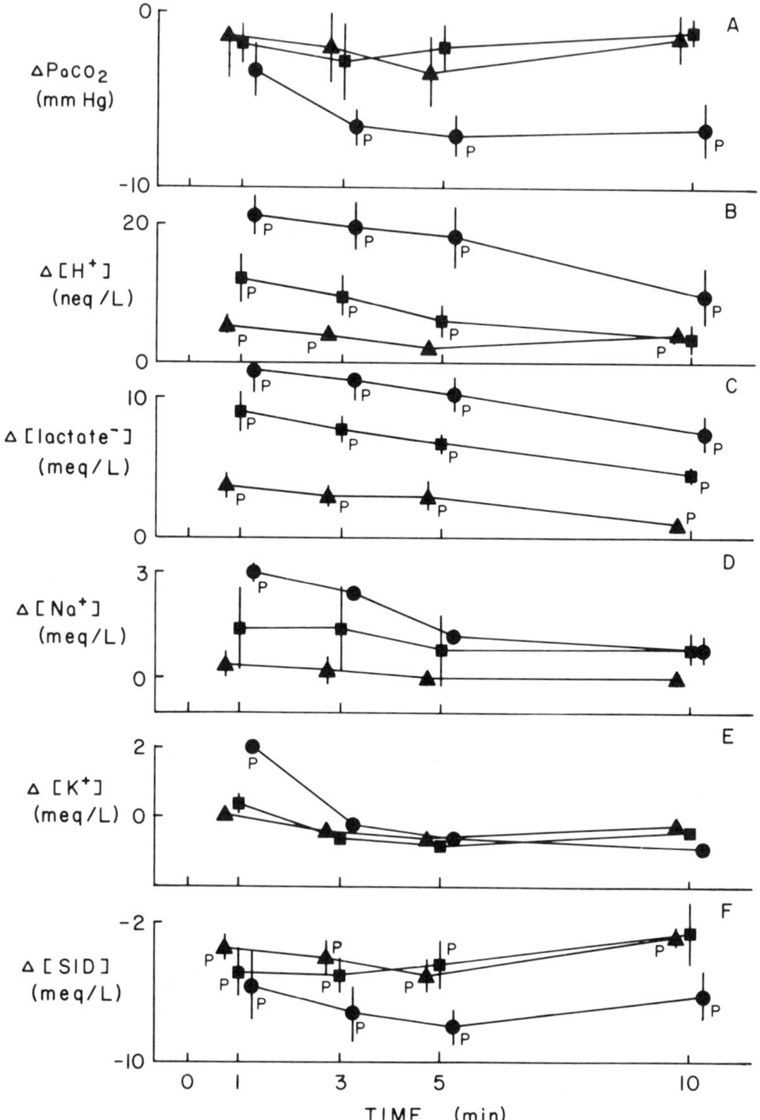

Figure 9 Changes in arterial CO_2 tension ($PaCO_2$), $[H^+]$, $[lactate^-]$, $[Na^+]$, $[K^+]$, and [SID] from predive values plotted against time after end of 1- (closed triangles), 2- (closed squares), and 4-min (closed circles) submergence. P indicates that the value is significantly different from the predive value. (From Shimizu and Jones, 1987.)

No direct measurements of acid-base balance have been made in voluntarily diving birds, though Millard et al. (1973) found only a slight reduction in the pH of penguin blood immediately following 20 to 30 min of diving activity. Woakes and Butler (1983) found that RQ increased from 0.84 at rest to 1.05 during diving activity in the tufted duck, indicating that excess carbon dioxide was being blown off during the interdive hyperventilation. This suggests that there is an acidosis in this species during voluntary diving. A gradual accumulation of [lactate$^-$] during voluntary diving could contribute to the stimulus to terminate a bout of diving in ducks.

C. Cardiorespiratory Control During Forced Submersion and Voluntary Dives

It has been known since 1913 that the cardiorespiratory response to forced submersion in the duck will occur after removal of suprabulbar structures of the CNS (Huxley, 1913a; Andersen, 1963; Gabbott and Jones, 1986). It would appear, then, that the cardiorespiratory responses to forced submersion are purely reflexogenic, and a considerable amount of time and effort has been spent trying to determine which afferent inputs contribute to the response, their relative importance, their interactions, and the efferent pathways by which they bring about the response. During voluntary dives, however, the variability of cardiorespiratory responses under various diving situations (e.g., Stephenson et al., 1986) and the occurrence of anticipatory changes in heart rate before the start and end of dives (Butler and Woakes, 1982b) indicate that suprabulbar and "psychogenic" neural influences may play an important role in naturally behaving animals (Gabbott and Jones, 1986; Furilla and Jones, 1987a).

Reflex apnea is the primary event to occur upon immersion in water, and it is maintained for the entire period of submersion, despite increasing stimulatory afferent neural inputs. Apnea is initiated by stimulation of receptors in the bill and upper respiratory tract (Bamford and Jones, 1974; Florin-Christensen et al., 1986), and these receptors are reported to be sensitive to mainly thermal stimuli, but also to mechanical and chemical stimuli in various species (Kitchell et al., 1959; Storey, 1968; Gregory, 1973; Bamford and Jones, 1974; Gottschaldt, 1974; Gottschaldt and Lansmann, 1974; Leitner and Roumy, 1974a,b; Leitner et al., 1974; Florin-Christensen et al., 1986). Afferent input from these receptors is conveyed by the opthalmic, maxillary, and mandibular branches of the trigeminal (V) nerves and also by the glottal branches of the glossopharyngeal (IX) nerves (Bamford and Jones, 1974). The receptors are slowly adapting, although Bamford and Jones (1974) found that their stimulation during forced head submersion would maintain apnea for only 2 min in Pekin and khaki Campbell ducks, *A. platyrhynchos* var., fitted with a tracheal cannula. Although largely ignored, it is also a possibility that postural reflexes initiate apnea during voluntary dives, when diving ducks assume a posture similar to that which elicits postural apnea in air, that is, dorsiflexion of the head (Huxley, 1913b,c; Paton, 1913, 1927; Koppanyi and Kleitman, 1927; Koppanyi and Dooley, 1928).

Several possible mechanisms for maintenance of apnea in intact birds can be suggested, but hard evidence is scarce. One old chestnut has been that respiratory sensitivity is lower in divers than in nondivers. Despite the conclusions of earlier studies (e.g., Orr and Watson, 1913; Dooley and Koppanyi, 1929), it is now generally accepted that the respiratory sensitivity to hypercapnia, hypoxia, and hypoxic hypercapnia is the same in diving and nondiving birds (Butler and Taylor, 1973, 1974, 1983; Milsom et al., 1981; Jones et al., 1985). The apparent insensitivity to hypercapnia and irregular breathing pattern (unchanged or decreased respiratory frequency and increase tidal volume) seen in some studies is due to the route of administration of the carbon dioxide (Dooley and Koppanyi, 1929; Jones et al., 1985). Avian intrapulmonary receptors are chemosensitive, rather than mechanosensitive (Fedde et al., 1974a,b), and the abnormal-breathing pattern that occurs during ventilation of high levels of carbon dioxide does not occur when carbon dioxide-sensitivity is tested by venous loading (Jones et al., 1985). In the latter situation, the ventilatory increase occurs as a result of elevations in both respiratory frequency and tidal volume. About 80% of the hypercapnic ventilatory response is due to stimulation of central chemoreceptors in the domestic duck (Milsom et al., 1981), whereas the carotid body chemoreceptors provide most of the ventilatory drive during hypoxia (Bouverot et al., 1979). In the absence of pulmonary afferent feedback (i.e., during apnea), the activity of central respiratory neurons is depressed as blood carbon dioxide increases in ducks, although not in chickens (Jones and Bamford, 1976). It is also possible that the increased peripheral chemoreceptor drive during apnea could reinforce, rather than oppose, apnea. Most diving birds (except penguins) dive in expiration, and it has been shown in cats that brief stimulation of the carotid body chemoreceptors and central chemoreceptors during expiration can enhance expiratory effort (Black and Torrance, 1971; Eldridge, 1976; Nye et al., 1981, 1983; Marek et al., 1985; Marek and Prabhakar, 1985). However, central chemoreceptor stimulation in expiration has also been reported to reduce expiratory effort (Hanson et al., 1978). If this is really so, then only if peripheral chemoreceptor input is dominant would this mechanism contribute to maintenance of apnea. Finally, most experiments involving forced submersion use fully conscious birds, and it is likely that cortical influences exert an inhibitory effect on respiration under these circumstances (Bamford and Jones, 1974; Florin-Christensen et al., 1986). Certainly, motivation is a powerful factor determining the breaking point during a voluntary breath hold in humans (Lin, 1982).

Reflex apnea is accompanied by cardiovascular adjustments during forced and voluntary submersion, the qualitative and quantitative characteristics of which depend upon the species in question and the precise conditions in which submersion occurs. Work on decerebrated Pekin ducks (Gabbott and Jones,

1986) indicates that the stereotyped response to forced submersion (the classic diving response) is probably a reflexogenic activation of widespread sympathetic and parasympathetic output, the selective distribution of blood to various organs being achieved by differences in the relative proportions of α- and β-receptors in the arteries supplying these organs and the different sensitivities of individual vascular beds to the dilating stimulus of local metabolite accumulation (Gabbott and Jones, in preparation). Maintenance of blood flow in cerebral and coronary circulations is probably a result of local vasodilator actions of blood gases or metabolites in these vascular beds (Grubb et al., 1977, 1978). Neurogenic vasoconstriction of large-diameter blood vessels in ducks (Folkow et al., 1966; Gooden, 1980), combined with their vasoconstrictor sensitivity to plasma norepinephrine (Gooden, 1980; Wilson and West, 1986) ensures a pronounced and maintained vasoconstriction during forced submergence, despite considerable accumulation of anaerobic metabolites in vessels supplying skeletal muscle and viscera. In concert with the increase in peripheral resistance during forced submersion is a reduction in cardiac output that is proportional to the fall in heart rate. There is little change in cardiac stroke volume, despite cardiac distension resulting from increased preload, because of the powerful negative inotropic influence of vagal efferent activity (Jones and Holeton, 1972). Cardiac output is almost exclusively under parasympathetic (vagal) control during forced submersion, as demonstrated by nerve section, cold blockade, and atropinization (Butler and Jones, 1968, 1971). A reduction in sympathetic tone may (Folkow et al., 1967) or may not (Butler and Jones, 1971) be involved.

The primary sensory afferent neural inputs during forced submersion arise from central and peripheral chemoreceptors, arterial baroreceptors, and upper respiratory tract receptors. Also important is a cessation of central respiratory neuron (CRN) activity and pulmonary afferent input which may "gate" input from the primary afferent receptors onto the efferent neurons (Lopez and Palmer, 1976). The gate is open when CRN and pulmonary afferent input are low, as during expiratory apnea, increasing the accessibility of cardiac vagal motoneurons and preganglionic sympathetic vasomotor neurons to input from the previously mentioned primary afferent receptors.

Recent research into the afferent control of the cardiovascular system (particularly heart rate) in aquatic birds has revealed some interesting differences, both interspecific differences in the response to any particular diving situation and differences within individuals when diving under different conditions. The cardiovascular response to forced submersion apparently is purely reflexogenic, requiring only peripheral afferent inputs and neural integration below the level of the midbrain (Gabbott and Jones, 1986). The onset of bradycardia in dabblers and penguins is gradual; in dabbling ducks, *A. platyrhynchos*, heart rate declines by approximately 50% after 25 to 30 s of head submersion (Butler and Jones, 1968; Mangalam and Jones, 1984). In diving ducks, cormorants, and

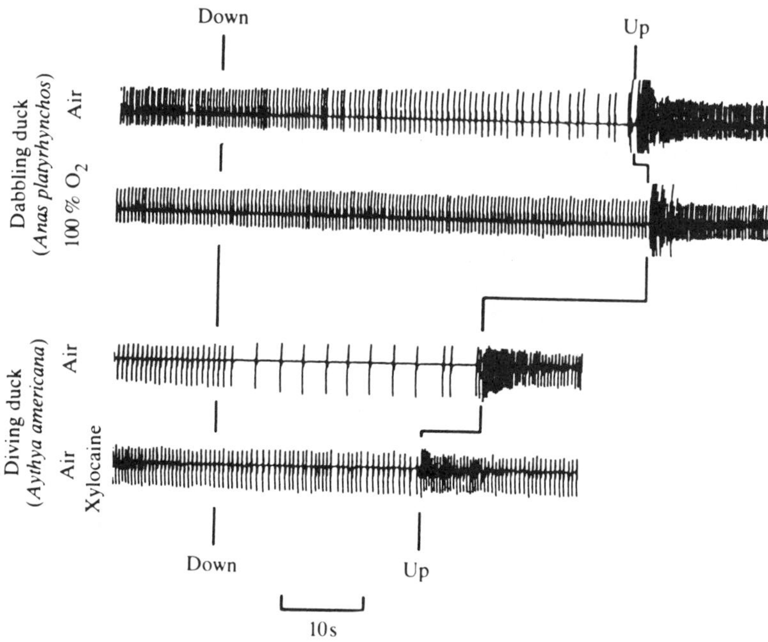

Figure 10 Traces showing ECG in restrained ducks before, during, and after forced submergence, illustrating differences in cardiac responses and their afferent control mechanisms in dabbling (top) and diving (bottom) ducks. The slowly developing bradycardia in dabbling ducks (upper trace) is abolished by breathing 100% O_2 before submergence (lower trace) illustrating the primary importance of chemoreceptor stimulation in response onset. The more rapidly developing bradycardia in diving ducks (upper trace), however, is primarily dependent upon the integrity of receptors in the bill and varies as shown by abolition of the response following application of local anesthetic to these receptors (lower trace). (From Furilla and Jones, 1986.)

the dipper, however, the development of bradycardia is relatively rapid; in the tufted duck, *A. fuligula*, for instance, heart rate declines by 50% within 5 s of head immersion (Butler and Woakes, 1982a). Underlying these differences in the manifestation of the response to forced submersion are differences in cardiac control mechanisms. In dabbling ducks and geese, bradycardia is reduced or delayed by breathing hyperoxic gases before submersion (Fig. 10; Cohn et al., 1968; Mangalam and Jones, 1984; Furilla and Jones, 1986), by perfusion of the carotid bodies with hyperoxic blood (Jones et al., 1982), or by denervation of the carotid bodies (Hollenberg and Uvnäs, 1963; Jones and Purves, 1970; Holm and Sorensen, 1972; Butler and Woakes, 1982; Lillo and Jones, 1982). Con-

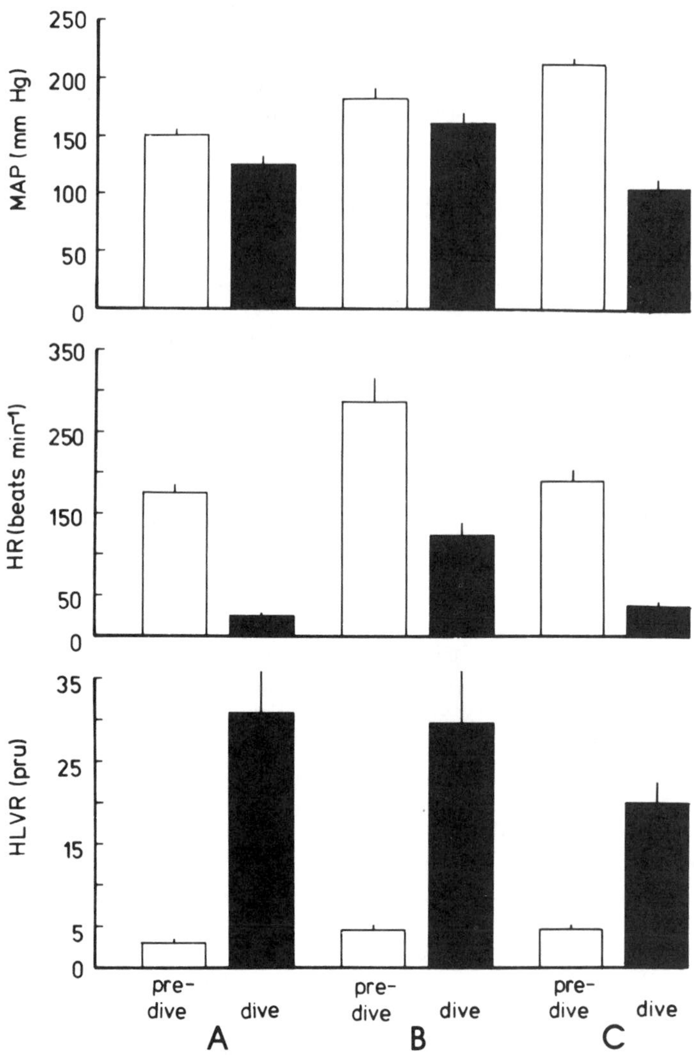

Figure 11 Mean (± SE) response to forced submergence in the Pekin duck, *A. platyrhynchos*: (A) intact animals; (B) after acute barodenervation (24 h after nerve section by snare withdrawal, 1–3 weeks postsurgery); (C) after chronic barodenervation (23 days post-nerve section). Open columns represent presubmergence values, closed columns represent values recorded after 2.5 min of immersion. (Adapted from Smith, 1987.)

versely, breathing hypoxic gas before submersion accentuates the bradycardia in the subsequent forced submersion (Cohn et al., 1968; Mangalam and Jones, 1984). In diving ducks and cormorants, however, manipulations of chemoreceptor activity have no effect on the onset of the rapidly developing bradycardia during forced submersion (Butler and Woakes, 1982a; Mangalam and Jones, 1984; Furilla and Jones, 1986).

In the redhead duck, *Aythya americana*, approximately 80% of the initial reduction in heart rate at the start of a forced dive is due to stimulation of receptors in the nasal passages (see Fig. 10; Furilla and Jones, 1986), and it is likely that a similar mechanism operates in the tufted duck, *A. fuligula* (Butler and Woakes, 1982a). In dabbling ducks, this nasal input is effective in reducing heart rate only if the predive rate exceeds 180 beats · min^{-1} (Jones et al., 1982) and otherwise is involved only in initiating apnea. In diving ducks, the cardiac chronotropic effect of chemoreceptor input is masked by that of nasal receptor input until enough time has passed for a sufficient depletion of PaO_2 and elevation of $PaCO_2$ to occur to excite the chemoreceptors, which seems to require 50 s of submersion in the tufted duck (Butler and Woakes, 1982a).

By means of pharmacological techniques, it was suggested that the baroreflex may be important in the development of bradycardia (Andersen and Blix, 1974; Blix et al., 1974), although this was not supported by Butler and Jones (1971), who employed similar methods. It has been shown that the baroreflex remains active, although the gain is reduced, in domestic ducks, *Anas boscas* (Millard, 1980), in contrast to the situation in the harbor seal, *Phoca vitulina*, in which the baroreflex gain is reported to increase during forced submergence (Angell-James et al., 1978).

Denervation of arterial baroreceptors has led to conflicting conclusions about their role during forced submersion in ducks (Jones et al., 1983). The effect of arterial baroreceptor deafferentiation on heart rate during forced submersion in dabbling ducks depends upon whether the animal has been recently denervated (1-2 days postoperative) or whether the denervation is longstanding (several weeks postoperative) (Jones, 1973; Jones et al., 1983). Bradycardia is markedly reduced in recently denervated ducks (Fig. 11), even when snares are used to section the nerves 1, or more, weeks after the operation, thereby eliminating the effects of surgical trauma (F. M. Smith and D. R. Jones, unpublished observations). Hind-limb vascular resistance (HLVR) during forced submergence is unaffected by acute barodenervation, indicating that peripheral resistance may not increase so much in other vascular beds during forced submersion, because the mean arterial pressure is unchanged, whereas the intensity of bradycardia is reduced (see Fig. 11). Thus, on the basis of these results, bradycardia would appear to result partly as a secondary reflex effect of increased peripheral resistance, as proposed by Blix and coworkers (Blix et al., 1974). However, a full bradycardia is observed in chronically denervated ducks. Here, peripheral resist-

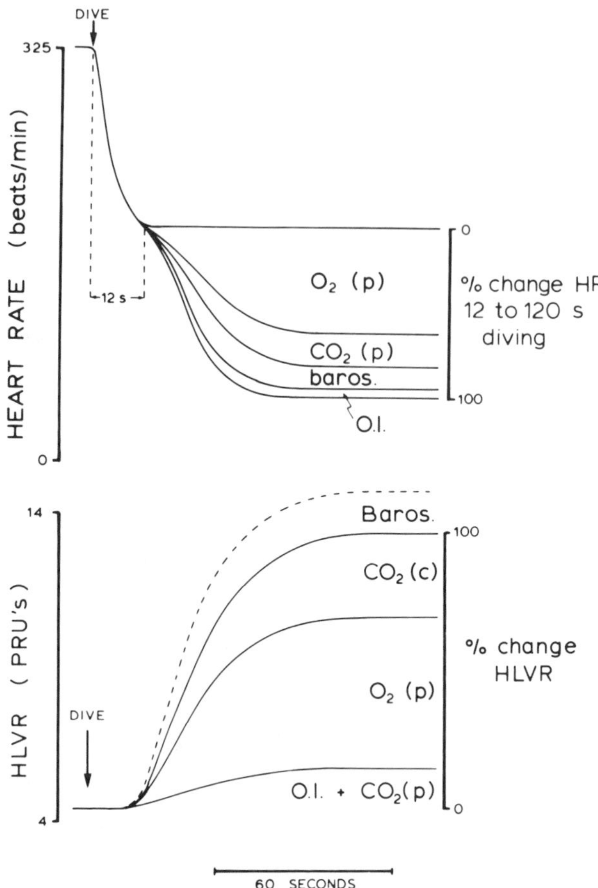

Figure 12 Assessment of the contribution of central (c) and peripheral (p) chemoreceptors to bradycardia and changes in hind-limb vascular resistance (HLVR) in ducks during the period from 12 to 120 s of forced submergence. The presumed contribution of baroreceptors (baros.) and other unidentified inputs (0.1) in accentuating the responses are also shown. (From Jones et al., 1982.)

ance (HLVR) increases by only half as much as it does in intact animals (see Fig. 11) so that in long-term barodenervates, blood pressure falls during forced submersion (Jones, 1973). Whether these changes in baroreflex effects with time after denervation are due to central neural reorganization of the dive response or to peripheral effector-related effects, is not yet known.

Jones et al. (1982) attempted to assess the relative contributions of the central and peripheral chemoreceptors and baroreceptors to the development of bradycardia and increase in HLVR in the white Pekin duck during forced submersion. By using cross perfusion between pairs of ducks, they estimated that approximately 85% of the total bradycardia and 67% of the increase in HLVR was due to stimulation of peripheral chemoreceptors (Fig. 12). A significant 30% of the increase in HLVR was the result of stimulation of central chemoreceptors, leaving only a minute influence of baroreceptors and other unidentified inputs on circulatory control. As noted earlier, the influence of nasopharyngeal receptor input will be the most significant input in diving ducks with respect to bradycardia, at least in the early part of a forced dive.

Control of the cardiovascular system during unrestrained diving activity is more complicated, as implied by the variability of the response under different situations (Stephenson et al., 1986; Furilla and Jones, 1987a). Although data are now sparse, apparently, at least in diving ducks, peripheral afferent inputs have a much smaller effect on heart rate during voluntary dives than they do during forced submersion. Abolition of nasal receptor input by local anesthesia removes only 10 to 30% of the initial reduction in heart rate at the start of voluntary dives (compared with 80% for forced submersion) in the redhead duck, *A. americana* (Fig. 13B) (Furilla and Jones, 1986). Carotid body chemoreceptor denervation (Butler and Woakes, 1982a) and breathing hyperoxic or hypoxic gas mixtures before diving have no effect on heart rate during voluntary dives of normal duration (see Figs. 8A and 13A) in redhead ducks, *A. americana*, and tufted ducks, *A. fuligula* (Furilla and Jones, 1986; P. J. Butler and R. Stephenson, unpublished observations). Similarly, chronic barodenervation has no effect on heart rate during voluntary dives in the redhead duck (see Fig. 13C; Furilla and Jones, 1987a). Interestingly, however, arterial baroreceptors do play an important role in the cardiac adjustments to voluntary diving by mallard ducks, *A. platyrhynchos*, that have been trained to dive, rather than dabble, for food (Furilla and Jones, 1987b). In intact mallards, the heart rate is adjusted to approximately 250 beats · min^{-1} during dives, regardless of predive heart rate (see Fig. 14A). This adjustment does not occur in chronic barodenervates (see Fig. 14B), although diving ability is not impaired (Furilla and Jones, 1987b).

It has been shown that diving ducks, *A. americana*, and *A. fuligula*, and Humboldt penguins, *Spheniscus humboldti*, are capable of evoking a full bradycardia, similar to that seen in forced submersion, during unrestrained dives when they find themselves unable to reach the surface (Butler and Woakes, 1984; Furilla and Jones, 1986; Stephenson et al., 1986). Although the onset (i.e., initial 2 s) of this bradycardia is unaffected, the subsequent reinforcement and maintenance of bradycardia is slowed after longstanding bilateral denervation of the carotid body chemoreceptors in the tufted duck (see Fig. 7; Butler and Stephenson, unpublished observations). However, breathing approximately 50% oxygen before the dives has no effect on the development of bradycardia during "trapped" dives in the redhead duck. Trapped heart rate, however, is higher on

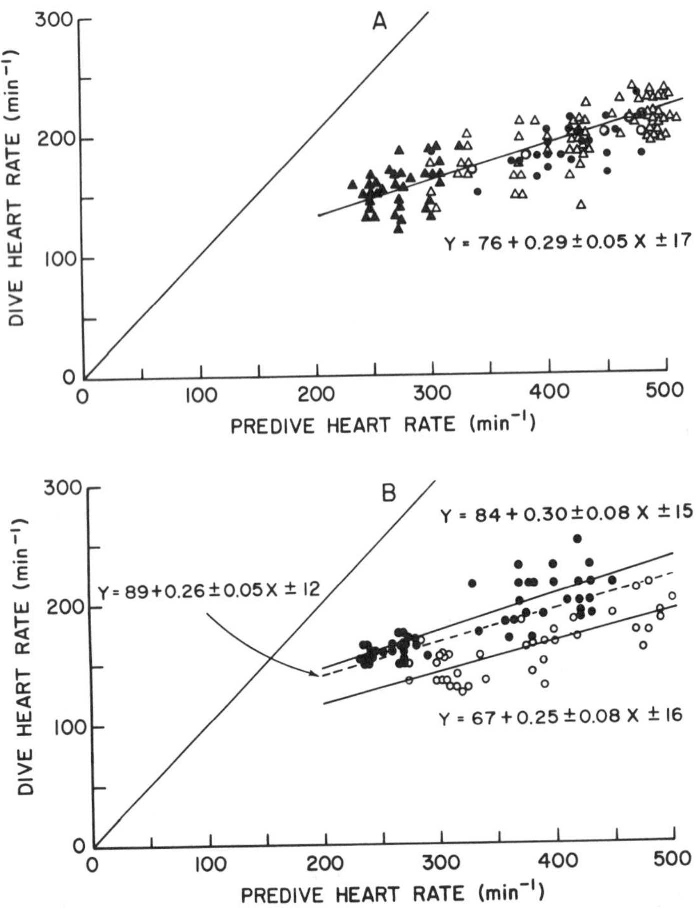

Figure 13 The relationships between predive heart rate and dive heart rate (after 2–5 s of voluntary submersion) in redhead ducks, *Aythya americana*, and lesser scaup, *A. affinis*: (A) From intact ducks (N = 5), before (open triangles) and after (closed triangles) β-blockade using propranolol. The regression equation was obtained using these data only. Also shown are data from four ducks breathing hypoxic ($< 16\%$ O_2; closed circles) and hyperoxic (50% O_2; open circles) gas mixtures. (B) Data from one female redhead duck during chase-induced dives before (open circles) and after (closed circles) local anesthesia of the nares. The dashed regression line represents data from this animal during spontaneous voluntary dives without anesthesia.

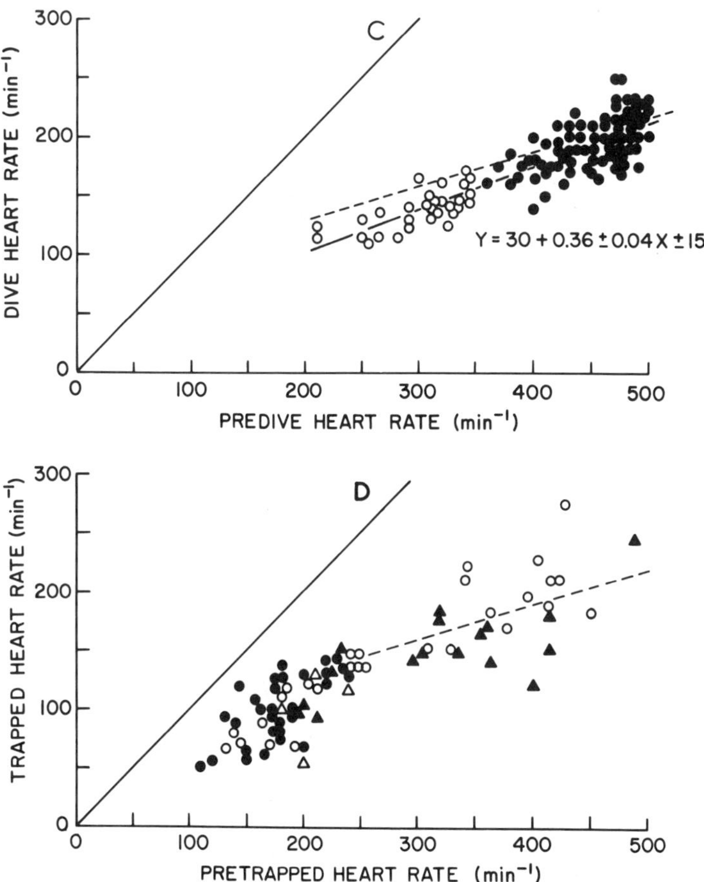

Figure 13 (continued) (C) Data from three ducks after chronic bilateral denervation of the arterial baroreceptors. The solid regression line is described by the equation and was obtained from data obtained before (closed circles) and after (open circles) β-blockade using propranolol. The broken line is from nondenervated ducks shown in (A). (D) The relationship between "trapped" and "pretrap" heart rate. Data are shown from intact animals that had breathed air before the dives (open circles), intact animals that had breathed O_2 before the dives (open circles), barodenervated ducks (closed triangles), and ducks with local anesthesia of the nares (open triangles). The dashed line represents the control data from intact ducks during normal voluntary dives shown in (A). In all figures the line through the origin represents the line of identity. (Adapted from Furilla and Jones, 1986; 1987a.)

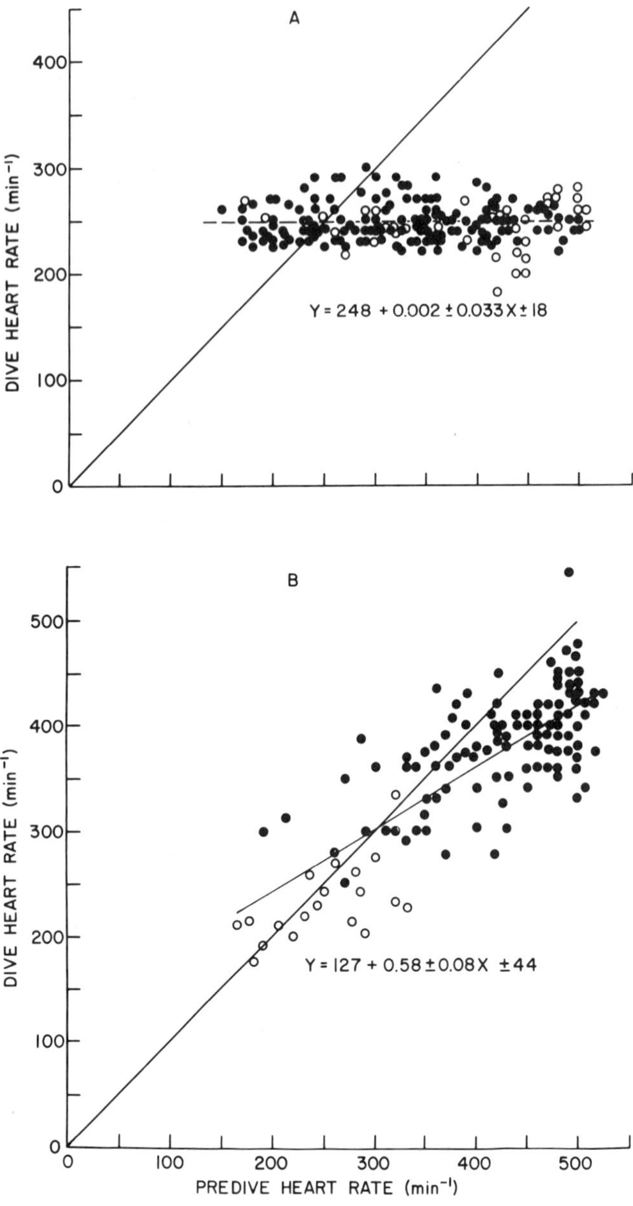

Figure 14 The relationship between predive and dive heart rate in the mallard (*A. platyrhynchos*): (A) during voluntary dives of two intact (closed circles) and one sham-operated (open circles) animals; (B) during voluntary dives of three barodenervated animals before (closed circles) and after (open circles) β-blockade using nadolol. The line of identity is shown in both diagrams. (From Furilla and Jones, 1987b.)

some occasions after breathing oxygen-enriched air compared with ducks that breathed normal air before diving, and these higher trapped heart rates are associated with higher pretrapped heart rates (see Fig. 13D; Furilla and Jones, 1987a). Barodenervation and anesthesia of the nares also apparently has no effect on development of bradycardia during trapped dives in the redhead duck (see Fig. 13D; Furilla and Jones, 1987a). Thus, the mechanisms controlling the onset and maintenance of bradycardia during such trapped dives remains unknown. The carotid body chemoreceptors may be partially involved, as they are during the more gradual development of bradycardia during long-distance ("extended") dives in the tufted duck (see Fig. 8B; P. J. Butler and R. Stephenson, unpublished observations). Another, as yet unexplored, afferent input during voluntary dives is that from the working muscles and moving joints (somatic reflex) which are known to have cardiovascular effects in mammals (e.g., McCloskey and Mitchell, 1972). Coupled with this is also the possibility of a "central command" component of cardiovascular control (e.g., Eldridge et al., 1985). Any cardioacceleratory effects that these mechanisms may have during voluntary dives, however, can obviously be overridden in a situation such as a trapped dive when oxygen conservation takes priority (Stephenson et al., 1986). It has been suggested that the central command mechanism represents the primary drive for both locomotion and the cardiorespiratory adjustments during exercise, whereas the feedback mechanism provides a fine modulation (Eldridge et al., 1985). The somatic reflex may be responsible for the entrainment of cardiorespiratory values with limb motion (e.g., Iscoe and Polosa, 1976), and in this connection, leg-beat frequency in freely diving tufted ducks is entrained to heart rate in a 1:1 ratio (Butler and Woakes, 1982b).

With the apparent reduction in influence of peripheral afferent inputs in cardiovascular control during voluntary dives, it is tempting to speculate that suprabulbar nervous influences are correspondingly greater. This has led to the current controversy over the role, if any, of the defense reaction during forced submersion and trapped dives. Basically, two opposing, but not necessarily mutually exclusive, hypotheses have been advanced: (1) that the oxygen-conserving response is directly stimulated by fear through activation of the "defense–arousal system," and (2) that the oxygen-conserving response is the basic reflex response to submersion, occurring independently of the defense–arousal system and is not fully expressed during unrestrained voluntary diving behavior.

Several authors, on the basis of a comparison of the response during forced and voluntary dives, have suggested that the classic diving response is a fear-induced artifact of the experimental conditions (e.g., Kanwisher et al., 1981; Smith and Tobey, 1983; Kanwisher and Gabrielsen, 1985). It has been claimed that a proportion of the response to forced submersion is the result of an orienting response or a passive defense reaction (Blix, 1985; Kanwisher and Gabrielsen, 1985), although evidence is mainly indirect and circumstantial and is, therefore, inconclusive. It has been observed that in restrained animals, pain, abrupt noise, or threatening gestures can elicit a typical bradycardia without submersion (e.g., Scholander, 1940; Irving et al., 1942; Elsner et al., 1966). Furthermore, a series of cardiovascular adjustments similar to those during forced submergence occurs in those birds and mammals that adopt a strategy of "freezing" or "playing dead" in response to a threatening stimulus (Gabrielsen et al., 1977; Butler and Woakes, personal communication). This response is characterized by physical immobility and reductions in heart rate, core body temperature, and rate of oxygen consumption (Smith et al., 1981). In view of the now well-established occurrence of cardiovascular–respiratory interactions (e.g., Daly, 1985), it is possible that during this "feigned death" response, immobility is the main determinant of survival. The reduction of respiratory movements may, therefore, represent the primary evoked response, the cardiovascular and metabolic adjustments occurring secondarily to this respiratory depression.

Several observations, however, do not support the contention that the forced submersion response is an artifact of fear. There are several documented cases in which the depth of "diving" bradycardia is reduced in struggling and stressed animals but more marked in quiet and calm animals (see Blix and Folkow, 1983). Furthermore, it was pointed out by Blix and Folkow (1983) "that the response is present also in decerebrate ducks, which are fairly difficult to scare," and Gabbott and Jones (1986) have shown that transection across the rostral mesencephalon below the (supposed) level of the hypothalmic defense areas has no effect on the bradycardia evoked by forced submergence (Fig. 15). In addition, nasal anesthesia in the redhead duck (Furilla and Jones, 1986) and denervation of the carotid body chemoreceptors or breathing oxygen before forced submergence in the domestic duck (Jones and Purves, 1970; Furilla and Jones, 1986) abolishes the bradycardia, suggesting that it is largely reflexogenic, although the strength of this latter argument is reduced by the recent finding that carotid body chemoreceptor activation can evoke a simulated defense reaction in the cat (Marshall, 1987).

The bradycardia evoked by forced submersion in dabbling ducks is susceptible to habituation (Gabrielsen, 1985; Gabbott and Jones, 1987), even in decerebrated ducks (G. R. J. Gabbott and D. R. Jones, unpublished observations). The response to forced submersion will also habituate in the redhead duck (Gabbott and Jones, unpublished observations), but in the tufted duck, the response evoked during trapped dives did not habituate after 26 trials in quick succession in three ducks (Stephenson, 198[illegible]).

It is possible that the response to normal voluntary dives is a habituated response and that, in a situation such as being trapped underwater, activation of suprabulbar structures, such as the defense areas, perhaps including the mesencephalic/hypothalamic "area A" described in ducks (Feigl and Folkow, 1963; Folkow and Rubinstein, 1965), may dishabituate the oxygen-conserving response and allow its full expression, thus, prolonging the period in which to find an escape route.

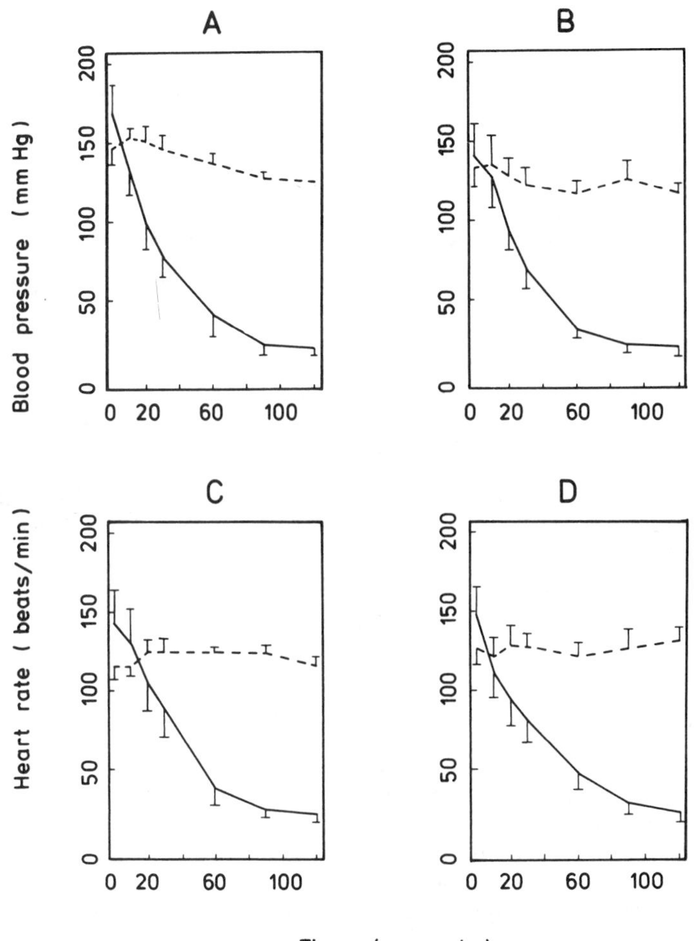

Figure 15 Mean (± SE) heart rate (solid lines) and arterial blood pressure (dashed lines) during forced dives of the Pekin duck, *A. platyrhynchos*: (A) intact animals; (B) after decerebration by aspiration of the cerebral hemispheres; (C) after reversible section of the brain stem by injection of local anesthetic at the rostral level of the mesencephalon; (D) after surgical transection of the rostral mesencephalon. (Adapted from Gabbott, 1985.)

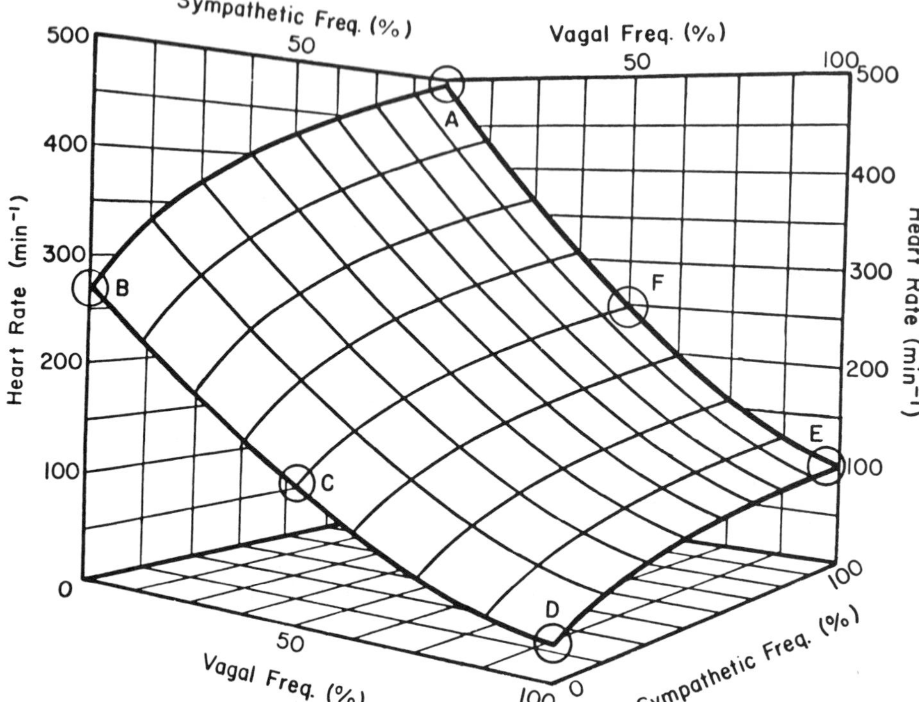

Figure 16 The relationship of heart rate to bilateral stimulation of the distal cut ends of the vagus and cardiac sympathetic nerves on the Pekin duck, *A. platyrhynchos.* 100% represents the frequency of stimulation above which no further changes in heart rate occurred. The heart rate resulting from a given level of vagal and sympathetic stimulation was plotted on "perspective" graph paper and the surface was drawn, by eye, to encompass all heart rates obtained in the stimulation experiments. Area B represents complete cardiac denervation, and area E maximal vagosympathetic stimulation. The effect of sympathetic stimulation at minimal and maximal vagal activity are represented by the lines A–B and D–E, respectively. Similarly, the effect of vagal stimulation at minimal and maximal sympathetic activity are represented by the lines B–D and A–E, respectively. See text for an explanation of points A–F relative to diving. (Reprinted from Furilla and Jones, 1987a.)

A possible explanation for at least some of the variability in heart rate observed during diving has recently been proposed by Furilla and Jones (1987a). After they had observed a close correlation between predive (or pretrapped) and dive (or trapped) heart rate in the redhead duck, *A. americana*, and lesser scaup, *A. affinis* (see Fig. 13), they investigated the efferent control of heart rate in the Pekin duck, *A. platyrhynchos*. By means of pharmacological blockade of vagal and cardiac sympathetic nerves (using atropine and propranolol, respectively) and by electrical stimulation of the distal cut ends of these nerves, a relationship between heart rate and normalized vagal and sympathetic nerve activities was obtained (Fig. 16). It is suggested, with reference to Fig. 16, that for diving ducks areas A, B, and C represent the vagosympathetic interplay that elicits predive heart rates in normal voluntary dives, voluntary dives after β-receptor blockade, and forced submersion, respectively, and that an approximately half maximal increase in vagal output produces the heart rates seen after 2 to 5 s of immersion (i.e., A–F, B–C, and C–D) (Furilla and Jones, 1987a). Changes in heart rate during all dabbles and dives, including the onset of the trapped response, could be interpreted in light of a similar 50% increase in vagal activity. The relationship, however, does not hold for voluntarily diving (rather than dabbling) mallard ducks (see Fig. 14; Furilla and Jones, 1987b).

On emersion, all birds hyperventilate, although the control mechanisms are still unclear. In ducks, maximum minute ventilation is reached in the first few seconds of recovery from a period of forced submergence (Bamford and Jones, 1976; Milsom et al., 1983), and the duration of hyperventilation appears to depend upon the duration of (or, more specifically, the degree of hypoxia reached during) the preceding dive (Lillo and Jones, 1982; Milsom et al., 1983). The duration of recovery hyperventilation is unaffected by carotid body denervation (Lillo and Jones, 1982), although tidal volume and, as a consequence, maximum minute ventilation, is markedly reduced.

Hyperventilation is augmented in the early stages of recovery by stimulation of the central and peripheral chemoreceptors (Lillo and Jones, 1982; Milsom et al., 1983), but it persists even after blood gas partial pressures have fallen below (for CO_2) and risen above (for O_2) normal levels (Shimizu and Jones, 1987). The mechanism that maintains this second phase of recovery is unknown. The intense hypoxemia developed during submersion is important for maximal hyperventilation, although hypoxia seems to have its effect through receptors other than the carotid body chemoreceptors (Milsom et al., 1983). It is possible that the role of hypoxia is indirect—acting through lactic acid accumulation. Infusion of sodium lactate has no effect on breathing, but lactic acid greatly enhances breathing and may provide the stimulus for the prolonged postdive hyperventilation (Shimizu and Jones, in preparation). Certainly, plasma anions remain unchanged from predive values during prolonged recovery, so [lactate$^-$] release during recovery would furnish the required reduction in strong ion differ-

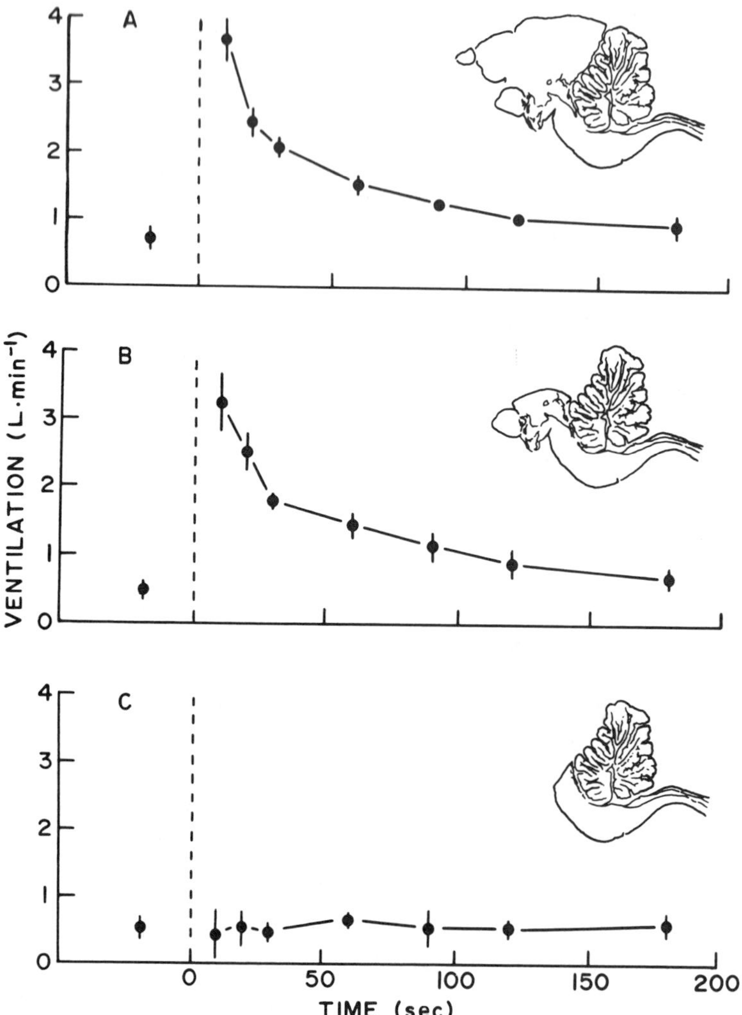

Figure 17 The effect of brain transection on breathing in the recovery period following 120 s of forced submergence in the Pekin duck, *A. platyrhynchos*: (A) intact animals; (B) decerebrate animals; (C) mesencephalic animals. The degree of surgical ablation is shown diagramatically in the midsagittal plane. The vertical dashed line indicates the end of submersion and the point left of this line on each graph represents presubmergence values. (From Jones and Furilla, 1987.)

ence to alter acid-base balance sufficiently to stimulate ventilation (see Fig. 9; Shimizu and Jones, 1987). Dodd and Milsom (1987) have shown that in ducks that breath hypercapnic gas mixtures for prolonged periods ventilatory control seems to be a single function of arterial pH.

The rapid onset of the recovery hyperventilation is dependent upon the integrity of the pulmonary afferent nerves in the mallard duck, the pattern of breathing being changed and initial minute ventilation reduced in pulmonary denervated ducks (Bamford and Jones, 1976; Butler and Taylor, 1983). Control mechanisms also appear to be dependent upon the integrity of the rostral midbrain, because transection at the thalamic level has no effect on breathing during recovery, whereas transection at the midcollicular level of the mesencephalon completely prevents any increase in minute ventilation upon emersion (Fig. 17; Gabbott, 1985).

The first breath following forced submersion initiates the cardiovascular recovery process, which is essentially a reversal of the submersion events, i.e., tachycardia and peripheral vasodilation (see Fig. 3). Mean arterial blood pressure may sometimes rise early in recovery, presumably a result of the failure of peripheral vasodilator mechanisms to keep pace with the rapid increases in cardiac output (Butler and Jones, 1971).

As with postdive hyperventilation, the full expression of the cardiovascular response upon emersion is primarily dependent upon the integrity of the afferent inputs from the intrapulmonary chemoreceptors (Bamford and Jones, 1976; Butler and Taylor, 1983). A "central irradiation" mechanism is also implicated by the fact that tachycardia (albeit reduced in intensity) will occur with the first voluntary breath terminating a dive in intact or lung-denervated domestic ducks, even if they are surfaced into air containing elevated P_{CO_2} (Bamford and Jones, 1976). On the other hand, lung-denervated ducks exhibit a much more markedly diminished cardiac chronotropic response to a single artificial inflation of the lungs during submergence (Bamford and Jones, 1976; Butler and Taylor, 1983).

The control of the circulation at the end of voluntary dives differs from that after forced submergences in that the heart rate often begins to increase in anticipation of the onset of respiration but before breathing has recommenced (Butler and Woakes, 1982b; Stephenson et al., 1986) (see Fig. 8B). It is likely that as yet unidentified suprabulbar nervous influences have a greater role in cardiac control during recovery from voluntary dives in birds.

VI. Epilogue

Aquatic birds have been used extensively to study the physiology of diving, and it is now clear that cardiovascular responses to submersion are extremely variable, depending upon the species under examination and the precise situation under which submergence takes place. There is still a paucity of data about the nature of responses to submergence in freely diving birds (basic observations of cardiac output, stroke volume, blood pressure, and blood flow distribution are yet to be made in free dives) and control mechanisms, particularly central nervous involvement, are largely unknown.

Current rapid advances in biotelemetry techniques encourage an optimistic outlook for the future in determination of qualitative and quantitative aspects of cardiorespiratory responses. Recently, some progress has been made in determining peripheral neural control mechanisms, but the real challenge to comparative physiologists in this field lies in understanding the central nervous mechanisms that apparently play a large part in behavioral and physiological control during diving in birds.

References

Andersen, H. T. (1959). Depression of metabolism in the duck during experimental diving. *Acta Physiol. Scand. 46*:234-239.

Andersen, H. T. (1963). The reflex nature of the physiological adjustments to diving and their afferent pathway. *Acta Physiol. Scand. 58*:263-273.

Andersen, H. T. (1965). Hyperpotassemia and electrocardiographic changes in the duck during prolonged diving. *Acta Physiol. Scand. 63*:292-295.

Andersen, H. T. (1966). Physiological adaptations in diving vertebrates. *Physiol. Rev. 46*:212-243.

Andersen, H. T., and Blix, A. S. (1974). Pharmacological exposure of components in the autonomic control of the diving reflex. *Acta Physiol. Scand. 90*:381-386.

Andersen, H. T., and Lövö, A. (1967). Indirect estimation of partial pressure of oxygen in arterial blood of diving ducks. *Respir. Physiol. 2*:163-167.

Andersen, H. T., Hustvedt, B. E., and Lövö, A. (1965). Acid-base changes in diving ducks. *Acta Physiol. Scand. 63*:128-132.

Angell-James, J. E., Daly, M. de B., and Elsner, R. (1978). Arterial baroreceptor reflexes in the seal and their modification during experimental diving. *Am. J. Physiol. 234*:H730-H739.

Baker, C. M. A., and Manwell, C. (1975). Penguin proteins: Biochemical contributions to classification and natural history. In *The Biology of Penguins*. Edited by B. Stonehouse. London, Macmillan, pp. 43-56.

Balasch, J., Palomeque, J., Palacios, L., Musquera, S., and Jimenez, M. (1974). Hematological values of some great flying and aquatic-diving birds. *Comp. Biochem. Physiol. 49A*:137-145.

Baldwin, J., Jardel, J.-P., Montague, T., and Tomkin, R. (1984). Energy metabolism in penguin swimming muscles. *Mol. Physiol. 6*:33-42.

Bamford, O. S., and Jones, D. R. (1974). On the initiation of apnoea and some cardiovascular responses to submergence in ducks. *Respir. Physiol. 22*: 199-216.

Bamford, O. S., and Jones, D. R. (1976). Respiratory and cardiovascular interactions in ducks: The effect of lung denervation on the initiation of and recovery from some cardiovascular responses to submergence. *J. Physiol. (Lond.) 259*:575-596.

Baudinette, R. V., and Gill, P. (1985). The energetics of "flying" and "paddling" in water: Locomotion in penguins and ducks. *J. Comp. Physiol. B. 155*: 373-380.

Baumann, F. H., and Baumann, R. (1977). A comparative study of the respiratory properties of bird blood. *Respir. Physiol. 31*:333-343.

Bellairs, A. d'A., and Jenkin, C. R. (1960). The skeleton of birds. In *Biology and Comparative Physiology of Birds*, Vol. 1. Edited by A. J. Marshall. New York, Academic Press, pp. 241-300.

Black, A. M., and Torrance, R. W. (1971). Respiratory oscillations in chemoreceptor discharge in the control of breathing. *Respir. Physiol. 13*:221-237.

Black, C. P., and Tenney, S. M. (1980). Oxygen transport during progressive hypoxia in high-altitude and sea-level water fowl. *Respir. Physiol. 39*:217-239.

Blix, A. S. (1985). Diving response of mammals and birds. In *Arctic Underwater Operations*. Edited by L. Rey. London, Graham and Trotman, pp. 73-79.

Blix, A. S., and Folkow, B. (1983). Cardiovascular adjustments to diving in mammals and birds. In *Handbook of Physiology*. The Cardiovascular System, Vol. 3. Edited by J. T. Shepherd and F. M. Abboud. Bethesda, American Physiology Society, pp. 917-945.

Blix, A. S., Gautvik, E. L., andRefsum, H. (1974). Aspects of the relative roles of peripheral vasoconstriction and vagal bradycardia in the establishment of the "diving reflex" in ducks. *Acta Physiol. Scand. 90*:289-296.

Bond, C. F., and Gilbert, P. W. (1958). Comparative study of blood volume in representative aquatic and nonaquatic birds. *Am. J. Physiol. 194*:519-521.

Bouverot, P., Douguet, D., and Sébert, P. (1979). Role of the arterial chemoreceptors in ventilatory and circulatory adjustments to hypoxia in awake Pekin ducks. *J. Comp. Physiol. B 133*:177-186.

Brodkorb, P. (1963). Birds from the upper Cretaceous of Wyoming. *Proc. 13th Int. Ornith. Congr.* pp. 55-70.

Brodkorb, P. (1971). Origin and evolution of birds. In *Avian Biology*. Vol. 1. Edited by D. S. Farner, J. R. King, and K. C. Parks. London, Academic Press, pp. 19-55.

Bryan, R. M., and Jones, D. R. (1980a). Cerebral energy metabolism in diving and nondiving birds during hypoxia and apnoeic asphyxia. *J. Physiol. (Lond.) 299*:323-336.

Bryan, R. M., and Jones, D. R. (1980b). Cerebral metabolism in mallard ducks during apneic asphyxia: The role of oxygen conservation. *Am. J. Physiol. 239*:R352-R357.

Butler, P. J. (1982). Respiratory and cardiovascular control during diving in birds and mammals. *J. Exp. Biol. 100*:195-221.

Butler, P. J. (1988). The exercise response and the "classical" diving response during natural submersion in birds and mammals. *Can. J. Zool. 66*:29-39.

Butler, P. J., and Jones, D. R. (1968). Onset of and recovery from diving bradycardia in ducks. *J. Physiol. (Lond.) 196*:255-272.

Butler, P. J., and Jones, D. R. (1971). The effect of variations in heart rate and regional distribution of blood flow on the normal pressor response to diving in ducks. *J. Physiol. (Lond.) 214*:457-479.

Butler, P. J., and Stephenson, R. (1987). Physiology of breath-hold diving: A bird's eye view. *Sci. Prog. (Oxford) 71*:439-458.

Butler, P. J., and Taylor, E. W. (1973). The effect of hypercapnic hypoxia, accompanied by different levels of lung ventilation, on heart rate in the duck. *Respir. Physiol. 19*:176-187.

Butler, P. J., and Taylor, E. W. (1974). Responses of the respiratory and cardiovascular systems of chickens and pigeons to changes in PaO_2 and $PaCO_2$. *Respir. Physiol. 21*:351-363.

Butler, P. J., and Taylor, E. W. (1983). Factors affecting the respiratory and cardiovascular responses to hypercapnic hypoxia in mallard ducks. *Respir. Physiol. 53*:109-127.

Butler, P. J., and Woakes, A. J. (1979). Changes in heart rate and respiratory frequency during natural behaviour of ducks, with particular reference to diving. *J. Exp. Biol. 79*:283-300.

Butler, P. J., and Woakes, A. J. (1982a). Control of heart rate by carotid body chemoreceptors during diving in tufted ducks. *J. Appl. Physiol. 53*:1405-1410.

Butler, P. J., and Woakes, A. J. (1982b). Telemetry of physiological variables from diving and flying birds. *Symp. Zool. Soc. Lond. 49*:107-128.

Butler, P. J., and Woakes, A. J. (1984). Heart rate and aerobic metabolism in Humboldt penguins, *Spheniscus humboldti*, during voluntary dives. *J. Exp. Biol. 108*:419-428.

Butler, P. J., Stephenson, R., and Woakes, A. J. (1986). Variability of the heart rate response during voluntary diving in the tufted duck, *Aythya fuligula*. *J. Physiol. (Lond.) 37*:69P.

Casler, C. L. (1973). The air-sac systems and buoyancy of the anhinga and double-crested cormorant. *Auk 90*:324-340.

Castellini, M. A., and Somero, G. N. (1981). Buffering capacity of vertebrate muscle: Correlations with potentials for anaerobic function. *J. Comp. Physiol. 143*:191-198.

Clarke, B. D., and Bemis, W. (1979). Kinematics of swimming penguins at Detroit zoo. *J. Zool. 188*:411-428.

Cohn, J. E., Krog, J., and Shannon, R. (1968). Cardiopulmonary responses to head immersion in domestic geese. *J. Appl. Physiol. 25*:36–41.

Cole, R. P. (1982). Myoglobin function in exercising skeletal muscle. *Science 216*:523–525.

Cole, R. P. (1983). Skeletal muscle function in hypoxia: Effect of alteration of intracellular myoglobin. *Respir. Physiol. 53*:1–14.

Cracraft, J. (1982). Phylogenetic relationships and monophyly of loons, grebes and hesperornithiform birds, with comments on the early history of birds. *Syst. Zool. 31*:35–56.

Daly, M. de B. (1985). Interactions between respiration and circulation. In *Handbook of Physiology*. The Respiratory System, Vol. 2. Edited by A. P. Fishman and A. B. Fisher. Bethesda, American Physiological Society, pp. 529–594.

Davis, R. W., Kooyman, G. L., and Croxall, J. P. (1983). Water flux and estimated metabolism of free-ranging Gentoo and Macaroni penguins at South Georgia. *Polar Biol. 2*:41–46.

Dehner, E. (1946). An Analysis of Buoyancy in Surface-Feeding and Diving Ducks. Ph.D. Thesis. Cornell University.

Dewar, J. M. (1924). *The Bird as a Diver*. London, H. F. & G. Witherby.

Dodd, G. A. A., and Milsom, W. K. (1987). Effect of H^+ versus CO_2 ventilation in the Pekin duck. *Respir. Physiol. 68*:189–201.

Dooley, M. S., and Koppanyi, T. (1929). The control of respiration in the domestic duck (*Anas boscas*). *J. Pharm. Exp. Ther. 36*:507–518.

Eldridge, F. L. (1976). Expiratory effects of brief carotid sinus nerve and carotid body stimulations. *Respir. Physiol. 26*:394–410.

Eldridge, F. L., Millhorn, D. E., Kiley, J. P., and Waldrop, T. G. (1985). Stimulation by central command of locomotion, respiration and circulation during exercise. *Respir. Physiol. 59*:313–337.

Eliassen, E. (1960). Cardiovascular responses to submersion asphyxia in avian divers. *Arbok. Univ. Bergen Mat. Naturvitensk Ser. 2*:1–100.

Elsner, R., Franklin, D. L., Van Citters, R. L., and Kenney, D. W. (1966). Cardiovascular defense against asphyxia. *Science 153*:941–949.

Fedde, M. R., Gatz, R. N., Slama, H., and Scheid, P. (1974a). Intrapulmonary CO_2 receptors in the duck. I. Stimulus specificity. *Respir. Physiol. 22*:99–114.

Fedde, M. R., Gatz, R. N., Slama, H., and Scheid, P. (1974b). Intrapulmonary CO_2 receptors in the duck. II. Comparison with mechanoreceptors. *Respir. Physiol. 22*:115–122.

Feduccia, A. (1980). *The Age of Birds*. London, Harvard University Press.

Feigl, E., and Folkow, B. (1963). Cardiovascular responses in "diving" and during brain stimulation in ducks. *Acta Physiol. Scand. 57*:99–100.

Florin-Christensen, J., Florin-Christensen, M., Corley, E. G., Garcia Samartino, L., and Affani, J. M. (1986). A novel receptive area of key importance for the onset of diving responses in the duck. *Arch. Int. Physiol. Biochim. 94*: 29-36.

Folkow, B., and Rubinstein, E. H. (1965). Effect of brain stimulation on "diving" in ducks. *Hvalradets Skr. 48*:30-41.

Folkow, B., Fuxe, K., and Sonnenschein, R. R. (1966). Responses of skeletal musculature and its vasculature during "diving" in the duck: Peculiarities of the adrenergic vasoconstrictor innervation. *Acta Physiol. Scand. 67*: 327-342.

Folkow, B., Nilsson, N. J., and Yonce, L. R. (1967). Effects of "diving" on cardiac output in ducks. *Acta Physiol. Scand. 70*:347-361.

Freeman, B. M. (1984). Appendix: Biochemical and physiological data. In *Physiology and Biochemistry of the Domestic Fowl*, Vol. 5. Edited by D. J. Bell and B. M. Freeman. London, Academic Press, pp. 407-424.

Furilla, R. A., and Jones, D. R. (1986). The contribution of nasal receptors to the cardiac response to diving in restrained and unrestrained redhead ducks (*Aythya americana*). *J. Exp. Biol. 121*:227-238.

Furilla, R. A., and Jones, D. R. (1987a). The relationship between dive and predive heart rates in restrained and free dives by diving ducks. *J. Exp. Biol. 127*:333-348.

Furilla, R. A., and Jones, D. R. (1987b). Cardiac responses to dabbling and diving in the mallard, *Anas platyrhynchos. Physiol. Zool. 60*:406-412.

Gabbott, G. R. J. (1985). Neural control of the Cardiac Response of the Pekin Duck (*Anas platyrhynchos*) to Forced Submersion. Ph.D. Thesis, University of British Columbia.

Gabbott, G. R. J., and Jones, D. R. (1986). Psychogenic influences on the cardiac response of the duck (*Anas platyrhynchos*) to forced submersion. *J. Physiol. (Lond.) 371*:71P.

Gabbott, G. R. J., and Jones, D. R. (1987). Habituation of the cardiac response to involuntary diving in diving and dabbling ducks. *J. Exp. Biol. 131*:403-415.

Gabrielsen, G. W. (1985). Free and forced diving in ducks: Habituation of the initial dive response. *Acta Physiol. Scand. 123*:67-72.

Gabrielsen, G., Kanwisher, J., and Steen, J. B. (1977). "Emotional" bradycardia: A telemetry study on incubating willow grouse (*Lagopus lagopus*). *Acta Physiol. Scand. 100*:255-257.

Giardina, B., Corda, M., Pellegrini, M. G., Condò, S. G., and Brunori, M. (1985). Functional properties of the hemoglobin system of two diving birds (*Podiceps nigricollis* and *Phalacroxorax carbonsinensis*). *Mol. Physiol.* 7:281-292.

Gooden, B. A. (1980). A comparison in vitro of the vasoconstrictor responses of the mesenteric arterial vasculature from the chicken and the duckling to nervous stimulation and to noradrenaline. *Br. J. Pharmacol. 68*:263-273.

Goodge, W. R. (1959). Locomotion and other behaviour of the dipper. *Condor 61*:4-17.

Gottschaldt, K.-M. (1974). The physiological basis of tactile sensibility in the beak of geese. *J. Comp. Physiol. 95*:29-47.

Gottschaldt, K.-M., and Lausmann, S. (1974). The peripheral morphological basis of tactile sensibility in the beak of geese. *Cell Tissue Res. 153*:477-496.

Gregory, J. E. (1973). A electrophysiological investigation of the receptor apparatus of the duck bill. *J. Physiol. (Lond.) 229*:151-164.

Grubb, B., Mills, C. D., Colacino, J. M., and Schmidt-Nielsen, K. (1977). Effect of arterial carbon dioxide on cerebral blood flow in ducks. *Am. J. Physiol. 232*:H596-H601.

Grubb, B., Colacino, J. M., and Schmidt-Nielsen, K. (1978). Cerebral blood flow in birds: Effect of hypoxia. *Am. J. Physiol. 234*:H230-H234.

Hanson, M. A., Nye, P. C. G., and Torrance, R. W. (1978). Sudden excitation of central chemoreceptors. *J. Physiol. (Lond.) 285*:54-55.

Harms, S. J., and Hickson, R. C. (1983). Skeletal muscle mitochondria and myoglobin, endurance, and intensity of training. *J. Appl. Physiol. 54*:798-802.

Harrison, J. G. (1964). Prematization of bone. In *A New Dictionary of Birds*. Edited by A. L. Thompson. London, Nelson, pp. 649-650.

Harvey, E. N., Barnes, D. K., McElroy, W. D., Whiteley, A. H., Pease, D. C., and Cooper, K. W. (1944a). Bubble formation in animals. I. Physical factors. *J. Cell. Comp. Physiol. 24*:1-22.

Harvey, E. N., Whiteley, A. H., McElroy, W. D., Pease, D. C., and Barnes, D. K. (1944b). Bubble formation in animals. II. Gas nuclei and their distribution in blood and tissues. *J. Cell. Comp. Physiol. 24*:23-34.

Hickson, R. C. (1981). Skeletal muscle cytochrome c and myoglobin, endurance, and frequency of training. *J. Appl. Physiol. 51*:746-749.

Ho, C. Y.-K., Prager, E. M., Wilson, A. C., Osuga, D. T., and Feeney, R. E. (1976). Penguin evolution: Protein comparisons demonstrate phylogenetic relationship to flying aquatic birds. *J. Mol. Evol. 8*:271-282.

Holle, J. P., Meyer, M., and Scheid, P. (1977). Oxygen affinity of duck blood determined by in vivo and in vitro technique. *Respir. Physiol. 29*:355-361.

Hollenberg, N. K., and Uvnäs, B. (1963). The role of cardiovascular response in the resistance to asphyxia of avian divers. *Acta Physiol. Scand. 58*:150-161.

Holm, B., and Sorensen, S. C. (1972). The role of the carotid body in the diving reflex in the duck. *Respir. Physiol. 15*:302-309.

Hou, L., and Liu, Z. (1984). A new fossil bird from Lower Cretaceous of Gansu and early evolution of birds. *Sci. Sin. 27*:1296-1303.

Huang, H., Sung, P. K., and Huang, T. (1974). Blood volume, lactic acid and catecholamines in diving response in ducks. *J. Formosan Med. Assoc. 73*: 203-210.

Hudson, D. M., and Jones, D. R. (1986). The influence of body mass on the endurance to restrained submergence in the Pekin duck. *J. Exp. Biol. 120*: 351-367.

Huxley, F. M. (1913a). On the reflex nature of apnoea in the duck in diving: I. The reflex nature of submersion apnoea. *Q. J. Exp. Physiol. 6*:147-157.

Huxley, F. M. (1913b). On the reflex nature of apnoea in the duck in diving: II. Reflex postural apnoea. *Q. J. Exp. Physiol. 6*:158-182.

Huxley, F. M.(1913c). On the resistance to asphyxia of the duck in diving. *Q. J. Exp. Physiol. 6*:183-196.

Irving, L. (1934). On the ability of warm-blooded animals to survive without breathing. *Sci. Mon. 38*:422-428.

Irving, L. (1939). Respiration in diving mammals. *Physiol. Rev. 19*:112-134.

Irving, L., Scholander, P. F., and Grinnell, S. W. (1942). The regulation of arterial blood pressure in the seal during diving. *Am. J. Physiol. 135*:557-566.

Iscoe, S., and Polosa, C.(1976). Synchronization of respiratory frequency by somatic afferent stimulation. *J. Appl. Physiol. 40*:138-148.

Johansen, K. (1964). Regional distribution of circulating blood during submersion asphyxia in the duck. *Acta Physiol. Scand. 62*:1-9.

Jones, D. R. (1973). Systemic arterial baroreceptors in ducks and the consequences of their denervation on some cardiovascular responses to diving. *J. Physiol. (Lond.) 234*:499-518.

Jones, D. R. (1987). The duck as a diver. In *Advances in Physiological Research.* Edited by H. McLennan, J. R. Ledsome, C. H. S. McIntosh, and D. R. Jones. New York, Plenum.

Jones, D. R., and Bamford, O. S. (1976). Open loop respiratory sensitivity in chickens and ducks. *Am. J. Physiol. 230*:861-867.

Jones, D. R., and Furilla, R. A. (1987). The anatomical, physiological, behavioral and metabolic consequences of voluntary and forced diving. In *Bird Respiration*. Edited by T. J. Seller. Boca Raton, CRC Press.

Jones, D. R., and Holeton, G. F. (1972). Cardiac output of ducks during diving. *Comp. Biochem. Physiol. 41A*:639-645.

Jones, D. R., and Purves, M. J. (1970). The carotid body in the duck and the consequences of its denervation upon the cardiac responses to immersion. *J. Physiol. (Lond.) 211*:279-294.

Jones, D. R., Bryan, R. M., West, N. H., Lord, R. H., and Clark, B. (1979). Regional distribution of blood flow during diving in the duck (*Anas platyrhynchos*). *Can. J. Zool. 57*:995-1002.

Jones, D. R., Milsom, W. K., and Gabbott, G. R. J. (1982). Role of central and peripheral chemoreceptors in diving responses of ducks. *Am. J. Physiol. 243*:R537-R545.

Jones, D. R., Milsom, W. K., Smith, F. M., West, N. H., and Bamford, O. S. (1983). Diving responses in ducks after acute barodenervation. *Am. J. Physiol. 245*:R222-R229.

Jones, D. R., Milsom, W. K., and Butler, P. J. (1985). Ventilatory responses to venous CO_2 loading by gut ventilation in ducks. *Can. J. Zool. 63*:1232-1236.

Jones, D. R., Furilla, R. A., Heieis, M. R. A., Gabbott, G. R. J., and Smith, F. M. (1988). Forced and voluntary diving in ducks: Cardiovascular adjustments and their control. *Can. J. Zool. 66*:75-83.

Kanwisher, J. W., and Gabrielsen, G. W. (1985). The diving response in man. In *Arctic Underwater Operations*. Edited by L. Rey. London, Graham and Trotman, pp. 81-95.

Kanwisher, J. W., Gabrielsen, G., and Kanwisher, N. (1981). Free and forced diving in birds. *Science 211*:717-719.

Keijer, E., and Butler, P. J. (1982). Volumes of the respiratory and circulatory systems in tufted and mallard ducks. *J. Exp. Biol. 101*:213-220.

Kessler, L. G., and Avise, J. C. (1984). Systematic relationships among waterfowl (*Anatidae*) inferred from restriction endonuclease analysis of mitochondrial DNA. *Syst. Zool. 33*:370-380.

King, A. S. (1966). Structural and functional aspects of the avian lungs and air sacs. *Int. Rev. Gen. Exp. Zool. 2*:171-267.

Kitchell, R. L., Ström, L., and Zotterman, Y. (1959). Electrophysiological studies of the thermal and taste reception in chickens and pigeons. *Acta Physiol. Scand., 46*:133-151.

Kooyman, G. L. (1975). Behaviour and physiology of diving. In *Biology of Penguins*. Edited by B. Stonehouse. London, Macmillan, pp. 115-137.

Kooyman, G. L., Drabek, C. M., Elsner, R., and Campbell, W. B. (1971). Diving behaviour of the emperor penguin, *Aptenodytes forsteri. Auk 88*:775-795.

Kooyman, G. L., Wahrenbrock, E. A., Castellini, M. A., Davis, R. W., and Sinnett, E. E. (1980). Aerobic and anaerobic metabolism during voluntary diving in Weddell seals: Evidence of preferred pathways from blood chemistry and behaviour. *J. Comp. Physiol. B 138*:335-346.

Kooyman, G. L., Davis, R. W., Croxall, J. P., and Costa, D. P. (1982). Diving depths and energy requirements of King penguins. *Science 217*:726-727.

Koppanyi, T., and Kleitman, N. (1927). Body righting and related phenomena in the domestic duck. *Am. J. Physiol. 82*:672-685.

Koppanyi, J., and Dooley, M. S. (1928). The cause of cardiac slowing accompanying postural apnoea in the duck. *Am. J. Physiol. 85*:311-332.

Lapennas, G. N., and Lutz, P. L. (1982). Oxygen affinity of sea turtle blood. *Respir. Physiol. 48*:59-74.

Leitner, L.-M., and Roumy, M. (1974a). Mechanosensitive units in the upper bill and in the tongue of the domestic duck. *Pflügers Arch 346*:141-150.

Leitner, L.-M., and Roumy, M. (1974b). Thermosensitive units in the tongue and skin of the duck's bill. *Pflügers Arch. 346*:151-155.

Leitner, L.-M., Roumy, M., and Miller, M. J. (1974). Motor responses triggered by diving and by mechanical stimulation of the glottis of the duck. *Respir. Physiol. 21*:385-392.

Lenfant, C., Kooyman, G. L., Elsner, R., and Drabeck, C. M. (1969). Respiratory function of the blood of the Adèlie penguin, *Pygoscelis adeliae. Am. J. Physiol. 216*:1598-1600.

Lillo, R. S., and Jones, D. R. (1982). Control of diving responses by carotid bodies and baroreceptors in ducks. *Am. J. Physiol. 242*:R105-R108.

Lopes, O. U., and Palmer, J. F. (1976). Proposed respiratory "gating" mechanism for cardiac slowing. *Nature 264*:454-456.

Lin, Y. C. (1982). Breath-hold diving in terrestrial mammals. In *Exercise and Sports Sciences Reviews*, Vol. 10. Edited by R. L. Terjung. Philadelphia, Franklin Press, pp. 270-307.

Lutz, P. L. (1980). On the oxygen affinity of bird blood. *Am. Zool. 20*:187-198.

Lutz, P. L., Longmuir, I. S., and Schmidt-Nielsen, K. (1974). Oxygen affinity of bird blood. *Respir. Physiol. 20*:325-330.

McCloskey, D. I., and Mitchell, J. H. (1972). Reflex cardiovascular and respiratory responses originating in exercising muscle. *J. Physiol. (Lond.) 224*: 173-186.

Maginnis, L. A. (1985). Blood oxygen transport in the house sparrow, *Passer domesticus. J. Comp. Physiol. B 155*:277-283.

Mangalam, H. J., and Jones, D. R. (1984). The effects of breathing different levels of O_2 and CO_2 on the diving responses of ducks (*Anas platyrhynchos*) and cormorants (*Phalacrocorax auritus*). *J. Comp. Physiol. B 154*: 243-247.

Manwell, C. (1958). Respiratory properties of the haemoglobin of two species of diving birds. *Science 127*:705-706.

Marek, W., and Prabhakar, N. R. (1985). Electrical stimulation of arterial and central chemosensory afferents at different times in the respiratory cycle of the cat: II. Responses of respiratory muscles and their motor nerves. *Pflügers Arch., 403*:422-428.

Marek, W., Prabhakar, N. R., and Loeschke, H. H. (1985). Electrical stimulation of arterial and central chemosensory afferents at different times in the respiratory cycle of the cat: I. Ventilatory responses. *Pflügers Arch. 403*: 415-421.

Marshall, J. M. (1987). Contribution to overall cardiovascular control of the chemoreceptor-induced altering/defence response. In *Neurobiology of the Cardiorespiratory System*. Edited by E. W. Taylor. Manchester, Manchester University Press.

Martin, L. D. (1983). The origin and early radiation of birds. In *Perspectives in Ornithology*. Edited by A. H. Brush and G. A. Clark, Jr. Cambridge, Cambridge Universtiy Press, pp. 291-238.

Millard, R. W. (1980). Depressed baroreceptor-cardiac reflex sensitivity during simulated diving in ducks. *Comp. Biochem. Physiol. 65A*:247-249.

Millard, R. W., Johansen, K., and Milsom, W. K. (1973). Radiotelemetry of cardiovascular responses to exercise and diving in penguins. *Comp. Biochem. Physiol. 46A*:227-240.

Miller, A. H. (1931). An auklet from the Eocene of Oregon. *Univ. Calif. Publ. Bull. Dept. Geol. Sci. 20*:23-26.

Milsom, W. K., Johansen, K., and Millard, R. W. (1973). Blood respiratory properties in some Antarctic birds. *Condor 75*:472-474.

Milsom, W. K., Jones, D. R., and Gabbott, G. R. J. (1981). On chemoreceptor control of ventilatory responses to CO_2 in anesthetized ducks. *J. Appl. Physiol. 50*:1121-1128.

Murphy, B., Zapol, W. M., and Hochachka, P. W. (1980). Metabolic activities of heart, lung, and brain during diving and recovery in the Weddell seal. *J. Appl. Physiol. 48*:596-605.

Murrish, D. E. (1970). Responses to diving in the dipper, *Cinclus mexicanus. Comp. Biochem. Physiol. 34*:853-858.

Nye, P. C. G., Hanson, M. A., and Torrance, R. W. (1981). The effect on breathing of abruptly stopping carotid body discharge. *Respir. Physiol. 46*:309-326.

Nye, P. C. G., Hanson, M. A., and Torrance, R. W. (1983). The effect of breathing of abruptly reducing the discharge of central chemoreceptors. *Respir. Physiol. 51*:109-118.

Olson, S. L. (1985). The fossil record of birds. In *Avian Biology*, Vol. VIII. Edited by D. S. Farner, J. R. King, and K. C. Parkes. London, Academic Press, pp. 79-238.

Orr, J. B., and Watson, A. (1913). Study of the respiratory mechanism in the duck. *J. Physiol. (Lond.) 46*:337-348.

Owre, O. T. (1967). Adaptations for locomotion and feeding in the anhinga and the double crested cormorant. *Ornithol. Monogr. 6*:1-138.

Pagés, T., and Planas, J. (1983). Muscle myoglobin and flying habits in birds. *Comp. Biochem. Physiol. 74A*:289-294.

Palacios, L., Palomeque, J., Riera, M., Pagés, T., Viscor, G., and Planas, J. (1984). Oxygen transport properties in the starling, *Sturnus vulgaris* L. *Comp. Biochem. Physiol. 77A*:255-260.

Paton, D. N. (1913). The relative influence of the labrinthine and cervical elements in the production of postural apnoea in the duck. *Q. J. Exp. Physiol. 6*:197-207.

Paton, D. N. (1927). Submergence and postural apnoea in the swan. *Proc. Rev. Soc. Edin. B 47*:283-293.

Pattengale, P. K., and Holloszy, J. O. (1967). Augmentation of skeletal muscle myoglobin by a program of treadmill running. *Am. J. Physiol. 213*:783-785.

Patton, J. C., and Avise, J. C. (1986). Evolutionary genetics of birds. IV. Rates of protein divergence in waterfowl (*Anatidae*). *Genetica 68*:129-143.

Pickwell, G. V. (1968). Energy metabolism in ducks during submergence asphyxia: Assessment by a direct method. *Comp. Biochem. Physiol. 27*: 455-485.

Portman, A. (1950). Squelette. In *Traite de Zoologie*, Vol. 15. Oiseaux. Edited by P. Grassé. Paris, Maison et Cie., pp. 78-107.

Raikow, R. J. (1970). Evolution of diving adaptations in the stifftail ducks. *Univ. Calif. Publ. Zool. 94*:1-52.

Raikow, R. J. (1973). Locomotor mechanisms in North American ducks. *Wilson Bull. 85*:295-307.

Raikow, R. J. (1985). Locomotor system. In *Form and Function in Birds*, Vol. 3. Edited by A. S. King and J. McLelland. London, Academic Press, pp. 57-147.

Reynafarje, B. (1962). Myoglobin content and enzyme activity of muscle and altitude adaptation. *J. Appl. Physiol. 17*:301-305.

Richardson, F. (1939). Functional aspects of the pneumatic system of the California brown pelican. *Condor 41*:13-17.

Scheipers, G., Kawashiro, T., and Scheid, P. (1975). Oxygen and carbon dioxide dissociation of duck blood. *Respir. Physiol. 24*:1-13.

Scholander, P. F. (1940). Experimental investigations on the respiratory function in diving mammals and birds. *Hvalradets Skr. 22*:1-131.

Scholander, P. F. (1960). Oxygen transport through hemoglobin solutions. *Science 131*:585-590.

Schorger, A. W. (1947). The deep diving of the loon and old-squaw and its mechanism. *Wilson Bull. 59*:151-159.

Shimizu, M., and Jones, D. R. (1987). Acid-base balance in ducks (*Anas platyrhynchos*) during involuntary submergence. *Am. J. Physiol. 252*:R348-R352.

Sibley, C. G., and Ahlquist, J. E. (1986). Reconstructing bird phylogeny by comparing DNAs. *Sci. Am. 254*:82-92.

Simpson, G. G. (1975). Fossil penguins. In *The Biology of Penguins*. Edited by B. Stonehouse. London, Macmillan, pp. 19-41.

Smith, F. M. (1987). Arterial Baroreceptor Control of the Circulation During Forced Dives in Ducks (*Anas platyrhynchos* var.). Ph.D. Thesis, University of British Columbia.

Smith, E. N., and Tobey, E. W. (1983). Heart-rate response to forced and voluntary diving in swamp rabbits, *Sylvilagus aquaticus. Physiol. Zool. 56*:632-638.

Smith, E. N., Sims, K., and Vich, J. F. (1981). Oxygen consumption of frightened swamp rabbits, *Sylvilagus aquaticus. Physiol. Zool. 56*:632-638.

Snyder, G. K., Byers, R. L., and Kayar, S. R. (1984). Effects of hypoxia on tissue capillarity in geese. *Respir. Physiol. 58*:151-160.

Spring, L. (1971). A comparison of functional and morphological adaptations in the common murre (*Uria aalge*) and thick billed murre (*Uria lomvia*). *Condor 73*:1-27.

Stephenson, R. (1987). The Physiology of Voluntary Diving Behaviour in the Tufted Duck (*Aythya fuligula*) and the American mink (*Mustela vison*). Ph.D. Thesis. University of Birmingham, U.K.

Stephenson, R., Butler, P. J., and Woakes, A. J. (1986). Diving behaviour and heart rate in tufted ducks (*Aythya fuligula*). *J. Exp. Biol. 126*:341-359.

Stewart, P. A. (1981). *How to Understand Acid-Base. A Quantitative Acid-Base Primer for Biology and Medicine*. New York, Elsevier North-Holland.

Stewart, P. A. (1983). Modern quantitative acid-base chemistry. *Can. J. Physiol. Pharmacol. 61*:1444-1461.

Storer, R. W. (1956). The fossil loon, *Colymboides minutus. Condor 58*:413-426.

Storer, R. W. (1960). Evolution in the diving birds. *Proc. 12th Int. Ornithol. Congr. 1958*, pp. 694-707.

Storer, R. W. (1971). Adaptive radiation of birds. In *Avian Biology*, Vol. I. Edited by D. S. Farner, J. R. King, and K. C. Parkes. London, Academic Press, pp. 149-188.

Storey, A. T. (1968). A functional analysis of sensory units innervating epiglottis and larynx. *Exp. Neurol. 20*:366-383.

Thomas, V. G. (1985). Myoglobin levels and mATPase activity in pectoral muscles of spruce and ruffed grouse (Aves: Tetraoninae). *Comp. Biochem. Physiol. 81A*:181-184.

Turner, D. L. (1986). The metabolic, cardiovascular and muscular responses of the tufted duck, *Aythya fuligula*, to exercise and the adaptations to training. M.Sc. (Qual.) Thesis. University of Birmingham, U.K.

Vandecasserie, C., Paul, C., Schnek, A. G., and Leónis, J. (1973). Oxygen affinity of avian hemoglobins. *Comp. Biochem. Physiol. 44A*:711-718.

Weber, R. E., Hemmingsen, E. A., and Johansen, K. (1974). Functional and biochemical studies of penguin myoglobin. *Comp. Biochem. Physiol. 49B*: 197-214.

Weinstein, G. N., Anderson, C., and Steeves, J. D. (1984). Functional characterization of limb muscles involved in locomotion in the Canada goose, *Branta canadensis. Can. J. Zool. 62*:1596-1604.

Wells, R. M. G. (1976). The oxygen affinity of chicken haemoglobin in whole blood and erythrocyte suspensions. *Respir. Physiol. 27*:21-31.

West, N. H. (1981). The effect of age and the influence of the relative size of the heart, brain and blood oxygen store on the responses to submersion in mallard ducklings. *Can. J. Zool. 59*:986-993.

Wilcox, H. H. (1952). The pelvic musculature of the loon, *Gavia immer*. *Am. Midl. Nat.* *48*:513-573.

Wilson, J. X., and West, N. H. (1986). Cardiovascular responses to neurohormones in conscious chickens and ducks. *Gen. Comp. Endocrinol.* *62*:268-280.

Wittenberg, J. B. (1970). Myoglobin-facilitated oxygen diffusion: Role of myoglobin in oxygen entry into muscle. *Physiol. Rev.* *50*:559-636.

Woakes, A. J., and Butler, P. J. (1983). Swimming and diving in tufted ducks, *Aythya fuligula*, with particular reference to heart rate and gas exchange. *J. Exp. Biol.* *107*:311-329.

Woakes, A. J., and Butler, P. J. (1986). Respiratory, circulatory and metabolic adjustments during swimming in the tufted duck, *Aythya fuligula*. *J. Exp. Biol.* *120*:215-231.

26

Diving Physiology
Man

SUK KI HONG

State University of New York
Buffalo, New York

I. Introduction

For centuries, man has been exploring the seabottom for foods, corals, and pearls, among others. Until rather recently, the only means to do so was breath-hold diving, which can be carried out without any equipment. However, both the duration and depth of such diving are limited and, subsequently, more sophisticated diving techniques have been developed in an attempt to prolong the diving time and to extend the depth of dive. These include air SCUBA (self-contained underwater breathing apparatus) or mixed-gas saturation dives. Using the latter technique, a successful dry (chamber) dive to a simulated depth of 686 m (69.6 ata) was conducted in 1981 at the F. G. Hall Laboratory of Duke University (Bennett et al., 1982). Although each of these diving techniques presents unique physiological problems, this chapter will deal only with the physiology of breath-hold diving.

A breath-hold dive is the simplest form of dive, practiced worldwide by perhaps millions of recreational divers. In addition, there are many thousands of professional divers who dive daily for a living. Examples of the latter group include Navy divers, women divers of Korea (Hae-Nyo) and Japan (ama), sponge divers in Greece, and pearl divers in the Tuamotu Archipelago. Intensive physiological studies have been conducted in some of these divers, especially Korean women divers, which contributed greatly to the understanding of the physiology of breath-hold diving.

Breath-hold diving imposes stresses to respiratory, cardiovascular, and thermoregulatory systems that limit the diving capability in terms of the depth and duration. Some of these stresses are caused by the act of breathholding, whereas others are attributed to water immersion, which is a prerequisite for actual (wet) divers. The magnitude of, and acclimatization to, each of these physiological stresses will be presented in this chapter.

II. Diving Pattern

Two types of breath-hold diving are found in professional divers of Korea and Japan: unassisted (cachido) and assisted (funado) (Hong and Rahn, 1967). Unassisted diving is conducted alone and is practiced by most of the recreational and professional divers. On the other hand, assisted diving represents a more sophisticated technique, practiced by more experienced divers. These divers carry a counterweight (about 13 kg) to assist descent to the bottom (where they release the weight and swim about); at the end of the dive helpers in a boat above pull them up with a rope. While the diver is resting alongside the boat between dives, the counterweight is pulled up by a helper.

The average diving pattern of these two types of divers is summarized in Table 1. Although these divers are capable of diving deeper, the average depth of dive is approximately 5 m for cachidos and 10 m for funados. The rates of descent and ascent are 0.6-0.8 m/s and 1.2-1.4 m/s, respectively, in cachidos and funados of both sexes wearing cotton bathing suits (without fins) (Hong et al., 1963; Park et al., 1983; Shiraki et al., 1985; Teruoka, 1932). Interestingly, male cachidos wearing wet suits (and fins) showed a selective increase in the descent rate to 1.1 m/s, comparable with that observed in female funados wearing cotton suits (Shiraki et al., 1985). Given these rates of descent and ascent and the average duration of a dive (30 s for cachidos and 60 s for funados), bottom time was estimated to be approximately 15 s and 30 s, respectively, for cachidos and funados. An analysis of the diving frequency indicated that cachidos make 60 dives per hour and funados 30 (Hong and Rahn, 1967), indicating that there is no difference in the total bottom time-per-hour between the two types of diving. Each dive is followed by a period of rest at the water surface (cachidos usually leaning over a float). On the average, the surface time/diving time ratio is approximately 1.0 in both types of diving.

Table 1 Average Diving Pattern of Korean and Japanese Professional Divers

	Diving velocity				
	Descent rate (m/s)	Ascent rate (m/s)	Diving depth (m)	Diving time (s)	Ref.
Female divers					
cachido (cotton suits)	0.6	0.6	5–10	30	Hong et al., 1963
cachido (wet suits)	0.6	0.8	5–10	30	Park et al., 1983
funado (cotton suits)	1.2	1.4	10–20	60	Teruoka et al., 1932
Male divers					
cachido (swim trunks)	0.7	0.7	5–10		Shiraki et al., 1985
cachido (swim trunks)	0.8	0.7	10–20		Shiraki et al., 1985
cachido (wet suits)	1.1	0.8	10–20	30	Shiraki et al., 1985

The longest diving time in sport competition to depths of 100 m was reported to be 3 min and 14 s by Jacques Mayol (Missiroli, 1983). On the basis of an oxygen store of 1600 ml in a human subject (Rahn, 1964) and the average oxygen consumption of 400 ml/min during a breath-hold dive, one would expect the theoretical maximal breath-hold diving time of 4 min. In other words, the average diving time of 30 to 60 s observed in Korean and Japanese divers is extremely conservative, and the occurrence of diving-related accidents in these divers is known to be extremely rare. On the other hand, Tuamotu (male) pearl divers are known to routinely engage in dives lasting 1.5 to 2.5 min and to show a high rate of accidents (Cross, 1965).

The maximal depth of diving is thought to be determined by the total lung capacity (TLC)/residual volume (RV) ratio, assuming that extrathoracic dead space volume is negligible. This is based on the premise that the lung volume cannot be compressed to the level below RV without developing thoracic barotrauma and, also, that the RV is a fixed entity that does not change during div-

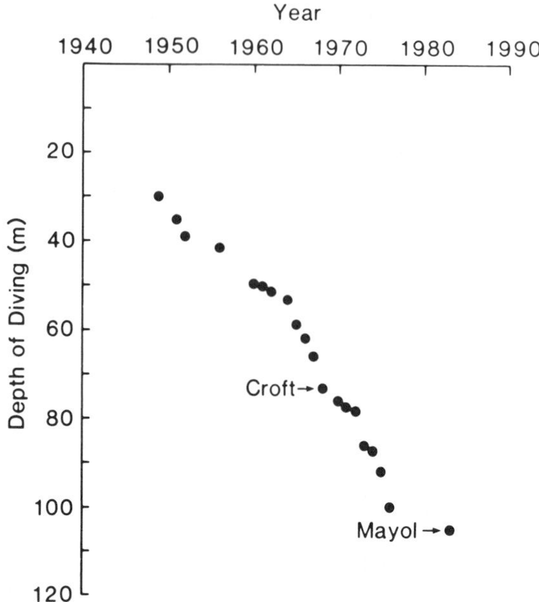

Figure 1 Maximal depth records for breath-hold diving during 1949–1983. [Depth records for 1949–1976 are from Mayol (1976); 1983 record to 105 m by J. Mayol from Missiroli (1983–1984).]

ing. On the average, Korean women divers descend after inhalation of air equivalent to 85% of the vital capacity (Hong et al., 1963), with the lung volume/RV ratio of 3.56 (4.06/1.14). This indicates that they can dive to a depth of 25 m (equivalent to 3.5 ata). In practice, however, they elect to dive to 5 to 10 m, again illustrating how conservative these divers are.

The concept of the theoretical maximal depth of breath-hold diving is, however, inconsistent with the depth records set by various divers. As shown in Figure 1, the depth reached by various breath-hold divers has been increasing linearly since 1949 (Mayol, 1976). The current depth record is held by Jacques Mayol who dived to 105 m in 1983 (Missiroli, 1983). The TLC/RV ratio of Jacques Mayol is 3.7 (7.22/1.88), based on the measurements made in the laboratory. In other words, the existing dogma would have predicted that his maximal depth of dive would be 27 m. Obviously, there is a flaw in the current concept!

The large difference between the predicted and actual maximal depths of dive may be explained if the RV decreases during diving. Schaefer et al. (1968) estimated the thoracic blood volume during the open-sea dive to 43 m, by using the impedance pneumograph, and found that about 1 L of blood was forced into the thorax during diving. Because the thoracic cage is rigid during breath-hold diving under the influence of hydrostatic compression, it may be surmised that such an increase in the intrathoracic blood volume should replace the equivalent volume of residual gas in the lung, resulting in a corresponding decrease in the RV. Therefore, on the basis of the report by Schaefer et al. (1968), one may speculate that Jacques Mayol's RV during diving was reduced to 0.88 L instead of 1.88 L. This would increase his maximal depth to 72 m (7.22/0.88 = 8.2), which is considerably greater than 27 m originally predicted by the TLC/RV ratio determined in the laboratory, but it is still shallower than the actual depth record of 105 m. However, a small additional increase in thoracic blood volume (by 250 ml) to further decrease his RV to 0.63 L could account for the current depth record (7.22/0.63 = 11.5). Although this consideration is still speculative, there is evidence to indicate that the RV must be decreased during diving. Craig (1968) reported that the subject (RV = 2.0 L) who was asked to dive following a full expiration was able to dive to a depth of 4.5 m without developing a significant difference between the ambient pressure at depth and the intrathoracic pressure. These results indicated to him that the subject's RV must have been compressed from 2.0 L at the surface to 1.4 L during diving.

III. Alveolar Gas Exchange

During a simple breath holding in air, both F_{AO_2} and P_{AO_2} decrease progressively because of continuous diffusion of O_2 from the lung into the blood across the alveolar epithelium, whereas both F_{ACO_2} and P_{ACO_2} increase curvilinearly because of diffusion of CO_2 from the blood into the lung. However, the time course of changes in alveolar O_2 and CO_2 concentrations and pressures during breath-hold diving is markedly different from this pattern. In a 40-s breath-hold dive to a depth of 10 m (2 ata), alveolar gas samples were obtained immediately before the dive (after inspiration of air equivalent to 85% of the vital capacity), at the time of arrival at 10 m depth (20 s), and immediately upon surfacing (40 s) (Hong et al., 1963). The results of analyses of these samples are shown in Fig. 2 (right panel), along with the comparable set of data obtained during a 90-s breath holding in air with TLC (left panel) (Hong et al., 1971).

The reason for the marked difference in alveolar gas profile between the two different breath-holding maneuvers is that the chest is compressed during descent and is then reexpanded during ascent. During descent, when the chest (and, hence, the lung volume) is compressed, the P_{AO_2} increases, whereas $P_{\bar{V}O_2}$ should not change appreciably, at least during the first 20 s (circulation time) of the dive. At a depth of 10 m, it is expected that P_{AO_2} should be increased to twofold that of the predive value of 120 torr. However, the actual value at 10 m depth was only 150 torr instead of 240 torr. This is due to the

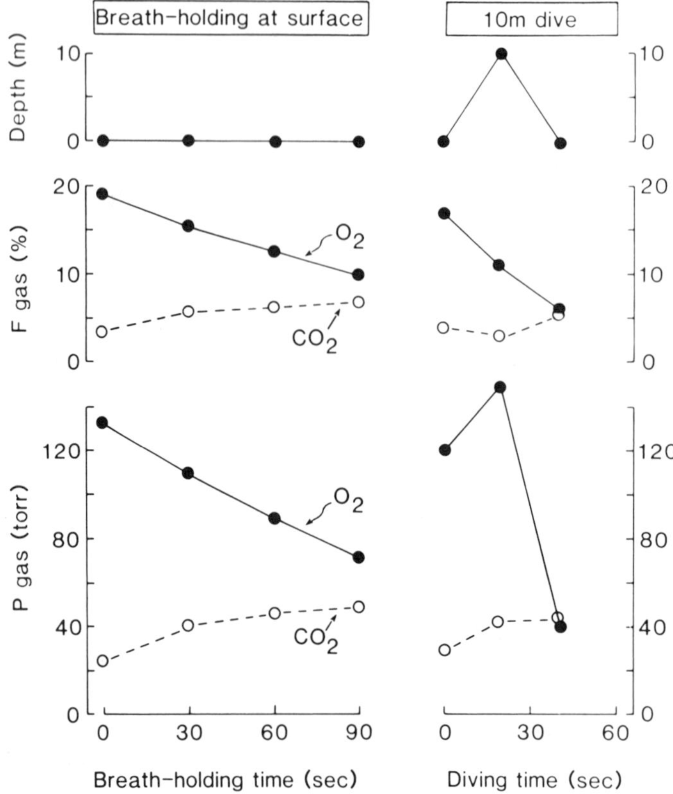

Figure 2 Time course of changes in alveolar O_2 and CO_2 concentrations (F) and pressures (P) during a 90-s breath holding at surface (left panel) and a 40-s breath-hold diving to 10 m (right panel). The dive profile is shown on top of the right panel. (Data from Hong et al., 1963, 1971.)

diffusion of O_2 from the lung into the blood during descent in the continuous presence of a favorable diffusion gradient, as reflected by a much lower F_{AO_2} (11%) at 10-m depth compared with a predive value of 16.7%. During ascent, the chest is reexpanded and P_{AO_2} now decreases rapidly, thereby decreasing the diffusion gradient. By the time the diver returned to the surface (40-s point), P_{AO_2} decreased to 40 torr, which is virtually the same as $P\bar{V}O_2$. In other words, the transfer of O_2 from the lung to the blood is severely affected during ascent. In fact, it is even possible to reverse the normal direction of O_2 transfer during a prolonged dive (Hong et al., 1963; Lanphier and Rahn, 1963; Teruoka, 1932). Olszowka and Rahn (1987) recently developed a computer model to analyze the time course of changes in P_{AO_2} and $P\bar{V}O_2$ during a 220-s dive to a depth of

100 m. According to their analysis, PAO_2 and $P\bar{V}O_2$ are 25 and 57 torr, respectively, at the end of the dive. These investigators also predicted that O_2 begins to be transferred from the mixed venous blood to the lung (i.e., the reversal of O_2 flux) at 173 s when the diver ascended to 40 m depth. It was further estimated that 58 ml (STPD) O_2 is transferred from the blood to the lung during ascent from 40-m depth to the surface.

Compression of the chest during descent also increases $PACO_2$ to a level greater than that of the blood PCO_2. Consequently, the normal direction of CO_2 transfer from the blood to the lung is now reversed and there is a net loss of CO_2 from the lung during descent. Therefore, large amounts of CO_2 are retained in the blood, with a resultant increase in blood PCO_2. It is also interesting that $PaCO_2$ is now greater than that of $P\bar{V}CO_2$, as long as CO_2 is diffusing into the blood. It is this retention of CO_2, with an attendant increase in PCO_2 of blood, that gives the signal to the diver to return to the surface. During ascent, CO_2 retained in the blood furing descent now leaves the blood for the lung as $PACO_2$ continuously decreases. However, not all CO_2 retained in the blood during descent is eliminated into the lung during ascent, and the process of excess CO_2 elimination continues even after the return to the surface.

Although there is no net transfer of N_2 between the lung and the blood under normal conditions at 1-atm environment, N_2 is transferred to the blood from the lung during descent along with O_2 and CO_2. However, the amount of N_2 transferred is rather small because of its very low solubility in plasma. This small amount of N_2 that enters the circulation and tissue during descent will now slowly leave during ascent. Because the amount of N_2 transferred from the lung to the blood during a breath-hold dive is small, there is no real danger for developing decompression sickness. However, it is theoretically possible to accumulate enough N_2 to develop signs of decompression sickness if the diver repetitively dives to considerable depths with very short surface intervals (Lanphier, 1965; Paulev, 1965).

A seemingly complicated pattern of alveolar gas exchange during a breath-hold dive may be summarized as follows: The transfer of O_2 from the lungs to the blood is not disturbed until ascent starts. It is during this ascending phase that the diver could encounter a critical state of hypoxia. The normal direction of CO_2 transfer from the lungs to the blood is reversed during descent, which results in a significant retention of CO_2 in the blood (hypercapnia). During ascent, the retained CO_2 is transferred to the lung. A small amount of N_2 also enters the circulation during descent, which is reversed during ascent.

The duration of a breath hold increases significantly when it is preceded by hyperventilation. Consequently, novice divers often hyperventilate to prolong the duration of breath-hold diving. However, Craig (1961a,b) convincingly demonstrated that an excessive hyperventilation before diving could exaggerate the degree of hypoxia during ascent.

Professional divers are engaged in a number of dives every day. For instance, a group of Japanese male cachido divers of Tsushima Island make nearly 200 dives on a typical summer day (Shiraki et al., 1985). Hence, these divers repetitively expose themselves to both hypoxic and hypercapnic stresses for years. Studies conducted on various groups of divers to examine if they have developed any acclimatization to these stresses did, indeed, show a reduced sensitivity of their ventilatory system to hypoxia in Japanese female funado divers (Honda et al., 1983) and in the U.S. Navy Submarine Escape Training Tank instructors (Schaefer, 1965). Similarly, a reduced sensitivity of the ventilatory system to a given hypercapnia has also been demonstrated in Korean women divers (Song et al., 1963) and in U.S. Navy divers (Schaefer, 1965).

IV. Cardiovascular Changes

The most important cardiovascular change during breath-hold diving is the development of bradycardia, which was observed in the duck more than a century ago. This bradycardia is thought to be a component of drastic cardiovascular adjustments to diving, subserving to conserve O_2 during diving, at least in diving animals, as described in previous chapters.

Scholander et al. (1962) were the first to demonstrate that human breath-hold divers, native men of the Torres Straight archipelago, developed bradycardia while diving for 45 to 60 s. They observed that all 19 divers decreased their heart rate to 40–50 beats/min within 20 to 30 s, which persisted in spite of considerable exercise under water. In a later study on Korean women divers, Hong et al. (1967) found that the degree of diving bradycardia is considerably greater in winter compared with summer and, also, that a virtually identical pattern of bradycardia develops even during a simple breath holding in water with only the face submerged. Furthermore, Moore et al. (1972) demonstrated the quantitative similarity of apneic bradycardia induced by whole-body immersion to that induced by face immersion alone. Evidently, neither the depth of diving nor the swimming exercise seems to contribute to the development of diving bradycardia. Whatever the mechanism underlying this bradycardia, the parasympathetic nerve seems to play a critical role because diving bradycardia in humans can be blocked by atropine (Heistad et al., 1968). It could be that inhibition of the respiratory center induced by the cessation of respiratory movements excites cardiac vagal motoneurons leading to bradycardia (Daly and Angell-Jones, 1979).

Most of the recent studies employed the breath-hold face immersion technique to determine the role of various factors modulating the bradycardic response. These factors may be divided into three major categories (Hong, 1987): neural, mechanical, and chemical. Neural factors include cold receptors and putative intrathoracic receptors, indicated by the potentiation of bradycardic

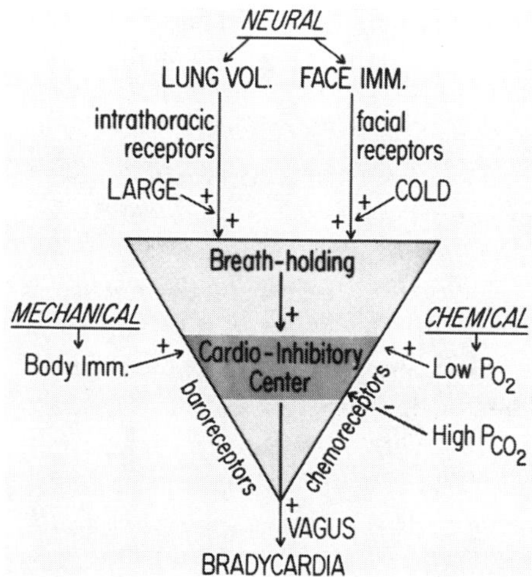

Figure 3 A schematic model of factors modulating diving bradycardia in humans. + indicates potentiation; – indicates attenuation of bradycardic response. Triangle symbolizes the different types of factors modulating the basic bradycardia accompanying apnea, per se. (From Hong, 1987.)

response by low water temperature and large lung volumes (Song et al., 1969). The mechanical factor seems to involve the baroreceptors, as suggested by the potentiation of bradycardia by a decrease in the intrathoracic pressure, which should increase the venous return and then decrease the heart rate through a baroreflex mechanism (Craig, 1965). Chemical factors involve the chemoreceptors, as indicated by either the potentiation of bradycardia by hypoxia or the attenuation by hypercapnia (Lin et al., 1983). A schematic model of these factors modulating diving bradycardia is shown in Figure 3.

Because the face immersion greatly potentiates the breath-hold bradycardia, many investigators attempted to determine if a certain region of the face potentiates the bradycardic response. However, the results obtained from different laboratories are conflicting. It is not even unequivocally established that the face needs to be wetted during face immersion to potentiate breath-hold bradycardia. Separating the face from water by thin plastic sheet either attenuated (Gooden et al., 1978) or had no significant effect (Moore et al., 1972) on the breath-hold bradycardia.

An important difference exists between humans and diving animals in the occurrence of cardiac arrhythmia during the breath-hold diving or face immersion. Diving animals are known to develop diving bradycardia without cardiac arrhythmias. However, the breath-hold bradycardia in humans is often associated with various types of cardiac arrhythmias. In Korean women divers, Hong et al. (1967) observed abnormal P waves and nodal rhythms, idioventricular rhythms, premature atrial beats, premature ventricular beats, and others. Moreover, the incidence of these arrhythmias was considerably higher in winter (72%)

than in summer (43%). Scholander et al. (1962) were also surprised to find in human professional divers a high incidence of arrhythmias developed during diving.

In diving animals engaged in protracted dives, the diving bradycardia is associated with an intense vasoconstriction and a marked reduction in the cardiac output (Anderson, 1966). Moreover, the arterial blood pressure remains unchanged. In the face of such a marked reduction in cardiac output, the blood flow to the brain and the heart appears to be preferentially maintained, whereas that to the muscle and the viscera is severely curtailed, thereby conserving O_2. In contrast, the breath-hold bradycardia in humans is accompanied by an increase in arterial blood pressure (Kawakami et al., 1967; Lin et al., 1983). Moreover, the cardiac output during breath holding, with or without face immersion, either remained unchanged (Hong et al., 1971; Lin et al., 1983), decreased by ~20% (Kawakami et al., 1967; Whayne et al., 1973), or increased by 14% (Paulev and Wettergvist, 1968). More recently, Bjertnaes et al. (1984) studied cardiovascular responses to face immersion and apnea during steady-state muscle exercise and reported that the cardiac output during the last half of breath-hold face immersion was reduced by 49%, whereas systemic vascular resistance increased by 200%. Moreover, these investigators found that myocardial O_2 demand determined by the heart rate–pressure double product decreased by 42% during breath-hold face immersion. However, they also noted that the rise in systemic vascular resistance is not closely adjusted to the reduction in cardiac output, and that the O_2-saving potential is reduced because of rise in cardiac afterloads.

In the only study that was conducted in human divers during dry and wet breath-hold diving (to a simulated depth of 20 m), Ferrigno et al. (1987) found that breath holding (at surface) with large lung volume increases intrathoracic pressure and caused a decrease in cardiac index. During compression, the cardiac index increased by 35% in the nonsubmerged and by 30% in the submerged conditions, which was attributed to a fall in intrathoracic pressure. As a result of the combination of the opposite effects of breath holding (at surface) and compression to 20 m, cardiac performance remained unchanged during the dive (relative to the surface control).

A most important question, namely whether or not the cardiovascular changes during breath-hold diving in humans also subserves to conserve O_2 as in diving animals cannot be unequivocally answered. Careful measurements of O_2 consumption before, during, and after breath-hold diving are critically needed to answer this question.

V. Body Heat Exchange

That the human body cools faster in water than in air of the same temperature is well recognized because the specific heat of water is 1000 times, and thermoductivity 25 times, greater than those of air. Although the thermal comfort zone (i.e., thermoneutral temperature) for a resting unclothed man immersed in water varies inversely with the subcutaneous fat thickness (SFT) of the subject, this value is generally reported to be 33 to 35°C (Craig and Dvorak, 1966; Smith and Hanna, 1975). Moreover, the critical water temperature (i.e., the lowest end of the zone of vasomotor regulation at which maximal peripheral vasoconstriction develops) is also as high as 29 to 33°C, depending upon SFT. Because the water temperature for divers is generally much lower, it is obvious that divers are exposed to considerable cold water stress.

The Korean women divers engage in daily diving work throughout the year. The temperature of these waters varies from about 27°C in midsummer to 10°C in midwinter. Until 1977, these divers, with small SFT of 0 to 2 mm, wore only a cotton bathing suit throughout the year and exposed themselves to the severe cold water stress. Field studies showed that they will stay in water until the rectal temperature falls to about 35°C when they feel extremely cold, develop violent shivering, and voluntarily terminate the diving work (Kang et al., 1965). These temperatures were reached in about 40 min and 20 min, respectively, in summer and winter. Their O_2 consumption in the water increased about 2.5 times during the summer and 3.5 times during the winter. Given these data, the cumulative extra heat loss per diving work shift was estimated to be 390 kcal (or ~10 kcal/min) in summer and 560 kcal (or ~30 kcal/min) in winter and indicate that the degree of cold stress is high, even during summer. In fact, the duration of a diving work shift is primarily determined by the seawater temperature, varying from 15 to 20 min in midwinter to 150 min in midsummer (Kang et al., 1963).

Since 1977, however, these divers have been wearing wet suits to avoid cold water stress, which extended the duration of diving work shift to 120 min even in midwinter (Park et al., 1983). Actual measurements of their body temperatures and O_2 consumption during diving work in the sea indicated that the rectal temperature decreased little, whereas the O_2 consumption increased only about twofold, even in midwinter (Kang et al., 1983), with the net heat loss estimated to be 260 kcal and 370 kcal in summer (180 min of working time) and winter (120 min of working time), respectively. In other words, the rate of heat loss in these protected (wet suit) divers is equivalent to 1.4 and 3.1 kcal/min, respectively, in summer and winter, which represent only about 10% of the corresponding values obtained earlier in traditional unprotected (cotton suit) divers.

Because these divers were continuously exposed to severe cold water stress before 1977, when they started wearing wet suits, extensive studies on their thermoregulatory functions were conducted during the 1960s to define the pattern of cold acclimatization, if indeed it occurs in humans. The following pattern was obtained (see a review by Hong, 1973): (1) a consistent, reversible increase in basal metabolic rate (BMR) in winter when the seawater temperature is lowest (i.e., metabolic acclimatization); (2) a very small (but significant) increase in O_2 consumption in response to exogenous norepinephrine in winter but not in summer, indicating that the development of nonshivering thermogenesis is not the main feature of cold acclimatization; (3) a lower critical water temperature (T_{cw}) at a comparable SFT in both summer and winter, indicating the elevation of shivering threshold (i.e., hypothermic acclimatization, most probably representing habituation); (4) a greater maximal body (thermal) insulation (I_{max}) at a comparable SFT in both summer and winter; (5) evidence for a more efficient countercurrent heat exchange system in the limbs; and (6) the maintenance of the lower finger skin temperature and blood flow ($\dot{Q}_{finger}$) during immersion of one hand in 6°C in water (i.e., vascular acclimatization). On the basis of these observations, it was concluded that Korean women divers before 1977 had definitely developed various types of acclimatization to cold as a result of repetitive exposure to cold water stress.

However, the definitive proof that these phenomena represent a true cold acclimatization was obtained in subsequent studies conducted during the early 1980s (Park et al., 1983). As stated earlier, contemporary Korean women divers have worn wet suits since 1977 to avoid the cold water stress. It was thus rationalized that these divers should begin to lose previously acquired cold acclimatization, providing us with an opportunity to study the time course of deacclimatization to cold water immersion. On the other hand, if the alterations of thermoregulatory function documented in traditional unprotected divers are not linked to the repetitive cold water stress, they should remain unchanged even after the adoption of wet suits. The results of studies on contemporary wet-suited divers may be summarized as follows: (1) the BMR did not undergo seasonal fluctuation (1980-1981) and was within the DuBois standard year around; (2) T_{cw} at a given SFT was still reduced by 2 to 3°C in 1980 but increased progressively to equal that of nondivers in 1982; (3) I_{max} at a given SFT was identical with nondivers (1980-1982); and (4) $\dot{Q}_{finger}$ during immersion of one hand in 6°C water was significantly lower in 1980 but slowly returned to controls in 1981-1982. The time course of cold deacclimatization thus was BMR, < 3 years; I_{max}, < 3 years; $\dot{Q}_{finger}$, 4 years; and T_{cw}, 5 years. More importantly, this longitudinal study provided further evidence that cold acclimatization did at one time exist in these diving women. However, it should be cautioned that, although the demonstration of cold acclimatization in these divers is important in terms of human biology, acclimatization (or habituation) to cold are rather ineffective as a real defense against long, slow cooling, particularly if accompanied by exercise (Hong et al., 1986).

References

Andersen, H. T. (1966). Physiological adaptation in diving vertebrates. *Physiol. Rev. 46*:212-243.

Bennett, P. B., Coggin, R., and McLeod, M. (1982). Effect of compression rate on use of trimix to ameliorate HPNS in man to 686 m. *Undersea Biomed. Res. 9*:335-351.

Bjertnaes, L., Hauge, A., Kjekshus, J., and Soyland, E. (1984). Cardiovascular responses to face immersion and apnea during steady state muscle exercise. A heart catheterization study on humans. *Acta Physiol. Scand. 120*:605-612.

Craig, A. B., Jr. (1961a). Underwater swimming and loss of consciousness. *J. Am. Med. Assoc. 176*:255-258.

Craig, A. B., Jr. (1961b). Causes of loss of consciousness during underwater swimming. *J. Appl. Physiol. 16*:583-586.

Craig, A. B., Jr. (1965). Effects of submersion and pulmonary mechanics on cardiovascular function in man. In *Physiology of Breath-Hold Diving and the Ama of Japan*. Edited by H. Rahn and T. Yokoyama. Washington, National Academy of Sciences–National Research Council, Publication 1341, pp. 295-302.

Craig, A. B., Jr. (1968). Depth limits of breath hold diving (an example of fennology). *Resp. Physiol. 5*:14-22.

Craig, A. B., Jr., and Dvorak, M. (1966). Thermal regulation during water immersion. *J. Appl. Physiol. 21*:1577-1585.

Cross, E. R. (1965). Taravana-diving syndrome in the Tuomotu diver. In *Physiology of Breath-Hold Diving and the Ama of Japan*. Edited by H. Rahn and T. Yokoyama. Washington, National Academy of Sciences–National Research Council, Publication 1341, pp. 207-219.

Daly, M. de B., and Angell-James, J. E. (1979). The diving response and its possible clinical implication. *Int. Med. 1*:12-19.

Ferrigno, M., Hickey, D. D., Liner, M. H., and Lundgren, C. E. G. (1987). Simulated breath-hold diving to 20 meters: Cardiac performance in man. *J. Appl. Physiol. 62*:2160-2167.

Gooden, B. A., Holdstock, G., and Hampton, J. R. (1978). The magnitude of the bradycardia induced by face immersion in patients convalescing from myocardial infarction. *Cardiovasc. Res. 12*:239-242.

Heistad, D. D., Abboud, F. M., and Eckstein, J. W. (1968). Vasoconstrictor response to simulated diving in man. *J. Appl. Physiol. 25*:542-549.

Honda, Y., Masuda, Y., Hayashi, F., and Yoshida, A. (1983). Differences in ventilatory responses to hypoxia and hypercapnia between assisted (funado) and non-assisted (kachido) breath-hold divers. In *Hyperbaric Medicine and Underwater Physiology*. Edited by K. Shiraki and S. Matsuoka. Kitakyushu, Japan, Program Committee of III UOEH Symposium, pp. 45-58.

Hong, S. K. (1973). Pattern of cold adaptation in women divers of Korea (ama). *Fed. Proc. 32*:1614-1622.

Hong, S. K. (1987). Breath-hold bradycardia in man: An overview. In *Proceedings of Workshop on the Physiology of Breath-Hold Diving*. Edited by C. Lundgren and M. Ferrigno. Bethesda, Undersea Medical Society, pp. 158-173.

Hong, S. K., Lin, Y. C., Lally, D. A., Yim, B. J., Kominami, N., Hong, P. W., and Moore, T. O. (1971). Alveolar gas exchanges and cardiovascular functions during breath holding with air. *J. Appl. Physiol. 30*:540-547.

Hong, S. K., and Rahn, H. (1967). The diving women of Korea and Japan. *Sci. 216*:34-43.

Hong, S. K., Rahn, H., Kang, D. H., Song, S. H., and Kang, B. S. (1963). Diving pattern, lung volumes, and alveolar gas of the Korean diving women (ama). *J. Appl. Physiol. 18*:457-465.

Hong, S. K., Rennie, D. W., and Park, Y. S. (1986). Cold acclimatization and deacclimatization of Korea women divers. *Exercise Sports Sci. Rev. 14*:231-268.

Hong, S. K., Song, S. H., Kim, P. K., and Suh, C. S. (1967). Seasonal observations on the cardiac rhythm during diving in the Korean ama. *J. Appl. Physiol. 23*:18-22.

Kang, B. S., Song, S. H., Suh, C. S., and Hong, S. K. (1963). Changes in body temperatures and basal metabolic rate of the ama. *J. Appl. Physiol. 18*: 483-488.

Kang, D. H., Kim, P. K., Kang, B. S., Song, S. H., and Hong, S. K. (1965). Energy metabolism and body temperature of the ama. *J. Appl. Physiol. 20*: 46-50.

Kang, D. H., Park, Y. S., Park, Y. D., Lee, I. S., Yeon, D. S., Lee, S. H., Hong, S. Y., Rennie, D. W., and Hong, S. K. (1983). Energetics of wet-suit diving in Korean women breath-hold divers. *J. Appl. Physiol. 54*:1702-1707.

Kawakami, Y., Natelson, B. H., and DuBois, A. B. (1967). Cardiovascular effects of face immersion and factors affecting diving reflex in man. *J. Appl. Physiol. 23*:964-970.

Lanphier, E. H. (1965). Application of decompression tables to repeated breath-hold dives. In *Physiology of Breath-Hold Diving and the Ama of Japan*. Edited by H. Rahn and T. Yokoyama. Washington, National Academy of Sciences–National Research Council, Publication 1341, pp. 227-236.

Lanphier, E. H., and Rahn, H. (1963). Alveolar gas exchange during breath-hold diving. *J. Appl. Physiol. 18*:471-477.

Lin, Y. C., Shida, K. K., and Hong, S. K. (1983). Effects of hypercapnia, hypoxia and rebreathing on heart rate response during apnea. *J. Appl. Physiol. 54*:166-171.

Lin, Y. C., Shida, K. K., and Hong, S. K. (1983). Effects of hypercapnia, hypoxia and rebreathing on circulatory response to apnea. *J. Apply. Physiol. 54*:172-177.

Mayol, J. (1976). Jacques Mayol–apnea a meno cento. *Frateli Fabbri Editori*, January, pp. 1-96.

Missiroli, di F. M. (1983-1984). Mayol a 105 metri. *Mondo Sommerso N271*: 32-37.

Moore, T. O., Lin, Y. C., Lally, D. A., and Hong, S. K. (1972). Effects of temperature, immersion, and ambient pressure on human apneic bradycardia. *J. Appl. Physiol. 33*:36-41.

Olszowka, A. J., and Rahn, H. (1987). Breath-hold diving. In *Hypoxia and Cold*. Edited by J. R. Sutton, C. S. Houston, and G. Coates. Praeger Scientific, pp. 417-428.

Park, Y. S., Rahn, H., Lee, I. S., Lee, S. I., Kang, D. H., Hong, S. Y., and Hong, S. K. (1983). Patterns of wet suit diving in Korean women breath-hold divers. *Undersea Biomed. Res. 10*:203-216.

Park, Y. S., Rennie, D. W., Lee, I. S., Park, Y. D., Paik, K. S., Kang, D. H., Suh, D. J., Lee, S. H., Hong, S. Y., and Hong, S. K. (1983). Time course of deacclimatization to cold water immersion in Korean women divers. *J. Appl. Physiol. 54*:1708-1716.

Paulev, P. (1965).Decompression sickness following repeated breath-hold dives. In *Physiology of Breath-Hold Diving and the Ama of Japan*. Edited by H. Rahn and T. Yokoyama. Washington, National Academy of Sciences–National Research Council, Publications 1341, pp. 221-226.

Paulev, P. E., and Wettergvist, H. (1968). Cardiac output during breath-holding in man. *Scand. J. Clin. Lab. Invest. 22*:115-123.

Rahn, H. (1964). Oxygen stores of man. In *Oxygen in the Animal Organism*. Edited by F. Dickens and E. Neil. New York, Macmillan, pp. 609-618.

Schaefer, K. E. (1965). Adaptation to breath-hold diving. In *Physiology of Breath-Hold Diving and the Ama of Japan*. Edited by H. Rahn and T. Yokoyama. Washington, National Academy of Sciences–National Research Council, Publication 1341, pp. 237-252.

Schaefer, K. E., Allison, R. D., Dougherty, J. H., Jr., Carey, C. R., Walker, R., Yost, R., and Parker, D. (1968). Pulmonary and circulatory adjustments determining the limits of depths in breath-hold dive. *Science 162*:1020-1023.

Scholander, P. F., Hammel, H. T., LeMessurier, H., Hemmingsen, E., and Garey, W. (1962). Circulatory adjustment in pearl divers. *J. Appl. Physiol. 17*: 184-190.

Shiraki, K., Konda, N., Sagawa, S., Park, Y. S., Komatsu, T., and Hong, S. K. (1985). Diving pattern of Tsushima male breath-hold divers (Katsugi). *Undersea Biomed. Res. 12*:439-452.

Smith, R. M., and Hanna, J. M. (1975). Skinfolds and resting heat loss in cold air and water. *J. Appl. Physiol. 39*:93-102.

Song, S. H., Kang, D. H., Kang, B. S., and Hong, S. K. (1963). Lung volumes and ventilatory responses to high CO_2 and low O_2 in the ama. *J. Appl. Physiol. 18*:466-470.

Song, S. H., Lee, W. K., Chung, Y. A., and Hong, S. K. (1969). Mechanism of apneic bradycardia in man. *J. Appl. Physiol. 27*:323-327.

Teruoka, G. (1932). Die Ama und Ihre Arbeit. *Arbeitsphysiologie 5*:239-251.

Whayne, T. F., Smith, N. T. Y., Eger, E. I. II., Stoelting, R. K., and Whitcher, C. E. (1972). Reflex cardiovascular responses to simulated diving. *Angiologia 23*:500-508.

AUTHOR INDEX

Numbers in brackets give the page on which the complete reference is listed.

A

C

D

E

F

G

H

I

K

L

M

N

O

P

S

T

W

Y

Z

SUBJECT INDEX

A

D

G

M

N

O

Q

R

U

V

W

X

Z